PHARMACOLOGY

We dedicate this book to the memory of Professor H. O. Schild. Under his authorship the textbook Applied Pharmacology, the predecessor of the present book, set a standard we have tried to maintain.

For Churchill Livingstone

Publisher: Laurence Hunter
Project Editor: Barbara Simmons
Copy Editor: Susan Beasley
Indexer: Laurence Errington
Production Controller: Nancy Arnott
Design Direction: Erik Bigland
Sales Promotion Executive: Marion Pollock

PHARMACOLOGY

H. P. Rang MB BS MA DPhil FRS
Director,
Sandoz Institute for Medical Research,
London;
Visiting Professor of Pharmacology,
University College, London

M. M. Dale MB BCh PhD
Senior Teaching Fellow,
Department of Pharmacology,
University of Oxford;
Honorary Lecturer,
Department of Pharmacology,
University College, London

J. M. Ritter MA DPhil FRCP
Professor of Clinical Pharmacology,
United Medical and Dental Schools
(Guy's and St Thomas's Hospitals),
London

THIRD EDITION

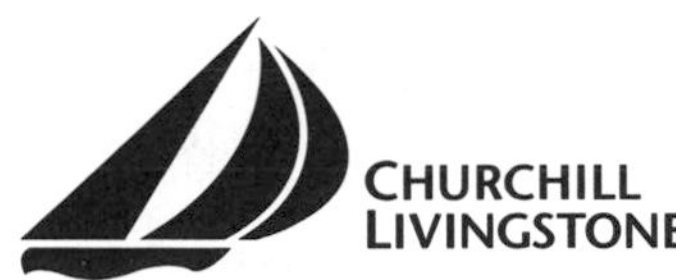

EDINBURGH LONDON NEW YORK PHILADELPHIA SAN FRANCISCO SYDNEY AND TORONTO 1996

CHURCHILL LIVINGSTONE

A Medical Division of Harcourt Brace and Company Limited

First edition 1987
Second edition 1991
Third edition 1995
Reprinted 1995
Reprinted 1996
Reprinted 1998

ISBN 0 443 050473

International Edition of 3rd edition
Reprinted 1995, 1996, 1998

ISBN 0 443 050864

British Library Cataloguing in Publication Data
A catalogue record for this book is available from the British Library.

Library of Congress Cataloging in Publication Data
A catalog record for this book is available from the Library of Congress.

The publisher's policy is to use **paper manufactured from sustainable forests**

Printed in the United States of America

Preface

For this third edition, as in the previous two, our approach has been not only to describe what drugs do but to emphasise the mechanisms by which they act – where possible at the cellular and molecular level. Therapeutic agents have a high rate of obsolescence and many are replaced each year; an appreciation of the mechanisms of action of the class of drugs to which a new agent belongs provides a good starting point for understanding and using the new compound intelligently.

In this edition, the clinical aspects of the book have been strengthened by the addition of a clinical pharmacologist as the third author. Furthermore, the therapeutic use of drugs has been given prominence by setting it out in easily identified pink 'clinical boxes'.

All chapters have been updated. As regards new material, we have taken into account not only new agents but also recent extensions of basic knowledge which presage further drug development. There are now new chapters on nitric oxide and on neurodegenerative disease and its treatment and there has been major revision of the sections on cardiovascular pharmacology, drugs acting on 5-HT-receptors, drug interactions, growth factors and cytokines, drug toxicity, and the course of HIV infection and approaches to its treatment. The sections on the general principles of how drugs act and on receptor pharmacology and signal transduction mechanisms have been updated and extended. As before, we have included chapters on measurement in pharmacology and on CNS transmitters as a basis for understanding the actions of drugs on the CNS. In addition, we have emphasised information which sheds new light on the aetiology and treatment of peptic ulcer, cyclo-oxygenases and the action of NSAIDs, and the biology of cancer, since there may well be a change in therapeutic practice in the first of these and rapid progress in new drug development in the latter two.

Inappropriate immune and inflammatory responses are involved in many if not most of the diseases which the clinician will meet, and the development of drugs to control these processes is a major concern of the pharmaceutical industry. Students of both pharmacology and medicine need to be aware of recent progress in these fields and we have therefore updated the sections on inflammation and allergy.

We have again incorporated short sets of key points, set off in red-outlined boxes throughout the text. These are not intended to be comprehensive summaries but rather to highlight pharmacological information which we consider important. We feel that inclusion of these boxes is of value because, with factual knowledge in pharmacology so extensive and expanding so rapidly, students can easily find the information load daunting.

As before, we have put emphasis on the chemical structures of those drugs for which knowledge of structure/activity relationships enhances appreciation of how the drugs act, and we have omitted many chemical structures which do not add to pharmacological understanding in favour of diagrams which do.

Pharmacology is a lively scientific discipline in its own right, with an importance beyond that of providing a basis for the use of drugs in therapy. We have therefore, where appropriate, included brief coverage of the use of drugs as probes for elucidating cellular and physiological functions, even when the compounds have no clinical uses.

It was gratifying to find that many readers found helpful the short summaries of relevant physiological and biochemical processes which we had placed at the beginning of many chapters to form a basis for the subsequent discussion of pharmacological actions; we have therefore retained and updated these. To cater for graduate students and university teachers who apparently found the previous editions useful, we have included fairly extensive sections on 'References and further reading' at the end of each chapter.

We are grateful to the readers who have written appreciative letters about the book and particularly to those who made constructive comments, which we have done our best to incorporate. Comments on the new edition will be welcome.

London 1995

H. P. Rang
M. M. Dale
J. M. Ritter

Acknowledgments

We would like to thank the following for their help and advice in the preparation of this edition; Dr Isobel Heyman, Professor J. Mandelstam, Dr P. J. Chowienczyk, Dr A. Dornhorst, Professor R. D. Rubens, Dr R. Botting, Dr L. G. Garland, Dr R. A. Coleman, Dr P. Blower, Dr G. Darby, Dr T. Peto, Dr G. Cook, Dr T. Cunnane, Dr K. Maynard, Dr K. G. H. Dyke, Mrs J. Andrews, Mrs E. A. Higgs, and the staff of the Royal Society of Medicine Library.

H. P. Rang
M. M. Dale
J. M. Ritter

Contents

GENERAL PRINCIPLES

1

HOW DRUGS ACT: GENERAL PRINCIPLES

Pharmacology can be defined as the study of the manner in which the function of living systems is affected by chemical agents. It is a rather young science, having first achieved independent recognition at the end of the nineteenth century in Germany. Long before this, of course, medical remedies based on herbs were in widespread use, but there was a surprising reluctance to apply anything resembling scientific principles to therapeutics. Even Robert Boyle, who laid the scientific foundations of chemistry in the middle of the seventeenth century, was content, when dealing with therapeutics (*A Collection of Choice Remedies*, 1692), to describe and recommend a hotchpotch of messes consisting of worms, dung, urine and the moss from a dead man's skull. It may be said, indeed, that therapeutics was scarcely influenced by science until the mid-nineteenth century, at which date Virchow dismissed the subject thus: 'Therapeutics is in an empirical stage cared for by practical doctors and clinicians, and it is by means of a combination with physiology that it must rise to be a science, which today it is not.' At that time, knowledge of the normal and abnormal functioning of the body was simply too incomplete to provide even a rough basis for understanding drug effects; at the same time there was a strong feeling that disease and death were semi-sacred subjects, appropriately dealt with by authoritarian, rather than scientific, doctrines. The history of malaria treatment shows how clinical practice could display an obedience to authority, and ignore what appear to be easily ascertainable facts. Cinchona bark was recognised as a specific and effective treatment, and a sound protocol for its use was laid down by Lind in 1765. In 1804, however, Johnson stated, on the basis of clinical practice in India, that cinchona bark was unsafe until the fever had subsided, and he recommended instead the use of large doses of calomel in the early stages. This advice, though murderous in practice, was generally acted upon for the next 40 years.

DRUGS IN MEDICINE

Repeated attempts were made to construct systems of therapeutics, many of which produced even worse results than pure empiricism. One of these was *allopathy*, espoused by James Gregory (1735–1821). The favoured remedies included blood-letting, emetics and purgatives, and these were used until the dominant symptoms of the disease were suppressed. Many patients died from such treatment, and it was in reaction against it that Hahnemann introduced the practice of *homoeopathy* in the early nineteenth century. The guiding principles of homoeopathy are:

- like cures like
- activity can be enhanced by dilution.

The system rapidly drifted into absurdity: for example, Hahnemann recommended the use of drugs at dilutions of $1:10^{60}$, equivalent to 1 molecule in a sphere the size of the orbit of Neptune.

Many other systems of therapeutics have come and gone, and the variety of dogmatic principles that they embodied have tended to hinder rather than advance scientific progress.*

Drugs have, for many years, been the most widely used form of therapeutic intervention available to doctors. Reliance on natural products, mainly from plants, predominated until, in the 1920s, synthetic chemicals were first introduced, and the modern pharmaceutical industry began to develop. Natural products are still important in some fields, notably chemotherapy (Ch. 35), but new synthetic chemicals are now the main source of new drugs. The last decade has seen the rapid emergence of biotechnology as a source of new therapeutic agents in the form of antibodies, enzymes and various regulatory proteins, including hormones, growth factors and cytokines. Very recently, the first human trials of gene therapy have begun, in which DNA is introduced into the genome of cells with the aim of correcting specific genetic or pathological defects (see Tolstoshev 1993). This trend will undoubtedly increase (see Weatherall 1991). The dividing line between these approaches and pharmacologically based therapeutics is an arbitrary one. In this book, only passing reference is made to biotechnologically based therapeutics.

Scientific understanding of drug action—the kind of understanding that enables us to predict the pharmacological effects of a novel chemical substance, or to design a chemical that will produce a specified therapeutic effect—is growing rapidly, but is still far from complete. Even so, certain generalisations are possible, and these are discussed in this chapter.

*Therapeutic systems whose basis lies outside the domain of science are, of course, very much alive today, and they are even gaining ground under the general banner of 'alternative' or 'holistic' medicine. Mostly they reject the 'medical model' which attributes disease to an underlying derangement of normal function which can be defined in biochemical or structural terms, detected by objective means, and influenced beneficially by appropriate chemical or physical interventions. They focus instead mainly on subjective malaise, which may be disease-associated or not. Abandoning objectivity in defining and measuring disease goes along with a similar departure from scientific principles in assessing therapeutic efficacy, with the result that principles and practices can gain acceptance without satisfying any of the criteria of validity that would convince a critical scientist, and that are required by law to be satisfied before a new drug can be introduced into therapy. As with electric hand-dryers, public acceptance has little to do with demonstrable efficacy; this is perhaps to be expected in a market economy.

To begin with, we should gratefully acknowledge Paul Ehrlich for insisting early in this century that drug action should be understood in terms of conventional chemical interactions between drugs and tissues, and for dispelling the idea that the remarkable potency and specificity of action of some drugs put them somehow out of reach of chemistry and physics and required the intervention of magical 'vital forces'. Although it is the case that many drugs produce actions in doses and concentrations so small that the dimensions assume an almost astronomical remoteness, low concentrations still involve very large numbers of molecules. Thus one drop of a solution of a drug at only 10^{-10} mol/l still contains about 10^{10} drug molecules, so there is no mystery in the fact that it may produce an obvious pharmacological response. Some bacterial toxins (e.g. diphtheria toxin) act with such precision that a single molecule taken up by a target cell is sufficient to kill it.

THE BINDING OF DRUG MOLECULES TO CELLS

One of the basic tenets of pharmacology is that drug molecules must exert some chemical influence on one or more constituents of cells in order to produce a pharmacological response. In other words, drug molecules must get so close to the molecules of which cells are made that the functioning of the cellular molecules is altered. Of course, the molecules in the organism vastly outnumber the drug molecules and if the drug molecules were merely distributed at random, the chance of interaction with any particular class of cellular molecule would be negligible. Pharmacological effects therefore require, in general, the non-uniform distribution of the drug molecule within the body or tissue, which is the same as saying that drug molecules must be 'bound' to particular constituents of cells and tissues in order to produce an effect. Ehrlich summed it up thus: '*Corpora non agunt nisi fixata*' (in this context, 'A drug will not work unless it is bound').*

*There are actually, if one looks hard enough, several exceptions to Ehrlich's dictum, drugs which act without being bound to any tissue constituent (for example osmotic diuretics, osmotic purgatives, antacids, heavy metal chelating agents). The principle remains true for the great majority, however.

Understanding the nature of these binding sites, and the mechanisms by which the association of a drug molecule with a binding site leads to a physiological response, constitutes the major thrust of pharmacological research. Most drugs produce their effects by binding, in the first instance, to protein molecules. There may be some exceptions to this. For example, the group of non-specific depressant substances, to which many general anaesthetics belong (see Ch. 26), have long been thought to produce their effects by an interaction with membrane lipid rather than with protein, though even this cherished theory is under strong attack from the protein lobby (see Franks & Lieb 1987). Apart from this, the only important exception to proteins as target sites is DNA, on which a number of antitumour and antimicrobial drugs act (Ch. 35), as well as mutagenic and carcinogenic agents (Ch. 43).

Protein targets for drug binding

Four kinds of regulatory proteins are commonly involved as primary drug targets, namely:

- enzymes
- carrier molecules
- ion channels
- receptors.

A few other types of protein (e.g. structural proteins such as tubulin, which specifically binds **colchicine**; Ch. 12) are known to function as drug targets, and it must be remembered that there exist many drugs whose sites of action have not yet been analysed in detail. Furthermore, many drugs are known to bind (in addition to their primary targets) to plasma proteins (see Ch. 4), as well as to cellular constituents, without producing any obvious physiological effect. Nevertheless, the generalisation that most drugs act on one or other of the four types of protein listed above serves as a good starting point.

Further discussion of the mechanisms by which such binding leads to cellular responses is given in Chapter 2.

A note on terminology

The term *receptor* tends to be used loosely, and can cause confusion. Some authors use it to mean *any* target molecule with which a drug molecule has to combine in order to elicit its specific effect, which can include any of the four types listed. Thus, the voltage-sensitive sodium channel of excitable membranes is sometimes referred to as the 'receptor' for local anaesthetics (see Ch. 34), or the enzyme dihydrofolate reductase as the 'receptor' for **methotrexate** (Ch. 36). In each case the drug molecule combines with and incapacitates the protein molecule, thus producing its effect. This is different from the situation where, for example, adrenaline acts on a receptor in the heart (see Ch. 7). In this case, the receptor molecule has no other function but to serve as a recognition site for catecholamines. When adrenaline binds to the receptor, a train of reactions is initiated (see Ch. 2), leading to an increase in force and rate of the heartbeat. The receptor produces an effect only when adrenaline is bound; otherwise it is functionally silent.* This, in general, is true of all hormone and neurotransmitter receptors. In this context, certain substances (*agonists*) can be said to 'activate' the receptors, and others (*antagonists*) may combine at the same site without causing activation. Receptors of this type form a key part of the system of chemical communication that all multicellular organisms use to coordinate the activities of their cells and organs. Without them we would be no better than a bucketful of amoebae. The distinction between agonists and antagonists only exists for receptors with this type of physiological regulatory role; we cannot usefully speak of 'agonists' for the noradrenaline carrier or for the voltage-sensitive sodium channel or for dihydrofolate reductase. In pharmacology it is best to reserve the term 'receptor' for interactions of the regulatory type, where the small molecule (*ligand*) may function either as an agonist or as an antagonist; in practice this limits use of the term to receptors which have a physiological regulatory function, and this usage will be observed in this book.** More details about the molecular nature of receptors, and the ways in which they influence cell function, are given in Chapter 2.

*Actually some receptors, such as the benzodiazepine receptor (Ch. 27) show resting activity, which can be either increased or decreased when a ligand molecule binds.

**We break our own rule in Chapter 15 by referring to the 'LDL receptor', a term in common usage to describe a macromolecule—not strictly a receptor according to our definition—which plays a key role in lipoprotein metabolism.

DRUG SPECIFICITY

For a drug to be in any way useful as either a therapeutic or a scientific tool, it must act selectively on particular cells and tissues. In other words it must show a high degree of *binding-site specificity*. Conversely, proteins that function as drug targets generally show a high degree of *ligand specificity*; they will recognise only ligands of a certain precise type, and ignore closely related molecules.

These principles of binding-site and ligand specificity can be clearly recognised in the actions of a mediator such as angiotensin (Ch. 14). This peptide acts strongly on vascular smooth muscle, and on the kidney tubule, but has very little effect on other kinds of smooth muscle, or on the intestinal epithelium. Other mediators affect a quite different spectrum of cells and tissues, the pattern in each case being determined by the specific pattern of expression of the protein receptors for the various mediators. On the other hand, a small chemical change, such as conversion of one of the amino acids in angiotensin from L- to D-form, or removal of one amino acid from the chain, can inactivate the molecule altogether, since the receptor fails to bind the altered form. The complementary specificity of ligands and binding sites is central to explaining many of the phenomena of pharmacology. One of the most exciting themes at the present time is the increasing understanding of protein structure and its relation to the remarkable powers of molecular recognition that many proteins (and particularly drug targets) possess. It is no exaggeration to say that the ability of proteins to interact in a highly selective way with other molecules—including other proteins—is the basis of living machines. Its relevance to the understanding of drug action will be a recurring theme in this book.

Finally, it must be emphasised that no drug acts with complete specificity. Thus histamine antagonists (Ch. 12), although they can be shown to have a higher affinity for histamine receptors than for other sites, produce many effects, such as sedation and prevention of vomiting, which do not appear to depend on histamine antagonism. In general, the lower the potency of a drug, and the higher the dose needed, the more likely it is that sites of action other than the primary one will assume significance. In clinical terms, this is often associated with the appearance of unwanted side effects, of which no drug is free.

The main thrust of pharmacological research in recent years has been to characterise, in molecular terms, the primary site of action of many different types of drug. The success of this approach has illuminated the mode of action of several important drugs whose actions were until recently not understood at all, only described. **Aspirin** is one example where, thanks to the work on prostaglandins by Vane and his colleagues (see Ch. 11), a multitude of apparently unrelated effects can now be explained in terms of inhibition of a single group of enzymes responsible for converting arachidonic acid to prostanoids. Similarly, the **benzodiazepines**, an important group of minor tranquillisers, are now known to act on specific sites in the brain, thereby potentiating the action of an inhibitory neurotransmitter (gamma-aminobutyric acid; see Ch. 24); the action of **morphine-like analgesics** (Ch. 31) has also been narrowed to specific receptor sites for these drugs, whose actions had been described in exhaustive physiological detail many years previously without any real insight into mechanism having been achieved.

Targets for drug action

- A drug is a chemical that affects physiological function in a *specific way*.
- Most drugs are effective because they bind to particular target proteins, namely:
  —enzymes
  —carriers
  —ion channels
  —receptors.
- Specificity is reciprocal: individual classes of drug bind only to certain targets, and individual targets recognise only certain classes of drug.
- No drugs are completely specific in their actions. In many cases, increasing the dose of a drug will cause it to affect targets other than the principal one, and lead to side effects.

RECEPTOR CLASSIFICATION

Where the action of a drug can be construed in terms of its combination with a special type of receptor, this provides a valuable means for classification and refinement in drug design. For example, by the mid-1960s, analysis of the numerous actions of histamine (see Ch. 11) showed that some of its effects (the H_1 effects, such as smooth muscle contraction) were strongly antagonised by the competitive histamine antagonists then known. Black and his colleagues, in 1970, suggested that the remaining actions of **histamine**, which included its powerful stimulant effect on gastric secretion, might represent a second class of histamine receptor. They tested this theory by preparing histamine analogues, some of which showed selectivity in stimulating gastric secretion while having only a weak effect on smooth muscle. By seeing which parts of the histamine molecule conferred this type of specificity, they were able to develop selective antagonists. Such antagonists proved to be potent in blocking gastric acid secretion and all of the other effects now classified as H_2 effects. A third type of histamine receptor (H_3) has recently been defined.

This example illustrates the principle of receptor classification based on pharmacological criteria—receptors being classified on the basis of the effects of particular drugs—which continues to be a valuable and widely-used approach. In recent years, however, new experimental approaches have revealed several different criteria on which to base receptor classification. The first of these was the direct measurement of ligand binding to receptors (see p. 13), which allowed many new receptor subclasses to be defined—subclasses only very dimly discernible from studies of drug effects. More recently, molecular cloning has revealed the amino acid sequence of many receptors (see Ch. 2), providing a completely new basis for classification at a much finer level of detail than can be reached through pharmacological analysis. Finally, analysis of the biochemical pathways that are activated in response to receptor activation (see Ch. 2) shows patterns that provide yet another basis for classification. The result of this data explosion has been that receptor classification has suddenly become very much more detailed, with a proliferation of receptor subtypes for all of the main types of ligand; more worryingly, alternative molecular and biochemical classifications began to spring up which were incompatible with the accepted pharmacologically defined receptor classes. Responding to this growing confusion, the International Union of Pharmacological Sciences (IUPHAR) has set up various expert working groups to produce agreed receptor classifications for the major types, taking into account the pharmacological, molecular and biochemical information available. These wise men have a hard task, and the results will be neither perfect nor final, but are essential to ensure a consistent terminology. To the student, this may seem an arcane exercise in taxonomy, generating much detail but little illumination; the tedious lists of drug names, actions and side effects that used to burden the subject are in danger of being replaced by exhaustive tables of receptors, ligands and transduction pathways. In this book, we have tried to avoid detail for its own sake, and include only such information on receptor classification as seems interesting in its own right, or is helpful in explaining the actions of important drugs. A useful summary of known receptor classes is now published annually (*Trends in Pharmacological Sciences, Receptor Supplement*).

QUANTITATIVE ASPECTS OF DRUG–RECEPTOR INTERACTIONS

An excellent account of the quantitative analysis of drug–receptor interactions is available for those seeking more detail than is given here (Kenakin 1987).

The first step in drug action on specific receptors is the formation of a reversible drug–receptor complex, the reactions being governed by the Law of Mass Action. Suppose that a piece of tissue, such as heart muscle or smooth muscle, contains a total number of receptors N_{tot}, for an agonist such as adrenaline. When the tissue is exposed to adrenaline at concentration x_A and allowed to come to equilibrium, a certain number N_A of the receptors will become occupied, and the number of vacant receptors will be reduced to $N_{tot} - N_A$. Normally the number of adrenaline molecules applied to the tissue in solution greatly exceeds N_{tot}, so that the binding reaction does not appreciably reduce x_A. The magnitude of the response produced by the adrenaline will be related (even if we do not know exactly how) to the number of receptors occupied, so it is useful to consider what quantitative relationship is predicted between N_A and x_A. The reaction can be represented by:

$$\underset{(x_A)}{\underset{\text{drug}}{\text{A}}} + \underset{(N_{tot}-N_A)}{\underset{\text{free receptor}}{\text{R}}} \underset{k_{-1}}{\overset{k_{+1}}{\rightleftharpoons}} \underset{(N_A)}{\underset{\text{complex}}{\text{AR}}}$$

The Law of Mass Action (which states that the

rate of a chemical reaction is proportional to the product of the concentrations of reactants) can be applied to this reaction.

$$\text{Rate of forward reaction} = k_{+1}x_A(N_{tot} - N_A) \qquad (1.1)$$

$$\text{Rate of backward reaction} = k_{-1}N_A \qquad (1.2)$$

At equilibrium the two rates are equal:

$$k_{+1}x_A(N_{tot} - N_A) = k_{-1}N_A \qquad (1.3)$$

The proportion of receptors occupied or 'occupancy', $p_A = N_A/N_{tot}$, which is independent of N_{tot}, is:

$$p_A = \frac{x_A}{x_A + k_{-1}/k_{+1}} \qquad (1.4)$$

Defining the equilibrium constant for the binding reaction, $K_A = k_{-1}/k_{+1}$, equation (1.4) can be written:

$$p_A = \frac{x_A}{x_A + K_A} \text{ or } p_A = \frac{x_A/K_A}{x_A/K_A + 1} \qquad (1.5)$$

This important result is known as the *Langmuir equation*, after the physical chemist who derived it to describe the adsorption of gases by metal surfaces.*

The equilibrium constant, K_A, is a characteristic of the drug and of the receptor; it has the dimensions of concentration and is numerically equal to the concentration of drug required to occupy 50% of the sites at equilibrium. (Verify from equation (1.5) that when $x_A = K_A$, $P_A = 0.5$.) The higher the *affinity* of the drug for the receptors, the lower will be K_A. Equation (1.5) describes the relationship between occupancy and drug concentration, and generates a characteristic curve known as a *rectangular hyperbola*, as shown in Figure 1.1A. It is common in pharmacological work to use a logarithmic scale of concentration; this converts the hyperbola to a symmetrical sigmoid curve (Fig. 1.1B).

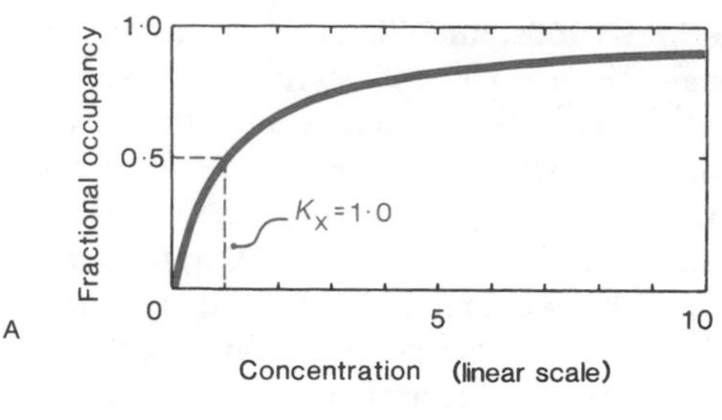

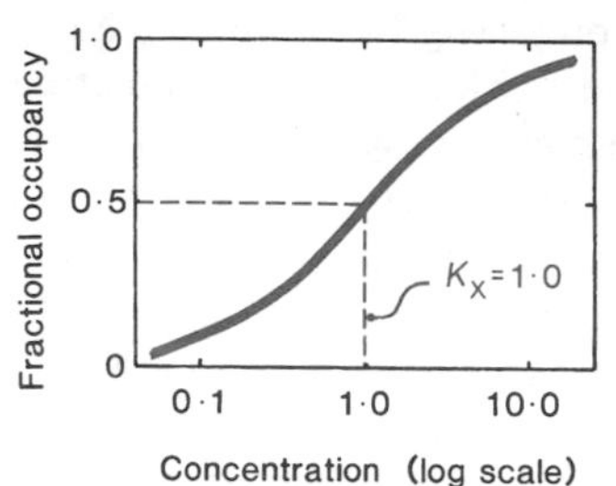

Fig. 1.1 Theoretical relationship between occupancy and ligand concentration, plotted according to equation (1.5). A. Plotted with a linear concentration scale, this curve is a rectangular hyperbola. **B.** Plotted with a logarithmic concentration scale, this is a symmetrical sigmoid curve.

AGONIST CONCENTRATION–EFFECT CURVES

It is now possible to measure directly the binding of drugs to their receptors in tissues (see p. 13) and to show that equation (1.5) is obeyed. Much more often it is a biological response, such as a rise in blood pressure, contraction or relaxation of a strip of smooth muscle in an organ bath, or the activation of an enzyme, that is actually measured and plotted as a *concentration–effect* or *dose–response curve*, as in Figure 1.2. These look similar to the theoretical concentration–occupancy curves in Figure 1.1B, and it is tempting to try to use such experimental curves to measure the affinity of agonist drugs for their receptors by making the assumption that the response produced is directly proportional to occupancy. This is, however, rarely valid, for in general the response is a complex, non-linear function of occupancy. For an integrated physiological response, such as a rise in arterial blood pressure produced by adrenaline, several different processes interact. **Adrenaline** (see Ch. 7) increases cardiac output and constricts some blood vessels while dilating others, and the change in arterial pressure itself evokes a reflex response which modifies the primary response to the drug. It is obviously unrealistic to expect that the final effect will be directly proportional to occupancy in this instance, and the same is true of most drug-induced effects.

A second difficulty in drawing inferences about agonist affinity from concentration–effect curves is

*It should actually have been named after A V Hill, the physiologist who derived it in 1909, but so many equations bear his name that it would be excessive to insist on adding another.

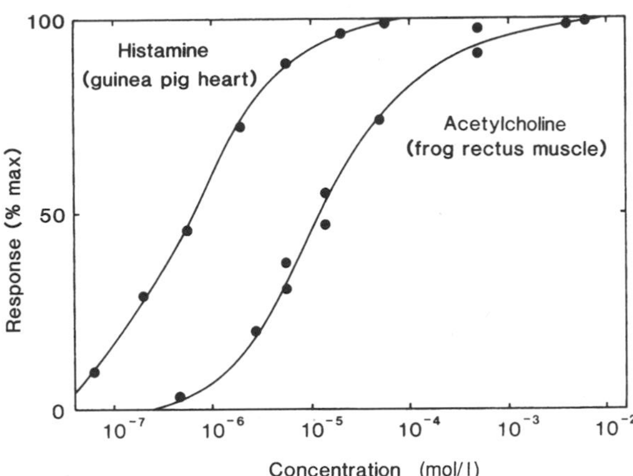

Fig. 1.2 Experimentally observed concentration–effect curves. Though the lines, drawn according to the binding equation (1.5), fit the points well, such curves do not give correct estimates of the affinity of drugs for receptors. This is because the relationship between receptor occupancy and response is usually non-linear.

that the concentration of the drug *at the receptors* is often not known, even though the concentration in the organ bath is simple to calculate. Thus agonists may be subject to rapid enzymic degradation or uptake by cells as they diffuse from the surface towards their site of action, and a steady state can be reached in which the agonist concentration at the receptors is very much less than the concentration in the bath. In the case of **acetylcholine,** for example, which is hydrolysed by cholinesterase present in most tissues (see Ch. 6), the concentration reaching the receptors can be less than 1% of that in the bath, and an even bigger difference has been found with **noradrenaline**, which is avidly taken up by sympathetic nerve terminals in many tissues (see Ch. 7). Thus, even if the concentration–effect curve looks just like a facsimile of the binding curve, as in Figure 1.2, it cannot be used directly to determine the affinity of the agonist for the receptors.

Binding of drugs to receptors

- Binding of drugs to receptors necessarily obeys the Law of Mass Action.
- At equilibrium, *receptor occupancy* is related to *drug concentration* by the *Langmuir equation.*
- The higher the *affinity* of the drug for the receptor, the lower the concentration range over which it will approach saturation of the receptors.
- The same principles apply when two or more drugs compete for the same receptors; each has the effect of reducing the apparent affinity for the other.

COMPETITIVE ANTAGONISM

Equation (1.5) describes the relationship between concentration and occupancy when a single drug is present. The treatment can easily be extended to describe the situation when two or more competing drugs are present. 'Competing' means that the receptor can bind only one drug molecule at a time. If the two drugs are designated A and B, the reactions can be represented as follows:

$$\underset{(x_A)}{A} + \underset{(N_{tot}-N_A-N_B)}{R} \underset{k_{-1A}}{\overset{k_{+1A}}{\rightleftharpoons}} \underset{(N_A)}{AR}$$

$$\underset{(x_B)}{B} + \underset{(N_{tot}-N_A-N_B)}{R} \underset{k_{-1B}}{\overset{k_{+1B}}{\rightleftharpoons}} \underset{(N_B)}{BR}$$

As before, at equilibrium, the forward and backward rates are equal:

$$k_{+1A}x_A(N_{tot} - N_A - N_B) = k_{-1A}N_A \qquad (1.6)$$

$$k_{+1B}x_B(N_{tot} - N_A - N_B) = k_{-1B}N_B \qquad (1.7)$$

Therefore:

$$p_A = \frac{x_A/K_A}{x_A/K_A + x_B/K_B + 1} \qquad (1.8)$$

Comparing this result with equation (1.5) shows that adding drug B (the competitive antagonist), as expected, reduces the occupancy by drug A, if the concentration of A is kept the same. Alternatively, the concentration of A may be increased (to x_A' say) so as to restore p_A, to the value reached in the absence of the antagonist, the ratio $r\ (= x_A'/x_A)$, by which the concentration will need to be increased, is given (from equations 1.5 and 1.8) by:

$$r = \frac{x_B}{K_B} + 1 \qquad (1.9)$$

If it is assumed that the response of the test system depends only on the agonist occupancy p_A' then it is predicted from the theory given above that the effect of the competitive antagonist on the response

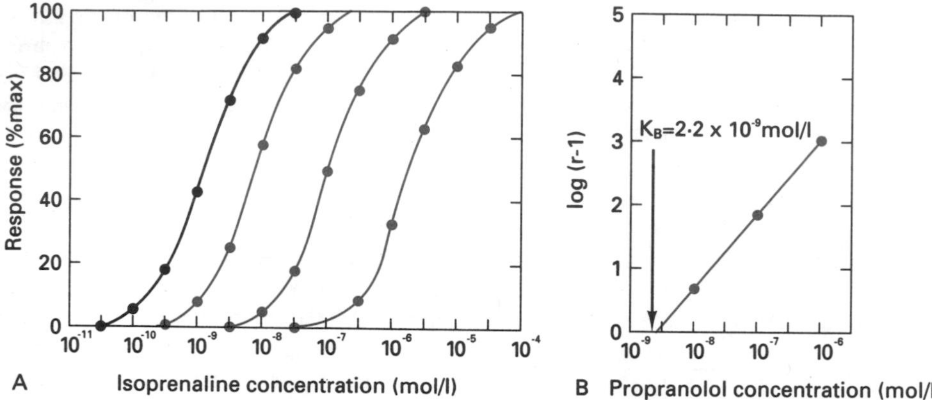

Fig. 1.3 Competitive antagonism of isoprenaline by propranolol measured on isolated guinea-pig atria. A. Concentration–effect curves at various propranolol concentrations (indicated on the curves). Note the progressive shift to the right without a change of slope or maximum. **B.** Schild plot (equation 1.10). The equilibrium constant (*K*) for propranolol is given by the abscissal intercept 2.2×10^{-9} mol/l. (Results from: Potter L T 1967 J Pharmacol 155: 91)

can also be overcome by increasing the agonist concentration *r*-fold. Equation (1.9) is therefore useful experimentally, because it should apply to measurements of biological responses as well as to direct measurements of agonist binding. Equation (1.9), which is often known as the *Schild equation* after its originator, predicts two characteristic properties of competitive antagonism:

- The dose ratio r depends *only* on the concentration and equilibrium constant of the antagonist, and not on the size of response that is chosen as a reference point for the measurements, nor on the equilibrium constant for the agonist. On a semilogarithmic plot of effect against concentration, therefore, the effect of the competitive antagonist will be to shift the curve to the right without changing its slope or maximum, a characteristic that can easily be tested experimentally.
- The dose ratio achieved should increase linearly with x_B, and the slope of a plot of $(r-1)$ against x_B is equal to $1/K_B$.* This relationship, being independent of the characteristics of the agonist, should be the same for all agonists that act on the same population of receptors.

These equations have been verified for many examples of competitive antagonism (Fig. 1.3). Equation (1.9) is often accurately obeyed up to dose ratios as high as 10 000, making it one of the most precisely obeyed relationships encountered in biology.

Competitive antagonism

- *Reversible competitive antagonism* is the commonest and most important type of antagonism, and has two main characteristics:
  - — in the presence of the antagonist, the agonist log concentration–effect curve is shifted to the right without change in slope or maximum, the extent of the shift being a measure of the dose *ratio*
  - — the dose ratio increases *linearly* with antagonist concentration; the slope of this line is a measure of the affinity of the antagonist for the receptor.
- Antagonist affinity, measured in this way, is widely used as a basis for receptor classification.

*Equation (1.9) can be expressed logarithmically in the form:

$$\log(r-1) = \log x_B - \log K_B \qquad (1.10)$$

Thus a plot of log $(r-1)$ against log x_B, usually called a *Schild plot*, should give a straight line with unit slope and an abscissal intercept equal to log K_B. A commonly used convention, analogous to the pH and pK notation, is to express antagonist potency as a pA_2 value; under conditions of competitive antagonism $pA_2 = -\log K_B$. Numerically, pA_2 is defined as *the negative logarithm of the molar concentration of antagonist required to produce an agonist dose ratio equal to 2.* As with pH notation, its principal advantage is that it produces simple numbers, a pA_2 of 6.5 being equivalent to $K_B = 3.2 \times 10^{-7}$ mol/l.

PARTIAL AGONISTS AND THE CONCEPT OF EFFICACY

In the discussion so far, drugs have been regarded either as *agonists*, which in some way 'activate' the receptor when they occupy it, or as *antagonists*, which cause no activation. However, the ability of a drug molecule to activate the receptor is actually a graded, rather than an all-or-nothing, property. If a series of chemically related agonist drugs acting on the same receptors is tested on a given biological system, it is often found that the maximal response (the largest response that can be produced by that drug in high concentration) differs from one drug to another. Generally, there are several agonists whose maximal response corresponds to the full response of the tissue (the largest response that the tissue is capable of giving). These drugs are known as *full agonists*, and those whose maximal response falls short of the full response are known as *partial agonists* (Fig. 1.4). The difference between them lies in the relationship between occupancy and response.

Figure 1.5 shows the relationship between occupancy and concentration for a drug whose equilibrium constant is 1.0 μmol/l. If the drug is a full agonist, it might produce a maximal response at about 0.2 μmol/l, the relationship between response and occupancy being shown in B (curve *a*). The situation for a partial agonist with the same affinity is also shown, the essential difference being that the response at any given occupancy is much smaller, so that it cannot produce a maximal response even at 100% occupancy. This can be expressed quantitatively in terms of *efficacy*, a parameter originally defined by Stephenson (1956) which describes the 'strength' of a single drug–receptor complex in evoking a response of the tissue. Subsequently, it was appreciated that characteristics of the tissue (e.g. the number of receptors that it possesses and the nature of the coupling between the receptor and the response; see Ch. 2), as well as of the drug–receptor complex, were important, and the concept of *intrinsic efficacy* was developed (see Kenakin 1987, 1989). The relationship between occupancy and response can thus be represented:

Characteristics of tissue

$$\text{Response} = f\left(\frac{\varepsilon N_{tot}\, x_A}{x_A + K_A}\right)$$

Characteristics of drug

In this equation, f represents the *transducer function* which describes the characteristics of the responding system; ε is the *intrinsic efficacy*, which is a characteristic of the drug–receptor complex. The importance of this formal representation is that it explains how differences in the transducer function and the density of receptors in different tissues can result in the same agonist, acting on what we believe to be the same receptor, appearing as a full agonist in one tissue and as a partial agonist in another. By the same token, the relative potencies of two agonists may be different in different tissues, even though the receptor is the same. Results of this kind have often been reported and interpreted as evidence for multiple types of receptor, but it has to be realised that agonist effects depend on more than just the receptor; in general, inferences about receptor classification are more safely based on studies with competitive antagonists (see above). A more detailed account of the formal analysis of drug–receptor interactions is given by Kenakin (1987).

It would be nice to be able to give a more concrete account of what efficacy means in physical terms, and to understand why one drug may be

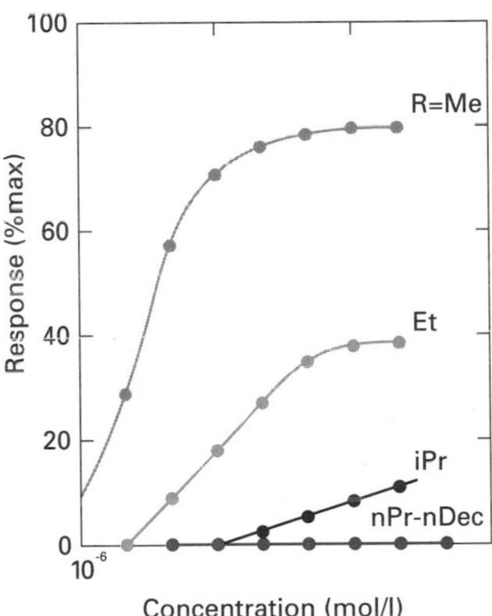

Fig. 1.4 Partial agonists. Concentration–effect curves for substituted methonium compounds on frog *rectus abdominis* muscle. The compounds were members of the decamethonium series (Ch. 6), R Me_2 $N^+(CH_2)_{10}$ N^+ Me_2 R. The maximum response obtainable decreases (i.e. efficacy decreases) as the size of R is increased. With R = nPr or larger, the compounds cause no response, and are pure antagonists. (Results from: Van Rossum J M 1958 Pharmacodynamics of cholinometic and cholinolytic drugs. St Catherine's Press, Bruges)

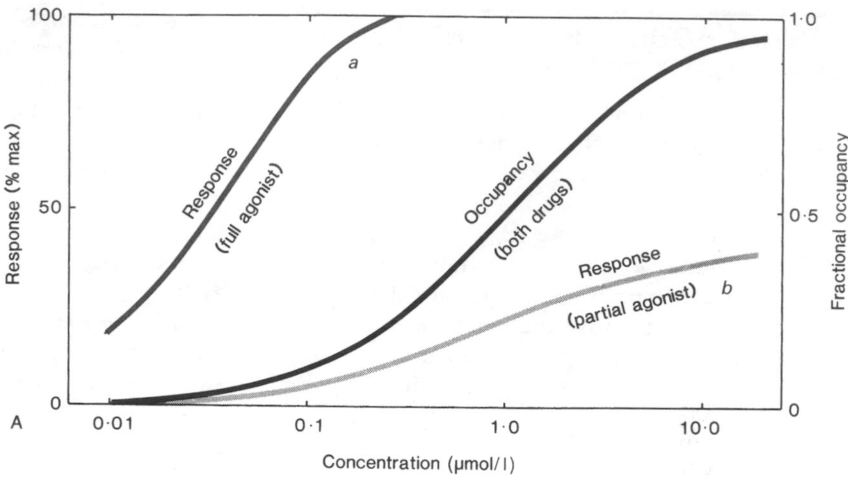

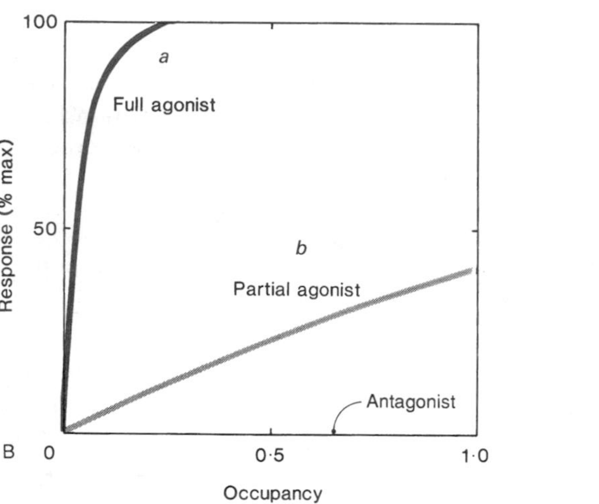

Fig. 1.5 Theoretical occupancy and response curves for full and partial agonists. A. The occupancy curve is for both drugs, the response curves *a* and *b* are for full and partial agonist respectively. **B.** The relationship between response and occupancy for full and partial agonist, corresponding to the response curves above. Note that curve *a* produces maximal response at about 20% occupancy, while curve *b* produces only a submaximal response even at 100% occupancy.

an agonist while another, chemically very similar, is an antagonist. As yet this cannot be done, but the simple scheme known as the *two-state model* (see Colquhoun 1973) shown in Figure 1.6 provides a starting point. It is envisaged that the receptor can exist in two states, 'resting' (*R*) and 'activated' ($R^{\star}$), either of which can bind a drug molecule, the equilibrium constants being K and $K^{\star}$ respectively. A shift in the equilibrium between these two states in favour of $R^{\star}$ initiates the response (see Ch. 2). Normally, when no ligand is present, the equilibrium favours the resting state. For binding of a drug molecule to shift the equilibrium in favour of $R^{\star}$ (in other words, for a drug to be an agonist), the necessary condition is that the drug should have a higher affinity for $R^{\star}$ than for R ($K > K^{\star}$). The larger the ratio $K/K^{\star}$, the greater the drug's efficacy. If $K = K^{\star}$, binding will leave the conformational equilibrium undisturbed, and the drug will be a pure competitive antagonist.*

This formalism is undoubtedly too simple, especially for receptors that act through more complex

*The two-state model can also account for the phenomenon of *inverse agonists*, which occurs with benzodiazepine receptors (Ch. 27) and calcium-channels (Ch. 14). For these two receptors, a range of ligands exists, some of which produce an agonist effect (increased sensitivity to GABA in the case of benzodiazepines; increased opening of voltage-sensitive calcium channels in the case of Ca^{2+} channel ligands); some act as competitive antagonists, while others produce the opposite effect (inverse agonists). It is postulated that these receptors, in the absence of any ligand, are distributed more or less equally between the two states, so that the equilibrium can be shifted in either direction, producing opposite effects, according to whether $K^{\star} > K$ or vice versa.

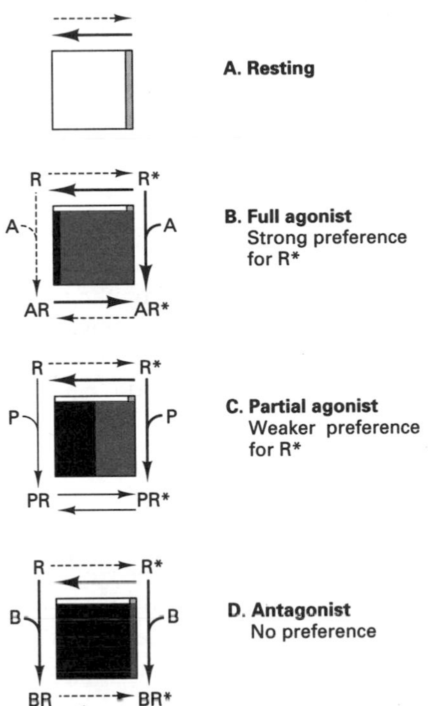

Fig. 1.6 Interpretation of efficacy in terms of binding preference of the ligand for the resting state (*R*) and the activated state (*R*) of the receptor. Black and dark pink blocks show the proportion of liganded receptors in the *R* and *R** conformations respectively, white and light pink blocks represent unoccupied receptors in the *R* and *R** conformations respectively. **A.** In the absence of ligand, the conformational equilibrium lies far towards *R*. **B.** A full agonist (*A*) binds much more strongly to *R** than to *R*, so among the liganded receptors (solid blocks), *AR** predominates over *AR*. Thus, when binding approaches saturation, virtually 100% of the receptors are in the *AR** compartment. **C.** A partial agonist (*P*) also shows a preference for *R**, but weaker. Thus, even at saturation, only a proportion of receptors exist as *PR**. **D.** An antagonist (*B*) binds no more strongly to *R** than to *R*, and therefore does not shift the equilibrium from the resting state even when binding approaches saturation. The fact that the receptors are occupied, however, prevents binding of an agonist.

transduction machinery (see Ch. 2). More elaborate models are discussed by Kenakin (1987).

Whatever its theoretical status, however, efficacy is a concept of great practical importance, since the ability of a drug to act as an agonist or antagonist on a particular type of receptor is often crucial for its therapeutic use.

Stephenson (1956), studying the actions of acetylcholine analogues in isolated tissues, found that many full agonists were capable of eliciting maximal responses at very low occupancies, often less than 1%. If a full response can occur when only a small fraction of the receptors is occupied, the system may be said to possess *spare receptors*, or a *receptor reserve*. This is often found among drugs that elicit smooth muscle contraction, but seems to be less important for other types of receptor-mediated response, such as secretion, smooth muscle relaxation or cardiac stimulation, where the effect is more nearly proportional to receptor occupancy. When we talk of spare receptors, this does not imply any actual subdivision of the receptor pool, but merely that the pool is larger than the number needed to evoke a full response. This surplus of receptors over the number actually needed might seem to be a somewhat profligate biological arrangement. In the context of the physiological role of receptors in mediating the actions of hormones and transmitters, however, it makes sense, because it means that a given number of agonist–receptor complexes, corresponding to a given level of biological response, can be reached with a lower concentration of hormone or neurotransmitter than would be the case if fewer receptors were provided. Economy of hormone or transmitter secretion is thus achieved at the expense of providing more receptors.

Agonists, antagonists and efficacy

- Drugs acting on receptors may be *agonists* or *antagonists*.
- Agonists initiate changes in cell function, producing effects of various types; antagonists bind to receptors without initiating such changes.
- Agonist potency depends on two parameters: *affinity* (i.e. tendency to bind to receptors) and *efficacy* (i.e. ability, once bound, to initiate changes which lead to effects).
- For antagonists, efficacy is zero.
- *Full agonists* (which can produce maximal effects) have high efficacy; *partial agonists* (which can produce only submaximal effects) have intermediate efficacy.

DIRECT MEASUREMENT OF DRUG BINDING TO RECEPTORS

Though the basic principles governing the binding of drugs to receptors, and the mode of action of competitive antagonists, were enunciated many years ago by A J Clark and others, it was not until the 1960s that the binding process was first studied directly, by the use of radioactive drug molecules. Such methods are now very widely used for investigating receptors of many different kinds. The main requirements for the method are that the radioactive ligand (which may be an agonist or antagonist for the receptors that are being studied) must bind with high affinity and specificity, must not be metabolised and can be labelled (usually with ^{3}H, ^{14}C or ^{125}I) to a sufficient specific radioactivity to enable minute amounts of binding to be measured. The usual procedure is to incubate samples of the tissue (or membrane fragments) with various concentrations of radioactive drug until equilibrium is reached. The tissue is then removed, or the membrane fragments separated by filtration or centrifugation, and dissolved in scintillation fluid for measurement of its radioactive content.

In such experiments there is invariably a certain amount of 'non-specific binding' (i.e. drug taken up by structures other than receptors) and it is important to choose the ligand and experimental conditions so that this component does not swamp out the specific binding. The amount of non-specific binding is estimated by repeating the experiment in the presence of a saturating concentration of a (non-radioactive) ligand that inhibits completely the binding of the radioactive drug to the receptors, leaving behind the non-specific component. This is then subtracted from the total binding to give an estimate of specific binding (Fig. 1.7).

If the specific binding follows the Langmuir equation (equation 1.5), the relationship between the amount bound (B) and ligand concentration (x) should be:

$$B = \frac{B_{max}x}{x + K} \qquad (1.11)$$

B_{max} is the total number of binding sites in the preparation (often expressed as pmol/mg protein) and K is the equilibrium constant (see equation 1.5). To display the results in linear form, equation (1.11) may be rearranged to:

$$\frac{B}{x} = \frac{B_{max}}{K} - \frac{B}{K} \qquad (1.12)$$

A plot of B/x against B (known as a Scatchard plot; Fig. 1.7) gives a straight line from which both B_{max} and K can be estimated. Statistically, this procedure is not without problems, and it is now usual to estimate these parameters by an iterative non-linear curve-fitting procedure running on a small computer.

Autoradiography can also be used to investigate the distribution of receptors in structures such as the brain, and direct labelling with ligands containing positron-emitting isotopes is now used to obtain images by *positron-emission tomography* (PET) of receptor distribution in vivo (Fig. 1.8). As the measurement of binding has become easier in many

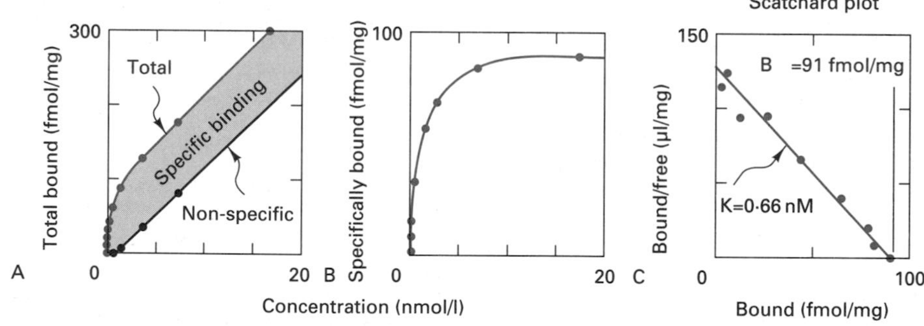

Fig. 1.7 Measurement of receptor binding (β-adrenoceptors in cardiac cell membranes). The ligand was ^{3}H-cyanopindolol, a derivative of pindolol (see Ch. 7). **A.** Measurements of total and non-specific binding at equilibrium. Non-specific binding is measured in the presence of a saturating concentration of a non-radioactive β-receptor antagonist, which prevents the radioactive ligand from binding to β-receptors. The difference between the two lines (light pink) represents specific binding. **B.** Specific binding plotted against concentration. The curve is a rectangular hyperbola (equation 1.11). **C.** Scatchard plot (equation 1.12). This gives a straight line from which the binding parameters K and B_{max} can be calculated.

instances than the measurement of pharmacological effects, 'receptors' are identified on the basis of binding measurements that have no clear connection with pharmacological effects. When combined with pharmacological studies, however, binding measurements have proved very valuable. It has, for example, been confirmed that the spare receptor hypothesis for muscarinic receptors in smooth muscle is correct; agonists are found to bind, in general, with rather low affinity, and a maximal biological effect occurs at low receptor occupancy. It has also been shown, in skeletal muscle and other tissues, that denervation leads to an increase in the number of receptors in the target cell, a finding that accounts, at least in part, for the phenomenon of denervation supersensitivity. More generally, it appears that receptors for many hormones and transmitters tend to increase in number, usually over the course of a few days, if the relevant hormone or transmitter is absent or scarce, and to decrease in number if it is in excess. The mechanism of these changes is not well understood, but the process represents an important cause of adaptation leading to gradual changes in responsiveness to drugs or hormones with continued administration (see p. 19).

Binding curves with agonists are more difficult to interpret than those with antagonists, since they often reveal an apparent heterogeneity among receptors. For example, agonist binding to muscarinic receptors (Ch. 6), and also to β-adrenoceptors (Ch. 7) suggests at least two populations of binding sites with different affinities (Fig. 1.9). This may be due to the fact that receptors can exist either unattached or coupled within the membrane to another macromolecule, the G-protein (see Ch. 2), which constitutes part of the transduction system through which the receptor exerts its regulatory effect. Antagonist binding does not show this complexity, probably because antagonists, by their nature, do not lead to the secondary event of G-protein coupling. Agonist affinity has, indeed, proved to be a very elusive parameter to measure, a fact which has led to a remarkable algebraic paperchase in the pharmacological literature, much admired by its followers.

DRUG ANTAGONISM

The situation commonly arises in pharmacology where the effect of one drug is diminished or com-

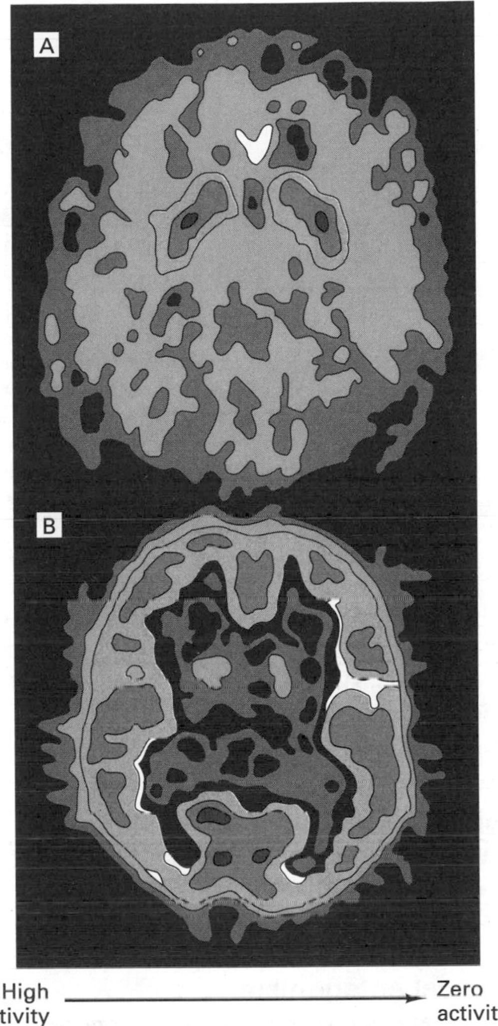

Fig. 1.8 Labelling of receptors in the living human brain. Images were obtained by positron-emission tomography (PET) scanning, after intravenous injection of receptor ligands labelled with the short-lived positron-emitting isotope, ^{11}C. The distribution of radioactivity, representing the labelling of receptors by the ligand, is plotted by computer over a horizontal section of the brain. **A.** Dopamine (D_2) receptors, labelled with ^{11}C-raclopride. The receptors are highly localised to the basal ganglia (see Ch. 30 for further details). **B.** Benzodiazepine receptors, labelled with ^{11}C-flumazenil. The receptors occur mainly in the cortex (see Ch. 27). (Figures kindly provided by Prof G Sedvall, Karolinska Institute, Stockholm)

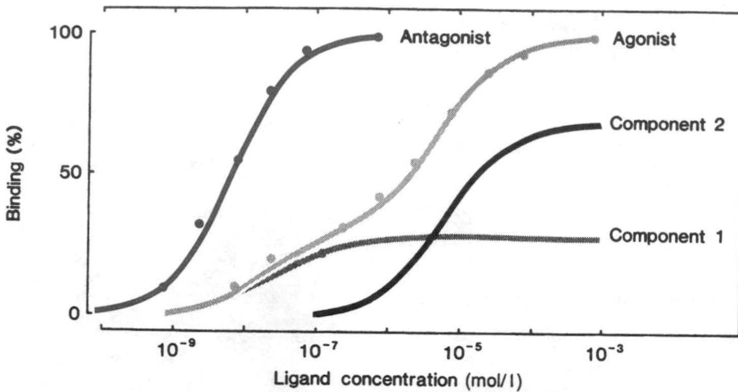

Fig. 1.9 Comparison of binding curves for muscarinic agonists and antagonists (brain membrane preparation). The antagonist binding curve (benzhexol) is well fitted by a single component (K = 8.3 μM). The agonist-binding curve (oxotremorine-M) is fitted by the sum of two separate components. Component 1 (K = 27 μmol/l) comprises 30% of the total sites, and component 2 (K = 5.9 μmol/l) comprises 70%. Such complex binding curves are common for agonists, and probably reflect the interaction of the receptor with other components of the transduction system. (Results from Birdsall N J M et al. 1978 Mol Pharmacol 14: 723)

pletely abolished in the presence of another. One mechanism, competitive antagonism, was discussed earlier; a more complete classification includes the following mechanisms:

- chemical antagonism
- pharmacokinetic antagonism
- antagonism by receptor block
- non-competitive antagonism, i.e. block of receptor–effector linkage
- physiological antagonism.

Chemical antagonism

Chemical antagonism refers to the uncommon situation where the two substances combine in solution, so that the effect of the active drug is lost. The most obvious example is the inactivation of heavy metals (lead, cadmium, etc.) whose toxicity is reduced by administration of a chelating agent (e.g. **dimercaprol**) which binds the metal ions tightly to form an inactive complex.

Pharmacokinetic antagonism

Pharmacokinetic antagonism describes the situation in which the 'antagonist' effectively reduces the concentration of the active drug at its site of action. This can happen in various ways. The rate of metabolic degradation of the active drug may be increased (e.g. the reduction of the anticoagulant effect of **warfarin** when an agent that accelerates its hepatic metabolism, such as **phenobarbitone**, is given; see Chs 3 and 42). Alternatively, the rate of absorption of the active drug from the gastrointestinal tract may be reduced, or the rate of renal excretion may be increased. Interactions of this sort are discussed in more detail in Chapter 42. They have a tendency to occur unexpectedly in clinical situations, and are a major preoccupation of clinical pharmacologists.

Antagonism by receptor block

Receptor-block antagonism involves two important mechanisms:

- reversible competitive antagonism
- irreversible, or non-equilibrium, competitive antagonism.

Reversible competitive antagonism has been discussed in some detail earlier in this chapter. Its key features are *surmountability*, expressed in the parallel shift of the agonist log concentration–effect curve without any reduction in the maximal response, and the *linear Schild plot* (see p. 10). These characteristics reflect the fact that the rate of dissociation of the antagonist molecules is sufficiently high that, on addition of the agonist, a new equilibrium is rapidly established. The agonist is effectively able to displace the antagonist molecules from the receptors, although the agonist, of course, has no power to evict a bound antagonist molecule, or vice versa. What happens, in fact, is that by occupying a proportion of the vacant receptors, the agonist reduces the rate of association of the antagonist molecules, so that the rate of dissociation temporarily exceeds that of association, and the overall antagonist occupancy falls.

Irreversible, or non-equilibrium, competitive antagonism occurs when the antagonist dissociates very slowly, or not at all, from the receptors, with the result that no change in the antagonist occupancy takes place when the agonist is applied.*

The fractional occupancy by the agonist is thus reduced in proportion to the fraction of receptors not occupied by the antagonist. Thus, if the fraction of receptors blocked by the antagonist is p_B, the agonist occupancy, p_A, is given by:

$$p_A = \frac{x_A}{x_A + K_A}(1 - p_B) \qquad (1.13)$$

This means that the antagonism is *non-surmountable* because no matter how high the agonist concentration, the agonist occupancy cannot exceed $(1 - p_B)$. The effect of reversible and irreversible antagonists is compared in Figure 1.10. In some cases (Fig. 1.11A), the theoretical effect is accurately reproduced, but the distinction between reversible and irreversible competitive antagonism (or even non-competitive antagonism; see below) is not always as obvious as the theoretical curves in Figure 1.10 would suggest. This is because of the phenomenon of spare receptors (see p. 13); if the agonist occupancy required to produce a maximal biological response is very small (say 1% of the total receptor pool), then it is possible to block irreversibly nearly 99% of the receptors without reducing the maximal response. The effect of a lesser degree of antagonist occupancy will be to produce a parallel shift of the log concentration–effect curve that is indistinguishable from reversible competitive antagonism (Fig. 1.11B). In fact, it was the finding that an irreversible competitive antagonist of histamine was able to reduce the sensitivity of a smooth muscle preparation to histamine nearly 100-fold without reducing the maximal response that first gave rise to the spare receptor hypothesis. Irreversible competitive antagonism occurs with drugs that possess reactive groups which form covalent bonds with the receptor. These are mainly used as experimental tools for investigating receptor function, and few are used clinically as receptor antagonists. Irreversible enzyme inhibitors which act similarly are clinically used, however, and include drugs such as aspirin (Ch. 12), omeprazole (Ch. 19) and monoamine oxidase inhibitors (Ch. 29).

*Some authors refer to this type of antagonism as non-competitive, but this term is best reserved for antagonism that does not involve occupation of the receptor site (see below).

Non-competitive antagonism

Non-competitive antagonism describes the situation where the antagonist blocks at some point the chain of events that leads to the production of a response by the agonist. For example, drugs such as **verapamil** and **nifedipine** prevent the influx of calcium ions through the cell membrane (see Ch. 14) and thus block, quite non-specifically, the contraction of smooth muscle produced by other drugs. As a rule, the effect will be to reduce the slope and maximum of the agonist log concentration–response curve as in Figure 1.10B though it is quite possible for some degree of rightward shift to occur as well. Many drugs, some of them thought until recently to act as competitive acetylcholine antagonists, have been found to produce a non-competitive block of the effects of acetylcholine on nicotinic receptors. Their effect appears to result from block of the cation-selective ionic channels that are controlled by these receptors (see Ch. 2) and an interesting point is that in many instances the blocking agent can act on the channel only after it has been opened by acetylcholine. The degree of block therefore increases if the agonist concentration is increased—the exact opposite of competitive antagonism. Drugs that work in this way include **hexamethonium** (a ganglion-blocking drug; see Ch. 6) and **tubocurarine** (a neuromuscular-blocking drug which has both competitive and non-competitive actions; see Ch. 6).

Physiological antagonism

Physiological antagonism is a term used loosely to describe the interaction of two drugs whose opposing actions in the body tend to cancel each other. For example, **noradrenaline** raises arterial pressure by acting on the heart and peripheral vessels, while **histamine** lowers arterial pressure by causing vasodilatation; the two drugs can be said

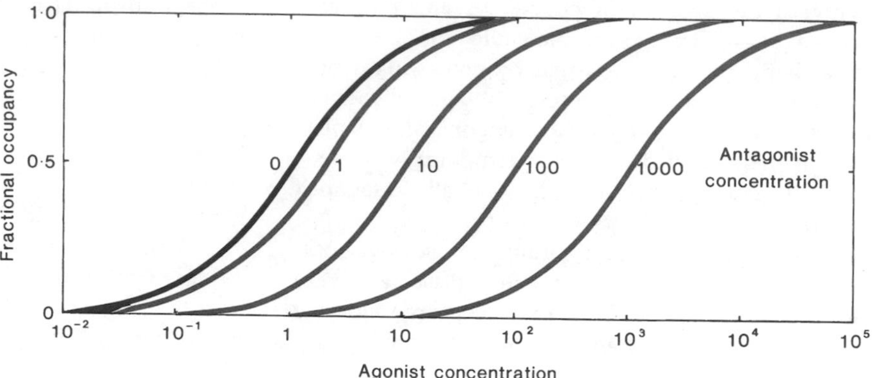

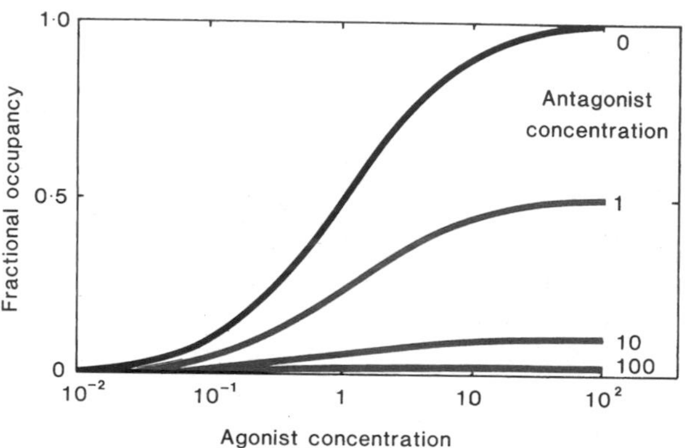

Fig. 1.10 Hypothetical agonist concentration–occupancy curves in the presence of reversible and irreversible competitive antagonists. The concentrations are normalised with respect to the equilibrium constants (i.e. 1.0 corresponds to a concentration equal to K, and results in 50% occupancy). **A.** Reversible competitive antagonism. **B.** Irreversible competitive antagonism.

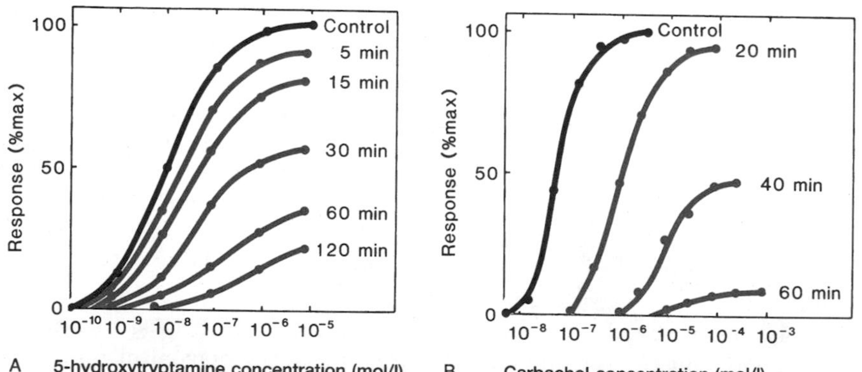

Fig. 1.11 Effects of irreversible competitive antagonists on agonist concentration–effect curves. A. Rat stomach smooth muscle responding to 5-hydroxytryptamine at various times after addition of methysergide (10^{-9} mol/l). **B.** Rabbit stomach responding to carbachol at various times after addition of dibenamine (10^{-5} mol/l). (After: (A) Frankhuijsen A L, Bonta I L 1974 Eur J Pharmacol 26: 220; (B) Furchgott R F 1965 Adv Drug Res 3: 21)

to act as physiological antagonists. It can be seen that the distinction between physiological and non-competitive antagonism is not a sharp one. Thus, if one drug lowers intracellular cAMP by inhibiting adenylate cyclase (see Ch. 2) and another has the opposite effect, the antagonism could be classified as either non-competitive or physiological. In practice, where two drugs act on separate cells or separate physiological systems to produce balancing actions, the term physiological antagonism is usually applied.

Drug antagonism

Drug antagonism occurs by various mechanisms:

- chemical antagonism (interaction in solution)
- pharmacokinetic antagonism (one drug affecting the absorption, metabolism or excretion of the other)
- competitive antagonism (both drugs binding to the same receptors); the antagonism may be reversible or irreversible
- non-competitive antagonism (the antagonist interrupts receptor–effector linkage)
- physiological antagonism (two agents producing opposing physiological effects).

DESENSITISATION AND TACHYPHYLAXIS

It is often found that the effect of a drug gradually diminishes when it is given continuously or repeatedly. *Desensitisation* and *tachyphylaxis* are synonymous terms used to describe this phenomenon which often develops in the course of a few minutes. The term *tolerance* is conventionally used to describe a more gradual decrease in responsiveness to a drug, taking days or weeks to develop, but the distinction is not a sharp one. The term *refractoriness* is also sometimes used, mainly in relation to a loss of therapeutic efficacy. *Drug resistance* is a term used to describe the loss of effectiveness of antimicrobial drugs. Many different mechanisms can give rise to this type of phenomenon, and they are rather poorly understood. They include:

- change in receptors
- loss of receptors
- exhaustion of mediators
- increased metabolic degradation
- physiological adaptation.

Change in receptors

Among receptors directly coupled to ionic channels, desensitisation is often rapid and pronounced. At the neuromuscular junction (Fig. 1.12A), there is evidence that the desensitised state is caused by a slow conformational change in the receptor, resulting in tight binding of the agonist molecule without the opening of the ionic channel (see Changeux et al 1987). A similar change has been described for

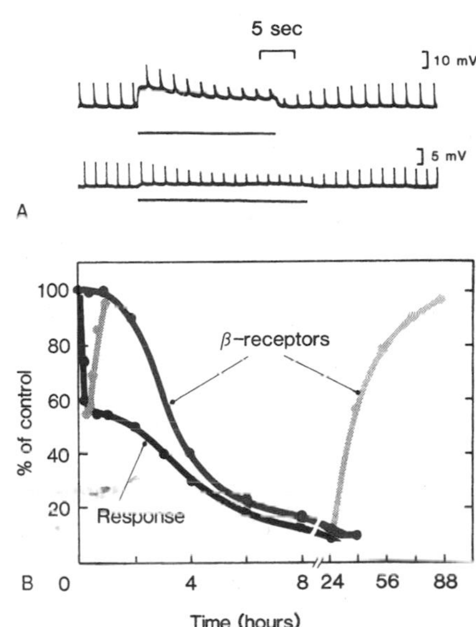

Fig. 1.12 Two kinds of receptor desensitisation. **A.** Acetylcholine at the frog motor endplate. Brief depolarisations (upward deflections) are produced by short pulses of ACh delivered from a micropipette. A long pulse (horizontal line) causes the response to decline with a time-course of about 20 seconds, due to desensitisation, and it recovers with a similar time-course. **B.** β-adrenoceptors of rat glioma cells in tissue culture. Isoprenaline (1 μM) was added at time zero, and the adenylate cyclase response and β-adrenoceptor density measured at intervals. The response declined rapidly at first, with no change in the number of adrenoceptors (early uncoupling phase of desensitisation); it then declined more slowly, concomitantly with a loss of receptors (late down-regulation phase). The grey and light pink lines show the recovery of the response and receptor density after the isoprenaline is washed out during the early or late phase. (From: (A) Katz B, Thesleff S 1957 J Physiol 138: 63; (B) Perkins J P 1981 Trends Pharmacol Sci 2: 326)

the β-adrenoceptor (Fig. 1.12B), which becomes, on desensitisation, unable to activate adenylate cyclase, though it can still bind the agonist molecule. It is believed that phosphorylation of a single serine residue may be responsible for this process (see Huganir & Greengard 1990).

Loss of receptors

In some cases, prolonged exposure to agonists results in the gradual reduction in the number of receptors as measured by drug-binding studies. This occurs with β-adrenoceptors (Fig. 1.12B) and appears to be a slower process than the 'uncoupling' from adenylate cyclase mentioned above. In studies on cell cultures, the number of β-adrenoceptors can fall to about 10% of normal in 8 hours in the presence of a low concentration of **isoprenaline**. Recovery to normal takes several days. Similar changes have been described for other types of receptor, including those for various peptides. It is believed that the vanishing receptors are taken into the cell by endocytosis of patches of the membrane. This type of elaborate regulatory mechanism appears to be common for hormone receptors, and has obvious relevance to the effects produced when drugs are given for extended periods. Receptor desensitisation can be exploited clinically, for example, in the use of gonadotrophin-releasing hormone (see Ch. 22) to treat endometriosis or prostatic cancer; given continuously, this paradoxically inhibits gonadotrophin release (in contrast to the normal stimulatory effect of the physiological secretion, which is pulsatile).

Exhaustion of mediators

In some cases, desensitisation is associated with depletion of an essential intermediate substance. Drugs such as **amphetamine**, which acts by releasing noradrenaline and other amines from nerve terminals (see Chs 7 and 24), show marked tachyphylaxis because the releasable stores of noradrenaline become depleted.

Increased metabolic degradation

Tolerance to some drugs, for example **barbiturates** (Ch. 27), occurs partly because repeated administration of the same dose produces a progressively lower plasma concentration. This also happens to an appreciable extent with ethanol. In general, the degree of tolerance that results is rather slight, and in both of these examples other mechanisms contribute to the substantial tolerance that actually occurs.

Physiological adaptation

Diminution of a drug's effect may occur because it is nullified by a homeostatic response. For example, diuretics which act by inhibiting carbonic anhydrase (see Ch. 18) produce only a transient diuresis because the acidosis that is produced reduces the loss of bicarbonate in the urine, and hence limits the diuresis. There are undoubtedly many more instances in which homeostatic responses operate in such a way as to modify or counteract drug effects, and if they occur slowly the result will be a gradually developing tolerance. It is a very common experience that many side effects of drugs, such as nausea or sleepiness, tend to subside even though drug administration is continued. We may assume that some kind of physiological adaptation is occurring, though little is known about the mechanisms involved.

REFERENCES AND FURTHER READING

Black J W, Jenkinson D H, Gerskowitch V P (eds) 1987 Perspectives on receptor classification. Liss, New York

Bouvier M, Hausdorff W P, De Blasi A, O'Dowd B F, Kobilka B K, Caron M G, Lefkowitz R J 1988 Removal of phosphorylation sites from the β-adrenergic receptor delays onset of agonist-promoted desensitization. Nature 333: 370–373

Changeux J-P, Giraudat J, Dennis M 1987 The nicotinic acetylcholine receptor: molecular architecture of a ligand-regulated ion channel. Trends Pharmacol Sci 8: 459–465

Colquhoun D 1973 The relationship between classical and cooperative models for drug action. In: Rang H P (ed) Drug receptors. Macmillan, London

Dolly J O, Barnard E A 1984 Nicotinic acetylcholine receptors: an overview. Biochem Pharmacol 33: 841–858

Franks N P, Lieb W R 1987 What is the molecular nature of general anaesthetic target sites. Trends Pharmacol Sci 8: 169–174

Huganir R L, Greengard P 1990 Regulation of neurotransmitter desensitization by protein phosphorylation. Neuron 5: 555–567

Kenakin T 1987 Pharmacologic analysis of drug–receptor interactions. Raven Press, New York

Kenakin T 1989 Challenges for receptor theory as a tool for drug and drug receptor classification. Trends Pharmacol Sci 10: 18–22

Lamble J W (ed) 1981 Towards understanding receptors. Elsevier, Amsterdam (A collection of articles published in Trends Pharmacol Sci)

Lamble J W (ed) 1982 More about receptors. Elsevier,

Amsterdam (A collection of articles published in Trends Pharmacol Sci)
Popot J L, Changeux J-P 1984 Nicotinic receptor of acetylcholine: structure of an oligomeric integral receptor protein. Physiol Rev 64: 1162–1239
Sibley D R, Lefkowitz R J 1985 Molecular mechanisms of receptor desensitization using the β-adrenergic receptor-coupled adenylate cyclase system as a model. Nature 317: 124–129
Stephenson R P 1956 A modification of receptor theory. Br J Pharmacol 11: 379–393
Taylor P, Lamble J W, Abbott A C 1984 Receptors again. Elsevier, Amsterdam (A collection of articles published in Trends Pharmacol Sci)
Tolstoshev P 1993 Gene therapy: concepts, current trials and future directions. Ann Rev Pharmacol Toxicol 32: 573–596
Weatherall D-J 1991 Gene therapy in perspective. Nature 349: 275–276

2

HOW DRUGS ACT: MOLECULAR ASPECTS

In Chapter 1, the general principles of drug action were discussed, but without much attention to how drugs act in a molecular sense. It is in the area of molecular pharmacology that the most rapid advances have been made in recent years. Jeremiahs may point out, with some justification, that very few useful new drugs have yet emerged from the application of knowledge about the molecular details of drugs and target molecules. To date, certainly, most new drugs have come, like off-the-peg suits, from projects in which many chemical analogues are screened to find one that fits, rather than being made-to-measure to fit precisely to the structure of a defined target. Drug design on a molecular basis is steadily gaining momentum, however, and no major drug company is ignoring its potential.

In this chapter we will first discuss the types of target proteins on which drugs commonly act, which were mentioned briefly in Chapter 1. Next, we will consider the main families of receptors which have been revealed by cloning and structural studies. Finally, we will discuss the various forms of receptor–effector linkage (often known as transduction mechanisms) through which receptors are coupled to systems that regulate cell function. The relationship that has recently become clear between the molecular structure of a receptor and its function in terms of linkage to a particular type of effector system, will be a principal theme. In this chapter, we go into more detail than is necessary for understanding today's pharmacology at a basic level, but we feel confident that tomorrow's pharmacology will rest heavily on the advances in cellular and molecular biology that are discussed here.

TARGETS FOR DRUG ACTION

The protein targets for drug action on mammalian cells (Fig. 2.1) can be broadly divided into:

- receptors
- ion channels
- enzymes
- carrier molecules.

These are discussed further in this chapter. Targets for chemotherapeutic drugs, where the aim is to suppress invading microorganisms or cancer cells, include DNA and cell wall constituents as well as proteins; they are described in Chapters 35–41.

Receptors

Receptors (Fig. 2.1A) can be regarded as the sensing elements in the system of chemical communications that coordinates the function of all the different cells in the body, the chemical messengers being hormones or transmitter substances. In some cases, for example benzodiazepine receptors (see Ch. 27) and cannabinoid receptors (Ch. 33), the receptor has been identified even though the presumed endogenous mediator has not, but in most cases, the endogenous mediator was discovered before the receptor was characterised pharmacologically. Many therapeutically useful synthetic drugs act, either as agonists or antagonists, on receptors for endogenous mediators. Some examples are given in Table 2.1.

There are four main types of receptor, classified

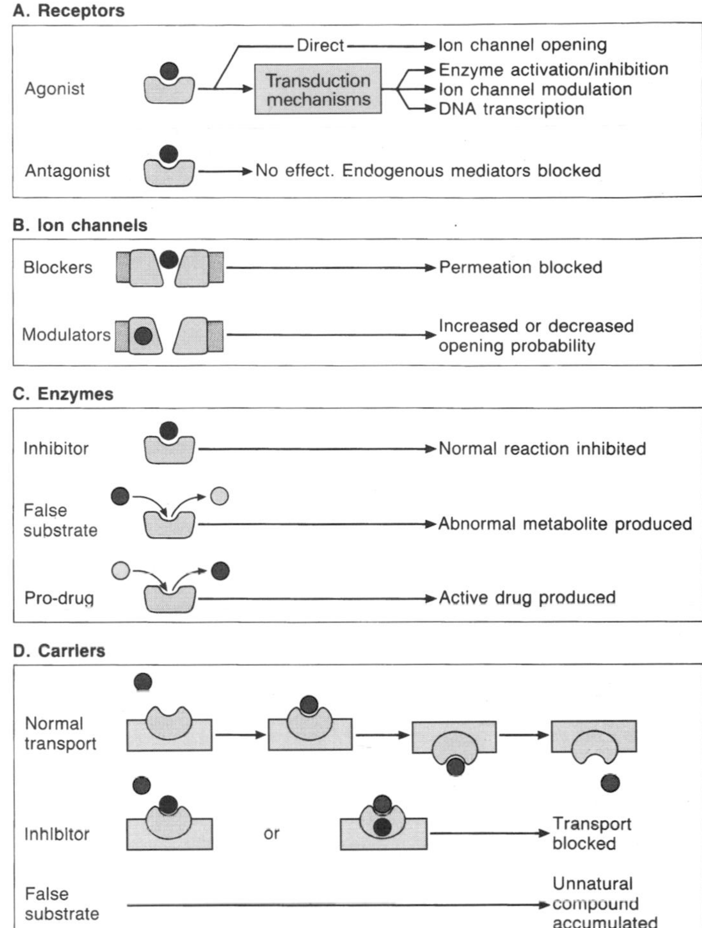

Fig. 2.1 Types of target for drug action.
A. Receptors. **B.** Ion channels.
C. Enzymes. **D.** Carrier molecules.

according to their molecular structure and the nature of the receptor–effector linkage; they are discussed in more detail later in this chapter.

Ion channels

Some ion channels (known as *ligand-gated* ion channels) are directly linked to a receptor, and open only when the receptor is occupied by an agonist. However, many other types of ion channel also serve as targets for drug action. In some cases the interaction is indirect, involving a G-protein and other intermediaries (see below), but there are also many examples where channel function is modulated by binding of drugs directly to parts of the channel protein. The simplest type of interaction involves a physical blocking of the channel by the drug molecule (Fig. 2.1B), exemplified by the blocking action of **local anaesthetics** on the voltage-gated sodium channel (see Ch. 34), or the blocking of sodium entry into renal tubular cells by the diuretic **amiloride** (see Ch. 18). More complicated examples of direct drug–channel interactions (i.e. where the drug binds to the channel protein itself) include the modulation of calcium channels by vasodilator drugs of the **dihydropyridine** type (see Ch. 14). In this case, the process of channel opening, which normally occurs in response to depolarisation of the membrane, may be inhibited or facilitated according to the structure of the dihydropyridine. The binding of the drug molecule thus influences the *gating* of the channel, a quite different mechanism from that of drugs which block *permeation* of the channel without greatly affecting its gating. Another example is that of the **benzodiazepine tranquillisers** (see

Table 2.1 Some examples of targets for drug action

Type of target	Effectors		Refer to
Receptors	**Agonists**	**Antagonists**	
Nicotinic ACh receptor	Acetylcholine Nicotine	Tubocurarine α-bungarotoxin	Ch. 6
β-adrenoceptor	Noradrenaline Isoprenaline	Propranolol	Ch. 7
Histamine (H_1 receptor)	Histamine	Mepyramine	Ch. 12
Histamine (H_2 receptor)	Impromidine	Ranitidine	Ch. 19
Opiate (μ-receptor)	Morphine	Naloxone	Ch. 31
5-HT_2 receptor	5-HT	Ketanserin	Ch. 8
Dopamine (D_2 receptor)	Dopamine Bromocryptine	Chlorpromazine	Ch. 28
Insulin receptor	Insulin	Not known	Ch. 20
Oestrogen receptor	Ethinylestradiol	Tamoxifen	Ch. 22
Progesterone receptor	Norethisterone	Danazol	Ch. 22
Ion channels	**Blockers**	**Modulators**	
Voltage-gated Na^+-channels	Local anaesthetics Tetrodotoxin	Veratridine	Ch. 34
Renal tubule Na^+-channels	Amiloride	Aldosterone	Ch. 18
Voltage-gated Ca^{2+}-channels	Divalent cations (e.g. Cd^{2+})	Dihydropyridines β-adrenoceptor agonists	Ch. 13 Ch. 7
Voltage-gated K^+-channels	4-aminopyridine		Ch. 34
ATP-sensitive K^+-channels	ATP	Cromokalim Sulphonylureas	Ch. 14 Ch. 20
GABA-gated Cl^--channels	Picrotoxin	Benzodiazepines	Chs 24, 27
Glutamate-gated (NMDA) cation channels	Dizocilpine Ketamine	Glycine	Ch. 24 Ch. 26
Enzymes	**Inhibitors**	**False substrates**	
Acetylcholinesterase	Neostigmine Organophosphates		Ch. 6
Choline acetyltransferase		Hemicholinium	Ch. 6
Cyclo-oxygenase	Aspirin		Ch. 12
Xanthine oxidase	Allopurinol		Ch. 12
Angiotensin-converting enzyme	Captopril		Ch. 14
Carbonic anhydrase	Acetazolamide		Ch. 18
HMG-CoA reductase	Simvastatin		Ch. 15
Dopa decarboxylase		Methyldopa	Ch. 7
Monoamine oxidase-A	Iproniazid		Ch. 29
Monoamine oxidase-B	Selegiline		Ch. 25
Dihydrofolate reductase	Trimethoprim Methotrexate		Ch. 37 Ch. 36
DNA polymerase	Cytarabine	Cytarabine	Ch. 36
Enzymes involved in DNA synthesis	Azathiaprine		Ch. 12
Enzymes of blood clotting cascade	Heparin		Ch. 16
Plasminogen*			Ch. 16
Carriers	**Inhibitors**	**False substrates**	
Choline carrier (nerve terminal)	Hemicholinium		Ch. 6
Noradrenaline uptake 1	Tricyclic antidepressants		Ch. 29
	Cocaine		Chs 7, 33
		Amphetamine	Ch. 7
		Methyldopa	Ch. 14

Table 2.1 (continued)

Type of target	Effectors	Refer to
Carriers continued	**Inhibitors** continued	
Noradrenaline uptake (vesicular)	Reserpine	Ch. 7
Weak acid carrier (renal tubule)	Probenecid	Ch. 18
$Na^+/K^+/2Cl^-$ co-transporter (loop of Henle)	Loop diuretics	Ch. 18
Na^+/K^+ pump	Cardiac glycosides	Ch. 13
Proton pump (gastric mucosa)	Omeprazole	Ch. 19

Note: Biochemical targets for drugs used in chemotherapy are discussed in Chapters 35–41
*Plasminogen activators: tissue plasminogen activator (TPA), APSAC

Ch. 27). These drugs bind to a region of the GABA-receptor/chloride channel complex (an example of a direct ligand-gated channel; see above). Most benzodiazepines act to facilitate the opening of the channel by the neurotransmitter GABA (see Ch. 24), but some are known that have the opposite effect, causing anxiety rather than tranquillity. In all of these examples, the structure of the protein forming the ionic channel has been determined by cloning, though the mechanism whereby ligand binding modulates the function of the channel is still not understood.

Another interesting example of drug action on ion channels concerns a special type of potassium channel in the membrane of the pancreatic β-cells, which secrete insulin when the plasma glucose concentration rises (see Ch. 20). These channels open when the intracellular ATP concentration drops (see Ashcroft 1988), and are blocked by drugs of the **sulphonylurea** class, which are used to treat diabetes (Ch. 20). Blocking these potassium channels causes the β-cell to depolarise, thus stimulating insulin secretion. The sulphonylureas do not appear to block the channel physically, but rather to modulate its gating, though the mechanism is not understood. The same type of channel occurs also in smooth muscle cells, and is the target for a new type of vasodilator drug (**cromokalim**; see Ch. 14) which selectively opens such channels and hyperpolarises the cells.

Ion channel modulation by drugs, acting directly on the channel or indirectly, is one of the most important mechanisms by which pharmacological effects are produced at the cellular level. The development of the patch-clamp technique (see below) which enables ion channel function to be observed with dramatic clarity and directness, has contributed greatly to understanding in this area in recent years.

Enzymes

Many drugs are targeted on enzymes (Fig. 2.1C). Most commonly, the drug molecule is a substrate analogue that acts as a *competitive inhibitor* of the enzyme, either reversibly (e.g. **neostigmine**, acting on acetylcholinesterase; Ch. 6), or irreversibly (e.g. **aspirin**, acting on cyclo-oxygenase; Ch. 12). Some of the more familiar examples are given in Table 2.1. Another type of interaction involves the drug as a *false substrate*, where the drug molecule undergoes chemical transformation to form an abnormal product which subverts the normal metabolic pathway. This occurs, for example, with the antihypertensive drug **methyldopa** (see Ch. 7), which mimics the noradrenaline precursor dopa, causing noradrenaline to be partly replaced by methylnoradrenaline, thus affecting the function of the sympathetic nervous system.

It should also be mentioned that drugs may require enzymic degradation to convert them from an inactive form, the *pro-drug* (see Ch. 4), to an active form. Examples are given in Table 4.4. Furthermore, as discussed in Chapter 43, certain types of drug toxicity require the enzymic conversion of the drug molecule to a reactive metabolite. As far as the primary action of the drug is concerned this is an unwanted side reaction, but it is of major practical importance.

Carrier molecules

The transport of ions and small organic molecules across cell membranes generally requires a carrier protein of some kind, since the permeating molecules are often too polar (i.e. insufficiently lipid soluble) to penetrate lipid membranes on their own. There are many examples of such carriers (Fig. 2.1D), including those responsible for the transport of glucose and amino acids into cells, the transport of ions and many organic molecules by the renal tubule, the transport of sodium and calcium ions out of cells and the uptake of neurotransmitter precursors (such as choline) or of neurotransmitters themselves (such as noradrenaline, 5-hydroxytryptamine, glutamate) by nerve terminals. Several neurotransmitter transporters have now been cloned. They form a well-defined structural family, distinct from the corresponding receptors (see Giros & Caron 1993). The carrier proteins embody a recognition site that makes them specific for a particular permeating species, and it is not surprising that these recognition sites can also be targets for drugs whose effect is to block the transport system. Some of the main examples are given in Table 2.1.

RECEPTOR PROTEINS

Isolation and characterisation of receptors

In the 1970s, pharmacology moved into a new phase when receptors, which had until then been treated largely as theoretical entities, began to emerge as biochemical realities, following the first successful receptor labelling experiments (see Ch. 1). If a tightly-bound radioactive ligand is available, this makes it possible to extract and purify the radioactively labelled receptor material. This approach was first used successfully on the nicotinic acetylcholine receptor (see Ch. 6), where advantage was taken of two natural curiosities. The first is that the electric organs of many fish, such as rays (*Torpedo* sp.) and electric eels (*Electrophorus* sp.) consist of modified muscle tissue in which the acetylcholine-sensitive membrane is extremely abundant, and these organs contain much larger amounts of acetylcholine receptor than any other tissue. Secondly, the venom of snakes of the cobra family contains polypeptides which bind with very high specificity to nicotinic acetylcholine receptors. These substances, known as α-toxins, can easily be labelled and used to assay the receptor content of tissues and tissue extracts. The best-known is **α-bungarotoxin**, which is the main component of the venom of the Malayan banded krait (*Bungarus multicinctus**). Treatment of muscle or electric tissue with non-ionic detergents brings the membrane-bound receptor protein into solution, and it can be purified by the technique of affinity chromatography in which a receptor ligand, bound covalently to the matrix of a chromatography column, is used to absorb the receptor and separate it from other substances in the extract. The receptor can then be eluted from the column by flushing it through with a solution containing an antagonist, such as gallamine. Similar approaches have now been used to purify a great many hormone and neurotransmitter receptors, as well as ion channels, carrier proteins and other kinds of target molecules.

The impact of molecular biology

Once a protein has been isolated and purified, it is usually possible to analyse the amino acid sequence of a short stretch, which enables the corresponding base sequence of the mRNA to be deduced (with some ambiguity, because of degeneracy in the

*Now officially an endangered species, threatened by scientists' demand for its venom. Evolution for survival can go one step too far.

The four main types of receptor

	Type 1	Type 2	Type 3	Type 4
Location	Membrane	Membrane	Membrane	Nucleus
Effector	Channel	Enzyme or channel	Enzyme	Gene transcription
Coupling	Direct	G-protein	Direct	Via DNA
Examples	nAChR $GABA_A$ receptor	mAChR Adrenoceptors	Insulin receptor ANF receptor	Steroid/thyroid receptor

genetic code). Oligonucleotide probes can then be synthesised and used to extract the full length DNA sequence by conventional *cDNA cloning* methods, starting from a cDNA library obtained from a tissue source rich in the receptor of interest. *Expression cloning* is an alternative strategy, which avoids the ambiguity of screening with oligonucleotide probes. It requires the use of a cDNA vector/host system that allows the production of the protein encoded by the cDNA. If these are expressed directly, for example in a bacterial cell, antibodies against the purified receptor protein may be used to detect clones carrying the correct cDNA. Otherwise, the cDNA may be transcribed artificially to produce mRNA, which is injected into a frog oocyte. The mRNA corresponding to the receptor protein is translated by the oocyte, and the protein is expressed on its surface, where its presence can be detected by recording changes in membrane potential or conductance in response to application of the relevant agonist. This technique, though laborious, has the advantage that the preliminary purification of the receptor protein is not necessary, and it has been widely used.

It is also possible to introduce foreign DNA into mammalian cell lines by transfection, and to monitor receptor expression by the appearance of specific ligand binding. This technique is often used to study the binding and pharmacological characteristics of the receptors that have been cloned by the approaches described above. In some cases it has been used as a cloning method itself (mainly for cytokine receptors), in conjunction with autoradiographic detection to identify the individual cells expressing the receptor.

Recently, cloning strategies which require neither protein purification nor expression systems, but only faith, have been enthusiastically embraced. These are based on anticipated sequence homologies between the receptor that is sought and those already known. A region of sequence homology allows, by the use of PCR (polymerase chain reaction) and RACE (rapid amplification of cDNA ends), replication of DNA molecules that contain that sequence. If the chosen sequence is, for example, one that is conserved in several dopamine receptors, what is amplified may well turn out to be another (novel) dopamine receptor, or it may turn out to be something quite different. There are several examples (e.g. the cannabinoid receptor; see Ch. 33) of unexpected receptors being found by accident in this way, and even more examples where 'orphan receptors'—receptor-like structures for which no functional ligand is known—have been cloned.

The main strategies currently used for receptor cloning are summarised in Figure 2.2.

The cloning of 'receptors' that have no pharmacological identity tends, in the short term at least, to produce some taxonomic confusion, but in the long term, molecular characterisation of receptors is essential. Barnard, one of the high priests of receptor cloning, is undaunted by the proliferation of molecular subtypes among receptors which pharmacologists had thought that they understood. He (Barnard 1988) quotes Thomas Aquinas: 'Types and shadows have their ending, for the newer rite is here.' The newer rite, he confidently asserts, is molecular biology. Not everyone fully agrees, however (see Black et al. 1987).

RECEPTOR FAMILIES: STRUCTURE AND SIGNAL TRANSDUCTION MECHANISMS

Receptors are clearly coupled to many different types of cellular effect, some of which may be very rapid, such as those involved in synaptic transmission, which in general occupy a millisecond time-scale. Other receptor-mediated effects, such as those produced by thyroid hormone or various steroid hormones, are very slow and occur over hours or days. There are also many examples of intermediate time-scales—catecholamines, for example, usually act in a matter of seconds, whereas many peptides take rather longer to produce their effects. Not surprisingly, very different types of linkage between the receptor occupation and the ensuing response are involved. In terms of both molecular structure and the nature of the transduction mechanism, we can distinguish four receptor types,* or *superfamilies* (see Figs 2.3 and 2.4):

*A fifth type of receptor has recently been identified, linked to the enzyme **guanylate cyclase** (see Goy 1991). Structurally, it resembles the tyrosine-kinase-linked receptors, with an extracellular agonist-binding domain linked through a single transmembrane helix to an intracellular catalytic domain. The hormones that act on these receptors belong to the class of **natriuretic peptides** (see Chs 13 and 14). The regulation of guanylate cyclase is described in more detail in Chapter 10.

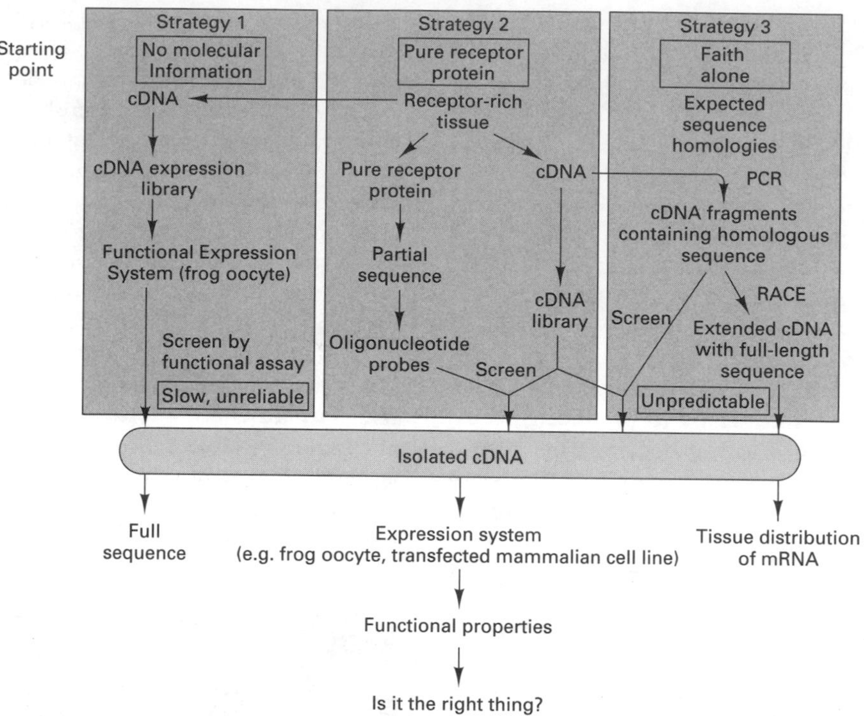

Fig. 2.2 Strategies for receptor cloning. *Strategy 1* starts from a cDNA library made from a receptor-rich tissue. mRNA clones from an expression library are injected into frog oocytes, which are then tested for induced sensitivity to the ligand in question. *Strategy 2* requires that the receptor protein is first purified and partially sequenced. From the inferred DNA sequence, oligonucleotide probes can be prepared for screening the cDNA library. This is a reliable strategy provided the pure protein is available. *Strategy 3* looks for sequence homologies with known receptors, and amplifies these by polymerase chain reaction (PCR). These fragments are then tested for binding to a cDNA library made from a receptor-rich tissue, in the hope of identifying receptor clones in the library. The results are unpredictable, and several 'orphan' receptors have been cloned by this approach. (RACE = rapid amplification of cDNA ends, a DNA amplification technique related to PCR)

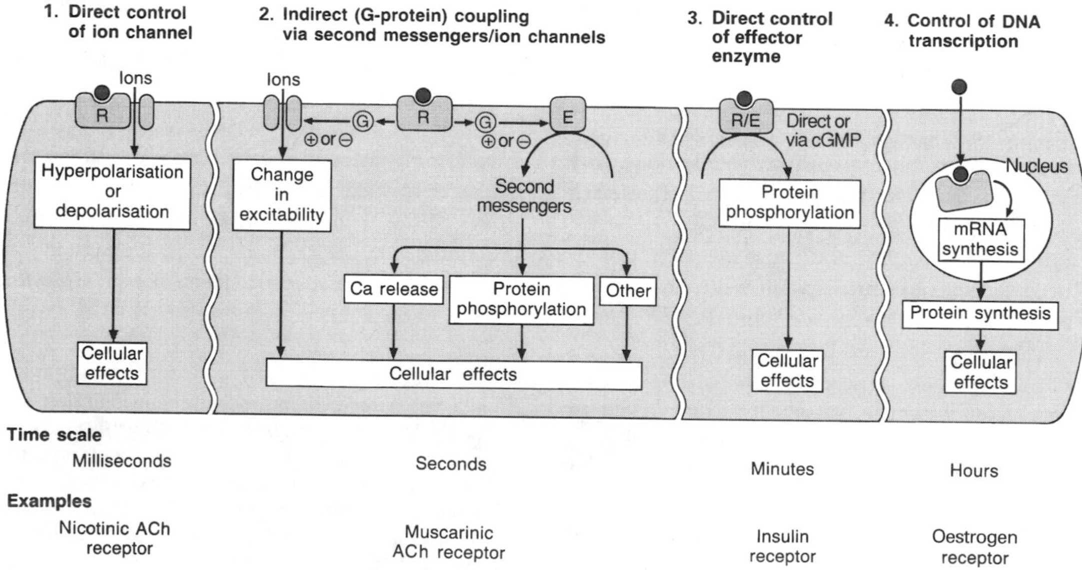

Fig. 2.3 Types of receptor–effector linkage. (R = receptor; G = G-protein; E = enzyme)

A. Direct ligand-gated channel type (type 1)

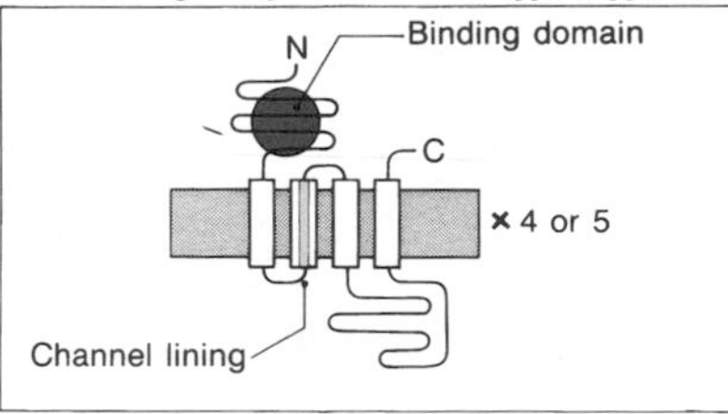

B. G-protein-coupled type (type 2)

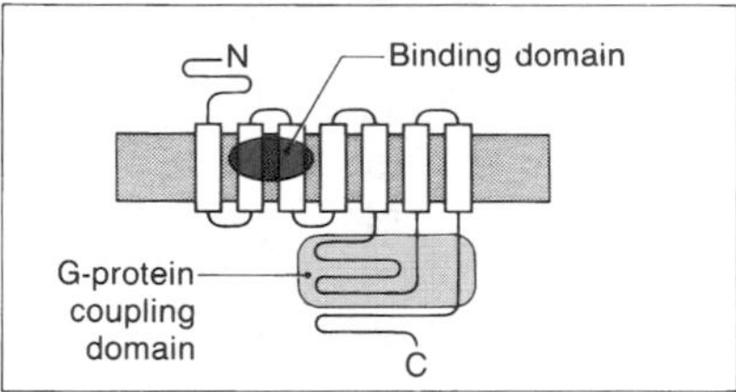

C. Tyrosine-kinase- /guanylate-cyclase-linked type (type 3)

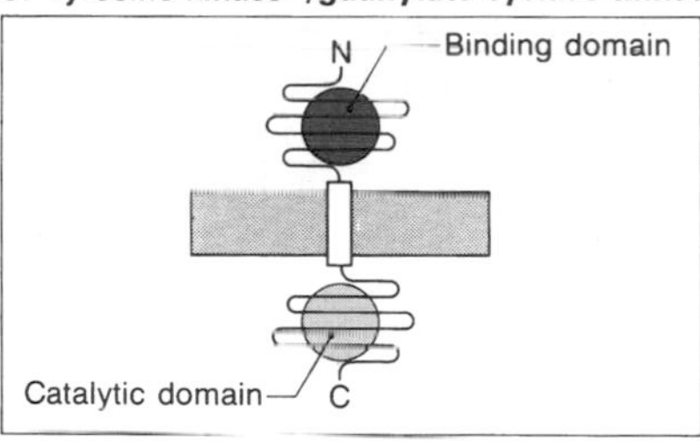

D. Intracellular steroid/thyroid type (type 4)

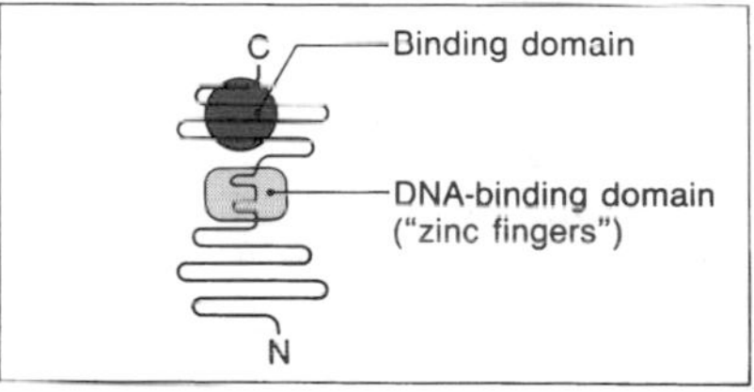

Fig. 2.4 General structure of four receptor superfamilies. The rectangular segments represent hydrophobic α-helical regions of the protein comprising approximately 20 amino acids, which form the membrane-spanning domains of the receptors. Receptors coupled directly to ion channels comprise 4–5 subunits of the type shown, the whole complex containing 16–20 membrane-spanning segments surrounding a central ion channel. **A.** Direct ligand-gated channel type* (type 1). **B.** G-protein-coupled type (type 2). **C.** Tyrosine-kinase- /guanylate-cyclase-linked type (type 3). **D.** Intracellular steroid/thyroid type (type 4).

*Recent evidence on the nicotinic acetylcholine receptor (Unwin 1993; see text) suggests that only one of the four helical segments in each subunit actually traverses the membrane, the other three forming a cluster in the extracellular region. Other ligand-gated channels have not yet been studied in such detail.

- *Type 1:* receptors for fast neurotransmitters, coupled directly to an ion channel, e.g. the nicotinic acetylcholine receptor (nAChR; see Ch. 6), the $GABA_A$ receptor (see Ch. 24), the glutamate receptor (see Ch. 24)
- *Type 2:* receptors for many hormones and slow transmitters, coupled to effector systems via a G-protein (see below), e.g. the muscarinic acetylcholine receptor (mAChR; see Ch. 6), noradrenergic receptors (see Ch. 7)
- *Type 3:* receptors for insulin and various growth factors, which are directly linked to tyrosine kinase (see Chs 20 and 21)
- *Type 4:* receptors for steroid hormones (see Ch. 21), thyroid hormone (Ch. 21) and other agents such as retinoic acid and vitamin D.

Receptors of the first three categories are all membrane proteins, whereas steroid receptors are soluble cytosolic or intranuclear proteins.

The molecular organisation of typical members of each of these four receptor superfamilies is shown in Figure 2.4. Though individual receptors show considerable sequence variation in particular regions, and the lengths of the main intracellular and extracellular domains also vary from one to another within the same family, the overall structural patterns are remarkably consistent. Indeed, no important exceptions have yet been discovered, and the identification of these superfamilies represents a major step forward in understanding how drugs act.

In the following section, we will discuss the structures and transduction mechanisms associated with each of these four receptor types in some detail. For many readers, this amount of detail may be unnecessary, but it is included because of the authors' conviction that the important discoveries made in this area during recent years will have a major influence on the future of pharmacology, and will shape the way in which new drugs are developed for therapeutic use.

RECEPTORS FOR FAST NEUROTRANSMITTERS

Molecular structure

The nicotinic acetylcholine receptor (see reviews by Changeux et al. 1992, Karlin 1993) is typical of the family of receptors for fast neurotransmitters, and it has been studied in more detail than any other receptor. The receptor consists of four different types

Receptor structure

- Many receptor proteins have been isolated and cloned.
- All membrane receptors possess extracellular ligand-binding domains. Their membrane-spanning segments consist of a 20–25 residue stretch of predominantly hydrophobic amino acids, forming an α-helix.
- Each of the four main classes consists of a protein superfamily whose members share a common architecture.

of subunit, termed α,β,γ,δ each of M_r 40–58 kDa. The oligomeric structure (α_2,β,γ,δ) possesses two acetylcholine-binding sites, each lying at the interface between one of the two α-subunits and its neighbour. Both must bind acetylcholine molecules in order for the receptor to be activated. This receptor is sufficiently large to be seen in electron micrographs, and Figure 2.5 shows a reconstruction, recently confirmed by a high resolution electron diffraction study (Unwin 1993) of the way in which it is thought to be inserted into the membrane. Evidence that the purified oligomer comprises both the receptor and the associated ionic channel which it controls comes from experiments in which the receptor protein has been inserted into artificial lipid bilayers, which then show an increased ionic conductance in the presence of acetylcholine or a similar agonist. Cloning has now revealed the complete sequence of all four subunits in a number of species. The four subunits of the ACh receptor show marked sequence homology, and analysis of the hydrophobicity profile, which determines which sections of the chain are likely to form membrane-spanning α-helices, suggests that they are inserted into the membrane as shown in Figure 2.4A. The whole receptor oligomer, with its five subunits, thus incorporates 20 separate membrane-spanning segments. Other receptors for fast transmitters, such as the $GABA_A$ receptor, the 5-HT_3 receptor (Ch. 8) and glutamate receptors are built on the same pattern (see Barnard 1992), and furthermore show considerable sequence homology with the nicotinic acetylcholine receptor, even though they are functionally quite different. Though the basic plan is constant, there are many sequence variations between receptors in different species, and in different locations in the same species. Thus, the nicotinic acetylcholine receptors found in different brain regions differ among themselves, and differ from the muscle receptor. Molecular heterogeneity within a single class of receptors has become a recurring theme as sequence data have accumulated, but its functional significance remains elusive. Some of the known pharmacological differences (e.g. sensitivity to blocking agents) that are known to exist between muscle and brain acetylcholine receptors are now known to correlate with specific sequence differences; however, as far as we know, all nicotinic acetylcholine receptors respond to the same physiological mediator and produce the same kind of

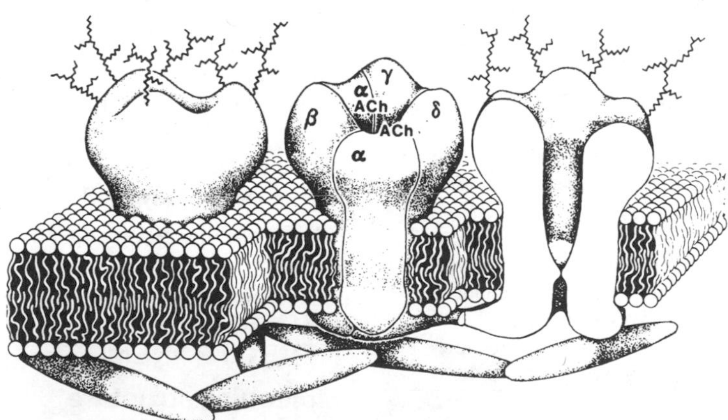

Fig. 2.5 Reconstruction of the nicotinic acetylcholine receptor (AChR). Drawing is based on electron microscopy and neutron scattering data from *Torpedo* electric organ membranes. The receptor and associated ion channel consists of five protein subunits (α_2, β, γ, δ), all of which traverse the membrane and surround a central pore. ACh binds to the α-subunits, and two ACh molecules must bind in order to open the channel. (From: Lindstrom et al. 1983 Cold Spring Harbour Symposium on Quantitative Biology 48: 89)

synaptic response, so why many variants should have evolved is still a puzzle.

The long extracellular N-terminal tails of the subunits have, in common with many membrane proteins, sugar residues coupled to particular amino acids (glycosylation), but these do not appear to be essential for function. The N-termini of the two α-subunits are believed to contain the acetylcholine-binding site, and there is evidence that one of the transmembrane helices (M2) from each of the five subunits may form the lining of the ion channel. The technique of site-directed mutagenesis, which enables short regions, or single residues, of the amino acid sequence to be altered, has been widely used to explore which domains of the receptor control what functions. Thus Galzi et al. (1992) found that a critical residue in the M2 helix controls the anion versus cation selectivity of the channel, and hence the distinction between inhibitory and excitatory transmitter receptors. Other mutations affect properties such as gating and desensitisation of ligand-gated channels. Exactly how the gating takes place is still not clear, though Unwin (1993) has shown that the five M2 helices that form the pore are sharply kinked inwards halfway through the membrane, forming a constriction. He suggests that they may snap to attention when acetylcholine is bound, thus opening the channel.

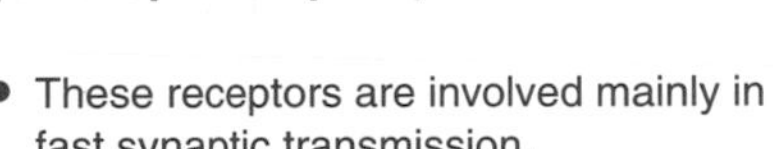

Receptors linked directly to ion channels (ionotropic receptors)

- These receptors are involved mainly in fast synaptic transmission.
- They are oligomeric proteins containing about 20 transmembrane segments arranged around a central aqueous channel.
- Ligand binding and channel opening occur on a millisecond time-scale.
- Examples include nACh, $GABA_A$, $5\text{-}HT_3$ receptors.

The gating mechanism

Receptors of this type control the fastest synaptic events in the nervous system, in which a neurotransmitter acts on the postsynaptic membrane of a nerve or muscle cell and transiently increases its permeability to particular ions. Most excitatory neurotransmitters such as acetylcholine at the neuromuscular junction (Ch. 6) or glutamate in the central nervous system (Ch. 24) cause an increase in sodium and potassium permeability. This results in a net inward current carried mainly by sodium ions, which depolarises the cell and increases the probability that it will generate an action potential. The action of the transmitter reaches a peak in a fraction of a millisecond, and usually decays within a few milliseconds. The sheer speed of this response implies that the coupling between the receptor and the ionic channel is a direct one, and the molecular structure of the receptor/channel complex (see above) agrees with this. It is known, for example, that purified acetylcholine receptors can function as ionic gates in completely artificial membranes, which rules out the involvement of any biochemical intermediates (in the cell or within the membrane) in the transduction process.

An experimental approach which made it possible for the first time to study the properties of individual receptor-operated ionic channels is the use of noise analysis, introduced by Katz & Miledi in 1972. Studying the action of acetylcholine at the motor endplate they observed that small random fluctuations of membrane potential were superimposed on the steady depolarisation produced by acetylcholine (Fig. 2.6). These fluctuations arise because, in the presence of an agonist, there is a dynamic equilibrium between open and closed ion channels. In the steady state, the rate of opening balances the rate of closing, but from moment to moment the number of open channels will show random fluctuations about the mean. By measuring the amplitude of these fluctuations, the conductance of a single ion channel can be calculated, and by measuring their frequency (usually in the form of a spectrum in which the noise power of the signal is plotted as a function of frequency) the average duration for which a single channel stays open (*mean channel lifetime*) can be calculated. In the case of acetylcholine acting at the endplate, the channel conductance is about 20 picosiemens (pS), which is equivalent to an influx of about 10^7 ions per second through a single channel under normal physiological conditions, and the mean lifetime is 1–2 milliseconds. The magnitude of the single channel conductance confirms that permeation occurs through a physical pore through the membrane, since the ion flow is too large to be compatible with a carrier mechanism. In studies with different acetycholine-like agonists it has usually been found that the channel conductances are all about the same,

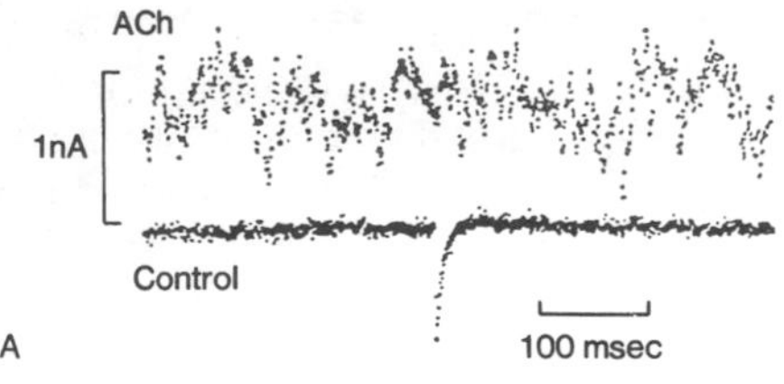

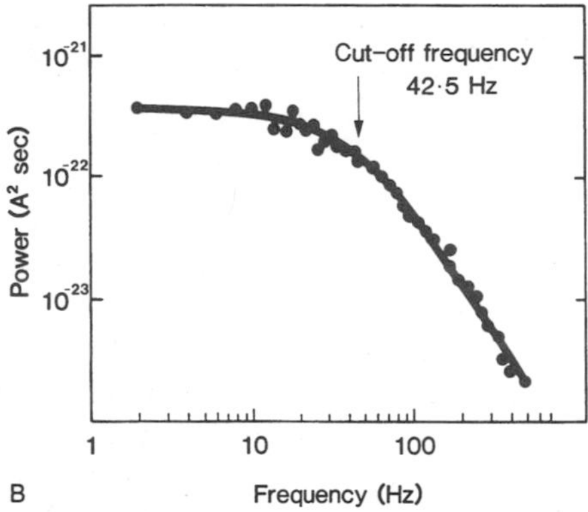

Fig. 2.6 Acetylcholine-induced noise at the frog motor endplate. A. Records of membrane current recorded at high gain under voltage-clamp. The upper noise record was recorded during the application of ACh from a micropipette. The lower record was obtained in the absence of ACh, the blip in the middle being caused by the spontaneous release of a packet of ACh from the motor nerve. The steady (DC) component of the ACh signal has been removed by electronic filtering, leaving the high frequency noise signal. **B.** Power spectrum of ACh-induced noise recorded in a similar experiment to that shown above. The spectrum is calculated by Fourier analysis and fitted with a theoretical (Lorentzian) curve which corresponds to the expected behaviour of a single population of channels whose lifetime varies randomly. The cut-off frequency (at which the power is half of its limiting low-frequency value) enables the mean channel lifetime to be calculated. (From: (A) Anderson C R, Stevens C F 1973 J Physiol 235: 655; (B) Ogden D C et al. 34 1981 Nature 289: 596)

whereas the mean channel lifetime varies. A simple scheme which accounts for these observations and also gives a physical explanation of efficacy for this type of drug response (see pp. 11–13) is as follows:

$$\underbrace{A + R \underset{k_{-1}}{\overset{k_{+1}}{\rightleftharpoons}} AR}_{\text{channel closed}} \underset{\alpha}{\overset{\beta}{\rightleftharpoons}} \underbrace{AR^{\star}}_{\text{channel open}} \qquad (2.1)$$

The conformation R*, representing the open state of the ion channel, is thought to be the same for all agonists, accounting for the finding that the channel conductance does not vary. Kinetically, the mean channel lifetime is determined mainly by the closing rate constant, α, and clearly varies from one drug to another. In this scheme, an agonist of high efficacy which activates a large proportion of the receptors that it occupies will be characterised by $\beta > \alpha$, whereas a drug of low efficacy will have the characteristic $\alpha > \beta$. For a pure antagonist, $\beta = 0$.

Studies on other transmitters that mediate fast synaptic responses show that although the ionic selectivity of the channel varies according to the nature of the synapse, as well as its conductance and mean lifetime, the basic mechanism of the scheme above appears to be quite general. The patch-clamp recording technique, devised by Neher & Sakmann, allows the very small current flowing through a single ionic channel to be measured directly (Fig. 2.7), and the results have fully confirmed the interpretation of channel properties based on noise analysis. This remarkable technique provides a view, unique in biology, of the physiological behaviour of individual protein molecules, and has given many new insights into the gating reactions and permeability characteristics of both the transmitter-operated channels discussed here (see Colquhoun 1987), and various voltage-gated channels (see Ch. 34). One surprising, and challenging, observation has been that some transmitters, most notably glutamate (see Ch. 24),

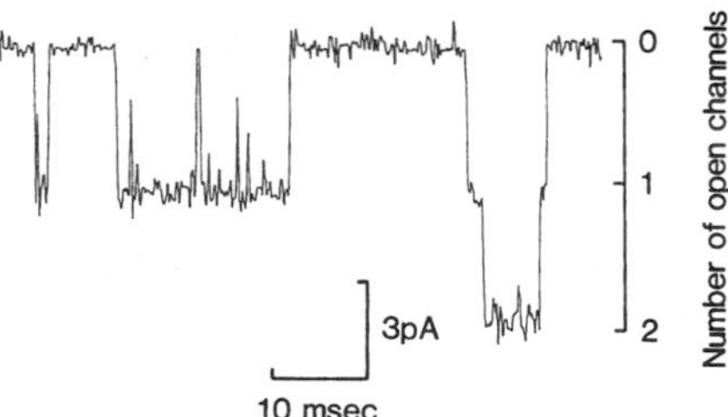

Fig. 2.7 Single acetylcholine-operated ion channels at the frog motor endplate recorded by the patch-clamp technique. The pipette, which was applied tightly to the surface of the membrane, contained 10 μmol/l ACh. The downward deflections show the currents flowing through single ion channels in the small patch of membrane under the pipette tip. Towards the end of the record two channels can be seen to open simultaneously. The conductance and mean lifetime of these channels agree well with indirect estimates from noise analysis (see Fig. 2.6). (Figure courtesy of D Colquhoun and D C Ogden)

cause individual channels to open to any one of several distinct conductance levels (Cull-Candy & Usowicz 1987), a finding which clearly necessitates some revision of the simple scheme above in which only a single open state, R*, is represented.

G-PROTEIN-COUPLED RECEPTORS

The G-protein-coupled receptor family comprises many of the receptors that are familiar to pharmacologists, such as muscarinic ACh receptors, adrenoceptors, dopamine receptors, 5-HT receptors, opiate receptors, receptors for many peptides, purine receptors and many others, including the chemoreceptors involved in olfaction (see Ronnett & Snyder 1992). For most of these, a variety of subtypes has been defined on pharmacological grounds. Many of these numerous receptors have been isolated and purified, and some have been cloned, revealing a remarkably coherent pattern of their molecular structure; it seems safe to predict that most or all of this large family will, like Greek amphitheatres, prove to be similar in their basic architecture.

Molecular structure

The first receptor of this type to be fully characterised was the β-adrenoceptor (Ch. 7; see review by O'Dowd et al. 1989), which was cloned by Dixon et al. (1986). At the time of writing, more than 50 such receptors have been cloned, and they keep coming. Most of the receptors consist of a single polypeptide chain of 400–500 residues whose general anatomy is shown in Figure 2.4B. They all possess seven transmembrane α-helices, similar to those of the channel-linked receptors discussed above, and these regions are the most highly conserved among the various receptors in this class. Both the extracellular amino terminus and the intracellular carboxy terminus vary greatly in length and sequence; another highly variable region is the long third cytoplasmic loop (Fig. 2.4B). The understanding of the function of receptors of this type owes much to detailed studies of a closely related protein, *rhodopsin*, which is responsible for transduction in retinal rods. This protein is abundant in rods, and therefore much easier to study than receptor proteins (which are anything but abundant); it is built on an identical plan to that shown in Figure 2.4 (see Stryer 1986) and also produces a response in the rod (hyperpolarisation, associated with a switching off of a sodium conductance) through a mechanism involving a G-protein. The most obvious difference is that a photon, rather than an agonist molecule, produces the response. In effect, rhodopsin can be regarded as incorporating its own inbuilt agonist molecule, namely retinal, which isomerises from the *trans* (inactive) to the *cis* (active) form when it absorbs a photon.

Site-directed mutagenesis experiments show that the long third cytoplasmic loop, part of which shows a high degree of conservation among these receptors, is the region of the molecule that couples to the G-protein, since deletion or modification of this section results in receptors that still bind ligands but cannot associate with G-proteins or produce responses. Usually, a particular receptor subtype couples selectively with a particular G-protein, and it has been shown that swapping, by genetic engineering, of the third cytoplasmic loop between different receptors alters their G-protein selectivity.

What is surprising is that the ligand-binding domain appears to reside not on the extracellular N terminal region, as with the ion-channel-coupled receptors (a region which, one might think, would be easily accessible to small hydrophilic molecules), but buried within the membrane on one or more of the α-helical segments (Fig. 2.8), similar to the slot occupied by retinal in the rhodopsin molecule (see review by Hibert et al. 1993). By single site mutagenesis experiments, considerable progress has recently been made in understanding the ligand-binding domain of these receptors, and it should soon be possible to design synthetic ligands based on knowledge of the receptor site structure—an important milestone for the pharmaceutical industry, which has relied up to now mainly on the structure of endogenous mediators (such as histamine) or plant alkaloids (such as morphine) for its chemical inspiration.

The sequence of these receptors includes certain residues (serine and threonine) mainly in the C-terminal cytoplasmic tail which appear to act as *phosphorylation sites* where specific kinase enzymes catalyse the coupling of phosphate groups. This has the effect of reducing the interaction of the receptor with the G-protein, and is probably important as a mechanism of agonist-induced desensitisation (see Ch. 1). Again, there are close parallels with the properties of rhodopsin.

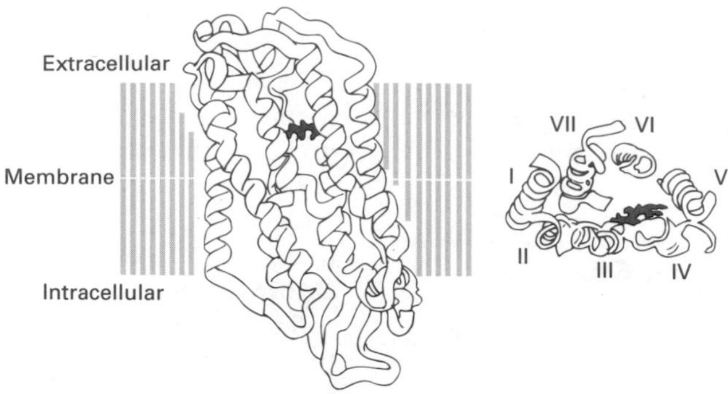

Fig. 2.8 Molecular model of a G-protein-coupled receptor (β-adrenoceptor) lying in the cell membrane, with a molecule of noradrenaline (red) lying in its binding site. The arrangement of the seven transmembrane helices (I–VII) is based on the crystal structure of bacterial rhodopsin. The docking site for the agonist molecule is shown lying among the helices. The particular amino acid side-chains (not shown) that interact with the agonist molecules have been discovered by selective mutagenesis experiments in which individual residues have been selectively mutated and the effect on agonist binding measured. Similar models are available for several different receptors. (Kindly provided by Dr C R Snell, Sandoz Institute for Medical Research)

G-PROTEINS AND THEIR ROLE

G-proteins represent the level of middle management in the organisational hierarchy, able to communicate between the receptors—choosy mandarins alert to the faintest sniff of their own particular hormone—and the effector enzymes or ion channels—the blue collar brigade that gets the job done without any questions about what kind of hormone authorised the process. As we all know, middle management is where the real power resides. They are the go-between proteins, but were actually called G-proteins because of their interaction with the guanine nucleotides, GTP and GDP. They are currently the object of much interest (see reviews by Neer & Clapham 1988, Ross 1989, Bourne et al 1990, Simon et al. 1991).

G-proteins consist of three subunits, α, β and γ (Fig. 2.9). Guanine nucleotides bind to the α-subunit, which has enzymic activity, catalysing the conversion of GTP to GDP. The β and γ subunits are very hydrophobic and remain associated as a βγ complex with the cytoplasmic surface of the membrane. G-proteins appear to be freely diffusible in the plane of the membrane, and it is a key aspect of their function that a single pool of G-protein in a cell can interact with several different receptors and effectors in an essentially promiscuous fashion. This has been convincingly demonstrated in experiments involving cell fusion in which receptors from one cell type can be shown to activate the G-proteins contributed from a different type of cell when the two are fused together. In the 'resting' state (Fig. 2.9), the G-protein exists as an unattached αβγ trimer, with GDP occupying the site on the α-subunit. When a receptor is occupied by an agonist molecule, a conformational change occurs, presumably involving the cytoplasmic domain of the receptor (Fig. 2.4B), causing it to acquire high affinity for αβγ. Association of αβγ with the receptor causes the bound GDP to dissociate and to be replaced with GTP (GDP/GTP exchange), which in turn causes dissociation of α-GTP from the βγ subunits. α-GTP is the 'active' form of the G-protein, which diffuses in the membrane and can associate with various enzymes and ion channels, causing activation or inactivation as the case may be. The process is terminated when the hydrolysis of GTP to GDP occurs through the GTPase activity of the α-subunit. The resulting α-GDP then dissociates from the effector, and reunites with βγ, completing the cycle. Attachment of the α-subunit to an effector molecule actually increases its GTPase activity, the magnitude of this increase

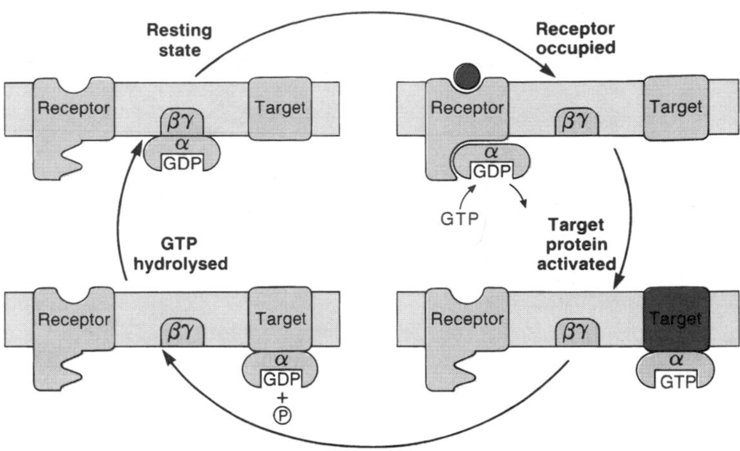

Fig. 2.9 The function of the G-protein. The G-protein consists of three subunits (α, β, γ), βγ serving to anchor the G-protein to the membrane. Coupling of the α-subunit to an agonist-occupied receptor causes the bound GDP to exchange with intracellular GTP; the α-GTP complex then dissociates from the receptor and interacts with a target protein (an enzyme such as adenylate cyclase, or an ion channel). The GTPase activity of the α-subunit is increased when the effector protein is bound, leading to hydrolysis of the bound GTP to GDP, whereupon the α-subunit reunites with βγ.

being different for different types of effector. Since GTP hydrolysis is the step that terminates the ability of the α-subunit to produce its effect, regulation of its GTPase activity by the effector protein means that the activation of the effector tends to be self-limiting. Mechanisms of this type in general result in amplification because a single agonist receptor complex can activate several G-protein molecules in turn, and each of these can remain associated with the effector enzyme for long enough to produce many molecules of product. The product (see below) is often a 'second messenger', and further amplification occurs before the final cellular response is produced.

How is specificity achieved so that a particular receptor controls only one kind of effector? With a common pool of promiscuous G-proteins linking the various receptors and effector systems in a cell it might seem that all specificity would be lost, but this is clearly not the case. For example, muscarinic ACh receptors and β-adrenoceptors, both of which are G-protein-coupled receptors found in cardiac muscle cells, produce opposite functional effects (Chs 6 and 7). The answer is not fully known (see Ross 1992, Milligan 1993), but an important factor is that G-proteins are not all identical, the α-subunit in particular showing considerable variability.* Thus, it is believed that there are three main varieties of G-protein (G_s, G_i and G_q); G_s and G_i produce, respectively, stimulation and inhibition of the enzyme adenylate cyclase (Fig. 2.10), and a similar bi-directional control operates on phospholipase C (see Linden & Delahunty 1989).

The α-subunits of these G-proteins differ in structure. One functional difference that has been useful as an experimental tool to distinguish which type of G-protein is involved in different situations, concerns the action of two bacterial toxins, *cholera toxin* and *pertussis toxin*. These toxins, which are enzymes, catalyse a conjugation reaction (ADP-ribosylation) on the α-subunit of G-proteins. Cholera toxin acts only on G_s, and it causes persistent activation. Many of the symptoms of cholera, such as the excessive secretion of fluid from the gastro-intestinal epithelium, are due to the uncontrolled activation of adenylate cyclase that occurs. Pertussis toxin acts on G_i in a similar way, but G_i seems to be more heterogeneous than G_s in both structure and function, so the functional effects of the toxin are not so clear-cut.

Many G-protein subtypes have now been characterised and cloned. They can be seen as a

*Simon et al. (1991) list 17 molecular variants of the α-subunit G_α, falling into four main classes. Having read this far, you will be unsurprised (though perhaps somewhat bemused) by this degree of molecular heterogeneity.

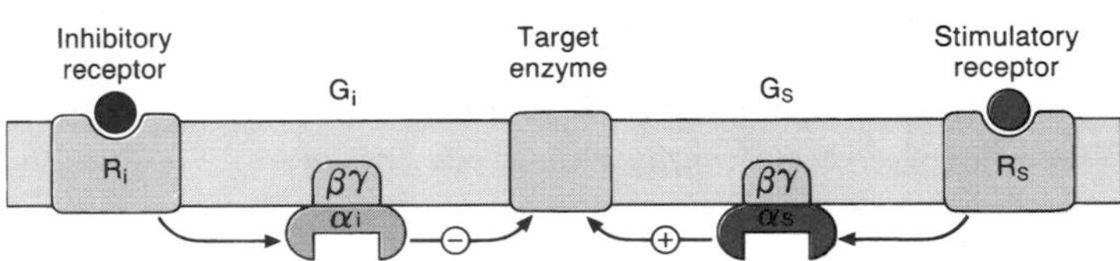

Fig. 2.10 Bidirectional control of AC by G_s and G_i. Heterogeneity of G-proteins allows different receptors to exert opposite effects on a target enzyme.

G-protein-coupled receptors

- All comprise seven membrane-spanning segments.
- One of the intracellular loops is larger than the others and interacts with the G-protein.
- The G-protein is a membrane protein comprising three subunits ($\alpha\beta\gamma$), the α-subunit possessing GTPase activity.
- When the trimer binds to an agonist-occupied receptor, the α-subunit dissociates and is then free to activate an effector (a membrane enzyme or ion channel). In some cases the $\beta\gamma$ subunit may be the activator species.
- Activation of the effector is terminated when the bound GTP molecule is hydrolysed, which allows the α-subunit to recombine with $\beta\gamma$.
- There are several types of G-protein, which interact with different receptors and control different effectors.
- *Metabotropic receptor* is the term used for G-protein-coupled receptors which operate through intracellular second messengers.
- Examples include mAChR, adrenoceptors and neuropeptide receptors.

system of intramembrane managers, dashing like stock exchange jobbers between receptors and effectors, controlling this microcosm but communicating very little with the world outside.

Targets for G-proteins

We have discussed the receptors and the G-proteins in some detail. What happens next? The pioneering studies on receptor–effector coupling, which led to the discovery of the role of G-proteins, focused on the regulation of a key membrane enzyme, *adenylate cyclase*, which was known to be activated by catecholamines in many different cells. It is now known that other membrane enzymes, such as *phospholipase C* and *phospholipase A_2*, as well as a variety of ion channels, are similarly controlled.

Three of these G-protein-coupled effector systems will now be considered in more detail. They are:

- the adenylate cyclase/cAMP system
- the phospholipase C/inositol phosphate system
- the regulation of ion channels.

The adenylate cyclase/cAMP system

The role of cAMP (cyclic 3′,5′-adenosine monophosphate) as a second messenger was first revealed by the work of Sutherland and his colleagues in the late 1950s. This discovery demolished at a stroke the barriers that existed between biochemistry and pharmacology, to the great benefit of both disciplines. There are now complete journals devoted to cAMP—a rare honour for a molecule. Cyclic-AMP is a nucleotide synthesised within the cell from ATP by the action of adenylate cyclase. It is produced continually and inactivated by hydrolysis to 5′-AMP, by the action of a family of enzymes known as phosphodiesterases. Many different drugs, hormones and neurotransmitters produce their effects by increasing or decreasing the catalytic activity of adenylate cyclase and thus raising or lowering the concentration of cAMP within the cell.

The regulatory effects of cAMP on cellular function are many and varied, including, for example, enzymes involved in energy metabolism, cell division and cell differentiation, ion transport, ion channel function, leading to changes in neuronal excitability, and the contractile proteins in smooth muscle. These varied effects are, however, all brought about by a common mechanism, namely the activation of various *protein kinases* by cAMP. These enzymes catalyse the phosphorylation of serine and threonine residues in different cellular proteins, using ATP as source of phosphate groups, and thereby regulate their function. Figure 2.11 shows the ways in which increased cAMP production in response to β-adrenoceptor activation affects the various enzymes involved in glycogen and fat metabolism in liver, fat and muscle cells. The result is a coordinated response in which stored energy in the form of glycogen and fat is made available as glucose to fuel muscle contraction.

Other examples of regulation by cAMP-dependent protein kinases include the increased activity of voltage-activated calcium channels in heart muscle cells (see Ch. 13); phosphorylation of these channels increases the amount of calcium entering the cell during the action potential, and thus increases the force of contraction of the heart.

In smooth muscle, cAMP-dependent protein kinase phosphorylates (thereby inactivating) another enzyme, *myosin-light-chain kinase*, which is required for contraction. This accounts for the smooth muscle relaxation produced by many drugs which increase cAMP production in smooth muscle (see Ch. 14).

As mentioned above, receptors linked to G_i rather than G_s inhibit adenylate cyclase, and thus reduce cAMP formation. Examples include certain types of muscarinic ACh receptor (e.g. the M_2 receptor of

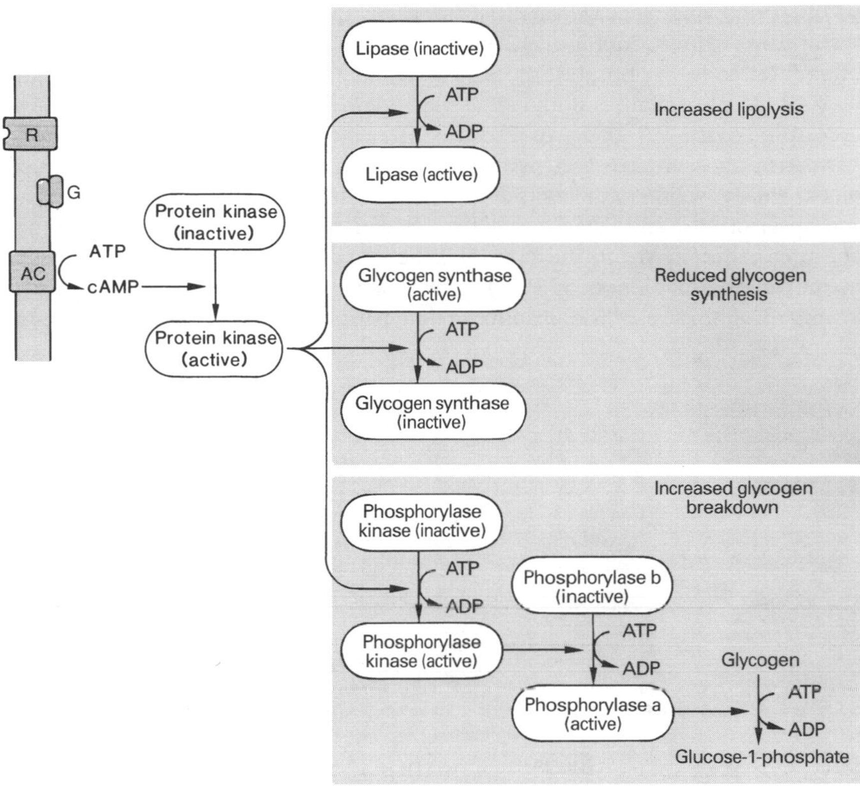

Fig. 2.11 Regulation of energy metabolism by cAMP.

cardiac muscle; see Ch. 6), α_2-adrenoceptors in smooth muscle (Ch. 7) and opioid receptors (see Ch. 31). Adenylate cyclase can be activated directly by certain agents, including forskolin and fluoride ions; these agents are used experimentally in studies on the role of the cAMP system.

cAMP is hydrolysed within cells by *phosphodiesterase*, an enzyme which is inhibited by drugs such as methylxanthines (e.g. **theophylline, caffeine**; see Chs 17 and 32). The similarity of some of the actions of these drugs to those of catecholamines probably reflects their common property of increasing the intracellular concentration of cAMP.

The phospholipase C/inositol phosphate system

The phosphoinositide system, an important intracellular second messenger system, was discovered by Michell and Berridge, biochemists working independently in the UK.

Michell noted in 1975 that with many hormones that produce an increase in free intracellular calcium concentration (which include, for example, muscarinic agonists and α-adrenoceptor agonists acting on smooth muscle and salivary glands, and vasopressin acting on liver cells) there was an accompanying increase in the rate of degradation of a class of minor membrane phospholipids, the phosphatidylinositols (Ptd Ins; see Fig. 2.12). Subsequently (see review by Berridge & Irvine 1984), it was found that one particular member of the Ptd Ins family, namely Ptd Ins $(4,5)P_2$ (PIP_2; Fig. 2.12), which has phosphate groups attached to the inositol ring, plays a key role. This phospholipid is the substrate for a membrane-bound enzyme, phospholipase C (PLC), which splits it into *diacylglycerol* (DAG) and *inositol (1,4,5)-triphosphate* ($InsP_3$), both of which function as second messengers as discussed below. The process of activation of phospholipase C by various agonists turns out to involve a G-protein (see Taylor & Merritt 1986, Sternweis & Smrka 1992), and to be essentially identical to the mechanism of adenylate cyclase activation described above, though different G-protein subtypes are involved. Phospholipase C can also be activated directly by receptors of the tyrosine kinase type (see above) through a quite separate mechanism, not involving a G-protein (see

p. 42). Following cleavage of PIP_2, the status quo is restored as shown in Figure 2.12. DAG is phosphorylated to form phosphatidic acid (PA), while the inositol (1)-phosphate is dephosphorylated and then recoupled with PA to form Ptd Ins once again. **Lithium**, an agent used in psychiatry (see Ch. 29) blocks this recycling pathway (see Fig. 2.12). The resynthesis of Ptd Ins takes some time because the enzymes required are in the cytosol rather than the membrane, so depletion of Ptd Ins may occur following an agonist response, leading to desensitisation (see p. 19).

The receptor-mediated activation of phospholipase A_2, leading to the production of arachidonic acid metabolites, appears to be basically similar to the activation of phospholipase C (see Axelrod et al. 1988). The role of arachidonic acid metabolites as mediators is discussed further in Chapter 11. It is of interest that arachidonic acid metabolites have recently been shown to function as intracellular messengers, controlling potassium channel function in certain neurons (Piomelli et al. 1987), in addition to their well-known role as local hormones communicating between cells. Recent evidence suggests

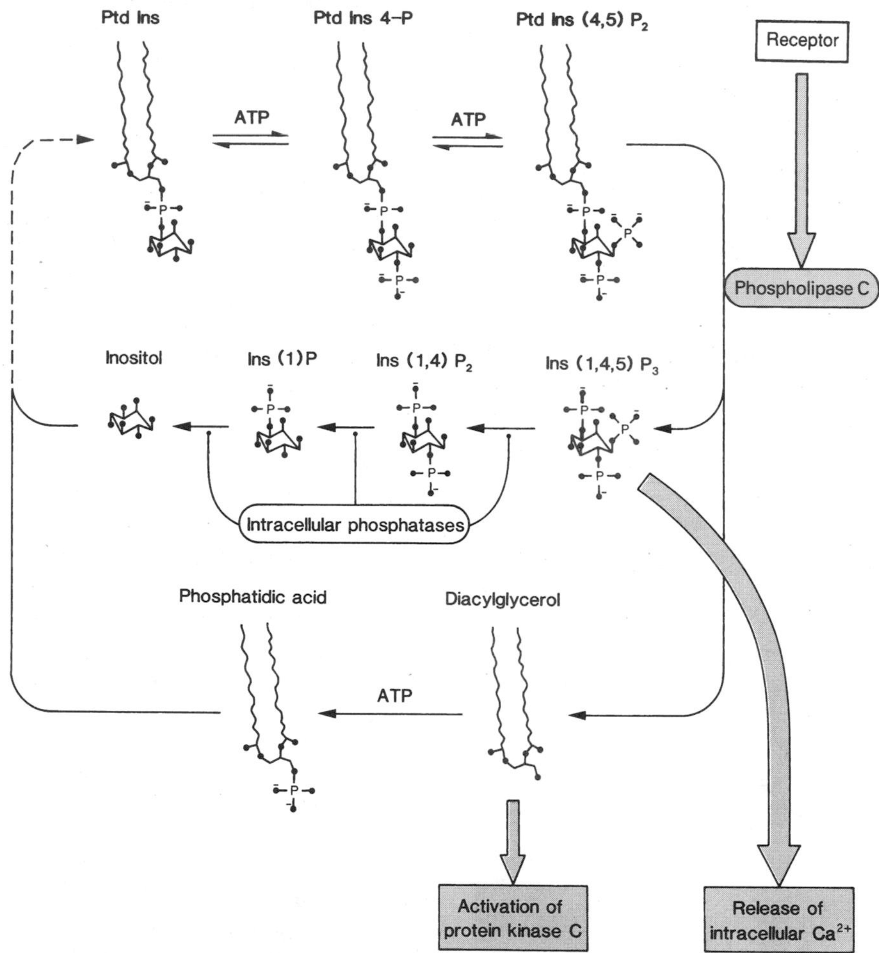

Fig. 2.12 The phosphatidylinositol cycle. Oxygen atoms (black or pink dots) and phosphorus atoms (P) are shown attached to the carbon skeleton. The agonist-activated enzyme phospholipase C acts on Ptd Ins $(4,5)P_2$ in the membrane to produce two second messengers: (1) inositol triphosphate, Ins $(1,4,5)P_3$, which is released into the cytosol; (2) diacylglycerol which remains in the membrane and activates protein kinase C, thus initiating various protein phosphorylation reactions. Dotted arrow indicates that intermediate steps occur in the process of resynthesis of Ptd Ins. Lithium blocks the recycling pathway.

that arachidonic acid itself may also function as an intracellular messenger.

Inositol phosphates and intracellular calcium. Inositol (1,4,5)-triphosphate acts very effectively to release calcium from intracellular stores, apparently by binding to a receptor on the membrane of the endoplasmic reticulum (the system of intracellular vesicles that sequesters and stores calcium, keeping the free intracellular calcium concentration normally very low—about 10^{-7} mol/l); $InsP_3$ is known to activate a calcium channel* in the endoplasmic reticulum, thereby releasing a flood of calcium into the cell and raising the free concentration 10- to 100-fold. (See Michell 1986, Fink et al. 1988, Berridge 1993.)

Two new techniques have been particularly important in unravelling the role of inositol phosphates and intracellular calcium as messengers controlling hormone responses. One is the measurement of free intracellular calcium concentration by the use of fluorescence indicators, such as Fura-2. This dye can be introduced into cells and used to report moment-to-moment changes in calcium concentration within a single cell, or even in parts of a cell. Figure 2.13 shows the signal recorded in this way from a sensory neuron in response to application of bradykinin, a peptide that causes excitation of these cells (see Ch. 31).

Another useful technique is intracellular perfusion of cells by means of tight-seal pipettes, which enables different substances that do not cross the cell membrane, such as $InsP_3$, to be introduced into a cell while the membrane potential or conductance of the cell is recorded, or while monitoring intracellular calcium. As a refinement, potential messenger substances can be introduced into cells in an inactive ('caged') form and activated by photolysis, using an intense light flash.

Subsequent to the discovery of Ins $(1,4,5)P_3$ as the major calcium-releasing messenger, a variety of other inositol phosphates have come on the scene (see Downes 1988) in which the phosphate groups appear to play a bewildering game of musical chairs around the inositol molecule, and much effort has gone into trying to identify a physiological role for some of these products. There is some evidence (see Downes 1988) that the tetraphosphate Ins $(1,3,4,5)P_4$ facilitates calcium entry through the cell membrane, thus helping to replenish the intracellular stores, but this remains controversial.

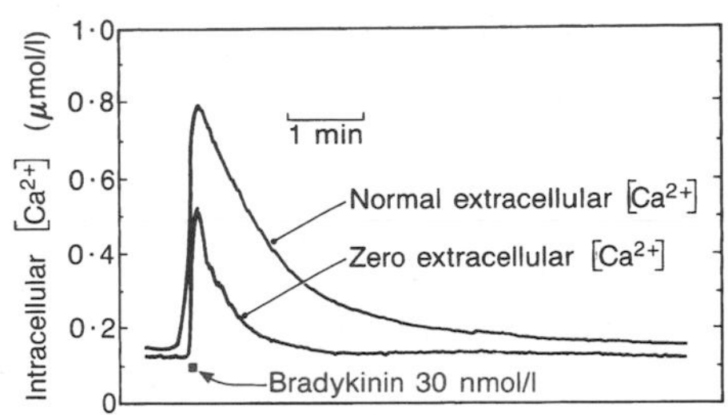

Fig. 2.13 Increase in intracellular calcium concentration in response to receptor activation. The records were obtained from a single rat sensory neuron grown in tissue culture. The cells were loaded with the fluorescent calcium indicator, Fura-2, and the signal from a single cell monitored with a fluorescence microscope. A brief exposure to the peptide bradykinin, which causes excitation of sensory neurons (see Ch. 31) causes a transient increase in $[Ca^{2+}]_i$ from the resting value of about 150 nmol/l. When calcium is removed from the extracellular solution, the bradykinin-induced increase in $[Ca^{2+}]_i$ is still present, but is smaller and briefer. The response in the absence of extracellular calcium represents the release of stored intracellular calcium, resulting from the intracellular production of $InsP_3$. The difference between this and the larger response when calcium is present extracellularly is believed to represent calcium entry through receptor-operated ion channels in the cell membrane. (Figure kindly provided by G M Burgess and A Forbes, Sandoz Institute for Medical Research)

The use of intracellular calcium monitoring in single cells has shown, in many instances, the surprising result that calcium release in response to agonists or $InsP_3$ injection does not occur continuously, but in a series of bursts (Fig. 2.14; see Rink & Jacob 1989, Berridge 1993). This is mainly due to the fact that calcium itself can, in many types of cell, act to open calcium channels in the endoplasmic reticulum, producing a delayed surge of calcium in response to the initial small release. This delayed feedback can give rise to an oscillatory response.

An increase in free intracellular calcium concentration occurs in many types of cell in response to a wide variety of agonists, and it is perhaps the most important pathway by which cellular effects are produced. For general reviews on intracellular calcium regulation see Campbell (1983), Blaustein

*You may wonder, with this talk of $InsP_3$ receptors controlling calcium channels, whether we have not come full circle back to receptor-operated ion channels; in all probability, we have, for the recent cloning of the $InsP_3$ receptor (Furuichi et al. 1989) suggests a structure reminiscent of our old friend the nicotinic acetylcholine receptor. ['Is this progress?' your authors wonder weakly.]

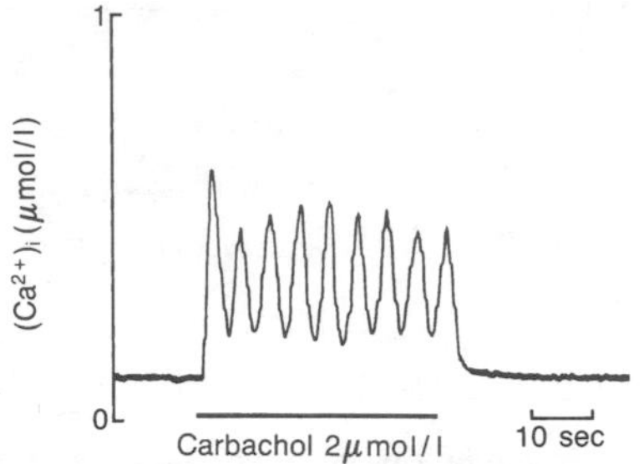

Fig. 2.14 Oscillations of intracellular calcium in response to an agonist. The recording was made from a single parotid gland cell, with Fura-2 as an intracellular calcium indicator, as in Figure 2.13. During the period indicated by the horizontal bar, the cell was exposed to 2 μmol/l carbachol (which elicits secretion from the salivary gland; see Ch. 6) which produced a sequence of regular oscillations in the intracellular calcium concentration. (From: Gray P T A 1988 J Physiol 406: 35–53)

(1988), Miller (1988), Berridge (1993). The range of cellular responses to increased intracellular calcium concentration is too broad to discuss in any detail. Examples that are of particular pharmacological importance include:

- smooth muscle contraction (Ch. 14)
- increased force of contraction of cardiac muscle (Ch. 13)
- secretion from exocrine glands and transmitter release from neurons (Chs 5 and 24)
- hormone release (Ch. 20)
- cytotoxicity (Ch. 45).

This list is far from complete. The actions of calcium depend on its ability to regulate the function of various enzymes, contractile proteins and ion channels. In many cases, *calmodulin* (see reviews in Cohen & Klee 1988), which is a ubiquitous cytosolic calcium-binding protein, acts as a go-between through which the action of calcium on various enzymes is mediated; the effects of calcium on ion channel function are probably direct.

Diacylglycerol and protein kinase C. The Ptd Ins response is involved in other ways besides regulating $[Ca^{2+}]_i$, for DAG directly affects the activity of a membrane-bound protein kinase, protein kinase C (PKC), and thus controls phosphorylation of serine and threonine residues of a variety of intracellular proteins (see Nishizuka 1984, 1986, 1988, Walaas & Greengard 1991). DAG, unlike the inositol phosphates, is highly lipophilic and remains within the membrane. It binds to a specific site on the protein kinase C molecule which is thought to migrate from the cytosol to the cell membrane in the presence of DAG, thereby becoming activated.* It is now known (see Nishizuka 1988) that at least six different types of PKC exist; they are distributed unequally in different cells and probably have different substrate specificities in terms of the proteins that are phosphorylated. They have in common the property of being activated by **phorbol esters** (highly irritant, tumour-promoting compounds produced by certain plants), which have been extremely useful in studying the functions of PKC. Interestingly, one of the subtypes is activated by arachidonic acid, which is a product of phospholipid hydrolysis by phospholipase A_2 (see above), so PKC activation can also occur with agonists that activate this enzyme. The physiological effects ascribed to PKC activation are many and varied (see Nishizuka 1986, who lists 45 proteins known then to be substrates). They include:

- release of hormones from many endocrine glands
- increases or decreases in neurotransmitter release and in neuronal excitability (mainly through effects on calcium and potassium channels)
- contraction or relaxation of smooth muscle
- inflammatory responses
- tumour promotion
- decrease in receptor sensitivity to agonists (i.e. receptor desensitisation)
- stimulation of ion transport by epithelia.

This very long list, along with many other types of response, underlines the importance of protein phosphorylation and dephosphorylation in regulating cell function. The members of the PKC family are, of course, not the only kinases that control this process. We have already discussed protein kinases that are regulated by cAMP and cGMP respectively, and another related group are the receptor-controlled tyrosine kinases that are discussed below. To make matters even more complicated, many of these kinases are highly sensitive to intracellular calcium, and may themselves be substrates for other kinases (e.g. the inactivation of myosin-light-chain kinase by cAMP-dependent kinase); furthermore, the substrates for phosphorylation include many of the receptors, channels and pumps that are involved in

*DAG can also arise from the action of another phospholipase (PLD) on phosphatidic acid.

calcium regulation. Additionally, there is evidence that G-protein-coupled receptors can modulate the activity of intracellular phosphatases, a heterogeneous family of enzymes which dephosphorylate many phosphoproteins (see Armstrong & White 1992). At this stage we have much data, but still too little understanding of how these systems interact in real life. There can be no doubt, though, that protein phosphorylation is a key mechanism through which many physiological mediators and drugs produce their effects.

The regulation of ion channels

In the last few years it has been found that G-protein-coupled receptors can control ion channel function by mechanisms that do not seem to involve any second messengers such as cAMP or inositol phosphates; instead, the G-protein interacts directly with the channel, presumably in the same way as it interacts with membrane enzymes responsible for second messenger synthesis. The first studies were concerned with cardiac muscle, but it now appears that this pattern of direct G-protein/channel interaction may be quite general (see reviews by Brown & Birnbaumer 1990, Hille 1992). The clearest examples come from studies on potassium channels. In cardiac muscle, for example, muscarinic ACh receptors are known to enhance K permeability (thus hyperpolarising the cells and inhibiting electrical activity; see Ch. 13). This effect requires functional G-proteins, which pass on the signal from the receptor to the channel. Similar mechanisms are believed to operate in neurons, where opiate analgesics reduce excitability by opening potassium channels (see Ch. 31). There is currently a dispute about whether the mechanism is of the kind shown in Figure 2.8 in which the free α-subunit controls the channel, or whether it is the βγ component. The latter is a heretical view in the face of the hardline G-protein orthodoxy which holds that the role of βγ is merely to act as chaperone to the flighty α-subunits, restraining them in the absence of hormone from rushing around the membrane and talking to every enzyme or channel protein within range. The controversy is not resolved, but it may turn out that βγ has the starring role in this small drama. Recent work suggests that βγ may also be the mediator responsible for activating protein kinase C in some cells.

The postulated roles of G-protein-coupled receptors in controlling enzymes and ion channels are summarised in Figure 2.15.

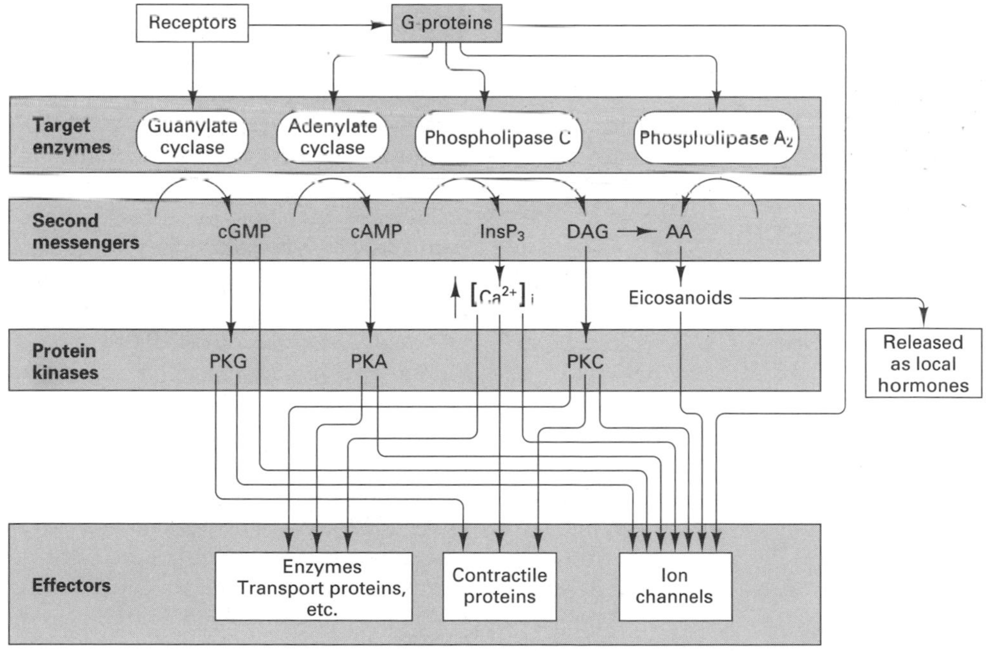

Fig. 2.15 G-protein and second messenger control of cellular effector systems.

Effectors controlled by G-proteins

Two key pathways are controlled by receptors, via G-proteins. Both can be activated or inhibited by pharmacological ligands, depending on the nature of the receptor and G-protein.

Adenylate cyclase/cAMP

- AC catalyses formation of the intracellular messenger, cAMP.
- cAMP activates various protein kinases which control cell function in many different ways by causing phosphorylation of various enzymes, carriers and other proteins.

Phospholipase C/inositol tris-phosphate/ diacylglycerol

- PLC catalyses the formation of two intracellular messengers, $InsP_3$ and DAG, from membrane phospholipid.
- $InsP_3$ acts to increase free cytosolic calcium by releasing calcium from intracellular compartments.
- Increased free calcium initiates many events, including contraction, secretion, enzyme activation and membrane hyperpolarisation.
- DAG activates protein kinase C, which controls many cellular functions by phosphorylating a variety of proteins.

Receptor-linked G-proteins also control:

- phospholipase A_2 (and thus the formation of arachidonic acid and eicosanoids)
- ion channels (e.g. K^+ and Ca^{2+} channels, thus affecting membrane excitability, transmitter release, contractility, etc.).

TYROSINE-KINASE- AND GUANYLATE-CYCLASE-LINKED RECEPTORS

Tyrosine-kinase-linked receptors are quite different in structure and function from either the channel-linked receptors or the G-protein-coupled receptors discussed above. They mediate the actions of a variety of growth factors, peptide mediators which stimulate mitogenesis (see Ch. 9), and also of insulin (see Ch. 20). For more detail, see reviews by Schlessinger & Ullrich (1992), Meakin & Shooter (1992), Taga & Kishimoto (1992). Guanylate-cyclase-linked receptors mediate the actions of certain peptides such as atrial natriuretic peptide (see Ch. 13).

The basic structure of these receptors is shown in Figure 2.4C. They comprise very large extracellular and intracellular domains, with about 400–700 residues in each. In the case of the insulin receptor, most of the extracellular domain is composed of a separate polypeptide chain which is linked by disulphide bonds to the chain that forms the trans-membrane and intracellular regions. In contrast, the growth factor receptors consist of a single long chain of over 1000 residues. The ligand-binding domain, as one would expect, shows very little sequence homology among members of this family, but the intracellular part is much more conserved, particularly in the region close to the membrane, which is believed to constitute an ATP-binding site—ATP being the source of the phosphate groups that become attached to tyrosine residues of a variety of proteins. The substrate-binding site is believed to lie further towards the end of the intracellular domain.

With only a single transmembrane helix linking the outer receptor domain with the inner kinase domain, a simple allosteric interaction seems unlikely as a mechanism by which the kinase activity responds to ligand binding. Instead, ligand binding generally leads to dimerisation of pairs of receptors (see Schlessinger & Ullrich 1992). The association of the two intracellular kinase domains allows an incestuous autophosphorylation of tyrosine residues in these two kinase domains to occur. The autophosphorylated tyrosine residues then serve as high affinity binding sites for various other intracellular proteins, which have in common a highly conserved sequence of about 100 amino acids, known as the SH2 domain (standing for Src-homology, since it was first identified in the Src oncogene product). Individual SH2-domain proteins, of which many are now known, bind very selectively to the phosphotyrosine residues of particular receptors, so the pattern of events triggered by particular growth factors is highly specific. The mechanism is summarised in Figure 2.16. What happens next varies greatly from receptor to receptor; some of these SH2-containing proteins are enzymes, including other protein kinases, and phospholipases. It is through activation of a specific subtype of phospholipase C that growth factors can initiate phospholipid breakdown, and thus cause $InsP_3$ formation and calcium release (see above). Other SH2-containing proteins are 'adaptors' which serve as a coupling between phosphotyrosine-containing proteins and a wide variety of other functional proteins, including many that are involved in the control of cell division and differentiation. Many growth factors are able to transform cells (i.e.

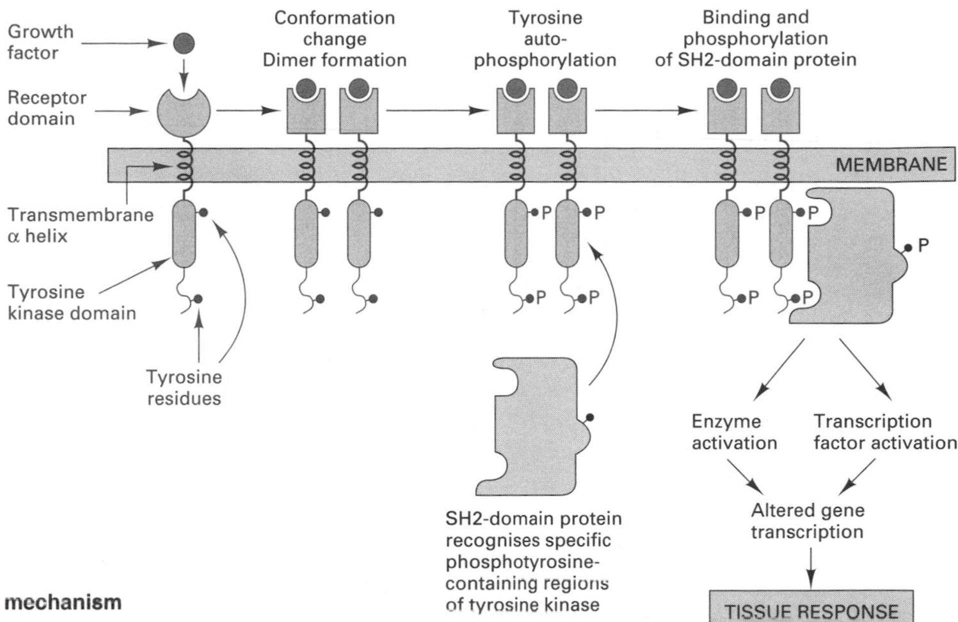

Fig. 2.16 Transduction mechanism of growth factor receptors.

enable them to divide indefinitely), and they generally do this by activating oncogenes. Their principal action, therefore, is to stimulate transcription of particular sections of the genome. The pathways responsible, involving receptor-controlled tyrosine phosphorylation and binding of various members of the SH2-containing protein family, play a key role in the control of growth, differentiation and intermediary metabolism. For more detail, see reviews by Carpenter (1992), Mayer & Baltimore (1993). The design of drug molecules that are either complementary to, or mimics of, the SH2 domain, as a strategy for treating many conditions, including cancers, immunological and metabolic disorders, holds great promise for the future.

Many cytokines (see Ch. 11) act on receptors similar in structure to the growth factor receptors, but lacking the intracellular tyrosine kinase domain. They nonetheless act by similar mechanisms, involving tyrosine phosphorylation and binding of SH2-domain proteins. It is thought that dimerisation of these receptors occurs when the cytokine binds, and this attracts a cytosolic tyrosine kinase unit to associate with the receptor dimer, initiating a similar cascade of reactions (see Taga & Kishimoto 1992).

It is interesting that the membrane-bound form of guanylate cyclase, the enzyme responsible for generating the second messenger cGMP in response to the binding of peptides such as atrial natriuretic peptide (ANP; see Chs 10 and 14), which intuitively one would have expected to resemble adenylate cyclase in its structure and regulation (see above), is similar in structure to the tyrosine kinase family (see Goy 1991). It is not known whether tyrosine phosphorylation is involved in the activation of the enzyme.

Tyrosine-kinase-linked receptors

- Receptors for various hormones (e.g. insulin) and growth factors incorporate tyrosine kinase in their intracellular domain.
- The receptors all share a common architecture, with a very large extracellular ligand-binding domain connected via a single α-helix to the catalytic region.
- Signal transduction generally involves dimerisation of receptors, followed by autophosphorylation of tyrosine residues. The phosphotyrosine residues act as acceptors for the SH2 domains of a variety of intracellular proteins, thereby allowing control of many cell functions.
- They are involved mainly in events controlling cell growth and differentiation, and act by regulating gene transcription.
- A few hormone receptors (e.g. ANF) have a similar architecture, and are linked to guanylate cyclase.

RECEPTORS THAT REGULATE DNA TRANSCRIPTION

The receptor-mediated regulation of DNA transcription is characteristic of steroid and thyroid hormones, and is quite different from the mechanisms described so far (see Evans 1988, Moore 1989, Laduron 1992 for recent reviews). One of the important advances of the past 20 years, initiated by the work of Jensen in Chicago, has been the recognition that the highly varied effects of different steroid drugs and hormones (which include numerous effects on the reproductive system, effects on the kidney causing salt and water retention, anti-inflammatory actions, etc.) all operate through the same basic mechanism, namely by stimulating transcription of selected genes (usually 50–100), leading to the synthesis of particular proteins and the production of cellular effects. The receptor for steroids is an intracellular protein located in the nucleus.* The basic structure of this family of receptors is shown in Figure 2.4D. They are large monomeric proteins of 400–1000 residues, containing a highly conserved region of about 60 residues in the middle of the molecule, which is believed to constitute the DNA-binding domain of the receptor. It contains two loops of about 15 residues each (*zinc fingers*), of which the knot consists of a cluster of four cysteine residues surrounding a zinc atom; these structures occur in many proteins that regulate DNA transcription, and the fingers are believed to wrap around the DNA helix. The hormone-binding domain lies downstream of this central region, while upstream lies a highly variable region which is responsible for controlling gene transcription.

The steroid molecule crosses the cell membrane readily, being highly lipid soluble, and binds to the receptor which is believed to unfold, thus exposing the normally buried DNA-binding domain. The receptor binds to certain well-defined regions of the nuclear DNA, known as hormone-responsive elements, which lie about 200 base pairs upstream from the genes that are regulated. An increase in RNA polymerase activity and the production of specific mRNA occur within a few minutes of adding the steroid, though the physiological response may take hours or days to develop. The different steroid hormones are able to activate different genes, and thus initiate completely different patterns of protein synthesis, and produce different physiological effects. For example, glucocorticoids enhance the production of lipocortin, which may account for their anti-inflammatory properties (see Ch. 12), whereas mineralocorticoids stimulate the production of various transport proteins that are involved in renal tubular function (see Ch. 18). Specificity at the DNA level seems to be a function of the amino-terminal and DNA-binding domain, rather than of the hormone-binding domain since chimaeric receptors consisting of the amino-terminus/DNA-binding part of one receptor (A) coupled to the hormone-binding part of another (B) will respond to hormone B but produce the effects associated with hormone A. More detail is given in the reviews mentioned above. Proteins resembling steroid receptors probably have much more general functions as transcriptional regulators. Thus, retinoic acid is an important regulator of embryonic development, and gradients of this substance arising during development play a key role in controlling the development of limbs and organs. It is known to act via a receptor of exactly the same type as we have been discussing, as is vitamin D which controls calcium metabolism (see Ch. 21). There are also, as with the tyrosine kinase receptors, several examples of oncogene products which appear to be surrogates of steroid or thyroid hormone receptors, but do not require hormone binding for activation (see Evans 1988).

Steroid receptors

- Ligands include steroid hormones, thyroid hormones, vitamin D and retinoic acid.
- Receptors are nuclear proteins, so ligands must first enter cells.
- Receptors consist of a conserved DNA-binding domain attached to variable ligand-binding and transcriptional control domains.
- DNA-binding domain recognises specific base sequences, thus activating particular genes.
- Pattern of gene activation depends on both cell type and nature of ligand, so effects are highly diverse.
- Effects are produced as a result of increased protein synthesis, and thus are slow in onset.

*Steroid receptors are often described as cytosolic because they were first discovered in the cytosolic compartment of homogenised cells. In life, they are confined to the nucleus.

There are a few exceptions to the general rule that steroids act by controlling protein synthesis. Aldosterone, in particular, produces rapid, non-genomic effects on renal function that appear to be mediated by a membrane receptor (see Wehling et al. 1993).

RECEPTORS AND DISEASE

Increasing understanding of receptor function in molecular terms has revealed a number of disease states directly linked to receptor malfunction, which may be either acquired or inherited. *Myasthenia gravis* (see Ch. 6), a disease of the neuromuscular junction, results from an autoimmune attack on nicotinic acetylcholine receptors. Inherited mutations of receptors for vasopressin and ACTH (see Chs 18 and 21) can result in resistance to these hormones. Conditions in which receptor mutations result in permanently switched-on effector mechanisms in the absence of agonist have also recently been described (see Lefkowitz 1993). One of these involves the receptor for thyrotrophin, producing continuous over-secretion of thyroid hormone; another involves the receptor for luteinising hormone, and results in precocious puberty. There is also a rare form of hypoparathyroidism, which appears to result from defective G-protein coupling of the parathyroid hormone receptor to adenylate cyclase.

REFERENCES AND FURTHER READING

Armstrong D L, White R E 1992 An enzymatic mechanism for potassium channel stimulation through pertussis-toxin-sensitive G proteins. Trends Neurosci 15: 403–408

Ashcroft F M 1988 Adenosine 5'-triphosphate-sensitive potassium channels. Annu Rev Neurosci 11: 97–118

Axelrod J, Burch R M, Jelsema C L 1988 Receptor-mediated activation of phospholipase A2 via GTP binding proteins: arachidonic acid and its metabolites as second messengers. Trends Neurosci 11: 117–123

Barnard E A 1988 Separating receptor subtypes from their shadows. Nature 335: 301–303

Barnard E A 1992 Receptor classes and the transmitter-gated ion channels. Trends Biochem Sci 17: 368–374

Berridge M 1993 Inositol trisphosphate and calcium signalling. Nature 361: 315–325

Berridge M J, Irvine R F 1984 Inositol trisphosphate, a novel second messenger in cellular signal transduction. Nature 312: 315–321

Black J W, Jenkinson D H, Gerskowitch V P 1987 Perspectives on receptor classification. Liss, New York

Blaustein M P 1988 Calcium transport and buffering in neurons. Trends Neurosci 11: 438–443

Bolton T B 1979 Mechanisms of action of neurotransmitters and other substances on smooth muscle. Physiol Rev 59: 606–718

Bourne H R, Sanders D A, McCormick F 1990 The GTPase superfamily: a conserved switch for diverse cell functions. Nature 348: 125–132

Brown A M, Birnbaumer L 1990 Ionic channels and their regulation by G protein subunits. Ann Rev Physiol 52: 197–213

Campbell A K 1983 Intracellular calcium; its universal role as regulator. John Wiley & Sons, Chichester

Carpenter G 1992 Receptor tyrosine kinase substrates: src homology domains and signal transduction. FASEB J 6:3283–3289

Changeux J-P, Galzi J-L, Devilliers-Thiery A, Bertrand D 1992 The functional architecture of the acetylcholine nicotinic receptor explored by affinity labelling and site-directed mutagenesis. Quart Rev Biophys 25: 395–432

Cohen P, Klee C B 1988 Calmodulin. Molecular aspects of cellular regulation, vol 5. Elsevier, Amsterdam

Colquhoun D 1987 Affinity, efficacy and receptor classification: Is the classical theory still useful? In: Black J W, Jenkinson D H, Gerskowitch V P (eds) Perspectives on receptor classification. Liss, New York

Cull-Candy S G, Usowicz M 1987 Multiple conductance channels activated by excitatory amino acids in cerebellar neurons. Nature 325: 525–528

Dixon R A F, Kobilka B K, Strader D, Benovic J, Dohlman H G, Frielle T, Bolanowski M A, Bennet C D, Rands E, Diehl R F, Mumford R A, Slater E, Sigal I S, Caron M G, Lefkowitz R J, Strader C D 1986 Cloning of the gene and cDNA for mammalian β-adrenergic receptor and homology with rhodopsin. Nature 321: 75–79

Downes C P 1988 Inositol phosphates: a family of signal molecules. Trends Neurosci 11: 336–338

Evans R M 1988 The steroid and thyroid hormone receptor superfamily. Science 240: 889–895

Fink L A, Kaczmarek L K 1988 Inositol polyphosphates regulate excitability. Trends Neurosci 11: 338–339

Fink L A, Connor J A, Kaczmarek L K 1988 Inositol trisphosphate releases intracellularly stored calcium and modulates ion channels in molluscan neurons. J Neurosci 8: 2544–2555

Furuichi T, Yoshikawa S, Miyawaki A, Wada K, Maeda N Mikoshiba K 1989 Primary structure and functional expression of the inositol 1,4,5-trisphosphate-binding protein. Nature 342: 32–38

Galzi J-L, Devilliers-Thiery A, Hussy N, Bertrand S, Changeux J-P, Bertrand D 1992 Mutations in the channel domain of a neuronal nicotinic receptor convert ion selectivity from cationic to anionic. Nature 359: 500–505

Giros B, Caron M G 1993 Molecular characteristics of the dopamine transporter. Trends Pharmacol Sci 14: 43–49

Goy M F 1991 cGMP: the wayward child of the cyclic nucleotide family. Trends Neurosci 14: 293–299

Grenningloh G, Rienitz A, Schmitt B, Methfessel C, Zensen M, Beyreuther K, Gundelfinger E D, Betz H 1987 The strychnine-binding subunit of the glycine receptor

shows homology with nicotinic acetycholine receptors. Nature 328: 215–220
Hibert M F, Trumpp-Kallmeyer S, Hoflack J, Bruinvels A 1993 This is not a G protein-coupled receptor. Trends Pharmacol Sci 14: 7–12
Hille B 1992 G Protein-coupled mechanisms and nervous signalling. Neuron 9: 187–195
Karlin A 1993 Structure of nicotinic acetylcholine receptors. Curr Opin Neurobiol 3: 299–309
Laduron P M 1992 Towards a genomic pharmacology: from membranal to nuclear receptors. Adv Drug Res 22: 108–148
Lefkowitz R J 1993 Turned on to ill effect. Nature 365: 603–605
Linden J, Delahunty T M 1989 Receptors that inhibit phosphoinositide breakdown. Trends Pharmacol Sci 10: 114–120
Majerus P W, Connolly T M, Deckmyn H, Ross T S, Bross T E, Ishii H, Bansal V S, Wilson D B 1986 The metabolism of phosphoinositide-derived messenger molecules. Science 234: 1519–1526
Mayer B J, Baltimore D 1993 Signalling through SH2 and SH3 domains. Trends Cell Biol 3: 8–13
Meakin S O, Shooter E M 1992 The nerve growth factor family of receptors. Trends Neurosci 12: 323–331
Michell R H 1986 Inositol lipids and their role in receptor function: history and general principles. In: Putney J W (ed) Phosphoinositides and receptor mechanisms. Alan Liss, New York
Miller R J 1988 Calcium signalling in neurons. Trends Neurosci 11: 415–419
Milligan G 1993 Mechanisms of multifunctional signalling by G protein-coupled receptors. Trends Pharmacol Sci 14: 239–244
Moore D 1989 Promiscuous behaviour in the steroid hormone receptor superfamily. Trends Neurosci 12: 165–168
Nahorski S R 1988 Inositol polyphosphates and neuronal calcium homeostasis. Trends Neurosci 10: 444–448
Neer E J, Clapham D E 1988 Roles of G-protein subunits in transmembrane signalling. Nature 333:129–134
Nishizuka Y 1984 The role of protein kinase C in cell surface signal transduction and tumour promotion. Nature 308: 693–698
Nishizuka Y 1986 Studies and perspectives of protein kinase C. Science 233: 305–312
Nishizuka Y 1988 The molecular heterogeneity of protein kinase C and its implications for cellular regulation. Nature 334: 661–665
O'Dowd B F, Lefkowitz R J, Caron M G 1989 Structure of the adrenergic and related receptors. Annu Rev Neurosci 12: 67–83
Piomelli D, Volterra A, Dale N, Siegelbaum S A, Kandel E R, Schwartz J H, Belardetti F 1987 Lipoxygenase metabolites of arachidonic acid as second messengers for presynaptic inhibition of *Aplysia* sensory cells. Nature 328: 38–43
Rink T J 1988 A real receptor-operated calcium channel? Nature 334: 649–650
Rink T J, Jacob R 1989 Calcium oscillations in non-excitable cells. Trends Neurosci 12: 3–46
Ronnett G V, Snyder S H 1992 Molecular messengers of olfaction. Trends Neurosci 15: 508–513
Rosen O M 1987 After insulin binds. Science 237: 1452–1458
Ross E M 1989 Signal sorting and amplification through G protein-coupled receptors. Neuron 3: 141–152
Ross E M 1992 Twists and turns in G-protein signalling pathways. Curr Biol 2: 517–519
Schlessinger J, Ullrich A 1992 Growth factor signalling by receptor tyrosine kinases. Neuron 9: 383–391
Simon M I, Strathmann M P, Gautam N 1991 Diversity of G proteins in signal transduction. Science 252: 802–808
Sporn M B, Roberts A B 1990 Growth factors and receptors. Handbook of experimental pharmacology, vol 95. Springer-Verlag, Berlin
Sternweis P C, Smrka A V 1992 Regulation of phospholipase C by G proteins. Trends Biochem Sci 17: 502–506
Stryer L 1986 Cyclic GMP cascade of vision. Annu Rev Neurosci 6: 87–119
Taga T, Kishimoto T 1992 Cytokine receptors and signal transduction. FASEB J 7: 3387–3396
Taylor C W, Merritt J E 1986 Receptor coupling to polyphosphoinositide turnover: a parallel with the adenylate cyclase system. Trends Pharmacol Sci 7: 238–242
Tsien R Y 1988 Fluorescence measurement and photochemical manipulation of cytosolic free calcium. Trends Neurosci 11: 419–424
Unwin N 1993 Nicotinic acetylcholine receptor at 9 Å resolution. J Mol Biol 229: 1101–1124
Walaas S I, Greengard P 1991 Protein phosphorylation and neuronal function. Pharm Rev 43: 299–349
Waterfield M D 1989 Epidermal growth factor and related molecules. Lancet 1: 1243–1246
Wehling M, Christ M, Gerzer R 1993 Aldosterone-specific membrane receptors and related non-genomic effects. Trends Pharmacol Sci 14: 1–4
Yarden Y, Ullrich A 1988 Growth factor receptor tyrosine kinases. Annu Rev Biochem 57: 443–478

3 MEASUREMENT IN PHARMACOLOGY

It is necessary to have reliable methods for measuring drug effects in order to be able to compare quantitatively the effects of different substances, or the same substance under different circumstances. It is also necessary to be able to measure the concentration of drugs and other active substances in, say, the blood or other body fluids. The first of these requirements is met by the techniques of bioassay. The second requirement is increasingly met by chemical techniques, but bioassay is necessary when the chemical identity of the active substance is unknown. In this chapter, the principles underlying the main types of bioassay are discussed, together with an account of some chemical methods that are particularly useful in pharmacology.

BIOASSAY

Bioassay is defined as the estimation of the concentration or potency of a substance by measurement of the biological response that it produces.

The uses of bioassay are:

- to measure the pharmacological activity of new or chemically undefined substances
- to measure the concentration of known substances
- to investigate the function of endogenous mediators
- to measure drug toxicity.

Clinical trials, used to assess the clinical effectiveness of drug treatments, embody the same principles as other types of bioassay, adapted to this special situation.

Bioassay is essential in the development of new drugs. The first stage in assessing a new compound is to compare its biological activity in various test systems with that of known compounds. The choice of suitable test systems for this preliminary bioassay is important and not always easy. The tests must be sufficiently simple and quick to be used routinely on numerous compounds, and they must also be as specific as possible for the type of biological activity that is being sought. This may be fairly obvious; local anaesthetic activity, for example, can be measured reliably by the ability of a substance to block action potential propagation in an isolated length of peripheral nerve. The results obtained in this way correlate well with activity in clinical use, so the test has good predictive value. In other cases, appropriate test systems are not at all obvious. When, for example, antipsychotic drugs are being sought, there is no single reliable test system. Many assays, on whole animals and on isolated systems, have been devised that give some indication of antipsychotic activity, but each will throw up false positive or negative results. Assessment of a new compound usually consists of carrying out a battery of such assays, and constructing a profile of activity. Clinical effectiveness, it is hoped, may appear to be associated with a particular pattern of activity in such a profile, rather than with activity in one particular test system.

In general, the less well we understand the mechanism of the therapeutic action of a drug, the more difficult it is to predict clinical effectiveness from the results of assays based on laboratory test systems.

In many cases, it is not until the point of actual clinical trial that it is known for certain whether the drug even possesses therapeutic activity of the kind required.

Bioassay is now rarely used for measurement of the concentration of known substances. *The British Pharmacopoeia* (1988), however, still lays down bioassay as the official method for estimating the activity of clinical preparations of a number of substances, such as **corticotrophin**, **insulin**, **vasopressin preparations** and **heparin**, as well as various vaccines and enzymes that are used therapeutically, all of which are prepared from biological material.

Acetylcholine was identified chemically as a neurotransmitter in 1933 (see Ch. 6), but only recently has it become possible to measure by chemical methods the minute amounts released by nerve terminals. Progress in studying acetylcholine release depended for many years on highly sensitive, but extremely laborious, bioassays. Chemical assays based on mass spectrometry and radio-enzymatic assays (see later) for acetylcholine have now, however, largely replaced bioassay.

Bioassay is indispensable in the study of new types of hormonal or other chemically mediated control systems. Mediators in such systems are usually first recognised by the biological effects that they produce, and it is only later that their chemical identity, and hence the possibility of using more direct chemical assay methods, is established. Sometimes (as in the discovery of the role of **dopamine** in the central nervous system; see Ch. 24) things happen the other way about, and a mediator is identified chemically before being shown to be functionally important. More often the first clue is the finding that a tissue extract or some other biological sample produces an effect on an assay system. For example, the ability of extracts of the posterior lobe of the pituitary to produce a rise in blood pressure and a contraction of the uterus was observed at the turn of the century. These actions were made the basis of quantitative assay procedures and a standard preparation of the extract was established by international agreement in 1935. By use of these assays it was shown that two distinct peptides were responsible, and they were eventually identified and synthesised in 1953. Biological assay had already revealed much about the synthesis, storage and release of the hormones, and was essential for their purification and identification. Though it is highly unlikely that future hormones and mediators will require 50 years of laborious bioassays before being chemically characterised,* bioassay remains crucial to such studies.

Bioassays on different test systems may be run in parallel to reveal the profile of activity of an unknown mediator. This was developed to an almost Baroque splendour in the work of Vane and his colleagues, who studied the generation and destruction of endogenous active substances, such as **prostanoids** (see Ch. 11) by the technique of cascade superfusion (Fig. 3.1). In this technique the sample is run sequentially over a series of test preparations chosen to differentiate between different active constituents of the sample. The pattern of responses produced identifies effectively the active material, and the use of such assay systems for 'on-line' analysis of biological samples has been invaluable in studying the production and fate of short-lived mediators such as prostanoids and the endothelium-derived relaxing factor (Ch. 10).

Measurement of the *therapeutic effectiveness* of drugs by clinical trials is an important and highly specialised form of biological assay. The need to use man as an experimental animal (particularly when the subjects are patients seeking medical advice, rather than selected volunteers) imposes many restrictions. Some of the basic principles involved in clinical trials are discussed later in this chapter.

Drug toxicity is measured in two distinct ways. In one kind of test, the ability of experimental animals to withstand large doses of the drug is assessed, the crudest such measurement being the *LD_{50} test*, a bioassay designed to measure the lethal dose in animals (see p. 57). The other kind of toxicity measurement involves the assessment of unwanted effects in man, either as part of a clinical trial whose primary purpose is to test therapeutic efficacy, or by adverse reaction monitoring which is designed to detect harmful effects when the drug is given therapeutically to large numbers of patients.

*Recently, a Japanese group (Yanagisawa et al. 1988) described in a single paper, regarded as something of a *tour de force*, the bioassay, purification, chemical analysis and synthesis, and DNA-cloning of a new vascular peptide, *endothelin* (see Ch. 14).

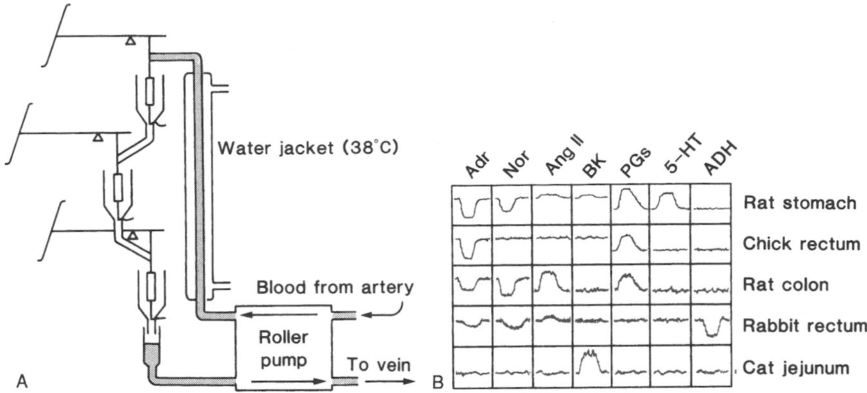

Fig. 3.1 Parallel assay by the cascade superfusion technique. A. Blood is pumped continuously from the test animal over a succession of test organs, whose responses are measured by a simple transducer system. **B.** The response of these organs to a variety of test substances (at 0.1–5 ng/ml) is shown. Each active substance produces a distinct pattern of responses, enabling unknown materials present in the blood to be identified and assayed. (Adr = adrenaline; Nor = noradrenaline; Ang II = angiotensin II; BK = bradykinin; PG = prostaglandin; 5-HT = 5-hydroxytryptamine; ADH = antidiuretic hormone) (From: Vane J R 1969 Br J Pharmacol 35: 209–242)

GENERAL PRINCIPLES OF BIOASSAY

This section is concerned with laboratory-based assays rather than with clinical trials or monitoring which are discussed later.

The use of standards

J H Burn wrote in 1950: 'Pharmacologists today strain at the king's arm, but they swallow the frog, rat and mouse, not to mention the guinea pig and the pigeon.' He was referring to the fact that the 'king's arm' had been long since abandoned as a standard measure of length, whereas drug activity continued to be defined in terms of dose needed to cause, say, vomiting of a pigeon or cardiac arrest in a mouse. A plethora of 'pigeon units', 'mouse units' and the like, which no two laboratories could agree on, contaminated the literature.* Even if two laboratories cannot agree—because their pigeons differ—on the activity in pigeon units of the same sample of an active substance, they should nonetheless be able to agree that preparation X is, say, 3.5 times as active as standard preparation Y on the pigeon test. Biological assays are therefore designed to measure the relative potency of two preparations, usually a *standard* and an *unknown*. The best kind of standard is, of course, the pure substance, but it is often necessary to establish standard preparations of various hormones, natural products and antisera against which laboratory samples can be calibrated, even though the standard preparations are not chemically pure.

The design of bioassays

Given the aim of comparing the activity of two preparations, a standard (S) and an unknown (U) on a particular preparation, a bioassay must provide an estimate of the dose or concentration of U that will produce the same biological effect as that of a known dose or concentration of S. As Figure 3.2 shows, provided that the log dose–effect curves for S and U are parallel, the ratio, M, of equiactive doses will not depend on the magnitude of response chosen. Thus, M provides an estimate of the potency ratio of the two preparations. It is worth noting that a comparison of the magnitude of the effects produced by equal doses of S and U does not provide an estimate of M, because the ratio of the effects

*More picturesque examples of absolute units of the kind that Burn would have frowned upon are the PHI and the mHelen. PHI, cited by Colquhoun (1971), stands for 'purity in heart index' and measures the ability of a virgin pure-in-heart to transform, under appropriate conditions, a he-goat into a youth of surpassing beauty. The mHelen is a unit of beauty, 1 mHelen being sufficient to launch 1 ship.

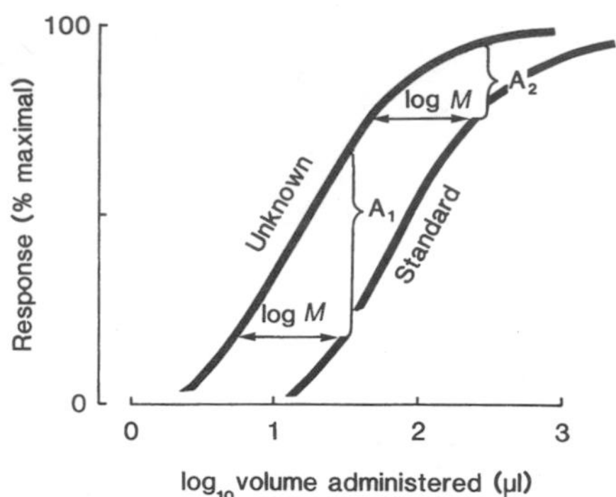

Fig. 3.2 Comparison of the potency of unknown and standard by bioassay. Note that comparing the magnitude of responses produced by the same dose (i.e. volume) of standard and unknown gives no quantitative estimate of their relative potency. (The differences, A_1 and A_2, depend on the dose chosen.) Comparison of equi-effective doses of standard and unknown gives a valid measure of their relative potencies. Since the lines are parallel, the magnitude of the effect chosen for the comparison is immaterial; i.e. log *M* is the same at all points on the curves.

produced by S and U will vary according to the dose chosen.

The main problem with all types of bioassay is that of biological variation, and the design of bioassays is aimed at:

- minimising variation
- avoiding systematic errors resulting from variation
- estimating the limits of error of the assay result.

Examples of the extent of biological variation encountered in two fairly typical bioassays are shown in Figure 3.3; in each case there is about a threefold range in the drug dose needed to produce a given biological response in the population of frogs or human subjects that were tested. In the examples shown in Figure 3.3, the distributions of individual effective doses (IED) are approximately symmetrical and correspond roughly to the normal distribution. The potency of the drug in such an assay is usually expressed in terms of the median value of the IED (known as the ED_{50} because it corresponds to the dose required to produce a response in 50% of the subjects tested). The ED_{50} can be read off the cumulative frequency distribution curve as shown in Figure 3.3B. If, as in Figure 3.3A and B, the distribution of IED values is nearly symmetrical, the mean IED for the population will agree quite closely with the ED_{50} (Fig. 3.3B).

Many different experimental designs have been proposed to maximise the efficiency and reliability of bioassays. Commonly, comparisons are based on analysis of dose–response curves, from which the matching doses of standard and unknown are calculated. Such calculations become much simpler if the dose–response curves are linear. In many cases this can be achieved (see Ch. 1) by using a logarithmic dose scale and restricting observations to the middle region of the log dose–effect curve, which is usually close to a straight line. The use of a logarithmic dose scale means that the curves for standard and unknown will normally be parallel, and the potency ratio (*M*) of the unknown, relative to the standard, is determined by the horizontal distance between the two curves (Fig. 3.2). Assays of this type are known as *parallel line assays*, and a convenient and simple design is the 2 + 2 assay, in which two doses of standard (S_1 and S_2) and two of unknown (U_1 and U_2) are used (Fig. 3.4). The doses are chosen to give responses lying on the linear part of the log dose–response curve. Within this design, the sequence of four doses, S_1, S_2, U_1, and U_2, is usually given as a series of *randomised blocks*, as in the record shown in Figure 3.4. The fact that each dose is repeated several times means that an inherent measure of the variability of the test system is available from this type of assay, and this can be used, by means of straightforward statistical analysis, to estimate the confidence limits of the final result.

In practice, most bioassays will give results whose 5% confidence limits lie within ± 20%, and many will do better than this.

The 2 + 2 assay also detects whether or not the two log dose–effect lines deviate significantly from parallelism. If the lines are not parallel, which may be the case if the assay is used to compare two drugs whose mechanism of action is not the same, it is not possible to define the relative potencies of S and U unambiguously in terms of a simple ratio. The experimenter must then face up to the fact that there are qualitative as well as quantitative differences between the two, so that comparison requires measurement of more than a single dimension of potency. An example of this kind of difficulty is met when diuretic drugs (Ch. 18) are compared. Some ('low ceiling') diuretics are capable of producing only a small diuretic effect, no matter how much is given; others ('high ceiling') can produce a very intense diuresis (described as 'torrential' by authors with vivid imaginations). A comparison of two such

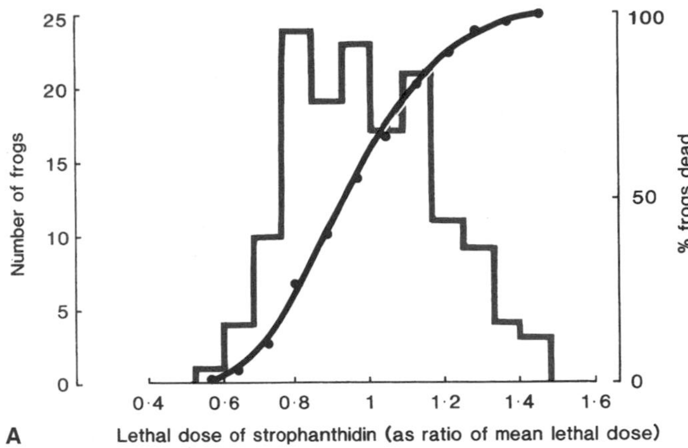

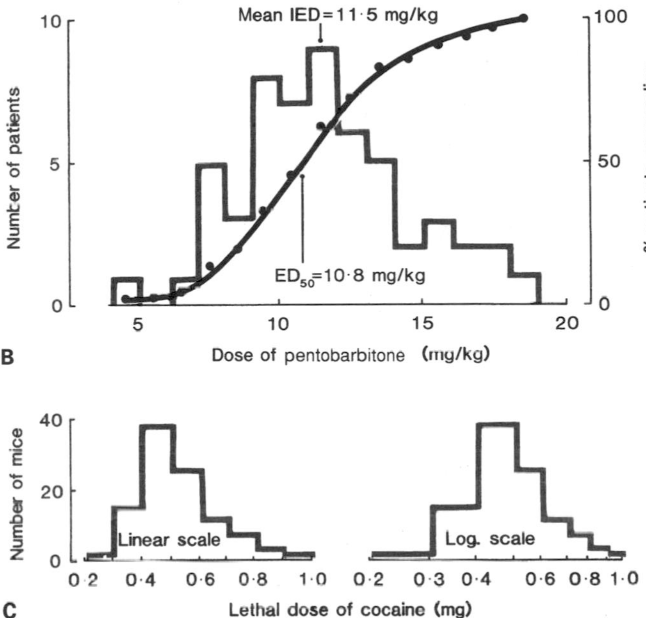

Fig. 3.3 Examples of biological variation. **A.** Histogram (left-hand ordinate) and cumulative frequency distribution (right-hand ordinate) of the lethal dose of a cardiac glycoside (strophanthidin) in frogs. The deviations extend roughly from 50% below the mean to 50% above. (Data from: Behrens 1929) **B.** Histogram and cumulative frequency distribution of the intravenous dose of pentobarbitone needed to cause a standard degree of drowsiness in obstetric patients. The scatter is rather greater than in A, presumably because the endpoint is less clearly defined. Note that the ED_{50} is not identical with the mean IED. **C.** Histograms of the lethal dose of cocaine in mice, plotted on linear and logarithmic concentration scales. Note that the linear scale gives a highly skewed distribution, whereas on a logarithmic scale it is roughly symmetrical. (Data from: Colquhoun D 1971 Lecture notes on biostatistics. Oxford University Press, Oxford)

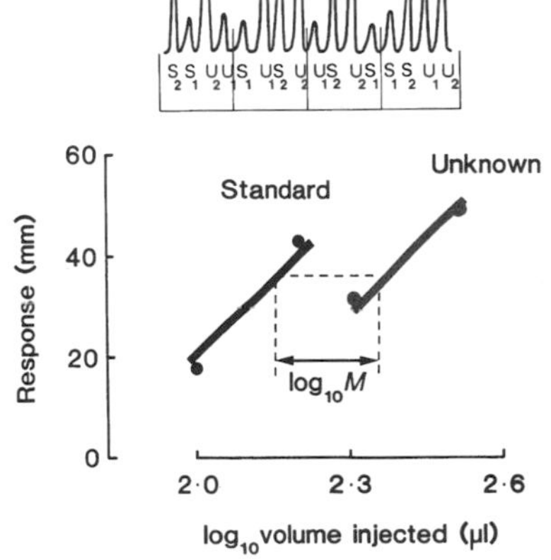

Fig. 3.4 Two-plus-two bioassay of an unknown versus a standard pituitary extract on an isolated rat uterus. Two doses of unknown (U_1 and U_2) and two standard (S_1 and S_2) were tested. They were chosen to give responses of similar magnitude, and with U_1/U_2 equal to S_1/S_2 for convenience in analysis. The four doses were tested in random order in each block (upper traces). The mean responses are shown below, with the calculated regression lines and potency ratio. In this assay $\log_{10} M = 0.20$; $M = 1.58$. Since the standard contained 400 mU/ml, the unknown was estimated as 400/1.58 = 252 mU/ml. Analysis of variance was used to calculate the 5% confidence limits (± 24 mU/ml) from the individual assay responses. (From: Holton P 1948 Br J Pharmacol 3: 278)

drugs requires not only a measure of the doses needed to produce an equal low-level diuretic effect, but also a measure of the relative heights of the ceilings.

Quantal and graded responses

The response used in an assay may be a *graded phenomenon*, such as a change in blood glucose concentration or contraction of a strip of smooth muscle or a change in the time taken for a rat to run a maze; it may also be *all-or-nothing*, such as death, loss of righting reflex or success in maze-running within a stipulated time. With the latter type of response, known as a *quantal response* because it either happens or it doesn't, the proportion of animals responding will vary according to the dose used, and the relationship between log dose and proportion of animals responding generally looks like Figure 3.3A. The shape and slope of such a curve is governed by the individual variation between animals—the more uniform the population, the steeper the curve. Therefore, the precision of assays based on quantal responses can be improved by using a uniform population of animals. With graded responses, the steepness of the dose–response curve is a property of the test system and has nothing to do with biological variation. Quantal responses can be used in essentially the same way as graded responses for the purposes of bioassay, though the appropriate statistical procedures are slightly different.

Bioassay

- Bioassay is the measurement of concentration or potency of a drug from the magnitude of the biological effect that it produces.
- Bioassay normally involves comparison of the *unknown* preparation with a *standard.* Estimates that are not based on comparison with standards are usually unreliable and vary from laboratory to laboratory.
- The parallel line assay is a widely used type of comparative bioassay, which allows the error limits of the assay result to be estimated.
- The biological response may be *quantal* (the proportion of tests in which a given all-or-nothing effect is produced) or *graded.* Different statistical procedures are appropriate in each case.

BIOASSAYS IN MAN

It is often useful to carry out bioassays in man when, for example, animal tests fail to predict human responses, or when the response is subjective and not measurable in animals. Furthermore, any drug that is intended for therapeutic use in man naturally has first to be tested in human subjects. Such tests are of two main types, namely:

- tests of pharmacological actions, potency, pharmacokinetic characteristics, side effects, etc. in normal subjects (termed *Phase I studies*) or small groups of patients (*Phase II studies*)
- tests of therapeutic efficacy in patients undergoing treatment, by the use of *clinical trials* (*Phase III studies*).

In principle, the use of human subjects for measurements of the first type is no different from the use of experimental animals, though in practice Ethical Committees associated with all medical research centres tightly control the type of experiment that can be done.

An example of the use of human subjects to compare two analgesic drugs (see Ch. 31) is shown in Figure 3.5. Though many animal tests have been devised (for example, measuring the effect of different doses of an analgesic drug on the mean time taken for groups of mice to jump off a surface heated to a mildly painful temperature), they often fail to predict accurately the subjective relief of pain in man. One method of measuring analgesia in man is to employ a graded stimulus, such as radiant heat, and determine the threshold at which pain is felt. It is generally agreed, however, that this type of artificial and superficial pain is quite different in quality and connotation from clinical pain and provides a relatively poor model. More useful assessments of analgesic drugs have, therefore, been developed on the basis of subjective reports of relief from persistent pain, such as that of malignant disease. Figure 3.5 shows a comparison of **morphine** and **codeine** in which a modified 2 + 2 design was used. Each of the four doses was given on different occasions to each of the four subjects, the order being randomised and both subject and observer being unaware of the dose given. Pain relief was assessed by questions from the trained observer, and the assay gave a precise comparison of the potencies of the two drugs, morphine turning out to be 13 times as potent as codeine. This, of course, does not prove its superiority, but merely shows that a smaller dose is needed to produce the same effect. Such a measurement is, however, an essential preliminary to assessing the relative therapeutic merits of the two drugs, for any comparison of other factors, such as side effects, duration of action, tolerance or dependence, needs to be done on the basis of doses that are equiactive so far as analgesia is concerned.

CLINICAL TRIALS

A clinical trial is a method for comparing objectively, by a prospective study, the results of two or more therapeutic procedures. It is important to realise that, until about 30 years ago, methods of treatment were chosen on the basis of clinical impression and personal experience rather than objective testing. Though many drugs, with undoubted effectiveness, remain in use without ever having been subjected to a controlled clinical trial, any new drug is now required to have been tested in this way before being licensed for general clinical use.*

General accounts of the principles and organisation of clinical trials are given by Harris & Fitzgerald (1970), Pocock (1983), Friedman et al. (1985). A clinical trial aims to compare the response of a *test group* of patients receiving a new treatment (A) with that of a *control group* receiving an existing 'standard' treatment (B). Treatment A might be a new drug or a new combination of existing drugs, or any other kind of therapeutic intervention such as a surgical operation, diet, physiotherapy and so on. The standard against which it is judged (treatment B) might be a currently used drug treatment or (if there is no currently available effective treatment) a placebo or no treatment at all.

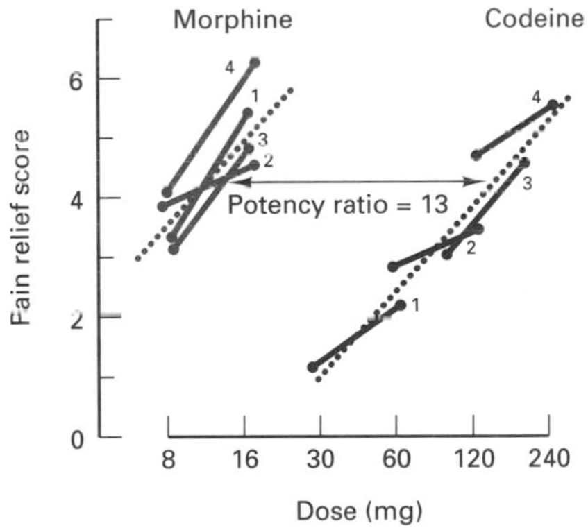

Fig. 3.5 Assay of morphine and codeine as analgesics in man. Each of four patients (numbered 1–4) was given, on successive occasions in random order, four different treatments (high and low morphine, and high and low codeine) by intramuscular injection and the subjective pain relief score calculated for each. The calculated regression lines (dotted) gave a potency ratio estimate of 13 for the two drugs. (After: Houde R W et al. 1965 In: Analgetics. Academic Press, New York)

The use of controls is crucial in clinical trials. Claims of therapeutic efficacy based on reports that, for example, 16 out of 20 patients receiving drug X got better within 2 weeks are of no value without a knowledge of how 20 patients receiving no treatment, or a different treatment, would have fared. Usually, the controls are provided by a separate group of patients from those receiving the test treatment, but sometimes a cross-over design is possible in which the same patients are switched from test to control treatment or vice versa, and the results compared. *Randomisation* (see p. 54) is essential to avoid bias in assigning individual patients to test or control groups. Hence, the randomised controlled clinical trial is now regarded as the essential tool for assessing clinical efficacy of new drugs.

Much concern has been expressed over the ethics of assigning patients at random to an untreated control group when the doctor in charge believes the test treatment to have advantages. However, the reason for setting up a trial is that existing anecdotal data or previous uncontrolled trials have failed to convince a substantial number of doctors that the treatment is superior, so for these doctors there is no ethical dilemma. If individual doctors are personally convinced that the treatment is beneficial, they should clearly avoid participating in a controlled trial. All would agree that all patients must be asked whether they are prepared to participate

*It is fashionable in some quarters to argue that to require evidence of efficacy of therapeutic procedures in the form of a controlled trial runs counter to the doctrines of 'holistic' medicine. This is a fundamentally anti-scientific view, for science advances only by generating predictions from hypotheses and by subjecting the predictions to experimental test. If a system of medicine is set up whose hypotheses are deemed to be immune to experimental test, then, like a religious doctrine, it lies outside the realm of science. This does not, of course, make it wrong, but it does make it incompatible with scientific medicine. One must view with great suspicion the suggestion that elements of both systems can be rationally combined without coming into fundamental conflict.

on the basis that they will be randomly and unknowingly assigned to either the treated or the control group.

Unlike the kind of bioassay that we have been considering up to this point, the clinical trial does not normally give any information about potency or the form of the dose–response curve, but merely compares the response produced by two stipulated therapeutic regimes. The investigator must decide in advance what dose to use and how often to give it, and the trial will only reveal whether the chosen regime performed better or worse than the control treatment. It will not say whether increasing or decreasing the dose would have improved the response; another trial would be needed to ascertain that. The basic question posed by a clinical trial is thus less sophisticated than that addressed by conventional bioassays. However, the organisation of clinical trials, with the problem of avoiding bias, is immeasurably more complicated, time-consuming and expensive than that of any laboratory-based assay.

Avoidance of bias

There are two main strategies that aim to minimise bias in clinical trials, namely:

- randomisation
- the double-blind technique.

If two treatments are being compared on a series of selected patients, the simplest form of randomisation is to allocate each patient to A or B by reference to a series of random numbers. If the number of patients is large enough, roughly equal numbers will be assigned to each group. In a small series, however, the groups could end up poorly matched, and a compromise solution is to split the series into blocks of, say, eight patients, each block consisting of four of A and four of B arranged in random order. Another difficulty with simple randomisation is that the two groups may turn out to be ill-matched with respect to a variable characteristic such as age or sex. The chance of serious mismatching of the groups obviously decreases as the size of the series increases. With small-scale trials, *stratified randomisation* is often used to avoid the difficulty. Thus the subjects might be divided into age categories, random allocation to A or B being used within each category. It is possible to treat two or more characteristics of the trial population in this way. Thus, if it were important to balance the groups with respect to age and sex, it might be necessary to define three age bands, each being split into males and females, making six strata in all. Severity of disease is another variable that is often incorporated into such stratification schemes. It will be appreciated that the number of strata can quickly become large, and the process is self-defeating when the number of subjects in each becomes too small. As well as avoiding error resulting from imbalance of groups assigned to A and B, stratification can also allow more sophisticated conclusions to be reached. B might, for example, prove to be better than A in a particular group of patients even if it is not significantly better overall.

The double-blind technique, which means that neither subject nor investigator is aware at the time of the assessment which treatment is being used, is intended to minimise subjective bias. It has been repeatedly shown that both participants, with the best will in the world, contribute to bias if they know which treatment is which, so the use of a double-blind technique is an important safeguard. It is not always possible, however. A dietary regime or a surgical operation, for example, cannot be disguised, and even with drugs, pharmacological effects may reveal to the patient what he is taking and predispose him to report accordingly.* In general, however, the use of a double-blind procedure, with precautions if necessary to disguise such clues as the taste or appearance of the two drugs, is an important principle.

The size of the sample

Both ethical and financial considerations dictate that the trial should involve the minimum number of subjects, and much statistical thought has gone into the problem of deciding in advance how many subjects will be required to produce a useful result. The results of a trial cannot, by their nature, be absolutely conclusive. This is because it is based on a sample of patients and there is always a chance that the sample was atypical of the population from which it came. Two types of erroneous conclusion

*The distinction between a true pharmacological response and a beneficial clinical effect produced by the knowledge (based on the pharmacological effects that the drug produces) that an active drug is being administered is not easy to draw, and we should not expect a clinical trial to resolve such a fine semantic issue.

are possible, referred to as *type I* and *type II errors.* A type I error occurs if a difference is found between A and B when none actually exists (false positive). A type II error occurs if no difference is found though A and B do actually differ (false negative). A major factor that determines the size of sample needed is the degree of certainty the investigator seeks in avoiding either type of error. The probability of incurring a type I error is expressed as the *significance* of the result. To say that A and B are different at the 0.05 level of significance means that the probability of obtaining a false positive result (i.e. incurring a type I error) is less than 1 in 20. For most purposes this level of significance is considered acceptable as a basis for drawing conclusions.

The probability of avoiding a type II error (i.e. failing to detect a real difference between A and B) is termed the *power* of the trial. We tend to regard type II errors more leniently than type I errors, and trials are often designed with a power of 0.8–0.9. To increase the significance and the power of a trial requires more patients. The second factor that determines the sample size required is the magnitude of difference between A and B that is regarded as clinically significant. For example, to show that a given treatment reduces the mortality in a certain condition by 10%, say from 50% (in the control group) to 40% (in the treated group) would require 850 subjects, assuming that we wanted to achieve a 0.05 level of significance and a power of 0.9. If we were content only to reveal a reduction by 20% (and very likely miss a reduction by 10%) only 210 subjects would be needed.

Meta-analysis

It is possible, by the use of the statistical technique known as *meta-analysis* or *overview analysis*, to combine the data obtained in several individual trials (provided each has been conducted according to a randomised design) in order to gain greater power and significance. This can be very useful in arriving at a conclusion on the basis of several published trials, of which some claimed superiority of the test treatment over the control while others did not. As an objective procedure, it is certainly preferable to the 'take-your-pick' approach to conclusion-forming employed by most human beings when confronted with contradictory data, but it suffers from unseen 'publication bias' since negative studies are generally considered less interesting, and are therefore less likely to be published, than positive studies.

Sequential trials

The purpose of sequential trials is to minimise the number of subjects used by computing the results continuously as the trial proceeds, and stopping it as soon as a result (at a predetermined level of significance) is achieved. In this type of trial, the subjects are usually paired, one subject receiving each treatment. (Alternatively, a cross-over design can be used in which each subject receives the treatments consecutively.) The result of each individual comparison is scored as *A better than B, B better than A*, or *no discernible difference*, and the analysis is performed graphically (Fig. 3.6). The example shown is a three-way comparison of **heroin, pholcodeine** and placebo used as cough suppressants in patients with chronic cough. Each patient was given the three treatments consecutively, in random order, and asked to rate them in order of effectiveness. The red line on the diagram represents the comparison between pholcodeine and heroin. If a subject preferred pholcodeine the line was extended upwards and to the right; if he preferred heroin the line was drawn downwards and to the right. Overall, the line was nearly horizontal, and after 24 subjects it crossed the boundary indicating that no significant difference could be demonstrated. The other two lines progress fairly steadily towards the boundaries indicating that both heroin (lower boundary) and pholcodeine (upper boundary) were better than the placebo. The position of the boundaries in such a diagram is calculated on the basis of the significance level and power required. In Figure 3.6 the significance was set at 0.05 and the power 0.95. Because of their simplicity and economy, sequential trials are widely used. They are not, as a rule, suitable where assessment of the result of treatment takes a long time (e.g. where death rates are being compared) since all the subjects will have been committed to the trial before any results are obtained.

Various 'hybrid' trial designs, which have the advantage of sequential trials in minimising the number of patients needed but do not require strict pairing of subjects, have been devised (see Friedman et al. 1985). Generally, they involve successive interim analyses of the accumulated data as the trial progresses, which allows the trial to be terminated as soon as a clear result is achieved. In a large-scale trial (Beta-blocker Heart Attack Trial Research Group 1982) of the value of long-term treatment with the β-adrenoceptor blocking drug **propranolol** (Ch. 7) following heart attacks, the interim results

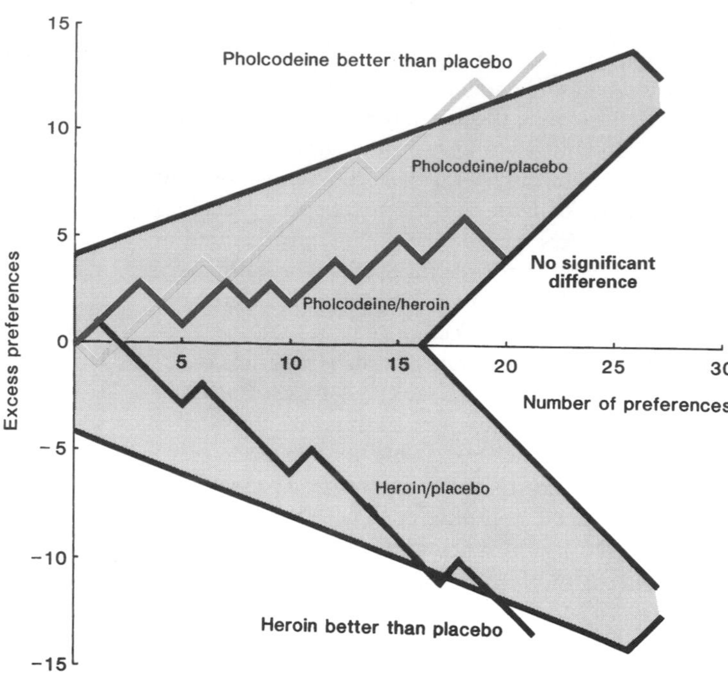

Fig. 3.6 Sequential clinical trial to compare pholcodeine, heroin and placebo as cough suppressants. Each of 27 patients was given, under double-blind conditions, the three treatments on successive occasions and asked to rank them in order of effectiveness. The stated preferences were then plotted on the diagram. The lines comparing either drug with placebo crossed the 0.05 significance limit after about 20 preferences had been expressed, showing both drugs to be significantly better than placebo. The line comparing heroin and pholcodeine failed to show a significant difference. The right-hand limit corresponds to power of 0.85 (i.e. a 15% chance that a real difference exists). (Redrawn from: Snell E S, Armitage P 1957, cited in Armitage P 1978 Sequential medical trials. Blackwell, Oxford)

showed a significant reduction in mortality which led to the early termination of the trial.

The organisation of clinical trials

The organisation of a clinical trial is liable to be a massive and expensive undertaking. A trial of the effectiveness of **urokinase** in the treatment of pulmonary embolism, carried out some years ago, may be taken as a typical example. The aim of the trial was to answer the simple question whether patients with pulmonary embolism (a common and dangerous consequence of prolonged bed-rest, in which venous thrombi forming in the legs come free and impact in the pulmonary artery) do better if treated with the fibrinolytic agent, urokinase, than with **heparin**. The trial involved 14 hospitals in the United States and was organised by a six-member Policy Board under which worked a dozen committees, panels and sub-committees concerned with different aspects of the study. As with all multi-centre trials, careful standardisation of diagnostic and investigative procedures was essential. A committee was set up to achieve this, and a visiting team had to be sent to each centre to ensure the necessary uniformity. In the course of 2 years, 160 patients entered the trial, having been selected on the basis of rigid diagnostic and age criteria. They were assigned at random to the two treatment groups—heparin (H) 78 patients, urokinase (U) 82 patients—and were subjected to elaborate investigative procedures to assess the severity and progress of the disease. The main results are summarised in Table 3.1, which shows that there were six deaths in the U group and seven in the H group, an insignificant difference. The incidence of bleeding complications and repeat emboli was also similar in the two groups. This example gives an idea of the scale of organisation needed to carry out a

Table 3.1 Trial of urokinase versus heparin treatment of pulmonary embolism

	Urokinase	Heparin
Number of patients	82	78
Deaths		
Day 1	1	2
Day 2–14	5	5
Total	6	7
Complications		
Bleeding		
Moderate	15	10
Severe	22	11
Recurrent pulmonary embolism	14	18

From: Urokinase pulmonary embolism trial (1973). Circulation 47 (supp. II)

satisfactory clinical trial on a relatively small group of patients to answer a simple and clear-cut question, and it also demonstrates the problem of detecting an improvement in mortality over the already low figure of 9% (in the heparin group). Because of the small number of events (death), the probability of a type II error is quite large, so a real difference between the two treatments cannot confidently be excluded.

Another large trial (Anturane Reinfarction Trial Research Group 1978) shows how easily things can go wrong. This huge trial involved 1620 patients at 26 research centres in the US and Canada, 98 collaborating researchers, and a formidable list of organising committees, including two independent audit committees to check that the work was being carried out in conformity with the strict protocols established. The conclusion was that the drug under test (sulphinpyrazone) reduced by 48.5% the mortality from repeat heart attacks in the 8-month period after a first attack, and could save many lives. The US Food and Drug Administration, however, refused to grant a licence for the use of the drug, criticising the trial as unreliable and biased in several respects. Their independent analysis of the data (Temple & Pledger 1980) showed the beneficial effect of the drug to be slight and insignificant. Further analysis and further trials, however, supported the original conclusion, but by then the efficacy of aspirin in this indication had been established, which curtailed the clinical use of sulphinpyrazone in heart disease.

Clinical trials

- A clinical trial is a special type of bioassay done to compare the clinical efficacy of a new drug or procedure with that of a known drug or procedure (or a placebo).
- Generally the aim is a straight comparison of unknown (A) with standard (B) at a single dose level. The result may be: 'B better than A', 'B worse than A', or 'No difference detected'. *Efficacy*, not *potency*, is compared.
- To avoid bias, clinical trials should be:
  - — randomised (assignment of subjects to A or B on a random basis)
  - — double-blind (neither subject nor assessor knows whether A or B is being used)
  - — controlled (comparison of A with B, rather than study of A alone).
- *Type I errors* (concluding that A is better than B when the difference is actually due to chance) and *type II errors* (concluding that A is no better than B because a real difference has escaped detection) can occur; the likelihood of either kind of error gets less as the sample size and number of end-point events is increased.
- *Sequential trials* are appropriate in some cases and provide a way of limiting the number of subjects studied.
- Clinical trials require very careful planning and execution and are inevitably expensive.

MEASUREMENT OF TOXICITY

Before any new compound is approved for testing in man, extensive toxicity testing is done in various animal species and with in vitro systems. The crudest type of toxicity test is the LD_{50} (Lethal Dose for 50% of a group of animals), in which various doses of the drug, estimated to cover the range from 0 to 100% lethality, are administered to groups of 10 animals. The mortality in each group within a fixed period of time (say 2 days) is determined and used to construct a curve relating fractional mortality to dose. Standard statistical procedures are available (see Colquhoun 1971) for estimating the LD_{50} from such data. This test, once regarded as *the* fundamental parameter defining chemical toxicity, is now largely discredited, particularly in relation to drugs intended for therapeutic use. The problems with it are:

- It measures only mortality and not sublethal toxicity.
- The LD_{50} varies widely between species and cannot be safely extrapolated to man.
- It measures only acute toxicity produced by a single dose, and not long-term toxicity.
- It cannot measure idiosyncratic reactions (i.e. reactions occurring at low dosage in a small proportion of subjects) though such reactions may be more relevant in practice than 'high dose' toxicity (see Chs 42 and 43).
- It requires the use of many animals, and entails suffering disproportionate to the knowledge gained.

An example of the weakness of the LD_{50} test as a measure of toxicity is shown in Figure 3.7. A single oral dose of **indomethacin** was given to groups of rats and the percentage mortality noted 24 hours and 14 days later. There was a nearly 30-fold difference in the LD_{50} according to the time at which the assessment was made, and a dose of indomethacin that was 100% lethal within 14 days caused no deaths within 24 hours. This example shows strikingly that the arbitrary choice of experimental conditions for the LD_{50} test can drastically alter the results obtained. The LD_{50} test is particularly inappropriate when used to assess the safety of substances such as food additives or cosmetics, where there is negligible likelihood of accidental poisoning. It is more appropriate for assessing the toxicity of industrial chemicals, such as insecticides, or of drugs that are likely to be taken in large overdose, though species differences greatly limit its usefulness even in these applications. A recent Home Office report on the LD_{50} test concluded that although some rough measure of acute toxicity in animals was needed for many substances, a simple 'limit' test, aimed at determining the effect on animals of the largest dose likely to be administered to a human being, was generally preferable. This principle has now been accepted by regulatory authorities in most countries; the elimination of the formal requirement for LD_{50} tests has considerably reduced the number of animals used for toxicity testing (see Paton 1993 for an account of the practical and ethical issues involved).

Toxicity takes many forms and cannot be measured purely in terms of increased mortality. The battery of tests through which potential new drugs are put during their development is designed to reveal many types of toxicity that are known to occur in man, and regulatory authorities require extensive and detailed studies of animal toxicity before they

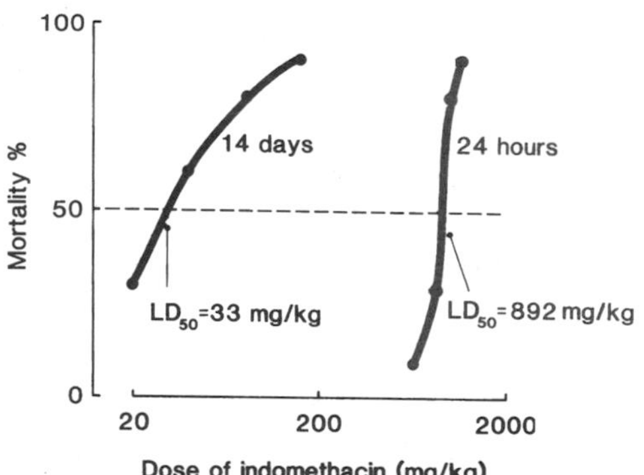

Fig. 3.7 Comparison of acute and chronic toxicity of indomethacin in mice. The LD_{50} measured 24 hours after dosing is 27 times larger than the LD_{50} measured at 14 days. Variability is also much less for the acute test, shown by the steeper red curve. (From: Beyer K H 1978 Discovery, development and delivery of new drugs. Spectrum Publications, Jamaica)

will grant a licence for testing in man and eventual sale of a new drug. Public opinion is inclined to demand the unattainable—namely that before any drug is released for widespread use, there is certainty that it will lack toxicity when used under clinical conditions. As Witts has pointed out, however: 'The final test of the safety of a drug is in fact its release for general use.' The only way that rare but serious toxicities can be detected is by clinical observation or by post-marketing surveillance (so-called *Phase IV studies*).

Two factors in particular make it unrealistic to expect studies on animals and human volunteers to serve as a complete safeguard against toxicity in clinical use. First, only such effects as are looked for are likely to be found. In 1960, when **thalidomide** was developed, the possibility of drug-induced foetal malformations (teratogenesis) had not yet been recognised, and the animal tests used at that time did not anticipate this form of toxicity; nor was there any likelihood of discovering it from studies on human volunteers. Discovery came only as a result of astute clinical detective work after the drug had been released and very successfully promoted. Once recognised, the effect can be tested for in animals and future disasters on the thalidomide scale* are highly unlikely. However, unsuspected types of toxicity will continue to appear, as exemplified by the syndrome of sclerosing peritonitis produced by **practolol** and the increased incidence of thrombotic disorders in women taking oral contraceptives.

Secondly, toxic effects may occur only in a very small proportion of patients. Thus an effect occurring in 1 in 1000 individuals will escape detection in a clinical trial on a few hundred patients, but may be of considerable clinical importance. For example, **phenylbutazone** (an anti-inflammatory drug; see Ch. 12) causes, as a rare side effect, aplastic anaemia, which has a high mortality. Phenylbutazone is estimated to kill 22 patients out of every million treated with the drug. It is obvious that such an infrequent event could not be discovered by any kind of preliminary trial in man. In common with other types of idiosyncratic reaction, it does not seem to become any more frequent if the dose of the drug is increased, thus would also escape detection in high-dose toxicity tests in animals.

*An estimated 10 000 children born with severe malformations. See Sjostrom (1972).

The recognition that animal studies and clinical trials by no means eliminate the risk of toxic effects when the drug is released for general clinical use has led to the development of various monitoring schemes which are intended to facilitate detection of toxicity. In the UK, the Committee on the Safety of Medicines runs a 'Yellow Card' scheme which relies on voluntary reporting by doctors of incidents that they think may be the result of adverse reactions to drugs. In Britain, over 15 000 such reports are received annually, and the aim is that classification of reported incidents by drug and by type of reaction will reveal rare forms of toxicity, such as the phenylbutazone example mentioned above. This type of surveillance was introduced in many countries shortly after the thalidomide tragedy and has been instrumental in drawing attention to several important types of drug toxicity. The dangers of high-oestrogen contraceptive pills, and of practolol (see above) were first detected in this way. Though useful, the Yellow Card system has serious weaknesses since it relies on voluntary reporting of incidents that are suspected to be drug related. There are moves to supplement it with systematic computerised monitoring of prescriptions of new drugs together with medical incidents occurring in those patients. Such a system would be expected to reveal a correlation between the use of a drug and the occurrence of a particular adverse reaction long before a doctor's suspicions might be aroused to the point of submitting a Yellow Card.

The function of monitoring is to sound an alarm; because of the haphazard origin of the data, it cannot by itself provide convincing evidence of toxicity. The next stage is therefore an epidemiological study designed to discover whether or not the incidence of the suspected type of reaction is actually enhanced in patients treated with the drug.

Therapeutic index

Ehrlich recognised that a drug must be judged not only by its useful properties, but also by its toxic effects, and he expressed the *Therapeutic Index* of a drug in terms of the ratio between the average minimum effective dose and the average maximum tolerated dose in a group of subjects, i.e.

$$\textit{Therapeutic Index} = \frac{\textit{Maximum non-toxic dose}}{\textit{Minimum effective dose}}$$

Unfortunately, the variability between individuals is not taken into account in this definition. Even if for any one subject there is a large margin between the maximum tolerated dose and minimum effective dose, individuals may vary widely in their sensitivity, so it is quite possible that the effective dose in some individuals will be toxic to others. A widely used definition which takes into account individual variation is:

$$\textit{Therapeutic Index} = LD_{50}/ED_{50}$$

Thus defined, Therapeutic Index gives some idea of the margin of safety in use of a drug, by drawing attention to the importance of the relationship between the effective and toxic doses, but it has obvious limitations and is therefore very rarely quoted as a number. Thus, it is not really a useful guide to the safety of a drug in clinical use. There are several reasons for this:

- LD_{50} is not a good guide to toxicity, since it is based only on mortality in animals. The kind of adverse effect that, in practice, limits the clinical usefulness of a drug is likely to be overlooked in the LD_{50} test.
- ED_{50} is often not definable, since it depends on what measure of effectiveness is used. Analgesic drugs, for example, may need to be given in different dosages according to the nature and severity of the pain. The ED_{50} for **aspirin** used for a mild headache would be much lower than the value for aspirin as an anti-rheumatic drug.
- Some very important forms of toxicity are *idiosyncratic* (i.e. only a small proportion of individuals are susceptible; see Ch. 42). In other cases, toxicity depends greatly on the clinical state of the patient. Thus, **propranolol** is dangerous to an asthmatic patient in doses that are harmless to a normal individual. More generally, we can say that wide individual variation (see Ch. 42) in either the effective dose or the toxic dose of a drug makes it inherently less predictable, and therefore less safe, though this is not reflected in the therapeutic index.

These shortcomings mean that therapeutic index is of little value as a measure of the clinical usefulness of a drug; **digoxin**, for example, used in treating cardiac failure for many years, has a notably low therapeutic index. Therapeutic index has rather more relevance as a measure of the impunity with which an overdose may be given. Thus, one reason why the **benzodiazepines** replaced **barbiturates** as hypnotic drugs (see Ch. 27) is that their therapeutic index is much greater, so they are much less likely to kill when taken in accidental or deliberate overdose. Ironically, though, **thalidomide**—probably the most harmful drug ever developed—was marketed specifically on the basis of its exceptionally high therapeutic index.

In summary, though therapeutic index expresses a valid general concept, it provides no measure of the actual usefulness of a drug. It is well to be suspicious of mathematically defined quantities that cannot be enumerated.

Therapeutic index

- Therapeutic index (= LD_{50}/ED_{50}) provides a very crude measure of the safety of any drug as used in practice.
- Its main limitations are:
  - —It is based on animal toxicity data, which may not reflect forms of toxicity that are important clinically.
  - —It takes no account of idiosyncratic toxic reactions.

CHEMICAL ASSAY METHODS

Until about 30 years ago, chemical assay methods were generally too insensitive to be of much use in pharmacology, but there are now several analytical methods whose sensitivity and specificity match or exceed that of bioassay. The most important of these techniques are:

- radioimmunoassay (RIA) and related types of saturation analysis
- various separation techniques involving chromatography and/or mass spectrometry, coupled with high-sensitivity detector systems to determine quantitatively the separated components
- photometric and fluorimetric techniques; a brief account of the principles is given here, but for more detail, specialised texts should be consulted
- electrometric techniques, which enable the local concentration of certain amine mediators to be determined directly in tissues with good time resolution.

RADIOIMMUNOASSAY (RIA)

RIA was first developed in 1959 for the assay of insulin. Detailed accounts are given by Patrono & Peskar (1987). The principle is simple (Fig. 3.8). The requirements are:

- an antibody which binds specifically and with high affinity the substance to be assayed
- a radioactively labelled version of the substance to be assayed
- a method for separating antibody-bound from free material in the solution.

Obtaining a suitable antibody is the most problematical part. Most drug molecules are not antigenic but can be made so by coupling them covalently to a protein such as serum albumin. When such a complex is injected, many different antibodies are produced, only a few of which will bind the drug molecule on its own with high affinity. Increasingly, monoclonal antibodies, which can be produced in large quantities in vitro, are being used for this purpose. It may not be necessary to use an antibody at all if another type of high-affinity binding protein is available. Thus, **thyroxine** can be assayed with thyroglobulin as the binding protein, and **steroids** can be assayed by means of the high-affinity receptor (see Ch. 2) to which they bind in cells. In this case the method is referred to as 'radioreceptor assay'.

Producing a radioactively labelled version of the substance to be assayed is usually straightforward. Most proteins and peptides can be labelled by substitution of ^{125}I into tyrosine residues without much loss of biological activity, and small molecules can often be labelled by synthesis from radioactive starting materials.

Efficient separation of the bound and free radioactivity in the assay mixture is essential. Many methods have been devised, including gel filtration and addition of activated charcoal or finely divided silicates to extract the free ligand. Alternatively, the antibody may be precipitated by addition of a suitable anti-IgG (double antibody method), or it may be covalently attached to a solid support (such as the wall of the assay tube), thus obviating the need for a separation step.

Enzyme immunoassay (EIA), also referred to as *enzyme-linked immunosorbent assay* (ELISA), is a variant of RIA in which the label used is an enzyme rather than a radioisotope (Fig. 3.8). In the simplest type of EIA, the enzyme-coupled derivative (E–X)

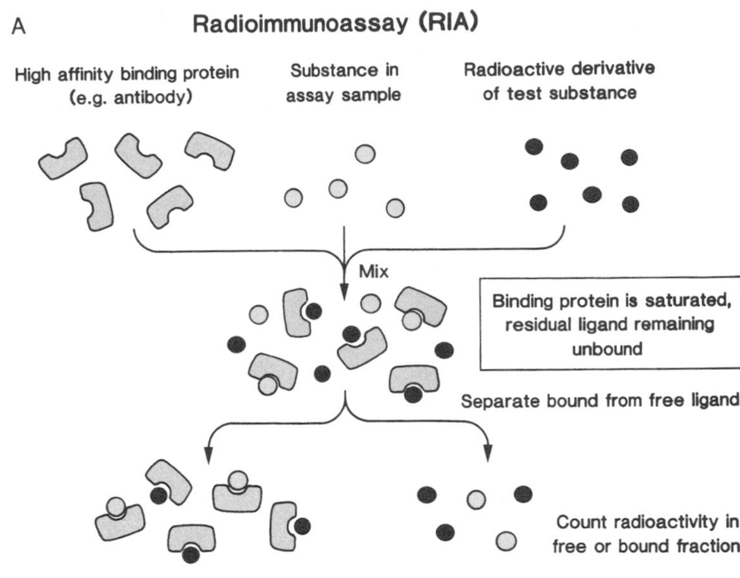

Fig. 3.8 The principle of immunoassay. A. With radioimmunoassay separation of the bound and free ligand is necessary before the final measurement. **B.** With enzyme-linked immunoassay separation is not needed, nor is any radioactive material used, so the technique is usually quicker and safer than radioimmunoassay.

of the substance to be assayed is prepared, by a covalent coupling reaction, and a standard quantity is added to the assay mixture together with antibody and the sample to be assayed. The amount of E–X that combines with Ab will depend on the amount of X in the sample. Usually, the enzymic activity of E–X–Ab is much less than that of E–X so that no separation step is required. All that is needed is a simple (usually photometric) measure of enzyme activity in the mixture. The more X is present, the greater the amount of free E–X and the greater the enzymic activity. This type of assay, known as EMIT (enzyme multiplied immunoassay technique), is used, for example, for the routine clinical monitoring of the antiepileptic drug **phenytoin** (Ch. 30). The drug can be coupled to glucose 6 phosphate dehydrogenase (G6PDH). Enzyme activity is lost when the complex binds to antibodies raised against phenytoin, and is very simply measured by a photometric technique. Many variants of the EIA principle have been devised (see Collins 1985), including the use of solid supports to which the antibody is attached. The amount of enzyme which sticks to the support depends on the concentration of drug or hormone present in the medium. The support is then washed and dipped into a reagent mixture that allows colourimetric monitoring of the enzyme activity. Home pregnancy test kits, based on the rise in urinary chorionic gonadotrophin in early pregnancy, are based on this principle. Immunoassays are widely used in research for measuring low levels of hormones and other mediators (e.g. insulin, neuropeptides, growth factors, cytokines, prostanoids, etc.) as well as clinically for measurement of the plasma concentration of drugs such as phenytoin and digoxin.

As with any assay method, the most important characteristics by which immunoassays have to be judged are *sensitivity* and *specificity*, both of which depend critically on the properties of the antibody. Immunoassays are among the most sensitive assay methods currently available (commonly able to detect as little as 10^{-15} moles), because antibody affinity is sufficiently high that effective competition between standard and sample occurs at very low concentrations.

Specificity is particularly important when the technique is used for assay of blood or tissue concentrations of drugs at various times after systemic administration, where metabolites of the parent compound are liable to cross-react in the assay. An example of an assay of very high specificity is shown in Figure 3.9. The assay was designed to measure the plasma concentration of **methotrexate**, a cytotoxic drug that very closely resembles the natural metabolite dihydrofolate (see Ch. 36). Figure 3.9 shows that the assay was about 1000 times as sensitive to methotrexate as to dihydrofolate, and even less sensitive to other folic acid derivatives.

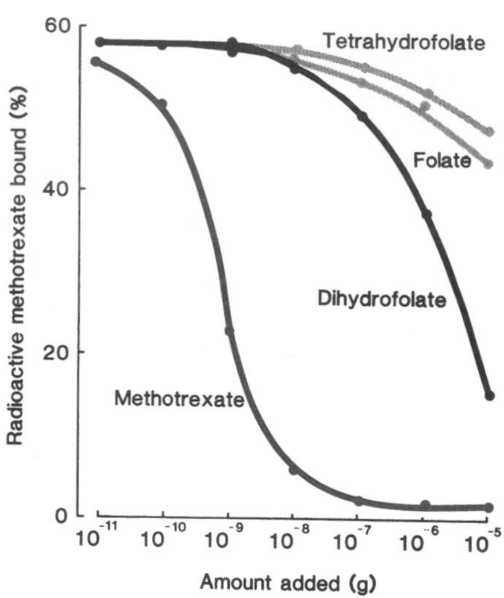

Fig. 3.9 Radioimmunoassay of the antitumour drug, methotrexate, in plasma. The antibody used in this assay was raised against a methotrexate–protein conjugate. It binds methotrexate with a very high affinity, enabling less than 1 ng to be assayed in a blood sample. Cross-reaction with folate derivatives, which occur endogenously and are chemically very similar to methotrexate, is slight. Dihydrofolate binds with less than 1/1000 the affinity of methotrexate, and the other two analogues even less. (Data from: Paxton J W et al. 1978 Clin Chem 24: 1534)

CHROMATOGRAPHIC TECHNIQUES

Chromatography provides a versatile repertoire of techniques for achieving separation of different chemical substances. Coupled with a detector of sufficient sensitivity, it provides the basis for many useful assay systems. The basic principle by which chemical separation is achieved is common to all types of chromatography. The *stationary phase* consists of particles of a substance such as resin, cellulose or alumina packed into a tube through which the *mobile phase* flows. The mobile phase is a liquid (usually an aqueous solution) or a gas, into which is introduced the sample containing the substances to be separated. Separation occurs because the stationary phase either binds, or selectively excludes, substances present in the sample. If binding occurs, for example in ion-exchange chromatography where the stationary phase possesses fixed negatively charged groups and the sample contains a basic substance, the sample will be retarded relative to the solvent as the solution flows through the column. The more tightly it is bound to the stationary phase the longer it will take to emerge. Many chemical factors, such as molecular size, pKa, hydrophobicity, etc., will affect the degree of binding, and hence separation of the different chemical species occurs as they pass through the column. In *gel filtration chromatography*, the column consists of a matrix of cross-linked carbohydrate whose interstices are sufficiently narrow that large molecules, such as proteins, are partly or completely excluded and remain confined to the mobile phase, thus passing more quickly through the column than smaller molecules, resulting in separation on the basis of molecular size.

Two technical advances, namely *gas chromatography* (GC) and *high-performance liquid chromatography* (HPLC) have greatly increased the speed and versatility of chromatographic assays for routine use.

In gas chromatography, the sample is volatilised and the gaseous medium passed through a narrow column of solid adsorbent at high temperature, which means that the diffusion rates are much higher than with liquid chromatography. For some applications, the emerging peaks can be analysed at very high sensitivity by means of on-line *mass spectrometry* (MS; see below), which provides exact chemical identification of the components of the mixture. This is a particularly powerful analytical technique, but too costly for most routine work.

In HPLC, the improvement over conventional liquid chromatography is brought about mainly by reducing the particle size of the stationary phase, and thus the diffusion distance, so speeding up equilibration between the two phases. HPLC avoids many of the drawbacks of GC and its greater range of applicability has led to its widespread use in pharmacology. Figure 3.10 shows the analysis of a sample of 'heroin' from an illicit dealer. Heroin itself (diacetylmorphine; peak 6) amounts to only about 40%, the rest consisting partly of hydrolysis products (morphine and monoacetylmorphine) and partly of other contaminants (mainly caffeine).

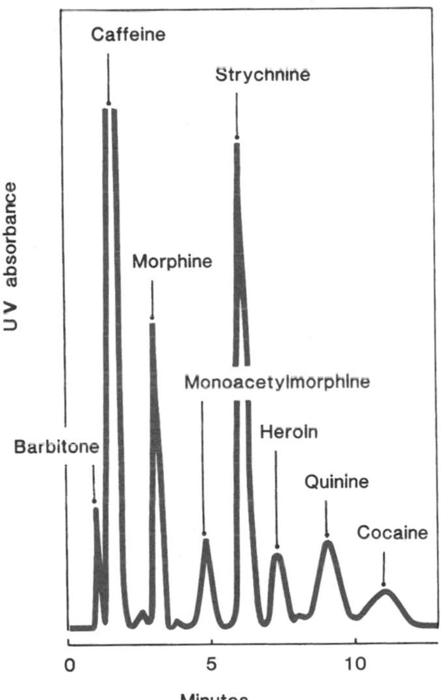

Fig. 3.10 HPLC analysis of materials found in illicit heroin samples. To obtain a quantitative estimate, standards must be tested to give a conversion factor relating concentration to UV absorbance. To estimate concentrations from the absorbance peaks, it is necessary to use a different calibration factor for each compound, based on its absorbance at the monitoring wavelength. In this example, the content of heroin is about 40%, even though the peak looks smaller than this.

MASS SPECTROMETRY

In a mass spectrometer the substance is converted to a volatile form, introduced into an evacuated chamber and then ionised. The resulting ions are accelerated in an electric field as a beam, which is deflected, usually by applying a transverse magnetic field. The degree of deflection of individual ions depends on the ratio of their mass to their charge (m/e ratio), those with the largest m/e ratio being deflected least. At the end of the instrument is a narrow slit through which a slice of the ion beam passes to a detector which measures its intensity at any moment. As the strength of the magnetic field is varied, so the beam of ions, separated according to their m/e ratios, sweeps across the detector slit in sequence to produce a spectrum, and the instrument can distinguish ions whose mass differs by much less than 1 dalton. Detectors can also be made extremely sensitive, allowing samples containing as little as 10^{-15} mole of the test substance to be assayed, a sensitivity that very few bioassays can match.

For most biological applications, the sample is first put through a GC column, the outlet of which is connected directly to the inlet of the mass spectrometer. This combined GCMS technique means that the sample is considerably purified before being subjected to MS analysis. Without this preliminary step, most biological samples would produce an uninterpretable forest of peaks because of the multitude of substances present. The GCMS technique is uniquely sensitive and selective, but too expensive and technically complex for most routine applications.

SPECTROPHOTOMETRY AND FLUORIMETRY

The fact that molecules can absorb energy from photons provides the basis for many analytical techniques that have found pharmacological application. In *absorption spectrophotometry*, a monochromatic light beam passes through a standard-sized cell containing the test solution. The fraction of light absorbed, which is estimated by comparing the intensity of the emergent beam with that of the incident beam, depends on:

- the nature of the absorbing compound
- its concentration and the length of the lightpath through the solution
- the wavelength of the light.

Because of the wavelength specificity of particular chemical groups, substances may be distinguished by the differing shapes of their absorption spectra, and this can be used to distinguish changes in a particular chemical component in a mixture. Where high sensitivity is not important, the simplicity of absorption spectroscopy is a great advantage. For many drugs the concentration needed to give a satisfactory absorption signal for assay purposes is in the range 3–30 μmol/l (roughly 1–10 μg/ml).

When a molecule absorbs a photon, the energy causes one of its electrons to move into an unstable higher energy state from which the molecule quickly recovers by releasing the energy in the form of another photon, of lower energy (i.e. longer wavelength) than the one that was absorbed. These emitted photons can be detected as fluorescence by a sensitive, wavelength-selective photomultiplier tube.

Fluorescence spectrophotometry (fluorimetry) is generally much more sensitive than absorption spectrophotometry (see Table 3.2) because only a minute fraction of the incident light needs to be absorbed to produce a detectable fluorescence signal. It is also somewhat more selective because both the absorption spectrum and the emission spectrum vary in shape (i.e. show maxima at different wavelengths) with different substances, so that discrimination between substances can be optimised by adjusting the wavelength of both the incident beam and the detector. In practice, the technique is most useful for compounds (e.g. most amine transmitters; see Chs 5 and 24) containing aromatic rings, since these give strong fluorescence signals.

Table 3.2 compares the sensitivities of absorption and fluorescence assays for some common drugs, and shows that therapeutic plasma concentrations are generally in the working range of fluorescence assays, but are often too low for absorption assays.

Chemical assay methods

- RIA is a highly sensitive and specific method applicable to many hormones and drugs, provided that a suitable antibody is available. Enzyme-linked variants are increasingly being used to provide simpler automated assays that do not involve radioactivity.
- Many drugs and drug metabolites can be measured in body fluids by HPLC and GCMS methods. These methods are usually technically complex, and often less sensitive than RIA, but do not require antibodies.
- Spectroscopic methods, especially fluorimetry, provide high-sensitivity detector systems which can often be used in conjunction with HPLC separation.
- Chemical methods have superseded bioassay for most routine purposes.
- Voltammetry is a special technique which can be used in vivo to obtain an immediate read-out of the local concentration of certain endogenous mediators, by means of a microelectrode introduced into the tissue.

Table 3.2 Sensitivity of absorbance and fluorescence assay

Drug	Approximate therapeutic plasma concentration (μmol/l)	Approximate sensitivity limits: Absorbance (μmol/l)	Approximate sensitivity limits: Fluorescence (μmol/l)
Aspirin	250	10	0.05
Chloroquine	0.4	7	0.15
Desmethylimipramine	0.2	15	0.4
Isoniazid	30	15	0.7
Methotrexate	0.8	4	0.04
Procainamide	20	10	0.04
Quinine	15	12	0.006
Tetracycline	5	8	0.05

Data from: Richens & Marks (1981)

Fluorescence assays may be made even more sensitive by chemically modifying the assay substance in order to enhance its fluorescence. Some substances, such as **noradrenaline** and **histamine**, are only weakly fluorescent, but can be assayed in tissues and body fluids after conversion to highly fluorescent condensation products. This has formed the basis of a widely used assay for measuring the catecholamine content of tissues and body fluids. With these and other important endogenous amines, the replacement of cumbersome bioassay methods by fluorimetric assays was essential before their tissue distribution and metabolism could be studied in detail.

VOLTAMMETRY

This measurement technique (see Stamford 1985) relies on the fact that certain mediator substances, particularly monoamines, are readily oxidised, and have different redox potentials. Application of a ramp-shaped voltage pulse (usually about 0.5 V) to a carbon fibre microelectrode exposed to the substance in question causes a current to flow, which suddenly increases as the redox potential is reached, and the current amplitude varies with the concentration of the substance. The measurement reflects the concentration at the tip of the electrode, and is made in a few milliseconds, so the method has exceptional temporal and spatial resolution, which has been useful in measurements of the release of transmitters such as noradrenaline, dopamine and 5-HT in discreet regions of the brain. Recently, it has been used to monitor the time-course of release of the contents of a single secretory vesicle from isolated mast cells (Alvarez de Toledo et al. 1993; see Ch. 5).

REFERENCES AND FURTHER READING

Alvarez de Toledo G, Fernandez-Chacon R, Fernandez J M 1993 Release of secretory products during transient vesicle fusion. Nature 363: 554–558

Anturane Reinfarction Trial Research Group 1978 Sulfinpyrazone in the prevention of cardiac death after myocardial infarction. N Engl J Med 298: 289–295

Armitage P 1978 Sequential clinical trials. Blackwell, Oxford

Beta-blocker Heart Attack Trial Research Group 1982 A randomised trial of propranolol in patients with acute myocardial infarction. 1. Mortality results. JAMA 247: 1707–1714

Bird I M 1989 High performance liquid chromatography: principles and clinical applications. Br Med J 299: 783–787

Burn J H, Finney D J, Goodwin L G 1950 Biological standardisation. Oxford University Press, Oxford

Collins W P (ed) 1985 Alternative immunoassays. John Wiley & Sons, Chichester

Colquhoun D 1971 Lectures on biostatistics. Oxford University Press, Oxford

Finney D J 1964 Statistical method in biological assay. Griffin, London

Friedman L M, Furberg C D, DeMets D L 1985 Fundamentals of clinical trials, 2nd edn. PSG Publishing, Littleton, Mass.

Harris E L, Fitzgerald J D (eds) 1970 The principles and practice of clinical trials. Churchill Livingstone, Edinburgh

Inman W H 1986 Monitoring for drug safety. 2nd edn. MTP Press, Dordrecht

Laska E M, Meisner M J 1987 Statistical methods and the applications of bioassay. Annu Rev Pharmacol 27: 385–397

Miller J N 1982 Developments in non-isotopic immunoassay. Nature 295: xiii

Paton W D M 1993 Man and mouse: animals in medical research. Oxford University Press, Oxford

Patrono C, Peskar B A 1987 Radioimmunoassay in basic and clinical pharmacology. Handbook of experimental pharmacology, vol 82. Springer-Verlag, Berlin

Paxton J W 1981 Development of radioimmunoassays for drugs. Methods Find Exp Clin Pharmacol 3: 105–117

Pocock S J 1983 Clinical trials. John Wiley & Sons, Chichester

Richens A, Marks V 1981 Therapeutic drug monitoring. Churchill Livingstone, Edinburgh

Schwarz D, Flamant R, Lellouch J 1980 Clinical trials. Academic Press, New York

Sjostrom N 1972 Thalidomide and the power of the drug companies. Penguin, London

Stamford J A 1985 In vivo voltammetry: promise and perspective. Brain Res Rev 10: 119–135

Temple R, Pledger G W 1980 The FDA's critique of the anturane reinfarction trial. N Engl J Med 202: 1488–1492

Watson J T 1976 Introduction to mass spectroscopy: biomedical, environmental and forensic applications. Raven Press, New York

Yalow R S 1980 Radioimmunoassay. Annu Rev Biophys Bioeng 9: 327–345

Yanagisawa M, Kurihara H, Kimura S, Tomobe Y, Kobayashi M, Mitsui Y, Yazaki Y, Goro K, Masaki T 1988 A novel potent vasoconstrictor peptide produced by vascular endothelial cells. Nature 332: 411–415

4

ABSORPTION, DISTRIBUTION AND FATE OF DRUGS

The action of any drug requires the presence of an adequate concentration in the fluid bathing the target tissue. In many cases the time-course of a drug's action simply reflects the time-course of the rise and fall of its concentration at its site of action. The exceptions to this are certain 'hit and run' drugs, whose effects remain after their concentration has dropped to zero. Examples are drugs that kill cells (such as cytotoxic alkylating agents like mustine) or render them incapable of division, or inactivate an enzyme or receptor irreversibly, such as aspirin, which inhibits cyclo-oxygenase by acetylating a serine residue in its active site (Ch. 12), or α-bungarotoxin, which binds essentially irreversibly to nicotinic receptors at the neuromuscular junction (Ch. 2). The relationship between the administration of a drug, the time-course of its distribution and the magnitude of the concentration attained in different regions of the body is discussed in this chapter. This part of pharmacology is termed *pharmacokinetics* (what the body does to the drug), to distinguish it from *pharmacodynamics* (what the drug does to the body). The distinction is useful, though the words cause dismay to etymological purists.

The two fundamental processes that determine the concentration of a drug at any moment and in any region of the body are:

- *translocation of drug molecules*
- *chemical transformation of drug molecules.*

It is only by the movement of molecules or by the formation or disappearance of molecules that the concentration of a drug in any given region can change. In the first part of this chapter we discuss these two basic processes, and in the second part we consider particular tissues and organs in more detail with emphasis on the different routes of administration and the different patterns of drug distribution that are possible. The third part sets out some quantitative principles that are helpful in interpreting pharmacokinetic data and in predicting how different drugs will behave in practice.

TRANSLOCATION OF DRUG MOLECULES

Drug molecules move around the body in two ways:

- by *bulk flow transfer* (i.e. in the bloodstream)
- by *diffusional transfer* (i.e. molecule-by-molecule, over short distances).

With bulk flow transfer, the chemical nature of the drug makes no difference. The cardiovascular system provides a very fast long-distance distribution system for all solutes irrespective of their chemical nature. In general, what distinguishes one drug pharmacokinetically from another are its *diffusional* characteristics, in particular its ability to cross non-aqueous diffusion barriers, which are composed of cell membranes that separate the various aqueous compartments of the body (i.e. plasma, interstitial fluid, intracellular fluid and transcellular fluid; see Fig. 4.10, p. 79). Aqueous diffusion must, of course, occur as part of the overall mechanism of drug transport, since it is this process that delivers drug molecules to and from the non-aqueous barriers. The rate of diffusion of a substance depends mainly on its molecular size, the *diffusion coefficient* for small molecules being inversely proportional to the square root of molecular weight. Thus, large molecules diffuse more slowly than small ones, but the variation with molecular weight is relatively slight. Most drugs fall within the molecular weight range 200–1000, and variations in aqueous diffusion rate have only a small effect on their overall pharmacokinetic behaviour (exceptions are some of the increasing number of macromolecular drugs synthesised by recombinant DNA technology rather than by organic synthesis, such as erythropoietin, interleukins, and various vaccines). Thus, for most purposes we can regard the body as a series of interconnected *well-stirred compartments* within each of which the drug concentration remains uniform. It is the movement between compartments, which generally involves the penetration of non-aqueous diffusion barriers, that determines where, and for how long, a drug will be present in the body after it has been administered. The analysis of drug movements with the help of a simple compartmental model is discussed in a later section (p. 94).

THE MOVEMENT OF DRUG MOLECULES ACROSS CELL BARRIERS

The barriers between aqueous compartments in the body consist of cell membranes. A single layer of membrane separates the intracellular from the extracellular compartments. An epithelial barrier, such as the gastrointestinal mucosa or renal tubule, consists of a layer of cells tightly connected to each other so that molecules must traverse two layers of membrane to pass from one side to the other. Vascular endothelium is more complicated. Capillaries are fenestrated in most tissues, the gaps in the endothelial cells being large enough to permit small molecules to cross by aqueous diffusion but too small to allow molecules exceeding about 30 000 molecular weight (i.e. most protein molecules) to pass through. In some organs, especially the central nervous system and the placenta, the capillary endothelium is continuous, and penetration by drug molecules involves the crossing of the endothelial cell membrane, an important feature that makes these vascular beds quite distinct from those of other organs and has major pharmaco-kinetic consequences.

In general, there are four main ways by which small molecules cross cell membranes (Fig. 4.1):

- by diffusing through the *lipid*
- by diffusing through *aqueous pores* that traverse the lipid
- by combination with a *carrier molecule* which acts as a ferry-boat across the lipid region of the membrane
- by *pinocytosis*.

Of these routes, diffusion through lipid and carrier-mediated transport are particularly important in relation to pharmacokinetic mechanisms. Diffusion through aqueous pores is unimportant in this context, since these pores (whose existence remains controversial) are probably too small in diameter (about 0.4 nm) to allow most drug molecules (which usually exceed 1 nm in diameter) to pass through, though they are believed to be the major route by which water and other small polar molecules (e.g. urea) traverse cell membranes. Pinocytosis involves the invagination of a part of the cell membrane and the trapping within the cell of a small vesicle containing extracellular constituents. The vesicle contents can then be released within the cell, or extruded from the other side of the cell. This mechanism appears to be important for the transport of some macromolecules (e.g. insulin, which crosses the blood–brain barrier by this process), but there is no evidence that it contributes appreciably to movements of small molecules. Mechanisms involving diffusion of molecules through lipid and carrier-

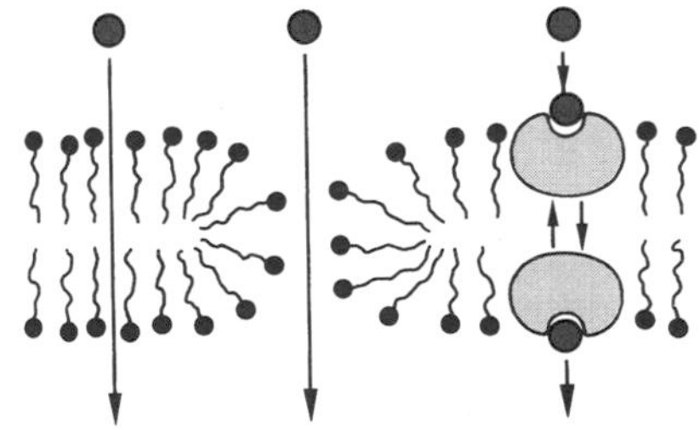

Fig. 4.1 The routes by which solutes can traverse cell membranes.

mediated transport will now be discussed in more detail; diffusion through aqueous pores and transport by pinocytosis will not be considered further.

Diffusion through lipid

Non-polar substances (i.e. substances with molecules in which electrons are uniformly distributed so that there is no separation of positive and negative charges) dissolve freely in non-polar solvents, such as lipids, and therefore penetrate cell membranes very freely by diffusion. The permeability coefficient, P, for a substance diffusing passively through a membrane is given by the number of molecules crossing the membrane per unit area, time and concentration difference across the membrane. It is clear that permeant molecules must be present within the membrane in sufficient numbers, and that they must be mobile within the membrane if rapid permeation is to occur. Thus two physicochemical factors contribute to P, namely solubility in the membrane (which can be expressed as a partition coefficient for the substance distributed between the membrane phase and the aqueous environment) and diffusivity, which is a measure of the mobility of molecules within the lipid and is expressed as a diffusion coefficient. Among different drug molecules the diffusion coefficient varies only slightly, as noted above, so the most important variable is the partition coefficient (see Fig. 4.2). Thus, there is a close correlation between lipid solubility and the permeability of the cell membrane to different substances. For this reason, lipid solubility is one of the most important determinants of the pharmacokinetic characteristics of a drug, and many properties, such as rate of absorption from the gut, penetration into the brain and other tissues, and duration of action can be predicted from knowledge of a drug's lipid solubility.

pH and ionisation

One important complicating factor in relation to membrane permeation is that many drug molecules are weak acids or bases and can therefore exist in both unionised and ionised form, the ratio of the two forms varying with pH. For a weak base, the ionisation reaction is:

$$BH^+ \overset{K_a}{\rightleftharpoons} B + H^+$$

and the dissociation constant pK_a is given by the Henderson–Hasselbalch equation:

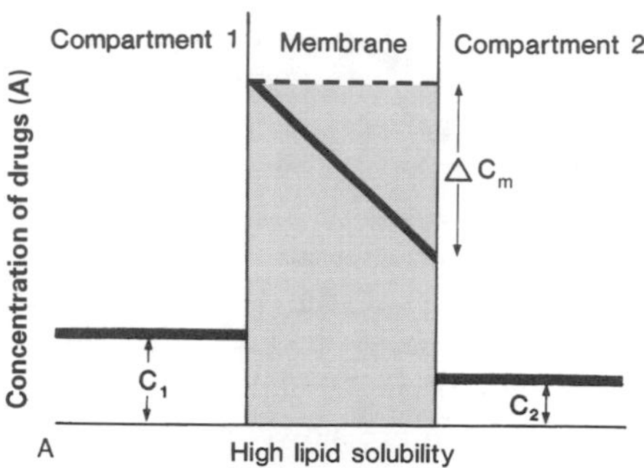

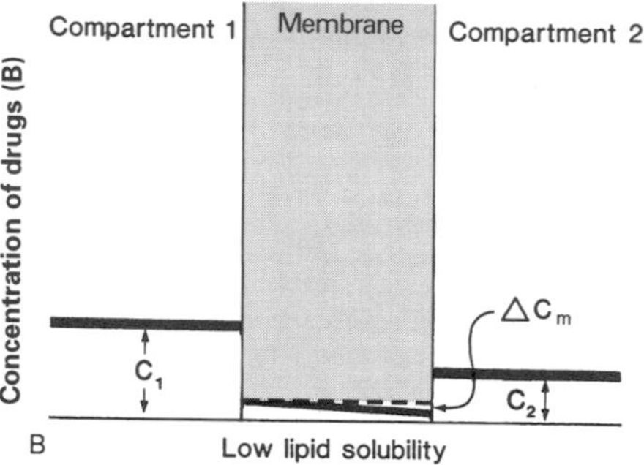

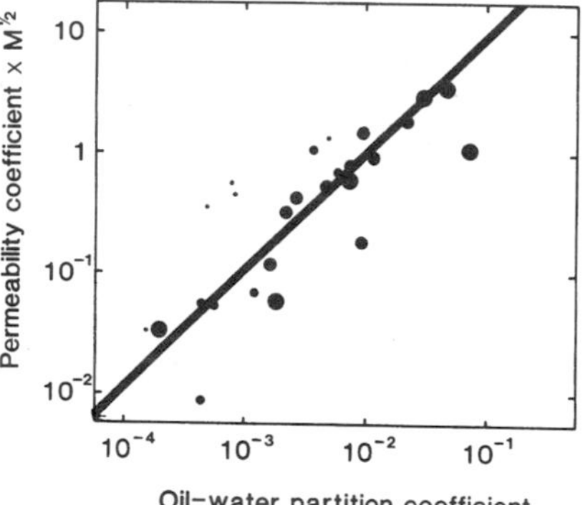

Fig. 4.2 The importance of lipid solubility in membrane permeation. A. and **B.** Figures show the concentration profile in a lipid membrane separating two aqueous compartments. A lipid-soluble drug (A) is subject to a much larger transmembrane concentration gradient (ΔC_m) than a lipid-insoluble drug (B). It therefore diffuses more rapidly even though the aqueous concentration gradient ($C_1 - C_2$) is the same in both cases. **C.** Permeability of plant cells to organic non-electrolytes of varying molecular volume (indicated by size of points). There is a linear relationship between $P \times M^{1/2}$ and lipid solubility, which applies irrespective of the molecular volume. The $M^{1/2}$-term corrects approximately for the variation of the free diffusion coefficient with molecular size. These data show that for organic non-electrolytes, permeation involves diffusion through lipid rather than traversing pores of a fixed size.

$$pK_a = pH + \log_{10}\frac{[BH^+]}{[B]}$$

For a weak acid:

$$AH \underset{}{\overset{K_a}{\rightleftharpoons}} A^- + H^+$$

$$pK_a = pH + \log_{10}\frac{[AH]}{[A^-]}$$

In either case the ionised species, BH^+ or A^- has very low lipid solubility and is virtually unable to permeate membranes except, rarely, where a specific transport mechanism exists. The lipid solubility of the uncharged species, B or AH, will depend on the chemical nature of the drug; for the majority of drugs the uncharged species is sufficiently lipid soluble to permit rapid membrane permeation, though there are exceptions (e.g. **aminoglycoside antibiotics**; see Ch. 37) where even the uncharged molecule is insufficiently lipid soluble to cross membranes appreciably. This is usually due to a preponderance of hydrogen-bonding groups, such as –OH, as in the sugar moiety in the aminoglycosides, that render the uncharged molecule hydrophilic.

pH partition and ion trapping

Ionisation affects not only the rate at which drugs permeate membranes, but also the steady-state distribution of drug molecules between aqueous compartments, if a pH difference exists between them. Figure 4.3 shows how a weak acid (e.g. **aspirin**, pK_a 3.5) and a weak base (e.g. **pethidine**, pK_a 8.6) would be distributed at equilibrium between three body compartments, namely plasma (pH 7.4), alkaline urine (pH 8) and gastric juice (pH 3). Within each compartment the ratio of ionised to unionised drug is governed by the pK_a and the pH of that compartment, according to the Henderson–Hasselbalch equation. It is assumed that the unionised species can cross the membrane, and therefore reaches an equal concentration in each compartment. The ionised species is assumed not to cross at all. The result is that at equilibrium the total (ionised + unionised) concentration of the drug will be different in each compartment, with an acidic drug being concentrated in the compartment with high pH, and vice versa (*ion trapping*). The theoretical concentration gradients produced by ion trapping can be very large if there is a large pH difference between compartments. Thus, aspirin would be concentrated more than fourfold with respect to plasma in an alkaline renal tubule, and about 6000-fold in plasma with respect to the acidic gastric contents. Such large gradients are, however, unlikely to be achieved in reality for two main reasons. Firstly, the assumption of total impermeability to the charged species is not realistic, and even a small permeability will considerably attenuate the concentration difference that can be reached. Secondly, body compartments rarely approach equilibrium. Neither the gastric contents nor the renal tubular fluid stands still, and the resulting flux of drug molecules has the effect of reducing the concentration gradients well below the theoretical equilibrium conditions. The pH partition mechanism none the less correctly explains some of the qualitative effects of pH changes in different body compartments on the pharmacokinetics of weakly acidic or basic drugs, particularly in relation to renal excretion and penetration of the blood–brain barrier. pH partition is not the main determinant of the site of absorption of drugs from the gastrointestinal tract. This is because the enormous absorptive surface area of the villi and microvilli in the ileum compared to the much smaller surface area in the stomach is of overriding importance. Thus, absorption of an acidic drug such as **aspirin** is promoted by drugs that accelerate gastric emptying (e.g. **metoclopramide**) and retarded by drugs that slow gastric emptying (e.g. **propantheline**), despite the fact that the acidic pH of the stomach contents favours absorption of weak acids. Values of pK_a for some common drugs are shown in Figure 4.4.

Some important consequences of the pH partition mechanism are:

- Urinary acidification will accelerate the excretion of weak bases and retard that of weak acids, while urinary alkalinisation will have the opposite effect.
- Increasing plasma pH (e.g. by administration of sodium bicarbonate) will cause weakly acidic drugs to be extracted from the central nervous system into the plasma. Conversely, reducing plasma pH (e.g. by administration of a carbonic anhydrase inhibitor such as **acetazolamide**; see p. 382) will cause weakly acidic drugs to become concentrated in the central nervous system, increasing their toxicity. This has practical consequences in choosing a means to alkalinise urine in treating **aspirin** overdose (see p. 383): either bicarbonate or acetazolamide causes increased

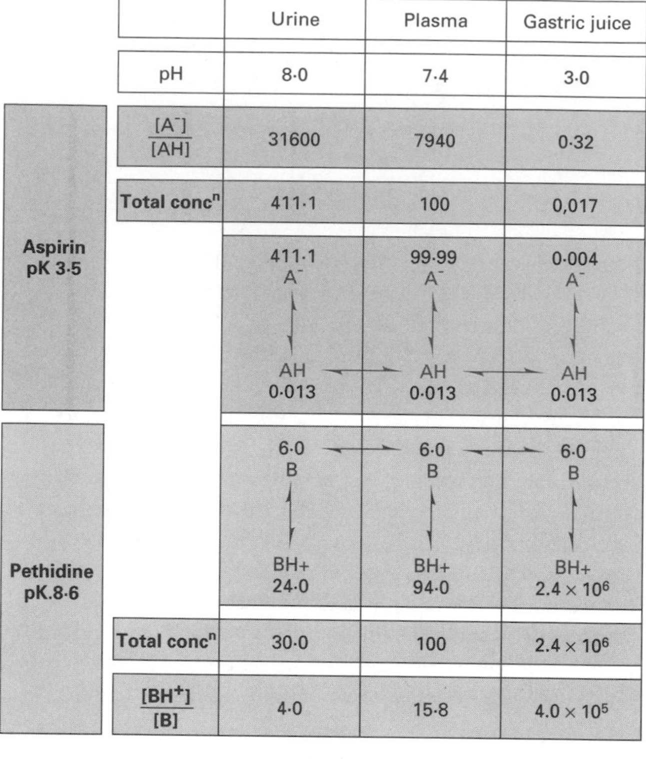

Urine
Plasma
Gastric juice
pH
8·0
7·4
3·0
Aspirin pK 3·5
[A⁻]/[AH]
31600
7940
0·32
Total concⁿ
411·1
100
0,017
411·1 A⁻
99·99 A⁻
0·004 A⁻
AH 0·013
AH 0·013
AH 0·013
Pethidine pK.8·6
6·0 B
6·0 B
6·0 B
BH+ 24·0
BH+ 94·0
BH+ 2.4 × 10⁶
Total concⁿ
30·0
100
2.4 × 10⁶
[BH⁺]/[B]
4·0
15·8
4.0 × 10⁵

Fig. 4.3 Theoretical partition of a weak acid (aspirin) and a weak base (pethidine) between aqueous compartments (urine, plasma and gastric juice) according to the pH difference between them. Numbers represent relative concentrations (total plasma concentration = 100). It is assumed that the uncharged species in each case can permeate the cellular barrier separating the compartments, and thus reaches the same concentration in all three. Variations in the fractional ionisation as a function of pH give rise to the large total concentration differences with respect to plasma.

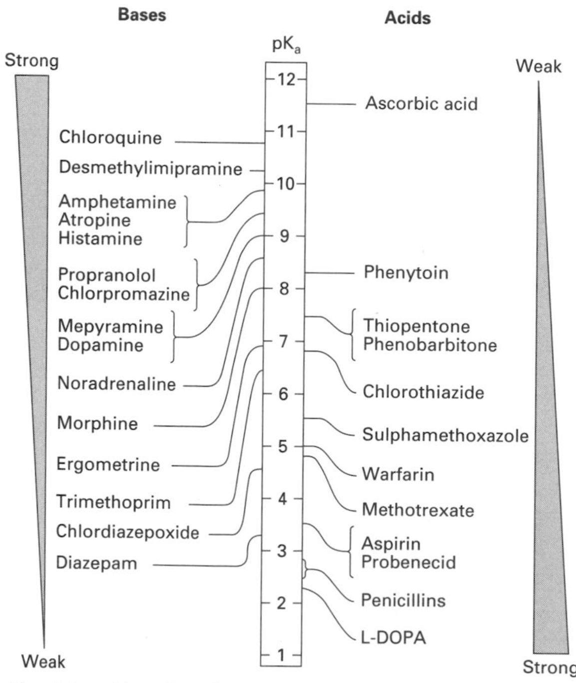

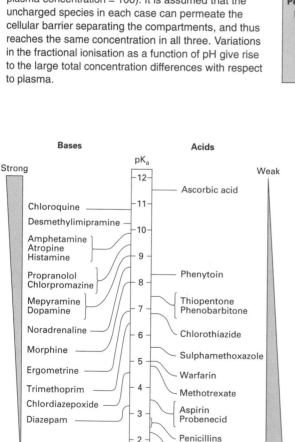

Fig. 4.4 pK_a values for some acidic and basic drugs.

urine pH and hence increased salicylate elimination, but bicarbonate is preferred since it reduces rather than increases distribution of salicylate to the central nervous system.

Carrier-mediated transport

Many cell membranes possess specialised transport mechanisms that regulate entry and exit of physiologically important molecules, such as sugars, amino acids, neurotransmitters and metal ions. Generally, such transport systems involve a carrier molecule, i.e. a transmembrane protein, which binds the transported molecule and conveys it to the other side of the membrane. Such systems may operate purely passively, without any energy source; in this case they merely facilitate the process of transmembrane equilibration of the transported species in the direction of its electrochemical gradient and the mechanism is called *facilitated diffusion*. Alternatively, they may be coupled to an energy source, either directly to ATP hydrolysis or indirectly to the electrochemical gradient of another species such as Na^+; in this case transport can occur against an electrochemical gradient and is called *active transport*. Carrier-mediated transport, because it involves a

Movement of drugs across cellular barriers

- To traverse cellular barriers (e.g. gastro-intestinal mucosa, renal tubule, blood–brain barrier, placenta), drugs have to cross lipid membranes.
- Drugs cross lipid membranes mainly (a) by passive diffusional transfer and (b) by carrier-mediated transfer.
- The main factor that determines the rate of passive diffusional transfer across membranes is a drug's lipid solubility. Molecular weight is a less important factor.
- Many drugs are weak acids or weak bases, whose state of ionisation varies with pH according to the Henderson–Hasselbalch equation.
- With weak acids or bases, only the uncharged species (the protonated form for a weak acid; the unprotonated form for a weak base) can diffuse across lipid membranes; this gives rise to pH partition.
- pH partition means that weak acids tend to accumulate in compartments of relatively high pH, whereas weak bases do the reverse.
- Carrier-mediated transport (e.g. in the renal tubule, blood–brain barrier, gastrointestinal epithelium) is important for some drugs that are chemically related to endogenous substances.

binding step, shows the characteristic of *saturation*. With simple diffusion the rate of transport increases directly in proportion to the concentration gradient, whereas with carrier-mediated transport the carrier sites become saturated at high ligand concentrations and the rate of transport does not increase beyond this point. *Competitive inhibition* of transport also occurs if a second ligand that binds to the carrier is present.

Carriers of this type are ubiquitous and many pharmacological effects are the result of interference with them. Thus, nerve terminals have transport mechanisms for accumulating specific neurotransmitters, and there are many examples of drugs that act by inhibiting these transport mechanisms (see Chs 6, 7 and 24). From a pharmacokinetic point of view, though, there are only a few sites in the body where carrier-mediated drug transport is important, the main ones being:

- the renal tubule
- the biliary tract
- the blood–brain barrier
- the gastrointestinal tract.

The characteristics of these transport systems are discussed later when patterns of distribution and elimination in the body as a whole are considered more fully.

In addition to the processes so far described that govern the transport of drug molecules across the barriers between different aqueous compartments, two additional factors have a major influence on drug distribution and elimination. These are:

- partition into body fat and other tissues
- binding to plasma proteins.

PARTITION INTO BODY FAT

Fat represents a large, non-polar compartment. On average, fat constitutes about 15% of body weight, and its volume is about 25% of that of the total body water, though these proportions are highly variable. Thus, if a non-polar drug molecule has a fat:water partition coefficient of 10, roughly 75% of the drug would, at equilibrium, be dissolved in the body fat, exerting no pharmacological action but forming a large reservoir of drug in communication with the plasma compartment. In practice this is important for only a few drugs, mainly because the effective fat:water partition coefficient is relatively low for most drugs. **Morphine**, for example, though quite lipid-soluble enough to cross the blood–brain barrier, has a lipid:water partition coefficient of only 0.4, so sequestration of the drug by body fat is of little importance. With **thiopentone**, on the other hand (fat:water partition coefficient approximately 10), accumulation in body fat is considerable, and has important pharmacokinetic consequences when the drug is used as an intravenous anaesthetic agent (Ch. 26).

The second factor that limits the accumulation of drugs in body fat is its low blood supply—less than 2% of the cardiac output. Thus drugs are delivered to body fat rather slowly, so that the theoretical equilibrium distribution between fat and body water is approached slowly. For practical purposes, therefore, partition into body fat is important following acute dosing only for a few highly lipid-soluble drugs (e.g. **general anaesthetics**; Ch. 26), as well as for chronic dosing with lipid-soluble drugs (e.g. **benzodiazepines**, Ch. 27, **probucol**, Ch. 15). Furthermore, there are some environmental contaminants (xenobiotics), such as insecticides, that are poorly metabolised and so if taken in over a period of time slowly accumulate in high concentration in body fat.

Body fat is not the only tissue in which drugs can accumulate. Some drugs (e.g. **mepacrine**, an antimalarial drug; see Ch. 40) have a high affinity for nucleic acid, and are strongly taken up by nuclei in hepatocytes. **Chloroquine**—another antimalarial drug (Ch. 40), used additionally to treat rheumatoid disease (Ch. 12)—has a high affinity for melanin and is taken up by tissues such as retina that are rich in melanin granules, accounting for its tendency to cause retinitis following overdose. **Tetracyclines** (Ch. 37) accumulate slowly in bones and teeth, because they have a high affinity for calcium, and should not be used in children for this reason. Very high concentrations of **amiodarone** (an antidysrhythmic drug; Ch. 13) accumulate in liver and lung as well as fat.

BINDING OF DRUGS TO PLASMA PROTEINS

Many drugs exist in plasma mainly in bound form at therapeutic concentrations. The fraction of drug that is free in aqueous solution can be as low as 1%, the remainder being associated with plasma protein. This binding can be demonstrated by various methods that enable free and bound drug to be separated. Thus, if the plasma is dialysed against a protein-free aqueous medium, the drug concentration in the protein-free compartment will be much lower than that in the plasma compartment because only the free drug molecules are able to cross the dialysis membrane. There are also spectroscopic and fluorescence techniques that distinguish between free and bound molecules on the basis of optical properties such as polarisation of emitted light.

The most important plasma protein in relation to drug binding is albumin, which binds many acidic drugs and a smaller number of basic drugs (see Table 4.1). Other plasma proteins, including β-globulin and an acid glycoprotein which, although present in much smaller amounts than albumin, is an acute phase protein that increases in disease (see Kremer, Wilting & Janssen 1988), have also been implicated in the binding of certain basic drugs, such as **chlorpromazine** and **quinine**.

Table 4.1 Some drugs that bind to plasma albumin

Drug	% bound at therapeutic concentration	% binding sites occupied
Diclofenac	99.5	< 1
Diazepam Warfarin	95–99	< 1
Amitriptyline Nortriptyline Chlorpromazine Imipramine Desmethylimipramine Indomethacin	90–95	< 1
Sulphisoxazole Tolbutamide Valproic acid	90–95	50–60
Phenytoin	90	3
Hydralazine	85–90	< 1
Quinine	70–90	< 1
Lignocaine	50	< 1
Aspirin	50	50

Drugs with high % bound will be susceptible to displacement. Drugs that occupy 50% or more of sites may cause effects by displacement of other drugs.

The amount of a drug that is bound to protein will depend on three factors:

- the free drug concentration
- its affinity for the binding sites
- the protein concentration.

As a first approximation, the binding reaction can be regarded as a simple association of the drug molecules with a finite population of binding sites, exactly analogous to drug–receptor binding (see Ch. 1).

$$\underset{\text{free drug}}{\mathrm{D}} + \underset{\text{binding site}}{\mathrm{S}} \rightleftharpoons \underset{\text{complex}}{\mathrm{DS}}$$

We would then expect a hyperbolic saturation curve if the amount bound is plotted against the free concentration (Fig. 4.5). Actually, the binding curve is usually more complex, because each albumin molecule has at least two binding sites for most drugs, but the general shape of the curve resembles

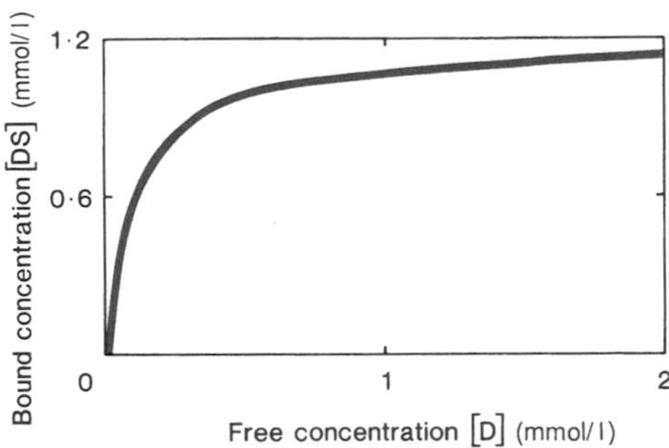

Fig. 4.5 Binding of drugs to protein. The relationship between the bound and the free concentrations is shown for a drug that binds to plasma albumin (total binding capacity 1.2 mmol/l) with an equilibrium constant of 0.1 mmol/l.

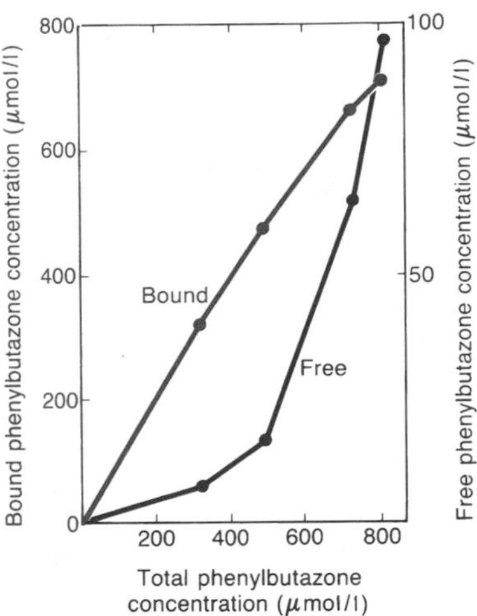

Fig. 4.6 Binding of phenylbutazone to plasma albumin. The graph shows the disproportionate increase in free concentration as the total concentration increases, due to the binding sites approaching saturation. (Data from: Brodie B, Hogben C A M 1957 J Pharm Pharmacol 9: 345)

Figure 4.5. The usual concentration of albumin in plasma is about 0.6 mmol/l (4 g/100 ml). With two sites per albumin molecule, the drug-binding capacity of plasma albumin would therefore be about 1.2 mmol/l. For most drugs the total plasma concentration required for a clinical effect is much less than 1.2 mmol/l (see Table 4.1), so the binding sites are far from saturation, and the concentration bound [DS] varies nearly in direct proportion to the free concentration [D]. Under these conditions the fraction bound, [DS]/([D] + [DS]), shown in Table 4.1, is independent of the drug concentration. However, some drugs, for example **tolbutamide** (Ch. 20) and some **sulphonamides** (Ch. 37), work at plasma concentrations at which the binding to protein is approaching saturation (i.e. on the flat part of the binding curve). This means that addition of more drug to the plasma will increase the free concentration disproportionately. Doubling the dose of such a drug can therefore more than double the free (pharmacologically active) concentration. This is shown for the anti-inflammatory drug **phenylbutazone** in Figure 4.6 (see also Ch. 12).

The existence of binding sites on plasma albumin for which many different drugs have an affinity means that competition can occur between them, so that administration of drug B can reduce the protein binding, and hence increase the free plasma concentration, of drug A. To do this drug B needs to occupy an appreciable fraction of the binding sites. Most of the drugs in Table 4.1 will not affect the binding of other drugs because they occupy, at therapeutic plasma concentrations, only a tiny fraction of the available sites, and it is only a few drugs (e.g. **sulphonamides**, Ch. 37) which occupy about 50% of the binding sites at therapeutic concentrations, that cause unexpected effects by displacing other drugs. The displaced drug need not occupy an appreciable fraction of the sites, so **diazepam**, for example, is appreciably displaced from protein-binding sites by **aspirin** (Chs 12 and 16), but not vice versa. Much has been made of the importance of binding interactions of this kind as a source of untoward drug interactions in clinical medicine, but a critical look at the evidence suggests

Binding of drugs to plasma proteins

- Plasma albumin is most important; β-globulin and acid glycoprotein also bind some drugs.
- Plasma albumin binds mainly acidic drugs (approximately two molecules per albumin molecule). Basic drugs may be bound by β-globulin and acid glycoprotein.
- Saturable binding sometimes leads to a non-linear relation between dose and free (active) drug concentration.
- Extensive protein binding slows drug elimination (metabolism and/or excretion by glomerular filtration).
- Competition between drugs for protein binding rarely leads to clinically important drug interactions.

that this type of competition is less important than was once thought (see Ch. 42).

DRUG DISPOSITION

We will now consider how the basic processes responsible for the translocation and distribution of drug molecules—diffusion, penetration of membranes, partition, and binding to protein—influence the overall behaviour of drug molecules in the body. Such drug disposition can be divided into four stages:

- absorption from the site of administration
- distribution within the body
- metabolic alteration
- excretion.

The main pharmacokinetic pathways are shown schematically in Figure 4.7.

DRUG ABSORPTION

ROUTES OF ADMINISTRATION

Absorption is defined as the passage of a drug from its site of administration into the plasma. It must therefore be considered for all routes of administration, except for the intravenous route. There are instances, such as the inhalation of a bronchodilator aerosol to treat asthma (Ch. 17), where absorption as just defined is not required for the drug to act, but in most cases the drug has to enter the plasma before it can reach its site of action, and has first to be absorbed.

The main routes of administration are:

- sublingual
- oral
- rectal
- application to epithelial surfaces (e.g. skin, cornea, vagina and nasal mucosa)
- inhalation
- injection
  —subcutaneous
  —intramuscular
  —intravenous
  —intrathecal.

Sublingual administration

Absorption directly from the oral cavity is sometimes useful (provided the drug does not taste too horrible) when a rapid response is required, particularly when the drug is either unstable at gastric pH or rapidly metabolised by the liver. **Glyceryl trinitrate** is an example of a drug that is often given sublingually (see Ch. 13). Drugs

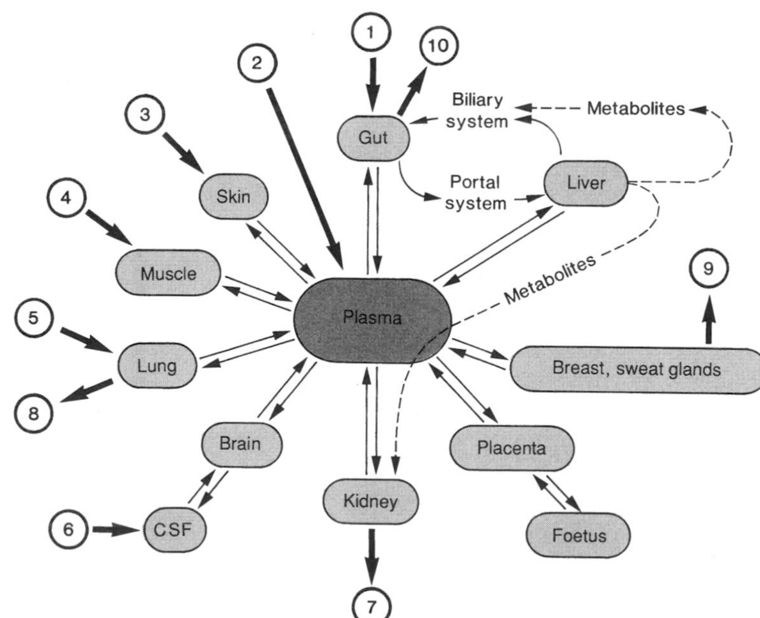

Fig. 4.7 The main routes of drug administration and elimination. Routes of administration: 1 = oral or rectal; 2 = intravenous; 3 = percutaneous; 4 = intramuscular; 5 = inhalation; 6 = intrathecal. Routes of elimination: 7 = urine; 8 = expired air; 9 = milk, sweat; 10 = faeces.

absorbed from the mouth pass straight into the systemic circulation without entering the portal system, and so escape first-pass metabolism (see below).

Oral administration

The great majority of drugs are taken by mouth and swallowed. In most cases little absorption occurs until the drug passes through the pyloric sphincter.

Drug absorption from the intestine

Measurements of drug absorption have shown that the basic mechanism is the same as for other epithelial barriers, namely passive transfer at a rate determined by the ionisation and lipid solubility of the drug molecules. Figure 4.8 shows the rate of absorption of a series of weak acids and bases as a function of pK_a. As expected, strong bases of pK_a 10 or higher are poorly absorbed, as are strong acids of pK_a less than 3, because they are fully ionised. Several clinically important drugs are strong bases, such as the muscle relaxants, **tubocurarine** and **suxamethonium** (Ch. 6), which are quaternary ammonium compounds and are poorly absorbed from the gastrointestinal tract. Muscle relaxants are used during anaesthesia (Ch. 6) and are always given intravenously. Other highly polar molecules, such as the **aminoglycoside antibiotics** and **vancomycin** (Ch. 37), are also very poorly absorbed. Vancomycin is used orally to eradicate toxin-forming *Clostridium difficile* from the gut in patients with pseudomembranous colitis (an adverse effect of treatment with broad-spectrum antibiotics due to appearance of this organism in the bowel), without causing systemic effects.

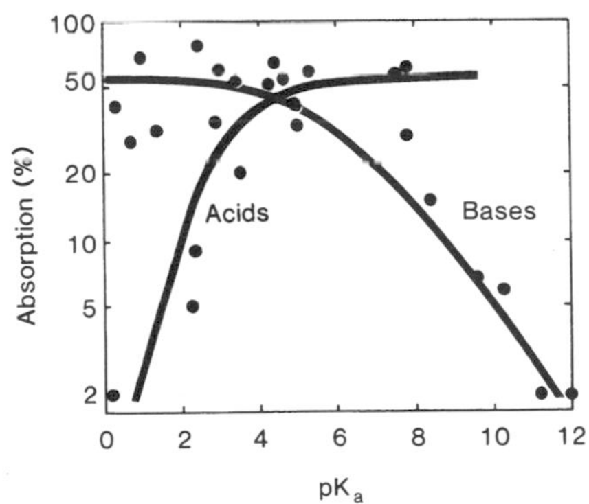

Fig. 4.8 Absorption of drugs from the intestine as a function of pK_a, for acids and bases. Weak acids and bases are well absorbed; strong acids and bases are poorly absorbed. (Redrawn from: Schanker L S et al. 1957 J Pharmacol 120: 528)

There are a few instances where intestinal absorption depends on carrier-mediated transport rather than simple lipid diffusion. Examples include **levodopa**, used in treating parkinsonism (see Ch. 30), which is taken up by the carrier that normally transports phenylalanine, and **fluorouracil** (Ch. 36), a cytotoxic drug that is transported by the system that carries the natural pyrimidines, thymine and uracil. Iron is absorbed via a specific carrier on the surface of mucosal cells in the jejunum, and calcium is absorbed by means of a vitamin D-dependent carrier system.

Factors affecting gastrointestinal absorption. As a rule, about 75% of a drug given orally is absorbed in 1–3 hours, but numerous factors can alter this, some physiological and some to do with the formulation of the drug. The main factors are:

- gastrointestinal motility
- splanchnic blood flow
- particle size and formulation
- physicochemical factors.

Gastrointestinal motility has a large effect. Many disorders (e.g. migraine and diabetic neuropathy) cause gastric stasis and slow drug absorption. Drug treatment can also affect motility, either reducing (e.g. drugs that block muscarinic receptors; see Ch. 6) or increasing it (e.g. **metoclopramide**, which speeds gastric emptying and is used in patients with migraine to facilitate absorption of analgesic (Ch. 8)). Excessively rapid movement of the gut contents can also impair absorption. A drug taken after a meal is often more slowly absorbed because its progress to the small intestine is delayed. There are exceptions, however, and several drugs (e.g. **propranolol**) reach a higher plasma concentration if they are taken after a meal, probably because food increases splanchnic blood flow.

Splanchnic blood flow is greatly reduced in hypovolaemic states, with a resultant slowing of drug absorption.

Particle size and formulation have major effects on absorption. In 1971, patients in a New York hospital were found to require unusually large maintenance doses of **digoxin** (Ch. 13). In a study on normal volunteers it was found that standard oral digoxin tablets from different manufacturers resulted in grossly different plasma concentrations (Fig. 4.9) even though the digoxin content of

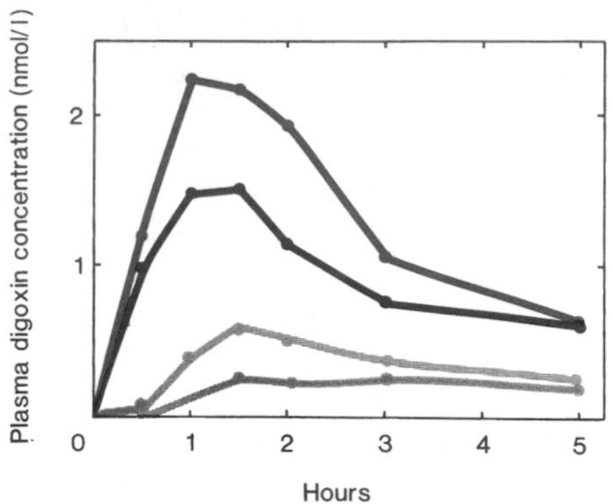

Fig. 4.9 Variation in oral absorption among different formulations of digoxin. The four curves show the mean plasma concentrations attained for the four preparations, each of which was given on separate occasions to four subjects. The large variation has caused the formulation of digoxin tablets to be standardised since this study was published. (From: Lindenbaum J et al. 1971 N Engl J Med 285: 1344)

the tablets was the same, because of differences in particle size. Because digoxin is rather poorly absorbed, small differences in the pharmaceutical formulation can make a large difference to the extent of absorption.

Pharmaceutical preparations are normally formulated to produce the desired absorption characteristics. Thus, capsules may be designed to remain intact for some hours after ingestion in order to delay absorption, or tablets may have a resistant coating to give the same effect. In some cases, a mixture of slow- and fast-release particles is included in a capsule to produce more sustained absorption. More elaborate pharmaceutical systems have been developed to deliver drugs at a constant rate throughout transit of the intestine, including various sustained-release preparations and osmotically driven 'mini-pumps' (see below, p. 96). Such preparations can reduce the frequency of dosing that is needed and reduce adverse effects related to high peak plasma concentrations following administration of a conventional formulation (e.g. flushing following a dose of the calcium channel antagonist **nifedipine**; Ch. 13). They may, however, have adverse effects due to the presence of high local concentrations of drug in the intestine (an osmotically released preparation of the anti-inflammatory drug **indomethacin** had to be withdrawn because it caused small bowel perforation), and are subject to variations in small bowel transit time that occur during ageing and with disease.

Physicochemical factors affecting drug absorption do so by influencing the state of the drug in the intestine. Thus **tetracycline** antibiotics bind strongly to calcium ions, and calcium-rich foods (especially milk) prevent their absorption (Ch. 37). Bile-acid-binding resins such as **cholestyramine** (used to treat hypercholesterolaemia; Ch. 15) bind several drugs, for example **digoxin** (Ch. 14), **warfarin** (Ch. 16), **thyroxine** (Ch. 21) and several antibiotics, and are administered at least 2 hours before or after other drugs for this reason.

Bioavailability. To get from the lumen of the small intestine into the systemic circulation a drug must not only penetrate the intestinal mucosa; it must also run the gauntlet of enzymes that may inactivate it in gut wall and liver. The term bioavailability is used to indicate the proportion of drug that passes into the systemic circulation after oral administration, taking into account both absorption and local metabolic degradation. It is a convenient term for making bland generalisations, but the concept creaks badly if attempts are made to use it with quantitative precision, or even to define it.* One problem is that it is not a characteristic solely of the drug preparation, since variations in enzyme activity of the gut wall or the liver, and in gastric pH or intestinal motility will all affect it. Because of this, one cannot speak strictly of the bioavailability of a particular preparation, but only of that preparation in a given individual on a particular occasion. Even with this caveat, the concept is of limited use because it relates only to the total proportion of the drug that reaches the systemic circulation, and ignores the time taken. Thus, if a drug is completely absorbed in 30 minutes, it will reach a much higher plasma concentration and have a more dramatic effect than the same drug absorbed over 6 hours. It is significant that one rarely sees a value assigned to 'bioavailability', and it is well to be wary of ostensibly measurable quan-

*The definition of bioavailability offered by the US Food and Drug Administration is: 'The rate and extent to which the therapeutic moiety is absorbed and becomes available to the site of drug action'. You may be forgiven for finding this confusing. The double use of 'and' gives the definition four possible meanings, two of which are obfuscated by the uncertain meaning of the phrase 'becomes available to the site of drug action'.

tities which are used impressionistically, but not actually given values. For these reasons, regulatory authorities—which have to make decisions about the licencing of products that are 'generic equivalents' of patented products—lay importance on evidence of bioequivalence, i.e. evidence that the new product behaves sufficiently similarly to the existing one to be substituted for it without causing clinical problems.

Rectal administration

Rectal administration is used either for drugs that are required to produce a local effect (e.g. anti-inflammatory drugs for use in ulcerative colitis), or to produce systemic effects. Absorption following rectal administration is often unreliable, but this route can be useful in patients who are vomiting or are unable to take medication by mouth (e.g. postoperatively). It is used to administer **diazepam** to children who are in *status epilepticus* (Ch. 30) in whom it is difficult to establish intravenous access. Often, though, the reasons for favouring the rectal route appear to be more cultural than pharmacological.

Drug absorption and bioavailability

- Drugs of very low lipid solubility, including those that are strong acids or bases, are generally poorly absorbed from the gut.
- A few drugs (e.g. levodopa) are absorbed by carrier-mediated transfer.
- Absorption from the gut depends on many factors, including:
  - — gastrointestinal motility
  - — gastrointestinal pH
  - — particle size
  - — physicochemical interaction with gut contents (e.g. chemical interaction between calcium and tetracycline antibiotics).
- Bioavailability is the fraction of an ingested dose of a drug that gains access to the systemic circulation. It may be low because absorption is incomplete, or because the drug is metabolised in the gut wall or liver before reaching the systemic circulation.
- Bioequivalence implies that if one formulation of a drug is substituted for another no clinically untoward consequences will ensue.

Application to epithelial surfaces

Cutaneous administration

In clinical practice, cutaneous administration is used mainly when a local effect on the skin is required (e.g. topically applied steroids). Appreciable absorption may nonetheless occur and lead to systemic effects.

Most drugs are absorbed very poorly through unbroken skin, because their lipid solubility is too low. However, a number of organophosphate insecticides (see Ch. 6), which must be able to penetrate an insect's cuticle in order to work, are absorbed through skin, and accidental poisoning among farm workers who get in the way of the crop sprayer is not uncommon. A case is recounted of a 35-year-old florist in 1932. 'While engaged in doing a light electrical repair job at a work bench he sat down in a chair on the seat of which some "Nico-Fume liquid" (a 40% solution of free nicotine) had been spilled. He felt the solution wet through his clothes to the skin over the left buttock, an area about the size of the palm of his hand. He thought nothing further of it and continued at his work for about fifteen minutes, when he was suddenly seized with nausea and faintness ... and found himself in a drenching sweat. On the way to hospital he lost consciousness.' He survived, just, and then four days later: 'On discharge from the hospital he was given the same clothes that he had worn when he was brought in. The clothes had been kept in a paper bag and were still damp where they had been wet with the nicotine solution.' The sequel was predictable. He survived again, but felt thereafter 'unable to enter a greenhouse where nicotine was being sprayed.' Some 60 years later, transdermal dosage forms of nicotine are being marketed to reduce the withdrawal symptoms that accompany stopping smoking (Ch. 34).

The use of such transdermal dosage forms, in which the drug is incorporated in a stick-on patch applied to an area of thin skin, is increasing, and several drugs—for example **glyceryltrinitrate**, used in angina (Ch. 13); **hyoscine** (Ch. 19), used to prevent seasickness; and **oestrogen**, used as hormone replacement following the menopause (Ch. 22), as well as nicotine—are now available in this form. Such patches produce a steady rate of delivery and offer several advantages, particularly ease of removal in case of unwanted effects. However, the method is suitable only for certain relatively lipid-soluble drugs, and such preparations are relatively expensive.

A few drugs, for example peptides related to the posterior pituitary hormone **antidiuretic hormone (ADH)** and to **gonadotrophin-releasing hormone** (see Ch. 21), are given as nasal sprays to avoid the need for frequent injections. These peptides are inactive when given orally, as they are quickly destroyed in the gastrointestinal tract, but enough is taken up from the nasal mucosa to provide a therapeutic effect.

Eye drops

Many drugs can be applied as eye drops, relying on absorption through the epithelium of the conjunctival sac to produce their effects. Adequate lipid solubility is necessary for absorption to occur. Thus, in treating glaucoma, a tertiary amine or uncharged form of anticholinesterase (e.g. **physostigmine**; see Ch. 6) works much better than a quaternary compound (e.g. **neostigmine**). Some systemic absorption occurs when eye drops are given, and can result in side effects (e.g. bronchospasm in asthmatic patients using **timolol** eye drops for glaucoma; see Ch. 7).

Administration by inhalation

Inhalation is the route used for volatile and gaseous anaesthetics (see Ch. 26). For these agents the lung serves as the route of both administration and elimination, and the rapid exchange that is possible as a result of the large surface area and blood flow makes it possible to achieve rapid adjustments of plasma concentration. The pharmacokinetic behaviour of inhalation anaesthetics is discussed more fully in Chapter 26.

Drugs used for their effects on the lung are also given by inhalation, usually as an aerosol. Bronchodilators, such as **salbutamol** (Ch. 17), are given in this way to achieve much higher concentrations in the lung than elsewhere in the body, thus minimising side effects. Though intended to act locally, drugs given by inhalation are usually partially absorbed into the circulation, and systemic side effects (e.g. tremor following salbutamol) can occur. Chemical modification of a drug may minimise such absorption. Thus **ipratropium**, a muscarinic receptor antagonist (Chs 6 and 17), is a quaternary ammonium ion analogue of atropine. It is used as an inhaled bronchodilator because its poor absorption minimises systemic adverse effects.

Cromoglycate, another anti-asthma drug (see Ch. 17), is insoluble in water and is inhaled as a dry powder dispersed as a fine cloud by means of a special device.

Endotracheal administration of drugs such as **atropine** or **adrenaline** (Ch. 13) is sometimes used in cardiac emergencies, the drug being given via an endotracheal tube. Rapid absorption, and rapid access of the drug to the heart via the pulmonary veins, as well as avoidance of the delay of venepuncture, may be advantageous in emergency situations.

Administration by injection

Intravenous injection is the fastest and most certain route of drug administration. If a single bolus injection is given, it produces a very high concentration of drug, which will first reach the right heart and lungs and then the systemic circulation. The actual peak concentration reaching the tissues depends critically on the rate of injection. Administration by steady intravenous infusion avoids the uncertainties of absorption from other sites. Drugs that are given intravenously include **heparin** (Ch. 16), **lignocaine** (when it is used as an antidysrhythmic drug; see Ch. 13), certain **anaesthetic agents** (Ch. 26), **ergometrine** (Ch. 22) and **diazepam** (Ch. 27).

Subcutaneous or *intramuscular injection* of drugs usually produces a faster effect than oral administration, but the rate of absorption depends greatly on the site of injection and on physiological factors, especially local blood flow.

The rate-limiting factors in absorption from the injection site are:

- diffusion through the tissue
- removal by local blood flow.

The importance of the former is shown by the powerful effect of hyaluronidase, an enzyme which breaks down the intercellular matrix. Adding hyaluronidase to the injection fluid increases the rate of diffusion through the interstitial space, and speeds up drug absorption.

Absorption from a site of injection may be increased by increasing local blood flow by the application of heat or massage. Local blood flow may be a critical factor if injections are given to patients with a failing peripheral circulation. Thus, if a patient were given a subcutaneous injection of **morphine** (Ch. 31) after severe trauma, absorption would be slow, resulting in inadequate analgesia; further doses might be given. When the circulation was restored a rapid and dangerous absorption of morphine would occur.

Methods for delaying absorption

It may be desirable to delay absorption either to reduce the systemic actions of drugs that are being used to produce a local effect, or to increase the duration of action of a drug by causing it to be absorbed slowly over a long period. Thus, the addition of **adrenaline** or **noradrenaline** to a solution of local anaesthetic reduces the absorption of the local anaesthetic into the general circulation, which usefully prolongs the anaesthetic effect, as well as reducing systemic toxicity.

Another method of delaying absorption from intramuscular or subcutaneous sites is to administer the drug in a relatively insoluble 'slow-release' form. This may be achieved by converting it into a poorly soluble salt, ester or complex which is injected either as an aqueous suspension or an oily solution. **Procaine penicillin** (Ch. 37) is a salt of penicillin which is only slightly water-soluble; when injected as an aqueous suspension it is slowly absorbed and exerts a prolonged action. Esterification of steroid hormones (e.g. **medroxyprogesterone acetate**, **testosterone propionate**; see Ch. 22) and antipsychotic drugs (e.g. **fluphenazine decanoate**; Ch. 28) increases their solubility in oil and in this way slows down their rate of absorption when they are injected in an oily solution.

The physical characteristics of a preparation may also be changed so as to influence its rate of absorption. Examples of this are the **insulin zinc suspensions** (see Ch. 20); insulin forms a complex with zinc, the physical form of which can be altered by varying the pH at which the reaction occurs. One form consists of a fine amorphous suspension which is relatively rapidly absorbed, and another consists of a suspension of large crystals which are slowly absorbed. These two preparations can be mixed to produce an immediate, but sustained, effect.

Another method used to achieve slow and continuous absorption of certain steroid hormones (e.g. **oestradiol**; Ch. 22) is the subcutaneous implantation of solid pellets. The rate of absorption is proportional to the surface area of the implant, so a flat pellet gives more uniform rate of absorption than a spherical one.

Intrathecal injection

Injection of a drug into the subarachnoid space via a lumbar puncture needle is used for some specialised purposes. **Methotrexate** (Ch. 36) is administered in this way in the treatment of certain childhood leukaemias that tend to spread to the central nervous system. Regional anaesthesia can be produced by injecting a **local anaesthetic** (see Ch. 34) intrathecally, and, recently, **opiate analgesics** (Ch. 31) have also been used successfully in this way. **Baclofen** (a GABA analogue, Ch. 24) has recently been administered in this way to minimise its adverse effects when treating patients with disabling muscle spasm caused by chronic neurological disease. Some antibiotic drugs cross the blood–brain barrier very slowly, and if essential may be given intrathecally to treat meningitis, but most cases of bacterial meningitis are caused by microorganisms that are sensitive to antibiotics such as **penicillin** (Ch. 37) and **chloramphenicol** that cross the blood–brain barrier adequately (at least when the meninges are inflamed) when given intravenously in appropriate doses, and the intravenous route is preferred in such cases.

DISTRIBUTION OF DRUGS IN THE BODY

BODY FLUID COMPARTMENTS

Body water is distributed into four main compartments as shown in Figure 4.10. The total body water as a percentage of body weight varies from 50–70%, being rather less in women than in men.

Extracellular fluid comprises the *blood plasma* (about 4.5% of body weight), *interstitial fluid* (16%) and *lymph* (1.2%). *Intracellular fluid* (30–40%) is the sum of the fluid contents of all cells in the body.

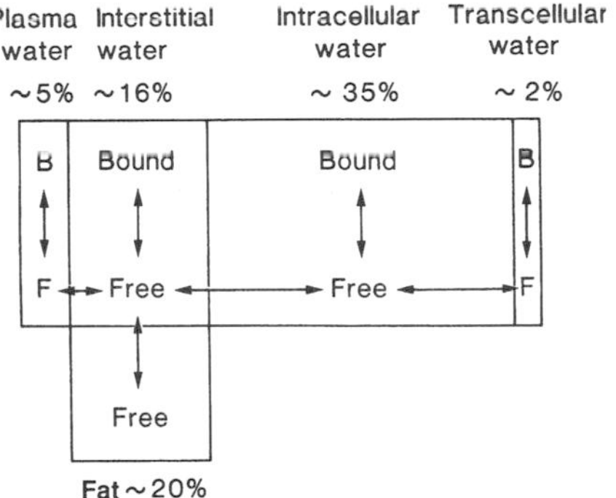

Fig. 4.10 The main body fluid compartments, expressed as a percentage of body weight. Drug molecules exist in bound or free form in each compartment, but only the free drug is able to move between the compartments.

Transcellular fluid (2.5%) includes the cerebrospinal, intraocular, peritoneal, pleural and synovial fluids and digestive secretions. The foetus may also be regarded as a special type of transcellular compartment. To enter the transcellular compartments from the extracellular compartment a drug must cross an epithelial barrier, such as the blood–brain barrier, which means that it has to be able to enter cells. This is especially important in relation to the brain, which is inaccessible to many systemically-acting drugs, including some antibiotics such as the **aminoglycosides**, whose lipid solubility is insufficient to allow penetration of the blood–brain barrier. However, inflammation, in the form of meningitis, can disrupt the integrity of the blood–brain barrier, allowing normally impermeant substances to enter the brain (Fig. 4.11), a fact that allows **penicillin** (Ch. 37) to be given systemically in the treatment of bacterial meningitis. Furthermore, some parts of the central nervous system, including the chemoreceptor trigger zone, are accessible to drugs that have not crossed the blood–brain barrier. This enables **domperidone**, a dopamine receptor antagonist (Ch. 28), to be used to prevent the nausea caused by dopamine agonists such as **apomorphine,** when these are used to treat advanced Parkinson's disease, without causing loss of efficacy by competition with dopamine receptors in the basal ganglia that are only accessible to drugs that have traversed the blood–brain barrier (Ch. 30).

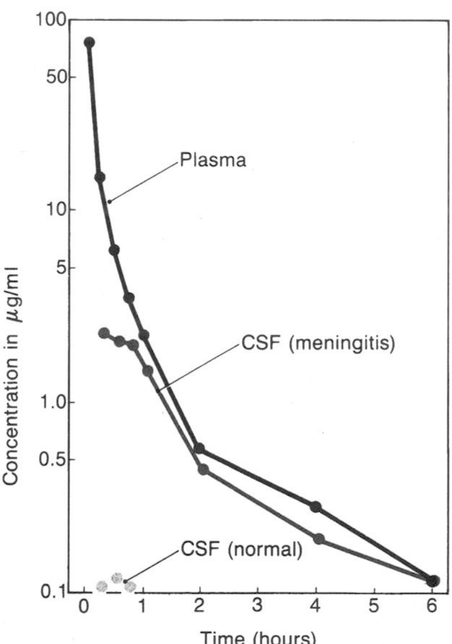

Fig. 4.11 Plasma and CSF concentrations of an antibiotic (thienamycin) following an intravenous dose (25 mg/kg). In normal rabbits, no drug reaches the CSF, but in animals with experimental *Esch. coli* meningitis, the concentration of drug in CSF approaches that in the plasma. (From: Patamasucon & McCracken 1973 Antimicrob Agents Chemother 3: 270)

Within each of these aqueous compartments, drug molecules usually exist both in free solution and in bound form; furthermore, drugs that are weak acids or bases will exist as an equilibrium mixture of the charged and uncharged forms, the position of the equilibrium depending on the pH (see p. 68).

The equilibrium pattern of distribution between the various compartments will thus depend on:

- permeability across tissue barriers
- binding within compartments
- pH partition
- fat:water partition.

Volume of distribution

The apparent volume of distribution, V_d, is defined as the volume of fluid required to contain the total amount, Q, of drug in the body at the same concentration as that present in the plasma, C_p.

$$V_d = \frac{Q}{C_p} \tag{4.1}$$

Values of V_d* have been measured for many drugs (Table 4.2). Some general patterns can be distinguished, but it is important to avoid identifying a given range of V_d too closely with a particular anatomical compartment. Thus insulin with a measured V_d similar to the volume of plasma water exerts its effects on muscle, fat and liver via receptors that are accessible to interstitial fluid (Ch. 20). Similarly, **atenolol** (Chs 7 and 14), a polar β-adrenoceptor antagonist with a V_d of only 0.16 l/kg body weight, can produce adverse effects on the

*The experimental measurement of V_d is complicated by the fact that the amount of drug present in the body, Q, does not stay constant (because of metabolism and excretion of the drug) during the time that it takes for it to be distributed among the various body compartments that contribute to the overall V_d. It therefore has to be calculated indirectly from a series of measurements of plasma concentrations as a function of time. On the basis of a two-compartment model (see p. 94), the distribution volume of each compartment can be calculated, but the validity of such estimates necessarily depends on the validity of the kinetic model used.

Table 4.2 Distribution volumes for some drugs compared with volume of body fluid compartments

Volume (litres/kg body weight)	Compartment	V_d (litres/kg body weight)	
0.05	Plasma	0.05–0.1	Heparin
			Insulin
		0.1–0.2	Warfarin
			Sulphamethoxazole
			Glibenclamide
			Atenolol
0.2	Extra-cellular fluid	0.2–0.4	Tubocurarine
		0.4–0.7	Theophylline
0.55	Total body water		Ethanol
			Neostigmine
			Phenytoin
		1–2	Methotrexate
			Indomethacin
			Paracetamol
			Diazepam
			Lignocaine
		2–5	Glyceryl trinitrate
			Morphine
			Propranolol
			Digoxin
			Chlorpromazine
		> 10	Nortriptyline
			Imipramine

central nervous system (e.g. nightmares) during chronic dosing.

Drugs confined to the plasma compartment

The plasma volume is about 0.05 l/kg body weight. A few drugs, such as **heparin** (Ch. 16), are confined to the plasma compartment because the molecule is too large to cross the capillary wall easily. More often, retention of a drug in the plasma following a single dose reflects strong binding to plasma protein (see Table 4.1). It is, nevertheless, the free drug in the interstitial fluid that exerts a pharmacological effect. Following repeated dosing, equilibration occurs and measured V_d increases. Some dyes, such as Evans blue, bind so strongly to plasma albumin that its distribution volume is used experimentally to measure plasma volume.

Drugs distributed in the extracellular compartment

The total extracellular volume is about 0.2 l/kg, and this is the approximate distribution volume for many polar compounds, such as **tubocurarine** (Ch. 6), **gentamicin** and **carbenicillin** (Ch. 37). These drugs cannot easily enter cells because of their low lipid solubility, and do not normally cross the blood–brain or placental barriers when used acutely. Distribution volumes in excess of the theoretical value of 0.2 l/kg result either from a limited degree of penetration into cells, or from binding of the drug in the extravascular compartment.

Distribution throughout the body water

Total body water represents about 0.55 l/kg, and this distribution volume is achieved by relatively lipid-soluble drugs that readily cross cell membranes such as **phenytoin** (Ch. 30), **ethanol** (Ch. 33) and **diazepam** (Ch. 37). Binding of the drug anywhere outside the plasma compartment, as well as partitioning into body fat, can increase V_d beyond the absolute value for total body water, and thus there are many drugs that give values well in excess even of the total body volume such as **morphine** (Ch. 31), **tricyclic antidepressants** (Ch. 27) and **haloperidol** (Ch. 28). Such drugs are *not* efficiently removed from the body by haemodialysis, which is therefore unhelpful in managing overdose with such agents. Drugs with a large distribution volume usually reach the brain and the foetus, as well as other transcellular compartments. This generalisation holds when the large volume of distribution is due to high lipid solubility. Exceptions occur among drugs with a large distribution volume as a consequence of extensive tissue binding. For example, the class III antidysrhythmic drug, **amiodarone** (Ch. 13) with V_d of 62 l/kg body weight accumulates to very high concentrations in fat, liver and lung, the lowest tissue concentrations occurring in brain and concentrations in foetal plasma being approximately 10% of those in maternal plasma.

REMOVAL OF DRUGS FROM THE BODY

The main routes by which drugs are removed from the body are:

- the kidneys
- the hepato-biliary system
- the lungs.

Drug distribution

- The major compartments are:
  —plasma (5% of body weight)
  —interstitial fluid (16%)
  —intracellular fluid (35%)
  —transcellular fluid (2%)
  —fat (20%).
- Volume of distribution (V_d) is defined as the volume of plasma that would contain the total body content of the drug at a concentration equal to that in the plasma.
- Drugs that are strongly protein-bound stay mainly in the plasma compartment (small V_d).
- Lipid-insoluble drugs are mainly confined to plasma and interstitial fluids; most do not enter the brain following acute dosing.
- Lipid-soluble drugs reach all compartments, and may accumulate in fat.
- For drugs that accumulate outside the plasma compartment (e.g. in fat, or by being bound to tissues) V_d may exceed total body volume.

Excretion via the lungs occurs only with highly volatile or gaseous agents, and the great majority of drugs leave the body in the urine. Some drugs are secreted into the bile via the liver, but in most cases reabsorption occurs from the intestine. There are, however, instances (e.g. **rifampicin**) where faecal loss accounts for the elimination of a substantial fraction of unchanged drug in healthy individuals, and faecal elimination of drugs such as **digoxin** that are normally excreted in urine becomes progressively more important in patients with advancing renal failure. Drugs are also excreted in secretions such as milk or sweat. These routes are quantitatively minor compared with renal excretion, although excretion into milk can sometimes have effects on a suckling child.

Lipophilic drugs are not eliminated efficiently as such by the kidney, because they are passively reabsorbed from tubular fluid as this becomes concentrated. Consequently, most lipophilic drugs are metabolised to more polar products that do not readily cross membrane barriers and so are excreted efficiently in urine. Drug metabolism occurs predominantly in the liver and results in metabolites that are more polar than the parent drug. In this section we consider first the main pathways of drug metabolism, and then factors that determine the rate of renal elimination.

DRUG METABOLISM

Gibson & Skett (1986) give a useful general account of drug metabolism.

Enzymatic modification of drug molecules usually abolishes their pharmacological activity; exceptions to this (see Table 4.4, p. 87) are discussed later in this chapter.

Metabolic alteration of drug molecules involves two kinds of biochemical reaction, which often (though not invariably) occur sequentially, known as *phase I* and *phase II* reactions.

Phase I reactions usually consist of oxidation, reduction or hydrolysis, and the products are often more reactive and sometimes more toxic than the parent drug; phase II reactions involve conjugation, which normally results in inactive compounds (although there are exceptions, for example the active sulphate metabolite of **minoxidil**, a potassium channel activator used to treat severe hypertension; Ch. 14). Phase I reactions often introduce a relatively reactive group, such as hydroxyl, into the

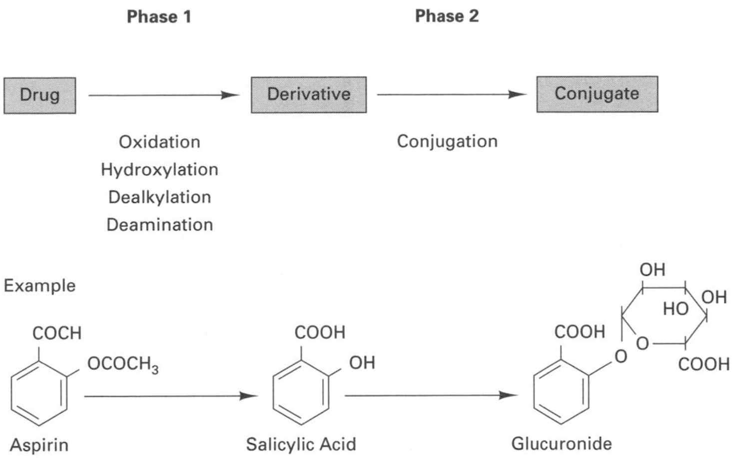

Fig. 4.12 The two phases of drug metabolism.

molecule (functionalisation). This functional group then serves as the point of attack for the conjugating system which attaches a larger substituent to it, such as a glucuronyl, sulphate or acetyl group (Fig. 4.12). Both stages normally decrease the lipid solubility of the substance, thus increasing the rate of renal elimination (see below), and the system of drug metabolising enzymes may be regarded as a non-selective detoxification system for ridding the body of a wide range of foreign substances.

Phase I and phase II reactions take place mainly in the liver, though there are some important exceptions of drugs that are metabolised in the plasma (e.g. hydrolysis of **suxamethonium** by plasma cholinesterase; see Ch. 6), in the lung (e.g. various **prostanoids**; see Ch. 11), or in the wall of the intestine (e.g. **tyramine**, **salbutamol**; Ch. 7). Within the liver the enzymes involved are intracellular. Many are attached to the smooth endoplasmic reticulum and they are often called 'microsomal' enzymes because, on homogenisation and differential centrifugation, the endoplasmic reticulum is broken into very small fragments that sediment only after prolonged high-speed centrifugation. To reach these metabolising enzymes in life, a drug must cross the hepatocyte plasma membrane. Polar molecules do this more slowly than non-polar molecules except where specific transport mechanisms exist, so for these drugs hepatic metabolism is in general less important, and a greater proportion is excreted unchanged in the urine.

Phase I reactions

Oxidative reactions, which include *hydroxylation* of nitrogen and carbon atoms, *N*- and *O-dealkylation* and *oxidative deamination* are catalysed by a complex enzyme system known as the *mixed function oxygenase* system, which resides on the smooth endoplasmic reticulum. Several enzymes are involved, the most important being *cytochrome P-450*, a haem protein which binds molecular oxygen as well as the substrate molecule and forms part of the electron transfer chain. Though the chemical end result may be different (e.g. hydroxylation, O-dealkylation or deamination) with different drugs, these reactions all start with a hydroxylation step catalysed by the P-450 system. This produces a reactive intermediate from which the end-product is derived (Fig. 4.13). The metabolism of **imipramine** (Fig. 4.14; see also Ch. 29) provides a typical example of how these reactions can combine to give rise to a whole family of metabolites.

The P-450 system has been studied in great detail and P-450 enzymes have several important functions (e.g. eicosanoid biosynthesis; Ch. 11) in addition to being the sentry system that first apprehends and incapacitates many foreign substances. It is estimated that 30–100 different subtypes (isoenzymes) exist, with differing substrate specificities and differing mechanisms controlling their expression (see Nebert & Gonzalez 1985, Gonzalez 1989).

Not all drug oxidation reactions involve the mixed function oxygenase system. For example, **ethanol** is metabolised by a soluble cytoplasmic enzyme, alcohol dehydrogenase. Other exceptions include the non-microsomal enzyme xanthine oxidase, which is involved in uric acid synthesis and the pathogenesis of gout (Ch. 12) and is also responsible

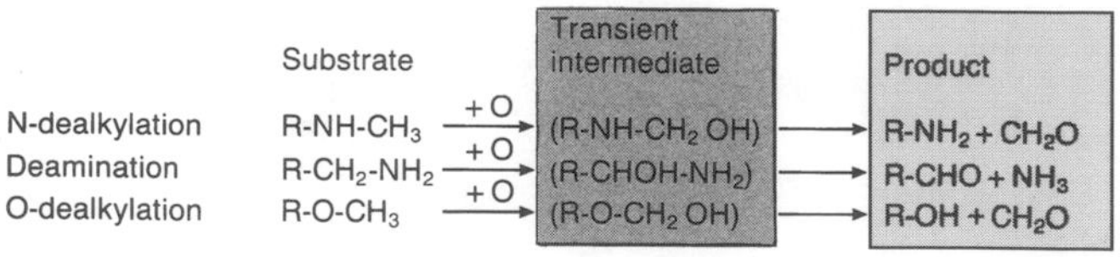

	Substrate		Transient intermediate		Product
N-dealkylation	R-NH-CH_3	+O →	(R-NH-CH_2 OH)	→	R-NH_2 + CH_2O
Deamination	R-CH_2-NH_2	+O →	(R-CHOH-NH_2)	→	R-CHO + NH_3
O-dealkylation	R-O-CH_3	+O →	(R-O-CH_2 OH)	→	R-OH + CH_2O

Fig. 4.13 Examples of phase I reactions.

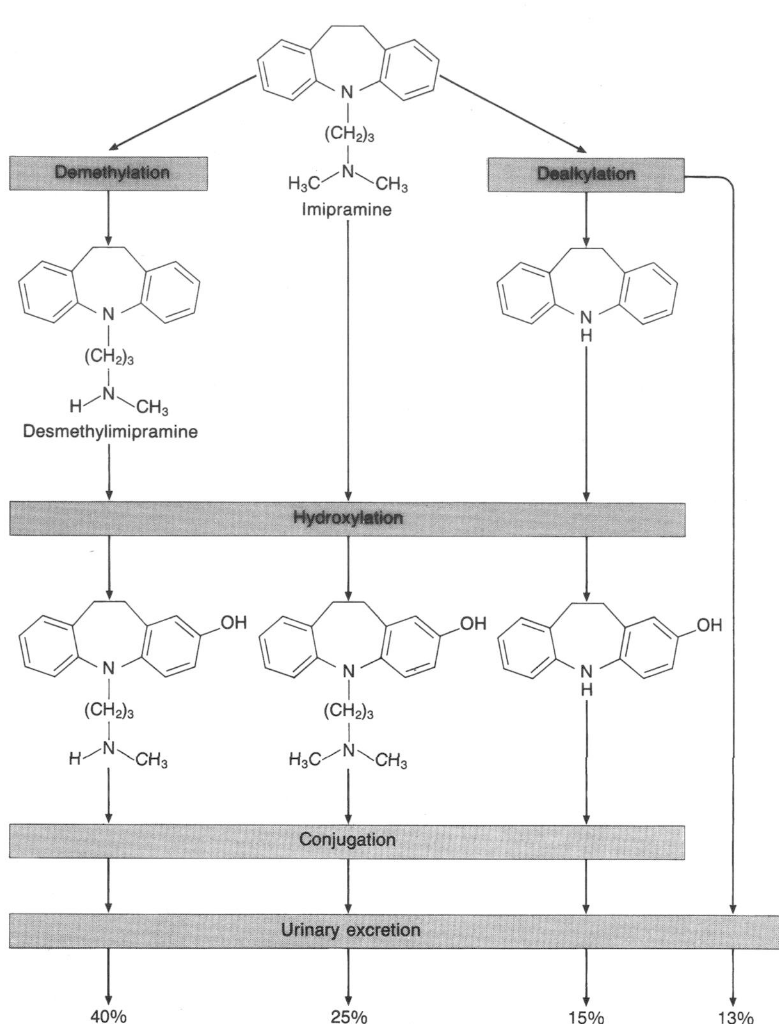

Fig. 4.14 The main routes of metabolism of imipramine. (From: Crammer J L et al. 1969 Psychopharmacologia 15: 207)

for inactivation of the cytotoxic drug **6-mercaptopurine** (Ch. 36), and monoamine oxidase which inactivates many biologically active amines (e.g. **noradrenaline, tyramine, 5-HT**; see Chs 7 and 29). These enzymes occur in many tissues besides the liver.

Reductive reactions are much less common than oxidative ones, but some are important. For example, the anticoagulant drug **warfarin** (Ch. 16) is inactivated by conversion of a ketone to a hydroxyl group. Glucocorticoids are still sometimes administered as ketones (e.g. **cortisone** and **prednisone**; see Ch. 21) which must be reduced to the corresponding hydroxy compounds in order to act (Table 4.4). These reductive reactions also involve microsomal enzymes.

Hydrolytic reactions do not involve hepatic microsomal enzymes, but occur in plasma and in many tissues. Both ester and amide bonds are susceptible to hydrolysis, the former more readily than the latter.

Phase II reactions

If a drug molecule has a suitable 'handle' (e.g. a hydroxyl, thiol or amino group), which may result from a phase I reaction or which the drug may possess anyway, it is susceptible to conjugation, i.e. attachment of a substituent group. The conjugate, which is almost always pharmacologically inactive (unlike the products of phase I reactions) and less lipid soluble than its precursor, is then excreted in the urine or in the bile.

The conjugates most commonly found are glucuronyl (Fig. 4.15), sulphate, methyl, acetyl, glycyl and glutathione (see Fig. 43.1). Glucuronide formation involves the formation of a high-energy phosphate compound, uridine diphosphate glucuronic acid (UDPGA), from which the glucuronic acid part is transferred to an electron-rich atom (N, O or S) on the substrate, forming an amide, ester or thiol bond. This is catalysed by an enzyme, UDP glucuronyl transferase, which has a very broad substrate specificity, so the reaction occurs with a wide variety of drugs and other foreign molecules.

Acetylation and methylation reactions occur with acetyl-CoA and S-adenosyl methionine, respectively, acting as the donor compounds. Many of these conjugation reactions occur in the liver, but other tissues, such as lung and kidney, are also sites of conjugation of some drugs. A number of important endogenous substances, such as bilirubin and adrenal corticosteroids, are conjugated by the same system. Glucuronide formation is the commonest conjugation reaction, reflecting the very broad substrate specificity of the enzyme, UDP-glucuronyl transferase. The highly polar nature of the glucuronic acid group means that the conjugates are usually pharmacologically inactive, and rapidly excreted.

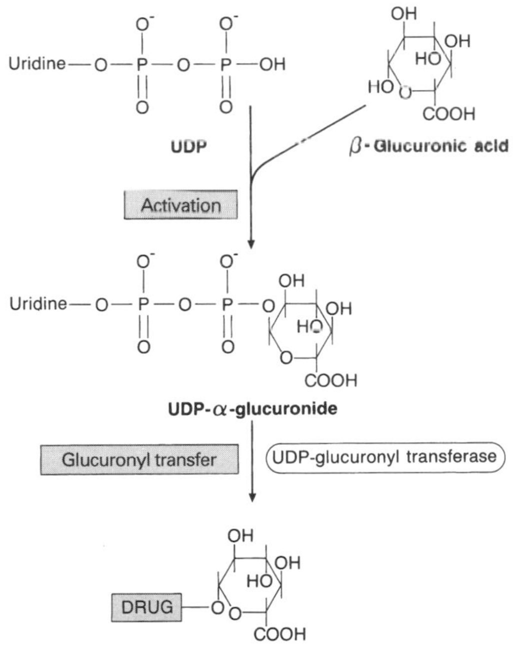

Fig. 4.15 The glucuronide conjugation reaction.

Induction of microsomal enzymes

A number of drugs such as **rifampicin** (Ch. 37), **ethanol** (Ch. 33), **carbamazepine** (Ch. 30), increase the activity of microsomal oxidase and conjugating systems when administered repeatedly. Many carcinogenic chemicals (e.g. **benzpyrene**) also have this effect, which can be substantial; Figure 4.16 shows a nearly 10-fold increase in the rate of benzpyrene metabolism two days after a single dose. The effect is referred to as induction, and it is the result of an increased synthesis of microsomal enzymes, rather than a change in the activity of existing enzyme molecules. Generally, the rate of metabolism of the inducing agent itself is increased, as well as that of various other compounds, and different agents vary in the pattern of induction that they produce. **Phenobarbitone** (Ch. 30) is a particularly versatile inducer, and it significantly increases the rate of degradation of many other

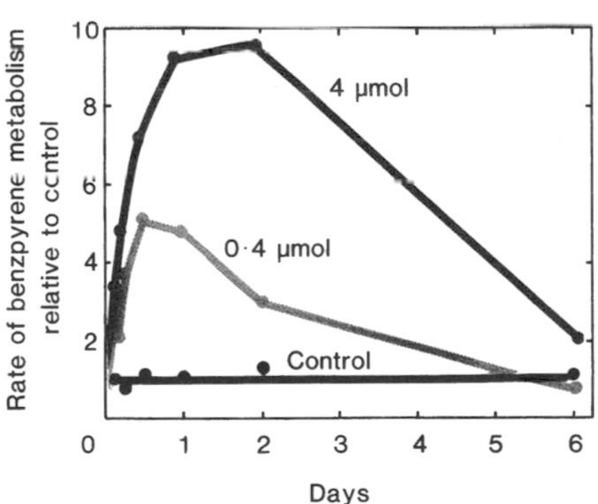

Fig. 4.16 Stimulation of hepatic metabolism of benzpyrene. Young rats were given benzpyrene (i.p.) in the doses shown, and the benzpyrene metabolising activity of liver homogenates measured at times up to 6 days. (From: Conney A H et al. 1957 J Biol Chem 228:753)

drugs (Ch. 42). Some insecticides, such as DDT, and other environmental contaminants also have a strong inducing effect. The pattern of enzyme induction is not the same for all inducing agents. Thus phenobarbitone and many related substances cause a non-selective increase in many microsomal enzymes (including glucuronyl transferases), whereas ethanol and polycyclic hydrocarbons such as benzpyrene and DDT produce more selective effects.

Enzyme induction, by accelerating phase I metabolism, can increase as well as decrease drug effects. There are drugs, for example **paracetamol** (Ch. 12), whose phase I metabolites are mainly responsible for their toxicity (see Ch. 43), and in these cases toxicity is increased following enzyme induction. The carcinogenic action of some polycyclic hydrocarbons is associated with increased hepatic formation of highly reactive oxidative products (e.g. epoxides) that can damage DNA.

The mechanism by which induction occurs is only partly understood (see Nebert & Gonzalez 1985). In common with the mechanism of steroid action (see Ch. 2), it clearly involves stimulation of gene transcription, leading to increased protein synthesis. It is suggested that the inducing agent may bind to a cytosolic receptor, which in turn binds to specific DNA sequences that are associated with the production of particular drug-metabolising enzymes.

First-pass (presystemic) metabolism

Some drugs are removed from the portal circulation very efficiently by the liver and metabolised, so that the amount reaching the systemic circulation is considerably less than the amount absorbed into the portal vein. A smaller number are metabolised in the wall of the intestine. This is known as the *first-pass effect* or *presystemic metabolism*, and it is significant for many clinically important drugs (Table 4.3).

Table 4.3 Drugs undergoing substantial presystemic elimination

Aspirin	Lignocaine
Chlormethiazole	Metoprolol
Chlorpromazine	Morphine
Dextropropoxyphene	Nortriptyline
Glyceryl trinitrate	Pethidine
Imipramine	Propranolol
Isosorbide dinitrate	Salbutamol
Levodopa	Verapamil

First-pass metabolism is generally a nuisance in practice, because:

- a much larger dose of the drug is needed when it is given orally than when it is given by other routes
- marked individual variations occur in the extent of first-pass metabolism of a given drug (see Ch. 42), which may produce a troublesome degree of unpredictability when such drugs are used orally.

Pharmacologically active drug metabolites

In some cases (see Table 4.4) the drug administered becomes biologically active only after it has been metabolised. Thus **azathioprine**, an immunosuppressant drug (Ch. 12), is metabolised to **mercaptopurine**, and **enalapril**, an angiotensin-converting enzyme inhibitor (Ch. 14), is hydrolysed to its active form **enalaprilat**. Such drugs, in which the parent compound lacks activity of its own, are known as *pro-drugs*. Metabolism can alter the pharmacological actions of a drug qualitatively. **Aspirin** powerfully inhibits some platelet functions and has anti-inflammatory activity (Ch. 12). It is hydrolysed to **salicylate** (Fig. 4.12), which has anti-inflammatory but not anti-platelet activity. In other instances, metabolites may have pharmacological actions similar to the parent compound (e.g. **benzodiazepines**, many of which form long-lived active metabolites that cause their effects to persist after the parent drug has disappeared). There are also cases in which metabolites are responsible for certain toxic effects. The liver toxicity of **paracetamol** is an example of this (see Ch. 43), as well as the nephrotoxicity of the antitumour drug, **cyclophosphamide** (see Ch. 36).

Stereoselectivity

Many clinically important drugs, such as **sotalol** (Ch. 13), **warfarin** (Ch. 16) and **cyclophosphamide** (Ch. 36), are mixtures of optical isomers, the components of which differ not only in their pharmacodynamic activity but also in their metabolism, which may follow completely distinct pathways. Several clinically important drug interactions involve stereospecific inhibition of metabolism of one drug by another (Ch. 42). In some cases, drug toxicity appears to be due mainly to one of the enantiomers, not necessarily the pharmacologically active one

Table 4.4 Some drugs that produce active or toxic metabolites

Inactive (pro-drugs)		Active		Toxic
	Heroin →	Morphine		
	Codeine →	Morphine		
	Propranolol →	4-hydroxypropranolol		
	Paracetamol →			N-acetyl-p-benzo-quinone imine
	Imipramine →	Desmethylimipramine		
	Amitriptyline →	Nortriptyline		
	Diazepam →	Nordiazepam →	Oxazepam	
Cortisone →		Hydrocortisone		
Prednisone →		Prednisolone		
Cyclophosphamide →		Phosphoramide mustard		
Chloral hydrate →		Trichloroethanol		
Azathioprine →		Mercaptopurine		
		Halothane →		Trifluoroacetic acid
		Sulphonamides →		Acetylated derivatives
		Methoxyflurane →		Fluoride
Enalapril →		Enalaprilat		
Zidovudine →		Zidovudine triphosphate		

Drug metabolism

- Phase I reactions: oxidation, reduction and hydrolysis:
  - — usually form more reactive products, sometimes toxic
  - — often involve mixed function oxidase system in which cytochrome P-450 plays a key role.
- Phase II reactions: conjugation (e.g. glucuronidation, glycine conjugation, sulphation, etc.) usually form inactive and readily excretable products.
- Induction of enzymes by other drugs and chemicals can greatly accelerate hepatic drug metabolism.
- Some drugs show rapid 'first-pass' hepatic metabolism, and thus poor oral bioavailability.

(see Trager & Testa 1985, Ariens 1986). Where practicable, regulatory authorities now urge that new drugs should consist of pure stereoisomers to avoid these complications.

RENAL EXCRETION OF DRUGS AND DRUG METABOLITES

Drugs differ greatly in the way that they are handled by the kidney, ranging from **penicillin** (Ch. 37), which is cleared from the blood almost completely on a single transit through the kidney, to **diazepam** (Ch. 27), which is cleared extremely slowly, so that the blood leaving the kidney contains almost as much drug as that entering it. The majority of drugs fall somewhere in between, and the products of phase I and phase II metabolism are nearly always cleared more quickly than the parent compound. There are three basic processes that account for these wide differences in renal excretion:

- glomerular filtration
- active tubular secretion or reabsorption
- passive diffusion across tubular epithelium.

Glomerular filtration

Glomerular capillaries allow drug molecules of molecular weight below about 20 000 to pass through into the glomerular filtrate. Plasma albumin (MW 68 000) is almost completely held back, but drugs—with the exception of macromolecular substances such as **heparin** (Ch. 16), **dextrans** and **protein hormones** (Ch. 21) and **growth factors** (Chs 11 and 23)—cross the barrier freely. If a drug binds appreciably to plasma albumin its concentration in the filtrate will be less than the total plasma concentration. If, like **warfarin** (Ch. 16), a drug is approximately 98% bound to albumin, the concentration in the filtrate is only 2% of that in plasma and clearance by filtration is correspondingly reduced.

Tubular secretion and reabsorption

Glomerular filtration is at most about 20% of renal plasma flow, and so leaves at least 80% of delivered drug to pass on to the peritubular capillaries of the proximal tubule where there are two independent and relatively non-selective carrier systems that transport drug molecules into the tubular lumen. One of these transports acidic drugs (as well as various endogenous substances, such as uric acid), the other system handles basic substances. Some of the more important drugs that are transported by these two carrier systems are shown in Table 4.5. The carriers can transport drug molecules against an electrochemical gradient, and can, therefore, reduce the plasma concentration nearly to zero. Since at least 80% of the drug delivered to the kidney is presented to the carrier, tubular secretion is potentially the most effective mechanism for drug elimination by the kidney. Unlike glomerular filtration, carrier-mediated transport can achieve maximal drug clearance even when most of the drug is bound to plasma protein.* **Penicillin** (Ch. 37), for example, though about 80% bound and therefore cleared only slowly by filtration, is almost completely removed by proximal tubular secretion, and its overall rate of elimination is very high.

Many of the drugs that are excreted by the kidney (Table 4.5) share the same transport system, and competition can occur between them. **Probenecid**, which was developed for the purpose of prolonging the action of penicillin by retarding its excretion, is an example. Probenecid is itself only slowly transported, but it competitively inhibits the transport of other drugs. It is usefully combined with **amoxycillin** (Ch. 37) in treating patients with gonorrhoea in whom efficacy following a single supervised administration is important. Probenecid also inhibits tubular reabsorption of uric acid (which relies on the same carrier), thereby increasing excretion of uric acid and lowering the plasma concentration of urate. It remains useful in the prophylaxis of gout in patients with this disorder who cannot take **allopurinol** (Ch. 12).

Table 4.5 Some drugs and related substances that are actively secreted into the proximal renal tubule

Acids	Bases
Acetazolamide	Amiloride
p-Aminohippuric acid	Dopamine
Aminosalicylic acid	Histamine
Cephaloridine	Mepacrine
Frusemide	Morphine
Glucuronic acid conjugates	Pethidine
Glycine conjugates	Quaternary ammonium compounds
5-Hydroxyindole acetic acid	Quinine
Indomethacin	Serotonin
Methotrexate	Tolazoline
Penicillins	Triamterene
Probenecid	
Renal radiocontrast media	
Salicylic acid	
Sulphate conjugates	
Sulphinpyrazone	
Thiazide diuretics	
Uric acid	

Diffusion across the renal tubule

As the glomerular filtrate passes through the renal tubule, water is progressively reabsorbed, the volume of urine emerging being only about 1% of that of the filtrate. If the tubule is freely permeable to drug molecules, the drug concentration in the filtrate will remain close to that in the plasma, and some 99% of the filtered drug will be reabsorbed passively. Drugs with high lipid solubility, and hence high tubular permeability, are therefore slowly excreted. If the drug is highly polar, and therefore of low tubular permeability, the filtered drug will not be able to leave the tubule, and its concentration will rise steadily until it is about 100 times as high in the urine as in the plasma. Drugs handled in this way include **digoxin**, and aminoglycoside antibiotics such as **gentamicin**. Many drugs, being weak acids or weak bases, change their ionisation with pH (see p. 68), and this can markedly affect renal excretion. The ion-trapping effect means that a basic drug will be more rapidly excreted in an acid urine, because the low pH within the tubule

*Because filtration involves isosmotic movement of both water and solutes, it will not affect the free concentration of drug in the plasma. Thus the equilibrium between free and bound drug will not be disturbed, and there will be no tendency for the bound drug to dissociate as the blood traverses the glomerular capillary. The rate of clearance of the drug by filtration is therefore reduced directly in proportion to the fraction that is bound. In the case of active tubular secretion, this is not so; secretion may be retarded very little even though the drug is mostly bound. This is because the carrier transports drug molecules unaccompanied by water. As free drug molecules are taken from the plasma, therefore, the free plasma concentration tends to fall. This causes a net dissociation of bound drug from the protein, so that effectively all of the drug, bound and free, is available to the carrier.

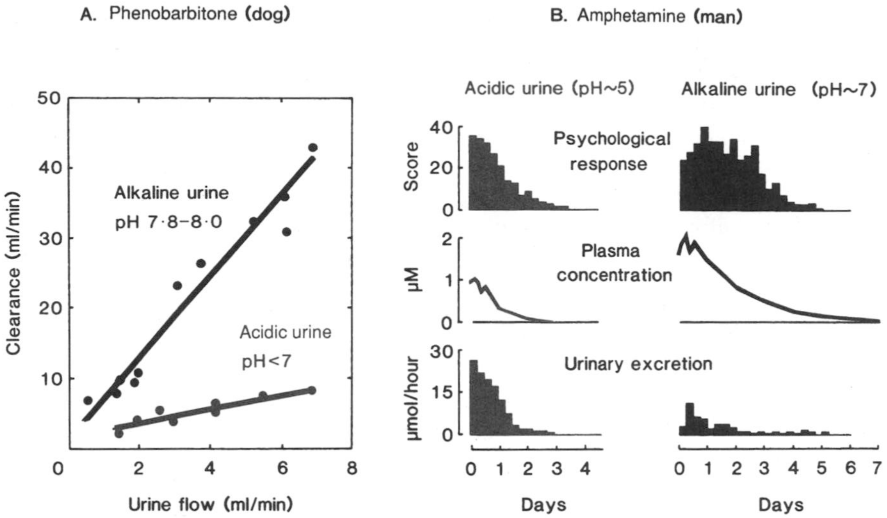

Fig. 4.17 The effect of urinary pH on drug excretion. A. Phenobarbitone clearance in the dog as a function of urine flow. Because phenobarbitone is acidic, alkalinising the urine increases clearance about fivefold. **B.** Amphetamine excretion in man. Acidifying the urine increases the rate of renal elimination of amphetamine, reducing its plasma concentration and its effect on the subject's mental state. (Data from: Gunne & Anggard 1974 In: Torrell T et al. (eds) Pharmacology and pharmacokinetics. Plenum, New York)

will favour ionisation and thus inhibit reabsorption. Conversely, an acidic drug will be most rapidly excreted if the urine is made alkaline.

These effects have some practical applications. Urinary alkalinisation, achieved by intravenous infusion of sodium bicarbonate (Ch. 18), is an effective way of accelerating the excretion of certain acidic drugs such as **barbiturates** (Ch. 30) or **aspirin** (Chs 12 and 16), and is employed in treating selected cases of drug overdose. Acidification of the urine accelerates excretion of basic drugs such as amphetamine (Fig. 4.17), although this is seldom used clinically. Alkalinisation of the urine has been used by athletes bent on illicit use of amphetamine to reduce its renal elimination, thus prolonging its effect and rendering its detection in urine more difficult (although this ruse is easily detected by checking urine pH).

Drug excretion expressed as clearance

Renal clearance, CL_r, is defined as the volume of plasma containing the amount of substance that is removed by the kidney in unit time. It is calculated from the plasma concentration, C_p, the urinary concentration, C_u, and the rate of flow of urine, V_u, by the equation:

$$CL_r = \frac{C_u V_u}{C_p} \tag{4.2}$$

The clearance of a substance depends, of course, on how it is handled by the processes of filtration, active secretion and passive diffusion; in relation to drug excretion, three special cases are relevant:

- A drug (e.g. **gallamine**; Ch. 6) that is completely filtered (i.e. not protein-bound), but neither reabsorbed nor secreted. This is the pharmacological equivalent of *inulin*, and its clearance will correspond to the glomerular filtration rate (about 120 ml/min in a young healthy adult).
- A drug that is completely removed (by active tubular secretion) during a single transit through the kidney. This is the pharmacological equivalent of *p-aminohippuric acid* (PAH) and its clearance will correspond to the renal plasma flow—about 700 ml/min. The nearest familiar example is **penicillin** (Ch. 37), though its clearance is lower than that of PAH.
- A drug that reaches equilibrium between plasma and urine by passive diffusion. If the drug is not ionised, or if the urinary pH is the same as that of plasma, the urinary concentration will equal the free plasma concentration; if the drug

is not protein-bound, the clearance will simply equal the rate of urine formation—usually about 1 ml/min but highly variable. For weak acids (e.g. **aspirin**; Chs 12 and 16) and bases (e.g. **morphine**; Ch. 31) this value will be multiplied by the pH partition factor (see Fig. 4.3), and it will also be reduced in proportion to the fraction of drug bound to plasma albumin.

Thus, the rate of renal clearance of drugs can vary very greatly, from less than 1 ml/min to the theoretical maximum of about 700 ml/min. The interpretation of these values in terms of the rate at which drugs are removed from the body, expressed as *plasma half-life*, is discussed in a later section.

As well as varying markedly from drug to drug, renal elimination varies considerably amongst individuals, and from time to time in the same individual, for reasons that are discussed in more detail in Chapter 42. For a small but important group of drugs (Table 4.6), which are not inactivated by metabolism, the rate of renal elimination is the main factor that determines their duration of action. These drugs have to be used with special care in individuals whose renal function may be impaired, including the elderly and patients who are suffering any severe acute illness.

Table 4.6 Drugs that are excreted largely unchanged in the urine

100–75%	Amiloride, frusemide, chlorothiazide, gentamicin, methotrexate, atenolol, digoxin, pyridostigmine
75–50%	Carbenicillin, benzylpenicillin, cimetidine, cephaloridine, oxytetracycline, neostigmine
~50%	Propantheline, tubocurarine

Elimination of drugs by the kidney

- Most drugs, except those highly bound to plasma protein, cross the glomerular filter freely.
- Many drugs, especially weak acids, are actively secreted into the renal tubule, and thus more rapidly excreted.
- Lipid-soluble drugs are passively reabsorbed by diffusion across the tubule, so are not efficiently excreted in the urine.
- Because of pH partition, weak acids are more rapidly excreted in alkaline urine, and vice versa.
- Several important drugs are removed predominantly by renal excretion, and are liable to cause toxicity in elderly persons and patients with renal disease.

The clearance concept is also useful in quantifying the rate of metabolic degradation of drugs, since this can be expressed in terms of the volume of plasma containing the amount of drug that is metabolised in unit time. Thus the overall rate of metabolism can be denoted by CL_{met}.

BILIARY EXCRETION AND ENTEROHEPATIC CIRCULATION

Liver cells transfer various substances from plasma to bile by means of transport systems similar to those of the renal tubule. In addition to acid- and base-handling systems, hepatocytes have a third mechanism that transports various uncharged molecules. Various hydrophilic drug conjugates (particularly glucuronides) are concentrated in bile and delivered to the intestine where the glucuronide is usually hydrolysed, releasing active drug once more; free drug can then be reabsorbed and the cycle repeated (enterohepatic circulation).

The effect of this is to create a 'reservoir' of recirculating drug that can amount to about 20% of total drug in the body and prolongs drug action. Examples where this is important include **digoxin** (Ch. 13), which is excreted in the bile in an unconjugated form, and **morphine** (Ch. 31), **chloramphenicol** (Ch. 37) and **ethinyloestradiol** (Ch. 22), which are transported as glucuronides. Several drugs are excreted to an appreciable extent in bile. **Vecuronium** (widely used as a non-depolarising muscle relaxant; Ch. 6) is an example of a drug that is excreted mainly unchanged in bile. **Rifampicin** (Ch. 37) is absorbed from the gut and gradually deacetylated, retaining its biological activity. Both forms are secreted in the bile, but the deacetylated form is not reabsorbed, so eventually most of the drug leaves the body in this form, in the faeces.

PHARMACOKINETICS

We have now discussed the various processes of absorption, distribution, metabolism and elimination of drugs that determine their overall kinetic behaviour. In this section a simple quantitative model is presented which provides a view of how the system will behave when these processes are operating simultaneously, and which will, in particular, enable us to predict the time-course of drug action (an extremely important characteristic from a clinical point of view).

SINGLE-COMPARTMENT MODEL

Consider first a highly simplified model of a human being, which consists of a single well-stirred compartment (of volume V_d) into which a quantity of drug Q is introduced rapidly by intravenous injection, and from which it can escape either by being metabolised or excreted (Fig. 4.18). The initial concentration, $C(0)$, will be Q/V_d. The concentration $C(t)$ at a later time t will depend on the rate of elimination of the drug. Most drugs exhibit first-order kinetics where elimination is directly proportional to drug concentration. Drug concentration then decays exponentially (Fig. 4.19), being described by the equation:

$$C(t) = C(0)\exp\frac{-CL_s}{V_d}.t \qquad (4.3)$$

where CL_s is the total clearance of the drug, equal to the sum of the clearance by metabolism and by renal excretion. Taking logarithms:

$$\ln C(t) = \ln C(0) - \frac{CL_s}{V_d}.t \qquad (4.4)$$

Thus, plotting $C(t)$ logarithmically against t yields a straight line with slope $-CL_s/V_d$. This slope is the *elimination rate constant*, k_{el}. The *half-life*, $t_{½}$, is an easily conceptualised parameter inversely related to k_{el}. It is the time taken for $C(t)$ to decrease by 50% and is equal to $\ln 2/k_{el}$ ($0.693/k_{el}$). The plasma half-life is therefore determined by the distribution volume V_d and clearance CL_s.

Effect of repeated dosage schedules

Usually drugs are given as repeated doses rather than single injections. A continuous infusion can be regarded as the extreme of a repeated dose schedule. In this case the plasma concentration increases until a steady-state concentration, *C(steady state)*, is reached where the rate of infusion, X, equals the rate of elimination. The rate of elimination is equal to $CL_s \cdot C(steady\ state)$, so that:

$$C(steady\ state) = \frac{X}{CL_s} \qquad (4.5)$$

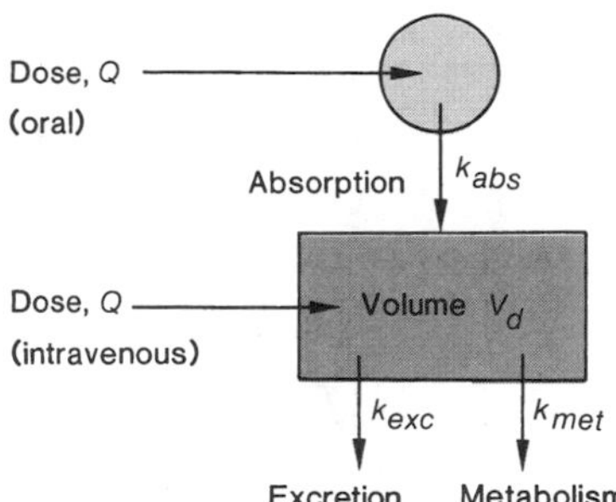

Fig. 4.18 Single-compartment pharmacokinetic model.

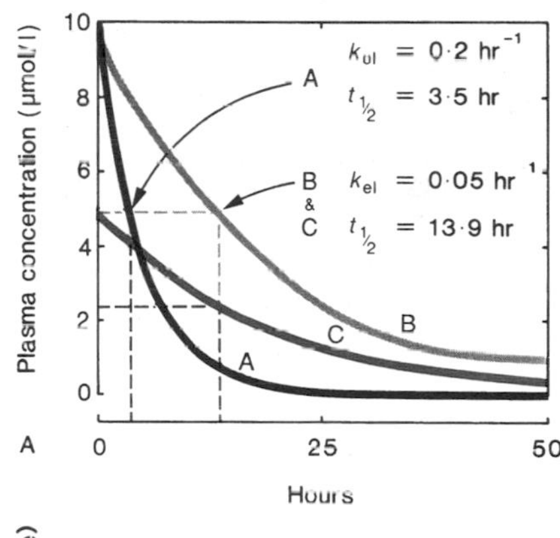

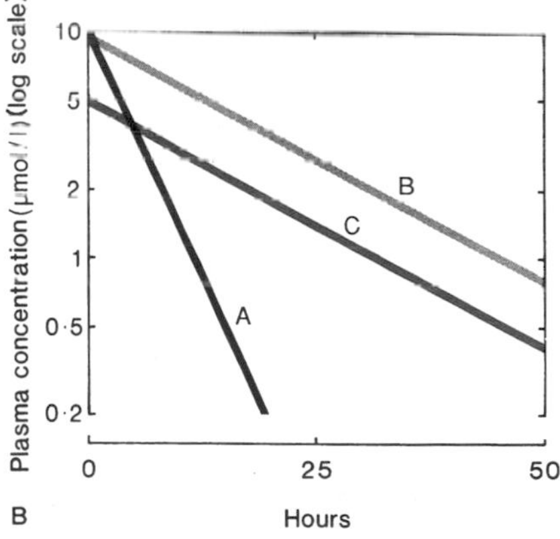

Fig. 4.19 Predicted behaviour of single-compartment model following intravenous drug administration at time 0. Drugs A and B differ only in their elimination rate constant, k_{el}. Curve C shows the plasma concentration time-course for a smaller dose of B. Note that t (indicated by broken lines) does not depend on the dose. **A.** Linear concentration scale. **B.** Logarithmic concentration scale.

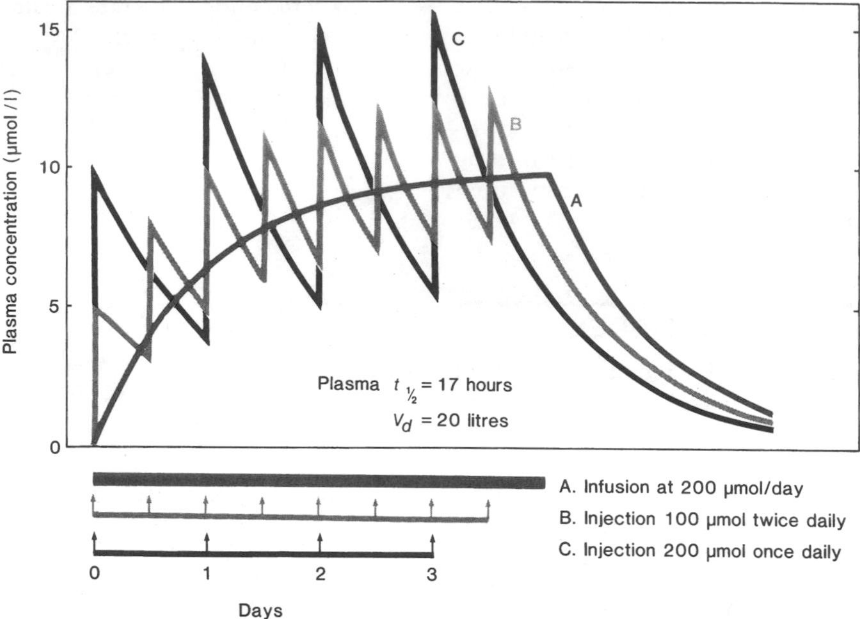

Fig. 4.20 Predicted behaviour of single-compartment model with continuous or intermittent drug administration. Smooth curve A shows the effect of continuous infusion for 4 days; curve B the same total amount of drug given in eight equal doses; and curve C the same total amount of drug given in four equal doses. Note that in each case a steady state is effectively reached after about 2 days (about 3 × $t_{1/2}$), and that the mean concentration reached in the steady state is the same for all three schedules.

The drug concentration approaches this steady-state value exponentially, with a half-time equal to $t_{1/2}$ (Fig. 4.20). Repeated injections (each of dose Q) give a more complicated pattern but the principle is the same. The concentration will rise to a mean steady-state concentration with an approximately exponential time-course but will oscillate (through a range Q/V_d). The smaller and more frequent the doses the more closely the situation approaches that of a continuous infusion and the smaller the swings in concentration. The exact dosage schedule, however, does not affect the *mean* steady-state concentration, nor the rate at which it is approached. In practice, a steady state is effectively achieved after 3 plasma half-times. Speedier attainment of the steady state can be achieved by starting with a larger dose. Such a *loading* dose is sometimes useful, for example when starting treatment of a patient with rapid atrial fibrillation with **digoxin** (Ch. 13). It must again be emphasised that the simple behaviour predicted for the single-compartment model only roughly corresponds to real life. Inclusion of other body compartments, particularly slowly-equilibrating ones such as body fat, will result in additional exponential components in the overall kinetic behaviour. Pharmacokinetic studies in man show that to produce a realistic simulation the inclusion of two or three compartments is often necessary (see later).

Effect of variation in rate of absorption

If a drug is absorbed slowly from the gut or from an injection site into the plasma, it is (in terms of a compartmental model) as though it were being injected slowly into the bloodstream. For the purpose of kinetic modelling, the transfer of drug from the site of administration to the central compartment can be represented approximately by a rate constant, k_{abs} (see Fig. 4.18). This assumes that the rate of absorption is directly proportional, at any moment, to the amount of drug still unabsorbed, which is at best a rough approximation to reality. The effect of slow absorption on the time-course of the rise and fall of the plasma concentration is shown in Figure 4.21. The curves show the effect of spreading out the absorption of the same total

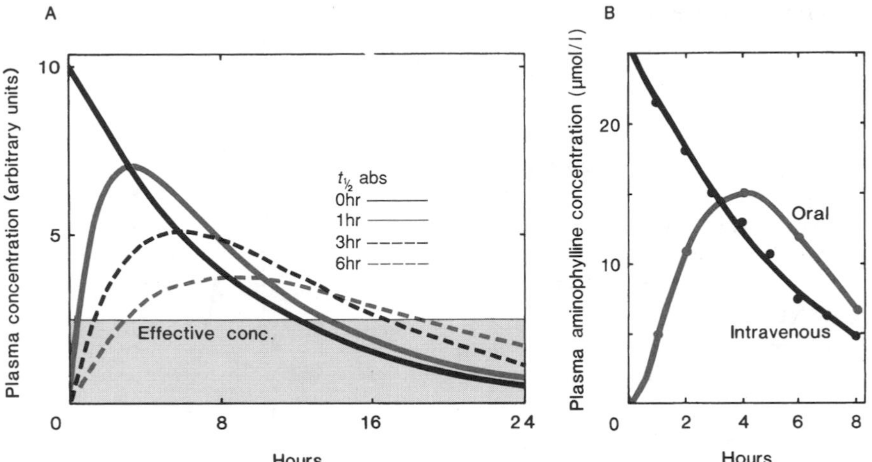

Fig. 4.21 The effect of slow drug absorption on plasma drug concentration.
A. Predicted behaviour of single-compartment model with drug absorbed at different rates from the gut or an injection site. The elimination half-time is 6 hours. The absorption half-times are marked on the diagram. (Zero indicates instantaneous absorption, corresponding to intravenous administration.) Note that the peak plasma concentration is reduced and delayed by slow absorption, and the duration of action somewhat increased. **B.** Measurements of plasma aminophylline concentration in man following equal oral and intravenous doses. (Data from: Swintowsky J V 1956 J Am Pharm Assoc 49: 395)

amount of drug over different periods of time. In each case, all of the drug is absorbed, but the peak concentration appears later and becomes lower and less sharp if absorption is slow. Once absorption is complete, the plasma concentration declines with the same half-time, irrespective of the rate of absorption.

It can be shown that, for the kind of pharmacokinetic model discussed here, the *area* under the plasma concentration–time curve (often abbreviated to AUC, for *Area Under the Curve*) is directly proportional to the total amount of drug introduced into the plasma compartment, irrespective of the rate at which it enters. Comparison of the AUC following oral and intravenous administration can therefore be used to determine the fraction of the oral dose that enters the bloodstream, and thus to measure *bioavailability* (see p. 76). Incomplete absorption, or destruction by first-pass metabolism before the drug reaches the plasma compartment, will mean that the AUC for oral administration will be smaller than that for intravenous administration, whereas changes in the *rate* of absorption will not affect it. Again it is worth noting that provided absorption is complete the relation between the rate of administration and the steady-state plasma concentration (equation 4.5) is unaffected by k_{abs}, though the size of the oscillation of plasma concentration with each dose will be reduced if absorption is slow.

MORE COMPLICATED KINETIC MODELS

So far we have considered a single-compartment pharmacokinetic model in which the rates of absorption, metabolism and excretion are all assumed to be directly proportional to the concentration of drug in the compartment from which transfer is occurring. This is a useful way to illustrate some basic principles, but is clearly a physiological oversimplification. The characteristics of different parts of the body, such as brain, body fat and muscle, are quite different in terms of their blood supply, partition coefficient for drugs and the permeability of their capillaries to drugs. These differences, which the single-compartment model ignores, can considerably affect the time-course of drug distribution and drug action, and much theoretical work has gone into the mathematical analysis of more complex models. Discussions can be found in specialised texts (e.g. Notari 1980). They are beyond the scope of this book, and perhaps also beyond the limit of what is actually useful, for the experimental data on pharmacokinetic properties of drugs are seldom accurate or reproducible enough to enable complex models to be tested critically.

The two-compartment model, which introduces a separate 'peripheral' compartment to represent the tissues, in communication with the 'central' plasma compartment, more closely resembles the real situation without involving excessive complications.

Two-compartment model

The two-compartment model is a widely-used approximation in which the tissues are lumped together as a peripheral compartment which drug molecules can enter and leave only via the central compartment (Fig. 4.22) which normally represents the plasma. For some drugs, however, which equilibrate particularly rapidly with extravascular compartments, some of these compartments may also be included in the central compartment. The effect of adding a second compartment to the model is to introduce a second exponential component into the predicted time-course of the plasma concentration, so that it comprises a fast and a slow phase. This pattern is often found experimentally, and is most clearly revealed when the concentration data are plotted semilogarithmically (Fig. 4.23). If, as is often the case, the transfer of drug between the central and peripheral compartments is relatively fast compared with the rate of elimination, then the fast phase (often called the *α-phase*) can be taken to represent the redistribution of the drug (i.e. drug molecules passing from plasma to tissues thereby rapidly lowering the plasma concentration). The plasma concentration reached when the fast phase is complete, but before any elimination has occurred, allows a measure of the combined distribution volumes of the two compartments; the half-time for

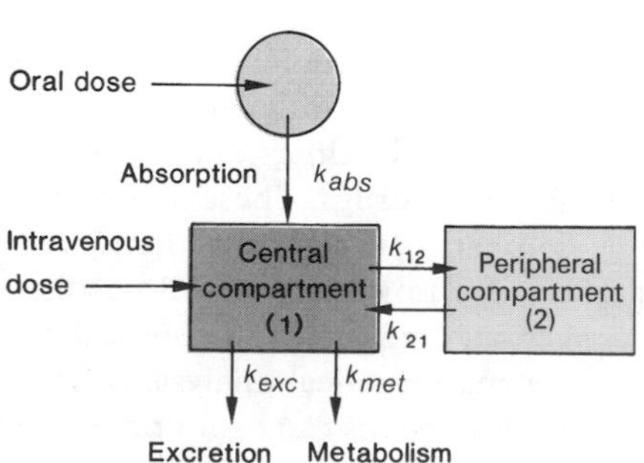

Fig. 4.22 Two-compartment pharmacokinetic model.

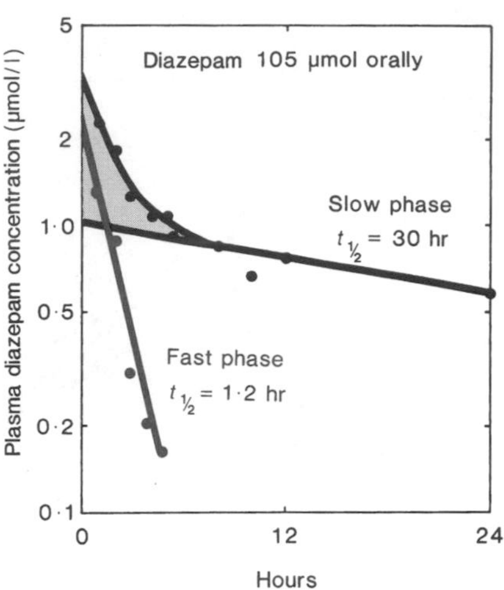

Fig. 4.23 Kinetics of diazepam elimination in man following a single oral dose. (The graph shows a semilogarithmic plot of plasma concentration versus time.) The experimental data (black symbols) follow a curve that becomes linear after about 8 hours (slow phase). Plotting the deviation of the early points (light red shaded area) from this line on the same coordinates (red symbols) reveals the fast phase. This type of two-component decay is consistent with the two-compartment model (Fig. 4.22) and is obtained with many drugs. (Data from: Curry S H 1980 Drug disposition and pharmacokinetics. Blackwell, Oxford)

the slow phase (the *β-phase*) provides an estimate of the rate constant for elimination, k_{el}. If a drug is rapidly metabolised, the α- and β-phases are not well separated and the calculation of V_d and k_{el} is not straightforward. Problems also arise with drugs (e.g. very fat-soluble drugs) for which it is unrealistic to lump all the peripheral tissues together, so caution is needed in the interpretation of such pharmacokinetic data.

It is important to realise that the addition of extra compartments to the basic model affects only the predicted time-course of drug action, and not the steady state. Thus the relation between plasma concentration and dose derived for the single-compartment model (equation 4.5) still applies.

Saturation kinetics

In a few cases where drugs are inactivated by metabolic degradation, such as **ethanol** (Ch. 33), **phenytoin** (Ch. 30) and **salicylate** (Ch. 12), the time-course of disappearance of drug from the plasma does not follow the exponential or bi-exponential pattern shown in Figures 4.19 and 4.23, but is initially linear (i.e. the drug is removed at a constant rate that is *independent* of plasma concentration). This is often called *zero-order kinetics* to distinguish it from the usual *first-order kinetics* which we have considered so far (terms that have their origin in chemical kinetic theory), though *saturation kinetics* is a better term. Figure 4.24 shows the

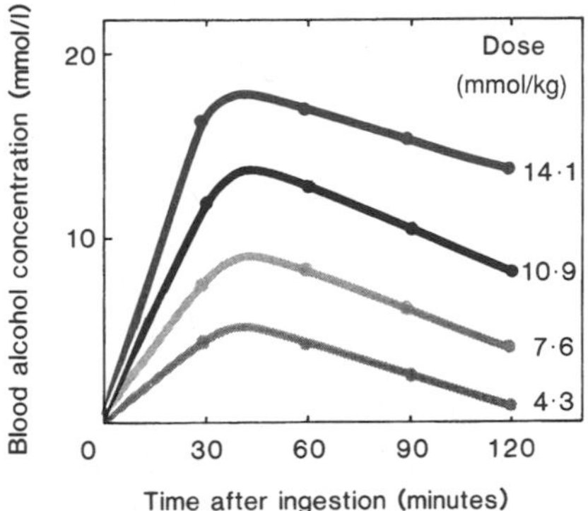

Fig. 4.24 Saturating kinetics of alcohol elimination in man. The blood alcohol concentration falls linearly rather than exponentially, and the rate of fall does not vary with dose. (From: Drew G C et al. 1958 Br Med J 2: 5103)

example of ethanol. It can be seen that the rate of disappearance of ethanol from the plasma is constant at about 4 mmol/l per hour irrespective of its plasma concentration. The explanation for this is that the rate of oxidation by the enzyme alcohol dehydrogenase reaches a maximum at low ethanol concentrations because of limited availability of the cofactor, NAD^+ (see Ch. 33).

Saturation kinetics can have several important consequences (see Fig. 4.25). One is that the duration of action is more strongly dependent on dose than is the case with drugs that do not show metabolic saturation. Another consequence is that the relationship between dose and steady-state plasma concentration is steep and unpredictable, and does not obey the proportionality rule implicit in equation 4.5 for non-saturating drugs. The maximum rate of metabolism sets a limit to the rate at which the drug can be administered, and if this rate is exceeded, the amount of drug in the body will, in principle, increase indefinitely and never reach a steady state (Fig. 4.25). This does not actually happen because there is always some dependence of

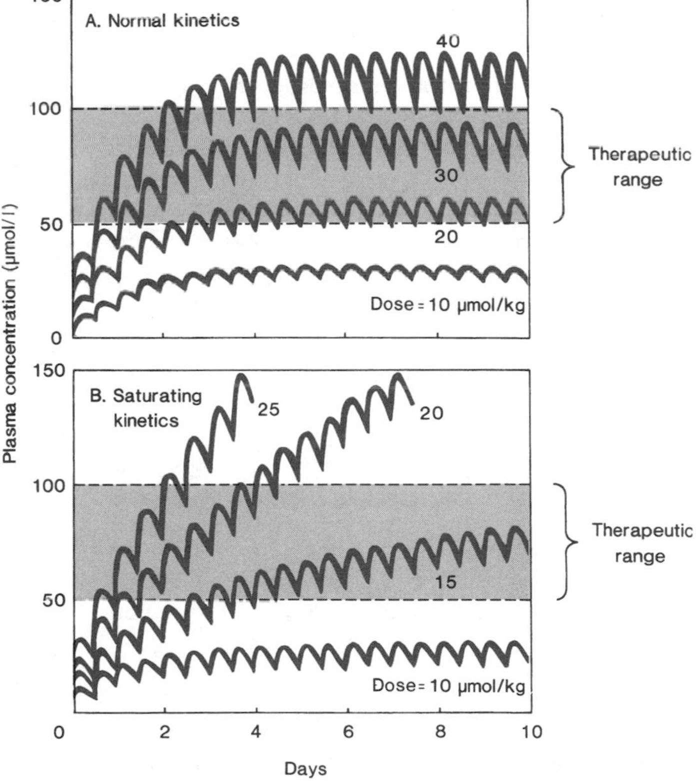

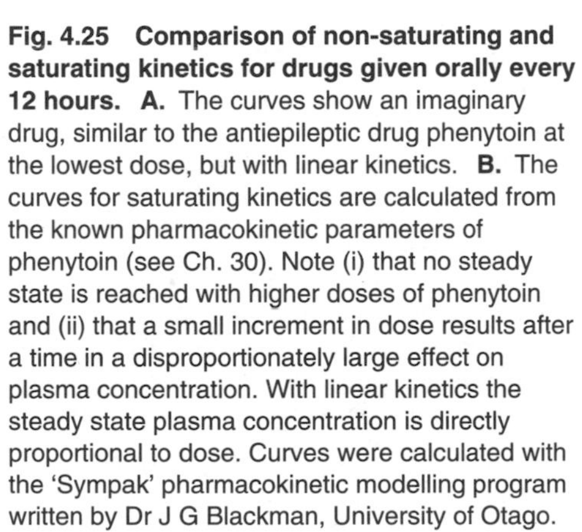

Fig. 4.25 Comparison of non-saturating and saturating kinetics for drugs given orally every 12 hours. A. The curves show an imaginary drug, similar to the antiepileptic drug phenytoin at the lowest dose, but with linear kinetics. **B.** The curves for saturating kinetics are calculated from the known pharmacokinetic parameters of phenytoin (see Ch. 30). Note (i) that no steady state is reached with higher doses of phenytoin and (ii) that a small increment in dose results after a time in a disproportionately large effect on plasma concentration. With linear kinetics the steady state plasma concentration is directly proportional to dose. Curves were calculated with the 'Sympak' pharmacokinetic modelling program written by Dr J G Blackman, University of Otago.

Pharmacokinetics

- For many drugs, disappearance from the plasma follows an exponential time-course characterised by the plasma half-life.
- Plasma half-life, in the simple case, is directly proportional to the volume of distribution, and inversely proportional to the overall rate of clearance.
- With repeated dosage or sustained delivery of a drug, the plasma concentration approaches a steady value within 3–5 plasma half-lives.
- A two-compartment model is often needed. In this case the kinetics become bi-exponential. The two components roughly represent the processes of transfer between plasma and tissues (α-phase) and elimination from the plasma (β-phase).
- Some drugs show non-exponential 'saturation' kinetics, with important clinical consequences, especially a disproportionate increase in steady-state plasma concentration when daily dose is increased, and disproportionately prolonged effects following increased doses.

the rate of elimination on the plasma concentration (usually because other, non-saturating metabolic pathways or renal excretion contribute significantly at high concentrations). Nevertheless, the steady-state plasma concentration of drugs of this kind varies with dose more widely and less predictably than it does with non-saturating drugs. Similarly, variations in the rate of metabolism (e.g. through enzyme induction) also produce disproportionately large changes in the plasma concentration. These problems are well recognised for drugs such as **phenytoin**, an antiepileptic drug (see Ch. 30) whose plasma concentration needs to be closely controlled to achieve an optimal clinical effect.

SPECIAL DRUG DELIVERY SYSTEMS

Several new approaches are being actively explored in an attempt to improve drug delivery (see Vaizoglu & Speiser 1982, Gregoriadis 1982, 1989, Prescott & Nimmo 1989 for reviews). They include:

- sustained-release preparations to avoid the need for frequent dosage
- pro-drugs
- antibody–drug conjugates
- packaging in liposomes.

Sustained-release preparations. Depot preparations of esterified phenothiazines (e.g. **fluphenazine undecanoate**) which are slowly hydrolysed, and whose antipsychotic action lasts for weeks after a single injection, are one example of sustained-release preparations which avoid the need for frequent dosage. Incorporation of drugs into injectable polymers, or conjugation with proteins, are other ways of achieving sustained release (see Prescott & Nimmo 1989). Osmotic mini-pumps can be swallowed to deliver drugs such as **metoprolol** or **nifedipine** at a constant rate during transit of the gastrointestinal tract are mentioned above (p. 76). More elaborately, implantable mini-pumps are being developed for administering **insulin**, and feedback control is even being incorporated with the aid of a glucose sensor so that the insulin delivery is adjusted to physiological needs.

Pro-drugs. Examples of pro-drugs are given in Table 4.4 (see also p. 86). Some of the examples in clinical practice confer no obvious benefits, and have been found to be pro-drugs only retrospectively, not having been designed with this in mind. However, some do have advantages. For example, the cytotoxic drug **cyclophosphamide** (see Ch. 36) becomes active only after it has been metabolised in the liver, and can therefore be taken orally without causing serious damage to the gastrointestinal epithelium. **Levodopa** is absorbed from the gastrointestinal tract and crosses the blood–brain barrier via an amino acid transport mechanism before conversion to active dopamine in nerve terminals in the basal ganglia (Ch. 24), whereas **dopamine** is administered intravenously for its effects on renal vasculature (Ch. 14). **Zidovudine** is phosphorylated to its active trisphosphate metabolite only in cells containing appropriate reverse transcriptase, hence conferring selective toxicity toward cells infected with the human immunodeficiency virus (Ch. 38). Other problems could theoretically be overcome by the use of suitable pro-drugs; for example instability of drugs at gastric pH, direct gastric irritation (aspirin was synthesised in the last century in a deliberate attempt to produce a pro-drug for salicylic acid that would be tolerable when taken by mouth), poor absorbability, failure of drug to cross blood–brain barrier and so on. Audus recently reviewed the influence of chemical and biological factors on brain uptake of drugs (Audus et al. 1992). Progress with this approach remains slow, however, and Albert (1965) warns the optimistic pro-drug designer '... he will have to bear in mind that an organism's normal reaction to a foreign substance is to burn it up for food.'

Antibody–drug conjugates. One of the aims of cancer chemotherapy is to improve the selectivity of cytotoxic drugs (see Ch. 36). One interesting possibility is to attach the drug to an antibody directed against a tumour-specific antigen, which will bind selectively to tumour cells. Such approaches look promising in experimental animals, but it is still too early to say whether they will succeed in man.

Packaging in liposomes. Liposomes are minute vesicles produced by sonication of an aqueous suspension of certain phospholipids. They can be filled with non-lipid-soluble drugs, which are retained until the liposome is disrupted. When injected, liposomes are mainly taken up by reticulo-endothelial cells, especially in the liver, and there is a possibility of achieving selective delivery of drugs (e.g. in hepatic amoebiasis or hepatic tumours) in this way. **Amphotericin**, an antifungal drug used to treat systemic mycoses (Ch. 39), is available in a liposomal formulation that is less nephrotoxic and better tolerated than the conventional form, albeit considerably more expensive. In the future, it may also be possible to direct drugs selectively by incorporating antibody molecules against specific tissue antigens into the surface of such particles, but this has yet to be proved in terms of clinical efficacy.

REFERENCES AND FURTHER READING

Albert A 1965 Selective toxicity, 3rd edn. Chapman & Hall, London

Ariens E J 1986 Chirality in bioactive agents and its pitfalls. Trends Pharmacol Sci 7: 200–205

Audus K L, Chikhale P J, Miller D W, Thompson S E, Borchadt R T 1992 Brain uptake of drugs: chemical and biological factors. Adv Drug Res 23: 1–64

Bundgaard H, Hansen A B, Kofod H 1982 Optimization of drug delivery. Munskgaard, Copenhagen

Caldwell J, Jakoby W B 1983 Biological basis of detoxification. Academic Press, London

Curry S H 1980 Drug disposition and pharmacokinetics. Blackwell, Oxford

de Leve L D, Piafsky K M 1983 Clinical significance of plasma binding of basic drugs. In: Lamble J W (ed) Drug metabolism and distribution. Elsevier, London

Gibaldi M 1984 Biopharmaceutics and clinical pharmacokinetics. Lea & Febiger, Philadelphia

Gibaldi M, Perrier D 1975 Pharmacokinetics. Dekker, New York

Gibaldi M, Prescott L 1983 Handbook of clinical pharmacokinetics. ADIS Health Service Press, Sydney

Gibson G, Skett P 1986 Introduction to drug metabolism. Chapman & Hall, London

Gonzalez F J 1989 The molecular biology of cytochrome P450s. Pharmacol Rev 40: 243–288

Gorrod J W, Beckett A H 1978 Drug metabolism in man. Taylor & Francis, London

Gregoriadis G 1982 Use of monoclonal antibodies and liposomes to improve drug delivery. Drugs 24: 261–266

Gregoriadis G 1989 Targetting of drugs: implications in medicine. In: Roerdink F H O, Kroon A M (eds) Drug carrier systems. John Wiley & Sons, Chichester

Juliano R L 1980 Drug delivery systems: characteristics and biomedical applications. Oxford University Press, Oxford

Jusko, W J, Gretch M 1976 Plasma and tissue protein binding of drugs in pharmacokinetics. Drug Metab Rev 5: 43

Kremer J M H, Wilting J, Janssen L M H 1988 Drug binding to human α-1-acid glycoprotein in health and disease. Pharmacol Rev 40: 1–47

Lamble J W (ed) 1983 Drug metabolism and distribution. Elsevier, Amsterdam

Nebert D W, Gonzalez F J 1985 Cytochrome P-450 gene expression and regulation. Trends Pharmacol Sci 16: 160–164

Notari R E 1980 Biopharmaceutics and clinical pharmacokinetics. Dekker, New York

Pardridge W M 1988 Recent advances in blood–brain barrier transport. Annu Rev Pharmacol Toxicol 28: 25–39

Prescott L F, Nimmo W S 1989 Novel drug delivery. John Wiley & Sons, Chichester

Richens A, Marks V 1981 Therapeutic drug monitoring. Churchill Livingstone, Edinburgh

Theorell P, Dedrick R L, Condliffe P G 1974 Pharmacology & pharmacokinetics. Plenum, London

Trager W F, Testa B 1985 Stereoselective drug disposition. In: Wilkinson G R, Rawlins M D (eds) Drug metabolism and disposition. MTP Press, Lancaster

Vaizoglu O, Speiser P 1982 'Intelligent' drug delivery systems. Trends Pharmacol Sci 3: 28–30

Wagner J G 1975 Do you need a pharmacokinetics model and, if so, which one? J Pharmacokinet Biopharm 3: 457

CHEMICAL MEDIATORS

5

CHEMICAL TRANSMISSION AND THE AUTONOMIC NERVOUS SYSTEM

The profusion of chemical signals by which cells in the body communicate with one another provides many opportunities for specific drug effects. This chapter concerns the process of chemical transmission in the peripheral nervous system, and the various ways in which the process can be pharmacologically subverted. In addition to *neurotransmission,* we also consider briefly the less clearly defined processes, collectively termed *neuromodulation,* by which many mediators and drugs exert control over the function of the nervous system. Many of the same mechanisms operate also in the central nervous system, and the same general principles apply, but the relative anatomical and physiological simplicity of the peripheral nervous system has made it the proving ground for most of the important discoveries about chemical transmission. These discoveries have been central to the understanding and classification of many major types of drug action, so it is apt to recount briefly how the subject first developed. An excellent account is given by Bacq (1975).

In the latter half of the nineteenth century, when experimental physiology became established as an approach to the understanding of living organisms, the peripheral nervous system, and particularly the autonomic nervous system, received a great deal of attention. The fact that electrical stimulation of nerves could elicit a whole variety of physiological effects—from blanching of the skin to arrest of the heart—presented a real challenge to comprehension, particularly of the way in which the signal was passed from the nerve to the effector tissue. In 1877, Du Bois Raymond was the first to put the alternatives clearly: 'Of known natural processes that might pass on excitation, only two are, in my opinion, worth talking about—either there exists at the boundary of the contractile substance a stimulatory secretion...; or the phenomenon is electrical in nature.' The latter view was more generally believed. In 1869 it had been shown that an exogenous substance, **muscarine**, could mimic the effects of stimulating the vagus nerve, and that **atropine** could inhibit the actions both of muscarine and of nerve stimulation. In 1905, Langley showed the same for **nicotine** and **curare** acting at the neuromuscular junction. These phenomena were generally ascribed, respectively, to stimulation and inhibition of the nerve endings, rather than to interference with a chemical transmitter.

Credit for suggesting, in 1904, that **adrenaline** might act as a chemical transmitter mediating the actions of the sympathetic nervous system goes to T R Elliot. The suggestion was coolly received, until J N Langley, the authoritarian Professor of Physiology at Cambridge at that time, suggested, a year later, that transmission to skeletal muscle involved the secretion by the nerve terminals of a substance related to nicotine.

One of the key observations for Elliot was that degeneration of sympathetic nerve terminals did not abolish the sensitivity of smooth muscle preparations to **adrenaline** (which the electrical theory predicted) but actually enhanced it. The hypothesis of chemical transmission was put to direct test by Dixon in 1907, who tried to show that vagus nerve stimulation released from a dog's heart into the blood a substance capable of inhibiting another heart. The experiment failed, and the atmosphere of scepticism discouraged Dixon from pursuing it.

Thus it was not until 1921, in Germany, that Loewi showed that stimulation of the vagosympathetic trunk to an isolated and cannulated frog's heart could cause the release into the cannula of a substance ('Vagusstoff') that, if the cannula fluid was transferred from the first heart to a second, would inhibit the second heart. This is a classic and much-quoted experiment that proved extremely difficult for even Loewi to perform reproducibly. In an autobiographical sketch, Loewi tells us that the idea of chemical transmission arose in a discussion that he had in 1903, but no way of testing it experimentally occurred to him until he dreamed of the appropriate experiment one night in 1920. He wrote some notes of this very important dream in the middle of the night, but in the morning could not read them. The dream obligingly returned the next night, and, taking no chances, he went to the laboratory at 3 a.m. and carried out the experiment successfully. Loewi's experiment may be, and was, criticised on numerous grounds (it could, for example, have been potassium rather than a neurotransmitter that was acting on the recipient heart), but a series of further experiments proved him to be right. His findings can be summarised as follows:

- Stimulation of the vagus caused the appearance in the perfusate of the frog heart of a substance capable of producing, in a second heart, an inhibitory effect resembling vagus stimulation.
- Stimulation of the sympathetic nervous system caused the appearance of a substance capable of accelerating a second heart. By fluorescence measurements, Loewi concluded later that this substance was adrenaline.
- **Atropine** prevented the inhibitory action of the vagus on the heart but did not prevent release of 'Vagusstoff'. Atropine thus prevented the effects, rather than the release, of the transmitter.
- When 'Vagusstoff' was incubated with ground-up frog heart muscle it became inactivated. This effect is due to enzymatic destruction of acetylcholine by cholinesterase.
- **Physostigmine** (eserine), which potentiated the effect of vagus stimulation on the heart, prevented destruction of 'Vagusstoff' by heart muscle, providing evidence that the potentiation is due to inhibition of cholinesterase which normally destroys the transmitter substance acetylcholine.

A few years later, in the early 1930s, Dale showed convincingly that acetylcholine was also the transmitter substance at the neuromuscular junction of striated muscle and at autonomic ganglia. One of the keys to Dale's success lay in the use of very highly sensitive bioassays, especially the leech dorsal muscle, for measuring acetylcholine release (see Ch. 3).

Chemical transmission at sympathetic nerve terminals was demonstrated at about the same time as cholinergic transmission and by very similar methods. Loewi's experiments on the frog heart had demonstrated the release of 'Acceleranstoff' when the sympathetic nerves were stimulated, but this work was strongly criticised. Cannon and his colleagues at Harvard first showed unequivocally the phenomenon of chemical transmission at sympathetic nerve endings, by experiments in vivo in which tissues made supersensitive to adrenaline by prior sympathetic denervation were shown to respond, after a delay, to the transmitter released by stimulation of the sympathetic nerves to other parts of the body. The chemical identity of the transmitter, tantalisingly like adrenaline, but not identical to it, caused a good deal of confusion for some years, until in 1946 von Euler showed it to be the non-methylated derivative, **noradrenaline**.

THE PERIPHERAL NERVOUS SYSTEM

The peripheral nervous system consists of the following principal elements:

- autonomic nervous system, which incudes the enteric nervous system
- somatic efferent system, innervating skeletal muscle
- somatic and visceral afferent system.

In this chapter we are concerned mainly with the autonomic nervous system, which for a long time occupied centre stage in the pharmacology of chemical transmission. Aspects of the somatic efferent system are considered in Chapter 6. It is becoming increasingly recognised that *afferent* nerves (particularly the non-myelinated nerves subserving nociceptive and other functions; see Ch. 31) also have important *effector* functions in the periphery, mediated mainly by neuropeptides (Ch. 9).

BASIC ANATOMY AND PHYSIOLOGY OF THE AUTONOMIC NERVOUS SYSTEM

The autonomic nervous system (see Gibbins 1990) consists of three main anatomical divisions, *sympathetic* and *parasympathetic* (see Fig. 5.1), and the *enteric nervous system* (see Furness & Costa 1987), consisting of the intrinsic nerve plexuses of the gastrointestinal tract, which is closely interconnected with the sympathetic and parasympathetic systems.

The autonomic nervous system conveys all of the outputs from the central nervous system to the rest of the body except for the motor innervation of skeletal muscle. The enteric nervous system has sufficient integrative capabilities to allow it to function in the absence of any input from the central nervous system, but the sympathetic and parasympathetic systems are essentially agents of the central nervous system, and cannot function without it. The autonomic nervous system is largely outside the influence of voluntary control. The main processes that it regulates are:

- contraction and relaxation of smooth muscle
- all exocrine and certain endocrine secretions
- the heartbeat
- certain steps in intermediary metabolism.

There is some argument about whether the term 'autonomic nervous system' should be extended to include the many afferent fibres that innervate viscera. From a pharmacological and functional point of view it is the efferent pathways that are distinctive, and the afferent fibres will not be discussed in this section.

The main difference between the autonomic and the somatic efferent pathways is that the former consists of two neurons arranged in series, whereas in the latter a single motoneuron connects the central nervous system to the skeletal muscle fibre (Fig. 5.2). The two neurons in the autonomic pathway are known respectively as *preganglionic* and *postganglionic* and they synapse in an *autonomic ganglion*, which lies outside the central nervous system and contains the nerve endings of preganglionic fibres and the cell bodies of postganglionic fibres.

The sympathetic preganglionic neurons have their cell bodies in the lateral horn of the grey matter of the thoracic and lumbar segments of the spinal cord, and the fibres leave the spinal cord in the

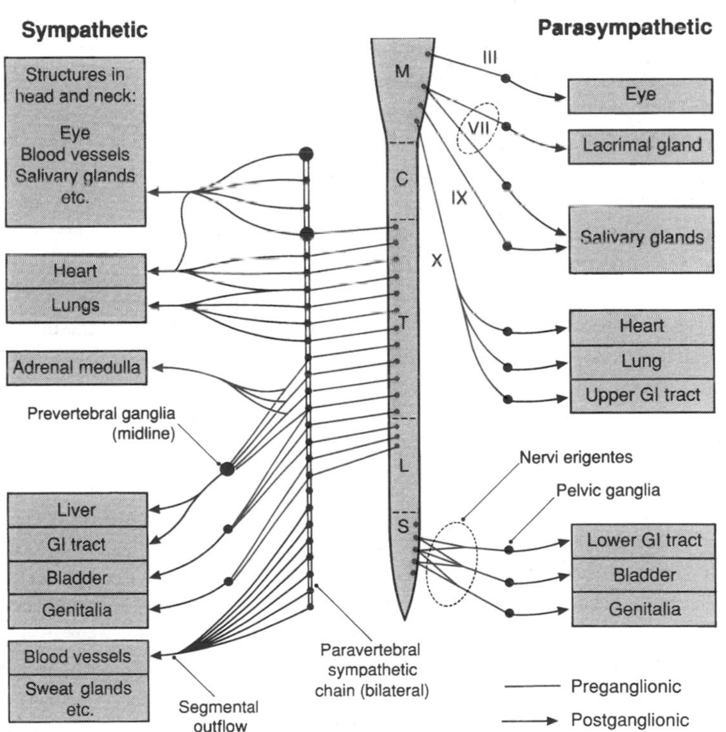

Fig. 5.1 Basic plan of the mammalian autonomic nervous system. (M = medullary; C = cervical; T = thoracic; L = lumbar, S = sacral)

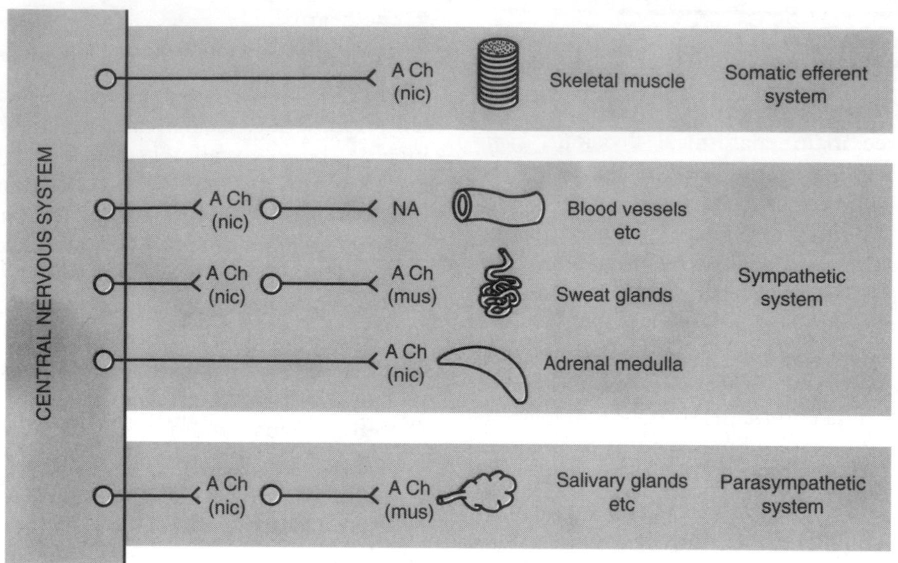

Fig. 5.2 Acetylcholine (ACh) and noradrenaline (NA) as transmitters in the peripheral nervous system. The two types of acetylcholine receptor, nicotinic (nic) and muscarinic (mus) (see Ch. 6), are indicated.

spinal nerves as *thoracolumbar sympathetic outflow.* Just outside the spinal cord they leave the spinal nerve as filaments that run to the *paravertebral chain* of sympathetic ganglia, which lies bilaterally on either side of the spinal column. These ganglia contain the cell bodies of the postganglionic sympathetic neurons, the axons of which rejoin the spinal nerve. Many of the postganglionic sympathetic fibres reach their peripheral destinations via the branches of the spinal nerves. Others, destined for abdominal and pelvic viscera, have their cell bodies in a group of unpaired *prevertebral ganglia* in the abdominal cavity. The only exception to the two-neuron arrangement is the innervation of the adrenal medulla, which secretes catecholamines in response to activity in the nerves supplying it. The cells of the adrenal medulla are, in effect, modified postganglionic sympathetic neurons, and the nerves supplying the gland are equivalent to preganglionic fibres.

The parasympathetic nerves emerge from two separate regions of the central nervous system. The *cranial outflow* consists of preganglionic fibres in certain cranial nerves, namely the oculomotor nerve (carrying parasympathetic fibres destined for the eye), the facial and glossopharyngeal nerves (carrying fibres to the salivary glands and the nasopharynx) and the vagus nerve (carrying fibres to the thoracic and abdominal viscera). The ganglia lie scattered in close relation to the target organs; the postganglionic neurons are very short compared with those of the sympathetic system. Parasympathetic fibres destined for the pelvic and abdominal viscera emerge as the *sacral outflow* from the spinal cord in a bundle of nerves known as the *nervi erigentes* (since stimulation of these nerves evokes erection of genital organs—a fact of some importance to those responsible for artificial insemination of livestock). These fibres synapse in a group of scattered pelvic ganglia, whence the short postganglionic fibres run to target tissues such as the bladder, rectum and genitalia. The pelvic ganglia carry both sympathetic and parasympathetic fibres, and the two divisions are not anatomically distinct in this region.

The enteric nervous system (Fig. 5.3; see Gershon 1981, Furness & Costa 1987) consists of the neurons whose cell bodies lie in the intramural plexuses in the wall of the intestine. It is estimated that there are more cells in this system than in the spinal cord, and functionally they do not fit simply into the sympathetic/parasympathetic classification. Incoming nerves from both the sympathetic and the parasympathetic systems terminate on enteric neurons, as well as running directly to smooth muscle, glands and blood vessels. Some of the neurons function as

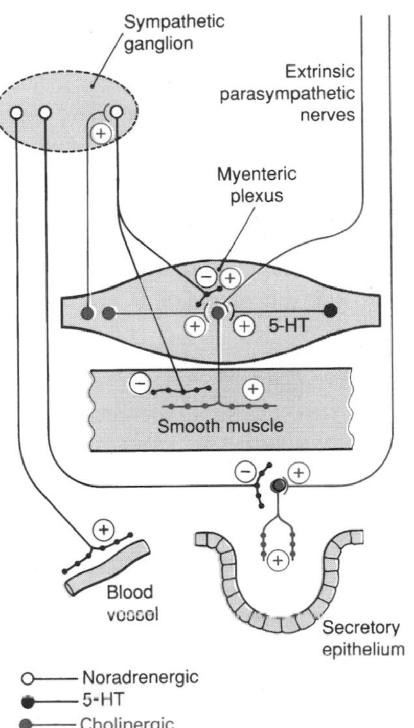

Fig. 5.3 Simplified diagram showing functional connections of the enteric nervous system. The main pathways involving acetylcholine, noradrenaline and 5-hydroxytryptamine are shown, but peptidergic nerves are not. There is actually an extensive network of peptide-releasing nerves in the enteric system; furthermore many neurons co-release peptides along with the conventional monoamine transmitters shown here. (See Furness & Costa 1987 for more details.)

mechanoreceptors or chemoreceptors, providing local reflex pathways that can control gastrointestinal function without external inputs. The enteric nervous system is pharmacologically more complex than the sympathetic or parasympathetic systems, involving many neuropeptide and other transmitters (such as 5-hydroxytryptamine) and is often described as a collection of 'little brains' outside the central nervous system, rather like those of many invertebrates. See Furness & Costa (1987) for a comprehensive account.

In some places (e.g. in the visceral smooth muscle of the gut and bladder and in the heart) the sympathetic and the parasympathetic systems produce opposite effects, but there are others where only one division of the autonomic system operates. The sweat glands and most blood vessels, for example, have only a sympathetic innervation, whereas the ciliary muscle of the eye has only a parasympathetic innervation. Bronchial smooth muscle has only a parasympathetic (constrictor) innervation (though its tone is highly sensitive to circulating adrenaline—acting probably on the constrictor innervation rather than on the smooth muscle directly). There are other examples, such as the salivary glands, where the two systems produce similar, rather than opposing, effects.

It is therefore a mistake to think of the sympathetic and parasympathetic systems as physiological opponents. Each serves its own physiological function and can be more or less active in a particular organ or tissue according to the need of the moment. Cannon rightly emphasised the general role of the sympathetic system in evoking 'fight or flight' reactions in an emergency, but emergencies are rare for most animals. The role of the autonomic nervous system in everyday life is to control specific functions from moment to moment (see Janig & MacLachlan 1992); the popular concept of a continuum from the extreme 'rest and digest' state (parasympathetic active, sympathetic quiescent) to the extreme emergency 'fight or flight' state (sympathetic active, parasympathetic quiescent) is a crude oversimplification.

Table 5.1 lists some of the more important autonomic responses in man.

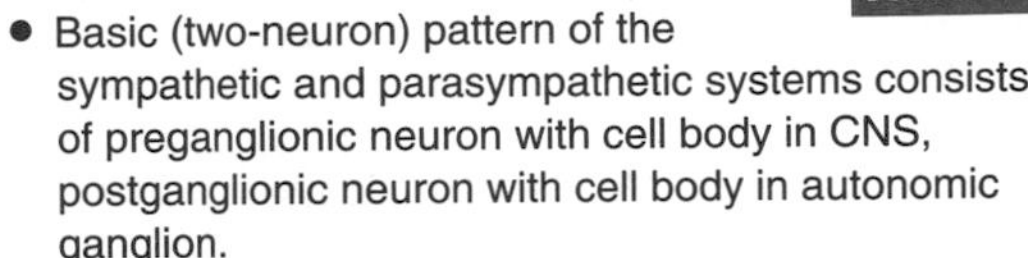

Basic anatomy of the autonomic nervous system

- Basic (two-neuron) pattern of the sympathetic and parasympathetic systems consists of preganglionic neuron with cell body in CNS, postganglionic neuron with cell body in autonomic ganglion.
- Parasympathetic system is connected to the CNS via:
  —cranial nerve outflow (III, VII, IX, X)
  —sacral outflow.
- Parasympathetic ganglia usually lie close to target organ.
- Sympathetic outflow leaves CNS in thoracic and lumbar spinal roots. Sympathetic ganglia form two paravertebral chains, plus some midline ganglia.
- The enteric nervous system consists of neurons lying in the intramural plexuses of the gastrointestinal tract. It receives inputs from sympathetic and parasympathetic systems, but can act on its own to control the motor and secretory functions of the intestine.

Table 5.1 The main effects of the autonomic nervous system

Organ	Sympathetic	Receptor type	Parasympathetic	Receptor type
Heart				
SA node	Rate ↑	β_1	Rate ↓	M_2
Atrial muscle	Force ↑	β_1	Force ↓	M_2
AV node	Automaticity ↑	β_1	Cond. vel. ↓ AV block	M_2 M_2
Ventricular muscle	Automaticity ↑ Force ↑	β_1	No effect	
Blood vessels				
Arterioles				
Coronary	Constriction	α		
Muscle	Dilatation	β_2	No effect	
Viscera Skin Brain	Constriction	α	No effect	
Erectile tissue Salivary gland	Constriction	α α	Dilatation	? M_3
Veins	Constriction Dilatation	α β_2	No effect	
Viscera				
Bronchi				
Smooth muscle	No sympathetic innervation, but dilated by circulating adrenaline	β_2	Constriction	M_3
Glands	No effect		Secretion	M_3
GI tract				
Smooth muscle	Motility ↓	α_1, α_2, β_2	Motility ↑	M_3
Sphincters	Constriction	α_2, β_2	Dilatation	M_3
Glands	No effect		Secretion Gastric acid secretion	M_3 M_1
Uterus				
pregnant	Contraction	α	Variable	
non-pregnant	Relaxation	β_2		
Male sex organs	Ejaculation	α	Erection	? M_3
Eye				
Pupil	Dilatation	α	Constriction	M_3
Ciliary muscle	Relaxation (slight)	β	Contraction	M_3
Skin				
Sweat glands	Secretion (mainly cholinergic)	α	No effect	
Pilomotor	Piloerection	α	No effect	
Salivary glands	Secretion	α, β	Secretion	M_3
Lacrimal glands	No effect		Secretion	M_3
Kidney	Renin secretion	β_2	No effect	
Liver	Glycogenolysis Gluconeogenesis	α, β_2	No effect	

Note: The receptor types given for the sympathetically and parasympathetically mediated responses are discussed more fully in Chapters 6 and 7.

TRANSMITTERS IN THE AUTONOMIC NERVOUS SYSTEM

The two main neurotransmitters that operate in the autonomic system are **acetylcholine** and **noradrenaline,** whose sites of action are shown diagrammatically in Figure 5.2. This diagram also shows the type of postsynaptic receptor with which the transmitters interact at the different sites. This

Physiology of the autonomic nervous system

- The autonomic system controls: smooth muscle (visceral and vascular); exocrine (and some endocrine) secretions; rate and force of the heart; certain metabolic processes (e.g. glucose utilisation).
- Sympathetic and parasympathetic systems have opposing actions in some situations (e.g. control of heart rate, gastrointestinal smooth muscle); but not in others (e.g. salivary glands, ciliary muscle).
- Sympathetic activity increases in stress (fight-or-flight response) whereas parasympathetic activity predominates during satiation and repose. Both systems exert a continuous physiological control of specific organs under normal conditions, when the body is at neither extreme.

receptor classification is discussed more fully in Chapters 6 and 7. Certain generalisations are valid:

- All motor nerve fibres leaving the central nervous system release acetycholine, which acts on nicotinic receptors (although in autonomic ganglia a minor component of excitation is due to activation of muscarinic receptors (see Ch. 6)).
- All postganglionic parasympathetic fibres release acetylcholine, which acts on muscarinic receptors.

Transmitters of the autonomic nervous system

- The principal transmitters are acetylcholine and noradrenaline.
- Preganglionic neurons are cholinergic, ganglionic transmission occurs via nicotinic ACh receptors (though excitatory muscarinic ACh receptors are also present on postganglionic cells).
- Postganglionic parasympathetic neurons are cholinergic, acting on muscarinic receptors in target organs.
- Postganglionic sympathetic neurons are mainly noradrenergic, though a few are cholinergic (e.g. sweat glands).
- Transmitters other than noradrenaline and acetylcholine (NANC transmitters) are also used extensively in the autonomic nervous system. NANC transmitters include nitric oxide, 5-HT, ATP, dopamine, GABA and several neuropeptides.
- Co-transmission may be a general phenomenon.

- All postganglionic sympathetic fibres (with one important exception) release noradrenaline, which may act on either α- or β-adrenoceptors (see Ch. 7). The exception, where transmission is due to acetylcholine acting on muscarinic receptors, is the sympathetic fibres supplying *sweat glands*. In some species, there is evidence for a cholinergic sympathetic nerve supply causing vasodilatation in skeletal muscle, but this does not exist in humans.

Acetylcholine and noradrenaline are the grandees among autonomic transmitters, and are central to understanding autonomic pharmacology. There is, however, an expanding retinue of chemical mediators known to be released by autonomic neurons (see below), whose functional significance is gradually becoming clearer.

TWO GENERAL PRINCIPLES OF CHEMICAL TRANSMISSION

Denervation supersensitivity

It is known, mainly from the work of Cannon on the sympathetic system, that if a nerve is cut and its terminals allowed to degenerate the structure supplied by it becomes supersensitive to the transmitter substance released by the terminals. Thus skeletal muscle, which normally responds to injected acetylcholine only if a large dose is given directly into the arterial blood supply, will, after denervation, respond by contracture to much smaller amounts. Other organs, such as salivary glands and blood vessels show similar supersensitivity to acetylcholine and noradrenaline when the postganglionic nerves degenerate, and there is evidence that pathways in the central nervous system show the same phenomenon.

Several mechanisms are known to contribute to denervation supersensitivity, but the extent and mechanism of the phenomenon varies from organ to organ. Reported mechanisms include the following:

- *Proliferation of receptors*. This is particularly marked in skeletal muscle, in which the number of acetylcholine receptors increases 20-fold or more after denervation; the receptors are no longer localised on the endplate region of the fibres. Elsewhere, much smaller increases in receptor number (about twofold) have often been reported, but there are examples where no change occurs.

- *Loss of mechanisms for transmitter removal.* At noradrenergic synapses the loss of neuronal uptake of noradrenaline contributes substantially to denervation supersensitivity. At cholinergic synapses a partial loss of cholinesterase occurs.
- *Increased postjunctional responsiveness.* In some cases the postsynaptic cells become supersensitive without a corresponding increase in the number of receptors. Thus, smooth muscle cells become partly depolarised and hyperexcitable, and this phenomenon contributes appreciably to their supersensitivity. The mechanism of this change and its importance for other synapses is not known.

Supersensitivity can occur, but is less marked, when transmission is interrupted by processes other than nerve section. Pharmacological block of ganglionic transmission, for example, if sustained for a few days, causes some degree of supersensitivity of the target organs, and long-term blockade of postsynaptic receptors also causes receptors to proliferate, leaving the cell supersensitive when the blocking agent is removed. Phenomena such as this are of importance in the central nervous system, where such supersensitivity can cause 'rebound' effects when drugs are given for some time and then stopped.

Dale's principle

Dale's principle, advanced rather tentatively by him in 1934, states, in its modern form: 'A mature neuron makes use of the same transmitter at all of its synapses.' Dale considered it unlikely that a single neuron could store and release different transmitters at different nerve terminals, and his view has been substantiated by physiological and neurochemical evidence. It is known, for example, that the axons of motor neurons have branches that synapse on interneurons in the spinal cord, in addition to the main branch that innervates skeletal muscle fibres in the periphery. The transmitter at both the central and the peripheral nerve endings is acetylcholine, in accordance with Dale's principle. The enzymes involved in transmitter synthesis are produced in the cell body and transported to the terminals by axonal transport. The enzymes, and the transmitter itself, are present throughout the cell, and not just at the terminals, and it is rather unlikely that different sets of enzymes, corresponding to different transmitters, could be directed selectively to particular terminals.

Various pieces of recent evidence have been held to refute the generality of Dale's principle (see Burnstock 1976, 1981). Thus, it has been shown that sympathetic neurons, during development, switch from being cholinergic to being noradrenergic. It has also been shown that nerves can synthesise and release more than one transmitter at a time (co-transmission; see p. 111). Though Dale's principle was framed before these complexities were discovered, it is not seriously undermined by them; there is still no example of a neuron known to release different transmitters at different terminals.

OTHER INTERACTIONS IN THE AUTONOMIC NERVOUS SYSTEM

Though the representation of the autonomic system in Figures 5.1 and 5.2 is basically correct and serviceable, it is oversimplified, particularly in the following two respects:

- Chemical mediators act on *presynaptic* terminals to influence transmitter release, as well as on postsynaptic structures.
- In addition to the classical pair of chemical transmitters—acetylcholine and noradrenaline—many others are involved, and very often the same nerve terminal releases more than one mediator (*co-transmission*).

Presynaptic effects of chemical mediators are an example of the type of phenomenon often described as *neuromodulation* (see Kaczmarek & Levitan 1987, Rand et al. 1987, Burnstock 1987) since the mediator acts to increase or decrease the efficacy of synaptic transmission without participating directly as a transmitter. Neuromodulation also operates on postsynaptic cells. Many neuropeptides, for example, affect membrane ion channels in such a way as to increase or decrease excitability, and thus control the firing pattern of the cell. Neuromodulation is a term with as many definitions as authors, and it is not possible to distinguish unequivocally, on functional, anatomical or biochemical grounds, exactly how a neurotransmitter differs from a neuromodulator. In general, though, neuromodulation involves slower processes (taking seconds to days) compared with neurotransmission (which occurs in milliseconds); furthermore, neuromodulation operates through elaborate cascades of intracellular messengers (Ch. 2), rather than directly on ligand-gated ion channels. Some aspects of this problem of terminology are discussed in Chapter 11.

Presynaptic interactions

The presynaptic terminals that synthesise and release transmitter in response to electrical activity in the nerve fibre are often themselves sensitive to transmitter substances and to other substances that may be produced locally in tissues (for reviews see Vizi 1979, Starke et al. 1989). Such presynaptic effects can act either to enhance or to inhibit transmitter release. Figure 5.4 shows the inhibitory effect of adrenaline on the release of acetylcholine (evoked by electrical stimulation) from the postganglionic parasympathetic nerve terminals of the intestine. It is now known that these nerve terminals are sensitive to noradrenaline as well as adrenaline, and that release of noradrenaline from nearby sympathetic nerve terminals can also inhibit release of acetylcholine. There is anatomical evidence showing that noradrenergic and cholinergic nerve terminals often lie close together in the myenteric plexus, so it is likely that the opposing effects of the sympathetic and parasympathetic systems result not only from the opposite effects of the two transmitters on the smooth muscle cells, but also from the inhibition of acetylcholine release by noradrenaline acting on the parasympathetic nerve terminals. A similar situation exists in the heart, where a mutual presynaptic inhibition has been demonstrated; noradrenaline inhibits acetylcholine release, as in the myenteric plexus, and acetylcholine also inhibits noradrenaline release. There is good evidence not only for the type of *heterotropic* interaction described above, where one neurotransmitter affects the release of another, but also for *homotropic* interaction, where the transmitter, by binding to *presynaptic autoreceptors*, affects the nerve terminals from which it is being released. There is evidence (see Rand et al. 1982, Starke et al. 1989) that this type of *autoinhibitory feedback* acts powerfully at noradrenergic nerve terminals. One of the strongest pieces of evidence is that the amount of noradrenaline released from tissues in response to repetitive stimulation of sympathetic nerves is increased 10-fold or more in the presence of an antagonist that blocks the presynaptic noradrenaline receptors (see Ch. 7). This suggests that the released noradrenaline can inhibit further release by at least 90%.

A similar state of affairs seems to exist at cholinergic nerve terminals as well, where release of transmitter can be increased considerably by antagonists that block the inhibitory action of acetylcholine on its own nerve terminals. In both the noradrenergic and cholinergic systems the presynaptic autoreceptors are pharmacologically distinct from the postsynaptic receptors (see Chs 6 and 7), so that it has been possible to develop drugs that act selectively, as agonists or antagonists, on the pre- or postsynaptic receptors.

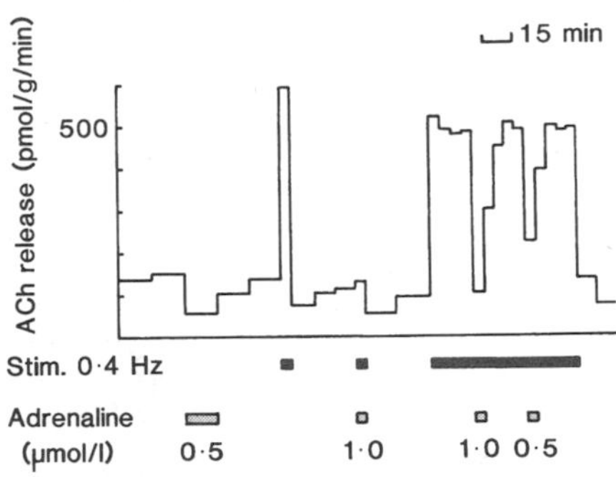

Fig. 5.4 Inhibitory effect of adrenaline on acetylcholine release from postganglionic parasympathetic nerves in the guinea-pig ileum. The intramural nerves were stimulated electrically where indicated, and the acetylcholine released into the bathing fluid determined by bioassay. Adrenaline strongly inhibits acetylcholine release. (From: Vizi 1979)

Cholinergic and noradrenergic nerve terminals respond not only to acetylcholine and noradrenaline, as described above, but also to other substances that may be present in tissues, including prostaglandins, purines (such as adenosine and ATP), dopamine, 5-hydroxytryptamine, gamma-aminobutyric acid (GABA), opioid peptides and many other substances. Evidence as to the physiological role and pharmacological significance of these multifarious interactions is incomplete, but there is no doubt that the simple description of the autonomic nervous system represented in Figure 5.2 is now a misleading oversimplification. Figure 5.5 shows some of the main presynaptic interactions that have been described between noradrenergic and cholinergic neurons of the autonomic nervous system, as well as showing some of the many chemical influences that are believed to regulate transmitter release from noradrenergic neurons.

The main mechanism by which presynaptic receptors regulate transmitter release is by affecting calcium entry into the nerve terminal (see Stjarne 1989). When a nerve terminal is depolarised by an

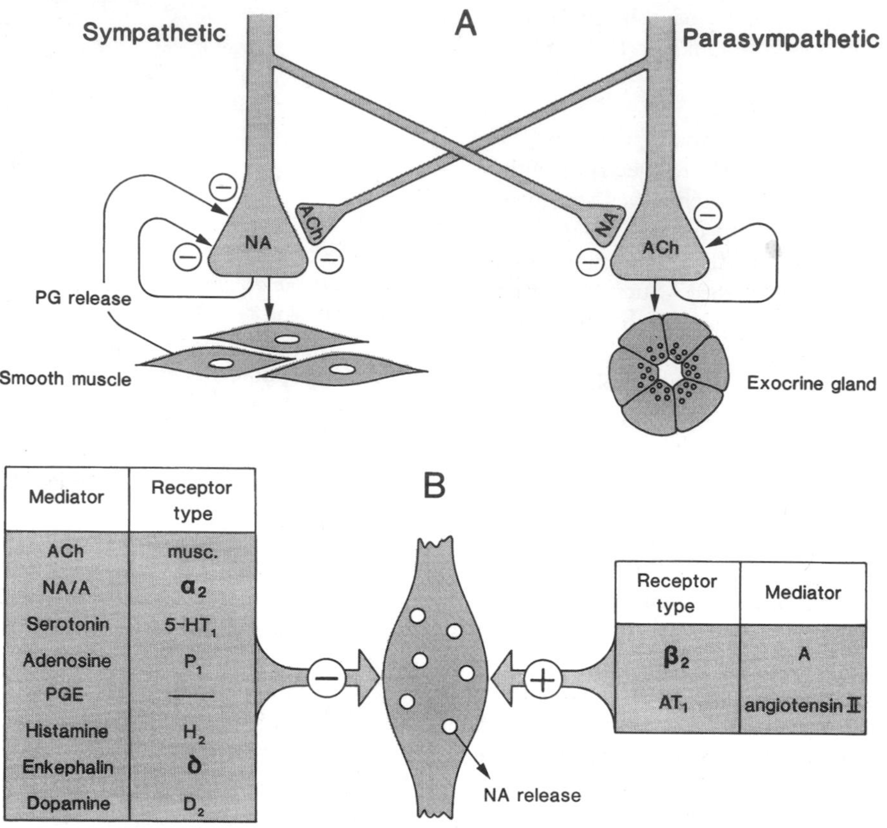

Mediator	Receptor type
ACh	musc.
NA/A	α_2
Serotonin	5-HT_1
Adenosine	P_1
PGE	——
Histamine	H_2
Enkephalin	δ
Dopamine	D_2

Receptor type	Mediator
β_2	A
AT_1	angiotensin II

Fig. 5.5 Presynaptic regulation of transmitter release from noradrenergic and cholinergic nerve terminals. A. Postulated homotropic and heterotropic interactions between sympathetic and parasympathetic nerves. **B.** Some of the known inhibitory and facilitatory influences on noradrenaline release from sympathetic nerve endings. (ACh = acetylcholine; A = adrenaline; NA = noradrenaline; PG = prostaglandin; PGE = prostaglandin E)

action potential, voltage-gated calcium channels open (see Fig. 5.10), and the resulting ingress of calcium is the trigger for transmitter-containing vesicles to discharge their contents into the synaptic cleft. Regulation of these calcium channels is mainly by phosphorylation (see Ch. 2). Most presynaptic receptors are of the G-protein-coupled type and are linked to phosphorylation events by either phospholipase C (which causes inhibition of calcium entry) or adenylate cyclase (which facilitates calcium entry). Other mechanisms may also contribute to presynaptic inhibition, such as an increased K^+-permeability, leading to hyperpolarisation of the terminal (analogous to the mechanism by which acetylcholine slows the heart; see Ch. 13), or impairment of the coupling between increased $[Ca^{2+}]_i$ and vesicle discharge (see Starke et al. 1989).

Postsynaptic modulation

Chemical mediators often act on postsynaptic structures, including neurons, smooth muscle cells, cardiac muscle cells, etc., in such a way that their excitability or spontaneous firing pattern is altered. In many cases, as with presynaptic modulation, the mechanisms appear to involve changes in calcium and/or potassium channel function mediated by a second messenger. We give only a few examples here:

- The slow excitatory effect produced by various mediators, including acetylcholine and peptides such as LHRH (see Ch. 22), on many peripheral and central neurons results mainly from a *decrease* in K^+-permeability. On the other hand, the inhibitory effect of various opiates is mainly due to *increased* K^+-permeability.

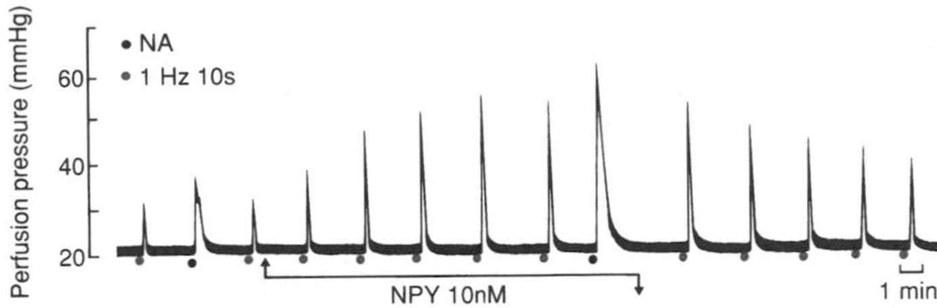

Fig. 5.6 Effect of neuropeptide Y (NPY) on noradrenergic transmission. Vasoconstriction (upward deflection) of the rabbit ear artery occurs in response to injections of noradrenaline (NA) (black symbols) or to a brief period of sympathetic nerve stimulation (red symbols). Infusion of a low concentration of NPY greatly increases the response to both. (From: Rand et al. 1987)

- Neuropeptide Y (NPY), which is released as a co-transmitter with noradrenaline at many sympathetic nerve endings and acts to enhance the vasoconstrictor effect of noradrenaline, thus greatly facilitating transmission (Fig. 5.6); the mechanism is not known.
- *Long-term potentiation* is a special and very long-lasting form of synaptic modulation associated with glutamate-mediated transmission in certain brain regions, and is believed to be important in memory. It is discussed further in Chapter 24.

Neuromodulation and presynaptic interactions

- As well as functioning directly as neurotransmitters, chemical mediators may regulate:
  —presynaptic transmitter release
  —neuronal excitability.
  Both are examples of neuromodulation, and generally involve second messenger regulation of membrane ion channels.
- Presynaptic receptors may inhibit or increase transmitter release, the former being more important.
- Inhibitory presynaptic autoreceptors occur on noradrenergic and cholinergic neurons, causing each transmitter to inhibit its own release (autoinhibitory feedback).
- Many endogenous mediators (e.g. GABA, prostaglandins, opioid and other peptides) as well as the transmitters themselves exert presynaptic control (mainly inhibitory) over autonomic transmitter release.

Transmitters other than acetylcholine and noradrenaline: NANC transmission

It was recognised many years ago that autonomic transmission in many organs could not be completely blocked by drugs that abolish responses to acetylcholine or noradrenaline, and it was acknowledged (though grudgingly) that other substances must be involved. The dismal but tenacious term *non-adrenergic non-cholinergic* (NANC) *transmission* was coined. The tide rapidly gathered strength when fluorescence and immunocytochemical methods showed that neurons, including autonomic neurons, contain many potential transmitters, often several in the same cell (see below). The abundance of possible mediators revealed by such studies (see Ch. 9) is in contrast to the number that are actually known to function physiologically as NANC transmitters or modulators in the periphery. Among these are *ATP*, *vasoactive intestinal peptide* (VIP), *neuropeptide Y* (NPY), gonadotrophin releasing hormone (GnRH; synonym LHRH), *5-hydroxytryptamine*, *γ-aminobutyric acid* (GABA) and *dopamine*. One of the most important NANC transmitters is nitric oxide whose recent discovery (see Ch. 10) has set off one of the most exciting pharmacological research trails in recent years. Table 5.2 summarises some well-documented examples of NANC transmitters.

Co-transmission

It is probably the rule rather than the exception that neurons release more than one transmitter or modulator (see Hokfelt et al. 1986, Furness et al. 1989), each of which interacts with specific receptors and produces effects, often both pre- and postsynaptically. We are only just beginning to understand the functional implications of this (see

Table 5.2 Examples of NANC transmitters and co-transmitters in the peripheral nervous system

Transmitter	Location	Function	Reference
Non-peptides			
ATP	Postganglionic sympathetic neurons (e.g. blood vessels, vas deferens)	Fast depolarisation/ contraction of smooth muscle cells	Review by Stjarne (1989)
GABA	Enteric neurons	Peristaltic reflex	Jessen et al. (1986)
5-HT			Gershon (1981)
Dopamine	Some sympathetic neurons (e.g. kidney)	Vasodilatation	Bell (1988)
NO	Pelvic nerves	Erection	see Ch. 10
NO	Gastric nerves	Gastric emptying	see Ch. 10
Peptides			
Neuropeptide Y (NPY)	Postganglionic sympathetic neurons (e.g. blood vessels)	Facilitates constrictor action of NA Inhibits NA release	Edvinsson et al. (1987)
Vasoactive intestinal peptide (VIP)	Parasympathetic nerves to salivary glands NANC innervation of airways smooth muscle	Vasodilatation Co-transmitter with ACh Bronchodilatation	Lundberg and Hokfelt (1983) Barnes (1987)
GnRH	Sympathetic ganglia	Slow depolarisation Co-transmitter with ACh	Jan and Jan (1983)
Substance P	Sympathetic ganglia Enteric neurons	Slow depolarisation Co-transmitter with ACh	Otsuka and Konishi (1983)
CGRP	Non-myelinated sensory neurons	Vasodilatation Vascular leakage Neurogenic inflammation	Foreman (1987) Saria et al. (1989)

Kupfermann 1991). The example of noradrenaline/ ATP co-transmission at the sympathetic nerve endings is shown in Figure 5.7, and the best-studied examples and mechanisms are summarised in Table 5.2 and Figure 5.8.

Faced with all this complexity, one might well ask: what can co-transmission achieve that could not be achieved with a single transmitter producing multiple effects via different receptors? One possibility is that one constituent of the cocktail (e.g. a

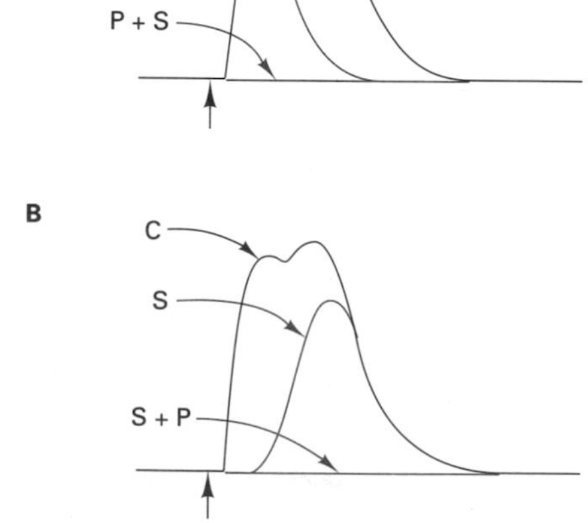

Fig 5.7 Noradrenaline/ATP co-transmission in the mouse vas deferens. Contractions of the tissue are shown in response to a single electrical stimulus causing excitation of sympathetic nerve endings. With no blocking drugs present (C), a twin-peaked response is produced. The late peak is blocked by the α_1-adrenoceptor antagonist, prazosin (P), while the early peak is selectively abolished by the ATP antagonist, suramin (S). The response is completely eliminated when both drugs are present (S + P).
(From: von Kugelglen & Starke 1991 Trends Pharmacol Sci 12: 319–324)

A. Presynaptic inhibition

Many noradrenergic and cholinergic terminals

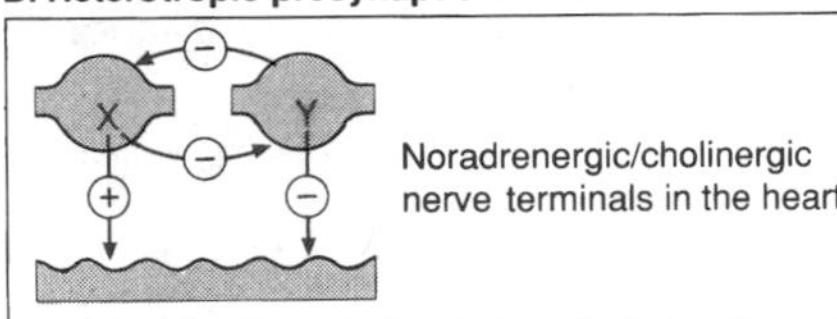

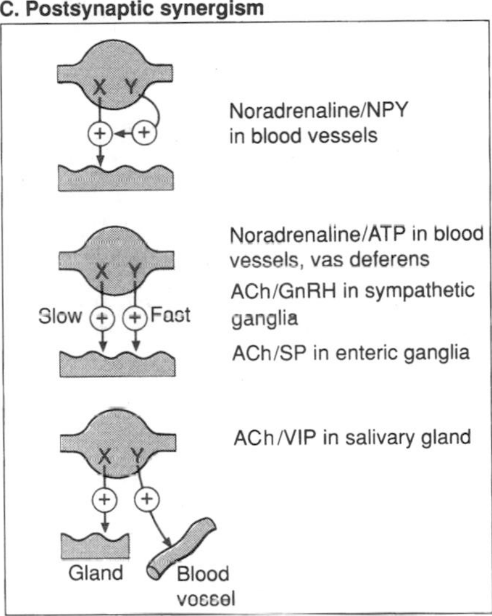

Fig. 5.8 Co-transmission and neuromodulation—some examples. A. Presynaptic inhibition. **B.** Heterotropic presynaptic inhibition. **C.** Postsynaptic synergism. (ACh = acetylcholine; NPY = neuropeptide Y; GnRH = gonadotrophin-releasing hormone = LHRH; SP = substance P; VIP = vasoactive intestinal peptide)

peptide) may be removed or inactivated more slowly than the other (e.g. a monoamine) and therefore reach targets further from the site of release, and produce longer-lasting effects. This appears to be the case, for example, with acetylcholine and GnRH in sympathetic ganglia (Jan & Jan 1983). Another possibility, which appears, for example, to operate with noradrenaline and NPY at sympathetic nerve terminals (see Stjarne 1989), is that the ratio of the two mediators released varies with stimulation frequency—higher frequencies releasing relatively more NPY. The implication is that differential release of one or other mediator may result from varying impulse patterns. Much remains to be discovered, and the advice given by Cooper et al. (1991) in a section entitled 'A reader's guide to peptide poaching' is worth repeating: 'Stay tuned, the data flow fast.' Not always quite as fast as the words, alas.

MECHANISMS OF TRANSMITTER RELEASE

The principal mechanism of transmitter release (see Fig. 5.9), in both the peripheral and central nervous systems, and also in many hormone-secreting cells, is *exocytosis*, whereby the transmitter is stored in intracellular vesicles, which fuse transiently with the cell membrane and discharge their contents, in response to an increase in the intracellular calcium concentration (see Nicholls et al. 1992). Though it has been studied in most detail for cholinergic and noradrenergic synapses, there is good evidence that other transmitters, including peptides, amino acids and purines, are all released in basically the same way. In neurons, the process is initiated by the arrival of an action potential, which depolarises

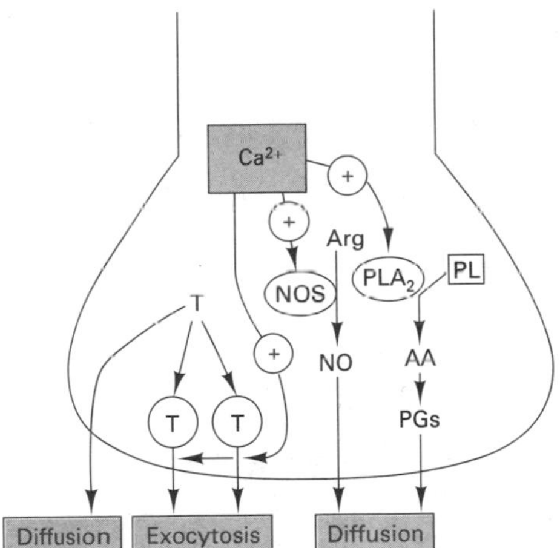

Fig. 5.9 Role of exocytosis and diffusion in mediator release. The main mechanism of release of monamine and peptide mediators is by Ca^{2+}-mediated exocytosis, but diffusional (or carrier-mediated) release from the cytosol also occurs. Nitric oxide (NO) and prostaglandins (PGs) are released by diffusion as soon as they are formed, from arginine (Arg) and arachidonic acid (AA) respectively, through the action of Ca^{2+}-activated enzymes, nitric oxide synthase (NOS) and phospholipase A_2 (PLA_2) (see Chs 10 and 11 for more details). T represents a conventional transmitter (e.g. acetylcholine, noradrenaline).

the membrane, thereby opening voltage-activated calcium channels and causing calcium to enter the cell. Evidence in favour of this mechanism comes from many sources, the most compelling being the early discovery, by Katz and his colleagues, that acetylcholine release at the neuromuscular junction is 'quantal' (i.e. occurs in discrete multimolecular packets), the direct observation of vesicle fusion during transmitter release, by rapid-freeze electron microscopy, and the correlation of release with sudden steps in the electrical capacitance of the membrane (as the vesicle fuses and increases the surface area of the cell). There is also biochemical evidence showing that, in addition to the transmitter, other constituents of the vesicles are released at the same time. If this neat and tidy picture of transmitter packets ready and waiting to pop obediently out of the cell in response to a puff of calcium seems a little too good to be true, rest assured that the picture is no longer quite so simple. Recently, for example, it has been shown that vesicles may fuse transiently with the cell membrane and release only part of their contents (see Neher 1993) before becoming disconnected. It is also known that monoamine transmitters can leak out of nerve endings from the cytosolic compartment, independently of vesicle fusion, partly by carrier-mediated transport; the functional significance of this is unknown.

There are now two important examples of mediator release, **nitric oxide** (see Bredt & Snyder 1992; Ch. 10) and **arachidonic acid metabolites** (e.g. prostaglandins; see Ch. 11), that do not involve vesicles and exocytosis, but rely on diffusion. The mediators are not stored, but escape from the cell as soon as they are synthesised. In both cases, the synthetic enzyme is activated by calcium, and the moment-to-moment control of the rate of synthesis depends on the intracellular calcium concentration. This kind of release is necessarily slower than the classical exocytotic mechanism, but in the case of nitric oxide, is fast enough for it to function as a true transmitter (see Chs 10 and 24).

Mechanisms of release of neurotransmitters and neuromodulators

- Most mediators are stored in presynaptic vesicles and released by exocytosis.
- Specialised synthetic enzymes and transport proteins are responsible for the uptake of precursors and synthesis and storage of individual mediators. These are often the targets for drugs that affect neurotransmission.
- Some important mediators (nitric oxide, prostaglandins) are synthesised 'on demand' and released by diffusion.
- Exocytosis, nitric oxide synthesis and prostaglandin synthesis are all activated by an increase in intracellular calcium concentration.

TERMINATION OF TRANSMITTER ACTION

Chemically transmitting synapses other than the peptidergic variety (Ch. 9) invariably incorporate a mechanism for rapidly disposing of the released transmitter, so that its action remains brief and localised. In most cases, a carrier-mediated transport mechanism exists in the presynaptic nerve membrane to recapture the transmitter; uptake by the postsynaptic cell, or by supporting cells such as glia, also plays a role. Cholinergic synapses (Ch. 6) are unusual in that the released acetylcholine is inactivated very rapidly in the synaptic cleft by acetylcholinesterase (Ch. 6). There is a family of these transporter proteins, each being specific for a particular transmitter (see Edwards 1992, Amara & Kuhar 1993). Several have now been isolated and cloned, and shown to belong to a distinct family, each molecule having 12 transmembrane helices. They all act as co-transporters of sodium ions, chloride ions and transmitter molecules, and it is the inwardly directed 'downhill' gradient for sodium that provides the energy for the inward 'uphill' movement of the transmitter. The simultaneous transport of several ions along with the transmitter means that the process generates a net current across the membrane, which can be measured directly, and used to monitor the transport process (Brew & Attwell 1988). Very similar mechanisms are responsible for other physiological transport processes, such as glucose uptake (Ch. 20) and renal tubular transport of amino acids. Since it is the electrochemical gradient for sodium ions that drives the inward transport of transmitter molecules, a reduction of this gradient can reduce or even reverse the flow of transmitter. This is probably not important under normal conditions, but when the nerve terminals are depolarised or abnormally loaded with sodium (e.g. in ischaemic conditions; see Attwell et al. 1993) the resulting non-vesicular release of transmitter (and prevention of the normal synaptic re-uptake mechanism) may play a significant role in the effects of ischaemia of tissues such as heart and brain (see Chs 13 and 25).

BASIC STEPS IN NEUROCHEMICAL TRANSMISSION—SITES OF DRUG ACTION

Figure 5.10 summarises the main processes that occur in a classical chemically transmitting synapse, and provides a useful basis for discussing the site of action of the many drugs that influence neurochemical transmission.

Though not all of these processes occur at all synapses, the scheme provides a useful basis for understanding the actions of the many different classes of drug, discussed in later chapters, which act by facilitating or blocking chemical transmission. Thus, all of the steps shown in Figure 5.10 (except for transmitter diffusion, step 8) can be influenced by drugs. For example, the enzymes involved in synthesis or inactivation of the transmitter can be inhibited by drugs, as can the transport systems responsible for the neuronal uptake of the transmitter or its precursor. In some cases the process can be changed in either direction. Thus, invasion of the nerve terminal by an action potential can be prevented by drugs such as local anaesthetics (Ch. 34), or enhanced by drugs such as 4-aminopyridine (Ch. 6). Similarly the receptors can be blocked or activated by exogenously applied drugs. The actions of the great majority of drugs that act on both the peripheral nervous system (Chs 6 and 7) and the central nervous system fit into this general scheme.

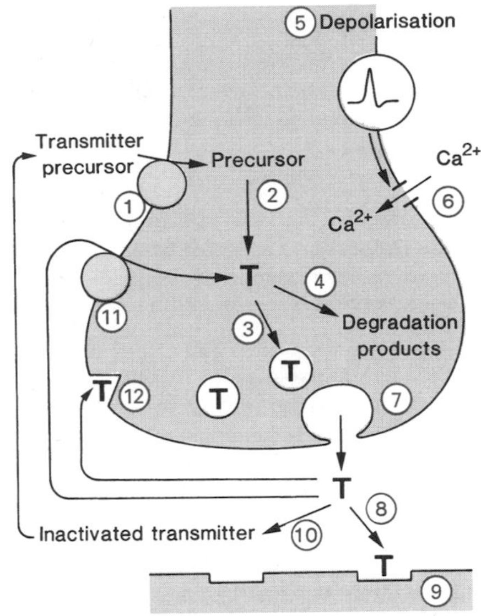

Fig. 5.10 The main processes involved in synthesis, storage and release of amine transmitters: 1 = uptake of precursors; 2 = synthesis of transmitter; 3 = storage of transmitter in vesicles; 4 = degradation of surplus transmitter; 5 = depolarisation by prolonged action potential; 6 = influx of Ca^{2+} in response to depolarisation; 7 = release of transmitter by exocytosis; 8 = diffusion to postsynaptic membrane; 9 = interaction with postsynaptic receptors; 10 = inactivation of transmitter; 11 = re-uptake of transmitter or degradation products; 12 = interaction with presynaptic receptors. These processes are well characterised for many transmitters (e.g. acetylcholine, noradrenaline, dopamine, 5-hydroxytryptamine), but may well differ significantly with other transmitters (e.g. amino acids, purines, peptides).

REFERENCES AND FURTHER READING

Amara S G, Kuhar M J 1993 Neurotransmitter transporters: recent progress. Ann Rev Neurosci 16: 73–93

Attwell D, Barbour B, Szatkowski M 1993 Non-vesicular release of neurotransmitter. Neuron 11: 401–407

Bacq Z M 1975 Chemical transmission of nerve impulses: a historical sketch. Pergamon Press, Oxford

Barnes P J 1987 Airway neuropeptides and asthma. Trends Pharmacol Sci 8: 24–27

Bell C 1982 Dopamine as a postganglionic autonomic neurotransmitter. Neuroscience 7: 1–8

Bell C 1987 Dopamine: precursor or neurotransmitter in sympathetically innervated tissues? Blood Vessels 24: 234–239

Bell C 1988 Dopamine release from sympathetic nerve terminals. Prog Neurobiol 30: 193–208

Bredt D S, Snyder S H 1992 Nitric oxide: a novel neuronal messenger. Neuron 8 3–11

Brew H, Attwell D I 1988 Electrogenic glutamate uptake is a major current carrier in the membrane of axolotl retinal ganglion cells. Nature 327: 707–709

Burnstock G 1972 Purinergic nerves. Pharm Rev 24: 509–581

Burnstock G 1976 Do some nerve cells release more than one transmitter? Neuroscience 1: 239–248

Burnstock G 1981 Review lecture. Neurotransmitters and trophic factors in the autonomic nervous system. J Physiol 313: 1–36

Burnstock G 1985 Purinergic mechanisms broaden their sphere of influence. Trends Neurosci 8: 5–6

Burnstock G 1987 Mechanisms of interaction of peptide and non-peptide vascular neuro-effector systems. J Cardiovasc Pharmacol 10 (Suppl 12): 574–581

Cooper J C, Bloom F E, Roth R H 1991 The biochemical basis of neuropharmacology. Oxford University Press, New York

Dunlap K, Fischbach G D 1981 Neurotransmitters decrease the calcium conductance activated by depolarisation of embryonic chick sensory neurons. J Physiol 317: 519–535

Edvinsson L, Hakanson R, Wahlestedt C, Uddman R 1987 Effects of neuropeptide Y on the cardiovascular system. Trends Pharmacol Sci 8: 231–235

Edwards R H 1992 The transport of neurotransmitters into synaptic vesicles. Curr Opin Neurobiol 2: 586–594

Foreman J C 1987 Peptides and neurogenic inflammation. Br Med Bull 43: 386–400

Furness J B, Costa M 1987 The enteric nervous system. Churchill Livingstone, Edinburgh

Furness J B, Morris J L, Gibbins I L, Costa M 1989 Chemical coding of neurons and plurichemical transmission. Annu Rev Pharmacol Toxicol 29: 289–306

Gershon M D 1981 The enteric nervous system. Annu Rev Neurosci 4: 227–272

Gibbins I L 1990 Peripheral autonomic nervous system. In: Paxinos G (ed) The human nervous system. Academic Press, San Diego

Hokfelt T, Fuxe K, Pernow B (eds) 1986 Coexistence of neuroactive substances in neurones: a new principle in chemical transmission. Progress in brain research. Elsevier, Amsterdam, vol 68

Jan Y N, Jan L Y 1983 A LHRH-like peptidergic neurotransmitter capable of 'action at a distance' in autonomic ganglia. Trends Neurosci 6: 320–325

Janig W, McLachlan E M 1992 Characteristics of function-specific pathways in the sympathetic nervous system. Trends Neurosci 15: 475–481

Jessen K R, Mirsky R, Mills J M 1986 GAGAergic neurons in the vertebrate peripheral nervous system. In: Erdo S L, Bowery N J (eds) GABAergic mechanisms in the mammalian periphery. Raven Press, New York

Kaczmarek L, Levitan I 1987 Neuromodulation. Oxford University Press, New York

Kalsner S 1982 The presynaptic receptor controversy. Trends Pharmacol Sci 8: 11–16

Kuffler S W, Nicholls J G, Martin A R 1984 From neuron to brain. Sinauer, New York

Kupfermann I 1991 Functional studies of cotransmission. Physiol Rev 71: 683–732

Lundberg J M, Hokfelt T 1983 Coexistence of peptides and conventional neurotransmitters. Trends Neurosci 6: 325–333

Neher E 1993 Secretion without full fusion. Nature 363: 497–498

Nicholls J G, Martin A R, Wallace B G 1992 From neuron to brain. Sinauer, Sunderland MA.

Otsuka M, Konishi S 1983 Substance P—the first peptide neurotransmitter? Trends Neurosci 6: 317–320

Pearse A G E 1983 The neuroendocrine division of the nervous system: APUD cells as neurones or paraneurones. In: Osborne N E (ed) Dale's principle and communication between neurones. Pergamon Press, Oxford

Rand M J 1992 Nitrergic transmission: nitric oxide as a mediator of non-adrenergic, non-cholinergic neuro-effector transmission. Clin Exp Pharmacol Physiol 19: 147–169

Rand M J, McCulloch M W, Story D F 1982 Feedback modulation of noradrenergic transmission. Trends Pharmacol Sci 3: 8–11

Rand M J, Majewski H, Wong-Dusting H, Story D F, Loiacono R E, Ziogas J 1987 Modulation of neuroeffector transmission. J Cardiovasc Pharmacol 10 (Suppl 12): S33–S44

Saria A, Yan Z, Wolf G, Loidolt D, Martling C R, Lundberg J M 1989 Control of vascular permeability and vascular smooth muscle in the respiratory tract by multiple neuropeptides. Acta Otorhinolaryngol 457 (Suppl): 25–28

Segal M 1983 Specification of synaptic action. Trends Neurosci 6: 118–121

Starke K, Gothert M, Kilbinger H 1989 Modulation of neurotransmitter release by presynaptic autoreceptors. Physiol Rev 69: 864–989

Stjarne L 1989 Basic mechanisms and local modulation of nerve impulse-induced secretion of neurotransmitters from individual sympathetic nerve varicosities. Rev Physiol Biochem Pharmacol 112: 4–137

Vizi E S 1979 Presynaptic modulation of neurochemical transmission. Prog Neurobiol 12: 181–290

6

CHOLINERGIC TRANSMISSION

This chapter is concerned mainly with cholinergic transmission in the periphery, and the way in which drugs affect it. Cholinergic mechanisms in the CNS and their relevance to dementia are discussed in Chapters 24 and 25.

The discovery of the pharmacological action of acetylcholine (ACh) arose from work on adrenal glands. Adrenal extracts were known to produce a rise in blood pressure owing to their content of adrenaline. In 1900, Reid Hunt found that after such extracts had been freed of adrenaline they produced a fall in blood pressure instead of a rise. He attributed the fall to their content of choline but at a later stage concluded that a more potent derivative of choline must be responsible. With Taveau he tested a number of choline derivatives and discovered that acetylcholine was some 100 000 times more active in lowering the rabbit's blood pressure. Although Hunt's studies suggested that acetylcholine may be a normal constituent of tissues, its physiological function was not apparent at that time and it remained for many years an interesting pharmacological curiosity.

MUSCARINIC AND NICOTINIC ACTIONS OF ACETYLCHOLINE

In a study of the pharmacological actions of acetylcholine carried out in 1914 Dale distinguished two types of activity which he designated as *muscarinic* and *nicotinic*. The muscarinic actions of acetylcholine are those that can be reproduced by the injection of **muscarine**, the active principle of the poisonous mushroom *Amanita muscaria*, and can be abolished by small doses of **atropine**. On the whole, muscarinic actions correspond to those of parasympathetic stimulation, as shown in Table 6.1. After the muscarinic effects have been blocked by atropine, larger doses of acetylcholine produce another set of effects, closely similar to those of **nicotine**. They include:

- stimulation of all autonomic ganglia
- stimulation of voluntary muscle
- secretion of adrenaline from the adrenal medulla.

The muscarinic and nicotinic actions of acetylcholine are demonstrated in Figure 6.1 in an experiment on the blood pressure of an anaesthetised cat. Small and medium doses of acetylcholine produce a transient fall in blood pressure due to arteriolar vasodilatation and slowing of the heart. Atropine abolishes these effects. A large dose of acetylcholine given after atropine produces nicotinic effects: an initial rise in blood pressure due to a stimulation of sympathetic ganglia and consequent vasoconstriction, and a secondary rise resulting from secretion of adrenaline.

Dale's classification was originally made on pharmacological grounds, but it has proved to correspond closely to the main physiological functions of acetylcholine in the body. The muscarinic actions correspond to those of acetylcholine released at

Table 6.1 Subtypes of muscarinic receptors

	M_1	M_2	M_3
Type	'Neural'	'Cardiac'	'Glandular'
Main locations	*Neural* CNS (cortex, hippocampus) Ganglia (enteric, autonomic) *Gastric* Parietal cells	*Cardiac* Atria Conducting tissue *Neural* Presynaptic terminals	Exocrine glands Smooth muscle Vascular endothelium
Effects			
Cellular	$\uparrow IP_3$, DAG Depolarisation Excitation (slow epsp) ($\downarrow G_k$)	$\downarrow$ cAMP Inhibition ($\uparrow G_k$, $\downarrow i_{Ca}$) Slow ipsp	$\uparrow IP_3$ Stimulation ($\uparrow [CA]_i$)
Functional	CNS excitation (? memory) Gastric acid secretion Gastrointestinal motility	Cardiac inhibition Presynaptic inhibition Neural inhibition	Secretion Smooth muscle contraction Vasodilatation (via NO)
Agonists	ACh CCh McNA343	ACh CCh	ACh CCh
Antagonists	Atropine Pirenzepine Dicyclomine	Atropine Gallamine AF-DX 116	Atropine HHSD*

*HHSD = hexahydrosiladifenol

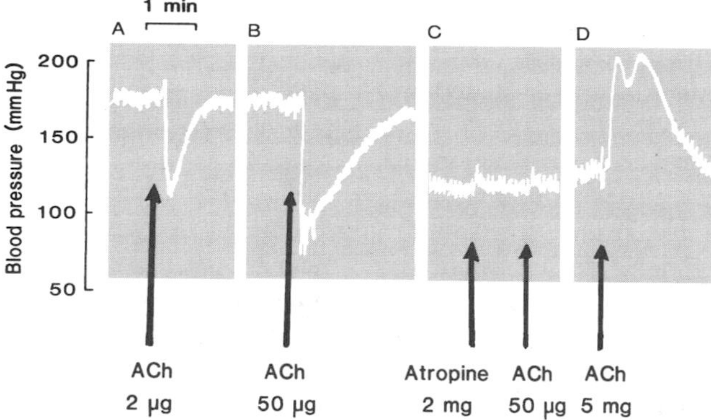

Fig. 6.1 Dale's experiment showing that acetylcholine produces two kinds of effect on the cat's blood pressure. Arterial pressure was recorded with a mercury manometer from a spinal cat. **A.** ACh causes a fall in blood pressure due to vasodilatation. **B.** A larger dose also produces bradycardia. Both A and B are muscarinic effects. **C.** After atropine (muscarinic antagonist) the same dose of ACh has no effect. **D.** Still under the influence of atropine, a much larger dose of ACh causes a rise in blood pressure (due to stimulation of sympathetic ganglia), accompanied by tachycardia, followed by a secondary rise (due to release of adrenaline from the adrenal gland). These effects result from its action on nicotinic receptors. (From: Burn J H 1963 Autonomic pharmacology. Blackwell, Oxford)

postganglionic parasympathetic nerve endings, with two significant exceptions:

- Acetylcholine causes generalised vasodilatation, even though most blood vessels have no parasympathetic innervation. This is an indirect effect: acetylcholine (like many other mediators) acts on vascular endothelial cells to release *endothelium-dependent relaxant factor* (EDRF, now identified as nitric oxide; see Ch. 10) which relaxes smooth muscle. The physiological function of this is uncertain, since acetylcholine is not normally present in circulating blood.
- Acetylcholine evokes secretion from sweat glands, which are innervated by cholinergic fibres of the sympathetic nervous system (see Table 5. 1). The nicotinic actions correspond to those of acetylcholine released at the ganglionic synapses of the sympathetic and parasympathetic systems, the motor endplate of voluntary muscle and the endings of the splanchnic nerves around the secretory cells of the adrenal medulla.

ACETYLCHOLINE RECEPTORS

Though Dale himself dismissed the concept of receptors as sophistry rather than science, his classification of the actions of acetylcholine provided the basis for distinguishing the two major classes of acetylcholine receptor. Within each class, there are further subdivisions. In the case of nicotinic receptors it has long been recognised that there are considerable pharmacological differences between the receptors of striated muscle fibres and those of autonomic ganglia. At least four subtypes of muscarinic receptor have been identified, and the targeting of drugs to specific subtypes has proved useful therapeutically.

NICOTINIC RECEPTORS

Nicotinic receptors occur peripherally at the neuromuscular junction and the ganglionic synapse, and also in the brain, where acetylcholine is a transmitter (Ch. 24). The molecular structure of these receptors (see Ch. 2) is very similar, but they differ pharmacologically (see Colquhoun et al. 1987), the differences being accounted for mainly by the existence of several variants of the α-, β- and γ-subunits (see Role 1992).

In general, agonists show rather little selectivity between ganglionic and neuromuscular receptors. One exception is **decamethonium** (see below), which is a potent depolarising agent (i.e. agonist) at the neuromuscular junction, but a weak antagonist on autonomic ganglia. Among antagonists there is strong selectivity. For example, **α-bungarotoxin** (see Ch. 2) blocks acetylcholine receptors at the neuromuscular junction at very low concentrations, but has no effect on autonomic ganglia. On the other hand, agents such as **mecamylamine** block ganglionic and CNS, but not neuromuscular, acetylcholine receptors. The role of nicotinic receptors in the central nervous system is discussed in Chapter 33.

MUSCARINIC RECEPTORS

Three main subclasses of muscarinic receptor have been characterised functionally (see Goyal 1989; Table 6.1). Gene cloning has so far actually revealed five distinct types (see Nathanson 1987, Bonner 1989), and the pharmacological classification given in Table 6.1 is bound to become more elaborate. M_1-receptors ('neural') are found mainly on CNS and peripheral neurons and gastric parietal cells. They are responsible for mainly excitatory effects, for example, the slow muscarinic excitation mediated by acetylcholine in sympathetic ganglia (Ch. 5) and similar excitation of central neurons. This excitation is produced by a decrease in K^+-conductance, which causes membrane depolarisation. Deficiency of this kind of acetylcholine-mediated effect in the brain is a possible cause of dementia (see Ch. 25). M_1-receptors are also involved in the increase of gastric acid secretion following vagal stimulation (see Ch. 19).

M_2-receptors ('cardiac') occur in the heart, and also on the presynaptic terminals of peripheral and central neurons. They exert inhibitory effects, mainly by increasing K^+-conductance and by inhibiting calcium channels (see Ch. 2). M_2-receptor activation is responsible for the vagal inhibition of the heart, as well as presynaptic inhibition in the central nervous system and periphery (Ch. 5).

M_3-receptors ('glandular/smooth muscle') have only recently been recognised as being distinct from M_2. They produce mainly excitatory effects, i.e. stimulation of glandular secretions (salivary, bronchial, sweat, etc.) and contraction of visceral smooth muscle. There are several examples of M_3-receptor-mediated relaxation of smooth muscle (mainly vascular), which are now known to result from the release of nitric oxide from neighbouring endothelial cells (Ch. 10). The cloned M_4-receptor does not occur in the periphery, but is confined to certain regions of the CNS.

The pharmacological classification of these receptor types relies on the existence of selective agonists and antagonists that can distinguish between them. Most agonists are non-selective, but one experimental compound, **McNA343,** is selective for M_1-receptors; **carbachol** is relatively inactive on these receptors. There is more selectivity amongst antagonists. Though most of the classical muscarinic antagonists (e.g. **atropine, hyoscine**) are non-selective, **pirenzepine** is selective for M_1-receptors. **Gallamine,** better known as a neuromuscular-blocking drug (see p. 133) is also a selective M_2-receptor antagonist, and recently other experimental drugs have been found that are selective for M_2- or M_3-receptors (Table 6.1).

Of the cloned muscarinic receptor subtypes, three are clearly identified with these pharmacological subtypes; the other two remain, for the time being, pharmacological orphans. All of them are Type 2 (G-protein-coupled) receptors (Ch. 2). The odd numbered members of the group (M_1, M_3, M_5) act through the inositol phosphate pathway (p. 37), while the even-numbered receptors (M_2, M_4) act by inhibiting adenylate cyclase and thus reducing intracellular cAMP (see Nathanson 1987, Goyal 1989).

Acetylcholine receptors

- Main subdivision is into nicotinic (nAChR) and muscarinic (mAChR) subtypes.
- nAChRs are directly coupled to cation channels, and mediate fast excitatory synaptic transmission at the neuromuscular junction, autonomic ganglia, and at various sites in the CNS. Muscle and neuronal nAChR differ in their molecular structure and pharmacology.
- mAChRs are G-protein-coupled receptors, causing:
  —activation of phospholipase C (hence formation of $InsP_3$ and DAG as second messengers)
  —inhibition of adenylate cyclase
  —activation of K^+-channels or inhibition of Ca^{2+}-channels.
- mAChRs mediate ACh effects at postganglionic parasympathetic synapses (mainly heart, smooth muscle, glands), and contribute to ganglionic excitation. They occur in many parts of the CNS.
- Three main types of mAChR occur:
  —M_1-receptors ('neural'), producing slow excitation of ganglia. They are selectively blocked by pirenzepine.
  —M_2-receptors ('cardiac'), causing decrease in cardiac rate and force of contraction (mainly of atria). They are selectively blocked by gallamine. M_2-receptors also mediate presynaptic inhibition.
  —M_3-receptors ('glandular'), causing secretion, contraction of visceral smooth muscle, vascular relaxation.
- All mAChRs are activated by ACh and blocked by atropine. There are also subtype-selective agonists and antagonists.

PHYSIOLOGY OF CHOLINERGIC TRANSMISSION

The physiology of cholinergic transmission is described in detail by Ginsborg & Jenkinson (1976) and Nicholls et al. (1992). The main ways in which drugs can affect cholinergic transmission are shown in Figure 6.2.

ACETYLCHOLINE SYNTHESIS AND RELEASE

Acetylcholine metabolism is well reviewed by Blusztajn & Wurtman (1983) and Parsons et al. (1993). Acetylcholine is synthesised within the nerve terminal from choline, most of which is taken up into the nerve terminal by a special choline transport system. This is in many ways similar to the carrier-mediated re-uptake mechanisms that exist for most non-peptide transmitters, such as noradrenaline (Ch. 7), 5-HT (Ch. 8) and amino acids (Ch. 24), but differs in that it transports choline but not acetylcholine, so it is not important in terminating the action of the transmitter. The concentration of choline in the blood and body fluids is normally about 10 μmol/l, but in the immediate vicinity of cholinergic nerve terminals it increases, probably to about 1 mmol/l, when the released acetylcholine is hydrolysed, and it appears that more than 50% of this choline is normally recaptured by the nerve terminals. Free choline within the nerve terminal is acetylated by a cytosolic enzyme, *choline acetyltransferase* (CAT), the source of the acetyl groups being acetyl-CoA.

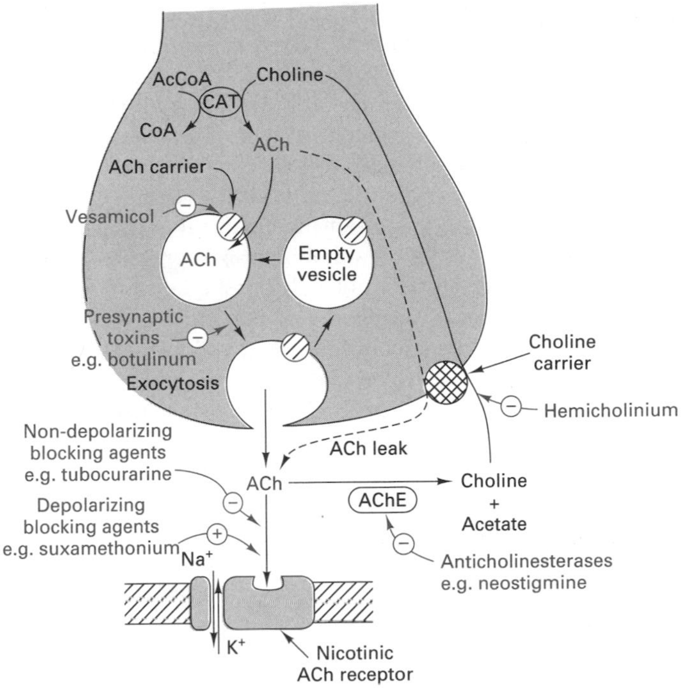

Fig. 6.2 Events and sites of drug action at a cholinergic synapse. ACh is shown acting postsynaptically on a nicotinic receptor controlling a ligand-gated cation channel (e.g. at the neuromuscular or ganglionic synapse). The main mechanism of release is by exocytosis, but some continuous leakage of cytosolic ACh occurs via the choline carrier (dotted line). This is detectable if acetylcholinesterase is inhibited, but is not directly involved in synaptic transmission. The main classes of drug that affect cholinergic transmission (see text) are shown in red.

The rate-limiting process in acetylcholine synthesis appears to be choline transport, the activity of which is regulated according to the rate at which acetylcholine is being released. Cholinesterase is present in the presynaptic nerve terminals and acetylcholine is continually being hydrolysed and resynthesised. Inhibition of the nerve terminal cholinesterase causes the accumulation of 'surplus' acetylcholine in the cytosol, which is not available for release by nerve impulses (though it appears to leak out via the acetylcholine carrier). Most of the acetylcholine synthesised, however, is packaged into synaptic vesicles, in which its concentration is very high (about 100 mmol/l), and from which, according to most authorities (though not all; see Dunant 1986, review by Oorschot & Jones 1987) release occurs by exocytosis.

The packaging of acetylcholine into vesicles occurs by an active transport process, which can be blocked by the experimental drug **vesamicol** (see Parsons et al. 1993), resulting in a slowly developing neuromuscular block. As at other chemically transmitting synapses, exocytosis occurs in response to calcium entry, which normally results from the depolarisation that occurs when an action potential arrives at the terminal. Following its release, the acetylcholine diffuses across the synaptic cleft* to combine with receptors on the postsynaptic cell. Some of it succumbs on the way to hydrolysis by cholinesterase, an enzyme that is bound to the basement membrane of the nerve terminal, which lies between the pre- and postsynaptic membranes. At fast cholinergic synapses (e.g. the neuromuscular and ganglionic synapses), but not at slow ones (smooth muscle, gland cells, heart, etc.), the released acetylcholine is hydrolysed very rapidly (within 1 ms), so that it acts only very briefly. At the neuromuscular junction, which is a highly specialised synapse, a single nerve impulse releases about 300 synaptic vesicles (altogether about three million acetylcholine molecules) from the nerve terminals supplying a single muscle fibre, which contain altogether about three million synaptic vesicles. Approximately two million acetylcholine molecules combine with receptors, of which there are about 30 million on each muscle fibre, the rest being hydrolysed without reaching a receptor. The acetylcholine molecules remain bound to receptors for, on average, about 2 ms, and are quickly hydrolysed after dissociating,

*At postsynaptic parasympathetic nerve terminals (e.g. those supplying intestinal smooth muscle) there is often no clearly defined 'synaptic cleft', such as exists at the neuromuscular or ganglionic synapse, and the transmitter may have to diffuse tens of microns to its site of action.

so that they cannot combine with a second receptor. The result is that transmitter action is very rapid and very brief, which is important for a synapse that has to initiate speedy muscular responses, and which may have to transmit signals at high frequency. Muscle cells are much larger than neurons, and require much more synaptic current to generate an action potential. Thus all of the chemical events happen on a larger scale than at a neuronal synapse: the number of transmitter molecules in a quantum, the number of quanta released, and the number of receptors activated by each quantum are all 10–100 times greater. Our brains would be uncontrollably jumpy if their synapses were built on the industrial scale of the neuromuscular junction.

Presynaptic modulation

Acetylcholine release is regulated by mediators, including acetylcholine itself, acting on presynaptic receptors, as discussed in Chapter 5. At post-ganglionic parasympathetic nerve endings, inhibitory M_2-receptors participate in autoinhibition of acetylcholine release (see Kilbinger 1984); other mediators, such as **noradrenaline**, also inhibit the release of acetylcholine (see Ch. 5). At the neuromuscular junction, on the other hand, presynaptic nicotinic receptors are believed to *facilitate* acetylcholine release (see Bowman et al. 1988), a mechanism that may allow the synapse to function effectively during prolonged high-frequency activity.

ELECTRICAL EVENTS IN TRANSMISSION AT CHOLINERGIC SYNAPSES

Acetylcholine, acting on the postsynaptic membrane of a nicotinic (neuromuscular or ganglionic) synapse, causes a large increase in its permeability to small cations, particularly to sodium and potassium ions, and to a lesser extent, calcium ions. Because of the large, inwardly directed electrochemical gradient for sodium ions across the cell membrane, an inflow of sodium ions occurs, causing depolarisation of the postsynaptic membrane. This transmitter-mediated depolarisation is called an *endplate potential* (epp) in a skeletal muscle fibre (see Ginsborg & Jenkinson 1976), or a *fast excitatory postsynaptic potential* (fast epsp) if it occurs in an autonomic neuron (see Skok 1980). In a muscle fibre the localised epp spreads to adjacent, electrically excitable parts of the muscle fibre; if its amplitude is sufficient to reach the threshold for excitation, an action potential is initiated, which propagates to the rest of the fibre and evokes a contraction.

In a nerve cell, depolarisation of the soma or a dendrite by the fast epsp causes a local current to flow. This depolarises the axon hillock region of the cell, from which, if the epsp is large enough, an action potential is initiated. Figure 6.3 shows that **tubocurarine**, a drug that blocks the action of acetylcholine on the postsynaptic membrane of the ganglion cell (see p. 133), reduces the amplitude of the fast epsp until it no longer initiates an action potential, though the cell is still capable of responding when it is stimulated antidromically. Most ganglion cells are supplied by several presynaptic axons, and it requires simultaneous activity in more than one to make the postganglionic cell fire. At the neuromuscular junction, where there is only one nerve fibre supplying each muscle fibre, the amplitude of the epp is normally more than enough to initiate an action potential—indeed transmission still occurs when the epp is reduced by 70–80% and is said to show a large *margin of safety* which means that fluctuations in transmitter release (e.g. during repetitive stimulation) do not affect transmission.

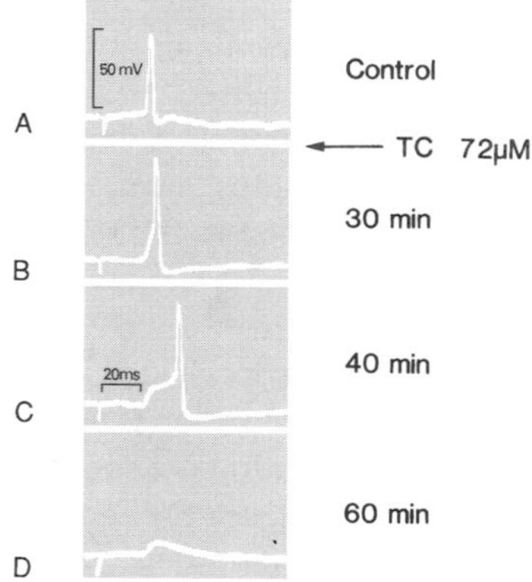

Fig. 6.3 Cholinergic transmission in an autonomic ganglion cell. Records were obtained with an intracellular microelectrode from a guinea-pig parasympathetic ganglion cell. The artefact at the beginning of each trace shows the moment of stimulation of the preganglionic nerve. Tubocurarine (TC), an acetylcholine antagonist, causes the epsp to become smaller. In record C it only just succeeds in triggering the action potential, and in D it has fallen below the threshold. Following complete block, antidromic stimulation (not shown) will still produce an action potential (cf. depolarisation block; Fig. 6.4). (From: Blackman J G et al. 1969 J Physiol 201: 723)

Transmission through autonomic ganglia is more complex than at the neuromuscular junction. Though the primary event at both is the occurrence of an epp or fast epsp resulting from the action of acetylcholine on nicotinic receptors, this is followed in the ganglion by a succession of much slower postsynaptic potential changes, whose physiological significance is not clear (see Karczmar et al. 1985). These comprise, according to most authors:

- A slow inhibitory postsynaptic potential (slow ipsp), which consists of a hyperpolarisation of the membrane lasting 2–5 seconds. An M_2-receptor-mediated increase in K^+-conductance is responsible in some ganglia, but other transmitters, such as dopamine and adenosine, have also been postulated.
- A slow epsp, which lasts for about 10 seconds. This is produced by acetylcholine acting on M_1-receptors, and thereby closing potassium channels.
- A late slow epsp, lasting for 1–2 minutes. This is thought to be mediated by a peptide co-transmitter, which may be substance P in some ganglia, and a GnRH-like peptide in others (see Ch. 5). Like the slow epsp, it is produced by a decrease in K^+-conductance.

Depolarisation block

Depolarisation block occurs at cholinergic synapses when the excitatory nicotinic receptors are *persistently* activated by nicotinic agonists, and it results from a decrease in the electrical excitability of the postsynaptic cell. This is shown in Figure 6.4. Application of **nicotine** to a sympathetic ganglion causes a depolarisation of the cell, which at first initiates action potential discharge. After a few seconds this discharge ceases, and transmission is blocked. The loss of electrical excitability at this time is shown by the fact that antidromic stimuli also fail to produce an action potential. The main reason for the loss of electrical excitability during a period of maintained depolarisation is that the voltage-sensitive sodium channels (see Ch. 34) become inactivated (i.e. refractory) and no longer able to open in response to a brief depolarising stimulus. The work of Burns & Paton (1951), on the neuromuscular-blocking action of decamethonium (see p. 135), elegantly demonstrated that it is membrane depolarisation *per se* that causes the transmission block, by showing that depolarisation induced electrically rather than pharmacologically also caused block and that restoration of the membrane potential (by passing current through the endplate region of the muscle fibres) was able to restore neuromuscular transmission in the presence of decamethonium.

A second type of effect is also seen in the experiment shown in Figure 6.4. After nicotine has acted for several minutes, the cell partially repolarises, and its electrical excitability returns, but, in spite

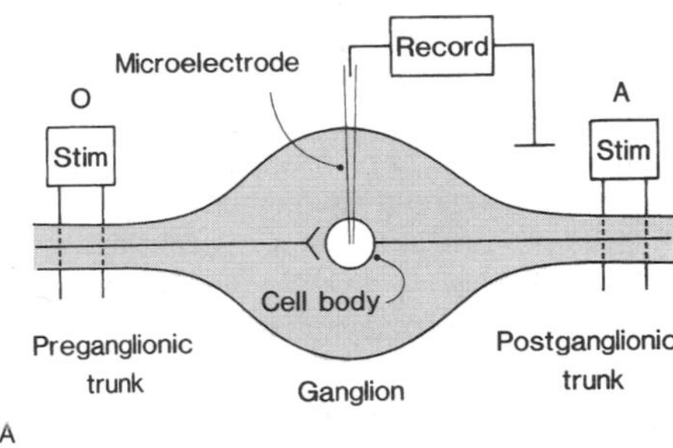

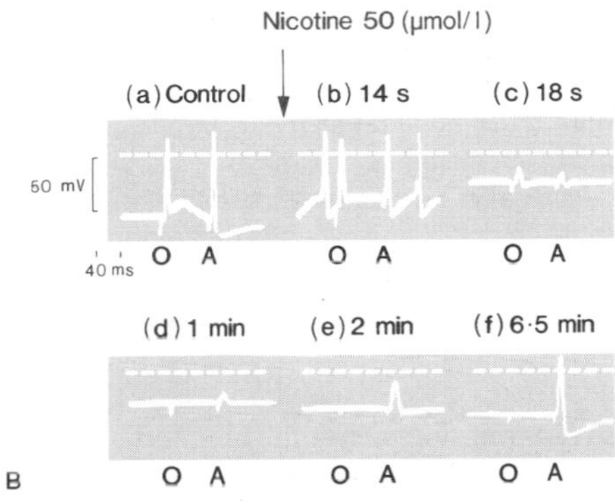

Fig. 6.4 Depolarisation block of ganglionic transmission by nicotine. A. System used for intracellular recording from sympathetic ganglion cells of the frog, showing the location of orthodromic (O) and antidromic (A) stimulating electrodes. Stimulation at O excites the cell via the cholinergic synapse, whereas stimulation at A excites it by electrical propagation of the action potential. **B.** The effect of nicotine: (a) Control records. The membrane potential is –55 mV (dotted line = 0 Mv) and the cell responds to both O and A. (b) Shortly after adding nicotine the cell is slightly depolarised, but still responsive to O and A. (c, d) The cell is further depolarised, to –25 Mv, and produces only a vestigial action potential. The fact that it does not respond to A shows that it is electrically inexcitable. (e, f) In the continued presence of nicotine, the cell repolarises, and regains its responsiveness to A, but is still unresponsive to O, because the ACh receptors are desensitised by nicotine. (From: Ginsborg B L, Guerrero S 1964 J Physiol 172: 189)

> **Cholinergic transmission**
>
> - ACh synthesis:
>   - Requires choline, which enters neuron via carrier-mediated transport.
>   - Acetylation of choline, utilising acetylCoA as source of acetyl groups, involves choline acetyl transferase (CAT), a cytosolic enzyme found only in cholinergic neurons.
>   - ACh is packaged into synaptic vesicles at high concentration by carrier-mediated transport.
> - ACh release occurs by Ca^{2+}-mediated exocytosis. At the neuromuscular junction, one presynaptic nerve impulse releases 100–500 vesicles.
> - At the NMJ, ACh acts on nAChR to open cation channels, producing a rapid depolarisation (endplate potential) which normally initiates an action potential in the muscle fibre. Transmission at other 'fast' cholinergic synapses (e.g. ganglionic) is similar.
> - At 'fast' cholinergic synapses, ACh is hydrolysed within about 1 ms by acetylcholinesterase, so a presynaptic action potential produces only one postsynaptic action potential.
> - Transmission mediated by mAChR is much slower in its time-course, and synaptic structures are less clearly defined. In most cases ACh functions as a modulator rather than as a direct transmitter.
> - Main mechanisms of pharmacological block: inhibition of choline uptake; inhibition of ACh release; block of postsynaptic receptors or ion channels; persistent postsynaptic depolarisation.

of this, transmission remains blocked. This type of secondary, non-depolarising block occurs also at the neuromuscular junction, where it is often referred to as *phase II block*, the initial phase of block caused by depolarisation being called *phase I*. The main factor responsible for phase II block appears to be *receptor desensitisation* (see Ch. 1). This causes the depolarising action of the blocking drug to subside, but at the same time the receptors become desensitised to acetylcholine, so that transmission fails for this reason.

EFFECTS OF DRUGS ON CHOLINERGIC TRANSMISSION

Drugs can influence cholinergic transmission either by acting on acetylcholine receptors or by affecting the release or destruction of endogenous acetylcholine (Fig. 6.2).

Drugs that act on acetylcholine receptors may:

- mimic the action of acetylcholine (e.g. cholinergic agonists, such as **muscarine, nicotine** and various synthetic analogues of acetylcholine)
- block the action of acetylcholine (e.g. cholinergic antagonists, such as **atropine, tubocurarine** and other agents that are specific for different types of acetylcholine receptor).

Drugs that affect the release or destruction of acetylcholine may:

- enhance the evoked release of acetylcholine (e.g. **4-aminopyridine** and related drugs, which affect the electrical properties of the presynaptic nerve terminals)
- inhibit cholinesterase, thereby increasing and prolonging the action of acetylcholine (e.g. **neostigmine**)
- inhibit acetylcholine release, by inhibiting synthesis (e.g. **hemicholinium**, which blocks choline uptake) or vesicular storage (e.g. **vesamicol**) or by inhibiting the release mechanism itself (e.g. **botulinum toxin, magnesium ion, aminoglycoside antibiotics**).

In the rest of this chapter we will consider the following groups of drugs, subdivided according to their physiological site of action:

- muscarinic agonists
- muscarinic antagonists
- ganglion-stimulating drugs
- ganglion-blocking drugs
- neuromuscular-blocking drugs
- anticholinesterases and other drugs that enhance cholinergic transmission.

MUSCARINIC AGONISTS

Structure–activity relationships

Muscarinic agonists, as a group, are often referred to as *parasympathomimetic* because the main effects that they produce in the whole animal resemble those of parasympathetic stimulation. The structures of the most important compounds are given in Table 6.2. This group includes acetylcholine itself and a number of closely related choline esters that are

Table 6.2 Muscarinic agonists

Drug	Structure	Receptor specificity		Hydrolysis by AChE
		Musc	*Nic*	
Acetylcholine		+++	+++	+++
Carbachol		++	+++	–
Methacholine		+++	+	++
Bethanechol		+++	–	–
Muscarine		+++	–	–
Pilocarpine		++	–	–
Oxotremorine		++	–	–

agonists at both muscarinic and nicotinic receptors. The reason for classifying them as muscarinic agonists is that they produce muscarinic responses at much lower concentrations than are needed to elicit nicotinic responses (see Fig. 6.1), and their limited therapeutic usefulness reflects their action on muscarinic receptors.

Acetylcholine itself (Table 6.2) is among the most potent agonists at both muscarinic and nicotinic receptors. The key features of the molecule that are important for its activity are:

- the quaternary ammonium group, which is strongly basic and bears a positive charge
- the ester group, which bears a partial negative charge.

Compounds such as choline, which possess the quaternary ammonium group but lack an ester bond, have only very weak activity. The presence of the ester group makes the molecule susceptible to hydrolysis by cholinesterase. Some modifications that can be made to the acetylcholine molecule without drastic loss of activity are shown in Table 6.2. The effects of these modifications are:

- to reduce the susceptibility of the compound to hydrolysis by cholinesterase

- to alter the relative activity on muscarinic and nicotinic receptors.

Substitution of the acetyl group by a carbamyl group yields **carbachol**, which has a similar potency to acetylcholine on both nicotinic and muscarinic receptors, but is not readily hydrolysed. Addition of a side-chain methyl group on the carbon atom produces **methacholine**, which acts selectively on muscarinic receptors but is rapidly hydrolysed. Combining these two modifications results in **bethanechol**, which is selective for muscarinic receptors and stable to hydrolysis.

Pilocarpine differs from the other drugs mentioned in being a partial agonist for many muscarinic responses, and it is also said to have a selective action in stimulating secretion from sweat, salivary, lacrimal and bronchial glands with relatively less effect on gastrointestinal smooth muscle and the heart compared with other muscarinic agonists.

Effects of muscarinic agonists

The main actions of muscarinic agonists are readily understood in terms of the parasympathetic nervous system.

Cardiovascular effects include cardiac slowing and a decrease in cardiac output. The latter action is due mainly to a decreased force of contraction of the atria, since the ventricles have only a sparse parasympathetic innervation and a low sensitivity to muscarinic agonists (see Table 6.1). Generalised vasodilatation also occurs (an NO-mediated effect that is not associated with a cholinergic innervation) and these two effects combine to produce a sharp fall in arterial pressure (Fig. 6.1). The mechanism of action of muscarinic agonists on the heart is discussed in Chapter 13.

Smooth muscle, other than vascular smooth muscle, contracts in response to muscarinic agonists. Peristaltic activity of the gastrointestinal tract is increased, which can cause colicky pain, and the bladder and bronchial smooth muscle also contract.

Exocrine glands are caused to secrete, leading to sweating, lacrimation, salivation and bronchial secretion. The combined effect of bronchial secretion and constriction can interfere with breathing.

Effects on the eye are of some importance. The parasympathetic nerves to the eye supply the *constrictor pupillae* muscle, which runs circumferentially in the iris, and the *ciliary muscle*, which adjusts the curvature of the lens (Fig. 6.5). Contraction of the ciliary muscle in response to activation of muscarinic receptors pulls the ciliary body forwards and inwards, thus relaxing the tension on the suspensory ligament of the lens, allowing the lens to bulge more and reducing its focal length. This parasympathetic reflex is thus necessary to accommodate the eye for near vision. The *constrictor pupillae* is important not only for adjusting the pupil in response to changes in light intensity, but also in regulating the intraocular pressure (see Leopold & Duzman 1986). Aqueous humour is secreted slowly and continuously by the cells of the epithelium covering the ciliary body, and it is removed continuously by drainage into the *canal of Schlemm* (Fig. 6.5) which runs around the eye close to the outer margin of the iris. The intraocular pressure is normally 10–15 mmHg above atmospheric, which keeps the eye slightly distended.

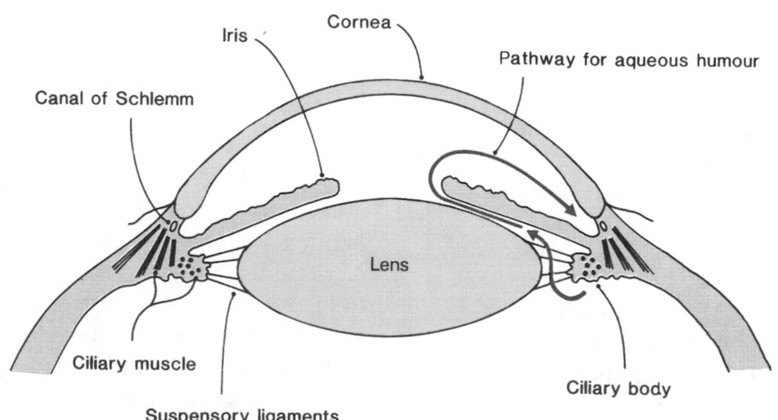

Fig. 6.5 The anterior chamber of the eye, showing the pathway for secretion and drainage of the aqueous humour.

Abnormally raised intraocular pressure (glaucoma) damages the eye and is one of the commonest preventable causes of blindness. In some individuals drainage of aqueous humour becomes impeded when the iris is dilated because folding of the iris tissue occludes the drainage angle, and the intraocular pressure rises for this reason. Activation of the *constrictor pupillae* muscle by muscarinic agonists will, in these circumstances, lower the intraocular pressure, though in a normal individual it will have little effect. The increased tension in the ciliary muscle produced by these drugs may also play a part in improving drainage by realigning the connective tissue trabeculae through which the canal of Schlemm passes.

Clinical use

The main use of muscarinic agonists is in treating glaucoma, by local instillation in the form of eye drops (see Leopold & Duzman 1986), although β-adrenoceptor antagonists (see Ch. 7) and/or surgery are generally preferred. **Pilocarpine** is the most effective as, being a tertiary amine, it can cross the conjunctival membrane. It is a stable compound whose action lasts for about 1 day.

A minor use is to stimulate bladder emptying (e.g. **carbachol, bethanechol**), when neurological disease or a surgical procedure has disturbed the normal emptying mechanism. It is important to exclude the possibility of bladder neck obstruction before using these drugs.

Unwanted effects

The side effects of muscarinic agonists are considerable, and they are generally poorly absorbed from the gastrointestinal tract, so they are now seldom used except in glaucoma. When a drug of this kind is needed for systemic use, **bethanechol**, which combines selectivity for muscarinic receptors with resistance to hydrolysis, is most often used. In principle, a selective M_2 agonist (yet to be discovered) would be useful for treating cardiac dysrhythmias without producing M_3-mediated side effects.

MUSCARINIC ANTAGONISTS

Muscarinic antagonists are often referred to as *parasympatholytic* because they selectively reduce or abolish the effects of parasympathetic stimulation. All of them are competitive antagonists of acetylcholine at muscarinic receptors. Their chemical structures (see Table 6.3) usually contain ester and basic groups in the same relationship as acetylcholine, but they have a much bulkier aromatic group in place of the acetyl group. The two naturally occurring compounds, **atropine** and **hyoscine**, are alkaloids found in solanaceous plants. The deadly nightshade (*Atropa belladonna*) contains mainly atropine, whereas the thorn apple (*Datura stramonium*) contains mainly hyoscine. **Homatropine** is synthesised from atropine and is pharmacologically very similar. These three compounds are all tertiary amines, largely ionised at physiological pH but sufficiently lipid soluble to be readily absorbed from the gut or conjunctival sac, and,

Table 6.3 Muscarinic antagonists, with acetylcholine for comparison

Drug	Structure
Acetylcholine (agonist)	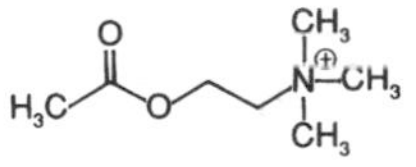
Atropine	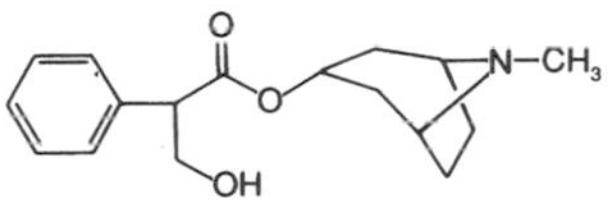
Atropine methonitrate	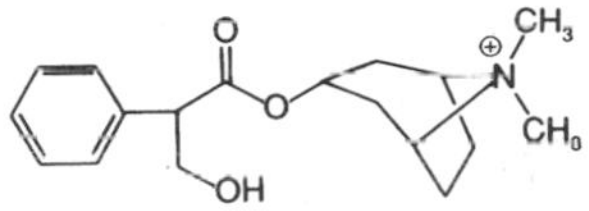
Hyoscine	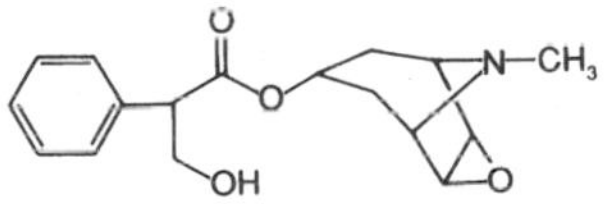
Dicyclomine	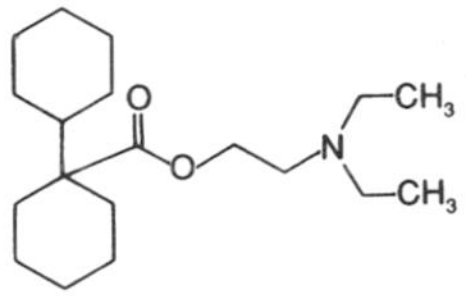
Cyclopentolate	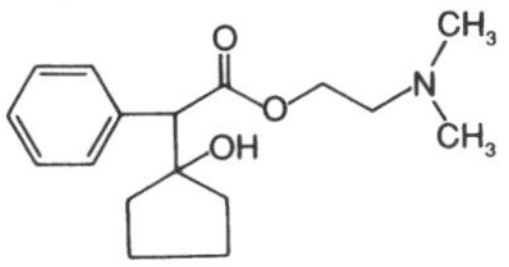
Pirenzepine	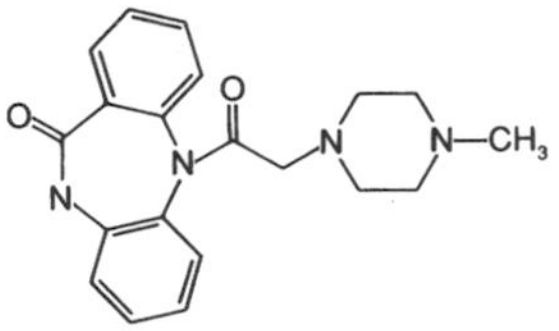

importantly, to penetrate the blood–brain barrier. Among synthetic muscarinic antagonists, the quaternary derivative of atropine, **atropine methonitrate**, has peripheral actions very similar to those of atropine but, because of its exclusion from the brain, lacks central actions. **Ipratropium**, another quaternary compound, is used by inhalation to produce bronchodilation. **Pirenzepine** is a relatively selective M_1-receptor antagonist.

Effects of muscarinic antagonists

All of the muscarinic antagonists produce basically similar peripheral effects, though some show a degree of selectivity, for example for the heart or the gastrointestinal tract, reflecting heterogeneity among muscarinic receptors (see p. 119).

The main effects of atropine are described below.

Inhibition of secretions. Salivary, lacrimal, bronchial and sweat glands are inhibited by very low doses of atropine, producing an uncomfortably dry mouth and skin. Gastric secretion is only slightly reduced.

Effects on heart rate. The first effect produced on the heart is, paradoxically, bradycardia, which results from a central action, increasing vagal activity. Slightly larger doses produce the expected tachycardia, due to block of cardiac muscarinic receptors. The tachycardia is modest, up to 80–90 beats/minute in man. This is because there is no effect on the sympathetic system, but only inhibition of the existing parasympathetic tone. The response of the heart to exercise is unaffected. Arterial blood pressure is unaffected, since most resistance vessels have no cholinergic innervation.

Effects on the eye. The pupil is dilated (mydriasis)* by atropine administration, and becomes unresponsive to light. Relaxation of the ciliary muscle causes paralysis of accommodation (cycloplegia), so that near vision is impaired. Intraocular pressure may rise; though this is unimportant in normal individuals, it can be dangerous in patients suffering from narrow-angle glaucoma.

Effects on the GI tract. Gastrointestinal motility is inhibited by atropine, though this requires larger doses than the other effects listed, and is not complete. This is because excitatory transmitters other than acetylcholine are important in normal function of the myenteric plexus (see Chs 5, 8 and 19). In pathological conditions in which there is increased gastrointestinal motility, atropine is rather more effective in causing inhibition. **Pirenzepine** inhibits gastric acid secretion in doses that do not affect other systems. **Dicyclomine** also affects gastrointestinal mobility selectively (see Ch. 19).

Effects on other smooth muscle. Bronchial, biliary and urinary tract smooth muscle are all relaxed by atropine. Reflex bronchoconstriction (e.g. during anaesthesia) is prevented by atropine, whereas bronchoconstriction caused by local mediators, such as histamine (e.g. in asthma) is unaffected (see Ch. 17). Though biliary and urinary tract smooth muscle are only slightly affected, probably because transmitters other than acetylcholine (see Ch. 5) are important in these organs, atropine and similar drugs commonly precipitate urinary retention in elderly men with prostatic enlargement.

Effects on the CNS. Atropine produces mainly excitatory effects on the central nervous system. At low doses this causes mild restlessness; higher doses cause agitation and disorientation. In *atropine*

Drugs acting on muscarinic receptors

Muscarinic agonists

- Important compounds include ACh, carbachol, methacholine, muscarine and pilocarpine. They vary in muscarinic/nicotinic selectivity, and in susceptibility to cholinesterase.
- Main effects are: bradycardia and vasodilatation (endothelium-dependent), leading to fall in blood pressure; contraction of visceral smooth muscle (gut, bladder, bronchi, etc.); exocrine secretions, pupillary constriction and ciliary muscle contraction, leading to decrease of intraocular pressure.
- Main use is in treatment of glaucoma (esp. pilocarpine).

Muscarinic antagonists

- Most important compounds are atropine, hyoscine, and pirenzepine.
- Main effects are: inhibition of secretions; tachycardia, pupillary dilatation and paralysis of accommodation; relaxation of smooth muscle (gut, bronchi, biliary tract, bladder); inhibition of gastric acid secretion (esp. pirenzepine); CNS effects (mainly excitatory with atropine; depressant, including amnesia, with hyoscine), including anti-emetic effect and anti-parkinsonian effect.

*The alluring quality of dilated pupils was well understood by fashionable women of the Italian Renaissance, whose cosmetic use of eye drops containing deadly nightshade berries led to the plant being called belladonna. Inability to see properly was evidently considered a price worth paying.

poisoning, which occurs mainly in young children who eat deadly nightshade berries, marked excitement and irritability result in hyperactivity and a considerable rise in body temperature, which is accentuated by the loss of sweating. These central effects are evidently the result of blocking muscarinic receptors in the brain, since they are opposed by anticholinesterase drugs such as **physostigmine**, which is an effective antidote to atropine poisoning. It is thus surprising that **hyoscine** has different central actions, causing marked sedation in low doses, though similar effects in high dosage. Hyoscine also has a useful anti-emetic effect, and is used in preventing motion sickness. Atropine, and other antimuscarinic drugs such as **benztropine** and **trihexyphenidyl** (an M_1 antagonist) also affect the extrapyramidal system, reducing the involuntary movement and rigidity of patients with Parkinson's disease (see Ch. 25).

The main uses of muscarinic antagonists are shown below.

Clinical uses of muscarinic antagonists

Cardiovascular
- Treatment of sinus bradycardia (e.g. after myocardial infarction; see Ch. 13): intravenous atropine.

Ophthalmic
- To dilate the pupil: e.g. tropicamide eye drops (relatively short-acting); cyclopentolate eye drops (long-acting).

Neurological
- Prevention of motion sickness; e.g. hyoscine, orally or transdermally.
- Parkinsonism (see Ch. 25), especially to counteract movement disorders caused by antipsychotic drugs (see Ch. 28): e.g. benzhexol, benztropine.

Respiratory
- Asthma (see Ch. 17): ipratropium by inhalation.
- Anaesthetic premedication to dry secretions; e.g. atropine, hyoscine by injection. Less commonly used nowadays since current anaesthetics are relatively non-irritant (see Ch. 26).

Gastrointestinal—to relax gastrointestinal smooth muscle ('antispasmodic' action) and suppress gastric acid secretion (see Ch. 19)
- To facilitate endoscopy and gastrointestinal radiology; e.g. hyoscine butylbromide intravenously.
- Irritable bowel syndrome, colonic diverticular disease; e.g. dicyclomine orally.
- Peptic ulcer disease; pirenzepine (M_1-selective, now less used since introduction of histamine H_2 antagonists).

DRUGS THAT STIMULATE AUTONOMIC GANGLIA

In addition to the agonists listed in Table 6.2 that act on both muscarinic and nicotinic receptors there are a few drugs that act selectively on nicotinic receptors; some of these affect both ganglionic and motor endplate receptors, but some show selectivity (see Kharkevich 1980).

Nicotine (Table 6.4), **lobeline** and **dimethylphenylpiperazinium** (DMPP) are three drugs that affect ganglionic nicotinic receptors preferentially. Nicotine and lobeline are tertiary amines found in the leaves of tobacco and lobelia plants respectively. Nicotine has a well-established place in pharmacological folklore as it was the substance on the tip of Langley's paint-brush which he found would stimulate muscle fibres when applied to the endplate region, and which caused him to postulate in 1905 the existence of a 'receptive substance' on the surface of the fibres (Ch. 5). Both of these substances affect the neuromuscular junction in concentrations only slightly greater than those that affect ganglia. DMPP is a synthetic compound that is selective for ganglionic receptors.

These substances are of no therapeutic value. They are used as experimental tools, and nicotine is, of course, important in relation to smoking (see Ch. 33). They cause complex peripheral responses associated with generalised stimulation of autonomic ganglia. The effects of nicotine on the gastrointestinal tract and sweat glands are familiar to neophyte smokers (see Ch. 33), though usually insufficient to act as an effective deterrent.

GANGLION-BLOCKING DRUGS

Ganglion block can occur by several mechanisms (see Brown 1980):

- *By interference with acetylcholine release*, as at the neuromuscular junction (see p. 124 and Ch. 5), and the same substances, namely **botulinum toxin**, **hemicholinium**, and **magnesium ion**, are effective in causing block. Skeletal muscle paralysis occurs at the same time as ganglion block, the latter being of little practical importance.
- *By interference with the postsynaptic action of acetylcholine*. All ganglion-blocking drugs of practical importance act by this mechanism, and are discussed in more detail below.

Table 6.4 Nicotinic receptor agonists and antagonists

Drugs	Main site	Type of action	Notes
Agonists			
Nicotine	Autonomic ganglia	Stimulation then block	No clinical uses
	CNS	Stimulation	For CNS effects, see Ch. 33
Lobeline	Autonomic ganglia	Stimulation	
	Sensory nerve terminals	Stimulation	
Suxamethonium	Neuromuscular junction	Depolarisation block	Used clinically as muscle relaxant
Decamethonium	Neuromuscular junction	Depolarisation block	No clinical use
Acetylcholine Carbachol			See p. 151
Antagonists			
Hexamethonium	Autonomic ganglia	Transmission block	No clinical use
Trimetaphan	Autonomic ganglia	Transmission block	Blood pressure lowering in surgery (rarely used)
Tubocurarine Gallamine Pancuronium Atracurium	Neuromuscular junction	Transmission block	Widely used as muscle relaxants in anaesthesia

- *By prolonged depolarisation.* **Nicotine** (see Fig. 6.4) can block ganglia, after initial stimulation, in this way, and so can acetylcholine itself if cholinesterase is inhibited so that it can exert a continuing action on the postsynaptic membrane. This type of block is much less important at the ganglionic synapse than at the neuromuscular junction (see p. 123).

Inhibitors of acetylcholine action

The major ganglion-blocking drugs all act by inhibiting the postsynaptic action of acetylcholine; they do not themselves cause depolarisation, and hence block transmission without causing initial stimulation. **Hexamethonium** (Table 6.4) was discovered by Paton & Zaimis in 1948. They investigated a series of methonium compounds of the same basic structure in which the length of the polymethylene chain was varied systematically, and found that the pharmacological actions of members of this series vary according to chain length. Compounds with five or six carbon atoms in the methylene chain linking the two quaternary groups produce ganglionic block; when the chain contains nine or ten carbon atoms (**decamethonium**) they produce neuromuscular block.

Hexamethonium, which was developed as an antihypertensive agent (see Ch. 14), is no longer in clinical use, though it is a valuable experimental tool. The only ganglion-blocking drug currently in clinical use is **trimetaphan** (Table 6.4), a very short-acting drug that can be administered as a slow intravenous infusion, for certain types of anaesthetic procedure that require controlled hypotension.

Mechanism of action of non-depolarising ganglion-blocking drugs

Hexamethonium blocks the response of the ganglion to acetylcholine or other ganglionic stimulants, but does not itself stimulate or depolarise the ganglion. Because of the structural similarity of the methonium series of compounds to acetylcholine it was originally believed that they act as competitive antagonists at the receptor sites. Recently, however, the action of many ganglion-blocking agents has been shown to result from a block, not of the receptor, but of the associated ion channel (see Fig. 6.6 and Ch. 2).

Tubocurarine (see p. 133) blocks ganglionic as well as neuromuscular transmission. On the ganglion its action is on the ionic channel, whereas at the neuromuscular junction it binds mainly to the receptor, with only a minor component of channel block.

Channel block as a mechanism for regulating

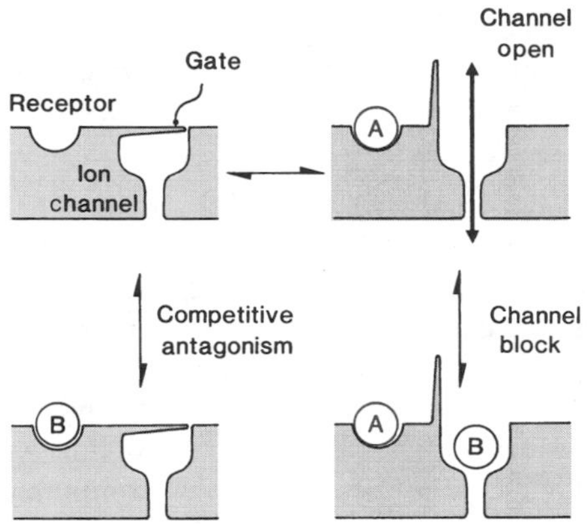

Fig. 6.6 Acetylcholine antagonism by receptor block (left) and channel block (right). Recent evidence favours the latter mechanism of action for many ganglion-blocking drugs. (A = ACh molecule; B = blocking molecule)

membrane excitability is discussed in relation to the heart (Ch. 13) and antiepileptic drugs (Ch. 30).

Effects of ganglion-blocking drugs

The effects of ganglion-blocking drugs are numerous and complex, as would be expected, since both divisions of the autonomic nervous system are blocked indiscriminately. Even large doses do not totally abolish transmission, because the excitatory action of the muscarinic receptors remains. The description by Paton of 'hexamethonium man' cannot be bettered:

> He is a pink-complexioned person, except when he has stood in a queue for a long time, when he may get pale and faint. His handshake is warm and dry. He is a placid and relaxed companion; for instance he may laugh but he can't cry because the tears cannot come. Your rudest story will not make him blush, and the most unpleasant circumstances will fail to make him turn pale. His collars and socks stay very clean and sweet. He wears corsets and may, if you meet him out, be rather fidgety (corsets to compress his splanchnic vascular pool, fidgety to keep the venous return going from his legs). He dislikes speaking much unless helped with something to moisten his dry mouth and throat. He is long-sighted and easily blinded by bright light. The redness of his eyeballs may suggest irregular habits and in fact his head is rather weak. But he always behaves like a gentleman and never belches or hiccups. He tends to get cold and keeps well wrapped up. But his health is good; he does not have chilblains and those diseases of modern civilization, hypertension and peptic ulcer, pass him by. He gets thin because his appetite is modest; he never feels hunger pains and his stomach never rumbles. He gets rather constipated so that his intake of liquid paraffin is high. As old age comes on, he will suffer from retention of urine and impotence, but frequency, precipitancy and strangury will not worry him. One is uncertain how he will end, but perhaps if he is not careful, by eating less and less and getting colder and colder, he will sink into a symptomless, hypoglycaemic coma and die, as was proposed for the universe, a sort of entropy death.

The most important effects are on the cardiovascular system and on visceral smooth muscle.

Effects on the cardiovascular system. A marked fall in arterial blood pressure results mainly from block of sympathetic ganglia, which causes arteriolar vasodilatation. Cardiac output falls slightly, but the main effect is to block cardiovascular reflexes. In particular, the venoconstriction, which occurs normally when a subject stands up from a sitting or lying position and which is necessary if the central venous pressure is to be prevented from falling sharply, is reduced. Standing thus causes a sudden fall in cardiac output and in arterial pressure (*postural hypotension*) that can cause fainting. Similarly, the vasodilatation of skeletal muscle during exercise is normally accompanied by vasoconstriction elsewhere (e.g. splanchnic area) produced by sympathetic activity. If this adjustment is prevented, the overall peripheral resistance falls and the blood pressure also falls (*post-exercise hypotension*).

Effects on the visceral smooth muscle. There is an inhibition of secretion and motility of all parts of the gastrointestinal tract, which leads to severe constipation. The peristaltic reflex, which can be elicited by raising the pressure within an isolated length of intestine, is inhibited by ganglion block. Bladder emptying is also inhibited, resulting in urinary retention, and the loss of autonomic reflexes causes impotence and failure of ejaculation.

Clinical use

Though ganglion-blocking drugs were the first really effective antihypertensive drugs (see Ch. 13), they had many serious side effects, and are now clinically

Drugs acting on autonomic ganglia

Ganglion-stimulating drugs
- Compounds include nicotine, DMPP.
- Both sympathetic and parasympathetic ganglia are stimulated, so effects are complex, including: tachycardia and increase of blood pressure; variable effects on gastrointestinal motility and secretions; increased bronchial, salivary and sweat secretions. Additional effects result from stimulation of other neuronal structures, including sensory and noradrenergic nerve terminals.
- Ganglion stimulation may be followed by depolarisation block.
- Nicotine also has important CNS effects.
- No therapeutic uses.

Ganglion-blocking drugs
- Compounds include hexamethonium, trimetaphan, tubocurarine (also nicotine; see above).
- Block all autonomic ganglia and enteric ganglia. Main effects: hypotension and loss of cardiovascular reflexes; inhibition of secretions; gastrointestinal paralysis; impaired micturition.
- Clinically obsolete, except for occasional use of trimetaphan to produce controlled hypotension in anaesthesia.

obsolete, with the exception of **trimetaphan**. This very short-acting drug is used in anaesthesia, in conjunction with a tilting operating table, to produce controlled hypotension, with the aim of minimising bleeding during certain kinds of surgery. The short action of trimetaphan means that it can be given as an intravenous infusion to produce minute-to-minute control of blood pressure.

NEUROMUSCULAR-BLOCKING DRUGS

The pharmacology of neuromuscular function is well reviewed by Bowman (1990) and Zaimis (1976).

Drugs can block neuromuscular transmission in three main ways:

- by inhibiting acetylcholine synthesis
- by inhibiting acetylcholine release
- by interfering with the postsynaptic action of acetylcholine. This category includes nearly all of the clinically useful drugs and may be further subdivided into:
  - — non-depolarising blocking agents, which act by blocking acetylcholine receptors (and, in some cases, also by blocking ion channels)
  - — depolarising blocking agents, which are agonists at acetylcholine receptors.

Drugs that inhibit acetylcholine synthesis

The steps in the synthesis of acetylcholine in the presynaptic nerve terminals are shown in Figure 6.2. The rate-limiting process appears to be the transport of choline into the nerve terminal, and the only important drugs that inhibit acetylcholine synthesis do so by blocking this step. A few compounds that inhibit choline acetyltransferase have been reported, but they are of low potency and specificity. Two drugs that inhibit choline transport are **hemicholinium** and **triethylcholine**, both of which are useful as experimental tools but have no clinical applications. Both of these compounds are chemically related to choline. Hemicholinium acts as a competitive inhibitor of choline uptake, but is not appreciably taken up itself. Triethylcholine, as well as inhibiting choline uptake, is itself transported and acetylated within the terminals, forming acetyltriethylcholine. This is stored in place of acetylcholine, and released as a false transmitter, but has no depolarising effect on the postsynaptic membrane.

An experimental drug, **vesamicol**, acts by blocking acetylcholine transport into synaptic vesicles, and produces a similar pattern of transmission block.

Drugs that inhibit acetylcholine release

Acetylcholine release by a nerve impulse involves the entry of calcium ions into the nerve terminal; the increase in $[Ca^{2+}]_i$ increases the rate of quantal release, probably by increasing the frequency of exocytotic events within the terminal (Fig. 6.2). Agents that inhibit the impulse itself (e.g. local anaesthetics; see Ch. 34) will obviously cause neuromuscular block, though they are not used for this purpose. Agents that inhibit calcium entry have a similar effect. These include **magnesium ion**, and various **aminoglycoside antibiotics** (e.g. streptomycin and neomycin; see Ch. 37). Intravenous magnesium salts were once used as anaesthetic agents, for the effect on transmitter release is a general one that affects central as well as peripheral synapses. Aminoglycoside antibiotics occasionally produce muscle paralysis as an unwanted side effect when used clinically. **Calcium antagonists** (see Ch. 14), which block calcium entry into smooth muscle and cardiac cells, have little effect on the release of neurotransmitters, because the calcium channels involved in transmitter release are distinct from those responsible for calcium entry into smooth muscle cells.

Two potent neurotoxins, namely **botulinum toxin** and **β-bungarotoxin** act specifically to inhibit acetylcholine release. Botulinum toxin is a protein produced by the anaerobic bacillus *Clostridium botulinum*, an organism that can multiply in preserved food, and can cause botulism, an extremely serious type of food poisoning. The potency of botulinum toxin is extraordinary. It is estimated that the minimum lethal dose in a mouse is less than 10^{-12} g, amounting to only a few million molecules. It binds tightly to cholinergic nerve terminals and it is calculated that no more than a few molecules need to be bound by each nerve terminal in order to inhibit acetylcholine release. Botulinum toxin belongs to the group of potent bacterial exotoxins that includes tetanus and diphtheria toxins. They possess two subunits, one of which binds to a membrane receptor and is responsible for cellular specificity. By this means the toxin enters the cell, where the other subunit exerts a toxic effect by inactivating specific enzymes; this involves an ADP-ribosylation reaction. Botulinum toxin is believed to inactivate actin, a protein involved in exocytosis, by this mechanism (see Aktories & Wegner 1989).

Botulinum poisoning causes progressive parasympathetic and motor paralysis, with dry mouth, blurred vision and difficulty in swallowing, followed by progressive respiratory paralysis. Treatment with antitoxin is effective only if given before symptoms appear, for once the toxin is bound its action cannot be reversed. Mortality is high, and recovery takes several weeks. Anticholinesterases and drugs that increase transmitter release (see p. 146) are ineffective in restoring transmission. Among the more spectacular outbreaks of botulinum poisoning was an incident on Loch Maree in Scotland in 1922 when all eight members of a fishing party died after eating duck pâté for their lunch. Their ghillies, consuming humbler fare no doubt, survived. The inn-keeper committed suicide.

Botulinum toxin, injected locally into muscles, is used to treat a form of persistent and disabling eyelid spasm (blepharospasm) as well as other types of local muscle spasm.

β-bungarotoxin is a protein contained in the venom of various snakes of the cobra family, and has a similar action to botulinum toxin. The same venoms also contain α-bungarotoxin (see Ch. 2) which blocks postsynaptic acetylcholine receptors, so these snakes evidently cover all eventualities as far as causing paralysis of their victims is concerned.

Drugs that act postsynaptically—non-depolarising blocking agents

In 1856, Claude Bernard showed that 'curare' causes paralysis by blocking neuromuscular transmission, rather than by abolishing nerve conduction or muscle contractility. In 1905, J N Langley suggested that it acts by combining with a 'receptive substance' at the motor endplate.

Chemistry and structure–activity relationships

'Curare' is a mixture of naturally occurring alkaloids found in various South American plants and used as arrow poisons by South American Indians. Many of these substances have neuromuscular-blocking activity, but the most important is **tubocurarine**, the structure of which was elucidated in 1935. Tubocurarine is still widely used in clinical medicine, but a number of synthetic drugs with very similar actions have been developed, the most important ones being **gallamine**, **pancuronium**, **vecuronium** and **atracurium**, which differ mainly in their duration of action. These substances are all quaternary ammonium compounds, which means that they are poorly absorbed and generally rapidly excreted. They also fail to cross the placenta, which is important in relation to their use in obstetric anaesthesia. The failure of tubocurarine to be absorbed when taken orally allowed it to be used safely in the hunting of animals for food.

Mechanism of action

Non-depolarising blocking agents all act as competitive antagonists (see Ch. 1) at the acetylcholine receptors of the endplate, and this largely accounts for their actions. The amount of acetylcholine released by a nerve impulse normally exceeds by several-fold what is needed to elicit an action potential in the muscle fibre. It is therefore necessary to block 70–80% of the receptor sites before transmission actually fails. When this happens it is still possible to record a small endplate potential in the muscle fibre though its amplitude fails to reach threshold (Fig. 6.7). In any individual muscle fibre transmission is all-or-nothing, so graded degrees of block represent a varying proportion of muscle fibres failing to respond. In this situation, where the amplitude of endplate potential in all of the fibres is close to threshold (just above in some, just below in others) small variations in the amount of transmitter released, or in the rate at which it is destroyed will have a large effect on the proportion of fibres contracting, so the degree of block is liable to vary according to various physiological circumstances (e.g. stimulation frequency, temperature, cholinesterase inhibition, etc.) which normally have relatively little effect on the efficiency of transmission.

In addition to blocking receptors, some of these drugs also block ion channels in a manner similar to the ganglion-blocking drugs, though this is probably of little importance in practice. Furthermore (see Bowman et al. 1988), some non-depolarising blocking agents also appear to block presynaptic autoreceptors, and thus inhibit the release of acetylcholine during repetitive stimulation of the motor nerve. This may play a part in causing the 'tetanic fade' seen with these drugs (see p. 136).

Effects of non-depolarising blocking drugs

The effects of non-depolarising neuromuscular-blocking agents are mainly due to motor paralysis, though some of the drugs also produce clinically significant autonomic effects. The first muscles to be affected are the extrinsic eye muscles (causing double vision) and the small muscles of the face, limbs and pharynx (causing difficulty in swallowing). Respiratory muscles are the last to be affected and the first to recover. A heroic experiment in 1947 in which a volunteer was fully curarised under artificial ventilation established this orderly paralytic march, and showed that consciousness and awareness of pain were quite normal even when paralysis was complete. The special characteristics of non-depolarising block, and the ways in which it differs from depolarisation block are described on page 136.

Unwanted effects

The main side effect of tubocurarine is a fall in arterial pressure, mainly due to ganglion block. An additional cause is the release of histamine from mast cells (see Ch. 11), which can also give rise to

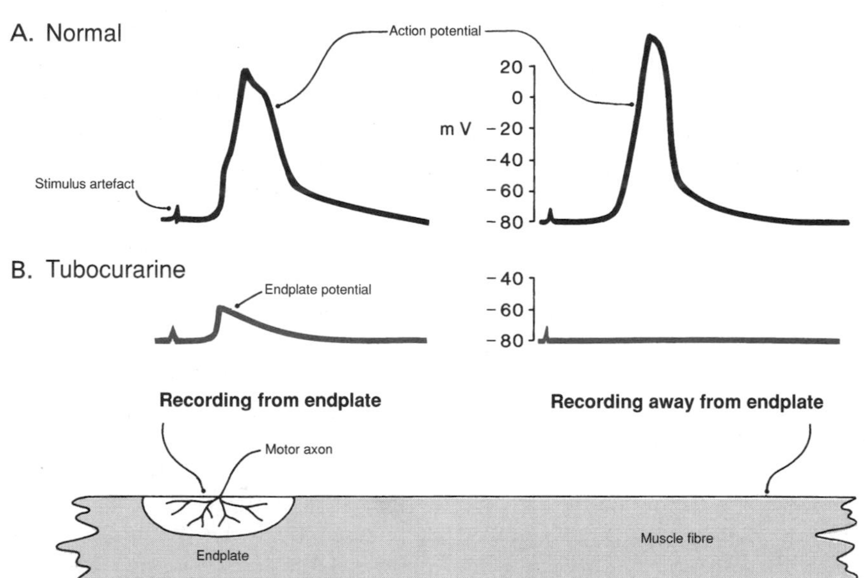

Fig. 6.7 The effect of tubocurarine on neuromuscular transmission.
A. Microelectrode recording at the endplate (left) normally shows a complex response to nerve stimulation, consisting of an endplate potential (epp), from the peak of which the action potential is initiated. The action potential is distorted by the local increase in conductance produced by the transmitter. Away from the endplate a simple propagated action potential is recorded. **B.** Tubocurarine reduces the epp amplitude, so that no action potential is generated.

bronchospasm in sensitive individuals. This is unrelated to nicotinic receptors, and is an effect common to many strongly basic drugs. The other non-depolarising blocking drugs, especially **vecuronium**, cause less ganglion block and histamine release than tubocurarine, and hence less hypotension. **Gallamine**, and to a lesser extent **pancuronium**, block muscarinic receptors, particularly in the heart, which results in tachycardia.

Drugs that act postsynaptically—depolarising blocking agents

This class of neuromuscular-blocking drugs was discovered by Paton & Zaimis in their study of the effects of symmetrical bisquaternary ammonium compounds. One of these, **decamethonium**, was found to cause paralysis without appreciable ganglion-blocking activity. Several features of its action showed it to be different from competitive blocking drugs such as tubocurarine. In particular it was found to produce a transient twitching of skeletal muscle (fasciculation) before causing block, and when it was injected into chicks it caused a powerful extensor spasm, whereas tubocurarine simply caused flaccid paralysis. In 1951 Burns & Paton showed that its action was to cause a maintained depolarisation at the endplate region of the muscle fibre, which led to a loss of electrical excitability (see p. 123), and they coined the term 'depolarisation block'. The reason for the curious extensor spasm produced in birds is that they possess a special type of skeletal muscle, rare in mammals, that has many endplates scattered over the surface of each muscle fibre. A drug that causes endplate depolarisation produces a widespread depolarisation in such muscles, resulting in a maintained contracture. In normal skeletal muscle, with only one endplate per fibre, endplate depolarisation is too localised to cause contracture on its own. Fasciculation occurs because the developing endplate depolarisation initially causes a discharge of action potentials in the muscle fibre. This subsides after a few seconds as the electrical excitability of the endplate region of the fibre is lost.

Decamethonium itself was used clinically but has the disadvantage of too long a duration of action. **Suxamethonium** (Table 6.4) is closely related in structure to both decamethonium and acetylcholine (consisting of two acetylcholine molecules linked by their acetyl groups). Its action is shorter than that of decamethonium because it is quickly hydrolysed by plasma cholinesterase. Suxamethonium and decamethonium act on the motor endplate just like acetylcholine (i.e. they are agonists that increase the cation permeability of the endplate). The difference is that decamethonium and suxamethonium, when given as drugs, diffuse slowly to the endplate and the concentration at the endplate persists for long enough to cause loss of electrical excitability. Acetylcholine, in contrast, when released from the nerve, reaches the endplate in very brief spurts and is rapidly hydrolysed in situ, so it never causes sufficiently prolonged depolarisation to result in block. If cholinesterase is inhibited, however (see p. 144), it is possible for the circulating acetylcholine concentration to reach a level sufficient to cause depolarisation block.

Comparison of non-depolarising and depolarising blocking drugs

The neuromuscular block produced by these two mechanisms differs in many characteristics, which are set out in Table 6.5. The most important distinction is that anticholinesterase drugs are very effective in overcoming the blocking action of competitive agents (Fig. 6.8). This is mainly because the released acetylcholine, protected from hydrolysis, can diffuse further within the synaptic cleft, and so gains access to a wider area of postsynaptic membrane than it normally would. The chances of an acetylcholine molecule finding an unoccupied receptor are thus increased. This diffusional effect seems to be of more importance than a truly competitive interaction, for it is unlikely that appreciable dissociation of the antagonist can occur in the short time for which the acetylcholine is present. With depolarisation block no reversal occurs with anticholinesterase drugs; indeed prolongation of the endplate potential can cause the block to be deepened slightly.

A mutual antagonism between competitive and depolarising drugs can be demonstrated (Fig. 6.8). Addition of tubocurarine to a muscle partly paralysed with suxamethonium will reduce the depolarisation, and, provided the tubocurarine concentration is not high enough to cause block in its own right, transmission will be restored. Similarly in a tubocurarine-blocked muscle the small depolarising effect of suxamethonium can bring the membrane potential closer to threshold, so that previously subthreshold endplate potentials exceed the threshold, and transmission is restored (Fig. 6.8).

Table 6.5 Comparison of effects of different types of neuromuscular block

Effect	Type of block Non-depolarising	Depolarising	Choline uptake inhibition
Effect of anticholinesterase	Block reversed	Block enhanced	No effect
Response to tetanus	Rapid fade	Sustained	Slow fade
Initial fasciculations	Absent	Present	Absent
Rate of onset	Fast (c. 1 min)	Fast (c. 30 s)	Slow
Effect of depolarising drugs*	Block reversed	Block enhanced	No effect
Effect of competitive antagonist*	Block enhanced	Block reduced	Block enhanced
Effect of choline	No effect	No effect	Block reversed
Effect of increased stimulation frequency	No effect	No effect	Block reversed
Effect in myasthenic patients	Blocking potency increased	Blocking potency reduced	Blocking potency increased

*In doses too small to affect transmission in normal muscle

A. Normal

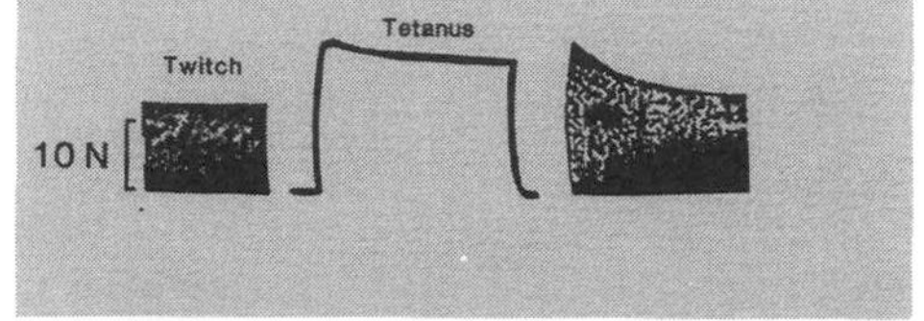

B. Competitive block

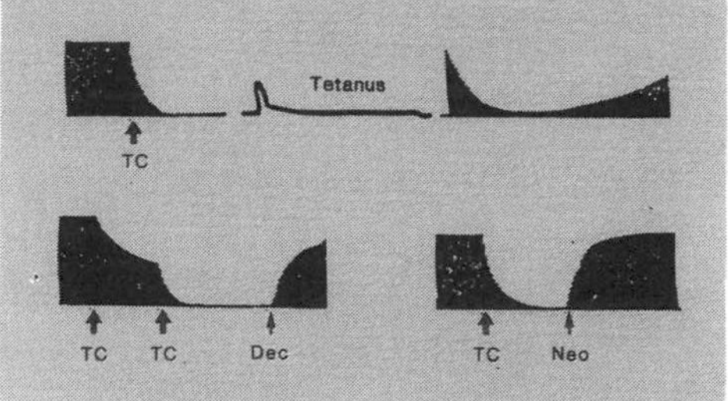

C. Depolarisation block

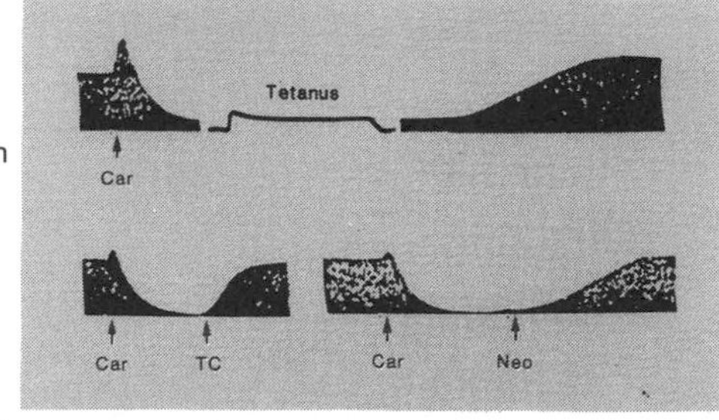

Fig. 6.8 Comparison of depolarising and non-depolarising (competitive) neuromuscular block. Contractions of the cat tibialis muscle were recorded in response to motor nerve stimulation. Twitches were produced by single stimuli delivered every 10 s (slow chart speed), tetani consisted of a 10-s train at 50 Hz (fast chart speed). **A.** Control records. The tetanus is well sustained, and is followed by slight post-tetanic potentiation of the twitch. This is due to a change in the contractile machinery of the muscle, not to facilitated neuromuscular transmission. **B.** Tubocurarine (TC) (0.6 μmol/kg) blocks the twitch completely. The tetanus is not sustained, and is followed by exaggerated post-tetanic potentiation. This is due to a post-tetanic increase in ACh release, which transiently overcomes the block. Tubocurarine block can be reversed by a depolarising drug (decamethonium; Dec) or an anticholinesterase (neostigmine; Neo). **C.** Depolarisation block produced by carbolonium (Car) (35 nmol/kg), a drug very similar to suxamethonium or decamethonium. There is initial enhancement of the twitch, associated with repetitive firing of the muscle fibres, and then block. The tetanus is reduced, but well sustained, and is not followed by post-tetanic potentiation. This is because increased ACh release is ineffective in overcoming depolarisation block. The block can be reversed by tubocurarine, but not by neostigmine. (Modified from: Bowman 1980)

The fasciculations seen with depolarising agents as a prelude to paralysis do not occur with competitive drugs. There appears to be a correlation between the amount of fasciculation and the severity of the *postoperative muscle pain* that is often produced by depolarising drugs, the mechanism of which is not clear.

Depolarising blocking agents are strikingly ineffective in patients with *myasthenia gravis.* In this disease (see p. 145) there are fewer receptors than normal at the endplate, so less depolarisation occurs. In contrast, these patients are hypersensitive to competitive blocking agents, because their margin of safety for transmission is reduced or absent.

'Tetanic fade' is a term used to describe the failure of muscle tension to be maintained during a brief period of nerve stimulation at a frequency high enough to produce a fused tetanus (about 50 Hz). In normal muscle tetanic fade is very slight, but in a muscle blocked with a non-depolarising drug it becomes very marked (Fig. 6.8). This is probably due mainly to the block of presynaptic nicotinic receptors, which normally serve to sustain transmitter release during a tetanus (see Bowman et al. 1988). Fade does not occur with depolarisation block. This difference forms the basis of a simple test used by anaesthetists to discover which type of block is present. Electrodes are used to stimulate a peripheral nerve, such as the ulnar nerve, through the skin, and muscle contraction is observed during a short period of tetanic stimulation.

Phase I and phase II block

With repeated or continuous administration, the action of depolarising drugs tends to change. Initially the block shows the physiological characteristics of depolarisation block, as described above (phase I), but later it takes on some of the properties associated with non-depolarising block (phase II). Thus the block becomes partially reversible by anticholinesterase drugs, and begins to show tetanic fade. The mechanism of this change is not very clear, but it probably results from *receptor desensitisation* produced by the continued presence of the depolarising drug. When this happens the membrane potential is partially restored (see Fig. 6.4), but at the same time the endplate sensitivity to acetylcholine will be reduced as with tubocurarine accounting for the change in mechanism of the block. The transition from phase I to phase II block has often been reported when large or repeated doses of suxamethonium are used clinically.

Unwanted effects and dangers of depolarising drugs

Suxamethonium, the only drug of current clinical importance in this group, can produce a number of important adverse effects which are described below.

Bradycardia. This is preventable by atropine and is probably due to a direct muscarinic action.

Potassium release. The increase in cation permeability of the motor endplates causes a net loss of potassium from muscle and, thus, a small rise in plasma potassium concentration (Fig. 6.9). In normal individuals this is not important, but in cases of trauma, especially burns, it may be. Figure 6.9 shows the greatly increased potassium release from muscles that have been paralysed by nerve injury. This increase occurs because of post-denervation spread of acetylcholine sensitivity to regions of the muscle fibre away from the endplates (see Ch. 5), so that a much larger area of membrane is sensitive to suxamethonium, and the resulting hyperkalaemia can be enough to cause serious ventricular dysrhythmia or even cardiac arrest.

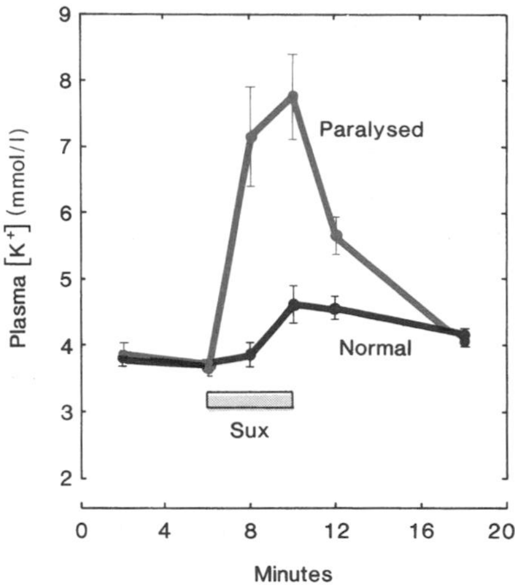

Fig. 6.9 Effect of suxamethonium on plasma potassium concentration in man. Blood was collected from veins draining paralysed and non-paralysed limbs of seven injured patients undergoing surgery. The injuries had resulted in motor nerve degeneration, and hence denervation supersensitivity of the affected muscles. (From: Tobey R E et al. 1972 Anaesthesiology 37: 322)

Increased intraocular pressure. This results from contracture of extraocular muscles (which are physiologically similar to avian muscles; see p. 135) applying pressure to the eyeball. It is particularly important to avoid this if the eyeball has been injured.

Prolonged paralysis. The action of suxamethonium given intravenously normally lasts for less than 5 minutes because the drug is hydrolysed by plasma cholinesterase. Its action is prolonged by various factors that reduce the activity of this enzyme:

- Genetic variants in which plasma cholinesterase is abnormal (see Ch. 42). Severe deficiency, enough to increase the duration of action to 2 hours or more, occurs in only about 1 in 2000 individuals. In a very few individuals, the enzyme is completely absent and the drug's effect lasts for many hours.

- Anticholinesterase drugs. The use of organophosphates to treat glaucoma (see p. 144) can inhibit plasma cholinesterase. Also, competing substrates for plasma cholinesterase (e.g. **procaine**, **propanidid**) can slow down suxamethonium hydrolysis.
- Neonates and patients with liver disease may have low plasma cholinesterase activity and show prolonged paralysis with suxamethonium.

Malignant hyperthermia. This is a rare congenital condition, determined by an autosomal dominant gene (see Ch. 42), which results in intense muscle spasm and a very sudden rise in body temperature when certain drugs are given. The most commonly implicated drugs are suxamethonium and halothane, though it can be precipitated by a variety of other drugs. The biochemical cause is uncertain. The condition carries a very high mortality (about 65%), and is treated by administration of **dantrolene**, a drug that inhibits muscle contraction by preventing calcium release from the sarcoplasmic reticulum.

Pharmacokinetic aspects

Neuromuscular-blocking agents are used mainly in anaesthesia to produce muscle relaxation. Though complete relaxation can be produced by anaesthetic drugs alone, the concentrations needed to obliterate spinal reflexes are high and it is much more satisfactory to produce paralysis by blocking neuromuscular transmission. The drugs are given intravenously, and act within about 30 seconds. Their duration of action varies considerably (Table 6.6, Fig. 6.10).

Table 6.6 Pharmacokinetic characteristics of neuromuscular-blocking drugs

Drug	Approximate duration (min)	Main route of elimination
Suxamethonium	3	Hydrolysis by plasma ChE
Tubocurarine	30	Hepatic 70%, Renal 30%
Gallamine	15	Renal > 95%
Pancuronium	60	Renal 80%
Vecuronium	15	Hepatic > 95%
Atracurium	10	Spontaneous hydrolysis in plasma

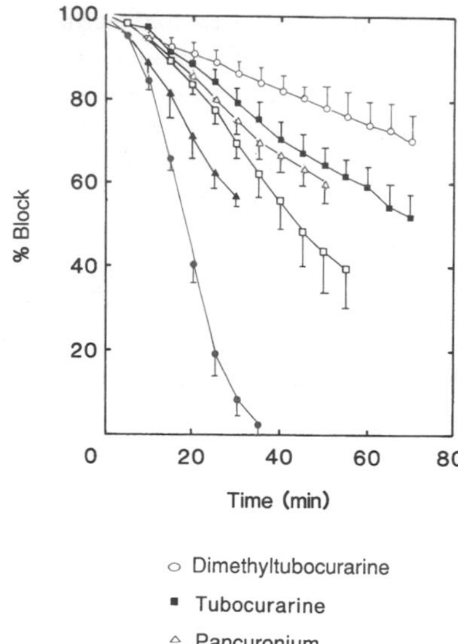

Fig. 6.10 Rate of recovery from various non-depolarising neuromuscular-blocking drugs in man. Drugs were given intravenously to patients undergoing surgery, in doses just sufficient to cause 100% block of the tetanic tension of the indirectly stimulated adductor pollicis muscle. Recovery of tension was then followed as a function of time. (From: Payne J P, Hughes R 1981 Br J Anaesth 53: 45)

Suxamethonium acts for about 3 minutes, being hydrolysed by plasma cholinesterase. It is used to produce transient paralysis for tracheal intubation or very brief procedures. Suxamethonium is also used to produce short-lasting paralysis in patients undergoing electroconvulsive therapy for depression (see Ch. 29). The paralysis reduces the risk of physical injury without diminishing the effectiveness of the treatment.

The non-depolarising blocking agents are, with the exception of **atracurium** (see below), metabolised by the liver or excreted unchanged in the urine, and their duration of action varies between about 10 and 60 minutes (Table 6.6). By this time the patient regains enough strength to cough and breathe properly, though residual weakness may persist for much longer. The route of elimination is important, since many patients undergoing anaesthesia have impaired renal or hepatic function, which, depending on the drug used, can enhance or prolong the paralysis to an important degree.

Gallamine, for example, normally has a rather short duration of action, but in patients with renal failure the paralysis may be dangerously prolonged.

Atracurium is a bisquaternary compound that was designed to be chemically unstable at physiological pH (splitting into two inactive fragments by cleavage at one of the quaternary nitrogen atoms), though indefinitely stable when stored at an acid pH. It has a shorter action than any of the other non-depolarising drugs, but more importantly its duration of action is unaffected by renal or hepatic function, and hence less variable than that of many other neuromuscular-blocking drugs. Because of the marked pH-dependence of its degradation, however, its action becomes considerably briefer during respiratory alkalosis caused by hyperventilation.

Neuromuscular-blocking drugs

- Substances that block choline uptake: hemicholinium, triethylcholine (neither used clinically).
- Substances that block ACh release: aminoglycoside antibiotics, botulinum toxin.
- Drugs used to cause paralysis during anaesthesia are:
  - — Non-depolarising neuromuscular-blocking agents: tubocurarine, gallamine, pancuronium, atracurium. These act as competitive antagonists at nAChR, and differ mainly in duration of action.
  - — Depolarising neuromuscular-blocking agents: suxamethonium.
- Important characteristics of non-depolarising and depolarising blocking drugs:
  - — Non-depolarising block is reversible by anticholinesterase drugs: depolarising block is not.
  - — Depolarising block produces initial fasciculations, and often post-operative muscle pain.
  - — Suxamethonium is hydrolysed by plasma cholinesterase, and is normally very short-acting, but may cause long-lasting paralysis in a small group of congenitally cholinesterase-deficient individuals.
- Main side effects: tubocurarine causes ganglion block, histamine release, hence hypotension, bronchoconstriction; suxamethonium may cause bradycardia, cardiac dysrhythmias due to K^+-release (especially in burned or injured patients), increased intraocular pressure, malignant hyperthermia (rare).

DRUGS THAT ENHANCE CHOLINERGIC TRANSMISSION

The most important drugs that enhance cholinergic transmission act either by inhibiting cholinesterase or by increasing acetylcholine release. In this chapter we discuss mainly the peripheral actions of such drugs; strategies for enhancing cholinergic transmission in the central nervous system, now of interest as possible treatments for senile dementia, are discussed in Chapter 25.

Distribution and function of cholinesterase

There are two distinct types of cholinesterase, namely *acetylcholinesterase* (AChE) and *butyrylcholinesterase* (BChE), closely related in molecular structure but differing in their distribution, substrate specificity and functions (see Chatonnet & Lockridge 1989). Both consist of globular catalytic subunits, which constitute the soluble forms found in plasma (BChE) and CSF (AChE). Elsewhere, the catalytic units are linked to collagen-like tails or to glycolipids, through which they are anchored, like a tethered bunch of balloons, to the cell membrane or the basement membrane at various sites, such as the erythrocyte and the motor endplate.

Acetylcholinesterase, otherwise known as *true cholinesterase*, is bound to the basement membrane in the synaptic cleft at cholinergic synapses, where its function is to hydrolyse the released transmitter. The enzyme is easily demonstrated histochemically (Fig. 6.11) by a technique in which acetylthiocholine is used as substrate and the resulting thiocholine used to form a sulphide precipitate with copper. The soluble form of AChE is also present in cholinergic nerve terminals, where it seems to have a role in regulating the free acetylcholine concentration, and from which it may be secreted; the function of the secreted enzyme is so far unclear. The membrane-bound form also occurs in unexpected places such as the erythrocyte, where its function is unknown. AChE is quite specific for acetylcholine; other closely related esters such as methacholine and acetylthiocholine are also good substrates, but most esters are not. Certain neuropeptides, such as substance P (Ch. 9) are inactivated by AChE, but it is not known whether this is of physiological significance.

Butyrylcholinesterase or *pseudocholinesterase* has a widespread distribution, being found in tissues

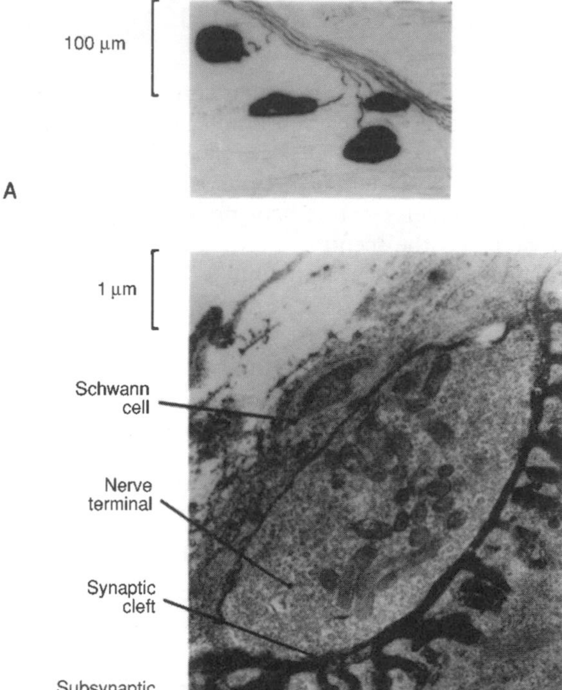

Fig. 6.11 Histochemical localisation of acetylcholinesterase at the mouse neuromuscular junction. A. Whole mount preparation showing individual motor axons (silver stained) terminating on AChe-stained endplates on separate muscle fibres. **B.** Electron micrograph showing staining of AChe in synaptic cleft. (Micrographs kindly provided by Prof L W Duchen)

such as liver, skin, brain and gastrointestinal smooth muscle, as well as in soluble form in the plasma. It is not particularly associated with cholinergic synapses, and has a broader substrate specificity than AChE. It hydrolyses butyrylcholine more rapidly than acetylcholine, as well as other esters, such as **benzoylcholine**, **procaine**, **suxamethonium** and **propanidid** (a short-acting anaesthetic agent; see Ch. 26). The function of this enzyme is not known, but the plasma enzyme is important in relation to the inactivation of the drugs listed above. Genetic variants of BChE occur (see Ch. 42), and these partly account for the variability in the duration of action of these drugs. The very short duration of action of acetylcholine given intravenously (see Fig. 6.1) results from its rapid hydrolysis in the plasma. Normally the activity of AChE and BChE keeps the plasma acetylcholine at an undetectably low level, so acetylcholine is strictly a neurotransmitter and not a hormone.

AChE and BChE belong to the class of *serine hydrolases*, which includes many proteases, such as trypsin. The active site of AChE comprises two distinct regions (Fig. 6.12), an anionic site that possesses a glutamate residue, and an esteratic site in which a histidine imidazole ring and a serine –OH group are particularly important. Catalytic hydrolysis occurs by a mechanism common to other serine hydrolases, whereby the acetyl group is transferred to the serine –OH group, leaving (transiently) an acetylated enzyme molecule and a molecule of free choline. Spontaneous hydrolysis of the serine acetyl group occurs rapidly, and the overall turnover number of AChE is extremely high (over 10 000 molecules of acetylcholine hydrolysed per second by a single active site).

Drugs that inhibit cholinesterase

Anticholinesterase drugs fall into three main groups according to the nature of their interaction with the active site, which determines their duration of action. Most of the clinically important drugs inhibit AChE and BChE about equally.

Short-acting anticholinesterases

The only important drug among the short-acting anticholinesterases is **edrophonium** (Table 6.7), a quaternary ammonium compound that binds to the anionic site of the enzyme only. The ionic bond formed is readily reversible and the action of the drug is very brief. It is used mainly for diagnostic purposes, since improvement of muscle strength by an anticholinesterase is characteristic of myasthenia gravis (see p. 145), but does not occur when muscle weakness is due to other causes.

Medium-duration anticholinesterases

The medium-duration anticholinesterases (Table 6.7) include **neostigmine** and **pyridostigmine,** which are quaternary ammonium compounds of clinical importance, and **physostigmine** (**eserine**), a naturally occurring tertiary amine, the effects of which on the autonomic nervous system were described many years before cholinergic transmission was understood. Physostigmine occurs naturally in the Calabar bean, extracts of which were once used as ordeal poisons to assess the guilt or innocence

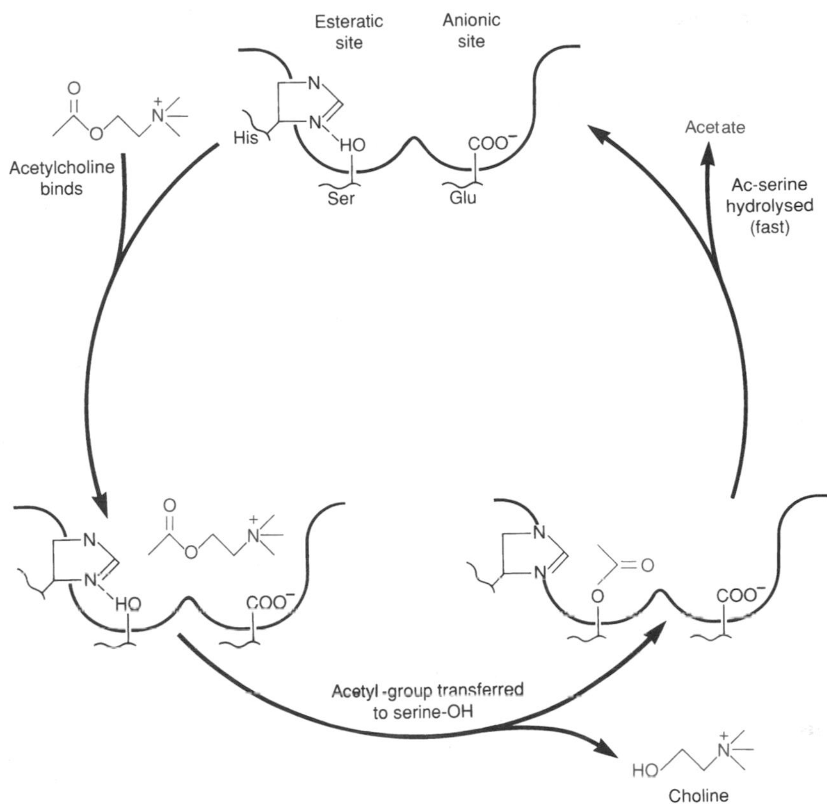

Fig. 6.12 Mechanism of acetylcholine hydrolysis by acetylcholinesterase.

of suspected criminals and heretics; death implied guilt.

These drugs all possess strongly basic groups, which bind to the anionic site, but are carbamyl, as opposed to acetyl, esters. Transfer of the carbamyl group to the serine –OH of the esteratic site occurs as with acetylcholine, but the carbamylated enzyme is very much slower to hydrolyse (Fig. 6.13), taking minutes rather than microseconds. The anticholinesterase drug is therefore hydrolysed, but at a negligible rate compared with acetylcholine, and the slow recovery of the carbamylated enzyme means that the action of these drugs is quite long-lasting.

Irreversible anticholinesterases

Irreversible anticholinesterases (Table 6.7) are pentavalent phosphorus compounds containing a labile group such as fluoride (in **dyflos**) or an organic group (in **parathion** and **ecothiopate**). This group is released, leaving the residue of the molecule attached covalently through the phosphorus atom to the serine –OH group of the enzyme (Fig. 6.13). Most of these organophosphate compounds, of which there are many, developed as war gases and pesticides as well as for clinical use, interact only with the esteratic site of the enzyme and have no cationic group. Ecothiopate is an exception in having a quaternary nitrogen group designed to bind also to the anionic site.

The inactive phosphorylated enzyme is usually very stable. With drugs such as dyflos no appreciable hydrolysis occurs, and recovery of enzymic activity depends on the synthesis of new enzyme molecules, a process that may take weeks. With other drugs such as ecothiopate slow hydrolysis occurs over the course of a few days, so that their action is not strictly speaking irreversible. Dyflos and parathion are volatile non-polar substances of very high lipid solubility, and are rapidly absorbed through mucous membranes and even through unbroken skin and insect cuticles; the use of these agents as war gases or insecticides relies on this property. The lack of a specificity-conferring quaternary group means that most of these drugs block other serine hydrolases

Table 6.7 Anticholinesterase drugs

Drug	Structure	Duration of action (long/med/short)	Main site of action	Notes
Edrophonium	HO–C₆H₄–N⊕(CH₃)₂–CH₂CH₃	S	NMJ*	Used mainly in diagnosis of myasthenia gravis. Too short-acting for therapeutic use.
Neostigmine	(H_3C)₂N–C(=O)–O–C₆H₄–N⊕(CH_3)₃	M	NMJ	Used i.v. to reverse competitive neuromuscular block. Used orally in treatment of myasthenia gravis. Visceral side effects.
Physostigmine	H(H₃C)N–C(=O)–O–(tricyclic, CH_3, N–CH_3, N–CH_3)	M	P	Used as eye drops in treatment of glaucoma.
Pyridostigmine	(H_3C)₂N–C(=O)–O–pyridinium–N⊕–CH_3	M	NMJ	Used orally in treatment of myasthenia gravis. Better absorbed than neostigmine, and has longer duration of action.
Dyflos	[(H_3C)₂CH–O]₂P(=O)F	L	P	Highly toxic organophosphate, with very prolonged action. Has been used as eye drops for glaucoma.
Ecothiopate	(H_3CCH₂O)₂P(=O)–S–CH₂CH₂–N⊕(CH_3)₃	L	P	Used as eye drops in treatment of glaucoma. Prolonged action; may cause systemic effects.
Parathion	(H_3CCH₂O)₂P(=S)–O–C₆H₄–NO_2	L	–	Converted to active metabolite by replacement of sulphur by oxygen. Used as insecticide, but commonly causes poisoning in man.

* NMJ = neuromuscular junction; P = postganglionic parasympathetic junction

(e.g. trypsin, thrombin) though their pharmacological effects result mainly from cholinesterase inhibition.

Effects of anticholinesterase drugs

The effects of cholinesterase inhibition are of three main types:

- effects on autonomic cholinergic synapses
- effects on the neuromuscular junction
- effects on the central nervous system.

Some organophosphate compounds can produce, in addition, a form of neurotoxicity not associated with cholinesterase inhibition.

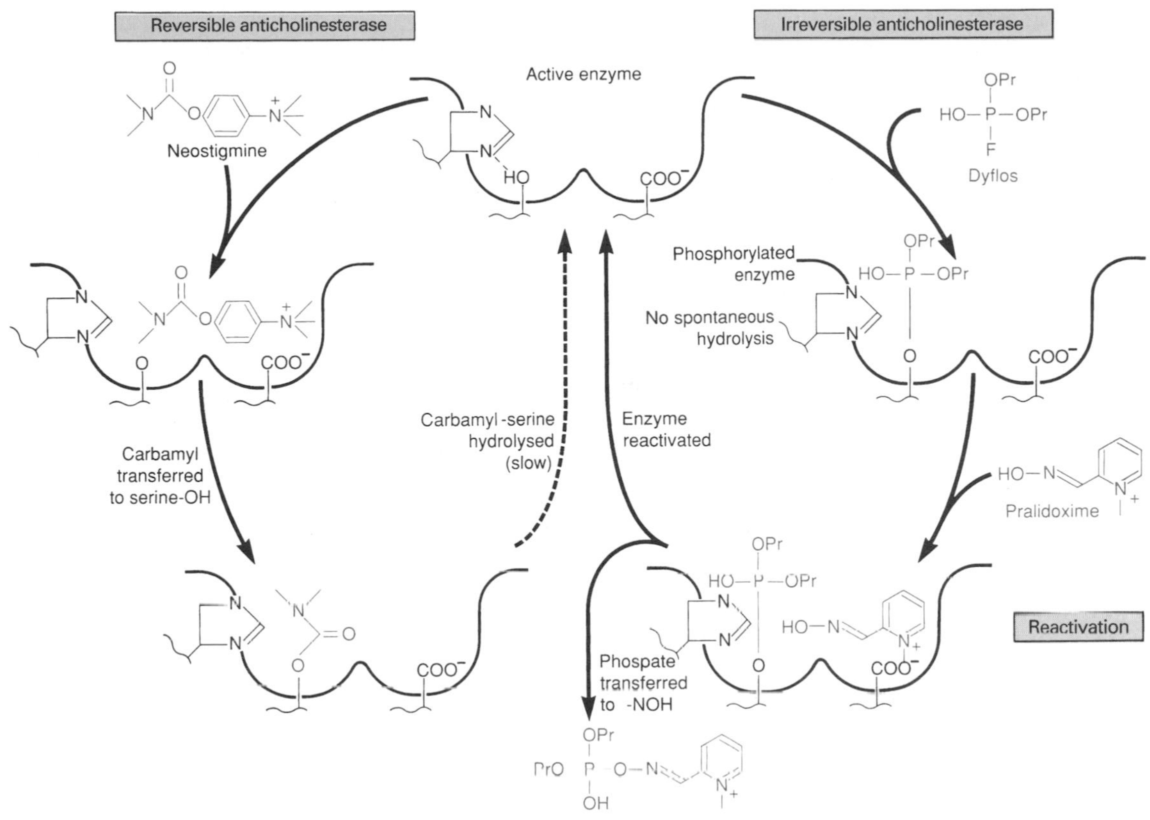

Fig. 6.13 Action of anticholinesterase drugs. *Reversible anticholinesterase* (neostigmine). Recovery of activity by hydrolysis of the carbamylated enzyme takes many minutes; *irreversible anticholinesterase* (dyflos); *reactivation of phosphorylated enzyme* by pralidoxime.

Effects on autonomic cholinergic synapses. These mainly reflect enhancement of acetylcholine activity at parasympathetic postganglionic synapses (i.e. increased secretions from salivary, lacrimal, bronchial and gastrointestinal glands, increased peristaltic activity, bronchoconstriction, bradycardia and hypotension, pupillary constriction, fixation of accommodation for near vision, fall in intraocular pressure). Large doses can stimulate, and later block, autonomic ganglia, producing complex autonomic effects. The block, if it occurs, is a depolarisation block and is associated with a build-up of acetylcholine in the plasma and body fluids. Neostigmine and pyridostigmine tend to affect neuromuscular transmission more than the autonomic system, whereas physostigmine and organophosphates show the reverse pattern. The reason is not clear, but therapeutic usage takes advantage of this partial selectivity.

Anticholinesterase poisoning (e.g. from contact with insecticides or war gases) causes severe bradycardia, hypotension and difficulty in breathing. Combined with a depolarising neuromuscular block, and central effects (see below), the result may be fatal.

Effects on the neuromuscular junction. The twitch tension of a muscle stimulated via its motor nerve is increased by anticholinesterases. Electrophysiological recording shows that this is associated with repetitive firing in the muscle fibre. Normally, the acetylcholine is hydrolysed so quickly that each stimulus initiates only one action potential in the muscle fibre. When cholinesterase is inhibited a single endplate potential lasts for long enough to produce a short train of action potentials in the muscle fibre, and hence greater tension. Much more important is the effect produced when transmission has been blocked by a competitive blocking agent, such as tubocurarine. In this case, addition of an anticholinesterase can dramatically restore transmission (Fig. 6.8). If a large proportion of the receptors is blocked, the majority of acetylcholine molecules will normally encounter, and be destroyed by, an AChE molecule before reaching a vacant receptor; inhibiting AChE will thus increase the number of acetylcholine molecules that will find their way to a vacant receptor, and thus increase the endplate potential so that it reaches threshold. In *myasthenia gravis* (see below) transmission fails because there are too few acetylcholine receptors, and cholinesterase inhibition improves transmission just as it does in curarised muscle.

In large doses, such as can occur in poisoning, anticholinesterases initially cause twitching of muscles. This is because spontaneous acetylcholine release can give rise to endplate potentials that reach the firing threshold, and may later cause a paralysis due to depolarisation block, which is associated with the build-up of acetylcholine in the plasma and tissue fluids.

Effects on the CNS. Tertiary compounds, such as physostigmine, and the non-polar organophosphates penetrate the blood–brain barrier freely and affect the brain. The result is an initial excitation, which can result in convulsions, followed by depression, which can cause unconsciousness and respiratory failure. These central effects result mainly from the activation of muscarinic receptors, and are antagonised by atropine. The potential use of brain-selective anticholinesterases to treat senile dementia is discussed in Chapter 25.

Neurotoxicity of organophosphates. Many organophosphates can cause a severe type of peripheral nerve demyelination, leading to slowly developing weakness and sensory loss. This is not a problem with clinically used anticholinesterases, but occasionally occurs with accidental poisoning. In 1931 an estimated 20 000 Americans were affected, some fatally, by contamination of fruit juice with an organophosphate insecticide, and other similar outbreaks have been recorded. The mechanism of this reaction is only partly understood, but it seems to result from inhibition of an esterase (not cholinesterase itself) specific to myelin.

The main clinical uses of anticholinesterases are summarised on page 145.

Cholinesterase reactivation

Spontaneous hydrolysis of phosphorylated cholinesterase is extremely slow, a fact that makes poisoning with organophosphates very dangerous. In 1955, Wilson developed a compound that can reactivate the enzyme by bringing into close proximity with the phosphorylated esteratic site an oxime group that is a sufficiently strong nucleophile for the covalent bond to be transferred to it from the serine –OH of the enzyme. This compound, **pralidoxime** (Fig. 6.13), also possesses a quaternary nitrogen atom so that it can bind to the anionic site. Its effectiveness in restoring cholinesterase activity in the plasma of a poisoned subject is shown in Figure 6.14. There are two drawbacks to its use as an antidote to organophosphate poisoning. The first is that within a few hours the phosphorylated enzyme undergoes a change ('ageing') that renders it no longer susceptible to reactivation, so that pralidoxime must be given early in order to work.

Cholinesterase and anticholinesterase drugs

- There are two main forms of cholinesterase (ChE): acetylcholinesterase (ACheE), which is membrane-bound, relatively specific for ACh, and responsible for rapid ACh hydrolysis at cholinergic synapses; butyrylcholinesterase (BChE) or pseudocholinesterase, which is relatively non-selective, and occurs in plasma and many tissues. Both enzymes belong to the family of serine hydrolases.
- Anticholinesterase drugs are of three main types: short-acting (edrophonium); medium-acting (neostigmine, physostigmine); irreversible (organophosphates, dyflos, ecothiopate). They differ in the nature of their chemical interaction with the active site of ChE.
- Effects of antiChE drugs are due mainly to enhancement of cholinergic transmission at cholinergic autonomic synapses and at the neuromuscular junction. AntiChEs that cross the blood–brain barrier (e.g. physostigmine, organophosphates) also have marked CNS effects. Autonomic effects include bradycardia, hypotension, excessive secretions, bronchoconstriction, gastrointestinal hypermotility, decrease of intraocular pressure. Neuromuscular action causes muscle fasciculation and increased twitch tension, and can produce depolarisation block.
- AntiChE poisoning may occur from exposure to insecticides or nerve gases.

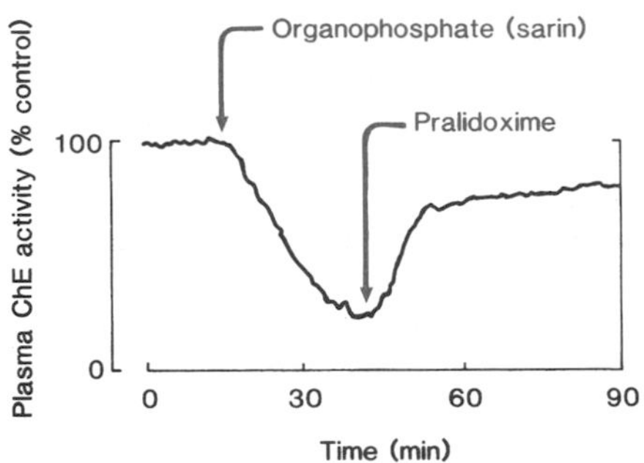

Fig. 6.14 Reactivation of plasma cholinesterase in a volunteer subject by intravenous injection of pralidoxime. (Redrawn from: Sim V M 1965 J Amer Med Ass 192: 404)

Clinical uses of anticholinesterases

- In anaesthesia; to reverse the action of non-depolarising neuromuscular blocking drugs; **neostigmine** intravenously.
  - —Neostigmine lacks central effects and causes fewer parasympathetic effects than other anticholinesterases; nevertheless, atropine is given routinely as a precaution.
- In the treatment of myasthenia gravis (see p 145); **neostigmine** or **pyridostigmine** orally.
  - —Pyridostigmine acts for slightly longer (3–6 h) than neostigmine (2–4 h).
  - —Muscarinic side effects tend to wear off with continued use.
  - —Excess use can produce a *cholinergic crisis* consisting of various muscarinic effects (salivation, gastrointestinal cramps, lacrimation, poor vision, etc.) together with muscle weakness, resulting presumably from depolarisation block. Injection of edrophonium may be used as a test to distinguish between this drug-induced weakness and the weakness of myasthenia itself; if the weakness transiently improves it is due to myasthenia and more anticholinesterase is indicated; if it gets worse the anticholinesterase dose should be reduced.
- In the treatment of glaucoma; **physostigmine** or **ecothiopate** as eye drops.
  - —Systemic side effects may occur, and plasma cholinesterase activity may be reduced, which can cause prolongation of the action of suxamethonium, if this is given concurrently.

Secondly, pralidoxime does not enter the brain, so cannot reverse the central effects of organophosphate poisoning.

Myasthenia gravis

The neuromuscular junction is a remarkably robust structure which very rarely fails, myasthenia gravis being one of the very few disorders that specifically affects it (see review by Drachman 1981, Graus & De Baets 1993). This disease affects about 1 in 2000 individuals, who show muscle weakness and increased fatigability resulting from a failure of neuromuscular transmission. Electrophysiological studies have shown that transmitter release is normal, but that the amplitude of the endplate potential is greatly reduced, so that it often fails to reach threshold. The tendency for transmission to fail during repetitive activity can be seen in Figure 6.15. Functionally, it results in the inability of muscles to produce sustained contractions, of which the

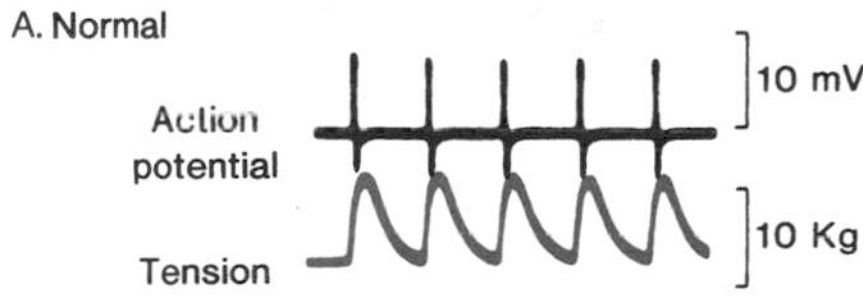

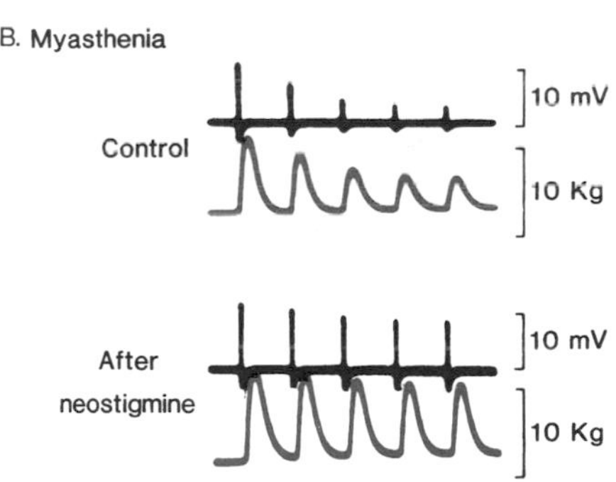

Fig. 6.15 Neuromuscular transmission in a normal and a myasthenic human subject. Electrical activity was recorded with a needle electrode in the adductor pollicis muscle, in response to ulnar nerve stimulation (3 Hz) at the wrist. **A.** In normal subject, electrical and mechanical response is well sustained. **B.** In myasthenic patient, transmission fails rapidly when nerve is stimulated. Treatment with neostigmine improves transmission. (From: Desmedt J E 1962 Bull Acad Roy Med Belg VII 2: 213)

characteristic drooping eyelids of myasthenic patients are a sign. The effectiveness of anticholinesterase drugs in improving muscle strength in myasthenia was discovered in 1931, long before the cause of the disease was known.

Studies with α-bungarotoxin binding revealed that in myasthenic muscle the number of receptors per endplate was, on average, only about one-third of normal. Before this it had been suspected that myasthenia had an immunological basis, for removal of the thymus gland (which often shows pathological changes in this disease) was frequently of benefit. An immunological explanation of the disappearance of receptors from the neuromuscular junction emerged in 1974, when the presence of antibody directed against the acetylcholine receptor protein was discovered in the serum of myasthenic patients (see Drachman 1994). It had earlier been found that immunisation of rabbits with purified acetylcholine receptor caused, after a delay, symptoms very similar to human myasthenia gravis. Myasthenia gravis can therefore be classified as an autoimmune disease, though the reason for the development of the immune response is still unknown.

The improvement of neuromuscular function by anticholinesterase treatment (shown in Fig. 6.15) can be dramatic. It occurs because any given acetylcholine molecule released into the synaptic cleft is less likely to be destroyed by an encounter with cholinesterase, and therefore more likely to reach one of the few remaining receptors. If the disease progresses too far, the number of receptors remaining may become too few to produce an adequate endplate potential, and anticholinesterase drugs will then cease to be effective.

Alternative approaches to the treatment of myasthenia are to remove circulating antibody by plasma exchange, which is transiently effective, or, for a more prolonged effect, to inhibit antibody production with steroids (e.g. **prednisolone**) or immunosuppressant drugs (e.g. **azathioprine**; see Ch. 12).

Other drugs which enhance cholinergic transmission

It was observed many years ago that tetraethylammonium, better known as a ganglion-blocking drug (see p. 129) could reverse the neuromuscular-blocking action of tubocurarine, and this was shown to be because it increases the release of transmitter evoked by nerve stimulation. About 10 years ago compounds of the aminopyridine group (see Ch. 34), which block K^+-channels, and thus prolong the action potential in the presynaptic nerve terminal, were found to act similarly, and to be considerably more potent and selective in their actions than tetraethylammonium. These drugs are not selective for cholinergic nerves, but increase the evoked release of many different transmitters, so have too many unwanted effects to be useful in treating neuromuscular disorders.

REFERENCES AND FURTHER READING

Aktories K, Wegner A 1989 ADP-ribosylation of actin by clostridial toxins. J Cell Biol 109: 1385–1387

Blusztajn J K, Wurtman R J 1983 Choline and cholinergic neurons. Science 221: 614–620

Bonner T I 1989 New subtypes of muscarinic acetylcholine receptors. Supplement to Trends Pharmacol Sci: 11–15

Bowman W C 1990 Pharmacology of neuromuscular function. Wright, Bristol

Bowman W C, Marshall I G, Gibb A J, Harborne A J 1988 Feedback control of transmitter release at the neuromuscular junction. Trends Pharmacol Sci 9: 16–20

Brown D A 1980 Locus and mechanism of action of ganglion blocking agents. In: Kharkevich D A (ed) Pharmacology of ganglionic transmission. Handbook of experimental pharmacology. Springer-Verlag, Berlin, vol 53: 185–235

Burns B D, Paton W D M 1951 Depolarisation of the motor end-plate by decamethonium and acetylcholine. J Physiol 115: 41–73

Chattonet A, Lockridge O 1989 Comparison of butyrlcholinesterase and acetylcholinesterase. Biochem J 260: 625–634

Colquhoun D, Ogden D C, Mathie A 1987 Nicotinic acetylcholine receptors of nerve and muscle: functional aspects. Trends Pharmacol Sci 8: 465–472

Drachman D B 1994 Myasthenia gravis. New Engl J Med 330: 1797–1810

Dunant Y 1986 On the mechanism of acetylcholine release. Prog Neurobiol 26: 55–92

Ginsborg B L, Jenkinson D H 1976 Transmission of impulses from nerve to muscle. In: Zaimis E J (ed) Neuromuscular junction. Handbook of experimental pharmacology. Springer-Verlag, Berlin, vol 42: 229–364

Goyal R K 1989 Muscarinic receptor subtypes: physiology and clinical implications. N Engl J Med 321: 1022–1029

Graus Y M, De Baets M H 1993 Myasthenia gravis: an autoimmune response against the acetylcholine receptor. Immunol Res 12: 78–100

Hunter J M 1987 Adverse effects of neuromuscular blocking drugs. Br J Anaesth 59: 46–60

Karczmar A G, Koketsu K, Nishi S 1985 Autonomic and enteric ganglia: transmission and its pharmacology. Plenum Press, New York

Kharkevich D A (ed) 1980 Pharmacology of ganglionic transmission. Handbook of experimental pharmacology. Springer-Verlag, Berlin, vol 53

Kilbinger H 1984 Presynaptic muscarinic receptors modulating acetylcholine release. Trends Pharmacol Sci 5: 103–105

Leopold I H, Duzman E 1986 Observations on the pharmacology of glaucoma. Annu Rev Pharmacol Toxicol 26: 401–426

Lindstrom J M, Seybold M E, Lennon V M, Whittingham S, Duane D 1976 Antibody to acetylcholine receptor in myasthenia gravis. Neurology 26: 1054–1059

Nathanson N M 1987 Molecular properties of the muscarinic acetylcholine receptor. Annu Rev Neurosci 10: 197–236

Newsom-Davis J, Vincent A, Wilcox N 1993 Autoimmune disorders of the neuromuscular junction. In: Lachmann P J, Peters D K, Rosen F S, Walport M J (eds) Clinical aspects of immunology. Blackwell, Oxford

Nicholls J G, Martin A R, Wallace B G 1992 From neuron to brain. Sinauer, Sunderland MA.

Oorschot D E, Jones D G 1987 The vesicle hypothesis and its alternatives: a critical assessment. In: Current topics in research on synapses. Liss, New York, vol 4: 85–122

Parsons S M, Prior C, Marshall I G (1993) Acetylcholine transport, storage and release. Int Rev Neurobiol 35: 279–390

Paton W D M 1954 The principles of ganglion block. Lectures on the scientific basis of medicine. Athlone Press, London, vol 2

Role L W 1992 Diversity in structure and function of neuronal nicotinic acetylcholine receptor channels. Curr Opin Neurobiol 2: 254–262

Skok V I 1980 Ganglionic transmission: morphology and physiology. In: Kharkevich D A (ed) Pharmacology of ganglionic transmission. Handbook of experimental pharmacology. Springer-Verlag, Berlin, vol 53: 9–39

Zaimis E 1976 Neuromuscular function. Handbook of experimental pharmacology. Springer-Verlag, Berlin, vol 42

7 NORADRENERGIC TRANSMISSION

The noradrenergic neuron is an important target for drug action, both as an object for investigation in its own right and as a point of attack for many clinically useful drugs. For convenience a table summarising much of the pharmacological information is given at the end of the chapter (Table 7.4), together with a short glossary of special terms relating to noradrenergic transmission.

CLASSIFICATION OF ADRENOCEPTORS

In 1896, Oliver & Schafer demonstrated that injection of extracts of adrenal gland caused a rise in arterial pressure. Following the subsequent isolation of adrenaline as the active principle, it was shown by Dale in 1913 that adrenaline causes two distinct kinds of effect, namely vasoconstriction in certain vascular beds (which normally predominates and causes the rise in arterial pressure) and vasodilatation in others. Dale showed that the vasoconstrictor component disappeared if the animal was first injected with an ergot derivative* (see p. 183), and noticed that adrenaline then caused a fall, instead of a rise, in arterial pressure. Dale, partly because of a disagreement with J N Langley, studiously avoided interpreting this result (which closely parallels his demonstration of the separate muscarinic and nicotinic components of the action of acetylcholine; see Ch. 6) in terms of a distinction between categories of receptor. Later pharmacological work, however, beginning with that of Ahlquist in 1948 showed clearly that several subclasses of adrenoceptor exist in the body. Ahlquist found that the rank order of the potencies of various catecholamines, including **adrenaline, noradrenaline** and **isoprenaline** (a synthetic catecholamine; see Fig. 7.1), fell into two distinct patterns, depending on what response was being measured. He postulated the existence of two kinds of receptor, α and β, defined in terms of agonist potencies as follows:

Receptor	Order of agonist potency
α	Noradrenaline > adrenaline > isoprenaline
β	Isoprenaline > adrenaline > noradrenaline

It was then recognised that certain ergot alkaloids,

*Dale was a new recruit in the laboratories of the Wellcome pharmaceutical company, and was responsible for checking the potency of adrenaline ampoules coming from the factory. He tested one batch at the end of a day's experimentation on a cat to which he had given an ergot preparation. Because the adrenaline had such an unexpected effect, he suggested that the whole expensive consignment should be destroyed. Unknown to him, the same sample was given to him again a few days later, and behaved perfectly normally. How Dale explained this to Wellcome's management is not recorded.

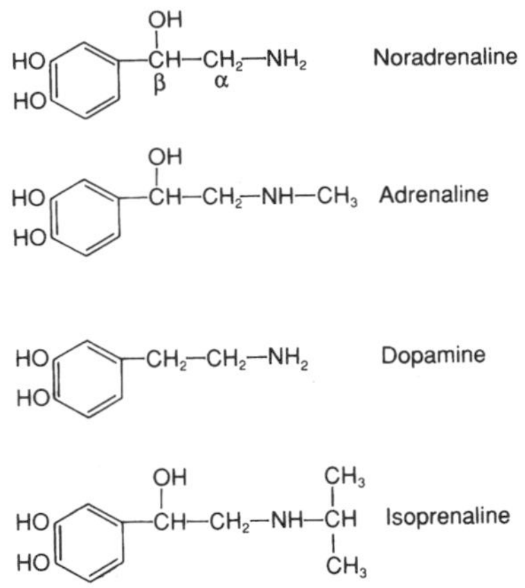

Fig. 7.1 Structures of the major catecholamines.

which Dale had studied, act as selective α-receptor antagonists, and that Dale's adrenaline reversal experiment reflected the unmasking of the β effects of adrenaline by α-receptor blockade. Various other α-receptor antagonists were known at that time, but selective β-receptor antagonists were not developed until 1955. The use of these selective antagonists confirmed Ahlquist's original classification, but also suggested the existence of further subdivisions of both α- and β-receptors. It was first shown by Lands and his colleagues that different β-adrenoceptor agonists differ in their relative potency in eliciting different types of β-receptor-mediated effects in different tissues; subsequent studies with agonists and antagonists have confirmed the existence of two main α-receptor subtypes and two main β-receptor

Table 7.1 Effects mediated by adrenoceptor subtypes

	Adrenoceptor			
Tissue	α_1	α_2	β_1	β_2
Smooth muscle				
Blood vessels	Constrict	Constrict		Dilate
Bronchi	Constrict			Dilate
GI tract				
Non-sphincter	Relax (hyperpolarisation)	Relax (presynaptic effect)		Relax (no hyperpolarisation)
Sphincter	Contract			
Uterus	Contract			Relax
Bladder				
Detrusor				Relax
Sphincter	Contract			
Seminal tract	Contract			Relax
Iris (radial)	Contract			
Ciliary muscle				Relax
Heart			Incr rate Incr force	
Skeletal muscle				Tremor
Liver	Glycogenolysis K^+ release			Glycogenolysis
Fat			Lipolysis (β_3-receptor)	
Nerve terminals				
Adrenergic		Decr release	Incr release	
Cholinergic (some)		Decr release		
Salivary gland	K^+ release		Amylase secretion	
Platelets		Aggregation		
Mast cells				Inhibition of histamine release
Second messengers	IP_3, DAG	↓cAMP	↑cAMP	↑cAMP

Table 7.2 Receptor specificity of adrenoceptor agonists and antagonists

	Adrenoceptor			
	α_1	α_2	β_1	β_2
Agonists				
Noradrenaline	+++	+++	++	+
Adrenaline	++	++	+++	+++
Isoprenaline	–	–	+++	+++
Phenylephrine	++	–	–	–
Methylnoradrenaline	+	+++	–	–
Clonidine	–	+++	–	–
Salbutamol	–	–	+	+++
Terbutaline	–	–	+	+++
Dobutamine	–	–	+++	+
Antagonists				
Phentolamine	+++	+++	–	–
Phenoxybenzamine	+++	+++	–	–
Ergotamine	++PA	++	–	–
Dihydroergotamine	++	++	–	–
Yohimbine	+	+++	–	–
Prazosin	+++	+	–	–
Indoramin	+++	+	–	–
Propranolol	–	–	+++	+++
Oxprenolol	–	–	+++PA	+++
Atenolol	–	–	+++	+
Butoxamine	–	–	+	+++
Labetalol	+	+	++	++

PA = partial agonist.

subtypes (Tables 7.1 and 7.2).* Cloning studies have shown that all of the adrenoceptors are G-protein-coupled receptors with seven transmembrane α-helical segments, and have revealed considerable molecular heterogeneity, even within the pharmacological classes listed in Table 7.1 (see Ruffolo et al. 1991; Summers & McMartin 1993).

Each of these pharmacological classes appears generally to be associated with a specific second messenger system (Table 7.1). Thus α_1-receptors are coupled to phospholipase C, and produce their effects mainly by the release of intracellular calcium; α_2-receptors are negatively coupled to adenylate cyclase, and reduce cAMP formation; all three types of β-receptor act by stimulation of adenylate cyclase. The major effects that are produced by these receptors, and the pattern of specificity among various agonists and antagonists are shown in Tables 7.1 and 7.2.

The distinction between β_1- and β_2-receptors is an important one, for β_1-receptors are found mainly in the heart, where they are responsible for the positive inotropic and chronotropic effects of catecholamines (see Ch. 13). β_2-receptors, on the other hand, are responsible for causing smooth muscle relaxation in many organs. The latter is often a useful therapeutic effect, while the former is more often harmful; consequently, considerable efforts have been made to find selective β_2 agonists, which would relax smooth muscle without affecting the heart, and selective β_1 antagonists, which would exert a useful blocking effect on the heart without at the same time blocking β_2-receptors in bronchial smooth muscle. The compounds listed in Table 7.2 are some of the results of these searches. Other experimental compounds that distinguish between the various adrenoceptor subtypes but are not yet available for clinical use are listed in the Receptor Nomenclature Supplement (1994). It is important to realise that the selectivity of these drugs is relative rather than absolute, and that the compounds listed, for example, as selective β_1 antagonists invariably have some action on β_2-receptors as well. Unfortunately, there are appreciable species differences, and the high degree of receptor specificity found for some agonists and antagonists in experiments on guinea-pig tissues in vitro has often not been borne out fully in measurements made on human subjects. Furthermore, it appears that both types of β-receptor contribute to some effects, such as the chronotropic action, with the relative contribution of each varying from species to species. The need to subdivide α-receptors arose when it was discovered in 1972 that catecholamines exert a presynaptic inhibitory effect (see Ch. 5), which is mediated by an α-receptor whose pharmacological specificity is different from that of the receptors responsible for the well-known effects of catecholamines. It was found, for example, that some agonists, such as **methylnoradrenaline** and **clonidine**, act selectively on presynaptic (α_2) receptors, as do certain antagonists, such as **yohimbine**, while other antagonists (e.g. **prazosin**) do not affect presynaptic receptors.

It was originally thought that the α_1/α_2 classification corresponded directly with the pre- or postsynaptic location of the receptors, but several exceptions to this rule are now known. Thus α_2-receptors occur on liver cells, platelets, smooth

*A third type of β-receptor (β_3) has recently been defined. It occurs mainly on fat cells, causing lipolysis.

Classification of adrenoceptors

- Main pharmacological classification into α- and β-subtypes, based originally on order of potency among agonists, later on selective antagonists.
- There are two main α-adrenoceptor subtypes (α_1, α_2) and three β-adrenoceptor subtypes (β_1, β_2, β_3). Cloning studies show that all are similar in structure, and belong to the superfamily of G-protein-coupled receptors.
- Second messengers: α_1-receptors activate phospholipase C, thus producing $InsP_3$ and DAG as second messengers; α_2-receptors inhibit adenylate cyclase, and thus decrease cAMP formation; all types of β-receptor stimulate adenylate cyclase.
- The main effects of receptor activation are:
  - —α_1-receptors—vasoconstriction, relaxation of gastrointestinal smooth muscle, salivary secretion and hepatic glycogenolysis
  - —α_2-receptors—inhibition of transmitter release (including NA and ACh release from autonomic nerves), platelet aggregation, contraction of vascular smooth muscle, CNS neurons
  - —β_1-receptors—increased cardiac rate and force, relaxation of gastrointestinal smooth muscle
  - —β_2-receptors—bronchodilatation, vasodilatation, relaxation of visceral smooth muscle, hepatic glycogenolysis and muscle tremor
  - —β_3-receptors—lipolysis.

muscle cells of blood vessels and CNS neurons, as well as on presynaptic nerve terminals in the CNS and periphery.

Partial agonist effects

Several drugs that act on adrenoceptors have the characteristics of partial agonists (see Ch. 1), i.e. they block receptors and thus antagonise the actions of full agonists, but also have a weak agonist effect of their own. Examples (see Table 7.2) include **ergotamine** (α_1-receptors) and **clonidine** (α_2-receptors). Some β-adrenoceptor blocking drugs (e.g. **alprenolol, oxprenolol**) cause, under resting conditions, an increase of heart rate, but at the same time oppose the tachycardia produced by sympathetic stimulation. This has been interpreted as a partial agonist effect, though there is evidence that mechanisms other than β-receptor activation may contribute to the tachycardia.

The possible clinical significance of partial agonists is discussed under the headings of individual drugs later in this chapter.

PHYSIOLOGY OF NORADRENERGIC TRANSMISSION

THE NORADRENERGIC NEURON

Noradrenergic neurons in the periphery are postganglionic sympathetic neurons, whose cell bodies lie in sympathetic ganglia. They generally have long axons that end in a series of varicosities strung along the branching terminal network (Fig. 7.2). These varicosities contain numerous synaptic vesicles, which are absent from other parts of the neuron, and they represent the sites of synthesis and release of noradrenaline. Fluorescence histochemistry, in which formaldehyde treatment is used to convert catecholamines to fluorescent quinone derivatives, shows clearly that noradrenaline is present at high concentration in these varicosities (Fig. 7.2). Noradrenergic neurons contain a population of characteristic large dense-cored vesicles which are the storage organelles for noradrenaline, which is released by exocytosis. In most peripheral tissues, the tissue content of noradrenaline closely parallels the density of the sympathetic innervation. With the exception of the adrenal medulla, sympathetic nerve terminals account for all of the noradrenaline content of peripheral tissues. Organs such as the heart, spleen, vas deferens, and some blood vessels are particularly rich in noradrenaline (5–50 nmol/g of tissue) and have been widely used for studies of noradrenergic transmission. Reviews on all aspects of noradrenergic neurons are available (see Trendelenburg & Weiner 1988, Fillenz 1990, Cooper et al. 1991).

NORADRENALINE SYNTHESIS

The biosynthetic pathway for noradrenaline synthesis is shown in Figure 7.3. The metabolic precursor for noradrenaline is **L-tyrosine**, an aromatic amino acid present in the body fluids, which is taken up (probably by a specific transport system) by noradrenergic neurons. **Tyrosine hydroxylase**, the enzyme which catalyses the conversion of tyrosine to **dihydroxyphenylalanine** (DOPA) is found only in catecholamine-containing cells, probably free in the cytosol. It is a rather selective enzyme; unlike

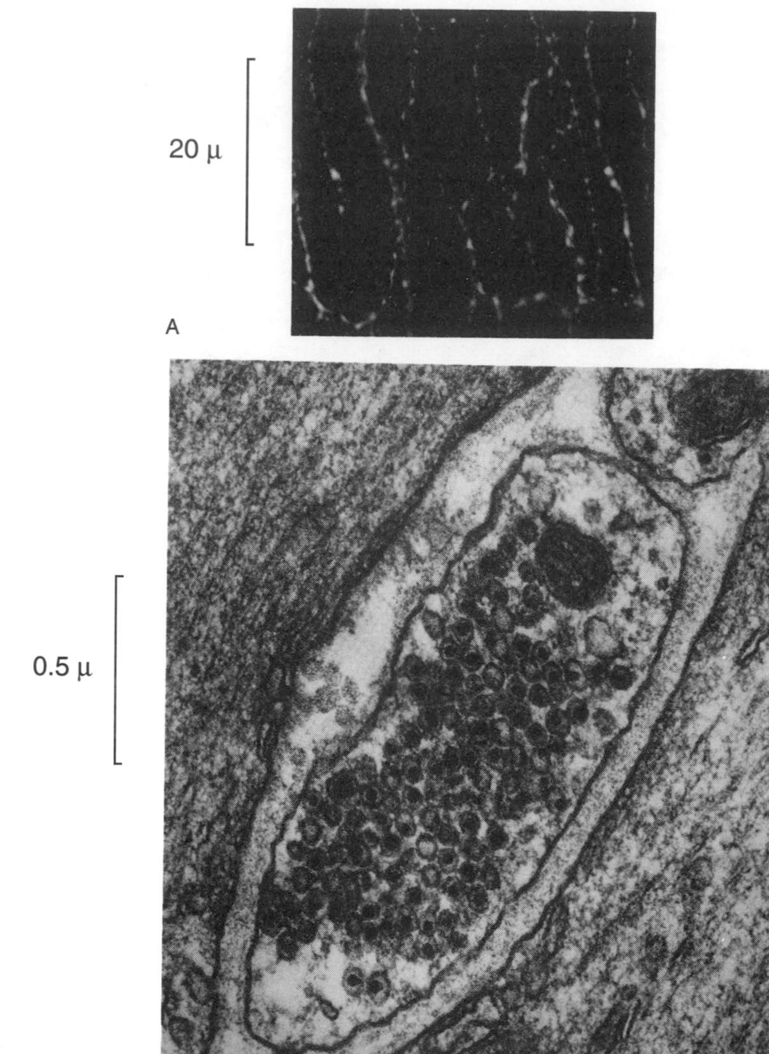

Fig. 7.2 Noradrenergic nerve terminals. A. Sheep mesenteric vein. Fluorescence microscopy following exposure to formaldehyde vapour. Varicosities containing noradrenaline (NA) can be seen along the path of individual nerve fibres. **B.** Transmission electronmicrograph of noradrenergic nerve terminal in mouse vas deferens, showing NA-containing vesicles with electron-dense core. (From: (A) Burnstock G 1970 In: Bulbring et al. (eds) Smooth muscle. Edward Arnold, London; (B) Furness J B et al. 1970 J Pharmacol Exp Ther 174: 111)

other enzymes involved in catecholamine metabolism, it does not accept indole derivatives as substrates, and so is not involved in 5-hydroxytryptamine metabolism. This first hydroxylation step is the main control point for noradrenaline synthesis. Tyrosine hydroxylase is inhibited by the end-product of the biosynthetic pathway, noradrenaline, and this provides the mechanism for the moment-to-moment regulation of the rate of synthesis; much slower regulation, taking hours or days, occurs by changes in the rate of production of the enzyme.

The tyrosine analogue **α-methyltyrosine** strongly inhibits tyrosine hydroxylase; it is used clinically in patients with the rare problem of inoperable phaeochromocytoma (see below), and may be used experimentally to block noradrenaline synthesis.

The next step, conversion of DOPA to dopamine, is catalysed by **DOPA decarboxylase**, an enzyme that is also found in the cytosol, but is by no means confined to catecholamine-synthesising cells. It is a relatively non-specific enzyme, and catalyses the decarboxylation of various other L-aromatic amino acids as well as L-DOPA, such as L-histidine and L-tryptophan, which are precursors in the synthesis of histamine and 5-HT, respectively. DOPA decarboxylase activity is not rate-limiting for noradrena-

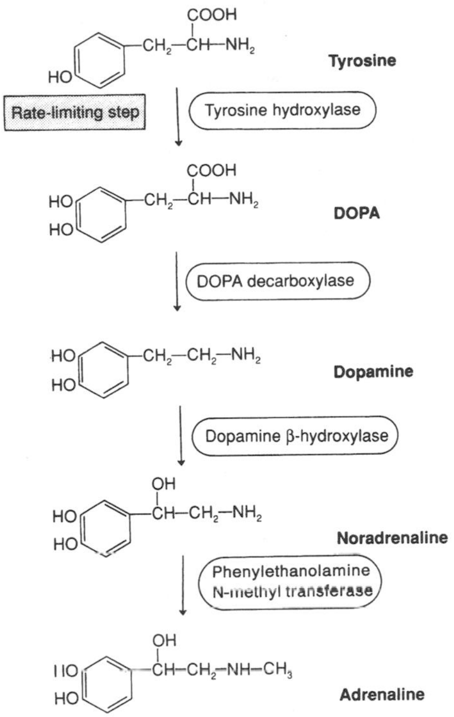

Tyrosine

Rate-limiting step — Tyrosine hydroxylase

DOPA

DOPA decarboxylase

Dopamine

Dopamine β-hydroxylase

Noradrenaline

Phenylethanolamine N-methyl transferase

Adrenaline

Fig. 7.3 Biosynthesis of catecholamines.

line synthesis, and the DOPA content of neurons is normally very low. Though various factors, including certain drugs, affect the enzyme, it is not an effective means of regulating noradrenaline synthesis.

Dopamine-β-hydroxylase (DBH) is also a relatively non-specific enzyme, but its distribution is restricted to catecholamine-synthesising cells. It is located in synaptic vesicles, probably in membrane-bound form. A small amount of the enzyme is released from noradrenergic nerve terminals in company with noradrenaline; this presumably represents enzyme that is in a soluble form within the vesicle, since there is evidence that the membrane proteins of the vesicle are retained when the vesicle discharges its contents by exocytosis. Unlike noradrenaline, the released DBH is not subject to rapid degradation or uptake, so its concentration in plasma and body fluids can be used as an index of overall sympathetic nerve activity.

Many drugs inhibit DBH, including copper-chelating agents and **disulfiram** (the main effect of which is to modify ethanol metabolism; see Chs 4 and 33). Such drugs can cause a partial depletion of noradrenaline stores and interference with sympathetic transmission.

Phenylethanolamine N-methyl transferase (PNMT) catalyses the N-methylation of noradrenaline to adrenaline. The main location of this enzyme is in the adrenal medulla, which contains a population of adrenaline-releasing (A) cells separate from the smaller proportion of noradrenaline-releasing (N) cells. The A cells, which appear only after birth, lie adjacent to the adrenal cortex, and there is evidence that the production of PNMT is induced by an action of the steroid hormones secreted by the adrenal cortex (see Chs 2 and 21). PNMT is also found in certain parts of the brain, where there is some evidence that adrenaline may function as a transmitter. In these sites, also, PNMT formation is sensitive to steroid hormones, providing a possible mechanism whereby these hormones can affect brain function.

Noradrenaline turnover can be measured under steady-state conditions by measuring the rate at which labelled noradrenaline accumulates when a labelled precursor, such as tyrosine or DOPA, is administered. The turnover time is defined as the time taken for an amount of noradrenaline equal to the total tissue content to be degraded and resynthesised. In peripheral tissues the turnover time is generally about 5–15 hours, but it becomes much shorter if sympathetic nerve activity is increased. Under normal circumstances the rate of synthesis closely matches the rate of release, so that the noradrenaline content of tissues is constant regardless of how fast it is being released.

NORADRENALINE STORAGE

Most of the noradrenaline in nerve terminals or chromaffin cells is contained in vesicles; only a little is free in the cytoplasm under normal circumstances. The concentration in the vesicles is very high (0.3–1.0 mol/l). Studies on isolated vesicles (chromaffin granules) have confirmed that they take up noradrenaline by a transport mechanism similar to the amine transporter responsible for noradrenaline uptake into the nerve terminal, but using a trans-vesicular proton gradient as its driving force (see Edwards 1992). Certain drugs, such as **reserpine** (see below), block this transport, and cause nerve terminals to become depleted of their noradrenaline stores. The vesicles contain two major constituents besides noradrenaline, namely ATP (about 4 molecules per molecule of noradrenaline) and a protein called chromogranin A. These substances are released along with noradrenaline, and it is generally assumed that a reversible complex, depending partly on the opposite charges on the molecules of noradrenaline and ATP, is formed within the vesicle. This would serve both to reduce the osmolarity of the vesicle contents and also to reduce the tendency of noradrenaline to leak out of the vesicles within the nerve terminal.

There is now considerable evidence (see von Kugelglen & Starke 1991) that ATP itself has a transmitter function at noradrenergic synapses, being responsible for the fast excitatory synaptic potential and the rapid phase of contraction produced by sympathetic nerve activity in many smooth muscle tissues.

NORADRENALINE RELEASE

The processes linking the arrival of a nerve impulse at a noradrenergic nerve terminal to the release of noradrenaline are basically the same as those at other chemically transmitting synapses (see Ch. 5, Stjarne 1989). Depolarisation of the nerve terminal membrane opens calcium channels in the nerve terminal membrane. Calcium enters the terminal, and, by mechanisms that are not well understood, promotes the fusion and discharge of synaptic vesicles. Studies on noradrenergic neurons and on the adrenal medulla have provided strong evidence in favour of the vesicular mechanism. Thus, the proportion of chromogranin, ATP and noradrenaline released is the same as that present in the vesicle (which would not occur if the vesicles were merely a reservoir of transmitter and not the immediate vehicle of release). It has also been found that immunologically distinctive constituents of the vesicle membrane appear on the outer cell membrane when release is evoked, as would be expected of an exocytotic mechanism. A surprising feature of the release mechanism at the varicosities of noradrenergic nerves is that the probability of release, even of a single vesicle, when a nerve impulse arrives at a varicosity, is very low (less than 1 in 50; see Cunnane 1984). A single neuron possesses many thousand varicosities, so one impulse leads to the discharge of a few hundred vesicles, scattered over a wide area. This contrasts sharply with the cholinergic synapse, where the release probability at a single bouton is high, but the boutons are few in number; the total release is similar, but it is sharply localised.

Regulation of noradrenaline release

It has recently been shown, by the work of Langer, Starke and others, that transmitter release can be controlled by a variety of substances that act on *presynaptic receptors* (see reviews by Starke et al. 1989, Langer 1981). Many different types of nerve terminal (cholinergic, noradrenergic, dopaminergic, 5-HT-ergic, etc.) are subject to this type of control, and many different mediators (e.g. acetylcholine, acting through muscarinic receptors, catecholamines acting through α- and β-receptors, prostaglandins, purine nucleotides, neuropeptides, etc.) can act on presynaptic terminals. It is now recognised that presynaptic modulation represents an important physiological control mechanism throughout the nervous system.

Of particular interest is the evidence suggesting that noradrenaline, by acting on presynaptic receptors, can regulate its own release, and also that of co-released ATP (see Ch. 5). This is believed to occur physiologically, so that released noradrenaline exerts a local inhibitory effect on the terminals from which it came—the so-called *auto-inhibitory feedback mechanism* (Fig. 7.4). The main evidence comes from studies of noradrenaline overflow in which the amount of radioactivity is measured in the effluent from an organ whose stores of noradrenaline have been previously labelled by infusion of tritiated noradrenaline. It was shown many years ago that α-receptor blocking drugs increase (by 10-fold or more in some tissues) the amount of noradrenaline overflow that occurs in response to sympathetic nerve stimulation. Overflow is also markedly affected by drugs (including many α-receptor antagonists) that inhibit the *re-uptake* of noradrenaline by nerve terminals (see p. 155). Even when this is allowed for, however, it seems that most of the increase in overflow is due to an increase in noradrenaline release, representing the loss of the normal feedback regulation. The magnitude of the change in noradrenaline overflow implies that this regulatory mechanism can, in some tissues, act to damp down noradrenaline release by 90% or more. Agonists or antagonists affecting these presynaptic receptors can, therefore, have large effects on sympathetic transmission. The physiological function of presynaptic autoinhibition in the sympathetic nervous system is still somewhat contentious, and there is evidence that, in most tissues, it is less influential than measurements of transmitter overflow would imply. Thus, although large changes in noradrenaline overflow occur when the feedback mechanism is interfered with pharmacologically, the associated

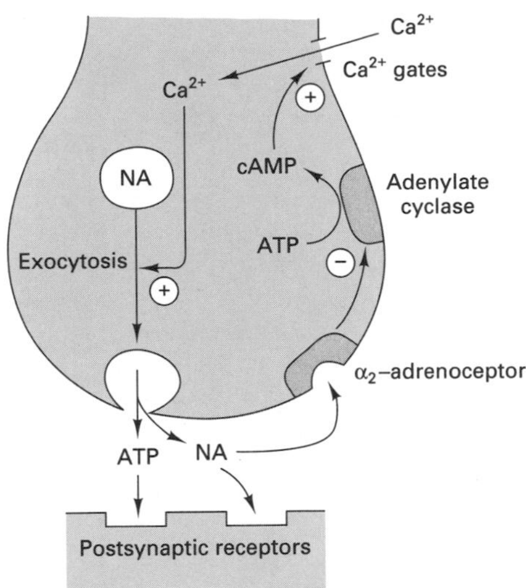

Fig. 7.4 Postulated feedback control of noradrenaline release. The presynaptic α_2-receptor inhibits adenylate cyclase, thereby reducing intracellular cAMP. cAMP acts to promote Ca^{2+} influx in response to membrane depolarisation and hence to promote the release of noradrenaline and ATP.

changes in the *tissue response* to sympathetic nerve activity are often rather small. This suggests that what is measured in overflow experiments may not be the physiologically important component of transmitter release.

The inhibitory feedback mechanism operates through α_2-receptors, and probably depends on inhibition of adenylate cyclase, and suppression of a particular type of calcium channel (the N-channel), which is believed to be important in transmitter release (see Lipscombe et al. 1989). It is interesting that sympathetic nerve terminals also possess β-receptors, coupled to activation of adenylate cyclase, which cause an increased noradrenaline release. Whether they have any physiological function is not yet clear.

UPTAKE AND DEGRADATION OF CATECHOLAMINES

Catecholamines differ markedly from acetylcholine in the way in which their action is terminated following release at the synapse. There is no synaptically located enzyme comparable with acetylcholinesterase that rapidly degrades catecholamines. Instead, reuptake of noradrenaline by noradrenergic nerve terminals, and by other cells, is the main mechanism by which the released transmitter is inactivated. Circulating adrenaline and noradrenaline are degraded enzymically, but much more slowly than acetylcholine. The two main enzymes responsible are both located intracellularly, so uptake into cells necessarily precedes metabolic degradation.

Uptake of catecholamines

Indirect evidence that sympathetic nerves can take up amines from the circulation and release them again as transmitter came originally from the work of Burn and his colleagues. In 1932 Burn found that the pressor effect of indirectly acting sympathomimetics (e.g. **tyramine**; see below) in whole animals was increased if the injection was preceded by injection of adrenaline, and he showed that this was because adrenaline was able to replenish the releasable amine stores of the nerve terminals. When tritiated noradrenaline became available, it was demonstrated that many tissues took it up rapidly from the circulation. Part of this uptake was shown to be by sympathetic neurons (for it disappeared when sympathetic nerves were allowed to degenerate), and the amine could be released again by sympathetic nerve stimulation. In a detailed study of noradrenaline uptake by isolated rat hearts, Iversen found that two distinct uptake mechanisms were involved, each of them having the characteristics of a saturable active transport system capable of accumulating catecholamines against a large concentration gradient. These two mechanisms, called *uptake 1* and *uptake 2*, correspond to neuronal and extra-neuronal uptake respectively. They have different kinetic properties as well as different substrate and inhibitor specificity, as summarised in Table 7.3.

The main differences are that uptake 1 is a high-affinity system with a relatively low maximum rate of uptake, whereas uptake 2 has low affinity for noradrenaline, but a much higher maximum rate. The substrate specificity is also different, uptake 1 being relatively selective for noradrenaline, whereas uptake 2 also accumulates adrenaline and isoprenaline. The effects of several important drugs that act on noradrenergic neurons depend on their ability either to inhibit uptake 1 or to enter the nerve terminal with its help (see Table 7.3). The uptake 1 transporter protein has recently been cloned and characterised (see Amara & Kuhar 1993, Trendelenburg 1991). It belongs to a family of neurotransmitter transporter proteins, which act as co-transporters of Na^+, Cl^- and the amine in question, using the

Table 7.3 Characteristics of uptake 1 and uptake 2

	Uptake 1	Uptake 2
Transport of noradrenaline (rat heart)		
V_{max} (nmol/g per min)	1.2	100
K_m (μmol/l)	0.3	250
Specificity	NA > A > ISO	A > NA > ISO
Location	Neuronal	Non-neuronal (smooth muscle, cardiac muscle, endothelium)
Other substrates	Methylnoradrenaline Dopamine 5-hydroxytryptamine Tyramine Adrenergic neuron blocking drugs (e.g. guanethidine)	(+)-noradrenaline Dopamine Serotonin Histamine
Inhibitors	Cocaine Tricyclic antidepressants (e.g. desipramine) Phenoxybenzamine Amphetamine	Normetanephrine Steroid hormones (e.g. corticosterone) Phenoxybenzamine

electrochemical gradient for Na^+ as a driving force (see Ch. 5). Thus changes in this gradient can alter, or even reverse, the operation of uptake 1, with marked effects on the availability of the released transmitter at postsynaptic receptors.

Metabolic degradation of catecholamines

Endogenous and exogenous catecholamines are metabolised mainly by two enzymes, *monoamine oxidase* (MAO) and *catechol-O-methyl transferase* (COMT). MAO occurs within cells, bound to the surface membrane of mitochondria. It is abundant in noradrenergic nerve terminals, but is also present in many other places, such as liver and intestinal epithelium. MAO converts catecholamines to their corresponding aldehydes, which, in the periphery, are rapidly metabolised by *aldehyde dehydrogenase* to the corresponding carboxylic acid (Fig. 7.5). In the case of noradrenaline this yields *dihydroxymandelic acid* (DOMA). MAO can also oxidise other monoamines, important ones being dopamine and 5-HT. It is inhibited by various drugs (see Table 7.4), which are used mainly for their effects on the central nervous system, where these three amines all have transmitter functions (see Ch. 24). These drugs have important side effects that are related to disturbances of peripheral noradrenergic transmission. Within sympathetic neurons MAO controls the content of dopamine and noradrenaline, and the releasable store of noradrenaline increases if the enzyme is inhibited. MAO occurs in two forms, MAO-A and MAO-B, which differ in their regional distribution, substrate specificity and susceptibility to inhibition by drugs (see Ch. 29). Noradrenaline and 5-HT are metabolised principally by MAO-A, whereas dopamine is a substrate for both forms. MAO inhibitors are discussed in more detail in Chapter 29.

The second major pathway for catecholamine metabolism involves methylation of one of the catechol –OH groups to give a methoxy derivative. COMT is a widespread enzyme that occurs in both neuronal and non-neuronal tissues. It acts on many different catechol-containing substrates, including the catecholamines themselves and the deaminated products, such as DOMA, that are produced by the action of MAO. O-methylation of noradrenaline gives rise to the metabolite *normetanephrine* (Fig. 7.5). When this product is acted on by MAO, or when DOMA is acted on by COMT, the product formed is *3-methoxy-4-hydroxymandelic acid* (VMA), which is the main final metabolite of adrenaline and noradrenaline. In patients with tumours of chromaffin tissue that secrete these amines (a rare cause of high blood pressure), the urinary excretion of VMA is markedly increased (Fig. 7.6). This increase forms the basis of a diagnostic test for this condition.

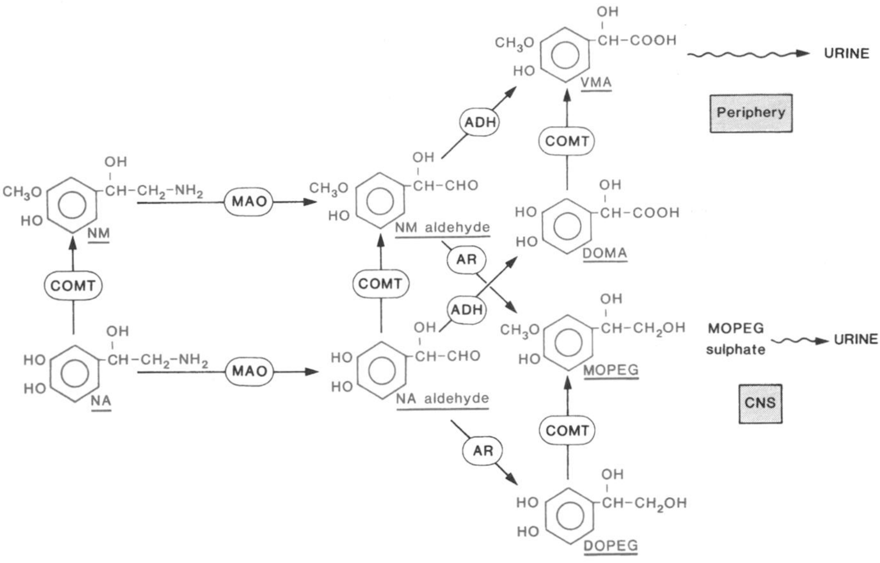

Fig. 7.5 The main pathways of noradrenaline metabolism in the brain and in the periphery. In the periphery, the oxidative branch (catalysed by ADH) predominates, giving VMA as the main urinary metabolite. In the brain, the reductive branch (catalysed by AR) predominates, producing MOPEG, which is conjugated to MOPEG sulphate before being excreted. (NA = noradrenaline; NM = normetanephrine; VMA = vanillylmandelic acid; DOMA = 3,4-dihydroxymandelic acid; MOPEG = 3-methoxy,4-hydroxyphenylglycol; DOPEG = 3,4-dihydroxphenylglycol; MAO = monoamine oxidase; COMT = catechol-O-methyl transferase; ADH = aldehyde dehydrogenase; AR = aldehyde reductase)

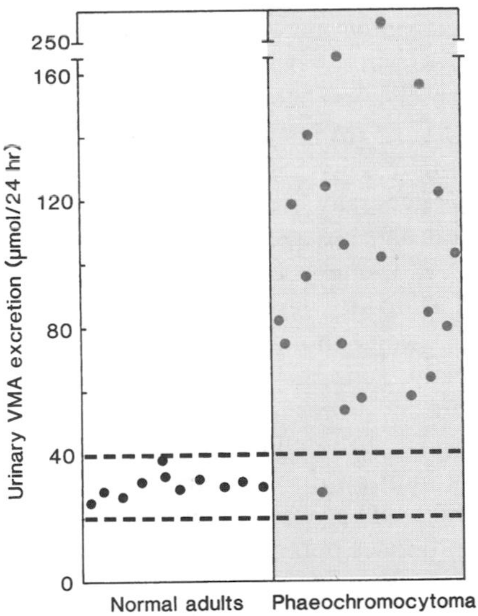

Fig. 7.6 Urinary excretion of vanillylmandelic acid (VMA) in normal subjects and patients with phaeochromocytoma. (After: Sandier M, Ruthven 1960 Adrenergic mechanisms. Churchill, London)

In the periphery, neither MAO nor COMT is primarily responsible for the termination of transmitter action, most of the released noradrenaline being quickly recaptured by uptake 1. Circulating catecholamines are usually inactivated by a combination of uptake 1, uptake 2 and COMT, the relative importance of these processes varying according to the agent concerned. Thus, circulating noradrenaline is removed mainly by uptake 1, whereas adrenaline is more dependent on uptake 2. Isoprenaline, on the other hand, is not a substrate for uptake 1, and is removed by a combination of uptake 2 and COMT.

The metabolism of noradrenaline in the central nervous system follows a different course (see Ch. 24 and Fig. 7.5). MAO is more important as a means of terminating transmitter action than it is in the periphery, and the resulting aldehydes are mainly reduced to the corresponding alcohols. The main excretory product of noradrenaline released in the brain is an ethyleneglycol derivative (MOPEG; see Ch. 24). Thus measurement of urinary VMA and

Noradrenergic transmission

- Transmitter synthesis:
  - — L-tyrosine is converted to DOPA by tyrosine hydroxylase (rate-limiting step). Tyrosine hydroxylase occurs only in catecholaminergic neurons.
  - — DOPA is converted to dopamine by dopa decarboxylase. Dopamine is converted to NA by dopamine β-hydroxylase (DBH), located in synaptic vesicles.
  - — In the adrenal medulla, NA is converted to adrenaline by phenylethanolamine N-methyl-transferase.
- Transmitter storage: NA is stored at high concentration in synaptic vesicles, together with ATP, chromogranin and DBH, all of which are released by exocytosis. Transport of NA into vesicles occurs by a reserpine-sensitive carrier. NA content of cytosol is normally low, due to monoamine oxidase in nerve terminals.
- Transmitter release occurs normally by Ca^{2+}-mediated exocytosis from varicosities on the terminal network. Non-exocytotic release occurs in response to indirectly acting sympathomimetic drugs (e.g. amphetamine) which displace NA from vesicles. NA escapes via uptake 1 (reverse transport).
- Transmitter action is terminated mainly by re-uptake of NA into nerve terminals. This uptake (uptake 1) is blocked by tricyclic antidepressant drugs.
- NA release is controlled by autoinhibitory feedback, mediated by α_2-receptors.
- Co-transmission occurs at many noradrenergic nerve terminals, ATP and neuropeptide Y being frequently co-released with NA. ATP mediates the early phase of smooth muscle contraction in response to sympathetic nerve activity.

MOPEG enables the central and peripheral release of noradrenaline to be quantified.

DRUGS ACTING ON ADRENOCEPTORS

STRUCTURE–ACTIVITY RELATIONSHIPS

The overall potency and receptor specificity of drugs that exert their effects by combining with adrenoceptors, depend on several factors:

- affinity for, and efficacy on, adrenoceptors
- interaction with neuronal uptake systems
- interaction with MAO
- interaction with COMT.

The relationship of these different factors with chemical structure is, not surprisingly, complex, but there are certain useful generalisations that can be made. The noradrenaline molecule can be modified in several different ways to yield compounds that interact with adrenoceptors (Fig. 7.7).

- Increasing the bulkiness of substituents on the N-atom produces compounds (**adrenaline, isoprenaline** and **salbutamol**) of relatively greater potency as β-agonists, and less susceptible to uptake 1 and MAO.
- Addition of an α-methyl group (**α-methylnoradrenaline, metaraminol**) increases α-receptor selectivity and also renders compounds resistant to MAO, though they remain susceptible to uptake 1.
- Removal of the β-OH group (**dopamine**) greatly reduces interaction with adrenoceptors. Most of the directly acting sympathomimetic amines and the β-receptor antagonists (though not all α-receptor antagonists) retain this critical –OH group.
- Substitution of the catechol –OH groups by similar electron-withdrawing groups, or their transfer to different ring positions (**salbutamol** and many β-receptor antagonists) render compounds resistant to COMT, but usually retaining their receptor activity. Substitution of catechol –OH groups generally yields compounds that are not substrates for uptake 1.
- Removal of one or both –OH groups (**tyramine, amphetamine, ephedrine**) abolishes affinity for receptors, though these compounds are still indirectly acting sympathomimetic amines, as they are substrates for uptake 1.
- Extension of the alkyl side chain, with isopropyl substitution on the N-atom, and modification of catechol –OH groups (**propranolol, oxprenolol,** etc.) produces potent β-receptor antagonists.

These general rules account fairly well for the properties of many directly and indirectly acting sympathomimetic drugs and for β-receptor antagonists. α-receptor antagonists are much more heterogeneous, however, and defy such generalisations.

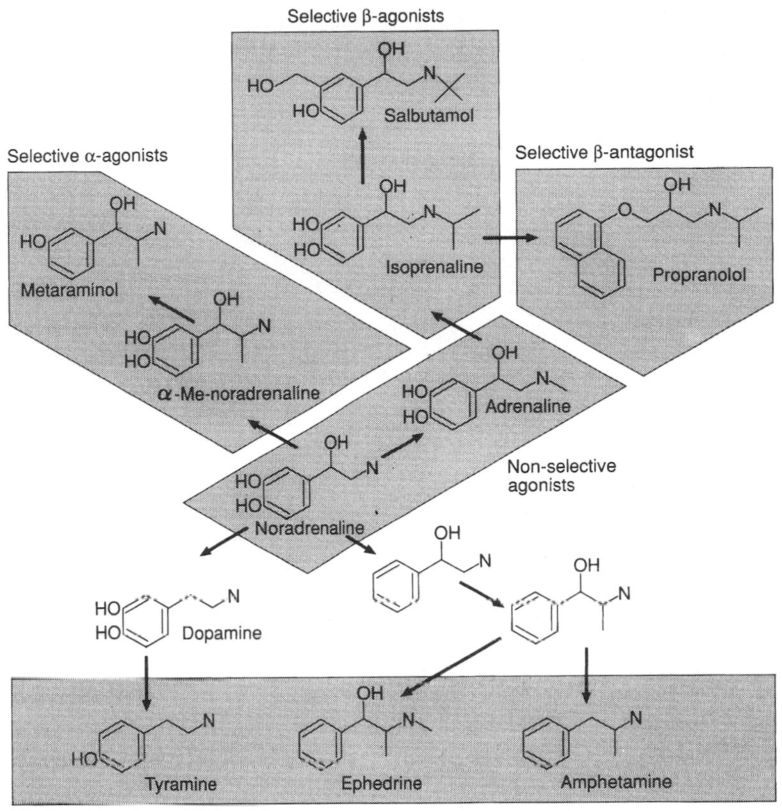

Fig. 7.7 Structure–activity relationships among catecholamines and related compounds.

ADRENOCEPTOR AGONISTS

Examples of the main types of adrenoceptor agonist are given in Table 7.2 and the characteristics of individual drugs are summarised in Table 7.4.

Actions

The major physiological effects mediated by different types of adrenoceptor are summarised in Table 7.1, and the more important ones are elaborated in this section.

Smooth muscle

All types of smooth muscle, except that of the gastrointestinal tract, contract in response to stimulation of α_1-adrenoceptors. Smooth muscle contraction caused by α-receptor stimulation results mainly from the release of intracellular calcium, through the action of the second messenger, inositol trisphosphate (see Ch. 2). There also appears to be an effect on the cell membrane, causing depolarisation and an increase in calcium permeability, which is often ascribed to the existence of receptor-operated channels (ROCs), though this is controversial. The resulting rise in the concentration of free intracellular calcium activates the contractile mechanism. When α-agonists are given systemically to experimental animals or man the most important action is on vascular smooth muscle, particularly in the skin and splanchnic vascular beds, which are strongly constricted. Large arteries and veins, as well as arterioles, are also constricted, resulting in decreased vascular compliance, increased central venous pressure and increased peripheral resistance, all of which contribute to an increase in systolic and diastolic arterial pressure. Some vascular beds (e.g. cerebral, coronary and pulmonary) are relatively little affected.

In the whole animal, baroreceptor reflexes are activated by the rise in arterial pressure produced by α-agonists, causing reflex bradycardia and inhibition of respiration.

Smooth muscle in the vas deferens, spleen capsule and eyelid retractor muscles (or nictitating membrane, in some species) is also stimulated by α-agonists and these organs are often used for pharmacological studies.

The α-receptors involved in smooth muscle contraction are mainly α_1 in type, though vascular smooth muscle possesses both α_1- and α_2-receptors. It appears that α_1-receptors lie close to the sites of release (and are mainly responsible for neurally mediated vasoconstriction), while α_2-receptors lie elsewhere on the muscle fibre surface, and are activated by circulating catecholamines (see McGrath 1983, McGrath & Wilson 1988).

Stimulation of β-receptors causes relaxation of most kinds of smooth muscle by a mechanism involving an increase in intracellular cAMP concentration (see Ch. 2). cAMP appears to cause relaxation by activating a protein kinase, which, in turn, phosphorylates and inactivates *myosin-light-chain kinase*, thereby inhibiting contraction (see Fig. 14.1). β-receptor activation also enhances Ca^{2+} extrusion, and so reduces the intracellular calcium concentration. It also affects intracellular calcium binding, though the mechanism is uncertain. Relaxation is usually produced by β_2-receptors, though the receptor that is responsible for this effect in gastrointestinal smooth muscle is not clearly β_1 or β_2. In the vascular system, β-mediated vasodilatation is particularly marked in skeletal muscle, but it can be demonstrated also in many other vascular beds.

The powerful inhibitory effect of the sympathetic system on gastrointestinal smooth muscle is produced by both α- and β-receptors, this tissue being unusual in that α-receptors cause relaxation in most regions. Part of the effect is due to stimulation of presynaptic α_2-receptors (see below), which inhibit the release of excitatory transmitters (e.g. acetylcholine) from intramural nerves, but there are also α-receptors on the muscle cells, stimulation of which hyperpolarises the cell (by increasing the membrane permeability to potassium), and inhibits action potential discharge. The sphincters of the gastrointestinal tract are contracted by α-receptor activation.

Bronchial smooth muscle is strongly dilated by activation of β_2-adrenoceptors, and selective β_2-agonists are important in the treatment of asthma (see Ch. 17). Uterine smooth muscle responds similarly, and these drugs are also used to delay premature labour.

Nerve terminals

Presynaptic adrenoceptors are present on both cholinergic and noradrenergic nerve terminals (see Ch. 5). The main effect is inhibitory, and is mediated through α_2-receptors, but a weaker facilitatory action of β-receptors on noradrenergic nerve terminals has also been described.

Heart

Catecholamines, acting on β_1-receptors, exert a powerful stimulant effect on the heart (see Ch. 13). Both the *heart rate* (*chronotropic effect*) and the *force of contraction* (*inotropic effect*) are increased, resulting in a markedly increased cardiac output and cardiac oxygen consumption. The *cardiac efficiency* (see Ch. 13) is reduced. Catecholamines can also cause *disturbance of the cardiac rhythm*, culminating in ventricular fibrillation. In normal hearts the dose required to cause marked dysrhythmia is greater than that which produces the chronotropic and inotropic effects, but in ischaemic conditions dysrhythmias are produced much more readily. Figure 7.8 shows the overall pattern of cardiovascular responses to catecholamine infusions in man, reflecting their actions on both the heart and vascular system.

Metabolism

Catecholamines encourage the conversion of energy stores (glycogen and fat) to freely available fuels (glucose and free fatty acids), and cause an increase in the plasma concentration of the latter substances. An increased production of gluconeogenic substrates (e.g. lactic acid, amino acids) from various peripheral tissues also occurs. The detailed biochemical mechanisms vary from species to species, but in most cases the effects on carbohydrate metabolism of liver and muscle (Fig. 7.9) are mediated through β_1-receptors (though hepatic glucose release can also be produced by α-agonists), and the stimulation of lipolysis is produced by β_3-receptors (see Summers & McMartin 1993). Adrenaline-induced hyperglycaemia in man is blocked completely by a combination of α- and β-antagonists but not by either on its own.

Other effects

Skeletal muscle is affected by adrenaline, acting on β_2-receptors, though the effect is far less dramatic than that on the heart. The twitch tension of fast-contracting fibres (white muscle) is increased by adrenaline, particularly if the muscle is fatigued,

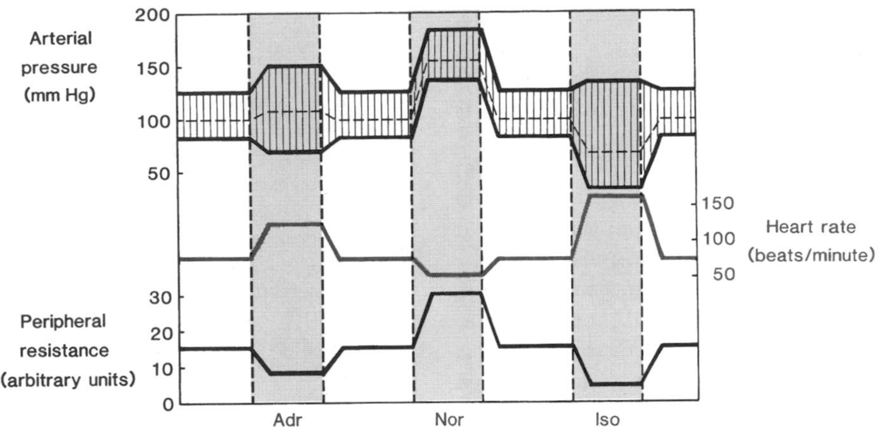

Fig. 7.8 Schematic representation of the cardiovascular effects of intravenous infusions of adrenaline, noradrenaline and isoprenaline in man. Noradrenaline (predominantly α-agonist) causes vasoconstriction and increased systolic and diastolic pressure, with a reflex bradycardia. Isoprenaline (β-agonist) is a vasodilator, but strongly increases cardiac force and rate. Mean arterial pressure falls. Adrenaline combines both actions.

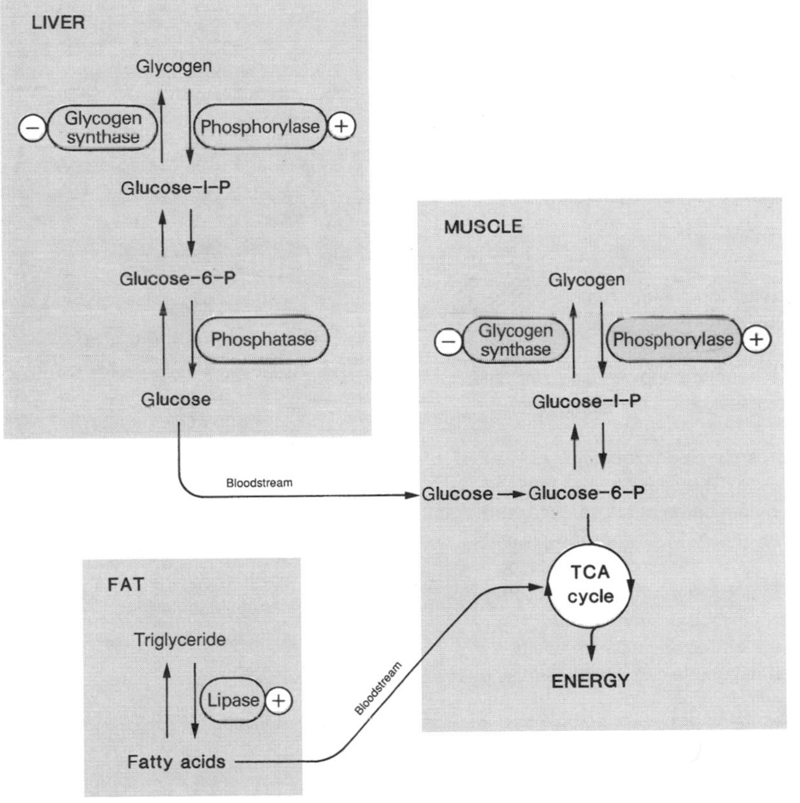

Fig. 7.9 Regulation of energy metabolism by catecholamines. The main enzymic steps that are affected by β-adrenoceptor activation are indicated by + and – signs, denoting stimulation and inhibition, respectively.

whereas the twitch of slow (red) muscle is reduced. These effects depend on an action on the contractile proteins, rather than on the membrane, and the mechanism is poorly understood. In man, **adrenaline** and other β_2-agonists cause a marked tremor, the shakiness that accompanies fear, excitement or the excessive use of β_2 agonists (e.g. **salbutamol**) in the treatment of asthma being examples of this. It probably results from an increase in muscle spindle discharge, coupled with an effect on the contraction kinetics of the fibres, these effects combining to produce an instability in the reflex control of muscle length. **β-receptor antagonists** are sometimes used to control pathological tremor.

Histamine release by human and guinea-pig lung tissue in response to anaphylactic challenge (see Ch. 11) is inhibited by catecholamines, acting apparently on β_2-receptors.

Lymphocytes are also sensitive to β-receptor agonists, both proliferation and lymphocyte-mediated cell killing being inhibited. The physiological and clinical importance of these effects has not yet been established.

Clinical use

The main clinical uses of adrenoceptor agonists are summarised opposite.

Adrenoceptor agonists

- Selective drugs exist for the four main adrenoceptor subtypes, α_1, α_2, β_1, and β_2; NA itself shows some selectivity for α- over β-adrenoceptors; adrenaline shows little selectivity.
- Selective α_1-agonists include phenylephrine, oxymetazoline.
- Selective α_2-agonists include clonidine, methylnoradrenaline. They cause a fall in blood pressure, partly by inhibition of NA release, and partly by a central action. Methylnoradrenaline is formed as a false transmitter from methyldopa, developed as a hypotensive drug (now obsolete).
- Selective β_1-agonists include dobutamine. Increased cardiac contractility may be useful clinically, but all β_1-agonists can cause cardiac dysrhythmias.
- Selective β_2-agonists include salbutamol, terbutaline, used mainly for their bronchodilator action in asthma.
- Dopamine has some action on β_1- and α-adrenoceptors, but acts also on specific dopamine receptors, causing renal vasodilatation.

Uses of adrenoceptor agonists

Cardiovascular system

- Cardiac arrest: **adrenaline** intravenously, or sometimes via an endotracheal tube.
- Cardiogenic shock (see Ch. 14): **dobutamine** (β_1-agonist) by intravenous infusion for its positive inotropic effect; low-dose **dopamine** to increase renal perfusion (via dopamine receptors in renal vasculature) and maintain glomerular filtration (see Ch. 18).
- Heart block: symptomatic heart block is treated by electrical pacing; β-agonists (**isoprenaline**) can be used temporarily while this is being arranged.

Anaphylactic reactions

- Acute anaphylactic (or type I hypersensitivity) reactions—sudden and sometimes life-threatening immunological reactions (see Chs 11 and 43), usually caused by bee stings or by hypersensitivity reactions to drugs (especially **penicillin**; see Ch. 34). The main effects are gross swelling of the skin and mucous membranes, which can obstruct breathing, and cardiovascular collapse due to vasodilatation. **Adrenaline** is the first-line treatment, usually injected intramuscularly; intravenous infusion requires close monitoring, usually in an intensive care unit.

Respiratory system

- Asthma (see Ch. 17): selective β_2-receptor agonists (**salbutamol**, **terbutaline**, **salmeterol**) by inhalation; salbutamol by intravenous infusion in severe attacks.
- Nasal decongestion: drops containing oxymetazoline or ephedrine for short-term use.

Miscellaneous indications

- Prolongation of local anaesthetic action (see Ch. 34): vasoconstrictor agents such as **adrenaline** can be injected with the local anaesthetic solution; it must not be injected into digits because of the risk of gangrene.
- Inhibition of premature labour (**salbutamol**).
- Miscellaneous indications for α_2-agonists (e.g. **clonidine**) include hypertension (Ch. 14), menopausal flushing, migraine prophylaxis (Ch. 8); efficacy is limited.

ADRENOCEPTOR ANTAGONISTS

The main drugs in the adrenoceptor antagonist category are listed in Table 7.2 and further information is given in Table 7.4. In contrast to the situation with agonists, most adrenoceptor antagonists are selective for α- or β-receptors, and many are also subtype selective.

ALPHA-ADRENOCEPTOR ANTAGONISTS

The main groups of α-adrenoceptor antagonists are:

- non-selective α-receptor antagonists
  - — haloalkylamines (e.g. **phenoxybenzamine**)
  - — other types, including imidazolines (e.g. **phentolamine**)
- α_1-selective antagonists (e.g. **prazosin, doxazosin, terazosin**)
- α_2-selective antagonists (e.g. **yohimbine, idazoxan**)
- ergot derivatives (e.g. **ergotamine, dihydro-ergotamine**). This group of compounds has many actions in addition to α-receptor block, and is discussed in Chapter 8. Their action on α-adrenoceptors is of pharmacological interest (see p. 148) but not used therapeutically.

Non-selective α-adrenoceptor antagonists

Haloalkylamines

The most important haloalkylamine compound is **phenoxybenzamine.** Haloalkylamines possess the same unstable N-chloroethyl group that occurs in the nitrogen mustards that are used in cancer chemotherapy (see Ch. 36). This group enables the drug to bind *covalently* to the receptor. Dissociation is extremely slow (>24 hours), since it requires cleavage of this covalent bond, and the pattern of antagonism produced is of the *irreversible competitive type* (see Ch. 1) in which the slope and maximum of the log concentration–effect curve for noradrenaline are reduced, in contrast to the effect of a reversible competitive antagonist. Phenoxybenzamine is not highly specific for α-receptors, and also antagonises the actions of acetylcholine, histamine and 5-hydroxytryptamine.

In man, phenoxybenzamine causes a fall in arterial pressure (because of block of α-receptor-mediated vasoconstriction) and postural hypotension. The cardiac output and heart rate are increased. This is a reflex response to the fall in arterial pressure, mediated through β-receptors. Blood flow through cutaneous and splanchnic vascular beds is increased, but effects on non-vascular smooth muscle are slight.

Other types

Phentolamine and **tolazoline** are very similar to phenoxybenzamine, except that they act as *reversible competitive antagonists*, and their action is short-lasting.

The uses of phenoxybenzamine and other α-receptor antagonists are described below, and summarised in Table 7.4. Though they all cause vasodilatation and a fall in blood pressure by blocking α_1-receptors, the concomitant block of α_2-receptors tends to increase noradrenaline release, which has the effect of enhancing the reflex tachycardia that occurs with any blood-pressure-lowering agent. Most sympathetic blocking agents cause an increase in gastrointestinal motility, and diarrhoea is a common side effect.

Labetalol is a mixed α- and β-receptor blocking drug, though clinically its effect on β-receptors predominates. Much has been made of the fact that it combines both activities in one molecule. To a pharmacologist, accustomed to putting specificity of action high on the list of pharmacological saintly virtues, labetalol may seem like a step backwards rather than forwards.

Alpha$_1$-selective antagonists

Prazosin was the first α_1-selective antagonist. Similar drugs with longer half-lives (e.g. **doxazosin, terazosin**), which have the advantage of allowing once-daily dosing, are now available. They are highly selective for α_1-receptors, and cause vasodilatation and fall in arterial pressure, but less tachycardia than occurs with non-selective α-receptor antagonists, presumably because they do not increase noradrenaline release from sympathetic nerve terminals. Cardiac output tends to decrease, as a result of the fall in central venous pressure due to dilatation of capacitance vessels, and the hypotensive effect is more dramatic than with non-selective α-receptor antagonists.

Alpha$_2$-selective antagonists

Yohimbine is a naturally occurring alkaloid; various synthetic analogues have been made, such as **idazoxan.** By blocking α_2-receptors, while sparing α_1-receptors, they increase noradrenaline release, and produce sympathomimetic effects in some organs. Blockade of postsynaptic α_2-receptors, which

α-adrenoceptor antagonists

- Most antagonists are α- or β-adrenoceptor selective (exception: labetalol).
- Drugs that block α_1- and α_2-adrenoceptors: phenoxybenzamine (irreversible haloalkylamine antagonist), phentolamine (reversible competitive antagonist). They were once used to produce vasodilatation in treatment of peripheral vascular disease, now largely obsolete.
- Selective α_1-antagonists include prazosin, doxazosin and terazosin, which are used in treating hypertension. Postural hypotension and impotence are unwanted effects.
- Yohimbine is a selective α_2-antagonist. It is not used clinically.

occurs in blood vessels and elsewhere, causes a block of sympathetic responses, so the overall effects are complex. Vasodilatation and a fall in blood pressure usually predominate, and its vasodilator effect has given yohimbine fame as an aphrodisiac (Dahl 1980). It is not employed therapeutically, but has proved useful in the experimental analysis of α-receptor subtypes.

General clinical uses and unwanted effects of α-adrenoceptor antagonists

The main uses of α-adrenoceptor antagonists are related to their cardiovascular actions, and are summarised below. They have been tried for many purposes, but have only limited therapeutic applications. In *hypertension*, non-selective α-blocking

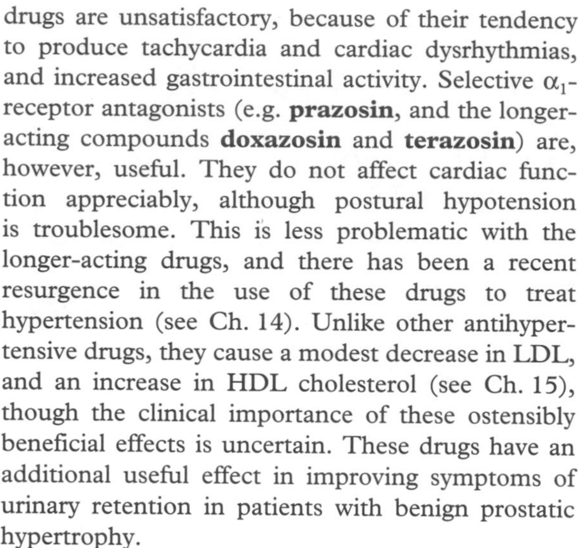

drugs are unsatisfactory, because of their tendency to produce tachycardia and cardiac dysrhythmias, and increased gastrointestinal activity. Selective α_1-receptor antagonists (e.g. **prazosin**, and the longer-acting compounds **doxazosin** and **terazosin**) are, however, useful. They do not affect cardiac function appreciably, although postural hypotension is troublesome. This is less problematic with the longer-acting drugs, and there has been a recent resurgence in the use of these drugs to treat hypertension (see Ch. 14). Unlike other antihypertensive drugs, they cause a modest decrease in LDL, and an increase in HDL cholesterol (see Ch. 15), though the clinical importance of these ostensibly beneficial effects is uncertain. These drugs have an additional useful effect in improving symptoms of urinary retention in patients with benign prostatic hypertrophy.

Phaeochromocytoma is a catecholamine-secreting tumour of chromaffin tissue, and one of the effects is to cause episodes of severe hypertension. A combination of α- and β-receptor antagonists is the most effective way of controlling the blood pressure. The tumour may be surgically removable, and it is essential to block α- and β-receptors before surgery is begun, to avoid the effects of a sudden release of catecholamines when the tumour is disturbed mechanically. A combination of α- and β-blocking drugs (e.g. **phenoxybenzamine** and **atenolol**), is effective for this purpose. It is desirable to use an irreversible α-receptor antagonist for this purpose because a large surge of adrenaline may overcome the block by a reversible antagonist. α-receptor blockade should be established before giving the β-receptor antagonist, to avoid the risk of paradoxically worsening the hypertension by blocking β-receptor-mediated vasodilatation while α-receptor-mediated vasoconstriction is still operative.

Uses of α-adrenoceptor antagonists

- Hypertension (see Ch. 14): α_1-selective antagonists. **Prazosin** is short-acting. Preferred drugs are longer-acting (e.g. **doxazosin**, **terazosin**), used either alone in mild hypertension, or in combination with other drugs (Ch. 14).
- Improvement of symptoms in some patients with benign prostatic hypertrophy.
- Phaeochromocytoma: phenoxybenzamine (non-selective irreversible α-receptor antagonist), used in conjunction with β-receptor antagonist in preparation for surgery.

BETA-ADRENOCEPTOR ANTAGONISTS

Beta-adrenoceptor antagonists comprise an important category of drugs. They were first discovered in 1958, ten years after Ahlquist had postulated the existence of β-adrenoceptors. The first compound, **dichloroisoprenaline**, was a simple derivative of isoprenaline in which both ring –OH groups were replaced by Cl-atoms. It has fairly low potency, and is a partial agonist. Further development led to **propranolol**, which is much more potent and a pure antagonist, with an equal blocking effect on

β_1- and β_2-receptors. The potential clinical advantages of drugs with some partial agonist activity, and/or with selectivity for β_1-receptors, led to the development of **practolol** (selective for β_1-receptors, but no longer used clinically because of its toxicity), **oxprenolol** and **alprenolol** (non-selective with considerable partial agonist activity), and **atenolol** (β_1-selective with no agonist activity). Many very similar drugs have been developed, and the characteristics of the most important compounds are set out in Tables 7.2 and 7.4. Most β-receptor antagonists are inactive on β_3-receptors, so do not affect lipolysis. **Labetalol** combines α- and β-blocking activity, but its effect on β-receptors predominates at low doses.

Actions

The pharmacological actions of β-receptor antagonists can be deduced from Table 7.1. The effects produced in man depend on the degree of sympathetic activity, and are slight in subjects at rest. The most important effects are on the cardiovascular system and on bronchial smooth muscle.

In a subject at rest, **propranolol** causes little change in heart rate, cardiac output or arterial pressure, but reduces the effect of exercise or excitement on these variables (Fig. 7.10). Drugs with partial agonist activity, such as **oxprenolol**, increase the heart rate at rest, but reduce it during exercise. Maximum exercise tolerance is considerably reduced in normal subjects, partly because of the limitation of the cardiac response, and partly because the β-mediated vasodilatation in skeletal muscle is reduced. Coronary flow is reduced, but relatively less than the myocardial oxygen consumption, so oxygenation of the myocardium is improved, an effect of importance in the treatment of *angina pectoris* (see Ch. 13). In normal subjects, the reduction of the force of contraction of the heart is of no importance, but it may have serious consequences for patients with heart disease (see below).

An important, and somewhat unexpected, effect of β-receptor antagonists is their *antihypertensive action* (see Ch. 14). Patients with hypertension (though not normotensive subjects) show a gradual fall in arterial pressure that takes several days to develop fully. The mechanism is complex, and involves the following:

- reduction in cardiac output
- reduction of renin release from the juxtaglomerular cells of the kidney
- a central action, reducing sympathetic activity.

Blockade of the facilitatory effect of presynaptic β-receptors on noradrenaline release (see p. 155) may also contribute to the antihypertensive effect. The antihypertensive effect of β-receptor antagonists is clinically very useful. Because reflex vasoconstriction is preserved, postural and exercise-induced

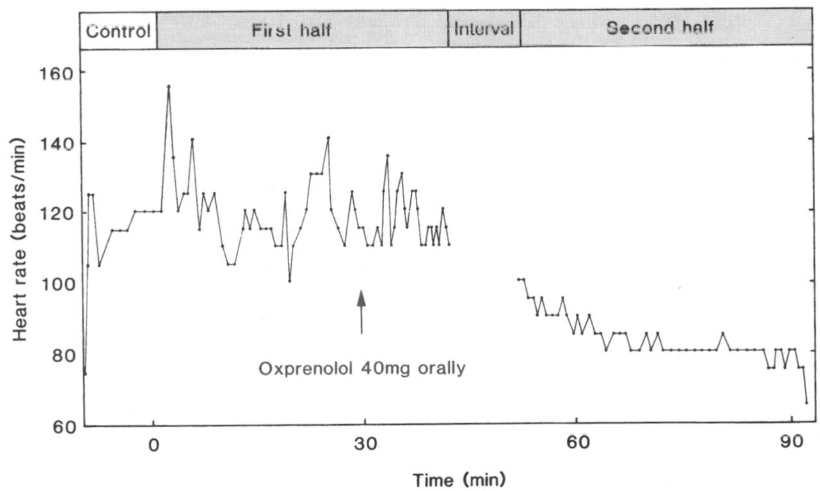

Fig. 7.10 Heart rate recorded continuously in a spectator watching a live football match, showing the effect of the β-adrenoceptor antagonist, oxprenolol. (From: Taylor S H, Meeran M K, 1973 In: Burley et al. (eds) New perspectives in beta-blockade. CIBA Laboratories, Horsham)

β-adrenoceptor antagonists

- β-adrenoceptor antagonists include propranolol, alprenolol, oxprenolol (non-selective between β_1 and β_2), atenolol (β_1-selective). Some (alprenolol, oxprenolol) have partial agonist activity, which some claim to be advantageous.
- Used mainly to treat hypertension, cardiac dysrhythmias, angina and myocardial infarction. They are also used to treat anxiety.
- Important hazards are bronchoconstriction, and bradycardia and cardiac failure (possibly less with partial agonists).
- Side effects include cold extremities, insomnia, depression.
- Many show rapid first-pass metabolism, hence poor bioavailability.
- Labetalol blocks both α- and β-receptors. It is used in hypertension.

hypotension (see Ch. 14) are much less troublesome than with many other antihypertensive drugs.

Many β-receptor antagonists have an antidysrhythmic effect on the heart, which is of clinical importance (see Ch. 13).

Airways resistance in normal subjects is only slightly increased by β-receptor antagonists, and this is of no consequence. In asthmatic subjects, however, non-selective β-receptor antagonists (such as **propranolol**) can cause severe bronchoconstriction, which does not, of course, respond to the usual doses of drugs such as **salbutamol** or **adrenaline.** This danger is less with β_1-selective antagonists, but none are so selective that this danger can be ignored.

In spite of the involvement of β-receptors in the hyperglycaemic actions of adrenaline, β-receptor antagonists cause only minor metabolic changes in normal subjects. They do not affect the onset of hypoglycaemia following an injection of **insulin**, but somewhat delay the recovery of blood glucose concentration. In diabetic patients, the use of β-receptor antagonists increases the likelihood of exercise-induced hypoglycaemia because the normal adrenaline-induced release of glucose from the liver is diminished. Also, sympathetic reflexes are an important cue by which hypoglycaemia is recognised; these symptoms are reduced by β-receptor antagonists, so hypoglycaemia is more likely to be unnoticed by the patient.

Uses of β-adrenoceptor antagonists

Cardiovascular system

- Hypertension (see Ch. 14). Mixed α- and β-receptor antagonist, **labetalol**, is often used in pre-eclamptic toxaemia (a form of hypertension occurring late in pregnancy).
- Angina pectoris (see Ch. 13).
- Following myocardial infarction (protection against dysrhythmias and repeated infarctions; see Chs 13 and 16).
- Cardiac dysrhythmias (Ch. 13).

Other uses

- Glaucoma: e.g. **timolol**, used as eye drops. Fewer side effects than anticholinesterases or muscarinic agonists (see Ch. 6).
- Thyrotoxicosis (see Ch. 21), as adjunct to definitive treatment (e.g. preoperatively).
- Anxiety states (see Ch. 27), to control somatic symptoms associated with sympathetic overactivity, such as palpitations and tremor.
- Migraine prophylaxis (see Ch. 8).
- Benign essential tremor (a familial disorder).
- The main drugs used are **propranolol**, **oxprenolol**, **alprenolol** and **atenolol**.
- The main risks and unwanted effects are:
  - — Bronchoconstriction—a serious hazard in asthmatic patients
  - — Cardiac failure
  - — Hypoglycaemia (with reduced awareness of hypoglycaemia in patients receiving insulin)
  - — Physical fatigue
  - — Cold extremities
  - — Bad dreams.

Clinical use

The main uses of β-receptor antagonists are connected with their effects on the cardiovascular system, and are discussed in Chapters 13 and 14. They are summarised above.

Unwanted effects

The main side effects of β-receptor antagonists are simply a consequence of their blocking action.

Bronchoconstriction. This is of little importance in the absence of airways disease, though it can be detected by measurement of forced expiratory rate. In asthmatic patients, this effect can be dramatic and life-threatening. It is also of clinical importance in patients with other forms of obstructive lung disease (e.g. chronic bronchitis, emphysema).

Cardiac failure. Patients with heart disease may rely on a degree of sympathetic drive to the heart to maintain an adequate cardiac output, and removal of this by blocking β-receptors will produce a degree of cardiac failure. In theory, drugs with partial agonist activity (e.g. **oxprenolol, alprenolol**) offer an advantage since they can, by their own action, maintain a degree of β_1-receptor activation, while at the same time blunting the cardiac response to increased sympathetic nerve activity or to circulating adrenaline. Clinical trials so far, however, have not shown a clear advantage of these drugs measurable as a reduced incidence of cardiac failure.

Hypoglycaemia. Glucose release in response to adrenaline is a safety device that may be important to diabetic patients and to other individuals prone to hypoglycaemic attacks. The sympathetic response to hypoglycaemia produces symptoms that are useful in warning patients of the urgent need for carbohydrate (usually in the form of a sugary drink). The use of β-receptor antagonists can be hazardous in these patients. There is a theoretical advantage in using β_1-selective agents, since glucose release from the liver is controlled by β_2-receptors.

Fatigue. Patients taking β-receptor blocking drugs often complain of fatigue, which is probably due to reduced cardiac output and reduced muscle perfusion in exercise.

Cold extremities. This results presumably from a loss of β-receptor-mediated vasodilatation in cutaneous vessels, and is a common side effect. Again, β_1-selective drugs ought to be less likely to produce this effect, but it is not clear that this is so in practice.

Other side effects associated with β-receptor antagonists are not obviously the result of β-receptor blockade. One is the occurrence of bad dreams, which occur mainly with highly lipid-soluble drugs such as propranolol, which enter the brain easily. A second is the serious *oculomucocutaneous syndrome* produced by **practolol.** This comprises lacrimal gland damage, leading to dryness of the cornea and sometimes blindness, together with sclerosing peritonitis, leading to digestive tract malfunction, and a skin rash. The cause of this reaction, which has led to the withdrawal of practolol from clinical use, is not known. It may well be immunological in origin, but this has not been conclusively shown.

DRUGS THAT AFFECT NORADRENERGIC NEURONS

Emphasis in this chapter is placed on peripheral sympathetic transmission. The same principles, however, are applicable to the central nervous system (see Ch. 24), where many of the drugs mentioned here also act.

DRUGS THAT AFFECT NORADRENALINE SYNTHESIS

Only a few clinically important drugs affect noradrenaline synthesis directly. Examples are **α-methyltyrosine**, which inhibits tyrosine hydroxylase and has been used in the treatment of phaeochromocytoma, and **carbidopa**, a hydrazine derivative of dopa, which inhibits dopa decarboxylase. Its main use is as an adjunct to treatment of parkinsonism with **L-dopa** (see Ch. 25). The peripheral side effects of L-dopa, which result from its conversion to dopamine and noradrenaline, are reduced by carbidopa, but, because the drug does not enter the brain, formation of dopamine in the brain, on which the therapeutic effectiveness of L-dopa depends, is not impaired.

An important indirect effect on noradrenaline synthesis is produced by **methyldopa**, a drug that is used in the treatment of hypertension (see Ch. 14). Methyldopa (Fig. 7.12) is taken up by noradrenergic neurons, where it is decarboxylated and hydroxylated to form the false transmitter, α-methyl-noradrenaline. This substance is not deaminated within the neuron by MAO and therefore tends to accumulate in larger quantities than noradrenaline, and displaces noradrenaline from the synaptic vesicles. The false transmitter is released in the same way as noradrenaline, but differs in two important respects in its action on adrenoceptors. α-methylnoradrenaline is somewhat less active than noradrenaline on α_1-receptors and thus is less effective in causing vasoconstriction. But it is more active on presynaptic (α_2) receptors, so the auto-inhibitory feedback mechanism operates more strongly than normal, thus reducing transmitter release below the normal levels. Both of these effects (as well as a central effect, probably caused by the same cellular mechanism) contribute to the hypotensive action.

Table 7.4 Summary of drugs that affect noradrenergic transmission

Type	Drug	Main action	Uses/function	Unwanted effects	Pharmacokinetic aspects	Notes
Sympathomimetic (directly acting)	Noradrenaline	α/β-agonist	Not used clinically. Transmitter at post-ganglionic sympathetic neurons, and in CNS. Hormone of adrenal medulla	Hypertension, vasoconstriction, tachycardia (or reflex bradycardia), ventricular dysrhythmias	Poorly absorbed by mouth. Rapid removal by tissues. Metabolised by MAO and COMT. Plasma $t_{½}$ ~ 2 min	
	Adrenaline	α/β-agonist	Asthma (emergency treatment), anaphylactic shock, cardiac arrest. Added to local anaesthetic solutions. Hormone of adrenal medulla	As noradrenaline	Given i.m. or s.c. As noradrenaline	See Chapter 17
	Isoprenaline	β-agonist (non-selective)	Asthma (obsolete). Not an endogenous substance	Tachycardia, dysrhythmias	Some tissue uptake, followed by inactivation (COMT). Plasma $t_{½}$ ~ 2 h	Now replaced by salbutamol in treatment of asthma (see Ch. 17)
	Dobutamine	$β_1$-agonist	Cardiogenic shock	Dysrhythmias	Plasma $t_{½}$ ~ 2 min. Given i.v.	See Chapter 13
	Saibutamol	$β_2$-agonist	Asthma, premature labour	Tachycardia, dysrhythmias, tremor, peripheral vasodilatation	Given orally or by aerosol. Mainly excreted unchanged. Plasma $t_{½}$ ~ 4 h	See Chapter 17
	Salmeterol	$β_2$-agonist	Asthma	As salbutamol	Given by aerosol. Long-acting	
	Terbutaline	$β_2$-agonist	Asthma	As salbutamol	Poorly absorbed orally. Given by aerosol. Mainly excreted unchanged. Plasma $t_{½}$ ~ 4 h	See Chapter 17
	Phenylephrine	$α_1$-agonist	Nasal decongestion	Hypertension, reflex bradycardia	Given intranasally. Metabolised by MAO. Short plasma $t_{½}$	
	Methoxamine	α-agonist (non-selective)	Nasal decongestion	As phenylephrine	Given intranasally. Plasma $t_{½}$ ~ 1 h	
	Clonidine	$α_2$-partial agonist	Hypertension, migraine	Drowsiness, orthostatic hypotension, oedema and weight gain, rebound hypertension	Well absorbed orally. Excreted unchanged and as conjugate. Plasma $t_{½}$ ~ 12 h	See Chapter 14
Sympathomimetic (indirectly acting)	Tyramine	NA release	No clinical uses. Present in various foods	As noradrenaline	Normally destroyed by MAO in gut. Does not enter brain	See Chapter 42

Table 7.4 (continued)

Type	Drug	Main action	Uses/function	Unwanted effects	Pharmacokinetic aspects	Notes
	Amphetamine	NA release, MAO inhibitor, uptake 1 inhibitor, CNS stimulant	Used as CNS stimulant in narcolepsy, also (paradoxically) in hyperactive children. Appetite suppressant. Drug of abuse	Hypertension, tachycardia, insomnia. Acute psychosis with overdose. Dependence	Well absorbed orally. penetrates freely into brain. Excreted unchanged in urine. Plasma $t_{1/2} \sim 12$ h, depending on urine flow and pH	See Chapter 32
	Ephedrine	NA release, β-agonist, weak CNS stimulant	Nasal decongestion	As amphetamine, but less pronounced	Similar to amphetamine	Contraindicated if MAO inhibitors are given
Adrenoceptor antagonists	Phenoxybenzamine	α-antagonist (non-selective, irreversible), uptake 1 inhibitor	Phaeochromocytoma	Hypotension, flushing, tachycardia, nasal congestion, impotence	Absorbed orally. Plasma $t_{1/2} \sim 12$ h	Action outlasts presence of drug in plasma, because of covalent binding to receptor
	Phentolamine	α-antagonist (non-selective), vasodilator	Rarely used	As phenoxybenzamine	Usually given i.v. Metabolised by liver. Plasma $t_{1/2} \sim 2$ h	Tolazoline is similar
	Prazosin	α_1-antagonist	Hypertension	As phenoxybenzamine, also drowsiness	Absorbed orally. Metabolised by liver. Plasma $t_{1/2} \sim 4$ h	Doxazosin, terazosin are similar but longer-acting. See Chapter 14
	Ergotamine	α-partial agonist, contracts uterus	Migraine	Vomiting, diarrhoea, gangrene, drowsiness, mental disturbances	Absorbed orally. Metabolised by liver. Plasma $t_{1/2} \sim 4$ h	See Chapter 8
	Yohimbine	α_2-antagonist	Not used clinically. Claimed to be aphrodisiac	Excitement, hypertension	Absorbed orally. Metabolised by liver. Plasma $t_{1/2} \sim 4$ h	Idazoxan is similar
	Propranolol	β-antagonist (non-selective)	Angina, hypertension, cardiac dysrhythmias, anxiety tremor, glaucoma	Bronchoconstriction, cardiac failure, cold extremities, fatigue and depression, hypoglycaemia	Absorbed orally. Extensive first-pass metabolism. About 90% bound to plasma protein. Plasma $t_{1/2} \sim 4$ h	Timolol is similar, and used mainly to treat glaucoma. See Chapter 13
	Alprenolol	β-antagonist (non-selective) (partial agonist)	As propranolol	As propranolol	Absorbed orally. Metabolised by liver. Plasma $t_{1/2} \sim 4$ h	Oxprenolol and pindolol are similar. See Chapter 13
	Practolol	β_1-antagonist	Hypertension, angina, dysrhythmias	As propranolol, also oculomucocutaneous syndrome	Absorbed orally. Excreted unchanged in urine. Plasma $t_{1/2} \sim 4$ h	Withdrawn from clinical use

Table 7.4 (continued)

Type	Drug	Main action	Uses/function	Unwanted effects	Pharmacokinetic aspects	Notes
	Metoprolol	β_1-antagonist	Angina, hypertension, dysrhythmias	As propranolol, less risk of bronchoconstriction	Absorbed orally. Mainly metabolised in liver. Plasma $t_{1/2} \sim 3$ h	Atenolol is similar. See Chapter 13
	Butoxamine	β_2-antagonist, weak α-agonist	No clinical uses			
	Labetalol	α/β-antagonist	Hypertension	Postural hypotension, bronchoconstriction	Absorbed orally. Conjugated in liver. Plasma $t_{1/2} \sim 4$ h	See Chapters 13 and 14
Drugs affecting noradrenaline synthesis	α-methyl-p-tyrosine	Inhibits tyrosine hydroxylase	Occasionally used in phaeochromocytoma	Hypotension, sedation		
	Carbidopa	Inhibits dopa decarboxylase	Used as adjunct to L-dopa, to prevent peripheral effects		Absorbed orally. Does not enter brain	See Chapter 30
	Methyldopa	False transmitter precursor	Hypertension	Hypotension, drowsiness, diarrhoea, impotence, hypersensitivity reactions	Absorbed slowly by mouth. Excreted unchanged or as conjugate. Plasma $t_{1/2} \sim 6$ h	See Chapter 14
	Reserpine	Depletes NA stores by inhibiting vesicular uptake of NA	Hypertension (obsolete)	As methyldopa. Also depression, parkinsonism, gynaecomastia	Poorly absorbed orally. Slowly metabolised. Plasma $t_{1/2} \sim 100$ h. Excreted in milk	Antihypertensive effect develops slowly, and persists when drug is stopped
Drugs affecting noradrenaline release	Guanethidine	Inhibits NA release. Also causes NA depletion, and can damage NA neurons irreversibly	Hypertension (obsolete)	As methyldopa. Hypertension on first administration	Poorly absorbed orally. Mainly excreted unchanged in urine. Plasma $t_{1/2} \sim 100$ h	Action prevented by uptake 1 inhibitors (see Ch. 4). Bethanidine and debrisoquin are similar.
Drugs affecting noradrenaline uptake	Imipramine	Blocks uptake 1. Also has atropine-like action	Depression	Atropine-like side effects. Cardiac dysrhythmias in overdose	Well absorbed orally. 95% bound to plasma protein. Converted to active metabolite (desmethylimipramine). Plasma $t_{1/2} \sim 4$ h	See Chapter 14. Desipramine and amitriptyline are similar. See Chapter 29
	Cocaine	Local anaesthetic. Blocks uptake 1, CNS stimulant	Rarely used local anaesthetic. Major drug of abuse	Hypertension, excitement, convulsions	Well absorbed orally	See Chapters 32 and 34
MAO inhibitors	Phenelzine	Inhibits MAO	Depression	Cheese reaction. Can cause hypotension	Well absorbed orally. Acetylated in liver	See Chapter 29

Other aspects of the pharmacology of methyldopa are discussed in Chapter 14.

A drug that subverts the machinery of the noradrenergic neuron in a particularly dramatic way is **6-hydroxydopamine**, which is identical with dopamine except that it possesses an extra ring –OH group. It is taken up selectively by noradrenergic nerve terminals, where it is converted to a reactive quinone, which destroys the nerve terminal, producing a 'chemical sympathectomy'. The cell bodies survive, and eventually the sympathetic innervation recovers. The drug is useful for experimental purposes, but has no clinical uses. If injected directly into the brain it selectively destroys those nerve terminals (i.e. dopaminergic and noradrenergic) that take it up, but it does not reach the brain if given systemically.

DRUGS THAT AFFECT NORADRENALINE STORAGE

The main drug that affects noradrenaline storage is **reserpine**, an alkaloid of complex chemical structure, bearing no obvious relationship to catecholamines. It comes from a shrub, *Rauwolfia*, which has been widely used in India for centuries as a medicine for the treatment of mental disorders. Reserpine, at very low concentration, blocks the transport of noradrenaline and other amines into synaptic vesicles, apparently by binding to the transport protein (see Edwards 1992). The transmitter accumulates instead in the cytoplasm, where it is degraded by MAO. The noradrenaline content of tissues thus drops to a low level, and sympathetic transmission is blocked. This effect is not confined to the periphery, nor to noradrenaline, for reserpine also causes depletion of 5-HT and dopamine from neurons in the brain in which these amines are transmitters (see Ch. 24). Reserpine, through its action on sympathetic nerve terminals, has some use as an antihypertensive drug (see Ch. 14), but its central effects, especially *depression*, which probably result from impairment of noradrenergic and 5-HT-mediated transmission in the brain (see Ch. 24) are a serious disadvantage.

Reserpine is a useful experimental drug for testing whether various physiological processes and drug effects require the presence of functional sympathetic nerve terminals.

DRUGS THAT AFFECT NORADRENALINE RELEASE

Drugs can affect noradrenaline release in four main ways:

- By preventing exocytosis from occurring in response to depolarisation of the nerve terminal (noradrenergic neuron blocking drugs).
- By evoking noradrenaline release in the absence of nerve terminal depolarisation (indirectly acting sympathomimetic drugs).
- By interacting with presynaptic receptors that inhibit or enhance depolarisation-evoked release (e.g. α_2-agonists, dopamine, prostaglandins, etc.). Effects mediated through α_2-adrenoceptors are discussed elsewhere in this chapter; the importance of the numerous other endogenous substances known to affect sympathetic nerve terminals is not clear at present. It is likely that these mechanisms are more important in the central than in the peripheral nervous systems.
- By increasing or decreasing available stores of noradrenaline (e.g. reserpine, see above; monoamine oxidase inhibitors). These drugs are discussed elsewhere in this chapter, and in Chapter 29, and are not considered further in this section.

Noradrenergic neuron blocking drugs

Noradrenergic neuron blocking drugs, of which **guanethidine** is the most important, were first discovered in the mid 1950s when alternatives to ganglion-blocking drugs, for use in the treatment of hypertension, were being sought.

The main effect of guanethidine is to inhibit the release of noradrenaline from sympathetic nerve terminals. It has little effect on the adrenal medulla, and none on nerve terminals that release transmitters other than noradrenaline. Drugs very similar to it include **bretylium**, **bethanidine**, and **debrisoquin**.

Actions

Drugs of this class reduce or abolish the response of tissues to sympathetic nerve stimulation, but do not affect (or may potentiate) the effects of injected noradrenaline. Their ability to block noradrenaline release can be demonstrated by measurement, for example, of the release of radioactivity from organs such as the spleen or vas deferens, in response to stimulation of the sympathetic nerves after the transmitter stores have been labelled by infusion of radioactive noradrenaline.

The mechanism of action of noradrenergic neuron blocking drugs is complex, but the following facts are known:

- They are selectively accumulated by noradrenergic nerve terminals. This occurs by means of uptake 1.
- Guanethidine is itself stored in synaptic vesicles (displacing noradrenaline), and released by nerve stimulation.
- Guanethidine and related drugs have some local anaesthetic activity, and impair impulse conduction in noradrenergic nerve terminals (Brock & Cunnane 1988).
- Guanethidine causes a slowly developing and long-lasting depletion of noradrenaline in sympathetic nerve endings, similar to the effect of reserpine. Inhibition of noradrenaline release occurs before this depletion has developed, but the depletion may have the effect of prolonging the blocking effect.
- The action of guanethidine is opposed by indirectly acting sympathomimetic drugs, such as amphetamine (see below). This may be because many of these drugs block uptake 1, or it may occur because they displace guanethidine, as well as noradrenaline, from storage sites in the synaptic vesicles.

Overall it seems most likely that the principal action of guanethidine involves its accumulation by the synaptic vesicles, which are then unable to fuse with the cell membrane in the normal way, so that exocytosis is prevented, but it is clear that the drug also has other effects, leading to transmitter depletion and block of impulse conduction.

Given in large doses, guanethidine causes structural damage to noradrenergic neurons, which is probably due to the fact that the terminals accumulate the drug in high concentration.

Guanethidine is no longer used clinically. Though extremely effective in lowering blood pressure, it produces severe side effects associated with the loss of sympathetic reflexes. The most troublesome are *postural hypotension*, *diarrhoea*, *nasal congestion* and *failure of ejaculation*. **Bretylium** is sometimes used to treat ventricular dysrhythmias resistant to other agents, during cardiac resuscitation (see Ch. 13); its mechanism of action in this setting is unknown. Guanethidine is very useful as an experimental tool to eliminate the effects of the sympathetic nervous system.

INDIRECTLY ACTING SYMPATHOMIMETIC AMINES

Mechanism of action and structure–activity relationships

The most important drugs in the indirectly acting sympathomimetic amine category are **tyramine**, **amphetamine** and **ephedrine**, all of which are structurally related to noradrenaline (Fig. 7.7). They each lack one or both of the catechol –OH groups, and thus have only weak actions on adrenoceptors, but sufficiently resemble noradrenaline to be transported into nerve terminals by uptake 1. Once inside the nerve terminals they cause displacement of noradrenaline from the vesicles into the cytosol, where some of it is degraded by MAO, while the rest escapes by carrier-mediated diffusion to act on postsynaptic receptors (Fig. 7.11). Exocytosis is not involved in the release process, so their actions do not require the presence of calcium. They are not

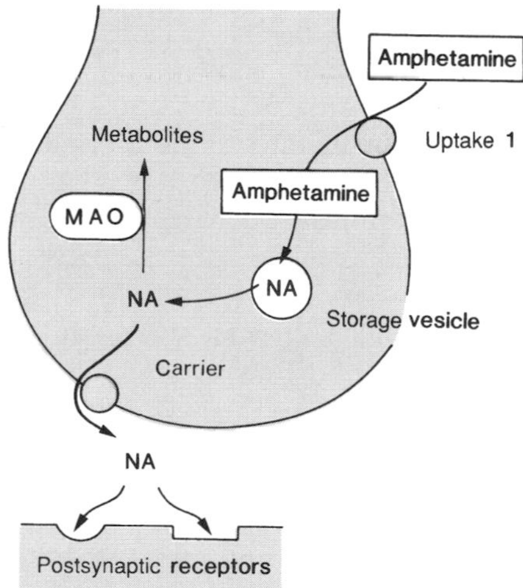

Fig. 7.11 The mode of action of amphetamine, an indirectly acting sympathomimetic amine. Amphetamine enters the nerve terminal via the NA carrier (uptake 1) and displaces NA from storage vesicles. Some of the NA is degraded by MAO within the nerve terminal and some escapes, via an exchange carrier, to act on postsynaptic receptors. Amphetamine also reduces NA re-uptake via uptake 1, so enhancing the action of the released NA. (NA = noradrenaline; MAO = monoamine oxidase)

completely specific in their actions, and act partly by a direct effect on adrenoceptors, partly by inhibiting uptake 1 (thereby enhancing the effect of the released noradrenaline), and partly by inhibiting MAO.

As would be expected, the effects of these drugs are strongly influenced by other drugs that modify noradrenergic transmission. Thus, **reserpine** or **6-hydroxydopamine** abolish their effects by depleting the terminals of noradrenaline. **MAO inhibitors**, on the other hand, strongly potentiate their effects by preventing breakdown, within the terminals, of the transmitter displaced from the vesicles. MAO inhibition particularly enhances the action of **tyramine** because this substance is itself a substrate for MAO. Normally dietary tyramine is destroyed by MAO in the gut wall and liver before reaching the systemic circulation. When MAO is inhibited this is prevented, and ingestion of tyramine-rich foods, such as cheese, can then provoke a sudden and dangerous rise in blood pressure. Inhibitors of uptake 1, such as **imipramine** (see below) interfere with the effects of indirectly acting sympathomimetic amines by preventing their uptake into the nerve terminals.

These drugs, especially **amphetamine**, have important effects on the central nervous system (see Ch. 32), which depend on their ability to release, not only noradrenaline, but also 5-HT and dopamine from nerve terminals in the brain. An important characteristic of the effects of indirectly acting sympathomimetic amines is that marked tolerance develops. Repeated doses of amphetamine or tyramine, for example, produce progressively smaller pressor responses. This is probably caused by a depletion of the releasable store of noradrenaline, since the response can be restored, in experimental animals, by infusion of noradrenaline, which has the effect of replenishing the releasable store. A similar tolerance to the central effects also develops with repeated administration, which partly accounts for the liability of amphetamine and related drugs to cause dependence.

Actions

The peripheral actions of the indirectly acting sympathomimetic amines closely resemble those of noradrenaline, namely *bronchodilatation*, *raised arterial pressure*, *peripheral vasoconstriction*, *tachycardia*, *increased force of myocardial contraction* and *inhibition of gut motility*, though they are longer lasting. The main central effects that occur, particularly with **amphetamine**, are:

- euphoria and excitement
- wakefulness and increased attentiveness
- loss of appetite
- in large doses, a schizophrenia-like syndrome with hallucinations and stereotyped behaviour.

These central actions are discussed further in Chapter 32. Because of them, amphetamine is no longer used as a peripheral sympathomimetic substance. **Ephedrine** has much less central action, though it can cause excitement and insomnia.

Legitimate clinical uses of indirectly acting sympathomimetic drugs are very limited. Amphetamines have some value in *narcolepsy* (an epilepsy-like condition in which patients suddenly and uncontrollably fall asleep), and possibly in treating *hyperactive children* (a controversial use, restricted to specialists). They are not indicated for treating depression or obesity. Ephedrine is still sometimes used as a nasal decongestant.

INHIBITORS OF NORADRENALINE UPTAKE

Neuronal re-uptake of released noradrenaline (uptake 1) is the most important mechanism by which its action is brought to an end. Many drugs inhibit this transport and thereby enhance the effects of both sympathetic nerve activity and injected noradrenaline. Uptake 1 is not responsible for clearing circulating adrenaline so these drugs do not affect responses to this amine.

The main class of drugs the primary action of which is inhibition of uptake 1 are the **tricyclic anti-depressants** (see Ch. 29), for example **desipramine**. These drugs have their major effect on the central nervous system, but also cause tachycardia and cardiac dysrhythmias which are a reflection of their atropine-like actions and peripheral effect on sympathetic transmission. **Cocaine**, a well-known local anaesthetic (Ch. 34), enhances sympathetic transmission, causing tachycardia and increased arterial pressure, by inhibiting uptake 1. Its central effects of euphoria and excitement (Ch. 33) are probably a manifestation of the same mechanism acting in the brain. It strongly potentiates the actions of noradrenaline in experimental animals or in isolated tissues provided the sympathetic nerve terminals are intact.

Many drugs that act mainly on other steps in sympathetic transmission also inhibit uptake 1 to some extent, presumably because the carrier molecule bears a steric relationship to other noradrenaline recognition sites, such as receptors and degradative enzymes. Examples include **amphetamine, phenoxybenzamine** and **guanethidine**.

Extraneuronal uptake (uptake 2), which is important in clearing circulating adrenaline from the bloodstream, is not affected by most of the drugs that block uptake 1. It is inhibited by **phenoxybenzamine**, however, and also by various **corticosteroids** (see Ch. 11). This action of corticosteroids may have some relevance to their therapeutic effect in conditions such as asthma, but it is not thought to be a major component of their effects.

The main sites of action of drugs that affect noradrenergic transmission are summarised in Figure 7.12.

DEFINITION OF TERMS RELATING TO NORADRENERGIC TRANSMISSION

Following is a list of important terms relating to noradrenergic transmission, and their definitions.

Noradrenergic: Term applied to a presynaptic neuron that releases noradrenaline as a transmitter. 'Adrenergic' is often used synonymously. The '...ergic' terminology was coined by Dale more than 50 years ago. Purists (Dale among them) have always insisted that it should be applied only to the presynaptic neuron, and deplore the tendency to use the word in other contexts (e.g. noradrenergic synapse, noradrenergic receptor, noradrenergic excitation, etc.).

Adrenoceptors: Receptors for adrenaline and noradrenaline. They are divided into α- and β-types, each of which has further subtypes denoted by numerical suffixes.

Noradrenergic neuron blocking agent: A distinct class of drugs which block noradrenergic transmission by inhibiting the release of noradrenaline from the nerve terminals. This group is quite distinct from adrenoceptor antagonists.

Catecholamine: A compound with a catechol nucleus (i.e. a benzene ring with two adjacent hydroxyl groups) and an amine-containing side chain. From a pharmacological point of view the most important catecholamines (see Fig. 7.1) are:

- *Noradrenaline*, the transmitter substance released by the majority of postganglionic sympathetic neurons (i.e. noradrenergic neurons).
- *Adrenaline*, a hormone secreted, along with noradrenaline, by the adrenal medulla. In mammals

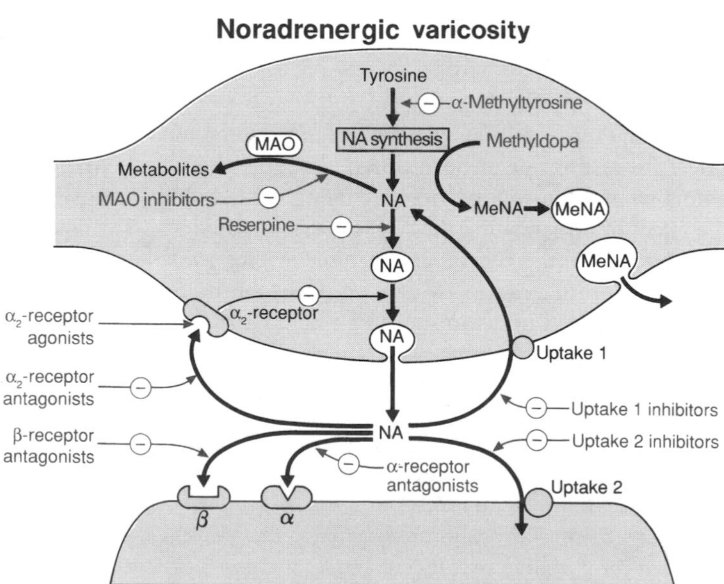

Fig. 7.12 Generalised diagram of a noradrenergic nerve terminal showing sites of drug action (in red).

Drugs acting on noradrenergic nerve terminals

- Drugs that inhibit NA synthesis include:
  - —α-methyltyrosine blocks tyrosine hydroxylase, not used clinically
  - —carbidopa blocks dopa decarboxylase and is used as adjunct to L-dopa treatment of parkinsonism to prevent peripheral decarboxylation; not much effect on NA synthesis.
- Methyldopa gives rise to false transmitter (methyl-NA) which is a potent α_2-agonist, thus causing powerful presynaptic inhibitory feedback (also central actions). Used as antihypertensive agent.
- Reserpine blocks carrier-mediated NA accumulation in vesicles, thus depleting NA stores and blocking transmission. Effective in hypertension, but may cause severe depression.
- Noradrenergic neuron blocking drugs (e.g. guanethidine, bretylium) are selectively concentrated in terminals by uptake 1, and block transmitter release, partly by local anaesthetic action. Effective in hypertension, but cause severe side effects (postural hypotension, diarrhoea, nasal congestion, etc.) so no longer used.
- 6-hydroxydopamine is selectively neurotoxic for noradrenergic neurons, because it is taken up and converted to a toxic metabolite. Used experimentally to eliminate noradrenergic neurons, not clinically.
- Indirectly acting sympathomimetic amines (e.g. amphetamine, ephedrine, tyramine) are accumulated by uptake 1 and displace NA from vesicles, allowing it to escape. Effect is much enhanced by MAO inhibition, which can lead to severe hypertension following ingestion of tyramine-rich foods by patients treated with MAO inhibitors.
- Drugs that inhibit uptake 1 include cocaine and tricyclic antidepressant drugs. Sympathetic effects are enhanced by such drugs.

adrenaline probably has no role as a peripheral neurotransmitter though it does in the brain.

- *Dopamine*, the metabolic precursor of noradrenaline and adrenaline. It functions as a neurotransmitter in its own right in many parts of the brain (see Ch. 24), and possibly also in the periphery.
- *Isoprenaline*, a synthetic derivative of noradrenaline that is not found in the body. It acts selectively on β-adrenoceptors.

Chromaffin cells: Catecholamine-containing non-neuronal cells derived from neural crest ectoderm. They are so called because they stain readily with various reagents that oxidise catecholamines to green or brown products. The largest group of chromaffin cells is in the adrenal medulla, but scattered cells are found in various tissues, including sympathetic ganglia, carotid and aortic bodies, and the wall of the intestine. *Phaeochromocytoma* and *carcinoid tumour* are examples of chromaffin cell tumours.

Sympathomimetic drug: A drug the effects of which resemble those of activity in the sympathetic nervous system. The term includes drugs that act directly on adrenoceptors in tissues, as well as those that act indirectly by evoking the release of noradrenaline from sympathetic nerve terminals. Some sympathomimetic amines are catecholamines, but by no means all.

REFERENCES AND FURTHER READING

Amara S G, Kuhar M J 1993 Neurotransmitter transporters: recent progress. Annu Rev Neurosci 16: 73–93

Angus J A, Korner P I 1980 Evidence against presynaptic adrenoreceptor modulation of cardiac sympathetic transmission. Nature 286: 288–291

Ariens E J, Simonis A M 1983 Physiological and pharmacological aspects of adrenergic receptor classification. Biochem Pharmacol 32: 1539–1545

Brock J A, Cunnane T C 1988 Studies on the mode of action of bretylium and guanethidine in post-ganglionic sympathetic nerve fibres. Naunyn-Schmiedeberg's Arch Pharmacol 338: 504–509

Bylund D B 1988 Subtypes of α-adrenoceptors: pharmacological and molecular biological evidence converge. Trends Pharmacol Sci 9: 356–361

Cooper J R, Bloom F E, Roth R H 1991 The biochemical basis of neuropharmacology. Oxford University Press, New York

Cunnane T C 1984 The mechanism of neurotransmitter release from sympathetic nerves. Trends Neurosci 7: 248–253

Dahl R 1980 My Uncle Oswald. Penguin, Harmondsworth

Edwards R H 1992 The transport of neurotransmitters into synaptic vesicles. Curr Opin Neurobiol 2: 586–594

Fillenz M 1990 Noradrenergic neurons. Cambridge University Press, Cambridge

Green A R, Costain D W 1981 Pharmacology and biochemistry of psychiatric disorders. J Wiley, New York

Hirst G D S, Nield T O 1980 Evidence for two populations of excitatory receptors for noradrenaline on arteriolar smooth muscle. Nature 283: 767–768

Langer S Z 1981 Presynaptic regulation of the release of catecholamines. Pharmacol Rev 32: 337–362

Lipscombe D, Kongsamut S, Tsien R W 1989 α-adrenergic inhibition of sympathetic neurotransmitter release mediated by modulation of N-type calcium channel gating. Nature 340: 639–642

McGrath J C 1983 The variety of vascular α-adrenoceptors. Trends Pharmacol Sci 4: 14–18

McGrath J C, Wilson V 1988 α-adrenoceptor subclassification by classical and response-related methods: same question, different answers. Trends Pharmacol Sci 9: 162–165

Molinoff P B 1984 α- and β-adrenergic receptor subtypes; properties, distribution and regulation. Drugs 28 (Suppl 2): 1–15

Receptor Nomenclature Supplement 1994 Trends Pharmacol Sci

Ruffolo R R, Nichols A J, Stadel J M, Hieble J P 1991 Structure and function of α-adrenoceptors. Pharm Rev 43: 475–505

Starke K 1977 Regulation of noradrenaline release through presynaptic receptor systems. Rev Physiol Biochem Pharmacol 77:1–124

Starke K, Göthert M, Kilbinger H 1989 Modulation of transmitter release by presynaptic autoreceptors. Physiol Rev 69: 864–989

Stjarne L 1989 Basic mechanisms and local modulation of nerve impulse-induced secretion of neurotransmitters from individual sympathetic nerve varicosities. Rev Physiol Biochem Pharmacol 112: 1–137

Story D F, McCulloch M W, Rand M J, Standford-Starr C A 1981 Conditions required for the inhibitory feedback loop in noradrenergic transmission. Nature 293: 62–65

Summers R J, McMartin L R 1993 Adrenoceptors and their second messenger systems. J Neurochem 60: 10–23

Trendelenburg U 1991 Functional aspects of the neuronal uptake of noradrenaline. Trends Pharmacol Sci 12: 334–338

Trendelenburg U, Weiner N 1988 Catecholamines. Handbook of experimental pharmacology. Springer-Verlag, Berlin, vol 90, parts 1 & 2

von Kugelglen I, Starke K 1991 Noradrenaline–ATP co-transmission in the sympathetic nervous system. Trends Pharmacol Sci 12: 319–324

8

OTHER PERIPHERAL MEDIATORS: 5-HYDROXYTRYPTAMINE AND PURINES

5-HYDROXYTRYPTAMINE

5-Hydroxytryptamine (5-HT) was originally discovered in 1948 when the identity of a vasoconstrictor substance released when blood is allowed to clot was being sought. It was originally called *serotonin*, a name that is still widely used, to denote its origin and biological action. It was subsequently found in the gastrointestinal tract and central nervous system, and shown to have an important role as a neurotransmitter, as well as functioning as a local hormone in the peripheral vascular system. It comes from many sources other than blood, and has many effects in addition to causing vasoconstriction, so serotonin is no longer a very appropriate name. This chapter deals with the metabolism, distribution and possible physiological roles of 5-HT in the periphery, and with the different types of 5-HT receptor and the drugs that act on them. Further information on the role of 5-HT in the brain, and its relationship to mental disorders and the actions of psychotropic drugs, is presented in Chapters 24, 28 and 29. More detailed information on 5-HT in the CNS and in the periphery can be found in Green (1985) and Fozard (1989).

DISTRIBUTION, BIOSYNTHESIS AND DEGRADATION

5-HT occurs in the highest concentrations in three situations in the body:

- *In the wall of the intestine.* About 90% of the total amount in the body is present in enterochromaffin cells, which are cells derived from the neural crest, similar to those of the adrenal medulla, that are interspersed with mucosal cells, mainly in the stomach and small intestine. Some 5-HT also occurs in nerve cells of the myenteric plexus, and there is good evidence that it functions there as an excitatory neurotransmitter (see Chs 5 and 19).
- *In blood.* 5-HT is present in high concentration in platelets, which accumulate it from the plasma by an active transport system, and release it when they aggregate at sites of tissue damage (see Ch. 16).
- *In the central nervous system.* 5-HT is a transmitter in the central nervous system (see Ch. 24) and is present in high concentrations in localised regions of the midbrain. Its functional role is discussed in Chapter 24.

The biosynthesis of 5-HT follows a pathway similar to that of noradrenaline (see Ch. 7), except that the precursor amino acid is *tryptophan* instead of tyrosine (Fig. 8.1). 5-HT is present in the diet, but most is metabolised before entering the bloodstream. Tryptophan is converted to *5-hydroxytryptophan* (in chromaffin cells and neurons, but not in platelets) by the action of *tryptophan hydroxylase* (an enzyme confined to 5-HT-producing cells). The 5-hydroxytryptophan is then decarboxylated to 5-HT, by a non-specific decarboxylase that acts on many other substrates, and is also involved in the synthesis of catecholamines (Ch. 7) and histamine (Ch. 11). Platelets (and neurons) possess a high affinity 5-HT uptake mechanism, and platelets become loaded with 5-HT as they pass through the intestinal circulation, where the local concentration is relatively high. The mechanisms of synthesis, storage, release and re-uptake of 5-HT are very similar to those of noradrenaline, and many drugs affect both processes indiscriminately (see Chs 7 and 29). Recent work has shown that 5-HT is often stored (in neurons and chromaffin cells) together with various peptide hormones, such as **somatostatin**, **substance P** or **vasoactive intestinal polypeptide** (VIP), and it is suggested that co-transmission (see Ch. 5) may be physiologically important.

Degradation of 5-HT (Fig. 8.1) occurs mainly through oxidative deamination, catalysed by *monoamine oxidase*, with the formation of an aldehyde; this is followed by oxidation to *5-hydroxyindoleacetic acid* (5-HIAA), the pathway being exactly analogous to that of noradrenaline catabolism (Fig. 7.5). 5-HIAA is excreted in the urine, and serves as an indicator of 5-HT production in the body. It is therefore useful in the diagnosis of *carcinoid syndrome* (see below). Some 5-HT is converted by methylation of the ring –OH group to 5-methoxytryptamine, this reaction being exactly analogous to the formation of normetanephrine from noradrenaline (Fig. 7.5). *5-methoxytryptamine* has actions of its own in the brain, and could be involved in some affective disorders (see Ch. 29).

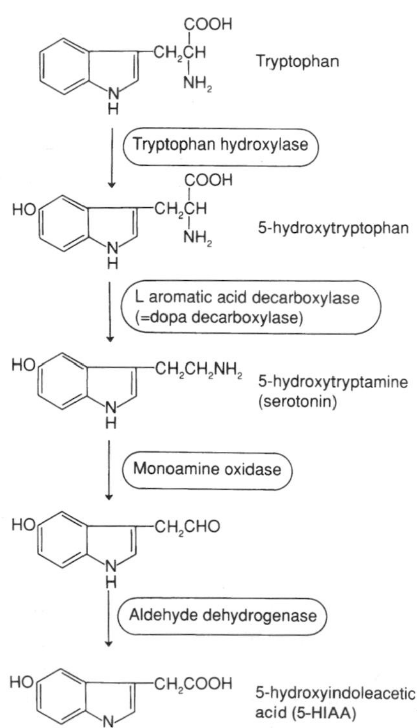

Fig. 8.1 Biosynthesis and metabolism of 5-HT.

Distribution, biosynthesis and degradation of 5-HT

- Structures rich in 5-HT are:
  - — gastrointestinal tract (chromaffin cells and enteric neurons)
  - — platelets
  - — central nervous system.
- Metabolism closely parallels that of noradrenaline.
- Formed from dietary tryptophan, which is converted to 5-hydroxytryptophan by tryptophan hydroxylase, then to 5-HT by a non-specific decarboxylase.
- 5-HT is transported into 5-HT-containing cells by a specific transport system.
- Degradation occurs mainly by MAO, forming 5-HIAA, which is excreted in urine.

PHARMACOLOGICAL EFFECTS

The actions of 5-HT are numerous and complex, and show considerable species variation. The main ones are described below.

Gastrointestinal tract. 5-HT causes increased gastrointestinal motility and contraction of isolated strips of intestine, this being partly due to a direct effect on the smooth muscle cells, and partly due to an indirect excitatory effect on enteric neurons. The peristaltic reflex, evoked by increasing the pressure within a segment of intestine, is mediated, partly at least, by the release of 5-HT from chromaffin cells in response to the mechanical stimulus. Chromaffin cells also respond to vagal stimulation by releasing 5-HT.

Smooth muscle elsewhere in the body (e.g. *uterus* and *bronchial tree*) is also contracted by 5-HT in many species, but only to a minor extent in man.

Blood vessels. Several effects are produced on the blood vessels, the overall effect varying according to the size of the vessel, and the prevailing sympathetic activity. Large vessels, both arteries and veins, are usually constricted by 5-HT, though the sensitivity varies greatly. This is a direct action on vascular smooth muscle cells, mediated through 5-HT_{2A} receptors (see below). 5-HT can also cause

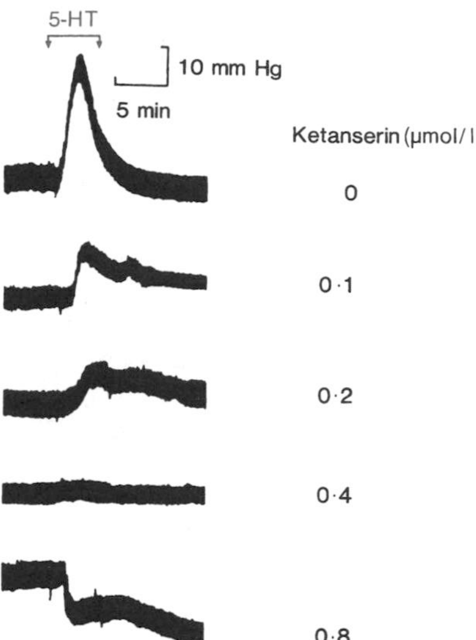

Fig. 8.2 Dual vascular effects of 5-HT. Dual effect of 5-hydroxytryptamine on blood vessels. The records show changes in the arterial perfusion pressure in a guinea-pig stomach preparation in response to 5-HT. The normal response to 5-HT is a strong vasoconstriction (*upper record*). Addition of increasing concentrations of the 5-HT_2-receptor antagonist, ketanserin, reduces the vasoconstriction and reveals a vasodilator effect (*lower trace*), which is probably mediated by 5-HT_1 receptors. (From: van Nueten J M et al. 1981 J Pharmacol Exp Ther 218: 217)

vasodilatation by several mechanisms, all operating through 5-HT_1 receptors: (1) by acting on endothelial cells to release nitric oxide which relaxes smooth muscle (see Ch. 10); (2) by inhibiting noradrenaline release from sympathetic nerve terminals; (3) possibly by a direct relaxant effect on smooth muscle cells. Thus 5-HT_2 receptors predominantly give rise to vasoconstriction, whereas 5-HT_1 receptors produce dilatation. When 5-HT_2 receptors are blocked by ketanserin (see Table 8.1) the vasodilator effect is revealed (Fig. 8.2).

In the microcirculation, 5-HT causes dilatation of arterioles, together with constriction of venules, with the result that capillary pressure rises and fluid escapes from the capillaries. 5-HT also has a direct effect on capillaries, rendering them more permeable to proteins, thus encouraging the formation of tissue fluid (Fig. 8.3).

If 5-HT is injected intravenously, the blood pressure usually first rises, due to the constriction of large vessels, and then falls, due to arteriolar dilatation and loss of blood volume.

Platelets. 5-HT causes platelet aggregation (see

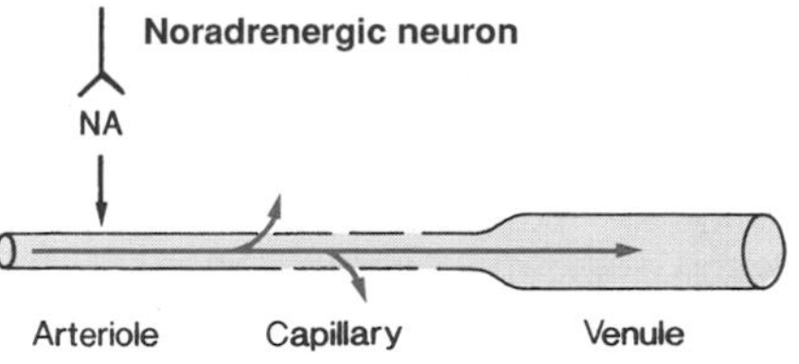

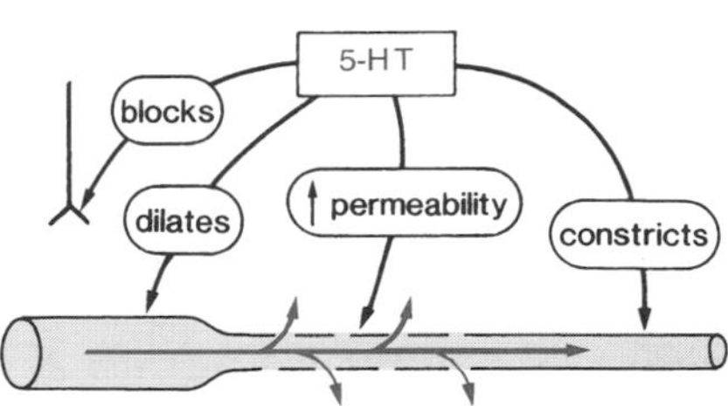

Fig. 8.3 Action of 5-HT on microvasculature. Four mechanisms are involved: (1) inhibition of NA release from sympathetic nerve terminals; (2) dilatation of precapillary vessels; (3) increase of capillary permeability; (4) constriction of postcapillary vessel. The dilatation is produced mainly through the release of nitric oxide from the vascular endothelium (see text).

Actions and functions of 5-HT

- Important actions are:
  - — increased gastrointestinal motility (direct excitation of smooth muscle and indirect action via enteric neurons)
  - — contraction of other smooth muscle (bronchi, uterus)
  - — mixture of vascular constriction (direct and via sympathetic innervation) and dilatation (endothelium dependent)
  - — platelet aggregation
  - — stimulation of peripheral nociceptive nerve endings
  - — excitation/inhibition of CNS neurons
  - — increased microvascular permeability.
- Postulated physiological and pathophysiological roles include:
  - — in periphery: peristalsis, vomiting, platelet aggregation and haemostasis, inflammatory mediator, sensitisation of nociceptors and microvascular control
  - — in CNS: many postulated functions, including control of appetite, sleep, mood, hallucinations, stereotyped behaviour, pain perception and vomiting.
- Clinical conditions associated with disturbed 5-HT function include migraine, carcinoid syndrome, mood disorders and anxiety (see Chs 27 and 29).

Ch. 16), and the platelets that collect in the vessel release more 5-HT. If the endothelium is intact, 5-HT release from adherent platelets causes vasodilatation, which helps to sustain blood flow; if it is damaged (e.g. by atherosclerosis), 5-HT causes constriction, and impairs blood flow further. These effects of platelet-derived 5-HT are thought to be important in vascular disease.

Nerve endings. 5-HT stimulates nociceptive (pain-mediating) sensory nerve endings. If injected into the skin it causes pain, and given systemically it elicits a variety of autonomic reflexes due to stimulation of afferent fibres in the heart and lungs, which further complicate the cardiovascular response. Nettle stings contain 5-HT, amongst other things.

Central nervous system. 5-HT excites some neurons and inhibits others, and also acts presynaptically to inhibit transmitter release from nerve terminals. Different receptor types and different membrane mechanisms mediate these effects (see Table 8.1; Bobker & Williams 1990). The role of 5-HT in the central nervous system is discussed in Chapter 24.

CLASSIFICATION OF 5-HT RECEPTORS

It has long been realised that the various actions of 5-HT are not all mediated by receptors of the same type, and various pharmacological classifications have come and gone. The amino acid sequence of many 5-HT receptor subtypes has now been determined by cloning (see Hartig 1989, Zifa & Fillion 1992), and considerable information has been gathered about the transduction mechanisms to which the receptors are coupled. Recently a summit meeting of 5-HT aficionados synthesised current knowledge of pharmacology, transduction mechanisms and cloning studies and delivered, with puffs of white smoke and much celebration, the latest version (Table 8.1; see Humphrey et al. 1993) of the classification. This recognises four main receptor types, 5-HT$_{1-4}$, types 1 and 2 being further subdivided.

5-HT$_1$ receptors occur mainly in the brain, the subtypes being distinguished on the basis of their regional distribution and their pharmacological specificity. Their neuronal effects are predominantly inhibitory (exerted both pre- and postsynaptically). 5-HT$_1$ receptors are G-protein-coupled receptors (Type 2; see Ch. 2) which are linked to inhibition of adenylate cyclase. The 5-HT$_{1A}$ subtype is particularly important in the brain, in relation to mood and behaviour (see Chs 24, 27 and 29). The 5-HT$_{1D}$ subtype, which is expressed in cerebral blood vessels, is believed to be important in migraine (see below), and is the target for the recently introduced anti-migraine drug, **sumatriptan**. These vessels are unusual in that vasoconstriction is mediated by 5-HT$_1$ receptors; in most vessels, 5-HT$_2$ receptors are responsible. The '5-HT$_{1C}$ receptor'—actually the first to be cloned—has now been officially declared non-existent, having been ignominiously reclassified as the 5-HT$_{2C}$ receptor when it was found be linked, not to adenylate cyclase, but to InsP$_3$ production.

5-HT$_2$ receptors are more important in the periphery than in the CNS. The effects of 5-HT on smooth muscle and platelets, which have been known for many years, are mediated by the 5-HT$_{2A}$ receptor, as are some of the behavioural effects of agents such as LSD (see Table 8.1 and Ch. 32). 5-HT$_2$ receptors are linked to phospholipase C, which catalyses phosphatidylinositol hydrolysis; 5-HT$_2$ agonists thus stimulate InsP$_3$ formation. The 5-HT$_{2A}$ subtype is functionally the most important, the others having a much more limited distribution and functional role. The role of 5-HT$_2$ receptors in normal physiological processes is probably a minor one, but it becomes more prominent in pathological conditions, such as asthma and vascular thrombosis (see Chs 16 and 17).

5-HT$_3$ receptors occur mainly in the peripheral nervous system, particularly on nociceptive sensory neurons (see Ch. 31), and on autonomic and enteric neurons, on which 5-HT exerts a strong excitatory effect. 5-HT itself evokes pain when injected locally, and when given intravenously elicits a fine display of autonomic reflexes, which result from excitation of many types of vascular, pulmonary and cardiac sensory nerve fibre. The physiological role of this receptor is not known, but it has been postulated that excitation of vascular sensory nerve terminals by 5-HT released from platelets may be involved in the pathogenesis of migraine (see below). 5-HT$_3$ receptors are exceptional in being directly linked to membrane ion channels (Type 1 receptors; Ch. 2), and do not involve any second messenger step in their transduction mechanism. 5-HT$_3$ receptors also occur in the brain, and blocking agents have an anxiolytic effect (see Ch. 27).

5-HT$_4$ receptors have recently been identified as a subclass distinct from 5-HT$_3$ receptors. Their main physiological role appears to be in the gastro-

Table 8.1 The main 5-HT receptor subtypes

Receptor	1A	1B	1D	2A	2B	2C	3	4
Location	CNS	CNS	CNS Blood vessels	CNS PNS Smooth muscle Platelets	Gastric fundus	CNS Choroid plexus	PNS CNS	PNS (GI tract) CNS
Main effects	Neuronal inhibition Behavioural effects: sleep, feeding, thermoregn, anxiety	Presynaptic inhibition Behavioural effects	Cerebral vasoconstn Behavioural effects: locomotion	Neuronal excitation Behavioural effects Platelet aggregation Smooth muscle contraction (gut, bronchi, etc.) Vasoconstn/ vasodiln	Contraction	CSF secretion	Neuronal excitation (autonomic, nociceptive neurons) Emesis Behavioural effects: anxiety	Neuronal excitation GI motility
Second messenger	Decr. cAMP	Decr. cAMP	Decr. cAMP	$InsP_3$/DAG	$InsP_3$/DAG	$InsP_3$/DAG	Ion channel	Incr. cAMP
Agonists	5-CT 8-OH-DPAT Buspirone (PA)	5-CT	5-CT Sumatriptan	α-Me-5-HT LSD (CNS)	α-Me-5-HT	α-Me-5-HT LSD	2-Me-5-HT Cl-Phenyl biguanide	5-methoxy-tryptamine Metoclopramide
Antagonists	Spiperone Methiothepin Ergotamine (PA)	Methiothepin Ergotamine (PA)	Methiothepin Ergotamine (PA)	Ketanserin Cyproheptadine Pizotifen (non-selective) LSD (periphery) Methysergide		Methysergide	Ondansetron Tropisetron Granisetron	

Abbreviations: 5-CT = 5-carboxamidotryptamine; 8-OH-DPAT = 8-hydroxy-2-(di n-propylamino)tetraline; α-Me-5-HT = α-methyl-5-HT; 2-Me-5-HT = 2-methyl-5-HT; PA = partial agonist.
For further details, see Zifa & Fillion 1992; Humphrey et al. 1993. Further main types (5-HT_5 and 5-HT_6, and subtypes (5-HT_{1E}) have recently been proposed.
The list of agonists and antagonists includes only the better-known compounds. Many new selective 5-HT receptor ligands, known only by code-numbers, are being developed.

intestinal tract, where they mediate the effect of 5-HT in stimulating peristalsis, though they also occur in the CNS.

DRUGS ACTING ON 5-HT RECEPTORS

Table 8.1 lists some of the selective agonists and antagonists for the different receptor types. Many of these compounds have been useful as experimental tools for defining the receptor subtypes; some of the newer compounds, such as the 5-HT_3 antagonists **ondansetron, tropisetron, granisetron** and the 5-HT_{1D} agonist **sumatriptan** are now in use as therapeutic agents; only a few established drugs (e.g. **cyproheptadine**) are thought to act principally on 5-HT receptors. It is, however, clear that many antidepressant drugs (see Ch. 29) act partly by affecting 5-HT metabolism or release, in addition to their actions on noradrenergic transmission. At the level of both transmitter metabolism and receptor interactions, there is much overlap between drug effects on the two systems, as is perhaps to be expected, since adrenoceptors and 5-HT receptors are now known to show considerable sequence homology. **Spiperone**, for example (Table 8.1), though selective for one type of 5-HT receptor, is a potent antagonist of dopamine and noradrenaline, and is better classified as a neuroleptic drug (Ch. 28).

Agonists

Sumatriptan is used in the treatment of migraine (see below). Selective 5-HT_{1A} agonists, such as 8-OH-DPAT (Table 8.1), are potent hypotensive agents, acting by a central mechanism, and may prove useful for this purpose.

Metoclopramide, a non-selective drug that acts on dopamine, as well as 5-HT receptors, is used clinically as an anti-emetic agent (Ch. 19). It acts mainly as a 5-HT_4 receptor agonist, to increase gastric peristalsis, and thus facilitate gastric emptying and removing the stimulus to vomiting.

Antagonists

'Classical' 5-HT antagonists form a group which are now known to act on the 5-HT_2 receptor. They include **methysergide, cyproheptadine** and **lysergic acid diethylamide** (LSD; Table 8.1). A newer compound of this type is **ketanserin,** which also blocks α-adrenoceptors. These drugs may be useful in treating vasospastic disorders, such as Raynaud's disease (see Ch. 14), but this is still controversial. Ketanserin is effective in lowering blood pressure, but it is uncertain whether this results from its 5-HT receptor-blocking action, or effects on α-adrenoceptors. The use of these drugs in migraine and carcinoid syndrome is discussed below.

Selective and potent 5-HT_3 receptor antagonists (e.g. **ondansetron, tropisetron**) have recently been developed (see Fozard 1989). These will be useful in elucidating the physiological role of 5-HT in the periphery, and are proving to be clinically useful as anti-emetic drugs, particularly in reducing the

5-HT receptors

- Four main types: 5-HT_1, 5-HT_2, 5-HT_3 and 5-HT_4. 5-HT_1 and 5-HT_2 receptors are further subdivided into A, B and C subtypes. Types 1, 2 and 4 are G-protein-coupled receptors; type 3 is a ligand-gated cation channel.
- 5-HT_1 receptors occur mainly in CNS (all subtypes) and some blood vessels (5-HT_{1D} subtype). Effects are neural inhibition and vasoconstriction. Act by inhibiting adenylate cyclase. *Specific agonists* include: sumatriptan (used in migraine therapy) and buspirone (used in anxiety). Ergotamine is a partial agonist. *Specific antagonists* include: spiperone, methiothepin and quipazine.
- 5-HT_2 receptors occur in CNS and many peripheral sites (especially blood vessels, platelets, autonomic neurons). Neuronal and smooth muscle effects are excitatory. Act through phospholipase C/inositol phosphate pathway. *Specific ligands* include LSD (agonist in CNS, antagonist in periphery). *Specific antagonists:* ketanserin, methysergide and cyproheptadine.
- 5-HT_3 receptors occur in peripheral nervous system, especially nociceptive afferent neurons and enteric neurons, and in CNS. Effects are excitatory, mediated via direct receptor-coupled ion channels. *Specific agonist:* 2-methyl-5-HT. *Specific antagonists:* ondansetron, tropisetron. Antagonists are used mainly as anti-emetic drugs, but may also be anxiolytic.
- 5-HT_4 receptors occur mainly in the enteric nervous system (also in CNS). Effects are excitatory, causing increased gastrointestinal motility. Act by stimulating adenylate cyclase. *Specific agonists* include metoclopramide (used to stimulate gastric emptying).
- Many new receptor-selective agonists and antagonists are being developed.

severe nausea and vomiting that occurs with many forms of cancer chemotherapy (see Chs 19 and 36)—a major advance, since this side effect is one of the main limiting factors in the effective use of chemotherapy.

Antagonism of 5-HT effects is also a property of various other drugs, such as **phenothiazines** and **butyrophenones** (which are antipsychotic drugs; see Ch. 28) and of drugs such as **pizotifen** and **ketotifen**. Pizotifen is used mainly in migraine prophylaxis (see p. 186); ketotifen has been claimed to be effective in asthma (see Ch. 17). These drugs are all non-selective in their actions, and it is uncertain whether 5-HT antagonism is important to their overall effects.

ERGOT ALKALOIDS

Ergot alkaloids constitute a hard-to-classify group of drugs that are used in medicine, many of which act on 5-HT receptors. Their actions are, however, complex and diverse. Ergot alkaloids occur naturally in a fungus (*Claviceps purpurea*) that infests cereal crops. Epidemics of ergot poisoning have occurred, and still occur, when contaminated grain is used for food. The symptoms produced include mental disturbances and intensely painful peripheral vasoconstriction, leading to gangrene, which came to be known in the Middle Ages as *St Anthony's fire*, because it was normally cured by a visit to the Shrine of St Anthony (which happened to be in an ergot-free region of France). Ergot contains many active substances, and it was a preoccupation with their complex pharmacological properties that led Dale to many important discoveries concerning acetylcholine, histamine and catecholamines.

Ergot alkaloids (Fig. 8.4) are molecules based on a complex aromatic acid, **lysergic acid**, and the different compounds in this group display many different types of pharmacological action. Chemically, they fall into two major categories, according to whether they possess an amine or an amino acid side-chain. Compounds with an amine side-chain include **lysergic acid diethylamide** (LSD; see Ch. 32), **methysergide** (Table 8.1) and **ergometrine**. Compounds with an amino acid side-chain include **ergotamine**, which acts on α-adrenoceptors and 5-HT_1 receptors, **dihydroergotamine**, and a semisynthetic compound, **bromocriptine**, which acts selectively on dopamine receptors (see Ch. 24). Ergometrine, which has a simple aliphatic side-chain, acts selectively on the smooth muscle of the uterus (see Ch. 22).

Actions

The ergot alkaloids all cause stimulation of smooth muscle, some being relatively selective for vascular smooth muscle, and others acting mainly on the uterus. In addition, the amino acid alkaloids affect catecholamine and 5-HT receptors in various ways. **Ergotamine** and **dihydroergotamine** are respectively a partial agonist and an antagonist at α-adrenoceptors; **bromocriptine** acts as an agonist on dopamine receptors, particularly in the central nervous system; **methysergide** is an antagonist at 5-HT_2 receptors.

The main pharmacological actions and uses of these drugs are summarised in Table 8.2. As one

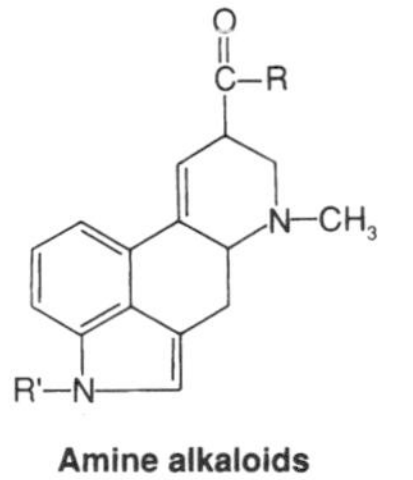

Amine alkaloids

	R	R′
Lysergic acid diethylamide (LSD)	$N(C_2H_5)_2$	H
Ergometrine	$NH.CH(CH_3)CH_2OH$	H
Methysergide	$NH.CH(CH_3)CH_2OH$	CH_3

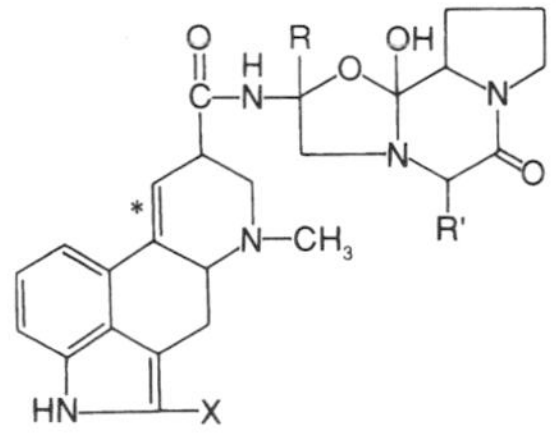

Amino acid alkaloids

	R	R′
Ergotamine	CH_3	CH_2-phenyl
Dihydroergotamine	CH_3	CH_2-phenyl (double bond* saturated)
Bromocriptine	$CH(CH_3)_2$	$CH_2.CH(CH_3)_2$ (Br at X)

Fig. 8.4 Structures of ergot alkaloids.

Table 8.2 Actions of ergot alkaloids

Drug	5-HT receptor	α-adrenoceptor	Dopamine receptor	Uterine contraction	Main uses
Ergotamine	**$5HT_1$ antag/PA**	PA (blood vessels)	– (emetic)	++	Migraine (acute attack)
Dihydro-ergotamine	$5HT_1$ antag/PA	Antagonist	–	+	Obsolete
Bromocriptine	–	Weak antagonist	**Agonist/PA**	–	**Parkinson's disease** (Ch. 25); **endocrine diseases** (Ch. 21)
Ergometrine	$5HT_1$ antag/PA	Weak agonist	Weak antagonist	**+++**	**Uterine contraction,** prevention of post-partum haemorrhage (Ch. 22)
Methysergide	**$5HT_2$ antag/PA**	–	–	–	**Carcinoid syndrome** Migraine (prophylaxis)

PA = partial agonist

would expect of drugs with so many actions, their physiological effects are complex, and rather poorly understood. Ergotamine, dihydroergotamine and methysergide are discussed here; further information on ergometrine and bromocriptine is given in Chapters 22, 24 and 25.

Vascular effects. When injected into an anaesthetised animal, **ergotamine** causes a sustained rise in blood pressure, caused by vasoconstriction. This effect is blocked by pure α-adrenoceptor antagonists such as phentolamine. At the same time as causing a rise in blood pressure, ergotamine reverses the pressor effect of adrenaline (see Ch. 7). The vasoconstrictor effect of ergotamine is responsible for the peripheral gangrene of St Anthony's fire, and probably also for some of the effects of ergot on the central nervous system. Methysergide and dihydroergotamine have much less vasoconstrictor effect.

Actions on 5-HT receptors. Methysergide is a potent 5-HT_2 receptor antagonist, whereas ergotamine and dihydroergotamine act selectively on 5-HT_1 receptors. Though generally classified as antagonists, they show partial agonist activity in some tissues, and this may account for their activity in preventing migraine attacks (see below).

Clinical use

The only use of ergotamine is in the treatment of attacks of migraine unresponsive to simple analgesics (see below). Methysergide is also sometimes used for migraine prophylaxis, but its main use is in treating the symptoms of carcinoid tumours (see below). All of these drugs can be used orally or by injection.

Unwanted effects

Ergotamine is very prone to cause nausea and vomiting, and it must be avoided in patients with peripheral vascular disease, because of its vasoconstrictor action. Methysergide also causes nausea and vomiting, but its most serious side effect, which restricts its clinical usefulness considerably, is retroperitoneal and mediastinal fibrosis, which can impair the functioning of the gastrointestinal tract, kidneys, heart and lungs. The mechanism of this is unknown, but it is noteworthy that similar fibrotic reactions also occur in carcinoid syndrome (see below) in which there is a high circulating level of 5-HT.

CLINICAL CONDITIONS IN WHICH 5-HT PLAYS A ROLE

In this section, we discuss two situations in which the peripheral actions of 5-HT are believed to be important, namely *migraine* and *carcinoid syndrome.* Further information is reviewed by Houston & Vanhoutte (1986). The possible role of 5-HT in vomiting, and the usefulness of 5-HT_3 antagonists in treating drug-induced emesis, are discussed in Chapter 19. Pharmacological interference with 5-HT-mediated transmission in the central nervous system is probably important in relation to the actions of many psychotropic drugs (see Ch. 24).

MIGRAINE AND ANTI-MIGRAINE DRUGS

Migraine is a common and unpleasant condition, the causation of which is not well understood (see Blau 1987, Moskowitz 1992). One commonly held view is that vascular changes are responsible, and that these are triggered by 5-HT release. The most common pattern of events in a migraine attack consists of an initial visual disturbance (the *aura*), in which the central area of the visual field is lost, and the surrounding area displays a jagged, flickering pattern. This visual disturbance is followed, about 30 minutes later, by a severe throbbing headache, starting unilaterally, often with photophobia, nausea and vomiting, which lasts for several hours.

Pathophysiology

There is much disagreement about whether the primary event in migraine is a humoral disturbance, leading to vascular responses which in turn disturb brain function and elicit pain, or a neurological disturbance originating in the brain or meninges, of which pain and vasomotor changes are consequences (see Blau 1987). The classical view (Woolf 1963) suggested that vascular abnormalities were the underlying cause, with an initial intracerebral vasoconstriction giving rise to the aura and visual disturbances, and an ensuing extracerebral vasodilatation phase causing the headache. This hypothesis has not, however, been generally supported by more recent blood flow studies involving non-invasive monitoring techniques in migraine patients (see Lauritzen 1987, Olesen et al. 1990, Moskowitz 1992, Ferrari & Saxena 1993).

The premonitory aura of migraine is indeed accompanied by a reduction of cerebral blood flow, though a similar reduction caused by other factors does not produce symptoms, suggesting that the vascular changes may accompany, rather than cause, the neurological symptoms. Furthermore, the vasoconstriction starts posteriorly and gradually spreads forwards over the rest of the hemisphere, suggesting a neural rather than a humoral cause. The blood flow slowly returns to normal after an hour or more, but there is no evidence for a secondary increase in blood flow suggestive of vasodilatation. Headache is believed to result from stimulation of sensory nerve terminals in the meninges or large arteries. Some studies (Friberg et al. 1991) have suggested that the headache phase is associated with widening of the middle cerebral artery on the side of the headache. Overall, however, there is no clear evidence suggesting that the headache is associated with vasodilatation, and the headache phase may begin before the initial vasoconstriction has even subsided. Thus, vascular changes are not established as the primary event in migraine.

A second hypothesis (see Lauritzen 1987) is that the underlying abnormality is neuronal, and is a process similar to cortical spreading depression. This is a dramatic, though poorly understood, phenomenon, which occurs in concussion, and is triggered off by local trauma to the cortex. The effect is to cause an advancing wave of profound neural inhibition, which progresses slowly over the cortical surface at a rate of about 2 mm/min. In the depressed area the ionic balance is grossly disturbed, with an extremely high extracellular potassium concentration, and the blood flow is reduced.

A third hypothesis (see Moskowitz 1992) suggests that migraine is initiated by activity in peptidergic nerve terminals in the meningeal vessels, leading to pain, which becomes reinforced by inflammatory changes caused by the released neuropeptides (neurogenic inflammation; see Ch. 9). There is evidence that one of these peptides is released into the meningeal circulation during a migraine attack. All of these theories have difficulty in explaining the link between the cerebral vasoconstriction associated with the aura, and the later extracerebral change which causes headache; the religious wars continue.

Whether one inclines to the view that migraine is a vascular disorder, a form of epilepsy, a platelet disorder, an inflammatory disease, a kind of spontaneous concussion, or just a bad headache, there is strong evidence to implicate 5-HT:

- There is a sharp increase in the urinary excretion of the main 5-HT metabolite, 5-HIAA, during the attack. The blood concentration of 5-HT falls, probably because of depletion of platelet 5-HT.
- Agents that release 5-HT (e.g. reserpine), when injected locally, cause migraine-like headache.
- Many of the drugs that are effective in treating migraine are 5-HT receptor agonists or antagonists (see Fozard 1982, 1987, Peatfield 1988). See page 187 for further information.

An uneasy compromise between the neurogenic and vascular theories (Fig. 8.5) suggests that a primary neuronal disturbance leads to hyperactivity of noradrenergic and 5-HT-releasing neurons in the

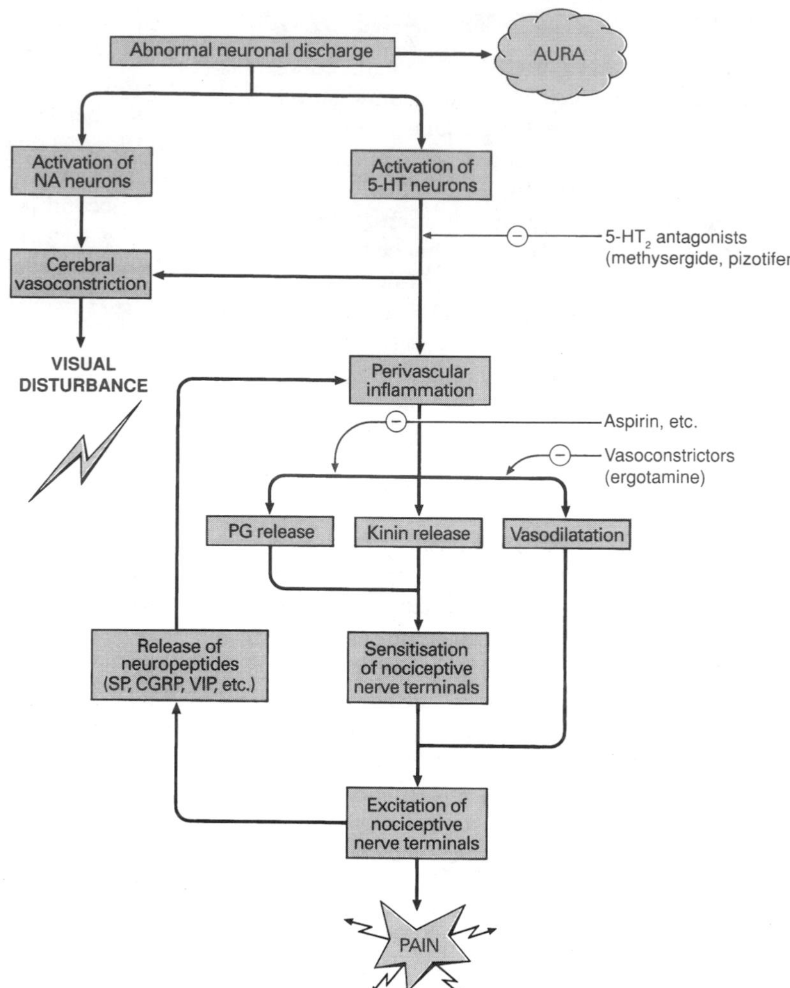

Fig. 8.5 Postulated pathogenesis of migraine. The initiating event is assumed to be an abnormal neuronal discharge, the cause and location of which is uncertain; it is probably set off by emotional or biochemical disturbances, but the details are unclear. An alternative view suggests that the primary event is excitation (cause unknown) of nociceptive nerve terminals in the meningeal vessels, leading to the cycle of neurogenic inflammation shown in the lower part of the diagram. (PG = prostaglandins; SP = substance P; CGRP = calcitonin gene related peptide; VIP = vasoactive intestinal peptide)

brainstem, causing intracerebral vasoconstriction. Release of 5-HT also leads to a local inflammatory response around the extracellular vessels, associated with the local release of other mediators, particularly bradykinin and prostaglandins (see Ch. 11). 5-HT and these other mediators act on, among other things, nociceptive nerve terminals (see Ch. 31), causing pain and also releasing a variety of neuropeptides, which further reinforce and prolong the pain response. It is suggested that afferent nerve terminals in the wall of blood vessels may become hypersensitive to vascular distension, thus accounting for the fact that many of the drugs that are effective are vasoconstrictors.

Anti-migraine drugs

The main drugs used to treat migraine are summarised on page 187. It is important to distinguish between drugs used to treat acute attacks of migraine (appropriate when the attacks are fairly infrequent, and prophylaxis is not justified) and drugs used for prophylaxis.

CARCINOID SYNDROME

Carcinoid syndrome (see Creutzfeld & Stockmann 1987) is a clinical state associated with malignant tumours of enterochromaffin cells, usually arising in the small intestine and metastasising to the liver. These tumours secrete, usually sporadically, a variety of hormones. 5-HT is the most important, but neuropeptides, such as substance P, and other agents, such as prostaglandins and bradykinin, are also produced. The sudden release of these sub-

Drugs used for migraine

Acute attack

- Simple analgesics, such as **aspirin** or **paracetamol**. May be given with **metoclopramide** to speed up absorption.
- **Ergotamine** ($5HT_{1D}$ receptor partial agonist). Various routes of administration (e.g. suppositories, sublingual tablets, oral spray) used to achieve absorption when patient is vomiting.
- **Sumatriptan** ($5HT_{1D}$ agonist) is highly effective, but expensive. Used instead of ergotamine. Contraindicated in patients with ischaemic heart disease because of tendency to cause coronary artery spasm. Given by mouth or subcutaneous injection. Short-acting (< 12 hours).

Prophylaxis (in cases with more than one severe attack per month)

- Pizotifen (adverse effects include weight gain, antimuscarinic effects).
- β-adrenoceptor antagonists (e.g. **propranolol**, **metoprolol**; see Ch. 7). Mechanism of action is not clear.
- Tricyclic antidepressants (e.g. **amitriptyline**; see Ch. 29). May be effective even though patients are not depressed.
- **Methysergide** ($5\text{-}HT_2$-receptor antagonist). Effective, but has dangerous and insidious adverse effects, especially retroperitoneal fibrosis and renal failure, so not generally used.
- α_2-adrenoceptor agonist (**clonidine**; see Ch. 7). Has been used, but efficacy is doubtful.
- Calcium antagonists (e.g. **dihydropyridines**, **verapamil**; see Ch. 14) cause headaches as a common side effect, but paradoxically may reduce frequency of migraine attacks. Mechanism of action is not clear.
- **Cyproheptadine** ($5\text{-}HT_2$-receptor antagonist, also has antihistamine and calcium antagonist actions) sometimes used in refractory cases.

stances into the bloodstream results in various unpleasant symptoms, including flushing, diarrhoea and bronchoconstriction, as well as hypotension, which may cause dizziness or fainting. Cardiac fibrosis also occurs, which can result in cardiac failure. The relationship of this to hormone secretion is not understood.

The syndrome is readily diagnosed by measuring the excretion of 5-HIAA, the main metabolite of 5-HT, in the urine, the level of which may increase 20-fold, and is raised even during periods when the tumour is asymptomatic.

$5\text{-}HT_2$ antagonists, such as **cyproheptadine**, are effective in controlling some of the symptoms of carcinoid syndrome. **Methysergide** is also effective, but is liable to cause retroperitoneal and cardiac fibrosis, a potentially serious side effect.

A complementary therapeutic approach is to use a long-acting analogue of somatostatin, namely **octreotide**, which suppresses hormone secretion from various neuroendocrine cells, including carcinoid cells (see Ch. 21).

PURINES

Purines, especially *adenosine*, and purine nucleotides, especially *ADP* and *ATP*, produce a wide range of pharmacological effects that are not directly related to their role in energy metabolism. It was shown in 1929 that adenosine injected into anaesthetised animals causes cardiac slowing, a fall in blood pressure, vasodilatation, and inhibition of intestinal movements, and it has since been suggested that adenosine or ATP is implicated in such physiological mechanisms as the regulation of coronary flow, 'antidromic' vasodilatation produced by retrograde stimulation of sensory nerves, platelet aggregation and peripheral transmission in the autonomic nervous system (see Ch. 5). For reviews, see Williams (1987), Stone, (1991a).

ATP AS A NEUROTRANSMITTER

The idea that such a work-a-day metabolite as ATP might be a member of the neurotransmitter elite was, for a long time, resisted, but there is now strong evidence in its favour. ATP is a transmitter in the periphery, both as a primary mediator (see Burnstock 1981, 1985, 1988, Evans et al. 1993) and as a co-transmitter in noradrenergic nerve terminals (see von Kugelglen & Starke 1991). ATP is known to be contained in synaptic vesicles of both noradrenergic and cholinergic neurons, and it has long been realised that many actions produced by stimulation of autonomic nerves are not due to acetylcholine or noradrenaline (see Ch. 5). These include effects such as relaxation of intestinal smooth muscle evoked by sympathetic stimulation, and contraction of the bladder produced by parasympathetic nerves. Burnstock and his colleagues have shown that ATP is released, in a calcium-dependent fashion, on nerve stimulation, and that exogenous ATP in general mimics the effects of nerve stimulation in various preparations. Furthermore, suramin, (developed many years ago for treating trypanosome infections) but recently shown to block ATP receptors, blocks these synaptic responses. Recent work has also shown ATP to function as a conventional 'fast' transmitter in the CNS and in autonomic ganglia (see Edwards & Gibb 1993). ATP has also been proposed as the transmitter responsible for the cutaneous vasodilatation caused by antidromic stimulation of sensory nerves, but there is also evidence favouring peptides, such as substance P, for this role.

The role of *intracellular* ATP in controlling membrane K^+-channels, and hence membrane potential, discussed in Chapter 14, is quite distinct from its transmitter function.

ATP receptors (P_2-purinoceptors)*

ATP receptors respond to various adenine nucleotides, generally preferring ATP to ADP or AMP. They fall into two main classes, P_{2X} and P_{2Y}, which are distinguished on the basis of their agonist selectivity. The fast transmitter function of ATP, including its vasoconstrictor function, is mediated by P_{2X}-receptors, which are blocked by suramin and a purine analogue, ANAPP3 (see Burnstock 1988). The use of these blocking agents has helped to clarify the physiological role of ATP. Its other actions are mediated through P_{2Y}-receptors, which are linked to various second messenger systems, and for which no specific antagonists are known. One important exception to the rule that P_2-receptors are relatively selective for ATP occurs in the platelet, which responds selectively to ADP. ADP causes platelet aggregation, the opposite effect to that of adenosine (see below), and its action is actually antagonised by ATP. ADP released from the vascular endothelium is believed to be an important factor promoting thrombosis (see Ch. 16).

Drugs acting selectively on ATP and ADP receptors have not yet been developed for clinical purposes.

*The original nomenclature referred to adenosine receptors as P_1-purinoceptors, and ATP receptors as P_2. P_1-receptors have now been renamed A_1 and A_2, but ATP receptors are still called P_2, and are divided into various subtypes, P_{2X}, P_{2Y}, etc.

ADENOSINE AS A MEDIATOR

Adenosine produces many pharmacological effects, both in the periphery and in the central nervous system (see below). There is evidence that it functions as a mediator in the central nervous system (see Phillis & Wu 1981, Stone 1991a). It is also likely that it has a physiological role in the periphery, but direct evidence for this is so far rather weak (see Williams 1987). Thus, many tissues produce adenosine, but mainly as a by-product of ATP breakdown; there does not seem to be a special synthetic mechanism for adenosine. It is probably not a true transmitter, for there is no evidence for vesicular storage of adenosine, nor of calcium-dependent release in response to stimulation in the brain or the periphery; it is released not only from neurons, but also from glia and other cells. It appears to be released through the operation of membrane transport systems (see Ch. 5). So far there are no potent antagonists of adenosine (though **theophylline** and other methylxanthines do have this action; see Ch. 17), and its role as a mediator remains unproven. It seems likely, however, that adenosine and ADP may function as local regulatory substances (e.g. in controlling blood flow), whose rate of production varies with the functional state of the tissue. Irrespective of the putative mediator role of adenosine and ADP, their pharmacological effects suggest that therapeutically useful drugs might be developed; hence the current active interest in adenosine pharmacology. Adenosine is destroyed or taken up within a few seconds when given intravenously, but longer-lasting analogues have been discovered which also show greater receptor selectivity. Adenosine uptake is blocked by **dipyridamole**, a vasodilator and antiplatelet drug (see Ch. 16). A possible role of adenosine in the heart, in relation to the phenomenon of 'ischaemic preconditioning' is discussed in Chapter 13.

Adenosine receptors and actions

The effects of *adenosine* are mediated by two distinct receptors, A_1 and A_2, linked, respectively, to the inhibition and stimulation of adenylate cyclase, thus reducing or increasing intracellular cAMP formation (see Stone 1991b, Collis & Hourani 1993). These adenosine receptors are not sensitive to nucleotides such as AMP, ADP or ATP. Methylxanthines, especially analogues of **theophylline** (Ch. 17) are A_1-receptor antagonists; however, they also increase cAMP by inhibiting phosphodiesterase, which probably accounts for most of their pharmacological actions independently of adenosine receptor antagonism. Certain derivatives of theophylline are claimed to show greater selectivity for A_1-receptors over phosphodiesterase.

The main effects of adenosine, and the receptors involved, are:

- Vasodilatation, including coronary vessels (A_2), except in the kidney, where A_1-receptors produce vasoconstriction. Adenosine infusion causes a fall in blood pressure.
- Inhibition of platelet aggregation (A_2).
- Block of cardiac AV conduction (A_1), and reduction of force of contraction.
- Bronchoconstriction, especially in asthmatic subjects (A_1). The anti-asthmatic effect of methylxanthines may partly reflect A_1-receptor antagonism.
- Stimulation of nociceptive afferent neurons, especially in the heart (A_2). Adenosine release in response to ischaemia has been suggested as a mechanism of anginal pain (Ch. 13).
- Inhibition of transmitter release at many peripheral and central synapses (A_1). In the central nervous system, adenosine generally exerts a pre- and postsynaptic depressant action. It reduces motor activity, depresses respiration, induces sleep, and reduces anxiety, all of which effects are the opposite of those produced by methylxanthines (Ch. 32).
- Neuroprotection, in cerebral ischaemia, probably through inhibition of glutamate release through A_1-receptors (see Rudolphi et al. 1992; Ch. 25).

Adenosine may be used, as intravenous bolus injections to suppress cardiac dysrhythmias (Ch. 13), based on its inhibitory effect on conduction. It is effective in converting paroxysmal supraventricular tachycardias to normal rhythm, and is safer than alternative drugs such as β-adrenoceptor antagonists or verapamil. This is because, although the force of contraction of the heart is reduced, the short duration of action of adenosine provides much closer control than can be achieved with other drugs. It must not be used in patients with heart block.

Otherwise adenosine is not used therapeutically, though longer-lasting A_1-receptor agonists may prove to be useful in various conditions (e.g. hypertension, ischaemic heart disease, stroke, diabetes, etc.).

Purines as mediators

- ATP functions as a neurotransmitter (or co-transmitter) at many peripheral neuro-effector junctions and also as a fast transmitter in the central nervous system. It also functions as an intracellular mediator, inhibiting the opening of membrane potassium channels.
- Adenosine affects many cells and tissues, including smooth muscle and nerve cells. It is not a conventional transmitter, but may be important as local hormone or modulator.
- ADP acts selectively on platelets, causing aggregation. This is important in thrombosis.
- ATP acts on two types of purinoceptor (P_2), one of which (P_{2X}) is a ligand-gated ion channel responsible for fast synaptic responses. The other (P_{2Y}) is coupled to various second messengers. Suramin blocks the P_{2X}-receptor.
- Adenosine acts through A_1- and A_2-receptors, coupled respectively to inhibition and stimulation of adenylate cyclase. A_1-receptors are blocked by xanthines, such as theophylline.
- The main effects of adenosine are:
  - — hypotension and cardiac depression
  - — inhibition of AV-conduction (anti-dysrhythmic effect)
  - — inhibition of platelet aggregation
  - — bronchoconstriction
  - — presynaptic inhibition in CNS (responsible for neuroprotective effect).
- Adenosine is sometimes used for its antidysrhythmic effect.

REFERENCES AND FURTHER READING

Bateman D N 1993 Sumatriptan. Lancet 341: 221–224
Blau J N (ed) 1987 Migraine. Chapman & Hall, London
Bobker D H, Williams J T 1990 Ion conductances affected by 5-HT receptor subtypes in mammalian neurons. Trends Neurosci 13: 169–173
Burnstock G 1981 Purinergic receptors. Chapman & Hall, London
Burnstock G 1985 Purinergic mechanisms broaden their sphere of influence. Trends Neurosci 8: 5–6
Burnstock G 1988 Sympathetic purinergic transmission

in small blood vessels. Trends Pharmacol Sci 9: 116–117

Collis M G, Hourani S M O 1993 Adenosine receptor subtypes. Trends Pharmacol Sci 14: 360–366

Creutzfeld W, Stockmann F 1987 Carcinoids and carcinoid syndrome. Amer J Med 82 (Suppl 58): 4–16

Edwards F A, Gibb A J 1993 ATP—a fast neurotransmitter. FEBS Letters 325: 86–89

Evans R J, Derkach V, Surprenat A 1993 ATP mediates fast synaptic transmission in mammalian neurons. Nature 357: 503–505

Ferrari M D, Saxena P R 1993 Clinical and experimental effects of sumatriptan in humans. Trends Pharmacol Sci 14: 129–133

Fozard J R 1982 Basic mechanism of anti-migraine drugs. Adv Neurol 33: 295–307

Fozard J R 1987 The pharmacological basis of migraine treatment. In: Blau J N (ed) Migraine. Chapman & Hall, London

Fozard J R (ed) 1989 The peripheral actions of 5-hydroxytryptamine. Oxford University Press, Oxford

Friberg L, Olesen J, Iversen H K, Sperling B 1991 Migraine pain associated with middle cerebral artery dilatation: reversal by sumatriptan. Lancet 338: 13–17

Green A R (ed) 1985 Neuropharmacology of serotonin. Oxford University Press, Oxford

Hartig P R 1989 Molecular biology of 5-HT receptors. Trends Pharmacol Sci 10: 64–69

Houston D S, Vanhoutte P M 1986 Serotonin and the vascular system: role in health and disease, and implications for therapy. Drugs 31: 149–163

Humphrey P P A, Feniuk W 1991 Mode of action of the anti-migraine drug sumatriptan. Trends Pharmacol Sci 12: 444–445

Humphrey P P A, Hartig P, Hoyer D 1993 A proposed new nomenclature for 5-HT receptors. Trends Pharmacol Sci 14: 233–236

Lauritzen M 1987 Cerebral blood flow in migraine and cortical spreading depression. Acta Neurol Scand Suppl 113: 140

Moskowitz M A 1992 Neurogenic versus vascular mechanisms of sumatriptan and ergot alkaloids in migraine. Trends Pharmacol Sci 13: 307–311

Olesen J, Friberg J, Olsen T S 1990 Timing and topography of cerebral blood flow, aura and headache during migraine attacks. Ann Neurol 28: 791–798

Peatfield R 1988 Drugs and the treatment of migraine. Trends Pharmacol Sci 9: 141–145

Phillis J W, Wu P H 1981 The role of adenosine and its nucleotides in central synaptic transmission. Prog Neurobiol 16: 187–239

Rudolphi K A, Schubert P, Parkinson F E, Fredholm B B 1992 Neuroprotective role of adenosine in cerebral ischaemia. Trends Pharmacol Sci 13: 439–445

Stone T W (ed) 1991a Adenosine in the nervous system. Academic Press, London

Stone T W (ed) 1991b Receptors for adenosine and adenine nucleotides. Gen Pharmacol 22: 25–31

von Kugelglen I, Starke K 1991 Noradrenaline–ATP co-transmission in the sympathetic nervous system. Trends Pharmacol Sci 12: 319–324

Williams M 1987 Purine receptors in mammalian tissues: pharmacology and functional significance. Annu Rev Pharmacol Toxicol 27: 315–345

Woolf H G 1963 Headache and other head pain. Oxford University Press, New York

Zifa E, Fillion G 1992 5-Hydroxytryptamine receptors. Pharm Rev 44: 401–458

9

PEPTIDES AS MEDIATORS

Much of pharmacology is based on signalling molecules that are of low molecular weight, and non-peptide in nature. What has become plain, mainly in the last 20 years, is that peptides are at least as important, and possibly much more so, as signalling molecules. Yet, the pharmacological manipulation of peptide signalling has yet to approach that of, say, the cholinergic, noradrenergic or 5-HT systems (Chs 6–8). Pharmacology, one could say, has some catching up to do.

Historically, there are two main reasons why pharmacology has a strong bias towards non-peptides. One is that the subject got started by analysing the actions of natural (mainly plant) products thought to have medicinal properties. Very few of these were peptides, and they did not, for the most part, interact with peptide signalling systems. The second reason is that the methodology required to study peptides has only recently been developed. The two key methodological advances are solid phase peptide synthesis, and the use of antibodies, both for radioimmunoassay (see Ch. 3) and for immunocytochemical localisation of peptides. These synthetic and analytical methods were unknown to chemists and pharmacologists until about 30 years ago, and very few were dogged enough to tackle peptide chemistry by classical methods.

In 1953, du Vigneaud made history, and earned a Nobel Prize, by determining the structure, and carrying out the synthesis, of **oxytocin**. This was the first peptide for which this was achieved and the first to be synthesised commercially for use in medicine. There were many other examples of mediators, for example substance P, bradykinin and angiotensin, which had been identified as peptides in the 1930s, but whose structure remained unknown for many years. Determination of their structure, and their chemical synthesis, was a major task; the structure of bradykinin was not known until 1960, while that of substance P was published in 1970. By contrast, the use of the newer, now routine, methods enabled endothelin (see Ch. 14, and below) to be fully characterised, synthesised and cloned within about a year, the complete information being published in a single paper (Yanagisawa et al. 1988).

The purpose of this chapter is to give an overview of the main characteristics of peptides as mediators, and to bring out the contrasts between peptide and non-peptide mediators. The pharmacology in this area is still sparse—a few saplings rather than a dense forest—and its therapeutic exploitation even sparser. But the saplings are multiplying fast, and many predict that peptide pharmacology is the coming therapeutic growth area, catalysed by the rapid developments in biotechnology and molecular biology. For readable and well-balanced views, with more detail than can be provided here, see Cooper et al. (1991), Hokfelt (1991). For still more detail, see Iversen et al. (1983), Krieger et al. (1984).

GENERAL PRINCIPLES OF PEPTIDE PHARMACOLOGY

ROLE OF MOLECULAR BIOLOGY

Because peptide structures are represented directly in the genome, molecular biology has been the key to most of the recent, dramatic, advances in knowledge. It is used in several ways:

- Cloning of peptide precursors (see below) has shown how various active peptides can arise from a single precursor protein.
- In some cases (e.g. calcitonin-gene-related peptide, CGRP) new peptides have been discovered.
- Cloning of peptide receptors (see Ch. 2). In general peptide receptors conform to the pattern of other receptors; there are no major surprises.
- The control of precursor synthesis can be studied by measuring mRNA, for which highly sensitive and specific assays have been developed. The technique of *in situ hybridisation* enables the location and abundance of the mRNA to be detected at high resolution.

These approaches are well summarised in recent reviews (Schwartz & Costa 1986, Eipper et al. 1986, Cooper et al. 1991).

STRUCTURE OF PEPTIDES

Endogenous peptide mediators typically consist of a linear chain of about 5–40 amino acids (Fig. 9.1), often with the C-terminus amidated, and with other post-translational modifications, such as glycosylation, acetylation, carboxylation, sulphation or phosphorylation of specific residues. They often contain intramolecular disulphide bonds, so that the molecule adopts a partially cyclic conformation. The conformation of peptides in solution is very ill-defined (see Milner-White 1989). Peptides of this size have mostly proved impossible to crystallise, which precludes the use of X-ray diffraction methods to study their conformation, and methods for examining conformational structure in solution, such as nuclear magnetic resonance spectroscopy, have generally shown these molecules to be highly flexible. To imagine them fitting into a receptor site in a precise 'lock-and-key' mode is to imagine that you can unlock your front door with a length of cooked spaghetti. This fact has greatly impeded the rational design of non-peptide analogues ('peptidomimetics') that mimic the structure of peptides and interact with peptide receptors, though considerable progress has been made recently (see below).

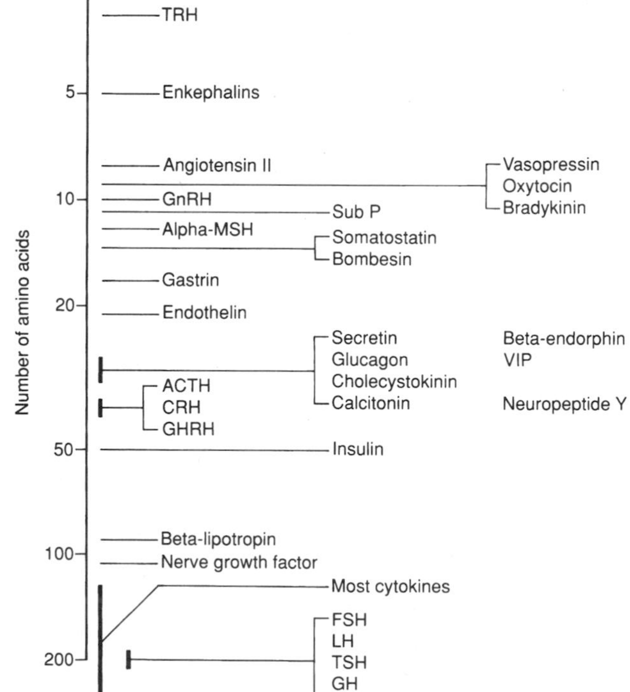

Fig. 9.1 Some typical peptide mediators. (TRH = thyrotrophin-releasing hormone; GnRH = gonadotrophin-releasing hormone; Sub P = substance P; Alpha-MSH = α-melanocyte-stimulating hormone; VIP = vasoactive intestinal peptide; ACTH = adrenocorticotrophic hormone; CRH = corticotrophin-releasing hormone; GHRH = growth hormone-releasing hormone; FSH = follicle-stimulating hormone; LH = luteinising hormone; TSH = thyroid-stimulating hormone; GH = growth hormone)

TYPES OF PEPTIDE MEDIATOR

The distinction between peptides and proteins is arbitrary, the cut-off point being at about 50 amino acids. The main source of peptide mediators in the body is the neuroendocrine system, with which this chapter is principally concerned, though there are also some important plasma-derived peptides, notably **angiotensin** (Ch. 14), and **bradykinin** (Ch. 11). The family of peptide mediators also includes **endothelin** (see Ch. 14), an extremely potent vasoconstrictor peptide released from vascular endothelial cells, and **atrial natriuretic peptide** (see Ch. 14). The soluble mediators of the immune system, known collectively as **cytokines**, are mainly larger proteins of 100 or more residues, and they are discussed in more detail in Chapter 11.

Growth factors, such as epidermal growth factor (EGF) and nerve growth factor (NGF), form another class of protein mediators, the main functions of which are to control cell division and differentiation.

Some of the most important examples of peptide and protein mediators are shown in Figure 9.1.

Peptides in the nervous system: comparison with conventional transmitters

There is a tendency to 'over-conceptualise' the role of peptides in the nervous system, as though they comprise a system of communication fundamentally different in its organisation and function from the conventional chemical transmitters. In most respects, however, neuropeptide-mediated transmission closely resembles transmission by classical non-peptide mediators. Thus, the mechanisms for vesicular storage and calcium-activated release (see Ch. 5) are essentially the same. Furthermore, the effects of peptides on target cells appear to involve exactly the same basic mechanisms—binding to receptors, activation of second messenger systems, etc.—as those involved in responses to non-peptides (see Ch. 2). As with other chemical mediators, their effects may be excitatory or inhibitory, pre- or postsynaptic, and exerted over short or long distances from the site of release. There are, however, certain monopolies of function between peptide and non-peptide mediators. For example, only non-peptides, such as acetylcholine, glutamate, glycine or GABA (see Chs 6 and 24), are so far known to serve as fast transmitters, with receptors directly linked to ion channels (see Ch. 2). It appears that peptides do not work in this way, but (along with many non-peptides) serve rather as 'neuromodulators' (Ch. 5). On the other hand, the ligands for tyrosine-kinase-linked receptors (see Ch. 2) are all peptides or proteins.

In summary, the similarities in function between peptide and non-peptide mediators are much more striking than the differences. The main difference is constitutional rather than functional, and stems from the fact that peptides, being gene products, represent variations on a single theme—a linear string of amino acids. Evolution, of course, plays many tunes on this theme, far more than are played on the structure of non-peptide mediators. As a result the number of known peptide mediators now greatly exceeds that of non-peptides. As Iversen pointed out in 1983: 'almost overnight, the number of putative transmitters in the mammalian nervous system has jumped from the ten or so monoamine and amino acid candidates to more than 40'. Since then, no new monoamine transmitters have appeared, but there are at least another 20 peptides.

There are a growing number of examples of co-transmission, namely the simultaneous release and postsynaptic action of two transmitters by the same neuron (see Ch. 5; Hokfelt 1991), in which one or both are peptides. In many cases, two or more peptides have been shown by immunocytochemistry to coexist in the same neuron (see Chan-Palay & Palay 1984), and in a few instances true co-transmission (involving co-release and demonstrable postsynaptic actions of both mediators) has been demonstrated. Two well-documented examples (see Ch. 5 and reviews by Hokfelt et al. 1986, Campbell 1987) are the parasympathetic nerves supplying salivary glands (where the secretory response is produced by acetylcholine and the vasodilatation partly by **vasoactive intestinal peptide**) and the sympathetic innervation to various tissues, which involves release of the vasoconstrictor **neuropeptide Y** in addition to noradrenaline.

The distinction between neuropeptides and peripherally acting hormones is useful, but not watertight. Thus, **insulin**, **angiotensin**, **atrial natriuretic peptide** and **bradykinin** are best known as hormones that are formed, released, and act, in the periphery. They are, however, also found in the brain, though their role there is uncertain. Similarly, endothelin was first discovered in blood vessels, but is now known to occur extensively in the brain as well.

Multiple physiological roles of peptides

In common with many non-peptide mediators, such as noradrenaline, dopamine, 5-HT or acetylcholine, the same peptides are often found, and presumably function as mediators, in several different parts of the body. Intriguingly, there often appears to be some connection between the effects of a peptide at different sites, in terms of coordinated physiological functions. Thus **angiotensin** acts on the cells of the hypothalamus to release **vasopressin**, which in turn causes water retention; it also acts elsewhere in the brain to promote drinking behaviour and to increase blood pressure by activation of the sympathetic system; in addition, it acts directly to constrict blood vessels. Each of these effects plays a part in the overall response of the body to water deprivation and reduced circulating volume. There are other examples of what appears to be an orchestrated functional response produced by the various actions of a single mediator, but there are many more examples where the multiple effects just seem to be multiple effects.

So far it cannot be claimed that the cataract of new information over the past 20 years has produced more than a fragmentary understanding of the functional role of neuropeptides.

Structure and function of peptide mediators

- Size varies from 3 to several hundred amino acids; conventionally, molecules of less than 50 residues are called peptides, larger molecules being proteins.
- Neural and endocrine mediators range in size from 3 to over 200 residues. Cytokines and growth factors are generally larger than 100 residues.
- Most known peptide mediators come from the nervous system and endocrine organs. However, some are formed in the plasma, and many occur at other sites (e.g. vascular endothelium, heart, cells of the immune system, etc.). The same peptide may occur in several places, and serve different functions.
- Small peptides act mainly on G-protein-coupled receptors, and act through the same second messenger systems as those used by other mediators. Cytokines and growth factors generally act through tyrosine-kinase-linked membrane receptors.
- Peptides frequently function in the nervous system as co-transmitters with other peptides or with non-peptide transmitters.
- The number of known peptide mediators now greatly exceeds that of non-peptides.

BIOSYNTHESIS OF PEPTIDES

Peptide structure is directly coded in the genome, in a way that the structure of, say, acetylcholine is not. It is in some ways simpler for a cell to produce a peptide than a conventional neurotransmitter. To do the latter, it must produce a series of carrier molecules (to collect the necessary precursors and store the product) and enzymes to perform the synthesis. To make a peptide (Fig. 9.2), it produces a precursor protein in which the peptide sequence is embedded, along with specific proteolytic enzymes that excise the active peptide, a process of sculpture rather than synthesis. The precursor protein is packaged into vesicles at the point of synthesis, and the active peptide is formed in situ ready for release. Thus there is no need for special uptake mechanisms for procuring the starting materials, and there are in general no mechanisms for recapturing released mediators, such as are important for noradrenergic transmission (see Ch. 7).

PEPTIDE PRECURSORS

Since the mid-1970s, cloning techniques have been used to define the structures of 30 or more peptide precursors (see review by Schwartz & Costa 1986). Once the peptide has been purified and its amino acid sequence determined, the corresponding cDNA can be synthesised and used to extract the full-length DNA coding for the protein in which the peptide sequence is embedded. The general pattern (see Burger 1988; Fig. 9.2) is that the precursor protein (the *preprohormone*), usually 100–250 residues in length, consists of an N-terminal *signal sequence*, followed by a variable stretch of unknown function, followed by a peptide-containing region in which several copies of active peptide fragments are contained. Often, several different peptides are found in one precursor, but sometimes there is only one in multiple copies. An extreme example occurs in the invertebrate *Aplysia*, in which the precursor contains more than 20 copies of the same short peptide. The signal peptide is strongly hydrophobic, and is important for insertion of the protein into the

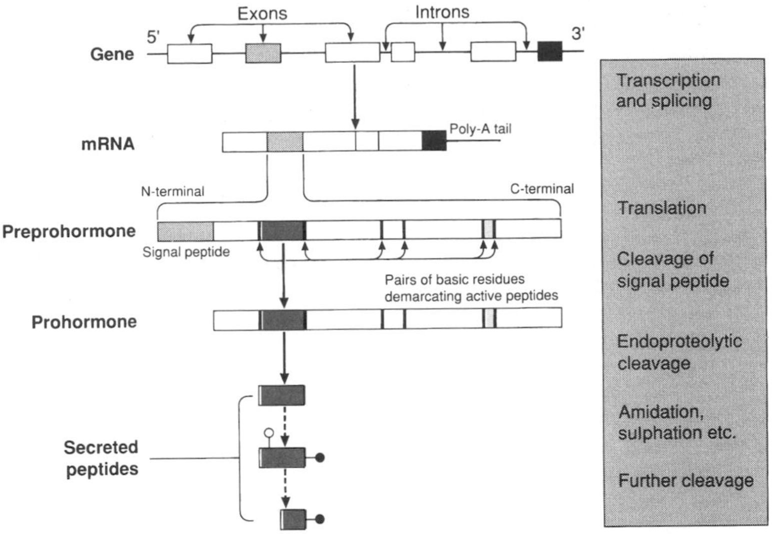

Fig. 9.2 Synthesis of a peptide mediator. The coding regions of the gene (exons) are transcribed and spliced to give rise to mRNA, segments of which are translated to produce the preprohormone. Cleavage of the N-terminal signal peptide produces the prohormone, from which endopeptidases excise peptide fragments. These may be active as such or they may undergo further post-translational processing (amidation, etc.).

endoplasmic reticulum; it is cleaved off at an early stage, to form the *prohormone*. The active peptides are usually demarcated within the prohormone sequence by pairs of basic amino acids (Lys–Lys or Lys–Arg), which are cleavage points for the various trypsin-like proteases that act to release the peptides. This endoproteolytic cleavage generally occurs before the peptides have been packaged in secretory vesicles. The enzymes responsible are known as *prohormone convertases*, of which two subtypes (PC1 and PC2) have been studied in detail (see Cullinan et al. 1991). Inspection of the prohormone sequence has often revealed likely cleavage points that demarcate unknown peptides. In some cases (e.g. CGRP; see below) new peptide mediators have been discovered in this way, but there are many examples where no function has yet been assigned. Whether they are, like strangers at a funeral, peptides waiting to declare their purpose, or merely functionless relics, remains a secret. There are also large stretches of the prohormone sequence lying between the active peptide fragments, for which no function is known. They may just be molecular rubbish, but few would bet on it.

DIVERSITY WITHIN PEPTIDE FAMILIES

Peptides commonly occur in families, with sequences and actions that are basically similar. Generally, as with opioid peptides or tachykinins (see below), the various related sequences are represented independently in the genome, but diversity can also arise at the stage of post-translational processing of the prohormone.

Gene splicing as a source of peptide diversity

Genes contain coding regions (exons) interspersed with non-coding regions (introns). The DNA forming the gene is initially transcribed *in toto* to form RNA (hnRNA), which is then *spliced* to remove the introns, and some of the exons, forming the mRNA that is translated. Control of the splicing process allows a measure of cellular control over the peptides that are produced. The best examples of this are **calcitonin/CGRP** and **substance P/substance K**.

The calcitonin gene codes for calcitonin itself (Ch. 21) and also for a completely dissimilar peptide, CGRP. Differential splicing allows cells to produce either procalcitonin (expressed in thyroid cells) or pro-CGRP (expressed in many neurons) from the same gene.

Substance P and substance K are two closely related tachykinins belonging to the same family (see below, Fig. 9.4) that are encoded on the same gene. Differential splicing results in the production of two precursor proteins—one of these includes both peptides, the other includes only substance P, and the ratio of the two varies widely between tissues. So far, the control of the splicing process is not well understood, but it is clearly an important regulatory mechanism.

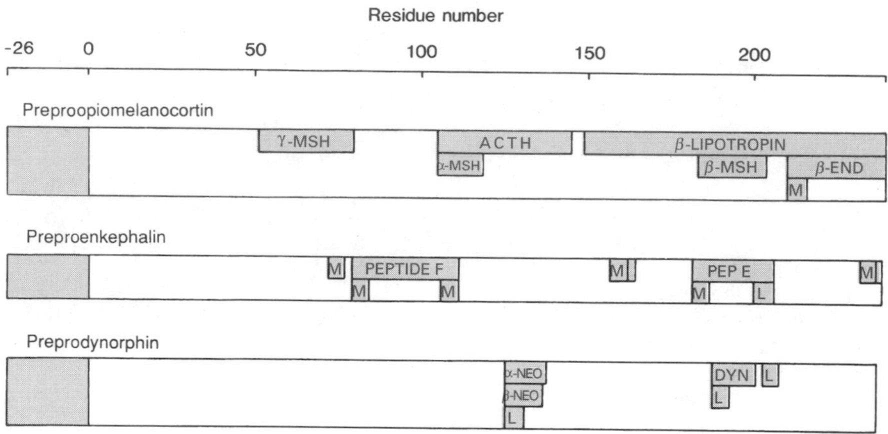

Fig. 9.3 Opioid precursors. Structures of the three opioid precursor proteins, showing the location of opioid and other peptides within the sequence. These contained peptides are bounded by pairs of basic amino acids, which form points of attack for enzymic cleavage. The signal peptide is shown as a shaded region. (MSH = melanocyte-stimulating hormone; ACTH = adrenocorticotrophic hormone; β-END = β-endorphin; M = methionine enkephalin; L = leucine enkephalin; DYN = dynorphin; NEO = neoendorphin)

Post-translational modifications as a source of peptide diversity

Many peptides, such as tachykinins and peptides related to ACTH (see Ch. 21) are converted enzymically to amides, by amidation at the carboxy terminus, and this is important for their biological activity. Another common pattern is for tissues to generate peptides of varying length from the same primary sequence, by the action of specific peptidases that cut the chain at different points. Thus *procholecystokinin* (pro-CCK) contains the sequences of at least five CCK-like peptides ranging in length from 58 to 4 amino acids, all with the same carboxy-terminal sequence. CCK itself (33 residues) is the main peptide produced by the intestine, whereas the brain produces mainly CCK-8. The opioid precursor, *prodynorphin,* similarly gives rise to several peptides with a common terminal sequence (see Fig. 9.3), the proportions of which vary in different tissues and in different neurons in the brain.

PEPTIDE ANTAGONISTS

Selective antagonists are known for the great majority of non-peptide receptors. In many cases they have come from nature (e.g. tubocurarine, atropine, strychnine, ergot derivatives), but synthetic chemistry has also succeeded in producing them in abundance, either by accident (e.g. phenothiazine neuroleptics) or by design (e.g. β-adrenoceptor antagonists, 5-HT_3 antagonists). In contrast, peptide antagonists are much rarer, and none, except for opiate antagonists (see Ch. 31) are yet in clinical use, though their therapeutic potential may be con-

Biosynthesis of peptides

- The genetically coded *preprohormone* is a large protein comprising a *signal sequence* (involved in transfer of the protein across the membrane) plus the *prohormone*, which contains the embedded sequences of one or more active peptides.
- The active peptides are produced intracellularly by selective enzymic cleavage, centred on pairs of adjacent Arg or Lys residues; in most cases the active peptides are stored (often in vesicles) in a releasable form.
- A single precursor gene may give rise to several peptides, either by selective DNA splicing before transcription, by selective cleavage of the prohormone, or by post-translational modification.
- There are many examples of closely related peptides, presumably produced by divergent evolution from a single gene, with different locations and physiological functions.

siderable. Recently, though, efforts to develop such compounds have begun to make progress. For many years, simple substitutions of natural L-amino acids in the peptide chain was the main approach to seeking antagonists, but this was rarely successful. Progress was made with substitution of unnatural amino acids, including D-amino acids, into the sequence; by this approach, antagonists to various peptides, such as substance P, angiotensin and bradykinin, can be produced. For reasons discussed below, however, such peptides are of little use therapeutically, so effort has gone into discovering non-peptides which bind to peptide receptors. One approach has been to modify the peptide backbone, while retaining as far as possible the disposition of the side-chain groups that are responsible for binding to the receptor. Such compounds, sometimes known as 'peptoids', have been developed for several peptide receptors. In other cases, the problem has yielded to brawn rather than brain, and non-peptide chemical leads have come from random chemical screening. Some of these have led to highly potent and selective compounds, which are currently under development as therapeutic agents, but understanding of what makes them recognisable by peptide receptors remains elusive, much to the frustration of medicinal chemists who would like to be able to design such compounds de novo. Examples of peptide mediators for which peptide or non-peptide antagonists are known are given in Table 9.1.

There remain many peptide mediators for which no antagonists are known, but the recent spate of successes in producing potent non-peptide antagonists from leads that have emerged from random screening has boosted hopes of developing therapeutic agents in what had seemed a rather sterile area.

PEPTIDES AS DRUGS

Some proteins, such as antibodies, cytokines, enzymes, clotting factors, etc., are used as therapeutic agents in specific conditions, and are invariably given by injection (see Table 9.2 for some examples; Bristow 1991 for further information). Smaller peptides are also used therapeutically, but, in general peptides make bad drugs; there are several reasons for this:

- They cannot be given orally, either because they

Table 9.1 Peptide antagonists

Mediator	Receptor types*	Antagonists: peptides or modified peptides	Antagonists: non-peptides	References
Angiotensin	AT_1	+ (saralasin, etc.)	+ (losartan and others)	Ch. 14 Timmermans et al. (1991)
Bradykinin	B_1, B_2	+ (des-Arg^9, Leu^8-BK, icatibant = HOE140)	–	Chs 11, 31 Bathon & Proud (1991) Kyle & Burch (1992)
Calcitonin gene-related peptide	CGRP	+ (CGRP$^{8-37}$)	–	
Cholecystokinin	CCK_A CCK_B	+ (CI-988)	+ (devazepide, lorglumide)	Woodruff & Hughes (1991)
Endothelin	ET_1, ET_2	+	+	Ch. 14
Opioid peptides	μ, δ, κ	+	+ (naloxone, etc.)	Ch. 31
Oxytocin/vasopressin	V_1, V_2, OT	+	+	Laszlo et al. (1991)
Tachykinins	NK_1, NK_2, NK_3	+ (Spantide II, GR 82334, MEN (10376, etc.)	+ (CP 96345, RP 67580, SR 48968, etc.)	Maggi et al. (1993)

*For further information on peptide receptor subtypes, see TIPS Receptor Nomenclature Supplement (1994).
Antagonists of larger peptide and protein mediators (e.g. insulin, cytokines, growth factors) are not known.

Table 9.2 Peptides and proteins as drugs

Drug	Use	Route
Peptides		
Captopril/enalapril (peptide-related)	Hypertension Heart failure (Ch. 14)	Oral
Vasopressin Desmopressin Lypressin	Diabetes insipidus (Ch. 20)	Intranasal, injection
Oxytocin	Induction of labour (Ch. 22)	Injection
GnRH analogues (e.g. buserelin)	Infertility, suppression of ovulation (Ch. 22) Prostate and breast tumours	Intranasal, injection
ACTH	Diagnosis of adrenal insufficiency (Ch. 21)	Injection
TSH/TRH	Diagnosis of thyroid disease (Ch. 21)	Injection
Calcitonin	Paget's disease of bone (Ch. 21)	Intranasal, injection
Insulin	Diabetes (Ch. 20)	Injection
Somatostatin, octreotide	Acromegaly, GI tumours (Ch. 21)	Intranasal, injection
Growth hormone	Dwarfism (Ch. 21)	Injection
Cyclosporin	Immunosuppression (Ch. 12)	Oral
F(ab) fragment	Digoxin overdose	Injection
Proteins		
Streptokinase, tissue plasminogen activator	Thromboembolism (Ch. 16)	Injection
Interferons	Tumour chemotherapy (Chs 12, 36)	Injection
Erythropoietin, G-CSF, etc.	Anaemia (Ch. 23)	Injection
Clotting factors	Clotting disorders (Ch. 16)	Injection
Antibodies, vaccines, etc.	Infectious diseases	Injection or oral

are hydrolysed in the gut or because they are not absorbed. (An important exception is **cyclosporin,** discussed in Ch. 12, which contains so many unnatural amino acids that no peptidase will touch it.)

- They are expensive to manufacture.
- They are usually quickly hydrolysed by plasma and tissue peptidases, and so have a short biological half-life, though there are exceptions to this.
- They do not penetrate the blood–brain barrier.

A list of clinically used peptides is given in Table 9.2 (see also Bristow 1991).

Peptides as drugs

- In spite of the large number of known peptide mediators, only a few peptides are, as yet, useful as drugs.
- In most cases, peptides:
  - —are poorly absorbed when given orally
  - —have a short duration of action because of rapid degradation in vivo
  - —fail to cross the blood–brain barrier
  - —are expensive to manufacture.
- In contrast to the situation with non-peptide mediators, relatively few peptide antagonists are known so far, but rapid progress is being made.

TWO IMPORTANT PEPTIDE FAMILIES

OPIOID PEPTIDES

In 1975, Hughes & Kosterlitz succeeded in isolating from the brain two pentapeptides, which compete strongly with morphine-like drugs for binding to receptors in the brain, and which have pharmacological actions closely resembling those of morphine itself. This outstanding work showed that the hitherto mysterious actions of morphine (see Ch. 31) stemmed from its ability to mimic the actions of a family of endogenous mediators, the opioid peptides. This very satisfying result fuelled the expectation that the discovery of other neuropeptides might similarly illuminate the actions of other types of drug that affect the central nervous system, and also point the way to the development of new and potentially useful drugs. In the event, neither expectation has been realised: morphine-like drugs remain the only class known to act by mimicking peptides, and, to date (not for want of trying), no non-peptide analogues with clinically useful effects have been modelled on known endogenous peptide structures. For a general review of opioid peptides, see Frederickson (1984).

Cloning studies have shown that opioid peptides, defined as peptides with opiate-like pharmacological effects, are coded by three distinct genes, whose products are respectively *preproopiomelanocortin* (POMC), *preproenkephalin* (or preproenkephalin A) and *preprodynorphin* (preproenkephalin B). Each of these precursors contains the sequences of a number of opioid peptides (Fig. 9.3). Hughes & Kosterlitz noticed that the sequence of met-enkephalin is contained within that of a pituitary hormone, β-lipotropin. At the same time, in other laboratories, three other peptides with morphine-like actions were discovered, α-, β- and γ-endorphin, which also comprised stretches of the β-lipotropin molecule. At first it was suspected that the enkephalins might be artefacts resulting from proteolytic fragmentation of larger mediators, but it soon became clear that they exist independently, and, indeed, that they actually come from other gene products, proenkephalin and prodynorphin, rather than from POMC itself. POMC serves as a source of ACTH, melanocyte-stimulating hormones (MSH) and β-endorphin, rather than enkephalin. The expression of the precursor proteins varies greatly in different tissues and brain areas. For example, POMC and its derived peptides are found mainly in the pituitary and hypothalamus, whereas enkephalins and their precursors are found throughout the central and peripheral nervous systems, and also in other organs such as the adrenal medulla. Studies with immunofluorescence show that these peptides and precursors are clearly restricted to individual cells, and distinct patterns of processing, leading to production of different peptides from the same precursor, can also be recognised in different tissues and brain areas. A review by Martinez & Potier (1986) lists 23 different POMC-derived peptides, all of which occur in the brain or pituitary, and all of which show biological activity. Not all of these are classed as opioid peptides, since many, related to ACTH or MSH, are not opiate-like in their actions. The mediators about which most is known are β-endorphin, met-enkephalin, leu-enkephalin and dynorphin. In the brain, β-endorphin occurs mainly in neurons that project from the hypothalamus to the thalamus and brainstem, while the enkephalins are found mainly in short interneurons, in many brain areas.

The actions of opioid peptides, like those of synthetic opiates (Ch. 31) are mediated by three distinct types of receptor, μ, δ and κ. β-endorphin and met-enkephalin act mainly on μ-receptors, leu-enkephalin on δ, and dynorphin on κ. They produce analgesia when injected locally into the brain, and their actions at a cellular level are mainly inhibitory. The pharmacological responses associated with the three receptor types, and the involvement of opioid peptides in pain and analgesia, are discussed in Chapter 31. The situation in which a family of non-peptide drugs mimics the actions of endogenous peptides appears to be unique to the opioid field. There is speculation that other types of drug, such as the benzodiazepine tranquillisers (Ch. 27) and the dihydropyridine calcium antagonists (Ch. 14) may also owe their actions to peptide mimicry, but the putative endogenous peptides remain elusive.

TACHYKININS

Substance P (SP) was discovered in 1931 by von Euler & Gaddum during an investigation of the biological activity of extracts of intestine and brain. They found that one of their samples showed activity to lower blood pressure and contract smooth muscle that was not due to acetylcholine, and its chemical properties suggested that it might be a peptide. Substance P (so called simply because of their sequential lettering system) was the first neuropeptide to be discovered, and is still much studied and much loved. In 1931 there was no simple way to purify or determine the structure of a peptide, and SP remained a pharmacological curiosity. Nearly 20 years later, Erspamer, who was looking for bioactive amines in marine animals, found another peptide, **eledoisin**, in a Mediterranean octopus, which had very similar actions to SP. He purified this from nearly two tons of octopus, and elucidated its sequence (Fig. 9.4). Encouraged, he did the same for some amphibian peptides, including **physalaemin**, which turned out to have very similar sequences. Erspamer called this family tachykinins (fast-acting) to distinguish them from bradykinin (see Ch. 11), which has a much slower action on smooth muscle. In 1970, SP was purified from hypothalamus, and its sequence showed that it clearly belonged to the tachykinin family (Fig. 9.4), which are characterised by the terminal sequence –Phe–X–Gly–Leu–Met–NH_2 (unblushingly referred to as the 'canonical sequence' by peptide pundits). More recently, two less-abundant mammalian tachykinins, **neurokinin A** (NKA, or substance K) and **neurokinin B**, have been discovered. As often happens in the peptide field, several groups converged on these substances, and called them by different names, causing a merry confusion. Detailed information on the tachykinins can be found in various reviews (Jessell 1983, Buck & Burcher 1986, Maggio 1988, Maggi et al. 1993).

Tissue distribution

Substance P and NKA, which are derived from the same gene (see above) are distributed similarly in the nervous system. In the brain, they are found especially in the substantia nigra and corpus striatum, suggesting a function in the motor system. The other main location of SP is in nociceptive primary afferent neurons (see Ch. 31) and enteric neurons. Nociceptive sensory neurons express many different neuropeptides, which are known to be released at both the central and the peripheral terminals when the neurons are activated. Release of SP, and possibly other neuropeptides, at the central terminals of nociceptive neurons, which are located in the superficial layers of the dorsal horn (Ch. 31), probably serves a transmitter role in the pain pathway (see Ch. 31). Release of peptides at the peripheral terminals of these neurons is thought to play a part in 'neurogenic inflammation' (see Lembeck 1983, Holzer 1988). SP-containing terminals are abundant in the walls of many blood vessels, including cerebral vessels, and it has been postulated that peptide release is involved in migraine and other types of headache (see Ch. 8). The enteric nervous system also contains many SP-neurons, including both visceral sensory neurons and interneurons (see Chs 5 and 19).

Actions, receptors and antagonists

Tachykinins elicit a wide range of responses on many types of cells, including neurons, smooth muscle, vascular endothelium, exocrine gland cells, mast cells and cells of the immune system (see review by Maggi et al. 1993), the overall pattern of effects being similar, though not identical, to the pattern seen with agents such as bradykinin (Ch. 11) or 5-HT (Ch. 8). Most types of smooth muscle, including that of the gastrointestinal tract and airways, contract in response to tachykinins; blood

Opioid peptides

Leu-enkephalin	Tyr	Gly	Gly	Phe	Leu												
Dynorphin A	Tyr	Gly	Gly	Phe	Leu	Arg	Arg	Ile	Arg	Pro	Lys	Leu	Lys	Trp	Asp	Asn	Gln
Met-enkephalin	Tyr	Gly	Gly	Phe	Met												
Beta-endorphin	Tyr	Gly	Gly	Phe	Met	+26 residues											

Tachykinins

Substance P	Arg	Pro	Lys	Pro	Gln	Gln	Phe	Phe	Gly	Leu	Met	NH_2	Mammalian
Substance K		His	Lys	Thr	Asp	Ser	Phe	Val	Gly	Leu	Met	NH_2	Mammalian
Neurokinin B		Asp	Met	His	Asp	Phe	Phe	Val	Gly	Leu	Met	NH_2	Mammalian
Eledoisin	pGlu	Pro	Ser	Lys	Asp	Ala	Phe	Ile	Gly	Leu	Met	NH_2	Amphibian
Physalaemin	pGlu	Ala	Asp	Pro	Asn	Lys	Phe	Phe	Gly	Leu	Met	NH_2	Amphibian

Fig. 9.4 Structures of opioid and tachykinin peptides, with common amino acids marked in light red.

vessels show a mixture of constrictor and dilator responses (endothelium-dependent; see Ch. 10), together with increased permeability, leading to oedema formation. Many neurons, including central and autonomic neurons, show a slow excitatory response. Intrathecal application of SP causes a scratching response in conscious animals, and may produce hyperalgesia, consistent with the postulated transmitter role of SP in the nociceptive pathway. Mast cells are activated, and release histamine, and various exocrine glands, including salivary glands, are also stimulated. In many systems, tachykinins have been shown to activate phospholipase C, which is coupled to the receptor via a G-protein (see Ch. 2), and the cellular responses result mainly from the formation of inositol phosphates, leading to the release of calcium within the cell. Receptor cloning (see Gerard et al. 1993) has shown that, as expected, tachykinin receptors belong to the general family of G-protein-coupled receptors described in Chapter 2.

The role of tachykinins in normal and pathophysiological processes is slowly becoming clearer through the use of specific antagonists (see below). There is now evidence to suggest that substance P is involved in the nociceptive pathway, and in various conditions with an inflammatory component, such as arthritis, asthma, hay fever, inflammatory bowel disease and migraine (see Maggi et al. 1993).

Pharmacological studies, mainly on smooth muscle preparations, in which the relative potencies of a range of tachykinins and tachykinin antagonists have been compared on different test systems (see Maggi et al. 1993) show that at least three receptor subtypes exist, NK_1, NK_2 and NK_3 (NK = neurokinin), and this has been confirmed by receptor cloning. The NK_1-receptor is preferred by SP (and also physalaemin), the NK_2-receptor by NKA (and by eledoisin), and the NK_3-receptor by NKB. Most of the known effects of tachykinins are mediated by NK_1- or NK_2-receptors, with much inter-species variation; less is known about NK_3-receptors, and their role seems to be more limited.

Modifications of the amino acid sequence of SP, the significant change being the incorporation of D-amino acids, led to the first generation of competitive antagonists (Rosell & Folkers 1982, Håkanson & Sundler 1985), in particular **spantide** (D-Arg[1] D-Trp[7,9] Leu[11]-SP), which acts selectively on the NK_1-receptor. More potent and selective peptide antagonists for NK_1- and NK_2-receptors quickly followed. In 1991, the first non-peptide tachykinin antagonist (CP 96345) made its appearance. This potent compound, which bears not the faintest chemical resemblance to substance P, was developed at the Pfizer laboratories from a lead which emerged from random screening. Other pharmaceutical companies were quick in pursuit, and there is now a profusion of both peptide and non-peptide tachykinin antagonists (see Table 9.1; Maggi et al. 1993), from which novel therapeutic agents for some of the conditions mentioned above can be expected in the near future.

Tachykinins

- The mammalian tachykinins comprise three related peptides, substance P, neurokinin A and neurokinin B.
- They occur mainly in the nervous system, particularly in nociceptive sensory neurons, enteric neurons and many regions of the brain.
- They are packaged and released as neurotransmitters, often in combination with other mediators.
- Tachykinins exert mainly excitatory effects on neurons, secretory cells and smooth muscle. They also cause vasodilatation and increase vascular permeability.
- Three distinct types of tachykinin receptor are known (NK_1, NK_2, NK_3), which are selective for the three endogenous tachykinins. Most of the known effects are mediated by NK_1- and NK_2-receptors.
- Several potent antagonists at NK_1- and NK_2-receptors have recently been discovered.
- Tachykinins may be involved in various disease states (e.g. pain, asthma, arthritis, headache), so tachykinin antagonists may soon become important therapeutically.

REFERENCES AND FURTHER READING

Bathon J M, Proud D J 1991 Bradykinin antagonists. Ann Rev Pharmacol Toxicol 31: 129–162

Buck S H, Burcher E 1986 The tachykinins: a family of peptides with a brood of 'receptors'. Trends Pharmacol Sci 7: 65–68

Burger E 1988 Peptide hormones and neuropeptides:

proteolytic processing of the precursor regulatory peptides. Arz Forsch 38: 754–761
Bristow A F 1991 The current status of therapeutic peptides and proteins. In: Hider R C, Barlow D (eds) Polypeptide and protein drugs. Ellis Horwood, Chichester
Campbell G 1987 Co-transmission. Annu Rev Pharmacol Toxicol 27: 51–70
Chan-Palay V, Palay S L (eds) 1984 Coexistence of neuroactive substances in neurones. J Wiley, New York
Cooper J R, Bloom F E, Roth R H 1991 Biochemical basis of neuropharmacology. Oxford University Press, New York
Cullinan W E, Day N C, Schafer M K, Day R, Seidah N G, Chretien M, Akil H, Watson S J 1991 Neuroanatomical and functional studies of peptide precursor-processing enzymes. Enzyme 45: 285–300
Eipper B A, Mains R E, Herbert E 1986 Peptides in the nervous system. Trends Neurosci 9: 463–468
Fredrickson R C A 1984 Endogenous opioids and related derivatives. In: Kuhar M J, Pasternak G W (eds) Analgesics: neurochemical, behavioral and clinical perspectives. Raven Press, New York
Gerard N P, Bao L, He X-P, Gerard C 1993 Molecular aspects of tachykinin receptors. Regulatory Peptides 43: 21–35
Håkanson R, Sundler F (eds) 1985 Tachykinin antagonists. Elsevier, Amsterdam
Hokfelt T 1991 Neuropeptides in perspective: the last ten years. Neuron 7: 867–879
Holzer P 1988 Local effector functions of capsaicin-sensitive sensory nerve endings: involvement of tachykinins, calcitonin gene-related peptide and other neuropeptides. Neuroscience 24: 739–768
Iversen L L, Iversen S D, Snyder SH (eds) 1983 Neuropeptides. Handbook of psychopharmacology. Plenum, New York, vol 16
Jessell T M 1983 Substance P in the nervous system. Handbook of psychopharmacology. Plenum, New York, vol 16
Krieger D T, Brownstein M J, Martin J B (eds) 1984 Brain peptides. Wiley, New York
Kyle D J, Burch R M 1992 Recent advances towards novel bradykinin antagonists. Drugs-Future 17: 305–312
Laszlo F A, Laszlo F, De Wied D 1991 Pharmacology and clinical perspectives of vasopressin antagonists. Pharm Rev 43: 73–108
Lembeck F 1983 Sir Thomas Lewis's nocifensor system, histamine and substance P containing afferent fibres. Trends Neurosci 6: 106–108
Maggi C A, Patacchini R, Rovero P, Giachetti A 1993 Tachykinin receptors and tachykinin receptor antagonists. J Auton Pharmacol 13: 23–93
Maggio J E 1988 Tachykinins. Annu Rev Neurosci 11: 13–28
Martinez J, Potier P 1986 Peptide hormones as precursors. Trends Pharmacol Sci 7: 139–147
Milner-White E J 1989 Predicting the biologically active conformations of short polypeptides. Trends Pharmacol Sci 10: 70–74
Rosell S, Folkers K 1982 Substance P antagonists; a new type of pharmacological tool. Trends Pharmacol Sci 5: 211–212
Schwartz J P, Costa E 1986 Hybridization approaches to the study of neuropeptides. Annu Rev Neurosci 9: 277–304
Swanson L W 1983 Neuropeptides new vistas on synaptic transmission. Trends Neurosci 6: 294–295
Timmermans P B M W M, Wong P C, Chiu A T, Herblin W F 1991 Nonpeptide angiotensin II receptor antagonists. Trends Pharmacol Sci 12: 55–62
Woodruff G N, Hughes J P 1991 Cholecystokinin antagonists. Ann Rev Pharmacol Toxicol 31: 469–501
Yanagisawa M, Kurihara H, Kimura S, Tomobe Y, Kobayashi M, Mitsui Y, Yazaki Y, Goto K, Masaki T 1988 A novel potent vasoconstrictor peptide produced by vascular endothelial cells. Nature 332: 411–415

10 NITRIC OXIDE

Nitric oxide (NO) is formed from oxygen and nitrogen in the atmosphere during lightning storms. Less dramatically, but with far-reaching biological consequences, it is also formed in an enzyme-catalysed reaction between *molecular oxygen* and *L-arginine* in cells and tissues of mammalian as well as of more primitive species. The convergence of several separate lines of research has led to the realisation within the past seven or eight years that NO acts as a signalling mechanism in the *cardiovascular* and *nervous* systems, has a role in *host defence* and is the endogenous activator of the soluble form of *guanylate cyclase* (see reviews by Moncada et al. 1991, Moncada & Higgs 1993). Not surprisingly, there has been an explosion of experimental work in the area at every level from the molecular to the clinical, and the picture is still changing rapidly.

Nitrogen and oxygen are neighbours in the periodic table, and NO shares several properties with O_2. In particular it combines with haem and other iron–sulphur groups with high affinity. This is important for many of its biological properties, including activation of guanylate cyclase and inactivation of NO by haemoglobin. NO possesses an unpaired electron in its outer shell, i.e. it is a free radical.

A physiological function of NO was first discovered in the vasculature when it was shown that the *endothelium-derived relaxing factor* described by Furchgott & Zawadzki in 1980 could be quantitatively accounted for by the formation of NO by endothelial cells (Fig. 10.1).

BIOSYNTHESIS OF NITRIC OXIDE AND ITS CONTROL

NO synthase (NOS) enzymes are central to the control of NO biosynthesis. Several isoforms have been isolated and purified. There is an essential distinction between *inducible* forms (expressed in response to pathological stimuli such as invading micro-organisms) and so-called '*constitutive*' forms of the enzyme that are present under physiological conditions. Table 10.1 summarises the properties of constitutive and inducible NOS. Induction is stimulated by bacterial lipopolysaccharide (LPS) and/or some of the cytokines synthesised in response to LPS, including interferon γ, tumour necrosis factor-α (TNF-α) and interleukin-1β (IL-1β) (see Ch. 11). Conversely, induction is inhibited by glucocorticoids (which do not influence constitutive NOS) and by several cytokines, including transforming growth factor-β (TGF-β), IL-4 and IL-10. Following induction, NOS activity rises and then falls again over a time-course of hours/days, one factor of importance in the decline in activity being irreversible feedback inhibition on NOS by NO itself.

The nitrogen atom in NO is derived from the terminal guanidino atoms of L-arginine, the oxygen coming from molecular O_2. There is currently disagreement as to whether substrate (L-arginine) availability is limited in endothelium under physiological conditions, although it may become so in some pathological states (e.g. hypercholesterolaemia; see below). Total concentrations of cytoplasmic L-arginine are higher than the Michaelis–Menten constant (Km) of L-arginine for NOS, but there may be a distinct pool of substrate accessible to enzyme, which can become depleted despite apparently plentiful total cytoplasmic arginine concentrations.

The activity of constitutive NOS isoforms is controlled by intracellular calcium/calmodulin (Fig. 10.2). NOS is stimulated in nervous tissue

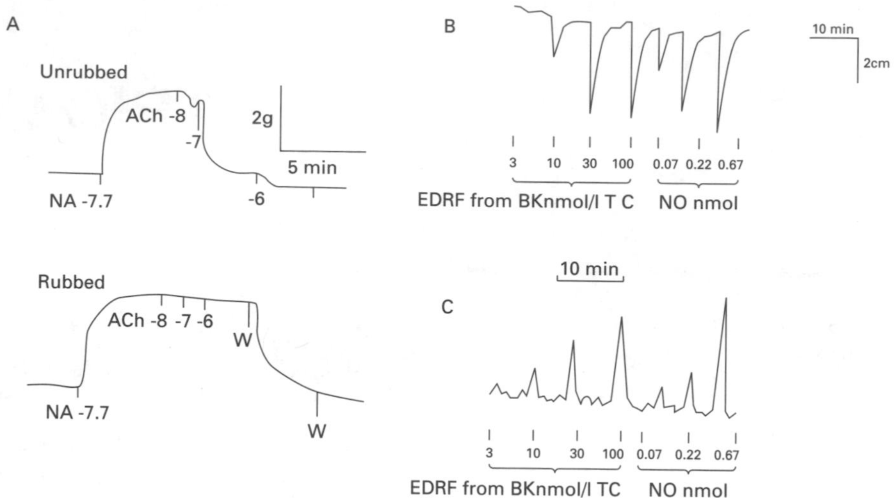

Fig. 10.1 Endothelium-derived relaxing factor is closely related to NO. A. Acetylcholine relaxes a strip of rabbit aorta pre-contracted with noradrenaline if the endothelium is intact, but not if it has been removed by gentle rubbing. The numbers are logarithms of molar drug concentrations. **B.** Endothelium-derived relaxing factor (EDRF) is released from a column of cultured endothelial cells by bradykinin (Bk 3–100 nmol) applied through the column of cells (TC) and relaxes a de-endothelialised precontracted bioassay strip, as does authentic NO. **C.** A chemical assay of NO based on chemiluminescence shows that similar concentrations of NO are present in the EDRF released from the column of cells as in equi-active authentic NO solutions. (From: (A) Furchgott R F, Zawadzki J V 1980 Nature 288: 373–376; (B and C) Palmer et al. 1987 Nature 327: 524–526)

Table 10.1 Properties of NOS

Constitutive	Inducible
Cytosolic	Cytosolic
NADPH-dependent	NADPH-dependent
Dioxygenase	Dioxygenase
Inhibited by L-arginine analogues	Inhibited by L-arginine analogues
Ca^{2+}/calmodulin dependent	Ca^{2+}/calmodulin independent
Picomoles NO released	Nanomoles NO released
Short-lasting release	Long-lasting release
Unaffected by glucocorticoids	Induction inhibited by glucocorticoids

(From: Moncada et al. 1991)

when cytoplasmic Ca^{2+} concentration ($[Ca^{2+}]_i$) rises following depolarisation and activation of voltage-gated Ca^{2+} channels or following influx of Ca^{2+} through receptor-operated channels when NMDA receptors are activated by **glutamate** (see Chs 24 and 25). The most important stimuli controlling endothelial NO synthesis under physiological conditions are probably *mechanical*, pulsatile flow and shear stress being important. In addition, endothelial cells possess receptors for a number of vasodilators including **acetylcholine, substance P, adenosine diphosphate** and **bradykinin** (Ch. 11), occupation of which increases $[Ca^{2+}]_i$ (see Ch. 2) and stimulates endothelial NO biosynthesis. Several of these (e.g. muscarinic acetylcholine receptors) are, however, unlikely to be physiologically important, although these agonists are very useful as experimental tools for investigating endothelial function.

Calcium ionophores (e.g. **A23187**) and polycations (e.g. **poly-L-lysine**) also cause endothelium-dependent relaxation, but operate by mechanisms that do not depend on occupation of specific receptors. Calcium ionophores cause transmembrane influx of Ca^{2+} into endothelial cells and release Ca^{2+} from intracellular stores. Poly-L-lysine partially neutralises negative charges on endothelial cell membranes and this may activate Ca^{2+}-permeable cation channels. A number of drugs with principal actions on other tissues (e.g. **propofol**, an intravenous anaesthetic agent (see Ch. 26), and **nebivolol**, a β-adrenoceptor antagonist) also release NO from endothelium by mechanisms that remain to be established. The resulting vasodilatation may contribute to their therapeutic or adverse effects.

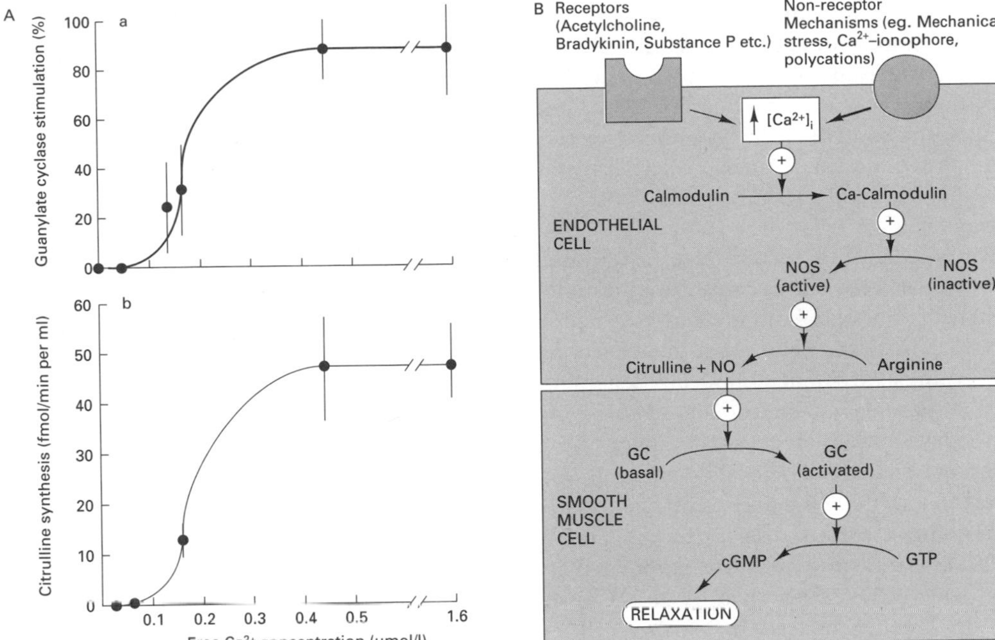

Fig. 10.2 Control of constitutive NOS by Ca^{2+}/calmodulin. **A.** Dependence on $Ca^{2+}$of NO and citrulline synthesis from L-arginine by rat brain synaptosomal cytosol. Rates of synthesis of NO from L-arginine were determined by stimulation of guanylate cyclase (a) or by synthesis of ^{3}[H]-citrulline from L-[^{3}H]arginine (b). **B.** A model of the regulation of guanylate cyclase in a smooth muscle cell by NO formed in a neighbouring endothelial cell (paracrine regulation). NO could also act on guanylate cyclase within the same (endothelial) cell (autocrine regulation). (From: (A) Knowles R G et al. 1989 Proc Natl Acad Sci USA 86: 5159–5162)

NO formation

- NO is synthesised from L-arginine and molecular O_2 by NO synthase (NOS).
- NOS exists in constitutive isoforms in vascular (especially endothelium) and nervous (CNS and NANC peripheral nerves) tissues, and in an inducible form. This is produced in response to cytokine (IL-1, TNF-α, etc.) stimulation in macrophages, neutrophils, vascular smooth muscle and endothelial cells. NOS are flavoproteins, contain tetrahydrobiopterin and have homology with cytochrome P-450 reductase. The constitutive enzymes are activated by Ca^{2+}/calmodulin and produce much smaller amounts of NO than does the induced enzyme.
- Brain NOS is present in CNS including specific neurons in cerebellum, hippocampus and olfactory lobes; and in NANC nerves including innervation to gastrointestinal tract, pelvic organs and trachea.
- Vascular NOS is present in platelets and renal mesangial cells in addition to endothelium.
- NO is unstable but can form more stable nitrosothiols. It is oxidised to nitrite and nitrate which are excreted in urine and provide an index of NO biosynthesis in humans receiving a low-nitrate diet.

DISTRIBUTION OF NITRIC OXIDE SYNTHASE

NADPH diaphorase (used empirically by neurohistochemists for many years) is a marker of NOS and there are now more specific immunocytochemical markers for different isoforms of NOS. These have shown that NOS enzymes are distributed in a wide variety of cells. The constitutive enzyme is present in platelets, renal mesangial cells, and osteoblasts and osteoclasts in addition to endothelium. NOS can be induced in macrophages and Kupffer cells, neutrophils, fibroblasts, vascular smooth muscle and endothelial cells. Brain NOS is present in numerous discrete sites including cerebellum, hippocampus and olfactory lobes, and the same isoform is present in peripheral nerves innervating gastrointestinal tract, pelvic organs, trachea and bladder and in the macula densa and adrenal glands.

NO activates guanylate cyclase (see below) and accumulated cGMP can be visualised by immunocytochemistry in vascular smooth muscle, neural and glial cells. These are believed to be targets on which NO synthesised in neighbouring cells acts. Consequently there is an anatomical relationship between the distribution of cells containing NOS and cells that accumulate cGMP. The match is not, however, perfect and there is evidence that guanylate-cyclase-containing neurons that are *not* closely related to NOS-containing cells are stimulated by carbon monoxide (CO) rather than by NO. Consequently, it has been proposed that CO is also a neuronal messenger (see Ch. 25).

DEGRADATION AND CARRIAGE OF NITRIC OXIDE

NO is highly reactive, but low concentrations are relatively stable in air, and when it is produced locally in the lung small amounts of NO escape degradation and can be detected in exhaled air. Elsewhere in the body, reactions of NO with ions and macromolecules such as haemoglobin can result either in its inactivation or, in some cases, in the formation of relatively stable NO-carrier intermediates that stabilise NO and permit it to act at a greater distance from its site of synthesis than would otherwise be possible (see below). Reaction of macromolecules with NO (nitrosylation) can result in cell damage and accounts for some of the effects of the large amounts of NO produced during host defence reactions and in some other pathological states. NO is oxidised to nitrite ion (NO_2^-) in tissue fluids, and then converted to nitrate (NO_3^-) in whole blood within 10–20 minutes.

NO diffuses freely across cell membranes, and diffusion is adequate to account for most of its local actions. The potential for action at a distance is, however, neatly demonstrated by *Rhodnius prolixus*, a blood-sucking insect that produces a salivary vasodilator/platelet inhibitor with the properties of a nitrovasodilator. This consists of a mixture of nitrosylated haemoproteins which bind NO in the salivary glands of the insect but subsequently release it in the tissues of its prey. The resulting local vasodilatation and inhibition of platelet activation presumably facilitates extraction of the bug's meal in liquid form. It is possible that analogous carrier mechanisms (e.g. cysteine- and/or –SH-containing proteins) operate in mammals, and allow NO to act at a distance from its site of biosynthesis.

EFFECTS OF NITRIC OXIDE

Some of the postulated effects of endogenous NO are shown in Table 10.2. Diseases in which excessive or inadequate effects of NO may be important are described below.

Biochemical and cellular aspects

Pharmacological effects of NO have been studied using NO gas dissolved in balanced salt solution that has been thoroughly deoxygenated by gassing with an inert gas such as helium. More conveniently, but less directly, various chemical donors of NO such as **sodium nitroprusside** (see below), **S-nitroso acetylpenicillamine** or **molsidomine** have been used as surrogates of NO. NO activates guanylate cyclase by combining with a haem group in the enzyme, and effects of low concentrations of NO are mediated by the resulting increase in cGMP.

NO could theoretically activate guanylate cyclase in the same cells that produce it—an *autocrine* effect. Indeed, it has been shown recently that endothelial NO production influences albumin permeability, implying an autocrine effect within the endothelium, and there is also evidence of an autocrine effect within platelets (see below). However, NO generally appears to function as a *paracrine* rather than as an autocrine mediator. It diffuses readily from sites of synthesis and activates guanylate cyclase in neighbouring cells. cGMP has actions on protein kinases, cyclic nucleotide phosphodiesterases, ion channels and possibly other proteins (Table 10.3). These effects lead to reduced $[Ca^{2+}]_i$ responses to contractile and pro-aggregatory agonists in, respectively, vascular smooth muscle and platelets, without markedly influencing basal $[Ca^{2+}]_i$. Additionally, NO causes hyperpolarisation of vascular smooth

Table 10.2 Postulated* roles of endogenous NO

System	Role		
	Physiological	Pathological	
		Excess production	Inadequate production or action
Cardiovascular			
Endothelium/vascular smooth muscle	Control of regional blood flow; ?control of blood pressure	Hypotension (septic shock)	Atherogenesis, thrombosis, vasospasm (e.g. in ? hypercholesterolaemia, ? diabetes mellitus, ? essential hypertension)
Platelets	? limitation of adhesion/aggregation		
Host defence			
Macrophages, neutrophil leucocytes	Defence against viruses, bacteria, fungi, protozoans, metazoan parasites		
Nervous			
Central	Neurotransmission; long-term potentiation; plasticity (? memory, appetite control, nociception)	Excitotoxicity (Ch. 24) (e.g. ischaemic stroke, Huntington's disease, AIDS dementia)	
Peripheral	Neurotransmission (e.g. gastric emptying, penile erection)		Hypertrophic pyloric stenosis ? Impotence in diabetes mellitus

*Evidence is incomplete (see Moncada & Higgs 1993).

Table 10.3 Mechanisms of action of cGMP

Primary targets	Mediator	Examples
Ion channels	(Direct)	Photoreceptor cells: opens cation channels Kidney: inhibits Na^+ channel
cGMP-dependent protein kinases	Phosphorylation	Snail neurons: increases Ca^{2+} current Smooth muscle: decreases $[Ca^{2+}]_i$ Platelets: decreases $[Ca^{2+}]_i$
cGMP-stimulated phosphodiesterase (II)	cAMP decrease	Heart: decreases Ca^{2+} current Hippocampus: decreases Ca^{2+} current
cGMP-inhibited phosphodiesterase (III)	cAMP increase	Smooth muscle: decreases $[Ca^{2+}]_i$ Platelets: decreases $[Ca^{2+}]_i$

(From: Garthwaite 1991)

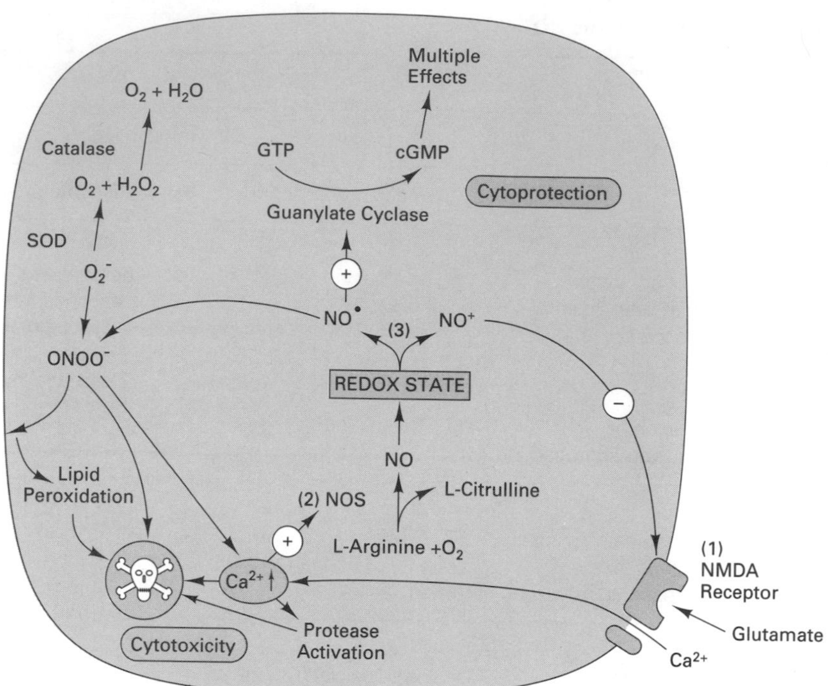

Fig. 10.3 Simplified scheme showing postulated mechanism whereby NO causes cytotoxicity or cytoprotection in nervous tissue. Glutamate increases Ca^{2+} entry via NMDA receptors (1). Ca^{2+}-calmodulin activates NOS (2) which leads to formation of NO, either as NO• or NO^+ (3), depending on the redox state of the cell. NO• reacts with O_2^- to form $ONOO^-$ which can cause lipid peroxidation and react with macromolecules leading to calcium overload and cell death. Superoxide dismutase (SOD) can prevent this by reducing O_2^- to oxygen and hydrogen peroxide which in turn is degraded by catalase. NO^+ feeds back on NMDA receptors by nitrosylating a sulphydryl group on the receptor leading to down-regulation and hence opposing further Ca^{2+} entry. The pathways are drawn as though they occurred within a single cell but NO can diffuse to neighbouring cells as well.

muscle in some circumstances as a consequence of K^+ channel activation.

When large amounts of NO are produced as a result of excessive stimulation of NMDA receptors in the brain, or of induction of NOS in the periphery, it can cause direct chemical effects as opposed to indirect physiological actions mediated via guanylate cyclase activation. As a free radical it is highly reactive, and reacts with many macromolecules and also with *superoxide anion* (O_2^-) (which is produced in activated leucocytes) to form *peroxynitrite radical* ($ONOO^-$), a potent oxidant which mediates some of the cytotoxic effects of NO. These are involved in host defence and in the neuronal destruction that occurs when there is excessive NO biosynthesis due to over-stimulation of NMDA receptors by glutamate (see Ch. 25). Paradoxically, NO is also cytoprotective under some circumstances due to its unusual redox properties (see Fig. 10.3).

Vascular effects

The endothelial L-arginine/NO pathway is a physiological vasodilator mechanism which influences peripheral vascular resistance and systemic blood pressure. It contributes to homeostasis in several regional vascular beds including the cerebral, pulmonary and coronary circulations. Increased endothelial NO generation may contribute to the generalised vasodilatation that occurs during pregnancy. cGMP inhibits cell proliferation, and basal endothelial NO biosynthesis may protect against atheroma (which is a proliferative response to injury; Ch. 15) and influence angiogenesis.

Platelets and leucocytes

NO potently inhibits adhesion and aggregation of platelets, neutrophil leucocytes and monocytes. The high concentration of haemoglobin in blood probably prevents endothelium-derived NO from affecting platelet function under normal conditions. NO biosynthesis within platelets themselves may, however, provide autocrine control when platelets are exposed to aggregating agents, although NOS within platelets is much harder to detect than in endothelium. Effects of nitrovasodilators on platelet aggregation and Ca^{2+} mobilisation are readily demonstrable in platelet suspensions in vitro. However, high concentrations of **nitroprusside** or **glyceryl trinitrate** are needed to affect platelets and a recent clinical trial (ISIS-IV) failed to demonstrate that addition of glyceryl trinitrate to standard therapy improved mortality in patients with acute coronary thrombosis.

Neuronal effects

NO has been proposed as the non-noradrenergic non-cholinergic (NANC) neurotransmitter in many tissues (e.g. rodent anococcygeus and bovine retractor penis; see Ch. 5). It causes adaptive relaxation of the stomach and relaxes the internal anal sphincter. NO has been implicated in the control of neuronal development and of synaptic plasticity in the central nervous system, as well as in appetite and nociception (see Ch. 31). It is produced postsynaptically in response to activation of receptors for excitatory amino acids (notably NMDA receptors; see Ch. 25). In view of these wide-ranging effects, a recent report that mice carrying a selective mutation in neuronal NOS (*'NOS gene knockout mice'*) are viable, fertile and not noticeably externally different from their wild-type or heterozygous litter mates, is somewhat disconcerting. Brain NOS was completely absent from the mutant mice but NOS neurons were intact. Brain NOS was also absent from peripheral NANC nerves. Interestingly, these mice have grossly distended stomachs with histologic appearances similar to those in hypertrophic pyloric stenosis (a human disease of unknown aetiology in which hypertrophy of the pylorus of the stomach causes obstruction to gastric outflow into the duodenum). Intriguingly, NOS is reported to be absent in pyloric tissue from babies with ideopathic hypertrophic pyloric stenosis, which occurs in approximately 1 in 150 male infants and can be fatal if not corrected surgically in infancy.*

*No doubt reports of staining of various tissues for the brain isoform of NOS from individuals who had hypertrophic pyloric stenosis corrected in infancy will soon appear, although the possibility that such individuals will turn out to be 'NOS gene knockout humans' may appear fanciful!

Actions of NO

- NO exerts effects by:
  - activating guanylate cyclase thereby indirectly influencing $[Ca^{2+}]_i$
  - cytotoxic effects via combination with superoxide anion to yield peroxynitrite anion
  - cytoprotective effects via vasodilatation and by down-regulation of NMDA receptors.
- Actions of NO include:
  - vasodilatation, and inhibition of platelet adhesion and aggregation
  - NANC effects including penile erection, nervous control of gastric and colonic function
  - CNS effects including possible influences on neuronal development, synaptic plasticity, memory, vision, nociception (note that these involve retrograde flow of information from postsynaptic to presynaptic structures)
  - host defence and cytotoxic effects including killing of pathogens and neuronal damage in stroke and possibly other neurodegenerative diseases.

Host defence and cytotoxicity

Cytotoxic and/or cytostatic effects of NO are important in non-specific host defence against numerous pathogens and tumour cells including bacteria, fungi, protozoa, and metazoan parasites. The antiviral effect of interferon γ is accounted for by induction of NOS. Neutrophils as well as monocytes produce NO after induction of NOS, and some stimuli to NO biosynthesis (e.g. **FMLP**; see Ch. 11) also cause neutrophil superoxide anion (O_2^-) production. $NO^\bullet$ reacts with O_2^- to yield cytotoxic peroxynitrite anion ($ONOO^-$) (see above and Fig. 10.3), which can destroy invading organisms, but if produced in excess can also damage the host. Other mechanisms of NO-induced cell damage include nitrosylation of nucleic acids and combination with haem-containing enzymes including those involved in cell respiration.

THERAPEUTIC USE OF NITRIC OXIDE AND NITRIC OXIDE DONORS

Nitric oxide

Inhalation of high concentrations of NO (as occurred when cylinders of nitrous oxide, N_2O, for anaesthesia were accidentally contaminated) causes acute pulmonary oedema and methaemoglobinaemia, but concentrations below 50 ppm do not appear to be toxic. NO at 5–300 ppm inhibits bronchoconstriction in guinea pigs, but the main action of inhaled NO is pulmonary vasodilatation. Two distinctive features make this action potentially therapeutically important. First, its action is *limited to the pulmonary circulation*. Second, since it is administered in inspired air it *acts preferentially on ventilated alveoli*.

These properties have raised hopes that inhaled NO may be therapeutically useful in disorders such as adult respiratory distress syndrome (see p. 363). This condition has a high mortality and is caused by diverse insults of which infection is the most common. It is characterised by intrapulmonary 'shunting' (i.e. pulmonary arterial blood entering the pulmonary vein without passing through capillaries in contact with ventilated alveoli) resulting in arterial hypoxaemia, and by acute pulmonary arterial hypertension. Inhaled NO is expected to cause vasodilatation specifically in ventilated alveoli, and thus reduce shunting; early experience with NO in this condition has been encouraging.

Nitric oxide donors

In contrast to the recent experimental use of NO as a therapeutic gas, **nitrovasodilators** have been used therapeutically for over a century. It is now appreciated that the common mode of action of these drugs, which are discussed in Chapters 13 and 14, is as a source of NO.

INHIBITION OF NITRIC OXIDE

Haemoglobin inhibits NO by virtue of avid binding to haem. This is probably important physiologically in limiting the actions of endothelium-derived NO to the immediately underlying vascular smooth muscle and preventing effects downstream through circulating blood. Haemoglobin has also been much used experimentally as an NO inhibitor, as have inhibitors of guanylate cyclase, although these are non-specific (e.g. *methylene blue*). Drugs that inhibit NOS by competition with L-arginine (e.g. **L-N monomethyl arginine** (**L-NMMA**)) have also been used experimentally, but additionally have promise as therapeutic drugs. Several analogues of L-arginine (Fig. 10.4) have activity of this kind. Some of these have been detected in human urine, especially from patients with renal failure, raising the possibility that they influence the L-arginine/NO pathway under physiological and pathological conditions.

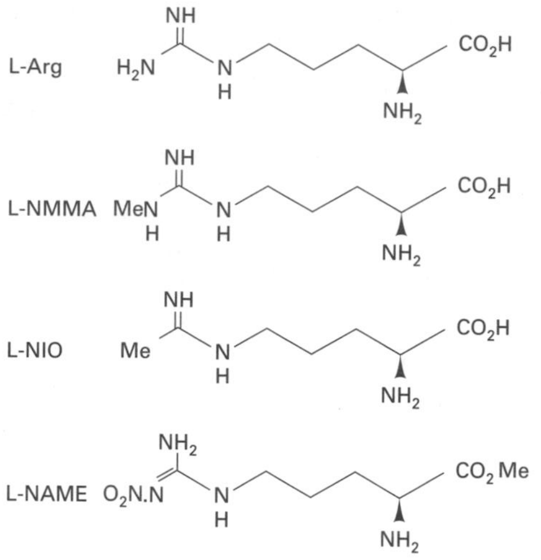

Fig. 10.4 L-arginine and some of its analogues that compete with it for NOS and inhibit NO formation. (L-arg = L-arginine; L-NMMA = N^G-monomethyl-L-arginine; L-NIO = N-iminoethyl-L-ornithine; L-NAME = N^G-nitro-L-arginine methyl ester)

Intravenous administration of L-NMMA increases blood pressure in several species including man. Increased blood pressure caused by L-NMMA in conscious rats is accompanied by vasoconstriction in renal, mesenteric, carotid and hindquarters vascular beds. Infusion of L-NMMA into human brachial artery causes vasoconstriction (Fig. 10.5). The implication is that *basal* release of NO occurs in this vascular bed under physiological conditions of flow and pulsatility, providing an active background vasodilator tone.

There is much interest on the part of the pharmaceutical industry in the possibility of selective inhibition of different forms of NOS. **N-iminoethyl-L-ornithine** (**L-NIO**) is a potent and irreversible inhibitor of NOS in activated macrophages. **7-nitroindazole** inhibits mouse cerebellar NOS and, following intraperitoneal administration, inhibits *nociception* without altering arterial blood pressure, suggesting that it may be selective for the brain constitutive NOS isoform at doses that do not inhibit endothelial NOS; it is not known if this results from a pharmacokinetic effect related to concen-

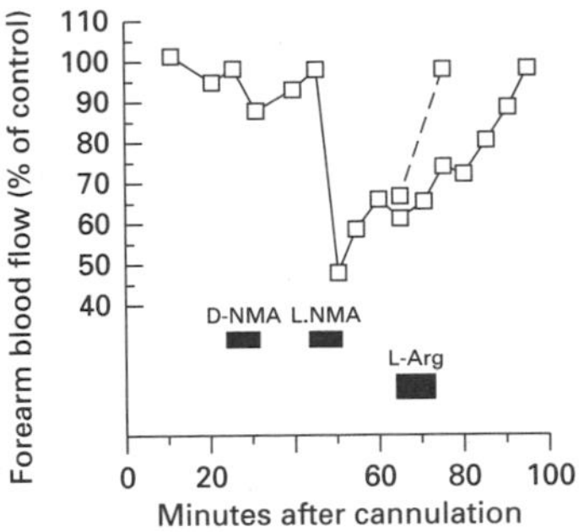

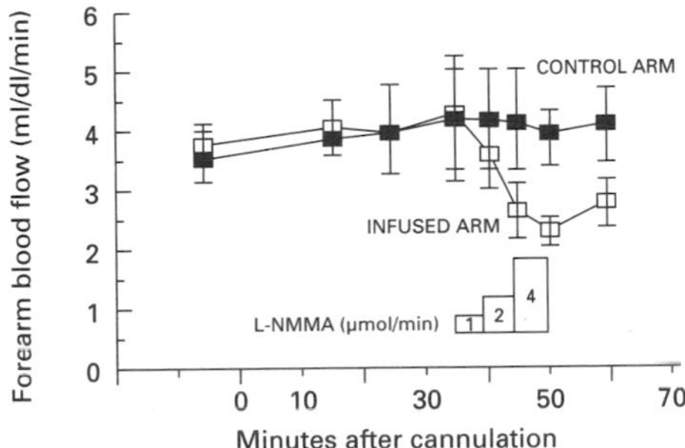

Fig. 10.5 Basal blood flow in the human forearm is influenced by basal NO biosynthesis. Brachial artery infusion of L-NMMA causes vasoconstriction which is not evident in the control (non-infused) arm. L-arginine accelerates recovery from such vasoconstriction (upper panel, dashed line). D-NMMA is ineffective. (From: Vallance et al. 1989 Lancet ii: 997–1000)

Inhibition of the L-Arginine/NO pathway

- Haemoglobin binds NO to haem.
- Methylene blue inhibits guanylate cyclase.
- Glucocorticoids inhibit biosynthesis of inducible (but not constitutive) NOS.
- Competition for substrate by arginine analogues, e.g. L-NMMA, L-NAME.
- Selective inhibitors of different NOS isoforms are being sought energetically.

tration within the central nervous system, or from different affinity for different isoforms of the enzyme.

CLINICAL CONDITIONS IN WHICH NITRIC OXIDE MAY PLAY A PART

The importance of abnormalities in the L-arginine/NO pathway as mechanisms of disease has been reviewed recently (Moncada & Higgs 1993). The wide distribution of NOS and diverse actions of NO have suggested that abnormalities in this pathway could be involved in the pathophysiology of numerous clinical disorders. Since NO is believed to participate in physiological as well as pathological processes, it is evident that either increased or reduced production could play a part in disease states, and hypotheses abound. Evidence is harder to come by but has been sought using various indirect approaches including:

- analysis of products of NO (NO_2^- and NO_3^-) or of its second messenger (cGMP) in urine
- measurement of vasoconstrictor effects of NOS inhibitors (e.g. **L-NMMA**)
- comparison of vascular responses to endothelium-dependent agonists (e.g. **acetylcholine**) with endothelium-independent agonists that work through the same effector mechanism (e.g. **nitroprusside**)
- study of histochemical appearances and pharmacological responses of tissue in vitro.

All such methods have limitations, and the dust is far from settled (see review by Lüscher, 1994). Nevertheless, it seems likely that the L-arginine/NO pathway will indeed prove to be a player in the pathogenesis of several important diseases. If so, it will open the door to new therapeutic approaches.

NO in pathophysiology

- NO is synthesised under both physiological and pathological circumstances.
- NO causes cytotoxic or cytoprotective effects depending on its redox state.
- Either reduced or increased NO production can contribute to disease processes.
- Under-production of neuronal NO is reported in babies with hypertrophic pyloric stenosis and adults with achalasia of the oesophagus. There is indirect evidence of reduced endothelial NO production in some patients with hypercholesterolaemia, essential hypertension and diabetes mellitus.
- Over-production of NO may be important in cerebral infarction and possibly other neurodegenerative diseases (e.g. AIDS dementia) as well as following sepsis.

We touch only briefly on these possibilities here and would caution the reader that not all of these exciting possibilities are likely to withstand the test of time! Some postulated pathological roles of excessive or reduced NO production are summarised in Table 10.2.

Inducible nitric oxide synthase

Septicaemia can lead to multiple organ failure. It is likely that whereas NO is of benefit in host defence early in this sequence, by contributing to microbial killing, subsequent excessive NO production can cause harmful hypotension. Chronic low-grade endotoxaemia occurs in patients with cirrhosis of the liver, many of whom are systemically vasodilated. Urinary excretion of cGMP is increased in such patients, so the vasodilatation may be caused by induction of NOS leading to increased vascular NO synthesis.

L-NMMA may be of therapeutic use in patients with severe hypotension and multiple organ failure secondary to sepsis: preliminary clinical experience has been encouraging, but considerable caution is needed because NO biosynthesis in this setting has some advantageous effects (microbial killing and preservation of splanchnic and renal blood flow). Animal models of sepsis suggest that the dose of inhibitor will be critical, with low doses of L-NMMA conferring benefit but higher doses increasing mortality.

Constitutive nitric oxide synthase

Vasculature

Vasodilator agonists (e.g. **acetylcholine**) have been used as experimental probes of the endothelial L-arginine/NO pathway, and provided evidence of abnormal endothelial responsiveness in several diseases. Endothelium-dependent vasodilators have effects (e.g. stimulation of prostaglandin biosynthesis and release of endothelium-derived hyperpolarising factor) additional to their action on NO production, complicating interpretation of such experiments. There is, nonetheless, suggestive evidence of reduced NO biosynthesis in patients with *hypercholesterolaemia* and some other disorders that predispose to atheromatous vascular disease including *diabetes mellitus* and *arterial hypertension*. Several groups have found that responses of forearm vasculature to brachial artery administration of acetylcholine are blunted relative to responses to nitroprusside in patients with hypertension but this has not been a universal experience, perhaps because of the considerable heterogeneity that exists in human essential hypertension. In hypercholesterolaemia there is not only evidence of blunted NO release in both forearm and coronary vascular beds but also evidence that this abnormality can be *corrected* by treating hyperlipidaemia or by supplementation with L-arginine, findings that strengthen the case for involvement of the L-arginine/NO pathway.

Endothelial dysfunction in diabetic patients with impotence occurs in tissue from the corpora cavernosum of penis studied in vitro,* as evidenced by blunted relaxation to **acetylcholine** despite preserved responses to **nitroprusside** (Fig. 10.6). Vasoconstrictor responses to intra-arterial **L-NMMA** are reduced in forearm vasculature of insulin-dependent diabetics, especially in patients with

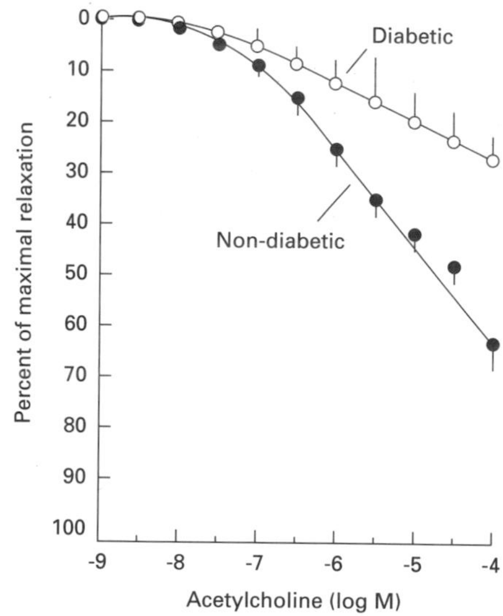

Fig. 10.6 Impaired endothelium-mediated relaxation of penile smooth muscle from diabetic men with impotence. Mean (±SE) relaxation responses to acetylcholine in corpora cavernosa tissue (obtained at the time of performing surgical implants to treat impotence) from 16 diabetic men and 22 non-diabetics. (Data from: Saenz de Tejada et al. 1989)

*Such tissue was obtained during surgical insertion of penile prostheses, a treatment for impotence now largely superseded by intracavernosal injection of papaverine or prostaglandin E_1; see Chapter 14.

traces of albumin in their urine (early evidence of glomerular endothelial dysfunction), suggesting that basal NO synthesis may be reduced throughout their circulation. By contrast, vasodilator responses to muscarinic agonists are not selectively impaired in such patients, so endothelial abnormalities in human diabetes mellitus are probably more subtle than in experimental animal models.

NO in therapeutics

- NO donors (e.g. nitroprusside and organic vasodilators) are well established in therapeutics (see Chs 13 and 14).
- Inhaled NO has therapeutic potential in adult respiratory distress syndrome but its effects on mortality are not known.
- Inhibition of NO biosynthesis (e.g. by L-NMMA) may be beneficial in patients with hypotension from multiple organ failure. It is a two-edged sword and dose will probably be critical.

Neuronal

Excessive NMDA receptor activation and consequent Ca^{2+} entry is believed to contribute to several forms of neurological damage including acute ischaemic stroke, head injury, epilepsy, and possibly also in AIDS dementia, Huntington's disease and Parkinson's disease. These are discussed in Chapter 25.

Clinical uses of NO donors and NO as a therapeutic gas, and of inhibition of the L-Arginine/NO system are summarised in the adjacent box.

REFERENCES AND FURTHER READING

Assreuy J, Cunha F Q, Liew F Y, Moncada S 1993 Feedback inhibition of nitric oxide synthase activity by nitric oxide. Br J Pharmacol 108: 833–837

Bredt D, Huang P, Dawson T, Fishman M, Snyder S 1993 Nitric oxide synthase gene knockout mice: molecular and morphologic characterization. Endothelium 1 (Suppl): s6

Chowienczyk P J, Watts G F, Cockcroft J R, Brett S E, Ritter J M 1994 Sex differences in endothelial function in normal and hypercholesterolaemic subjects, Lancet 344: 305–306

Elliott T G, Cockcroft J R, Groop P-H, Viberti G C, Ritter J M 1993 Inhibition of nitric oxide synthesis in forearm vasculature of insulin dependent diabetic patients. Clin Sci 85: 687–693

Garthwaite J 1991 Glutamate, nitric oxide and cell–cell signalling in the nervous system. Trends Neurol Sci 14: 60–67

Gustafsson L E, Leone A M, Persson M G, Wiklund N P, Moncada S 1991 Endogenous nitric oxide is present in the exhaled air of rabbits, guinea-pigs and humans. Biochem Biophys Res Commun 181: 852–857

Karupiah G, Xie Q, Buller M L, Nathan C, Duarte C, MacMicking J D 1993 Inhibition of viral replication by interferon-γ-induced nitric oxide synthase. Science 261: 1445–1448

LüScher T F 1994 The endothelium and cardiovascular disease – a complex relation. N Engl J Med 330: 1081–1083

McCall T B, Feelisch M, Palmer R M J, Moncada S 1991 Identification of N-iminoethyl-L-ornithine as an irreversible inhibitor of nitric oxide synthase in phagocytic cells. Br J Pharmacol 102: 234–238

Mearin F, Mourelle M, Guarner F 1993 Patients with achalasia lack nitric oxide synthase in the gastro-oesophageal junction. Eur J Clin Invest 23: 724–728

Moncada S, Higgs A 1993 Mechanisms of disease: the L-arginine-nitric oxide pathway. N Engl J Med 329: 2002–2012

Moncada S, Palmer R M J, Higgs E A 1991 Nitric oxide: physiology, pathophysiology and pharmacology. Pharmacol Rev 43: 109–142

Moore P K, Babbedge R C, Wallace P, Gaffen Z A, Hart S L 1993 7-Nitroindazole, an inhibitor of nitric oxide synthase, exhibits anti-nociceptive activity in the mouse without increasing blood pressure. Br J Pharmacol 108: 296–297

Rajfer J, Aronson W J, Bush P A, Dorcy F J, Ignarro L J 1992 Nitric oxide as a mediator of relaxation of the corpus cavernosum in response to non-adrenergic, non-cholinergic neurotransmission. N Engl J Med 326: 90–94

Ribiero J M C, Hazzard J M H, Nussenzveig R H, Champagne D E, Walker F A 1993 Reversible binding of nitric oxide by a salivary haem protein from a blood sucking insect. Science 260: 539–541

Saenz de Tejada I, Goldstein I, Azadzoi K, Krane R J, Cohen R A 1989 Impaired neurogenic and endothelium-mediated relaxation of penile smooth muscle from diabetic men with impotence. N Engl J Med 320: 1025–1030

Snyder S H 1993 Janus faces of nitric oxide. Nature 364: 577

Vallance P, Leone A, Calver A, Collier J, Moncada S 1992 Accumulation of endogenous inhibitor of nitric oxide synthesis in chronic renal failure. Lancet 339: 572–575

Vanderwinden J-M, Mailleux P, Schiffmann S N, Vanderhaeghen J-J, De Laet M-H 1992 Nitric oxide synthase activity in infantile hypertrophic pyloric stenosis. N Engl J Med 327: 511–515

Vanhoutte P M 1993 Other endothelium-derived vasoactive factors. Circulation 87 (Suppl V): V9–V17

11
LOCAL HORMONES, INFLAMMATION AND ALLERGY

Definitions of some terms applied to chemical mediators

The word *hormone*, as introduced by Bayliss & Starling, referred to a chemical substance which was secreted, without benefit of duct, directly into the bloodstream and which acted at long range, often slowly, on distant organs or tissues. When the role of some chemical substances in nervous transmission was established, *neurotransmitters* were held to be different from hormones in that they were released by neurons, not endocrine glands, and acted rapidly, briefly and at short range on an adjacent neuron or target cell. However, these tidy categories conferred a spurious order on the classification of the body's chemical messengers; in terms of defining them and understanding their function(s) we have recently moved from orderly inexactitude towards a disorderly precision.

It was realised several years ago that some substances which were not neurotransmitters nevertheless acted briefly at short range on adjacent target cells (e.g. histamine from mast cells), and these were classed as *local hormones* or *paracrine secretions*; and one must now consider as local hormones the *autocrine secretions*, which act on the cells which secrete them, as, for example, many cytokines do. It has also become clear that some substances defined as true hormones in the Bayliss & Starling sense (e.g. insulin), as well as some substances categorised initially as 'local hormones' (e.g. 5-hydroxytryptamine in platelets) are also neurotransmitters in the CNS (see Ch. 25); and conversely that neurons in what is indubitably a part of the CNS—the hypothalamus—release peptides and possibly amino acids into the bloodstream for action on distant target cells (see Ch. 21).

Further complexity has been added to the problem of defining these terms by the finding that many of the substances, including several considered as being hormones (e.g. insulin, corticotrophin, chorionic gonadotrophin and somatostatin), as well as others regarded as neurotransmitters (acetylcholine, catecholamines) are found in unicellular organisms such as protozoa and bacteria. Some of these agents are also known to have biological effects in these organisms. For example, adrenaline stimulates adenylate cyclase in protozoa (an effect blocked by propranolol), and opioid peptides alter the behaviour of amoebae (an effect blocked by naloxone).

It seems to be the case that the basic biochemical mechanisms involved in cell-to-cell communication arose very early in evolution and have been highly conserved; and that in higher organisms these basic elements have been adapted for more complex communication requirements. Whether a mammalian cell responds to a chemical messenger will depend partly on whether the cell expresses the appropriate receptor and partly on its situation, i.e. on whether it is easily accessible to the perfusing plasma or in close apposition to a neuron or a secreting cell.

The chemical messengers themselves can be used differently in different circumstances.

It is evident that in classifying the physiologically active chemical substances in man, the original concept of separate categories of hormones and transmitters, as defined originally, has given way to the idea of a spectrum of agents in which there are substances which are predominantly neurotransmitters at one end (e.g. acetylcholine) and substances which are predominantly hormones at the other (e.g. the sex steroids), with a range of substances in between in which these characteristics may overlap. Operational definitions are necessary, rather than definitions based on rigid, separate categories. Many of the intermediate substances may be considered to be *local hormones* or *paracrine secretions*.

The first part of this chapter deals with the ways in which cells and chemical messengers interact when the body is under threat from an invading pathogen (disease-causing organism; see Ch. 35) or other type of injury. The process to be considered is the *inflammatory reaction*. When the process has been outlined, the chemical substances, which are thought to act as local hormones in this context, are dealt with in more detail. Many mediators that are important in the context of inflammation (e.g. histamine and the prostaglandins) also have other functions in the body, which are also discussed. Drugs which modify the action of the cells and mediators involved in these reactions are dealt with in Chapter 12.

Consideration of the term 'local hormone'

- 'Hormones', 'neurotransmitters' and 'local hormones' (also termed 'autocoids' or 'paracrine secretions') were once considered to be separate categories in terms of function and locus of action, but it is now clear that these categories overlap.
- Most chemical mediators in the body can be considered to be part of a spectrum, with substances which are predominantly neurotransmitters at one end (e.g. acetylcholine) and substances which are predominantly hormones at the other (e.g. sex steroids).
- The chemical mediators of inflammation are intermediates in this spectrum and are considered to be *paracrine secretions* or *local hormones*.

THE ACUTE INFLAMMATORY REACTION AND THE IMMUNE RESPONSE

A mammalian organism which has to deal with an invasion by a pathogen can call on a prodigious array of powerful defensive responses and the result of the deployment of these constitutes the *acute inflammatory reaction*. The importance of the defensive responses is shown by the fact that when they are lacking (as for example in AIDS) or are suppressed by drugs, organisms which are not normally pathogens can, and often do, cause disease. However, in some circumstances these defensive responses may be brought into play inappropriately against innocuous substances from outside the body (e.g. pollen) or against the tissues of the body itself, and the responses themselves may then produce damage and may indeed constitute part of the disease process (either acutely as, for example, in anaphylaxis, or chronically as, for example, in asthma or rheumatoid arthritis, see Ch. 12, or in atherosclerosis, see Ch. 15). It is for these sorts of conditions that anti-inflammatory or, in some cases, immunosuppressive drugs may be required. Chemical mediators control or modulate these defensive responses of the host, and an understanding of the action of drugs which affect inflammation, and the development of improved anti-inflammatory agents, both depend on an appreciation of the way in which the cells and the mediators of inflammation interact with each other. An outline of these interactions is given below. This topic is covered in detail in Dale, Foreman & Fan (1994). The outline given here will of necessity be a very general one, but a specific example, to which most of the events described will apply, is a local staphylococcal infection causing an acute inflammatory reaction, i.e. a boil. The *innate reactions* (reactions which do not involve an immunological mechanism) will be described first, and then consideration will be given to how these reactions are sharpened and made more selective by the *specific immunological response*. Finally we shall consider briefly the outcome of the acute inflammatory response—either healing or progress to chronic inflammation.

It should be noted that there are many 'backup' systems, so that any one response can be produced in several ways, which is important for a reaction which has survival value.

The inflammatory reaction

- The term 'inflammatory reaction' refers to the events which occur in the tissues in response to an invading pathogen (disease-causing organism).
- It consists of immunologically specific reactions as well as various innate reactions, which have no immunological basis.
- These reactions are protective, i.e. they have survival value, but if inappropriately deployed they are deleterious.
- The outcome can be healing with or without scarring or, if the pathogen persists, chronic inflammation.
- Many of the diseases that need drug treatment involve inflammatory processes. Understanding of the action and therefore the use of anti-inflammatory and immunosuppressive drugs necessitates an understanding of the inflammatory reaction.

At the macroscopic level, the inflamed area is *reddened*, *swollen*, *hot* and *painful*, and there is *interference* with, or *alteration* of, *function*. Examples of this latter characteristic are the spasm of bronchiolar smooth muscle which occurs in asthma, or the restriction of movement in an inflamed joint.

INNATE REACTIONS

In terms of what is happening locally within the tissues, the changes can be divided into *vascular* and *cellular* events. Mediators are generated both from plasma and from cells during the vascular events, and these mediators in turn modify and regulate the vascular and cellular events.

VASCULAR EVENTS AND THE MEDIATORS DERIVED FROM PLASMA

The vascular events involve an initial *dilatation* of the small arterioles resulting in *increased blood flow*; this is followed by slowing and then *stasis* of the blood, an *increase in the permeability* of the post-capillary venules and *exudation* of fluid. The vasodilatation is brought about by various mediators produced by the interaction of the microorganism with tissue cells (histamine, prostaglandins E_2 and I_2, and so on). Some of these mediators (e.g. histamine and platelet-activating factor) are also responsible for the initial phase of increased vascular permeability. Neutrophil association with the walls of the postcapillary venules contributes to the later phase of increased vascular permeability.

The fluid exudate contains a variety of mediators which influence the cells in the vicinity, and the blood vessels themselves. These include the components for four enzyme cascades:

- the complement system
- the coagulation system
- the fibrinolytic system
- the kinin system.

The exudate is carried by lymphatics to local lymph glands or lymphoid tissue where the products of the invading microorganism may be instrumental in initiating an immune response.

The *complement system* is an enzyme cascade with nine major components, designated C1 to C9 (see Sim 1994 for more detail). Activation of the cascade can be initiated by substances derived from microorganisms, such as yeast cell walls, endotoxins, etc. This pathway of activation is termed 'the alternative pathway' (Fig. 11.1). (The 'classical pathway' involves antibody and is dealt with below.) One of the main events is the enzymic splitting of *C3* which gives rise to various peptides, one of which, *C3a* (termed an 'anaphylatoxin'), can stimulate mast cells to secrete chemical mediators, and can also directly stimulate some smooth muscle, while another, *C3b* (termed an 'opsonin'), can attach to the surface of a microorganism and facilitate its ingestion by white blood cells (see below). Enzymic action on a later component, *C5*, releases *C5a* which—in addition to causing release of mediators from mast cells—is powerfully chemotactic (i.e. acts as a chemical attractant) for white blood cells, and also activates them. The actions of these complement-derived mediators are considered below. Assembly of the last components in the sequence (*C5* to *C9*) on the cell membranes of certain bacteria leads to the lysis of these organisms (see Ch. 35). Hence, complement can mediate the destruction of invading bacteria or damage multicellular parasites; but it may sometimes cause injury to the host's own cells. The main event in the complement cascade—the splitting of C3—can also be brought about directly, by the principal enzymes of the coagulation and fibrinolytic cascades, thrombin and plasmin, respectively, and by enzymes released from white blood cells.

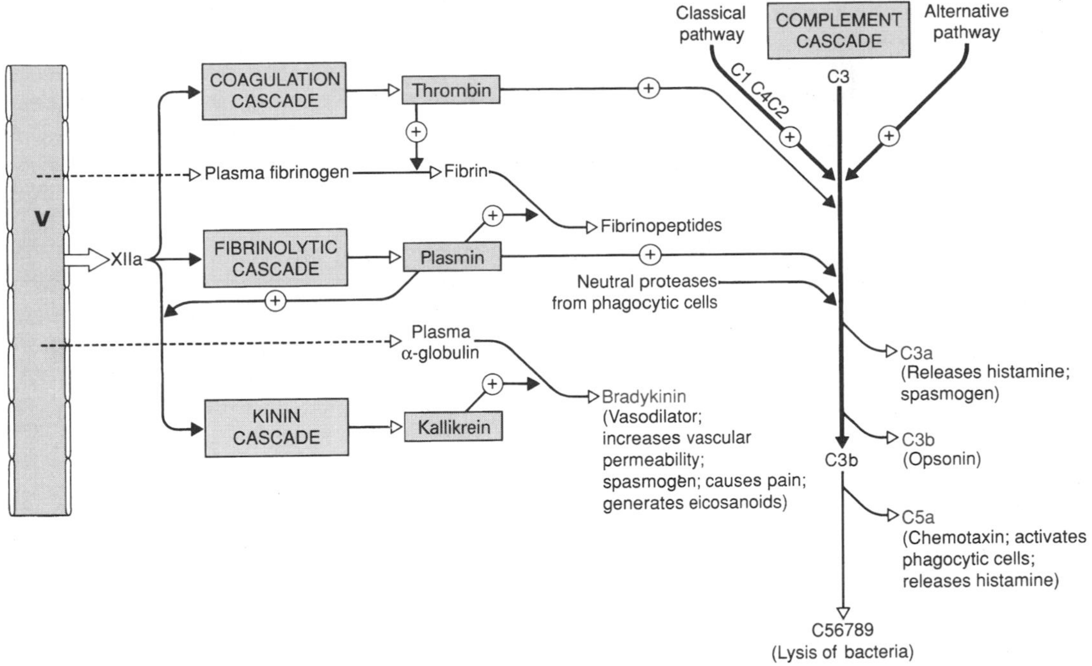

Fig. 11.1 Diagram showing the four enzyme cascades which are activated when plasma leaks out into the tissues as a result of the increased vascular permeability in an area of inflammation. Mediators generated are shown in dark pink. Complement components are indicated by Cl, C2, etc. When plasmin is formed it tends to increase kinin formation and decrease the coagulation cascade. (V = postcapillary venule) (Adapted from: Dale, Foreman & Fan 1994)

The *coagulation system* and the *fibrinolytic system* are described in Chapter 16. Factor XII is activated to XIIa (e.g. by collagen), and the end product is fibrin, which when laid down in the tissues during a host/pathogen interaction can serve to limit the extension of the infection. The main enzyme of the coagulation system, thrombin, is involved in the activation of the complement and kinin systems (Fig. 11.1) and, indirectly, in fibrinolysis (see Ch. 16).

The *kinin system* is another enzyme cascade; it results in the production of several mediators of inflammation, in particular bradykinin (Fig. 11.1) which is dealt with in more detail on page 238.

CELLULAR EVENTS

Of the cells involved in inflammation, some (vascular endothelial cells, mast cells and tissue macrophages) are normally present in tissues, while others (platelets and leucocytes) gain access from the blood. These latter, the *leucocytes*, are actively motile cells and are of two classes:

- *polymorphonuclear cells* (cells with many-lobed nuclei), which are subdivided into *neutrophils*, *eosinophils* and *basophils*, according to the staining properties of the granules in their cytoplasm. These may also be referred to as *granulocytes*.
- *mononuclear cells* (or cells with single-bodied nuclei), which are subdivided into *monocytes* and *lymphocytes*.

Mast cells

Mast cells are capable of secreting or generating mediators which can modify vascular and cellular reactions and also affect some of the plasma factors. The mast cell membrane has receptors both for a special class of antibody (IgE) and for complement components C3a and C5a. The cell can be activated to secrete mediators through these receptors and also by direct physical damage.

One of the main substances released by the mast cells is histamine (see below, p. 226); others are heparan or heparin (see Ch. 16), leukotrienes (p. 235), PGD_2 (p. 233), platelet-activating factor (p. 237), and some interleukins (p. 242). For a simple overview of mast cells, see Foreman (1994).

Polymorphonuclear leucocytes (polymorphs)

Polymorphs are the first of the blood leucocytes to enter the area of the inflammatory reaction (Fig. 11.2). They adhere to the vascular endothelial cells, a process which requires the interaction between adhesion molecules on the endothelial cell (e.g. the selectin and ICAM (intercellular adhesion molecule) families) with corresponding molecules on the neutrophil (e.g. the integrin family) (see Wilkinson 1994). The neutrophils then actively migrate through the wall of the vessel to the site of the invading pathogen, attracted by chemicals termed 'chemotaxins'—some released by the microorganism, such as formyl-Met–Leu–Phe; some produced locally, such as C5a (see above), leukotriene B_4 (p. 235) and various chemokines (see below, p. 241). Neutrophils are capable of engulfing, killing and digesting microorganisms. They, and the eosinophils, have receptors on their membranes for the complement product, C3b, which acts as an 'opsonin' (see above), i.e. it forms a link between polymorph and invading bacterium. (A more effective link may be made by antibody; see below.) The killing process involves, among other things, activation of a 'respiratory burst', during which there is a marked increase of oxygen consumption and the generation of toxic oxygen products. Neutrophils contain within their granules (some of which are similar to the lysosomes of other cells) a variety of digestive enzymes which can break down virtually all the components of most microorganisms. Many of these enzymes work optimally at the low pH found in lysosomes. Neutrophils can in some circumstances actively secrete the contents of their granules, including neutral proteases which work optimally at the pH of body fluids. When the neutrophil is inappropriately activated, the toxic oxygen products and neutral proteases can cause damage to the host's own tissues. For an overview, see, Muid, Twomey & Dale (1994).

Eosinophils have similar capacities to neutrophils and, in addition, are armed with a number of potent granule constituents which, when released extracellularly, can damage multicellular parasites (e.g. helminths). They include eosinophil cationic protein, a peroxidase, the eosinophil major basic protein and a neurotoxin. The eosinophil is now considered to be of primary importance in the pathogenesis of the late phase of asthma, in which its granule proteins cause damage to bronchiolar epithelium (see p. 358 and Fig. 17.3).

Basophils are very similar in many respects to mast cells.

Monocytes/macrophages

The monocytes enter the area at a later stage of the reaction, several hours after the polymorphs. Adhesion to endothelium and migration into the tissue follow a pattern similar to that of the neutrophil (see above), though chemotaxis of monocytes involves additional chemokines, for example *MCP-1*, which, reasonably enough, stands for 'monocyte chemoattractant protein-1' and *RANTES* which (wait for it—immunological nomenclature has excelled itself

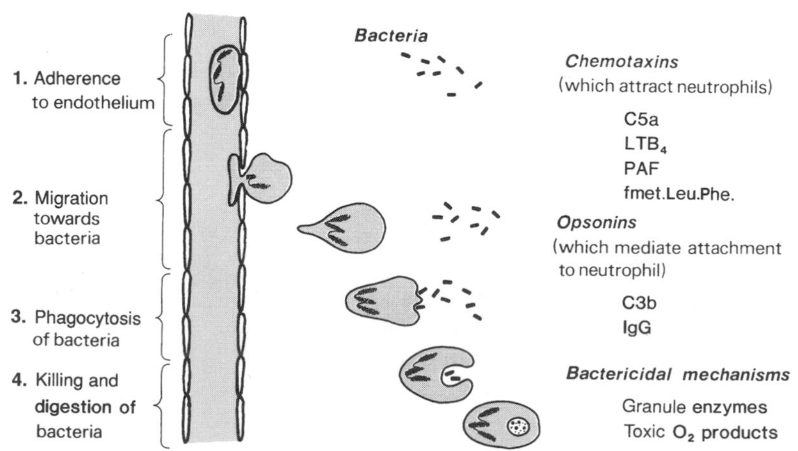

Fig. 11.2 Simplified diagram of the interaction of mediators and neutrophil leucocytes in an acute inflammatory reaction. Adherence involves interaction between the adhesion molecules on the endothelial cell and those on the neutrophil. (V = postcapillary venule; LTB_4 = leukotriene B_4; PAF = platelet-activating factor; C5a and C3b are complement components; fMet.Leu.Phe is a bacterial peptide; IgG = immunoglobulin G)

here) stands for '**r**egulated upon **a**ctivation, **n**ormal **T** cell **e**xpressed and **s**ecreted'.

In the tissues, monocytes become transformed into macrophages (literally 'big eaters', as compared to the polymorphs which were originally called microphages or 'little eaters'). Similar cells, all belonging to the mononuclear phagocyte system, are normally present in various tissues, probably all derived originally from blood-borne monocytes. The macrophage has a remarkable range of abilities, being not only a Jack of all trades but also master of many. With T cells, macrophages are crucial in the killing of virus-infected cells. In areas of inflammation they engulf tissue debris and dead cells as well as microorganisms, and they generate microorganism-destroying toxic oxygen metabolites. They are virtually chemical mediator factories and can produce and secrete not only enzymes, but complement components, eicosanoids (see p. 229), nitric oxide (Ch. 10), the 'tissue factor' which starts the extrinsic pathway of the coagulation cascade (Ch. 16), as well as various other coagulation factors, interferons (p. 243), a fibroblast-stimulating factor, pyrogens and a variety of cytokines which activate endothelial cells and other leucocytes. They are important in repair processes, and when stimulated by **glucocorticoids**, they secrete a lipocortin (a polypeptide which modulates the inflammatory response; see Ch. 21). For an overview of macrophage function, see Davies (1994).

Vascular endothelial cells

The vascular endothelial cells—originally considered as passive lining cells—are now known to play an active part in inflammation. The endothelial cells in the small arterioles, by secreting nitric oxide, which causes relaxation of the underlying smooth muscle (see Ch. 10), have a role in vasodilatation and thus in the delivery of plasma and blood cells to the area of inflammation, while the cells of the postcapillary venules have a regulatory role in the flow of exudate and thus in the delivery of plasma-derived mediators (see Fig. 11.1). On the luminal surface, a vascular endothelial cell expresses several adhesion molecules (the ICAM and selectin families; see above, p. 218) as well as a variety of receptors amongst which are those for histamine, acetylcholine, interleukin-1, etc. In addition to nitric oxide, the cells can synthesise and release the vasodilator agent, prostacyclin (p. 233), the vasoconstrictor agent, endothelin (Ch. 14), plasminogen activator (Ch. 16), platelet-activating factor (p. 237), and several cytokines (p. 242). For a simple overview of endothelial cell function in inflammation, see Fan & Dale (1994); for the role of the endothelial cell in *angiogenesis*, i.e. the growth of new blood vessels (which occurs in repair processes, chronic inflammation and cancer), see Fan (1994).

Platelets

Platelets are involved primarily in coagulation and thrombotic phenomena (see Ch. 16, p. 342) but may also play a part in inflammation. They have low affinity receptors for IgE and are believed to contribute to the first phase of asthma (Fig. 17.3). In addition to generating thromboxane A_2 and platelet-activating factor (Ch. 16), they can generate free radicals and pro-inflammatory cationic proteins. Platelet-derived growth factor contributes to the repair processes which follow inflammatory responses or damage to blood vessels.

MEDIATORS DERIVED FROM CELLS

When inflammatory cells are stimulated or damaged, another major mediator system is called into play—the *eicosanoids* (p. 229). Most of the current anti-inflammatory drugs act, at least in part, by interfering with synthesis of the eicosanoids. Other important inflammatory mediators derived from

The innate components of the inflammatory reaction

- The innate (non-immunological) components of the inflammatory reaction consist of vascular events and cellular events.
- Mediators are derived both from plasma and from cells, and in turn modify the vascular and cellular events.
- Vascular events:
  - — vasodilatation
  - — increased vascular permeability with exudation. The fluid exudate contains the components of enzyme cascades, the main ones being the kinin system and the complement system, both of which give rise to inflammatory mediators.
- Cellular events:
  - — stimulation of release of mast cell mediators by complement components
  - — accumulation in the tissues of white blood cells in response to chemo-attractant molecules
  - — engulfment and killing of microorganisms by phagocytic white blood cells.

cells are *histamine*, *platelet-activating factor* and the *cytokines* (the term 'cytokine' refers to a group of peptide cell regulators which includes lymphokines, interleukins, interferons; see p. 241). *Neuropeptides* are released from sensory neurons and contribute to inflammatory reactions in some tissues; for example substance P and the tachykinins produce smooth muscle contraction, mucus secretion and so on, and calcitonin gene-related peptide is a potent vasodilator. (See Chs 9, 14, 17 and 31.)

Before describing these mediators, we must consider the process which makes the innate components of the inflammatory response to invading pathogen immeasurably more efficient—the specific immunological response.

THE SPECIFIC IMMUNOLOGICAL RESPONSE

The specific immunological response to an invading organism makes the host's defensive response not only substantially more efficient but more *specific* for the invading pathogen. It is a complex response, detailed consideration of which is beyond the scope of this book. A simplified version of the immune response will be given here, stressing only those aspects which are relevant for an understanding of anti-inflammatory and immunosuppressant drugs. (For more detailed coverage, see Roitt 1994.)

The key cells are the *lymphocytes*. Their functions can be considered to involve two phases: an *induction phase* and an *effector phase*. The effector phase consists of two components: a humoral (antibody-mediated) component and a cell-mediated component.

Lymphocytes are divided into two main groups:

- *B cells*, which are responsible for antibody production (Fig. 11.3)
- *T cells*, which are important in the induction phase and are responsible for cell-mediated reactions (Fig. 11.4).

During the induction phase, T cells are involved

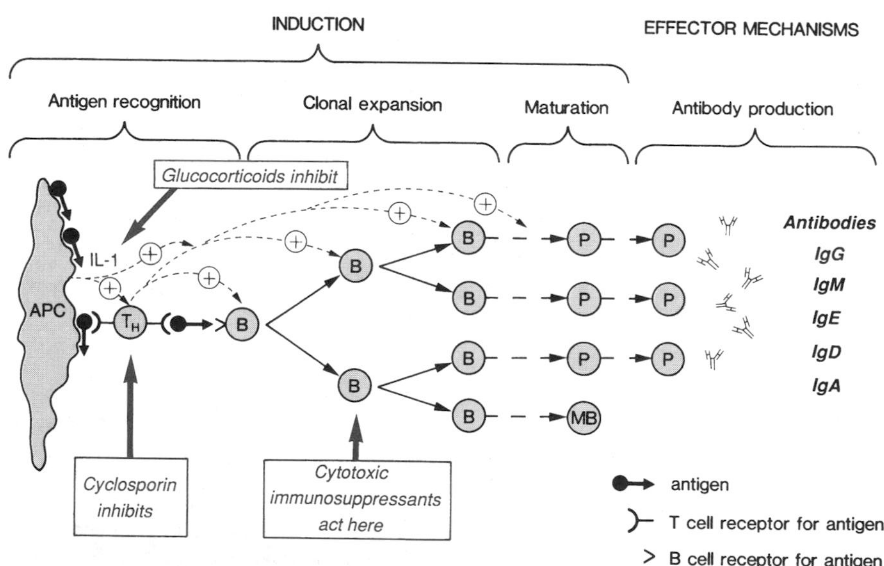

Fig. 11.3 Simplified diagram of induction of antibody-mediated immune response and the sites of action of immunosuppressant drugs. T cell factors (IL-2, IL-4, IL-5, IL-6) control the proliferation and maturation of B cells. The T_H cells are CD4+, i.e. they have the CD4 surface antigen; in addition to activating B cells, they release interleukins which stimulate eosinophil and mast cell production and the generation of IgE. (APC = antigen-presenting cell; T_H = T helper lymphocyte; B = B lymphocyte; IL = interleukin; P = plasma cell; MB = memory B cell; Ig = immunoglobulin)

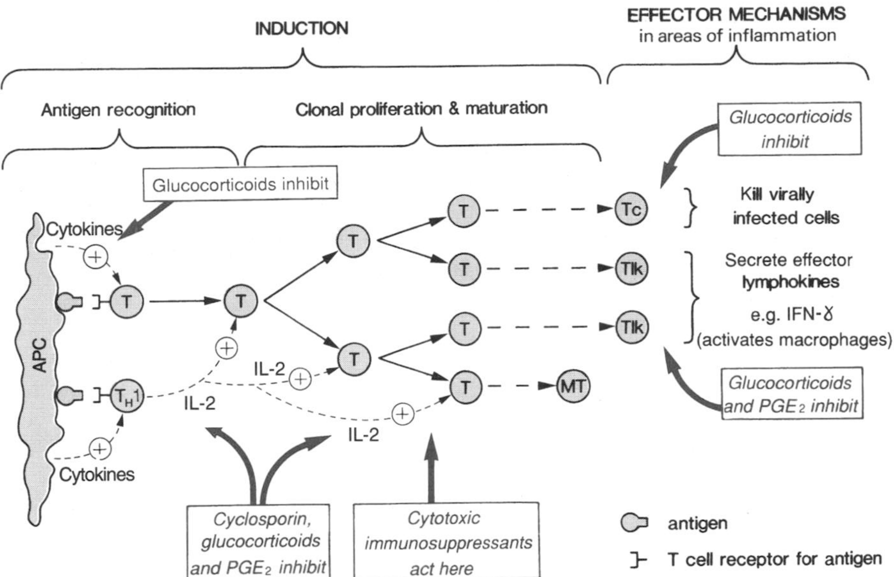

Fig. 11.4 Simplified diagram of induction of cell-mediated immune response and the sites of action of anti-inflammatory and immunosuppressant drugs. Other factors involved in the proliferation and maturation of T cells not shown here are IL-7 (from bone marrow stroma), IL-4 (from a subset of T cells) and tumour necrosis factor (from macrophages and other T cells). The T_H and Tlk cells possess CD4 surface proteins, and the Tc cells possess CD8 surface proteins. (APC = antigen-presenting cell; T = T cell; Tc = cytotoxic T cell; Tlk = lymphokine-secreting T cell (also referred to as inflammatory T cell); IL = Interleukin; MT = memory T cell; PG = prostaglandin; IFN-γ = interferon gamma)

in complex ways with B cells and other T cells. They may assist these cells ('helper/inducer T cells' or 'T_H cells') or inhibit them ('suppressor T cells').

On first contact with an antigen (foreign protein or polysaccharide), the lymphocytes which 'recognise' it start to divide, giving rise to a large clone of cells which all have the capacity to recognise and respond to that antigen. These either differentiate into plasma cells which go on to produce antibodies (if they are B cells) or are involved in cell-mediated immune responses (if they are T cells). Others will form an increased population of antigen-sensitive memory cells; a second exposure to the antigen will then result in a much multiplied response.

The induction and regulation of the immune response

The events involved in the induction and regulation of the immune response are very complex and are not yet entirely understood. A simplified outline of the main interactions between cells and mediators is given in Figures 11.3 and 11.4.

Antigenic molecules (e.g. bacterial products from the site of an infection, or experimentally injected proteins) reach the local lymph nodes via the lymphatics. In the nodes, the antigen is presented to lymphocytes on the surface of large dendritic cells called *antigen-presenting cells* (APCs), which are in some respects similar to macrophages. The APCs not only present antigen to lymphocytes but also release a peptide, *interleukin-1*, a cytokine which facilitates the response of these cells. (Interleukin-1 is also an important mediator in certain sorts of chronic inflammation; see p. 241.)

The *induction of antibody-mediated responses* varies with the type of antigen. Some types of antigen are presented directly to B cells by APCs. However, with most antigens, a cooperative process between T helper cells and B cells is necessary (Fig. 11.3). This process involves simultaneous recognition by T helper cells and B cells of different parts of the antigen molecule, by means of specific receptors, accompanied by the release of soluble factors from the T helper cell. These factors enable that clone of B cells to proliferate and subsequently to mature into antibody-producing cells (plasma cells). Interleukin-1 from APCs is involved in both the direct B cell response and the T helper/B cell response to antigen.

The *induction of cell-mediated immune responses* is still more complex and even less well understood. It is thought to occur as follows: T cells with specific receptors for antigen are activated by the antigen presented on APCs, facilitated by interleukin-1 (Fig. 11.4). These T cells then release *interleukin-2*, a cytokine which causes proliferation of other T cells on which interleukin-2 receptors have been induced. The resulting effector T cells may be cytotoxic cells or lymphokine-producing cells (also called inflammatory T cells).

Monoclonal antibodies have defined certain surface protein markers on T lymphocytes: both suppressor and cytotoxic T cells carry the CD8 marker, while helper T and lymphokine-producing T cells carry CD4. It is the loss of CD4-positive cells which is the basis of the immune deficiency in AIDS.

The **anti-inflammatory steroids** (see Ch. 21) and the immunosuppressive drug, **cyclosporin** (see Ch. 12), affect the events at the stage of interleukin-2 production and action. The cytotoxic **immunosuppressive drugs** (see Ch. 12) inhibit the proliferative phase of both B and T cells. Eicosanoids (see below) are believed to play a part in controlling these processes. For example, prostaglandins of the E series inhibit lymphocyte proliferation, probably by inhibiting the release of interleukin-2.

The effector phase of the immune response

The effector phase has two wings:

- the humoral immune response
- the cell-mediated immune response.

The humoral immune response involves antibodies and is effective in the fluid phases of the blood and the fluid phases of the tissues. However, antibodies cannot reach and deal with pathogens when these are within cells; cell-mediated immune mechanisms have evolved to deal with this.

The humoral response: antibodies and B lymphocytes

Antibodies are γ-globulins (immunoglobulins) which have two functions:

- to 'recognise' and interact specifically with particular antigens, i.e. proteins or polysaccharides foreign to the host
- to activate one or more of the host's defence systems.

The foreign substances may be part of an invading organism (the coat of a bacterium) or may be released by such an organism (a bacterial toxin), or they may be materials introduced experimentally in the laboratory in studies of the immune response (e.g. the injection of egg albumin into the guinea pig).

In simple terms, an antibody is a Y-shaped protein molecule in which the arms of the Y (the 'Fab' portions) are the recognition sites for specific antigens, and the stem of the Y (the 'Fc' portion) activates host defence mechanisms. B lymphocytes, the cells which are responsible for antibody production, 'recognise' foreign molecules by means of receptors on their surfaces, the receptor being essentially the immunoglobulin which that B cell clone will eventually produce. The mammalian organism possesses a vast number of clones of B cells producing different antibodies with recognition sites for different antigens. It is a miraculous fact that we come equipped with the ability to make antibodies that can recognise and react with virtually all foreign molecules which we are likely to encounter during our lifetime.

The ability to make antibodies has survival value; children born without this ability suffer repeated infections—pneumonia, skin infections, tonsillitis, etc. Before the days of antibiotics, they died in early childhood, and even today they require regular replacement therapy with immunoglobulin (see Ch. 12).

There are five classes of antibodies—IgG, IgM, IgE, IgA and IgD—which differ from each other in certain structural respects. (See Roitt 1994 for details.)

Antibodies markedly improve the host's response to an invading pathogen. Apart from their ability to interact *directly* with invading pathogens such as viruses or with bacterial toxins, thus impairing their capacity for damage, antibodies can multiply many-fold the effectiveness and specificity of the host's defence reaction in several ways, as follows:

Antibodies and the complement sequence. When antibodies react with antigenic material on the pathogen, the antigen–antibody reaction leads to the exposure, on the Fc portion, of a binding site for complement. This results in activation of the complement sequence with its biological repercussions—production of anaphylatoxin (C3a), chemotactic factor (C5a) and opsonin (C3b), and eventually the development of lytic potential (p. 216 and Figs 11.1 and 11.2). This route to C3 activation is referred to as 'the classical pathway' because it was investigated first. (The route outlined on page 216, initiated by microbial products such as endotoxin, is referred to as the 'alternative pathway' and was very probably developed much earlier in evolution.) The classical pathway provides an especially selective way of activating complement in response to a particular pathogen, since the antigen–antibody reaction which initiates it constitutes not only a highly specific recognition event but occurs in close association with the pathogen. The lytic property of complement can be used therapeutically: monoclonal antibodies and complement together can be used to clean bone marrow of cancer cells as an adjunct to chemotherapy or radiotherapy (see Ch. 36). Complement lysis is also implicated in the action of **anti-lymphocyte immunoglobulin** (p. 263).

Antibodies and the ingestion of bacteria. Antibodies can attach to the particular antigenic moieties on the surface of microorganisms which have been 'recognised' by their Fab portions, leaving the Fc part of the molecule projecting. Phagocytic cells (neutrophils and macrophages) have receptors on their membranes for these projecting Fc portions of antibody. Antibody thus forms a very specific link between microorganism and phagocyte and is more effective than C3b as an opsonin in facilitating phagocytosis (see Fig. 11.2).

Antibodies and cellular cytotoxicity. In some cases, for example in the case of parasitic worms, the invader may be too big to be ingested by phagocytes. In vitro studies show that antibody may still form a link between parasite and the host's white cells (in this case, eosinophils), which are then able to damage or kill the parasite by surface or extracellular actions.

Antibodies and mast cells or basophils. Mast cells and basophils have receptors for certain sorts of antibody (IgE), which can thus become attached to the cell membrane. When antigen reacts with this cell-fixed antibody, the whole panoply of pharmacologically active mediators is secreted. A complex reaction such as this, found widely throughout the animal kingdom, is unlikely to have been developed and retained during evolution unless it had survival value for the host. However, its precise biological significance in defence is not clear, though it may be of importance in association with eosinophil activity, in reactions against parasitic worms. When inappropriately triggered by substances not inherently damaging to the host, it is implicated in certain types of allergic reaction (see below and Ch. 17).

The cell-mediated immune response: T lymphocytes

T cells move into an inflammatory area by a process similar to that described for neutrophils and macrophages, namely interaction between adhesion molecules on both the endothelial cell and the lymphocyte.

The lymphocytes involved in cell-mediated responses are both cytotoxic T cells (Tc) and inflam-

The specific immunological response

- The specific immunological response vastly improves the effectiveness of the innate, non-immunological responses.
- The effector phase of the specific immunological response consists of an antibody component (mediated by B lymphocytes) and a cell-mediated component (mediated by T lymphocytes).
- Antibodies provide:
  - —neutralisation of some viruses and of some bacterial toxins
  - —more selective activation of the complement cascade
  - —more effective ingestion of microorganisms
  - —more effective attachment to multicellular parasites, facilitating their killing.
- Cell-mediated reactions involve:
  - —Tc cells (CD8-positive T cells) interacting with and killing virus-infected cells
  - —Tlk cells (CD4-positive T cells) interacting with macrophages, and releasing cytokines, such as gamma–interferon, which enable macrophages to kill intracellular pathogens such as the tubercle bacillus.
- Inappropriately deployed immune reactions are termed hypersensitivity reactions; these underlie the autoimmune diseases, i.e. diseases due to immune reactions directed at the host's own tissues.
- Anti-inflammatory drugs and immunosuppressive agents are used when the normally protective inflammatory and/or immune responses are inappropriately deployed.

matory (i.e lymphokine*-releasing) T cells (see Fig. 11.4).

When a mammalian cell is infected by an intracellular pathogen, there are two aspects to the resulting immune response. The first step, signalling that the cell is infected, is the expression on the cell surface of peptides derived from the pathogen; this is accomplished by transporter molecules, which are proteins coded for by the major histocompatibility complex (MHC) of genes. The second step is the recognition of the peptide–MHC complex by receptors on particular T cells. In the case of virally infected cells (which can be any of the cells in the body) the virus–MHC complex is recognised by the CD8 proteins on CD8-positive T cells—the cytotoxic T cells; these Tc cells then destroy the virus-infected cell.

Something similar happens with those intracellular pathogens within macrophages (e.g. the tubercle bacillus) which resist the normal macrophage killing mechanisms. The complex of MHC molecule plus bacterial peptide on the cell surface is recognised by a subset of CD4-positive T cells**—the inflammatory T cells (Tlk cells); these interact with the macrophage, generating lymphokines—such as interferon-γ—which confer on the macrophage the ability to kill the bacillus. It is the loss of these CD4-positive T cells in AIDS patients that makes them so susceptible to tuberculosis.

The specific immunological response, cell-mediated or humoral, is thus superimposed on the immunologically non-specific vascular and cellular reactions described previously, making them not only markedly more effective but much more ***specific*** *for particular invading organisms.* An important aspect of the specific immunological response is that the clone of lymphocytes which are programmed to respond to the antigens of the invading organism is greatly expanded after the first contact with the organism, and now contains 'memory cells'. Thus, subsequent exposure results in a greatly accelerated and more effective response. In some cases the response becomes so prompt and so efficient that, after the first exposure which initiates the specific immune response, some microorganisms can virtually never gain a foothold in the host's tissues again. Immunisation procedures make use of this fact.

*The term 'lymphokine' is used by some authorities to refer to cytokines released by lymphocytes.

**Dendritic cells and macrophages also carry surface CD4 proteins.

SYSTEMIC RESPONSES IN INFLAMMATION

In addition to the local changes in an inflammatory area, there are often various general responses such as a rise in temperature (see p. 248) and an increase in blood leucocytes, termed 'leucocytosis' (or neutrophilia if the increase is in the neutrophils only). There is also an increase in certain plasma proteins termed 'acute phase proteins'. These include C-reactive protein, α_2-macroglobulin, fibrinogen (see Fig. 11.1), α_1-antitrypsin, and some complement components. C-reactive protein binds to certain microorganisms and the resulting complex activates complement.

UNWANTED INFLAMMATORY AND IMMUNE RESPONSES

The responses described above can, in some circumstances, be inappropriately triggered by substances which are innocuous. It is when this happens that it becomes necessary to use **anti-inflammatory** or **immunosuppressive drugs**. Unwanted immune responses are termed *allergic* or *hypersensitivity reactions* and have been classified into four types.

Type 1: Immediate or anaphylactic hypersensitivity

Type I hypersensitivity occurs when antigenic material that is not in itself noxious (such as grass pollen, products from dead house-dust mites, certain foodstuffs or some drugs) evokes the production of antibodies of the IgE type, which fix to mast cells. Subsequent contact(s) with the material causes the release of histamine (p. 226), platelet-activating factor (p. 237), eicosanoids (p. 229), and cytokines (p. 241) from mast cells. The effects may be localised to the nose (hay fever), the bronchial tree (the initial phase of asthma), the skin (urticaria) or the gastrointestinal tract. In some cases the reaction is more generalised and produces anaphylactic shock.

Roughly speaking, this type of hypersensitivity

represents mainly inappropriate deployment of the processes outlined above in the section entitled 'Antibodies and mast cells or basophils' in the discussion of the humoral immune response (see p. 223). Some important unwanted effects of drugs are due to anaphylactic hypersensitivity responses (see Ch. 43). For a simple overview see Lichtenstein (1993).

Type II: Antibody-dependent cytotoxic hypersensitivity

Type II hypersensitivity occurs when the mechanisms outlined above (in the section entitled 'Antibodies and cellular cytotoxicity'; see p. 223) are directed against cells within the host, which are, or which appear to be, foreign; for example after incompatible blood transfusions or the alteration of the host's cells by drugs. The antigens form part of the surface of these cells and evoke antibodies. The antigen–antibody reaction initiates the complement sequence (with its repercussions) and can provide a basis for the attack by killer cells.

Examples of this latter class are the alteration by drugs of polymorphs which may lead to agranulocytosis (see Ch. 43), and of platelets which may lead to thrombocytopenic purpura (Ch. 16). Class II reactions are implicated in some types of autoimmune* thyroiditis (e.g. Hashimoto's disease; see Ch. 21).

Type III: Complex-mediated hypersensitivity

Type III hypersensitivity occurs when antibody reacts with *soluble* antigen. The antigen–antibody complexes can activate complement (see above) or attach to mast cells and stimulate the release of mediators (see above). An experimental example of type III hypersensitivity is a reaction termed the '*Arthus*' *reaction*, which occurs if a foreign protein is injected subcutaneously into a rabbit or guinea pig which has a high concentration of circulating antibody against that protein. The area becomes red and swollen 3–8 hours later. This is because the antigen–antibody complexes settle in the small blood vessels, complement is activated, and neutrophils are attracted and activated (by C5a) to generate toxic O_2 products and secrete enzymes. Mast cells are also stimulated by C3a to release mediators. Damage caused by this process is involved in serum sickness, in the reaction to mouldy hay, known as 'farmer's lung', and in certain types of autoimmune kidney and arterial disease. Type III hypersensitivity is also implicated in lupus erythematosus (a chronic, autoimmune inflammatory disease of connective tissue).

Type IV: Cell-mediated hypersensitivity

The prototype of type IV hypersensitivity is the *tuberculin reaction*—the reaction seen when proteins derived from cultures of the tubercle bacillus are injected into the skin of a person who has been sensitised to the bacillus by a previous infection or by immunisation. After 24 hours, the area becomes reddened and thickened. An 'inappropriate' cell-mediated immune response (see above, p. 223) has been stimulated and there has been infiltration of mononuclear cells and the release of various cytokines. Cell-mediated hypersensitivity is the basis of the reaction seen with some rashes (e.g. in mumps and measles) and with mosquito and tick bites. It is also important in the skin reactions to drugs or industrial chemicals (see Ch. 43), and in these cases the chemical combines with proteins in the skin to form the 'foreign' substance which evokes the cell-mediated immune response. A substance acting in this way is called a *hapten*.

In essence, inappropriately deployed T cell activity underlies all types of hypersensitivity, being the initiating factor in Types I, II and III and being involved in both the initiation and effector phase in Type IV.

The hypersensitivity reactions given above are the basis of the *autoimmune* diseases, which constitute many of the diseases seen in clinical medicine. For a simple overview, see Steinman (1993). Some examples of autoimmune conditions have been given above; other examples, held to have a marked component of cell-mediated hypersensitivity, are rheumatoid arthritis (p. 256), multiple sclerosis, insulin-dependent diabetes (p. 409).

Immunosuppressive drugs and/or **glucocorticoids** are employed as part of the treatment of some autoimmune diseases, and the use of cytokines and of antibodies to T cell surface antigens (e.g. the CD4 receptor) is being explored.

*Autoimmune diseases are diseases caused by the host's immune system attacking his/her own tissue; i.e. they are due to inappropriately deployed immune responses.

THE OUTCOME OF THE INFLAMMATORY RESPONSE

After this outline of the specific immune response, one needs to return to a consideration of the host–pathogen interaction—the local acute inflammatory response. It should be clear that this may consist of the innate, immunologically non-specific vascular and cellular events described initially, together with a varying degree of participation of the specific immunological response (either humoral or cell-mediated) the degree depending on several factors such as the nature of the pathogen and the organ or tissue involved. What is the final result of the interaction? If the pathogen has been dealt with adequately there may be complete healing and the tissue may be virtually normal thereafter. If there has been damage (death of cells, pus formation, ulceration), repair is usually necessary and may result in scarring. If the pathogen persists, the condition is likely to proceed to *chronic* inflammation, a slow smouldering reaction which continues for months or even years and involves destruction of tissue as well as local proliferation of cells and connective tissue. The principal cell types found in areas of chronic inflammation are *mononuclear* cells and abnormal cells derived from macrophages. In areas of healing and chronic inflammation there is angiogenesis (growth of new blood vessels) and also greatly increased activity of *fibroblasts* which lay down fibrous tissue. (For a simple overview of angiogenesis, see Fan 1994). The response to some microorganisms has the characteristic of chronicity from the start; examples are syphilis, tuberculosis and leprosy.

The components of the chronic inflammatory response to microorganisms are also seen in many if not most chronic autoimmune conditions.

Mediators of importance in healing, repair processes and chronic inflammatory reactions are, amongst others, platelet-derived growth factor (p. 342), transforming growth factor (see Table 11.2), and various fibroblast growth factors.

MEDIATORS OF INFLAMMATION AND ALLERGY

In the highly complex repertoire of reactions which constitutes the host response to invading pathogen, the precise role of the different mediators has not been completely clarified. Adequate assessment of the role of a putative mediator requires that the substance considered should fulfil certain criteria, modified from those outlined by Sir Henry Dale in 1933 for neurotransmitters.

A simple overview of these criteria and the degree to which the known inflammatory mediators fulfil them is considered by Dale (1994).

The mediators of pharmacological significance will be described below. Drugs which affect the inflammatory and immune responses will be considered in the next chapter.

HISTAMINE

Most of the early studies on the biological actions of this amine were carried out by Sir Henry Dale and his colleagues. Dale had shown that a local anaphylactic reaction (a Type I or 'immediate hypersensitivity reaction'; see above) was the result of an antigen–antibody reaction in sensitised tissue, and he subsequently demonstrated that histamine could largely mimic both the in vitro and in vivo anaphylactic responses. Feldberg and his co-workers showed that histamine was indeed released when antigen interacted with sensitised tissues, and later Riley & West identified the tissue mast cell as the main store of body histamine. After the first generation of antihistamine drugs was produced, following the work of Bovet and his co-workers, it became clear (as a result of careful quantitative studies by Schild) that there were two types of histamine receptor in the body and that this first generation of antihistamine drugs affected only one type—the H_1-receptors. The second type, termed H_2-receptors and important particularly in gastric acid secretion, was unaffected. Black and his colleagues, following up this classification proposed by Schild, developed the second generation of antihistamine drugs—the H_2-receptor antagonists. Subsequently, Sir James Black was awarded the Nobel prize for his work on H_2-receptors (and β-receptors; Ch. 7). More recently, evidence for the existence of a third type of histamine receptor—the H_3-receptor—has been produced by Arrang et al. (1983).

Synthesis and storage

Histamine is a basic amine, 2-(4-imidazolyl)-ethylamine (see Table 11.1a), and is formed from histidine by histidine decarboxylase. It is found in most tissues of the body, but is present in high concentrations in the lungs and the skin and in particularly high concentrations in the gastrointestinal tract. At the cellular level, it is found largely in mast cells and basophils, but non-mast-cell histamine occurs in the brain where it may be implicated in the activity of histaminergic neurons (see Ch. 24). The basophil content of the tissues is negligible—except in certain parasitic infections and hypersensitivity reactions (p. 224)—and basophils form only 0.5% of circulating white blood cells.

In mast cells and basophils, histamine is held in intracellular granules in a complex with an acidic protein and a heparin of high molecular weight, termed macroheparin. Together these comprise the matrix of the granule in which the basic molecule histamine is held by ionic forces. The molar ratio for histamine, heparin and protein in mast cells is 1:3:6 and the histamine content is approximately 0.1–0.2 pmol per mast cell, and 0.01 pmol per basophil.

Release

Histamine is released from mast cells by a secretory process during inflammatory or allergic reactions. As explained earlier in this chapter, stimuli include the interaction of complement components C3a and C5a with specific receptors on the cell surface, or the interaction of antigen with cell-fixed IgE antibodies. The secretory process is initiated by a rise in intracellular calcium. This follows cross-linking of receptors which initiates an increase in calcium permeability and a release of calcium from intracellular stores (see Ch. 2). Some neuropeptides, such as substance P, release histamine, though the concentrations required are fairly high. Various basic drugs, such as **morphine** and **tubocurarine** release histamine by non-receptor action.

Agents which increase cAMP formation (e.g. **β-adrenoceptor agonists**; see Ch. 7) inhibit histamine secretion, so it seems that, in these cells, cAMP-dependent protein kinase is an intracellular 'braking' mechanism. Replenishment of the histamine content of mast cell or basophil, after secretion, is a slow process which may take days or weeks, whereas turnover of histamine in the gastric 'histaminocyte' is very rapid.

Histamine is metabolised by histaminase and/or by the methylating enzyme imidazole N-methyltransferase.

Sensitivity to the effects of histamine varies between tissues and between species. The guinea pig is very sensitive and the mouse very insensitive to this agent. Human sensitivity lies between these two extremes.

Histamine receptors

Histamine produces its action by an effect on specific histamine receptors, which are of three main types, H_1, H_2 and H_3, distinguished by means of selective antagonist drugs. Some details of the actions of antagonist and agonist drugs used to investigate and define the three types of histamine receptor are given in Tables 11.1a and 11.1b. Selective antagonists at H_1-, H_2- and H_3-receptors are **mepyramine**, **cimetidine** and **thioperamide** respectively. Selective agonists for H_2- and H_3-receptors are **dimaprit** and **(R)α-methyl histamine** respectively; there are, as yet, no specific, selective agonists for H_1-receptors.

Histamine H_1 antagonists have clinical uses (see Chs 12 and 19), as do histamine H_2 antagonists (Ch. 19), but at present agents acting at H_3-receptors are used only as research tools.

H_1-receptors are found in human and guinea-pig bronchial muscle, and in guinea-pig ileum; stimulation causes contraction of the muscle. The histamine receptors in all these different tissues can be shown to have the same affinity for H_1 antagonists (such as **mepyramine**; Ch. 12), the antagonism being competitive and specific (see Ch. 1 and below). Histamine itself is the most potent agonist (Table 11.1a). H_1-receptors are linked to transduction systems which increase intracellular Ca^{2+} (see Ch. 2).

H_2-receptors are found in the acid-secreting cells in the stomach (Ch. 19), in rat uterus and in the heart; stimulation causes, respectively, gastric acid secretion, relaxation of the uterus and increased atrial rate. Agents such as cimetidine (see below) are specific competitive antagonists at these receptors (see Fig. 19.3). The most potent H_2 agonist is **impromidine** but it is also a very potent antagonist on H_3-receptors. H_2-receptors are linked to transduction systems which involve activation of adenylate cyclase and increased cyclic AMP (see Ch. 2). The H_2-receptor has been cloned.

H_3-receptors are associated mainly if not entirely with neural tissue, predominantly at presynaptic sites. Their activation results in inhibition of the release of a variety of neurotransmitters.

Table 11.1a Details of some agonist drugs used to define the three types of histamine receptors*

Drug	Structure	Relative activity in vitro (histamine 100%)		
		H_1-receptors (ileum contraction)	H_2-receptors (stimulation of atrial rate)	H_3-receptors (histamine release from brain tissue)
Histamine	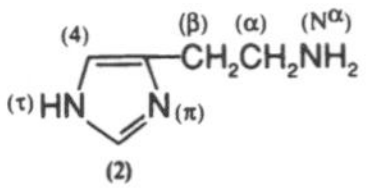 (4) (β) (α) ($N^{α}$) $CH_2CH_2NH_2$ (τ) HN N (π) (2)	**100**	100	100
Dimaprit	$NH_2-C(=NH)-S(CH_2)_3N(CH_3)_2$	< 0.0001	**71**	0.0008
(R) α-methylhistamine	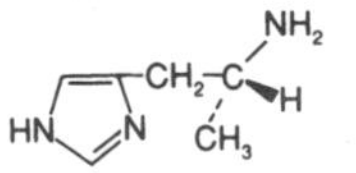 HN N $CH_2-C(NH_2)(H)CH_3$	0.49	1.02	**1550**

Table 11.1b Details of some antagonist drugs used to define the three types of histamine receptors*

Drug	Structure	H_1 (K_B M)	H_2 (K_B M)	H_3 (K_B M)
Mepyramine	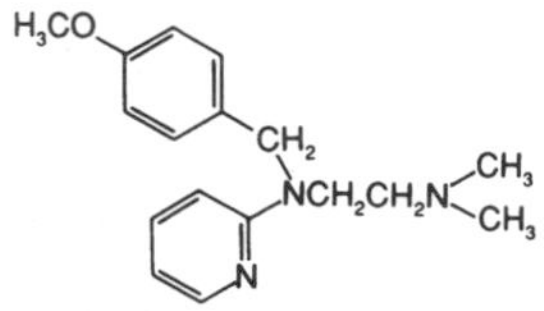 H_3CO, CH_2, $NCH_2CH_2N(CH_3)_2$, N	**0.4×10^{-9}**	–	$> 3 \times 10^{-6}$
Cimetidine	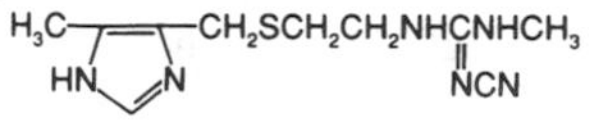 H_3C, HN N, $CH_2SCH_2CH_2NHCNHCH_3$ ‖ NCN	4.5×10^{-4}	**0.8×10^{-6}**	3.3×10^{-5}
Thioperamide	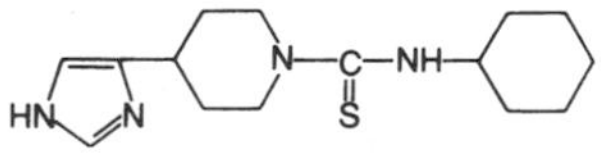 HN N, N–C(=S)–NH–	$> 10^{-4}$	$> 10^{-5}$	**4.3×10^{-9}**

*Data derived from Black J W et al 1972 Nature 236: 385–390; Ganellin C R 1982 In: Ganellin C R, Parson M E (eds) Pharmacology of histamine receptors. pp. 11–102; Arrang J M et al 1987 Nature 327: 117–123; van der Werf J F, Timmerman H 1989 Trends Pharmacol Sci 10: 159–162

Actions

Gastric secretion

Histamine stimulates the secretion of gastric acid by action on H_2-receptors. In clinical terms, *this is the most important action of histamine,* since it is implicated in the pathogenesis of peptic ulcer. It is considered in detail in Chapter 19.

Smooth muscle effects

Histamine, acting on H_1-receptors, causes contractions of the smooth muscle of the ileum, the bronchi and bronchioles, and the uterus.

The effect on the ileum is not as marked in man as it is in the guinea pig; the response of this latter tissue to histamine is the basis of the standard bioassay for histamine, familiar to students of experimental pharmacology. Bronchiolar constriction by histamine is also more marked in guinea pigs than in man, though histamine may be one of many factors causing reduction of air-flow in the first phase of bronchial asthma (see Ch. 17 and Fig. 17.3).

Uterine muscle in most species is contracted. In humans this is only significant if a massive release of histamine is produced by anaphylaxis during pregnancy, since this may lead to abortion.

Cardiovascular effects
Histamine dilates blood vessels by an action on H_1-receptors in man and by a combined action on H_1- and H_2-receptors in some experimental animals; the effect may be partly endothelium-dependent. It increases the rate and the output of the heart by action on cardiac H_2-receptors; this is a direct effect which may be coupled to an indirect, reflex response if there is a fall in blood pressure.

Injected intradermally, histamine causes a reddening of the skin and a wheal with a surrounding flare. This combination of effects was described by Sir Thomas Lewis over 50 years ago and was termed the 'triple response'. The reddening is due to vasodilatation of the small arterioles and precapillary sphincters, and the wheal is due to increased permeability of the postcapillary venules. These effects are mainly due to activation of H_1-receptors. (Contrary to popular belief and the statements in some pathology textbooks, histamine does not increase *capillary* permeability. Its locus of action in increasing permeability is on the postcapillary *venules*, as was clearly demonstrated by Majno & Palade and their colleagues in 1961.) The flare is due to an 'axon reflex' which involves stimulation of sensory nerve fibres and the passage of antidromic impulses through neighbouring branches of the same nerve with release of a vasodilator mediator, probably a peptide (Chs 10 and 14).

Itching
Itching occurs if histamine is injected into the skin or applied to a blister base, and is due to stimulation of sensory nerve endings.

It will be clear from the above that histamine is capable of producing many of the effects of inflammation and hypersensitivity—vasodilatation, increased vascular permeability and the spasm of smooth muscle—and it has long been thought to be one of the major mediators of acute inflammation. It is surprising therefore that histamine H_1 antagonists do not have much effect on the acute inflammatory response per se. It is probable that histamine is a mediator of importance only in some sorts of type I hypersensitivity reaction, such as allergic rhinitis and urticaria. The use of H_1 antagonists in these and other conditions is dealt with in Chapter 12.

The main pathophysiological role of endogenous histamine is as a stimulant of gastric acid secretion by an action on H_2-receptors (Ch. 19).

As regards the understanding of histamine action on H_3-receptors, the research work of medicinal chemists and pharmacologists has, at present, run far ahead of that of neurophysiologists, and the physiological significance of H_3-receptor activation has yet to be established.

For a simple overview of histamine, see Dale & Foreman (1994).

Histamine

- Histamine is a basic amine, stored in mast cells and basophils.
- It is held in granules with macroheparin, and secreted when complement components C3a and C5a interact with specific receptors, or when antigen interacts with cell-fixed IgE.
- It produces effects by acting on H_1-, H_2- or H_3-receptors on target cells.
- The main actions in humans (and the receptors involved) are:
  - —stimulation of gastric secretion (H_2)
  - —contraction of most smooth muscle other than that of blood vessels (H_1)
  - —cardiac stimulation (H_2)
  - —vasodilatation (H_1)
  - —increased vascular permeability (H_1).
- Injected intradermally it causes the 'triple response': local *vasodilatation* and *wheal* by direct action of blood vessels, and surrounding *flare* due to vasodilatation resulting from an 'axon' reflex in sensory nerves releasing a peptide mediator.
- The main pathophysiological roles of histamine are:
  - —as a stimulant of gastric acid secretion (treated with H_2-receptor antagonists)
  - —as a mediator of type 1 hypersensitivity reactions such as urticaria and hay fever (treated with H_1-receptor antagonists).
- The full physiological significance of H_3-receptors is not clear.

EICOSANOIDS

Eicosanoids, unlike histamine, are not found preformed in the tissues; they are generated de novo from phospholipids. They are implicated in the control of many physiological processes and are among

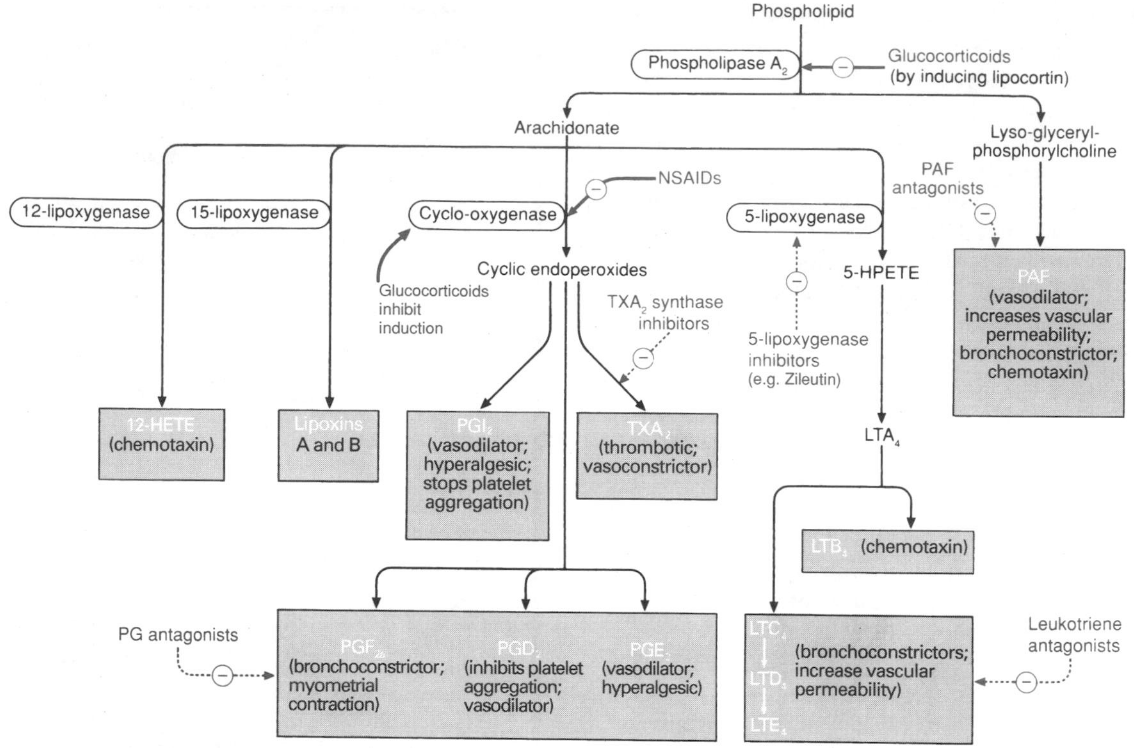

Fig. 11.5 Summary diagram of mediators derived from phospholipids and their actions, and the sites of action of anti-inflammatory drugs. The arachidonate metabolites are 'eicosanoids'. Established drugs are shown with full thickness arrows, drugs still under test with dashed arrows. The glucocorticoids inhibit transcription of the gene for cyclo-oxygenase-2, which is induced in inflammatory cells by inflammatory mediators.The effects of PGE_2 depend on which of the three receptors for this prostanoid are activated; see text. (PG = prostaglandin; PGI_2 = prostacyclin; TX = thromboxane; LT = leukotriene; HETE = hydroxyeicosatetraenoic acid; HPETE = hydroperoxyeicosatetraenoic acid; PAF = platelet-activating factor; NSAIDs = non-steroidal anti-inflammatory drugs; see Ch. 12)

the most important mediators and modulators of the inflammatory reaction (Fig. 11.5).

Interest in eicosanoids arose in the 1930s after reports that semen contained a substance which contracted uterine smooth muscle. The substance was believed to originate in the prostate and was saddled with the misnomer, *prostaglandin*. More than two decades later it became clear that prostaglandin was not just one substance but a whole family of compounds. In the 1960s, two prostaglandins (PGE and $PGF_{2\alpha}$) were isolated in crystalline form and their structures elucidated by Bergstrom & Samuelsson. Subsequently, several more prostaglandins were found to be generated in tissue, and it was shown that these compounds were derived from *arachidonate*. In the early 1970s, Vane advanced the hypothesis that inhibition of prostaglandin synthesis was the mechanism of action of aspirin-like drugs. Later, intermediate substances in the synthetic pathway—two unstable cyclic endoperoxides (see Fig. 11.8)—were isolated and identified, and two rather different compounds derived from these intermediates were discovered—*thromboxane A_2* by Hamberg et al. and *prostacyclin* by Moncada & Vane and their colleagues. Still later, the elucidation by Hamberg et al. of a different pathway of arachidonate metabolism, resulting in the production of the *leukotrienes*, led to a further understanding of the role of arachidonate metabolites in physiological and pathological processes. In 1982, Bergstrom, Samuelsson and Vane received the Nobel Prize for Medicine for their work in this area.

Structure and biosynthesis

The main source of the eicosanoids is *arachidonic acid* (5,8,11,14-eicosatetraenoic acid), a 20-carbon unsaturated fatty acid containing four double bonds (hence '*eicosa*' referring to the 20 carbon atoms, and '*tetraenoic*' referring to the 4 double bonds). Arachidonic acid is found esterified in the phospholipids, usually in the 2 position (Fig. 11.6) and to a lesser extent in the glycerides of cell membranes. The principal eicosanoids are the *prostaglandins*, the *thromboxanes* and the *leukotrienes*, though other derivatives of arachidonate, for example the *lipoxins*, are also produced. (The term *prostanoid* will be used here to encompass both prostaglandins and thromboxanes.) The initial and rate-limiting step in eicosanoid synthesis is the liberation of arachidonate, either in a one-step process or a two-step process. The one-step process involves phospholipase A_2 (Fig. 11.6); the two-step process (Fig. 11.7) involves either phospholipase C and then diacylglycerol lipase, or phospholipase D then phospholipase A_2. Phospholipase D has been shown to be important in signal transduction in phagocytic cells. Note that there are two forms of phospholipase A_2 (PLA_2)—one found intracellularly in the cytosol, and one present in the extracellular fluids. It is mainly the intracellular form which is implicated in the generation of inflammatory mediators, and its action can give rise not only to arachidonic acid and thus the eicosanoids, but also to lyso-glyceryl-phosphorylcholine (lyso-PAF), which is the precursor of another powerful mediator of inflammation—*platelet-activating factor* (see Figs 11.5 and 11.2).

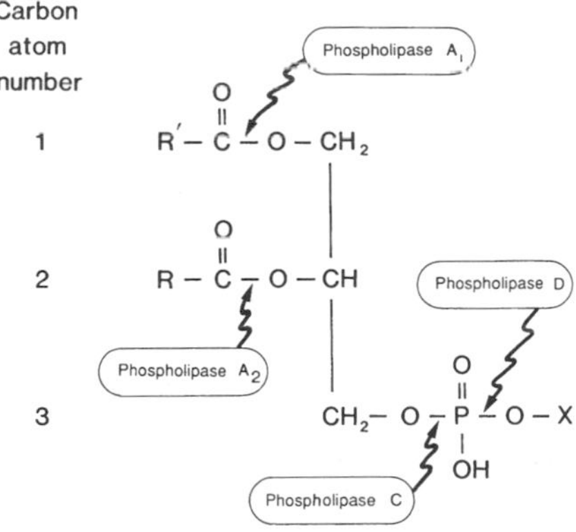

Fig. 11.6 Outline of structure of phospholipids and site of action of phospholipases—indicating how arachidonate can be released by a one-step process. The numbering of the carbon atoms in the glycerol 'backbone' is given on the left. Unsaturated fatty acids, such as arachidonic acid, are usually located at R on the 2nd carbon. This figure shows O-acyl residues on carbon atoms 1 and 2, but O-alkyl residues can occur (see Fig. 11.11). (X = choline, ethanolamine, serine, inositol or hydrogen)

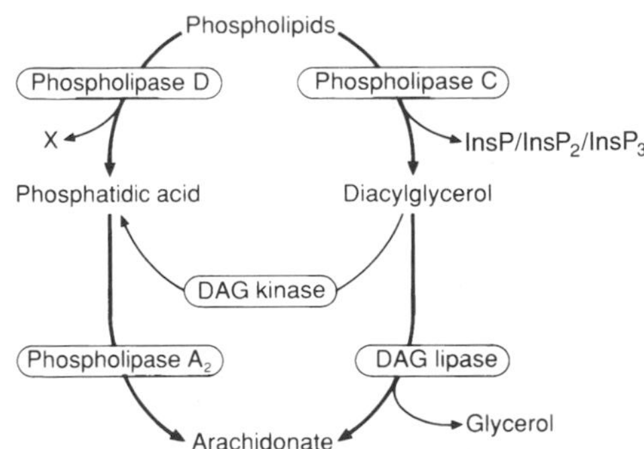

Fig. 11.7 Pathways of release of arachidonate from phospholipids by two-step processes. (InsP = inositol phosphate; DAG = diacyglycerol) (See also Fig. 11.6 and Fig. 2.12.)

Many stimuli can liberate arachidonic acid, and they vary with the cell type, for example thrombin in platelets, C5a in neutrophils, bradykinin in fibroblasts and antigen–antibody reactions on mast cells. General cell damage also starts the process.

The free arachidonic acid is metabolised by several pathways—by one of two fatty acid cyclo-oxygenases (see below) which initiate the biosynthesis of the prostaglandins and thromboxanes, and by various lipoxygenases (p. 234) which initiate the synthesis of the leukotrienes, the lipoxins and other compounds (Figs 11.5, 11.8 and 11.9). For a simple overview of the eicosanoids see Salmon & Higgs (1994).

The anti-inflammatory action of the **gluco-corticoids** (Ch. 21) is due largely to inhibition of *induction* of cyclo-oxygenase. These drugs may also stimulate production of the inhibitor lipocortin (Fig. 11.5).

The anti-inflammatory action of the **non-steroidal anti-inflammatory drugs** is due mainly to the fact that they inhibit the action of one of the fatty acid cyclo-oxygenases (Figs 11.5 and 11.8). Other compounds which act selectively on the cyclo-oxygenase induced in inflammatory cells or at specific sites of eicosanoid synthesis (e.g. inhibitors of 5-lipoxygenase, and thromboxane synthetase) are under test, as are specific antagonists of the prostaglandins and leukotrienes (Fig. 11.5.)

The products of the cyclo-oxygenase pathway: the prostanoids

Cyclo-oxygenase (COX) exists in two forms—COX-1

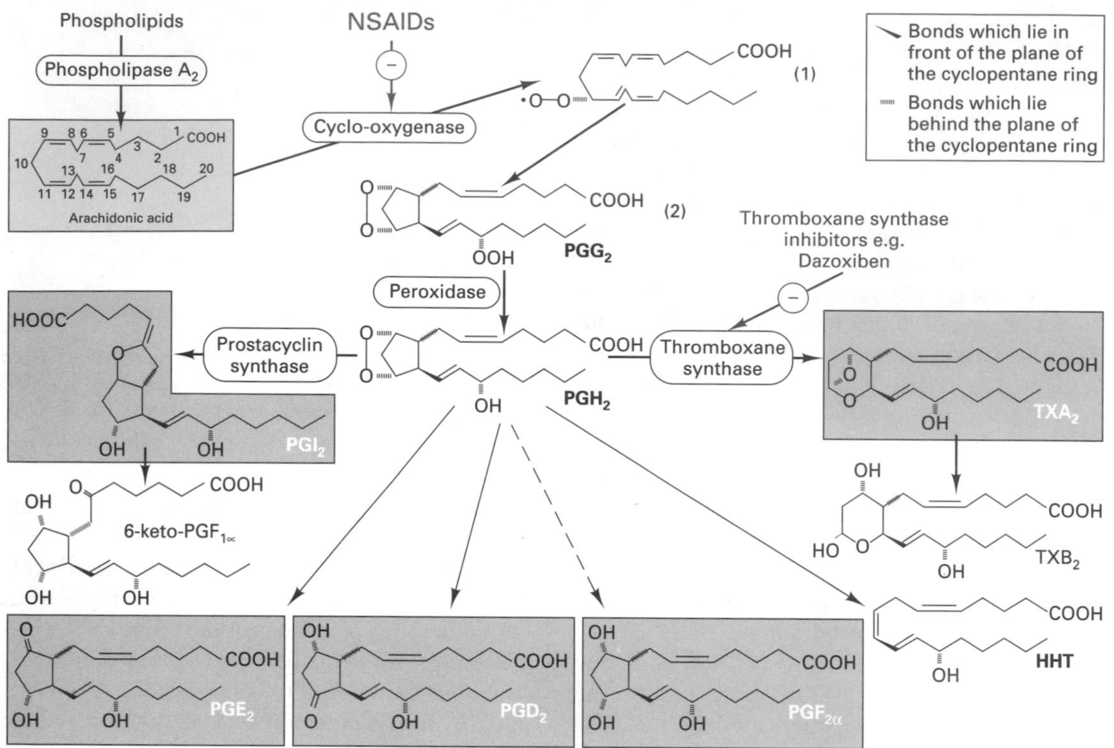

Fig. 11.8 The biosynthesis of prostaglandins, prostacyclin and thromboxane from arachidonate. Solid lines indicate known enzymic reactions, and dotted lines the transformations not known to be enzymic. Compounds with biological action are shown in boxes. There are two forms of cyclo-oxygenase (COX): one (COX–I) is constitutive and occurs in most cell types, and the other (COX–II) is induced in inflammatory cells by inflammatory stimuli. The current NSAIDs act mainly on COX-I. (PG = prostaglandin; TX = thromboxane; NSAIDs = non-steroidal anti-inflammatory drugs)

Mediators derived from phospholipids

- The main phospholipid-derived mediators are the eicosanoids (prostanoids and leukotrienes) and platelet-activating factor.
- The eicosanoids are derivatives of arachidonate which can be released from phospholipid by phospholipase (PL) action, either in one step by PLA_2, or by two steps—PLC then diacylglycerol lipase. Arachidonate can be metabolised either by one of two cyclo-oxygenases to give rise to various prostanoids, or by 5-lipoxygenase to give rise to various leukotrienes.
- Platelet-activating factor (PAF) is derived from phospholipid by PLA_2 giving rise to lyso-PAF which is acetylated to give PAF.

and COX-2. COX-1 is found in most cells as a constitutive enzyme (i.e. it is always present) and it is thought that the prostanoids it produces are involved in normal homeostasis (e.g. regulating vascular responses and coordinating the actions of circulating hormones). COX-2 is induced in inflammatory cells by an inflammatory stimulus. This has relevance for the mechanism of action of present and future **NSAIDs**.

Cyclo-oxygenase is found bound to the endoplasmic reticulum. It has two actions:

- an endoperoxide synthase action that first oxygenates arachidonate (step 1 in Fig. 11.8), followed by cyclisation to give the *cyclic endoperoxide* PGG_2 (step 2 in Fig. 11.8)

- a peroxidase action that converts PGG_2 to another *cyclic endoperoxide*, PGH_2 (see Fig. 11.8).*

Subsequent steps in arachidonate metabolism differ in different cells. In platelets, the pathway leads to *thromboxane* A_2 synthesis, in vascular endothelium it leads to *prostacyclin* synthesis and in macrophages it leads mainly to synthesis of *prostaglandin* E_2 (PGE_2). Mast cells synthesise PGD_2.

The confusing nomenclature of the eicosanoids derives from the fact that the names of the first two prostaglandins were based on the separation procedure—PG*E* partitioned into *E*ther, and PG*F* into the phosphate buffer (*F*osfat in Swedish). PG*A* and PG*B* (which are artefacts) were so called because of their stability or otherwise in *acids* and *bases*. Thereafter other letters of the alphabet were filled in. The subscripts refer to the number of double bonds; thus PGE_2 has two double bonds. The Greek letter subscript, the α in $PGF_{2\alpha}$, refers to the orientation of the hydroxyl above or below the plane of the ring. PGE_2, PGI_2, PGD_2, TXA_2 and $PGF_{2\alpha}$ are the most important products of the cyclo-oxygenase pathway. If the cyclo-oxygenase acts on eicosatrienoic acid instead of arachidonic acid, the resulting prostanoids have only a single double bond, for example PGE_1. For a simple overview of the eicosanoids, see Salmon & Higgs (1994).

Catabolism of the prostanoids

Several intracellular enzymes are involved in inactivation of the prostaglandins. After carrier-mediated uptake there is rapid inactivation by 'prostaglandin-specific' enzymes, then slow inactivation by general fatty-acid-oxidising enzymes. The metabolites of the prostaglandins are excreted in the urine. The prostaglandin-specific enzymes are present in high concentration in the lung, and 95% of infused PGE_2, PGE_1 or $PGF_{2\alpha}$, is inactivated on first passage. The $t_{½}$ of most prostaglandins in the circulation is less than 1 minute.

PGI_2 is not taken up into cells by the transport system in the lung, and thus survives passage through the lung. However, it is very short-lived ($t_{½} < 5$ min), being hydrolysed to 6-keto $PGF_{1\alpha}$ (Fig. 11.8).

Thromboxane A_2 hydrolyses rapidly to the biologically inactive TXB_2 ($t_{½} = 30$ sec).

Prostanoid receptors

A classification of prostanoid receptors has been proposed by Coleman et al (1993). Using data of the rank order of potency of five natural prostanoids on a range of different preparations, five main prostanoid receptors have been defined, one each for the natural prostanoids, PGD_2, $PGF_{2\alpha}$, PGI_2, TXA_2 and PGE_2, termed DP-, FP-, IP-, TP- and EP-receptors respectively. Synthetic analogues of the natural prostanoids support and extend this classification, which has been further confirmed as some receptor antagonists have become available. Data obtained with the synthetic compounds have led to the proposal that there are three subgroups of receptors for PGE_2—termed EP_1, EP_2 and EP_3. Binding studies have also provided supportive evidence for this classification. For a simple overview see Coleman (1994).

Actions of the prostanoids

The prostanoids affect most tissues, having a bewildering variety of effects. The fact that there is marked species variability in the response of different tissues has made information from experiments confusing and has compounded the difficulties of unravelling the pharmacological actions of these agents. Nevertheless, the general actions of the prostanoids can now be expressed in terms of their actions on their respective receptors as follows.

The action of PGD_2 on DP-receptors causes vasodilatation, inhibition of platelet aggregation, relaxation of gastrointestinal muscle, uterine relaxation, modification of release of hypothalamic/pituitary hormones. (Its bronchoconstrictor effect is due to an action on TP-receptors.) Signal transduction involves adenylate cyclase and an increase in cAMP (Ch. 2).

The action of $PGF_{2\alpha}$ on FP-receptors causes myometrial contraction in humans (see Ch. 22), luteolysis in some species (e.g. cattle) and bronchoconstriction in other species (cats and dogs). (The

*An autocatalytic mechanism is believed to be involved in the action of cyclo-oxygenase. The enzyme first produces a lipid peroxide—the formation of a peroxy radical at C11, compound (1) in Figure 11.8. This is followed by isomerisation, and also introduction of a hydroperoxy group at C15 to give PGG_2, compound (2) in Figure 11.8. It has been said that the lipid peroxide enhances the subsequent reactions of the enzyme, and that the continued presence of this (or other peroxides) is needed to sustain cyclo-oxygenase activity (although excess peroxide can inactivate the enzyme). (See Lands 1981.)

receptors involved in $PGF_{2\alpha}$-mediated release of gonadotrophins and prolactin are not yet known.) Signal transduction involves $InsP_3$ generation and increase of cytosolic $[Ca^{2+}]_i$.

The action of PGI_2 (prostacyclin) on IP-receptors causes vasodilatation, inhibition of platelet aggregation (see Ch. 16), renin release and natriuresis via effects on tubular reabsorption of Na^+. Signal transduction involves adenylate cyclase and an increase in cAMP.

The action of TXA_2 on TP-receptors causes vasoconstriction, platelet aggregation (see Ch. 16) and bronchoconstriction (the last more marked in guinea pig than in man). Signal transduction involves $InsP_3$ generation and increase of cytosolic $[Ca^{2+}]_i$.

The actions of PGE_2 are as follows:

- On EP_1-receptors it causes contraction of bronchial and gastrointestinal smooth muscle—the transduction mechanisms being $InsP_3$ generation and increase of cytosolic $[Ca^{2+}]_i$.
- On EP_2-receptors it causes bronchodilatation, vasodilatation, stimulation of intestinal fluid secretion and relaxation of gastrointestinal smooth muscle—the transduction mechanisms being activation of adenylate cyclase and an increase in cAMP.
- On EP_3-receptors it causes contraction of intestinal smooth muscle, inhibition of gastric acid secretion (see Ch. 19 and Fig. 19.2), increased gastric mucus secretion, inhibition of lipolysis, inhibition of autonomic neurotransmitter release and stimulation of contraction of the pregnant human uterus (Ch. 22)—the transduction mechanisms being inhibition of adenylate cyclase and a decrease in cAMP.

Actions of PGE_2 for which the receptor type is not yet known include the production of fever, inhibition of T cell proliferation (see Fig. 11.4), inhibition of macrophage activation, stimulation of release of adrenal steroids and of erythropoietin release from the kidney.

The role of the prostanoids in inflammation

The inflammatory response is always accompanied by the release of prostanoids, so they are certainly present at inflammatory sites, the predominant product being PGE_2, though PGI_2 can also be found. In areas of acute inflammation PGE_2 and PGI_2 are generated by the local tissues and blood vessels, and mast cells release PGD_2. In chronic inflammation, cells of the monocyte–macrophage series also release PGE_2.

The prostanoids have a sort of Yin-Yang action in inflammation—stimulating some responses and decreasing others as follows.

PGE_2, PGI_2 and PGD_2 are powerful *vasodilators* in their own right and synergise with other inflammatory vasodilators such as histamine and bradykinin. It is this combined dilator action on precapillary arterioles which contributes to the redness and increased blood flow in areas of acute inflammation. These prostanoids do not directly increase the permeability of the postcapillary venules, but they potentiate this effect of histamine and bradykinin. Similarly, they do not themselves produce pain, but *potentiate* the effect of bradykinin by sensitising afferent C fibres (see Ch. 30). The anti-inflammatory effects of the **NSAIDs** are due largely to inhibition of these actions of the prostaglandins.

Prostaglandins of the E series are also implicated

Prostanoids

- The term 'prostanoids' encompasses the prostaglandins (PGs) and the thromboxanes (TXs).
- Cyclo-oxygenase acts on arachidonate to produce cyclic endoperoxides (PGG_2, PGH_2).
- These can give rise to:
  - — PGI_2 (prostacyclin) predominantly from vascular endothelium; it acts on IP-receptors. Main effects: vasodilatation and inhibition of platelet aggregation.
  - — TXA_2 predominantly from platelets; it acts on TP-receptors. Main effects: platelet aggregation and vasoconstriction.
  - — PGE_2. Main effects: on EP_1-receptors—contraction of bronchial and GIT smooth muscle; on EP_2-receptors—relaxation of bronchial, vascular and GIT smooth muscle; on EP_3-receptors—inhibition of gastric acid secretion, increased gastric mucus secretion, contraction of pregnant uterus and of GIT smooth muscle, inhibition of lipolysis and of autonomic neurotransmitter release. PGE_2 is a mediator of fever.
  - — $PGF_{2\alpha}$ acts on FP-receptors which are found in smooth muscle and corpus luteum. Main effects in humans: contraction of uterus.
  - — PGD_2, derived particularly from mast cells, acts on DP-receptors. Main effects: vasodilatation and inhibition of platelet aggregation.

in the production of fever. High concentrations are found in the CSF in infections, and there is evidence that the increase in temperature generated by endogenous fever-inducing agents such as IL-1 is mediated by PGE_2. The antipyretic action of **NSAIDs** (Ch. 12) is due partly to inhibition of the synthesis of PGE_2 in the hypothalamus.

In addition to the pro-inflammatory mediator function mentioned above, prostaglandins have been shown to have a significant anti-inflammatory modulator role on inflammatory cells, *decreasing* their activities. Thus PGE_2 decreases lysosomal enzyme release and the generation of toxic oxygen metabolites from neutrophils and histamine release from mast cells. It also inhibits macrophage activation, lymphocyte activation (Fig. 11.4) and the generation and secretion of some cytokines.

Several prostanoids are available for clinical use (see below).

Clinical use of prostanoids

The main established uses are as follows:

- Gynaecological and obstetrical (see Ch. 22 for details):
  - — for termination of pregnancy: dinoprostone (PGE_2) given by extra-amniotic route; gemeprost given by vagina as pessary
  - — for induction of labour: dinoprostone locally in the vagina
  - — for postpartum haemorrhage: carboprost (if no response to other oxytocics).
- Gastrointestinal:
  - — to prevent gastric and duodenal ulcers in patients taking NSAIDs: misoprostol (a stable analogue of PGE_2) can be used (see Ch. 19 for details).
- Cardiovascular:
  - — For the treatment of congenital malformations of the heart in neonates, the purpose being to maintain the patency of the *ductus arteriosus* prior to surgical correction of the congenital defect: **alprostadil** (a preparation of PGE_1) is used, given by intravenous infusion.
  - — To inhibit platelet aggregation during haemodialysis: a short-acting PGI_2 preparation, **epoprostenol**, ($t_{½}$ 3 min) is used by infusion if heparin is contraindicated (see Ch. 16). Also used for treatment of primary pulmonary hypertension.

The products of the lipoxygenase pathways: the leukotrienes

The lipoxygenases, soluble enzymes located in the cytosol, are found in lung, platelets, mast cells and white blood cells. The main enzyme in this group is 5-lipoxygenase—the first enzyme in the biosynthesis of the *leukotrienes* ('leuko' because they are found in white cells and 'trienes' because they contain a conjugated triene system of double bonds; see Fig. 11.9). On cell activation this enzyme translocates to the cell membrane where it becomes associated with a protein termed the 'five-lipoxygenase activating protein' (FLAP), which is necessary for leukotriene synthesis in intact cells. The 5-lipoxygenase adds a hydroperoxy group to C5 in arachidonic acid (Fig. 11.9). The next step in the pathway is the synthesis of *leukotriene* A_4 (LTA_4). This compound may be converted enzymically to LTB_4 and is also the precursor for an important class of cysteinyl-containing leukotrienes—LTC_4, LTD_4, LTE_4 and LTF_4 (also referred to as the sulphidopeptide leukotrienes). The first three of this latter group together constitute 'slow reacting substance of anaphylaxis (SRS-A)', a substance shown many years ago to be generated in guinea-pig lung during anaphylaxis. LTB_4 is produced mainly by neutrophils, and the cysteinyl-leukotrienes mainly by eosinophils, mast cells, basophils and macrophages.

Lipoxins and other active products are also produced from arachidonate (Fig. 11.9).

Metabolism of the leukotrienes

LTB_4 can be converted to 20-hydroxy-LTB_4 by a unique membrane-bound P-450 enzyme which occurs in the neutrophil, and then futher oxidised to 20-carboxy-LTB_4. LTC_4 and LTD_4 are metabolised to LTE_4 which is excreted in the urine.

Actions and receptors* of the leukotrienes

***LTB_4*.** LTB_4 acts on specific LTB_4-receptors defined by selective agonists and antagonists, the transduction mechanism being $InsP_3$ generation and increase of cytosolic $[Ca^{2+}]_i$. It is a powerful chemotactic agent for both neutrophils and macrophages (see Fig. 11.2), acting in picogram amounts. On neutrophils, it also causes up-regulation of the membrane adhesion molecules and increases the

*It is suggested that receptors for the leukotrienes be termed LT-receptors—bLT for the class exemplified by LTB_4 and cLT for the cysteinyl-leukotrienes.

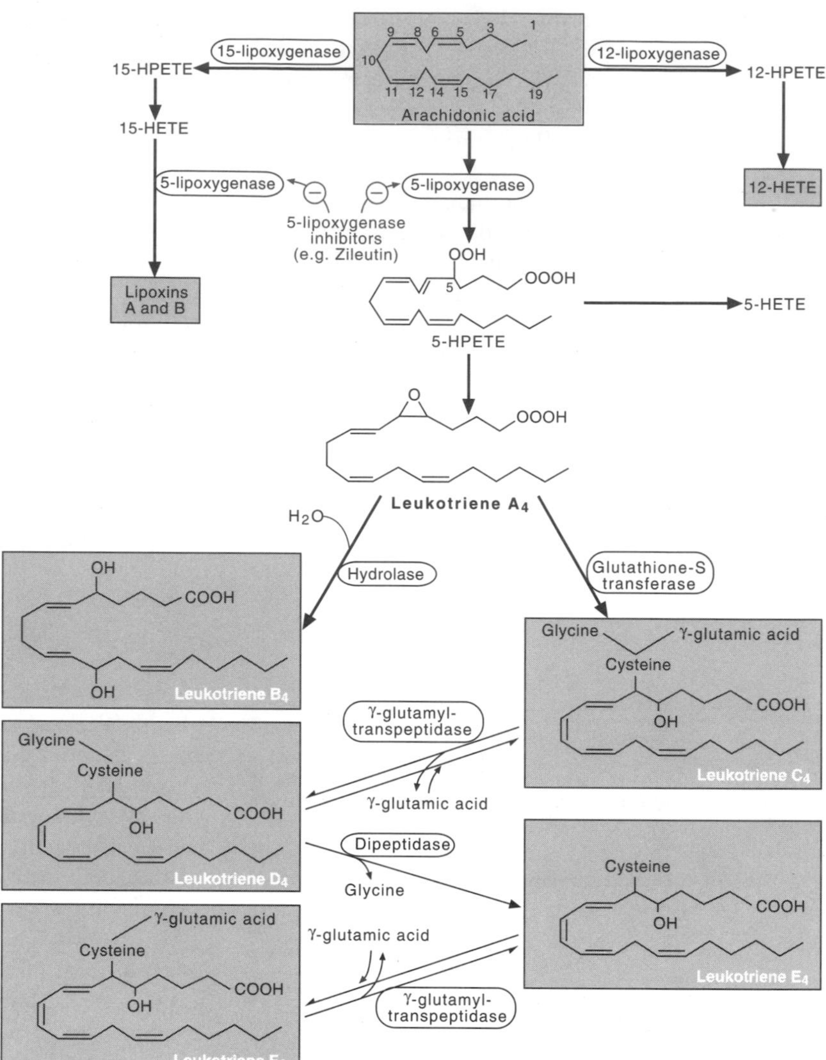

Fig. 11.9 The biosynthesis of leukotrienes from arachidonic acid. It is not clear whether LTF_4 occurs in vivo. Compounds with biological action are shown in grey boxes. (HETE = hydroxy-eicosatetraenoic acid; HPETE = hydroperoxyeicosatetraenoic acid)

production of toxic oxygen products and the release of granule enzymes. On macrophages and lymphocytes it stimulates proliferation and cytokine release.

Cysteinyl-leukotrienes. On the basis of the rank order of potency, there appear to be receptors for both LTD_4 and LTC_4, but there are few specific agonists for either compound. However, specific receptors for LTD_4 have been defined on the basis of selective antagonists.

Cysteinyl-leukotrienes have actions on:

- *The respiratory system.* They are potent spasmogens causing dose-related contraction of human bronchiolar muscle in vitro. LTE_4 is less potent than LTC_4 and LTD_4, but its effect is much longer lasting. All cause an increase in mucus secretion. Given by aerosol in vivo to human volunteers they cause marked reduction in specific airway conductance and in maximum expiratory flow rate, the effect being more protracted than that produced by histamine (Fig. 11.10).
- *The cardiovascular system.* Small amounts of LTC_4 or LTD_4 given intravenously cause a rapid, short-lived fall in blood pressure, and significant constriction of small coronary resistance vessels. Given subcutaneously they are equipotent with histamine in causing wheal and flare. Given topi-

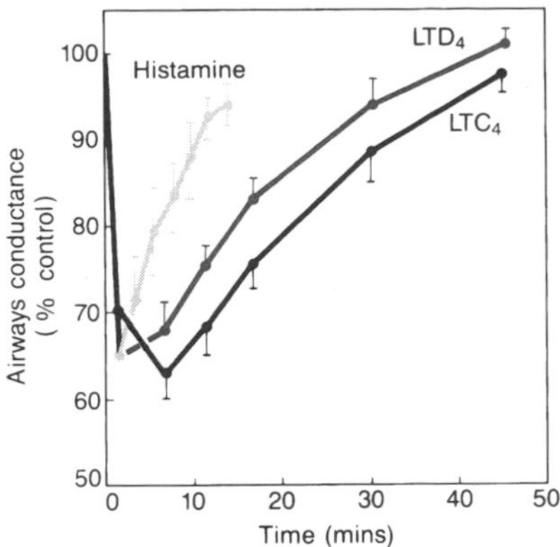

Fig. 11.10 The time-course of action on specific airways conductance of the cysteinyl-leukotrienes and histamine, in six normal subjects. Specific airways conductance was measured in a constant volume whole body plethysmograph and the drugs were given by inhalation. (From: Barnes P J, Piper P J, Costello J K 1984 Thorax 39: 500)

cally in the nose, LTD_4 increases nasal blood flow and increases local vascular permeability.

The role of leukotrienes in inflammation

LTB_4 can be found in inflammatory exudates and is present in the tissues in many inflammatory conditions, including rheumatoid arthritis, psoriasis (a chronic skin disease) and ulcerative colitis. The cysteinyl-leukotrienes are present in the sputum of chronic bronchitis in amounts which are biologically active. On antigen challenge they are released from samples of human asthmatic lung in vitro and into nasal lavage fluid in vivo in subjects with allergic rhinitis. There is evidence that they contribute to the underlying bronchial hyper-reactivity in asthmatics and it is thought that they are among the main mediators of both the early and late phases of asthma (p. 355, Fig. 17.2). An LTD_4 antagonist, **accolate,** has shown promise in the treatment of asthma (see Ch. 17.). It is also possible that cysteinyl-leukotrienes have a role in the cardiovascular changes of acute anaphylaxis.

Agents which inhibit the enzymes that generate the leukotrienes—5-lipoxygenase inhibitors—are under development as anti-asthmatic agents (e.g. **zileutin**; see Ch. 17) and anti-inflammatory agents. For a simple review, see McMillan & Walker (1992).

Leukotrienes (LTs)

- 5-lipoxygenase acts on arachidonate to give 5-HPETE which is converted by a dehydrase to LTA_4. This can be converted to either LTB_4 or to a series of cysteinyl-leukotrienes, LTC_4, LTD_4 and LTE_4, which have amino acids incorporated in their structure.
- LTB_4, acting on specific receptors, causes adherence, chemotaxis and activation of polymorphs and monocytes, and stimulates proliferation and cytokine production from macrophages and lymphocytes.
- The cysteinyl-leukotrienes cause:
  - — contraction of bronchial muscle
  - — vasodilatation in most vessels, but coronary vasoconstriction.
- LTB_4 is an important mediator in all types of inflammation; the cysteinyl-leukotrienes are of particular importance in asthma.

PLATELET-ACTIVATING FACTOR (PAF)

Platelet-activating factor, which is also variously termed *PAF-acether* and *AGEPC* (acetyl-glyceryl-ether-phosphorylcholine), is a biologically active lipid which can produce effects at exceedingly low concentrations (less than 10^{-10} mol/l). The name platelet-activating factor is misleading, since PAF has actions on a variety of different target cells and is believed to be an important mediator in both acute and persisting allergic and inflammatory phenomena. For a simple review see Page (1994).

PAF (Fig. 11.11) is derived from its precursor, acyl-PAF, by phospholipase A_2 activity, resulting in

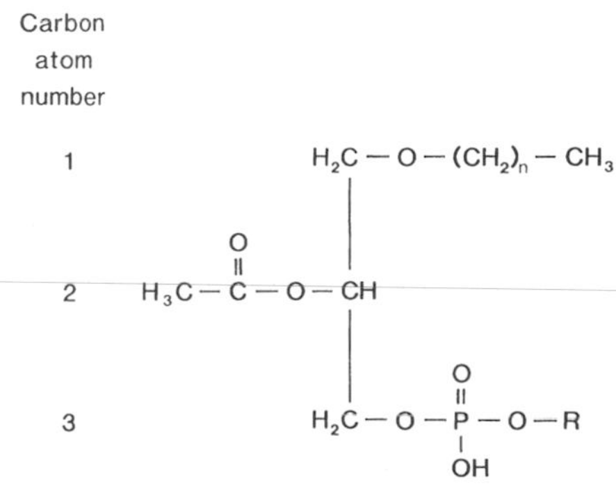

Fig. 11.11 The structure of PAF (platelet-activating factor). An O-alkyl residue is attached to carbon atom 1 (cf. Fig. 11.6). It may be hexadecyl or octadecyl; compounds containing either of these have PAF activity. (R = choline)

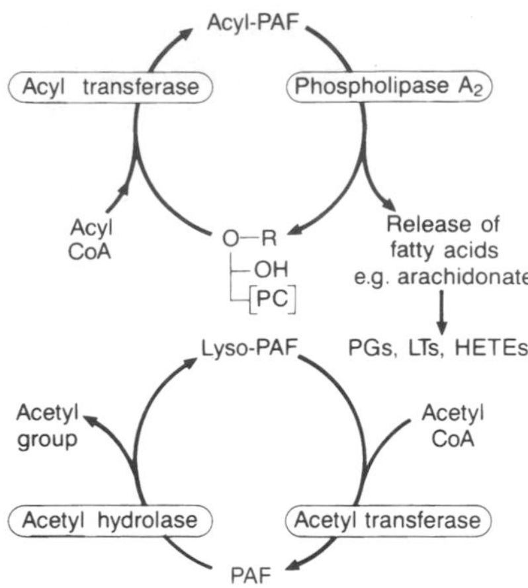

Fig. 11.12 The synthesis and breakdown of platelet-activating factor (PAF). (PC = phosphorylcholine; PG = prostaglandin; LT = leukotriene; HETE = hydroxyeicosatetraenoic acid)

'lyso-PAF' which is then acetylated to give PAF, which in turn can be deacetylated to lyso-PAF (Fig. 11.12).

Sources of PAF

PAF is generated and released from most inflammatory cells when these are stimulated. Thus it is released from neutrophil polymorphs on phagocytosis of opsonised particles, from activated macrophages and eosinophils, from mast cells and basophils on interaction with antigen and from platelets on stimulation with thrombin. Inflammatory cells have all the enzymes necessary both for the synthesis and inactivation of PAF, and an increase in cytosolic calcium in these cells is involved in stimulation of the synthesis and subsequent breakdown of this agent.

Actions

Acting on specific receptors, PAF has a wide range of pathophysiological actions and is capable of producing many of the phenomena of inflammation. In doses of 0.02–200 pmol injected locally, it produces not only local *vasodilatation* and thus erythema, but also *increased vascular permeability* and wheal formation. Higher doses produce *hyperalgesia*. It is a potent *chemotaxin* for polymorphs and monocytes and is important in *recruiting eosinophils* into the bronchial mucosa in the late phase of asthma (Fig. 17.2). It can stimulate activation of phospholipase A_2 with generation of eicosanoids.

On platelets, it causes *shape change* and the release of the contents of dense granules and of α_1 and α_2 granules. This effect is associated with metabolism of arachidonate and thromboxane A_2 generation and is important in haemostasis and thrombosis (see Ch. 16). PAF is also a *spasmogen* on both bronchial and ileal smooth muscle; its spasmogenic activity for human bronchial muscle may be due either to PLA_2 activation with resultant generation of cysteinyl-leukotrienes and/or be dependent on the presence of platelets.

The anti-inflammatory actions of the **glucocorticoids** are due, at least in part, to inhibition of PAF synthesis by virtue of the inhibitory effect of lipocortin on phospholipase A_2 (Fig. 11.5).

Competitive antagonists of the actions of PAF and/or specific inhibitors of lyso-PAF acetyl transferase could well be useful anti-inflammatory drugs. The former have been under test as anti-asthmatic agents (see Ch. 17).

Platelet-activating factor (PAF)

- PAF is released indirectly from many activated inflammatory cells by PLA_2 activity and acts on specific receptors in many cell types.
- Pharmacological actions: causes vasodilatation, increases vascular permeability, is chemotactic for leucocytes (especially eosinophils), activates leucocytes, activates and aggregates platelets and is spasmogenic for smooth muscle.
- It is a mediator in many types of inflammation and is implicated in bronchial hyper-responsiveness and in the delayed phase of asthma.

BRADYKININ

Bradykinin and the closely related peptide *kallidin* are vasoactive peptides formed by the action of enzymes on protein substrates termed *kininogens*. Information on these peptides derived originally from two separate lines of research. Werle and his colleagues described *kallikrein*, an enzyme in urine, that acts on serine proteins to liberate kallidin that causes a fall in blood pressure. Independently, Rocha e Silva and his co-workers showed that certain snake venoms, when incubated with serum, gave rise to a hypotensive substance which also caused a slow contraction of certain smooth muscle preparations. Because of this slow action it was called *bradykinin*. The two substances are now known to be virtually identical (see Fig. 11.14), kallidin possessing one additional amino acid.

Source and formation of bradykinin

An outline of the formation of bradykinin is given in Figure 11.13. Prekallikrein is present in plasma as the inactive precursor of the enzyme kallikrein. The substrate is *kininogen*—a plasma α-globulin. There are two forms of kininogen in plasma: high-molecular-weight kininogen (M_r 110 000) and low-molecular weight kininogen (M_r 70 000). Prekallikrein can be converted to the active enzyme (which is a serine protease) in a variety of ways. One of the physiological activators, particularly in the context of inflammation, is Hageman factor (factor XII of the blood clotting sequence; see Ch. 16 and Fig. 11.1).

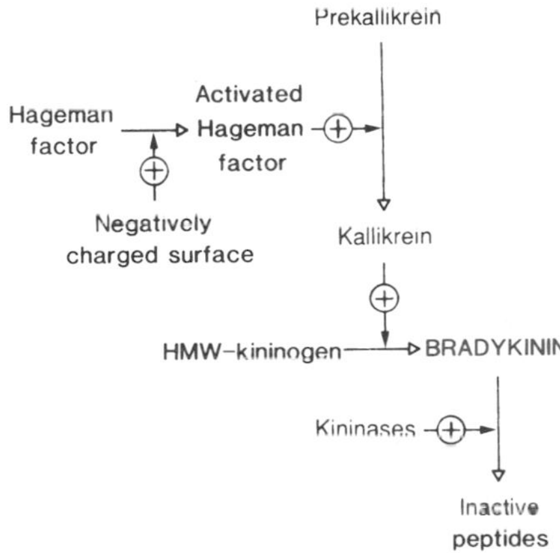

Fig. 11.13 The generation and breakdown of bradykinin. HMW-kininogen = high-molecular-weight kininogen; this substance probably acts both as a substrate for kallikrein and as a cofactor in the activation of prekallikrein.

Hageman factor is normally in inactive form in the plasma and is activated by contact with surfaces having a negative charge, such as collagen, basement membrane, bacterial lipopolysaccharides, urate crystals and so on. As a result of the increased vascular permeability which occurs in inflammation, Hageman factor, prekallikrein and the kininogens leak out of the vessels with the plasma. Contact with the negatively charged surfaces promotes the interaction of prekallikrein and Hageman factor, and this leads to kinin generation, bradykinin being clipped out of the high-molecular-weight kininogen molecules by the enzyme, which acts at two sites to release the nonapeptide (Fig. 11.14). Kallikrein can also activate the complement system, and can convert plasminogen to plasmin (see Fig. 11.1 and Ch. 16).

In addition to the plasma kallikrein described above, there are other kinin-generating kallikreins found in pancreas, salivary glands, colon and skin. Tissue kallikreins act on both high- and low-molecular-weight kininogens and generate mainly kallidin.

Inactivation of bradykinin

The main enzymes which inactivate bradykinin and related kinins are called *kininases* (Figs 11.13 and 11.14). One of these, *kininase II*, is the same as *angiotensin-converting enzyme* (see Ch. 14). This is a peptidyl dipeptidase which removes the two C-terminal amino acids from the kinin (Fig. 11.14). The enzyme is bound to the luminal surface of endothelial cells and is found mostly in the lung. It also cleaves the two C-terminal amino acids from the inactive peptide, angiotensin I, converting it to the active vasoconstrictor peptide, angiotensin II (see Chs 14 and 18). Thus, the enzyme inactivates a vasodilator and activates a vasoconstrictor. The affinity of the enzyme for kinins is two orders of magnitude higher than the affinity of the enzyme for angiotensin.

Kinins are also inactivated by the less specific *kininase I*, a carboxypeptidase present in serum (Fig. 11.14). It removes the C-terminal arginine from bradykinin generating des-Arg^9-bradykinin, which is a specific agonist at one of the two main classes of bradykinin receptor (see below).

Actions and role of bradykinin in inflammation

Bradykinin (Bk) causes vasodilatation and increased vascular permeability. Its vasodilator action is partly due to the fact that, in acting on endothelial cells, it stimulates PLA_2, generating PgI_2 (Fig. 11.5), and also causes release of nitric oxide (Chs 10 and 14). It is a potent pain-producing agent (Ch. 31), an effect which is potentiated by the prostaglandins.

Bradykinin is *spasmogenic* for several types of smooth muscle including that of the intestine and the uterus; bronchial muscle is also contracted in some species. The contraction is slow and sustained in comparison with that produced by histamine.

The pathophysiological function of bradykinin is still a matter of conjecture. The release of brady-

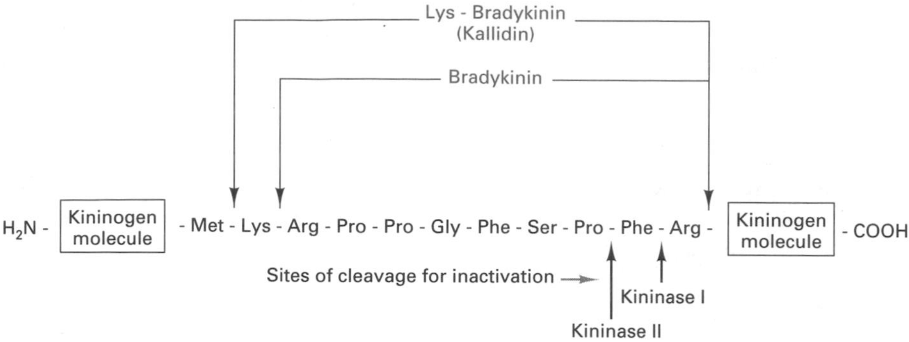

Fig. 11.14 Structure of bradykinin and some bradykinin antagonists. The sites of proteolytic cleavage for formation of kallidin and bradykinin by kallikrein from HMW-kininogen are shown in the upper half of the figure; the sites of cleavage for bradykinin inactivation are shown in the lower half. The B_2-receptor antagonist, icatibant (Hoe 140), has a pA_2 of 9, and the competitive B_1-receptor antagonist, des-Arg Hoe 140, has a pA_2 of 8. The Hoe compounds contain unnatural amino acids: Thi, D-Tic, and Oic, which are analogues of phenylalanine and proline.

kinin by tissue kallikrein may be of importance in controlling blood flow to certain exocrine glands, and thus influencing the secretions of the glands. It is known to stimulate ion transport and fluid secretion by various epithelia, including that of the intestine, the airways and the gall bladder. Excessive bradykinin production is probably a factor in causing diarrhoea in many gastrointestinal disorders, and in stimulating nasopharyngeal secretion in allergic rhinitis. It also plays a part in pancreatitis.

On the basis of experimental observations, it is capable of producing many of the phenomena seen in the inflammatory reaction—pain, vasodilatation, increased vascular permeability and spasm of smooth muscle, but its role in inflammation and allergy has not been clearly defined, not least because its effects are often part of a complex cascade of events which includes other mediators.

Bradykinin receptors

There is more than one type of bradykinin (Bk) receptor; B_1 and B_2 subtypes are currently recognised, and the existence of other subtypes has been proposed. The effects mediated by B_1 and B_2 receptors are very similar.

The characterisation of the B_1-receptor is based on the fact that Bk_{1-8} (des-Arg-Bk, which is left after kininase I action; see Fig. 11.14) is active only on a small subset of bradykinin-sensitive tissues, and that its effect is antagonised by the selective antagonists, Leu^8Bk_{1-8} and des-Arg Hoe 140 (pA_2:8; Fig. 11.14). B_1-receptors are often not seen when isolated tissues are first set up, but appear to be synthesised and expressed slowly over several hours. A similar process of induction is believed to occur during persistent inflammatory reactions.

The B_2-receptor is a catch-all category, consisting of virtually all bradykinin receptors which are not B_1 and subsuming most of the effects of bradykinin. B_2-receptors are not activated by Bk_{1-8}. B_2-receptors desensitise rapidly after activation. B_2-receptors have now been cloned and they belong to the family of G-protein-coupled receptors. Selective B_2-receptor antagonists, for example **icatibant** (Hoe 140, pA_2:9; see Fig. 11.14), have recently been developed (reviewed by Regoli et al. 1990, Cuthbert 1994). Such agents could well prove to be of value not only as investigative tools but also in the therapy of various disease states; for example some allergic conditions, carcinoid syndrome (see Ch. 8, p. 186), some gastrointestinal disorders and, possibly, also in acute pancreatitis (in which kinins released by pancreatic kallikrein contribute to the severe pain and the fluid exudation into the peritoneal cavity).

Bradykinin (Bk)

- Bradykinin is a nonapeptide. It is clipped out of kininogen, a plasma α-globulin, by a proteolytic enzyme, kallikrein.
- It is converted by kininase I, to an octapeptide, Bk_{1-8} (des-Arg-Bk), which is inactivated by angiotensin-converting enzyme in the lung.
- Pharmacological actions:
  - vasodilatation (largely endothelial cell-dependent, due both to generation of NO and activation of PLA_2 with release of PGI_2)
  - increased vascular permeability
  - stimulation of pain nerve endings
  - stimulation of epithelial ion transport and fluid secretion in airways and GIT
  - contraction of intestinal and uterine smooth muscle.
- There are two main subtypes of Bk receptors: B_1 and B_2; most Bk effects in humans are due to action on B_2-receptors.
- There are selective competitive antagonists for both B_1-receptors (des-Arg Hoe 140; pA_2:8) and B_2-receptors (icatibant, pA_2:9). Such antagonists could have therapeutic use.

CYTOKINES

Cytokines were once considered by many pharmacologists to be beyond the pale of respectable pharmacology—messy, ill-defined molecules whose actions were not only confusing, but were different when studied in different laboratories. Their very structures appeared to vary according to the method of extraction used, and each masqueraded under a plethora of different names. But recombinant DNA technology has revolutionised the situation and cytokines can now be produced in pure form and the range of their individual activities can be properly established. Some order has even been produced in the diffuse and chaotic nomenclature.

Cytokines* are peptides produced mainly from macrophages and lymphocytes but also from other leucocytes, endothelial cells and fibroblasts; they function as regulators of inflammatory and immune reactions and some are involved in multiplication and differentiation of cells and in repair processes. They are not produced constitutively but are synthesised *de novo* on cell activation. Most act locally by paracrine and/or autocrine mechanisms; exceptions being IL-1 (see below) and TNF-α (Table 11.2). On the target cell, cytokines act on specific, high affinity receptors, which, in most cases, are up-regulated in the cell when it is stimulated.

In addition to their own direct actions on cells, some cytokines induce formation of other cytokines (which could constitute a necessary amplification cascade), some induce the receptors for other cytokines, and some have complicated synergistic or antagonistic interactions with other cytokines. Cytokines have been likened to a complex signalling language with the final response of a particular cell involved being determined by a number of different messages received concurrently at the cell surface. The details of the functioning of this complex cytokine network are not yet fully understood. However, it is becoming clear that they are important pathophysiological mediators and have been shown to be implicated in the pathogenesis of numerous disease states.

The main cytokines, together with their principal actions, are listed in Table 11.2. Some cytokines thought to be of particular importance in inflammatory and immune conditions—the interleukin-1 family and the interferons—are considered in more detail below; the colony-stimulating factors are considered in Chapter 23. For simple reviews of cytokines, see Nicod (1993) and Hamblin (1994).

INTERLEUKIN-1 (IL-1)

Interleukin-1 is the term given to a family of three cytokines consisting of two active, *agonist* agents, IL-1α, IL-1β and an endogenous IL-1-receptor *antagonist* (IL-1ra). Interleukin-1 molecules are produced in infection and injury or on antigenic challenge, the primary source being the activated macrophage. IL-1α remains cell-associated and is active mainly during cell-to-cell contact, while the soluble IL-1β is the predominant form in biological fluids. On target tissues, all interleukin-1 molecules act on specific receptors, two of which have been cloned.

Several metabolic and physiological effects of interleukin-1 molecules have been reported (release of pituitary hormones, increased REM and decreased slow-wave sleep), but their main actions relate to their role as mediators or modulators of

*The term 'cytokine' subsumes the term 'lymphokine', a term which refers to a cytokine released from lymphocytes, and the term 'chemokine' is used for a cytokine which is chemotactic for leucocytes.

Table 11.2 Cytokines and their main actions

Agent	Main actions
IL-1	See text for details
IL-2	Stimulates proliferation and maturation of T_H cells (Fig. 11.4) and production of T_H cell cytokines that control the proliferation and differentiation of B cells (Fig. 11.3); induces TNF-α
IL-3 (a.k.a. multi-CSF; see Fig. 23.10)	Acts on the pluripotent haemopoietic stem cell to promote the development of granulocytes, macrophages, megakaryocytes, mast cells, erythroid cells (see Ch. 23, Fig. 23.10); activates eosinophils
IL-4	Promotes proliferation and maturation of B cells (also eosinophils and mast cells); inhibits the production of IL-1 and TNF by macrophages
IL-5	Promotes proliferation of B cells and eosinophils
IL-6	Promotes proliferation and differentiation of B cells; activates stromal bone marrow cells to produce colony-stimulating factors (Fig. 23.10); acts as a pyrogen (i.e. raises body temperature)
IL-7	Promotes proliferation of B cell progenitors
IL-8	Chemotactic for neutrophils; activates macrophages
IL-9	Enhances mast cell growth
IL-10	Inhibits clonal expansion of T cells
TNF-α and -β (tumour necrosis factor-α and -β)	On endothelial cells, it induces prostacyclin synthesis (see Ch. 16, p. 342), expression of adhesion molecules (see p. 219), synthesis of cytokines; it activates and induces expression of adhesion molecules on, and is chemotactic for, neutrophils and macrophages; it activates fibroblasts, osteoclasts and chondrocytes; TNF-α causes fever and release of acute phase proteins (see p. 224)
TGF-β (transforming growth factor-β)	Is a trophic regulator of cell proliferation and differentiation, and important in repair processes; involved in angiogenesis and in the organisation of extracellular matrix deposition; chemotactic for monocytes
PDGF (platelet-derived growth factor(s))	Cause proliferation of fibroblasts, vascular endothelial cells, smooth muscle (see Ch. 16, p. 342); implicated in angiogenesis (see p. 226), atherosclerosis (Ch. 16) and possibly in chronic asthma (Ch. 17)
IFN-γ (interferon-γ)	Induces expression of major histocompatibility complex proteins in macrophages; activates monocytes/macrophages; see text for more detail
GM-CSF (granulocyte-macrophage-colony-stimulating factor)	Is important in haemopoiesis (Ch. 23, Fig. 23.10); chemotactic for neutrophils; activates neutrophils and macrophages
β-chemokines	MIP-1α (monocyte-inflammatory protein-1α) and MCPs (monocyte chemotactic proteins) are chemotactic for monocytes and basophils, and MIP-1α is also chemotactic for lymphocytes; RANTES (**R**egulated upon **A**ctivation, **N**ormal **T** cell **E**xpressed and **S**ecreted!) is chemotactic for memory lymphocytes, monocytes, and eosinophils (see p. 218)

IL = interleukin
Cytokines not specified above are the growth factors—platelet-derived growth factor (see Ch. 16, p. 342) and epidermal growth factor—and the colony-stimulating factor, G-CSF, (which, along with GM-CSF, is important in haemopoiesis; see Ch. 23). Data from: Hamblin (1994), Davies (1994), Panayi (1994), Fan & Dale (1994); see also Arai et al. (1990)

immune and inflammatory responses. It is these actions which will be dealt with here. In the description below, the term IL-1 will be used for the active, agonist interleukin-1 molecules.

Actions of IL-1

IL-1 has a wide range of different effects on different cell types:

- It is of prime importance in the induction of the immune response, facilitating the responses of both B and T cells to antigen (see p. 221 and Figs 11.3 and 11.4).
- On vascular endothelial cells it increases synthesis of leucocyte adherence factors (see above, p. 219), stimulates NO production (Ch. 10), releases PDGF (see Table 11.2), and activates PLA_2 thus inducing synthesis of prostanoids and PAF (p. 237).
- It stimulates fibroblasts to proliferate and to synthesise collagen and to generate collagenase.
- It regulates the systemic inflammatory response —stimulating the synthesis of acute phase proteins and the increase in blood neutrophils, and causing fever by altering the set-point of temperature in the hypothalamus (see above, p. 224).
- It induces other cytokines—IL-2, the interferons, IL-3, IL-6, and, in the bone marrow, some colony-stimulating factors.
- It stimulates catabolism in certain tissues—wasting of muscle, bone resorption and degradation of cartilage.

It synergises with tumour necrosis factor α (TNF-α) for many of its actions, and its synthesis is stimulated by TNF-α. For a simple overview of IL-1, see Henderson (1994).

IL-1 is clearly of importance in combating pathogenic organisms; given to experimental animals, it reduces mortality from bacterial and fungal infections. However, as with other mediators of inflammatory and immune mechanisms, inappropriate production and action can be damaging to the host. Thus IL-1 is implicated in the pathogenesis of rheumatoid arthritis, inflammatory bowel disease and septic shock and there is also evidence for its involvement in chronic myelogenous leukaemia, insulin-dependent diabetes, osteoporosis and atherosclerosis. The pathogenesis of several other autoimmune diseases—for example autoimmune thyroiditis, psoriasis (a chronic skin disease)—has been linked to IL-1. (For an overview, see Dinarello & Wolff 1993.) A local imbalance between IL-1 and the endogenous IL-1-**r**eceptor **a**ntagonist, IL-1ra, may underlie the development and progress of some of these conditions.

The therapeutic effects of **glucocorticoids** (Ch. 21) in rheumatoid arthritis and other chronic inflammatory and autoimmune diseases may well involve inhibition of both IL-1 production and IL-1 activity. **Gold compounds** (used to treat arthritis; Ch. 12) also decrease IL-1 production. However, the effect of the glucocorticoids on IL-1 is complex because these agents also decrease production of PGE_2 and PGI_2 which down-regulate IL-1 synthesis in macrophages.

INTERFERONS

Interferons are a group of inducible cytokines synthesised in response to viral and other stimuli. There are three classes of interferon (IFN), termed IFN-α, IFN-β and IFN-γ. IFN-α is not a single substance but a family of 15 proteins with similar activities.

All interferons can be induced by other cytokines such as IL-1, IL-2, tumour necrosis factor, colony-stimulating factors. IFN-α and IFN-β are produced in many cell types—macrophages, fibroblasts, endothelial cells, osteoblasts, etc., being strongly induced by viruses, and less strongly by other microorganisms and bacterial products.

IFN-γ, also termed immune interferon, is produced mainly in antigen-activated T cells in inflammatory and autoimmune conditions, and it has a central role in controlling immune responses.

Actions of interferons

All interferons have antiviral activity, and all can induce fever and possess antitumour effects in vitro. In addition, IFN-γ has the following actions:

- induction of the expression of the major histocompatibility molecules (MHC I and II) that are involved in antigen presentation to T cells (see above, p. 223)
- induction of the expression on granulocytes of Fc receptors (important in phagocytosis; see above, p. 223)
- activation of macrophages
- promotion of differentiation of myeloid cells
- modulation of cytokine synthesis.

The production of interferon-γ during infections is beneficial in that it assists in overcoming the

Cytokines

- Cytokines are peptide regulators of inflammatory and immune reactions.
- Substances considered as cytokines include interleukins 1 to 10, the interferons, tumour necrosis factor, platelet-derived growth factor, transforming growth factor-β, the chemokines and the colony-stimulating factors.
- They act in a complex interconnecting network on leucocytes, vascular endothelial cells, mast cells, fibroblasts, haemopoietic stem cells and osteoclasts, controlling proliferation, differentiation and/or activation through autocrine or paracrine mechanisms.
- IL-1 is an important inflammatory mediator and is believed to be implicated in several important chronic inflammatory/autoimmune diseases such as rheumatoid arthritis.
- The three interferons (α, β and γ) have antiviral activity and interferon-γ has significant immunoregulatory function.

infection, but at the same time it can promote some autoimmune conditions.

Clinical use of interferons

Interferons are being used in cancer therapy (Ch. 36) and to treat virus infections (Ch. 38). Interferon-γ is undergoing trials for the therapy of hepatitis, leishmaniasis and leprosy, and interferon-β is showing promise in the treatment of multiple sclerosis.

Potential therapies based on cytokine manipulation

Modification of IL-2 function

High affinity IL-2-receptors are expressed only transiently during antigen-triggered clonal proliferation of lymphocytes. Antibodies (chimeras of mouse and human IgG) against a portion of the IL-2-receptor and complexes of IL-2 with toxins (e.g. diphtheria toxin) have both shown promise in IL-2-receptor-expressing leukaemias and lymphomas, and in some T-cell-dependent autoimmune diseases such as rheumatoid arthritis and early insulin-dependent diabetes.

Modification of IL-1 function

The endogenous antagonist to the IL-1 receptor (IL-1ra) has been cloned and is being evaluated in the treatment of conditions in which IL-1 is known to be implicated in tissue damage.

Inhibitors of the synthesis and release of IL-1 have shown efficacy in animal models of inflammation.

REFERENCES AND FURTHER READING

Arnaout M A 1990 Structure and function of the leukocyte adhesion molecules. Blood 75: 1037–1050

Arai K, Lee F, Miyajima A et al. 1991 Cytokines: coordinators of immune and inflammatory responses. Annu Rev Biochem 59: 783–836

Arrang J M, Garbarg M, Schwartz J C 1983 Autoinhibition of brain histamine release mediated by a novel class (H_3) of histamine receptor. Nature 302: 832–834

Arrang J M, Garbarg M et al. 1987 Highly potent and selective ligands for histamine H_3 receptors. Nature 327: 117–123

Balkwill F R 1989 Interferons. Lancet 1: 1060–1063

Balkwill F R, Burke F 1989 The cytokine network. Immunol Today 10: 299–304

Black J W, Duncan W A M, Durant G J et al. 1972 Definition and antagonism of histamine H_2-receptors. Nature 236: 385–390

Borden E C 1992 Interferons—expanding therapeutic roles. N Engl J Med 326: 1491–1493

Braquet P, Touqui L, Shen T Y, Vargaftig B 1987 Perspectives in platelet-activating factor research. Pharmacol Rev 39: 97–145

Coleman R A, Humphrey P A, Kennedy I, Lumley P 1984 Prostanoid receptors: the development of a working classification. Trends Pharmacol Sci 5: 303–306

Coleman R A, Humphrey P A et al. 1993 Prostanoid receptors: their function and classification. In: Vane J, O'Grady J (eds) Therapeutic applications of prostaglandins. Edward Arnold, London, ch 2: 15–36

Dale M M, Foreman J C, Fan T-P (eds) 1994 Textbook of immunopharmacology, 3rd edn. Blackwell Scientific Publications, Oxford
- Bronchud M H, Dexter T M: Leucocytosis. ch 19: 232–241
- Coleman R: Eicosanoid receptors. ch 12: 143–154
- Cuthbert A W: Kinins. ch 14: 170–178
- Dale M M: Summary of section on mediators. pp 206–207
- Dale M M, Foreman J C: Histamine. ch 10: 123–130
- Davies P: Macrophages. ch 5: 64–74
- Fan T-P: Angiogenesis. ch 23: 260–268
- Fan T-P D, Dale M M: The vascular endothelial cell. ch 8: 87–106
- Foreman J C: Mast cells and basophil leucocytes. ch 2: 21–34
- Foreman J C: Pyrogenesis. ch 21: 242–251
- Hamblin A S: Cytokines. ch 15: 179–192
- Henderson B: Interleukin-1. ch 16: 193–199
- Muid R E, Twomey B M, Dale M M: The neutrophil leucocyte. ch 3: 35–48

Page C P: The platelet. ch 4: 49–54
Panayi G S 1994 Lymphocytes Chapter 7 pp. 75–86
Richards C D, Gauldie J: The acute-phase protein response. ch 24: 269–276
Salmon J A, Higgs G A: The eicosanoids: generation and actions. ch 11: 131–142
Sim E: Complement. ch 13: 155–169
Wardlaw AJ, Moqbel R, Kay A B: The eosinophil leucocyte. ch 4: 55–63
Williams T J: Vascular changes in inflammation and mechanisms of oedema formation. ch 17: 211–217
Wilkinson P C: Cellular accumulation and inflammation. ch 19: 218–231

Dinarello C A 1993 Modalities for reducing interleukin activity in disease. Trends Pharmacol Sci 14: 155–158

Dinarello C A, Wolfe SM 1993 The role of interleukin-1 in disease. N Engl J Med 328:106–113

Duff G W 1989 Peptide regulatory network in nonmalignant disease. Lancet 1: 1432–1435

Editorial 1994 IgE declares war on parasites. Lancet 343: 309–310

Editorial 1991 Kinins and their antagonists. Lancet 338: 287–288

Folkman J, Klagsburn M 1987 Angiogenic factors. Science 235: 442–447

Ganellin C R, Parsons M E (eds) 1982 Pharmacology of histamine receptors. Wright, Bristol, p 481

Giles H 1990 More selective ligands of eicosanoid receptor subtypes improve prospects in inflammatory and cardiovascular research. Trends Pharmacol Sci 11: 301–304

Glaser K B, Mobilio D et al. 1993 Phospholipase A_2 enzymes: regulation and inhibition. Trends Pharmacol Sci 14: 92–98

Hamblin A, Brennan F 1989 Cytokines. Trends Pharmacol Sci 10: 299–304, centrefold chart

Hill S J 1990 Distribution, properties, and functional characteristics of three classes of histamine receptor. Pharmacol Rev 42: 46–81

Jaffe H S, Bucalco L R, Sherwin S A 1992 Anti-infective applications of interferon-gamma. Marcel Dekker, New York

Janeway C A 1993 How the immune system recognises invaders. Scientific American 269: 48–55

Kincade P W 1993 Sticking to the point. Nature 361: 15–16 (This article is on cytokines and adhesion molecules)

Lands W E 1981 Actions of anti-inflammatory drugs. Trends Pharmacol Sci 2: 78–80

Lewis R A, Austen K F, Soberman R J 1990 Leukotrienes and other products of the 5-lipoxygenase pathway. N Engl J Med 323: 645–655

Lichtenstein L M 1993 Allergy and the immune system. Scientific American 269: 84–93

Liew F Y 1993 Video cytokine. Nature 365: 402

Mahan M J 1994 Revealing bacterial infection strategies. Lancet 343: 869–870

McLean A 1994 Regulation with RANTES. Lancet 343: 189–190

McMillan R M, Walker E R H 1992 Designing therapeutically effective 5-lipoxygenase inhibitors. Trends Pharmacol Sci 13: 323–330

Nicod L P 1993 Cytokines 1: overview. Thorax 48: 660–667

Nossal G J V 1993 Life, death and the immune system. Scientific American 269: 20–31

Paul W E 1993 Infectious diseases and the immune system. Scientific American 269: 56–65

Powrie F, Coffman R L 1993 Cytokine regulation of T cell function: potential for therapeutic intervention. Trends Pharmacol Sci 14: 164–168

Proud D, Kaplan A P 1988 Kinin formation: mechanisms and role in inflammatory disorders. Annu Rev Immunol: 6: 49–83

Regoli D, Rhaleb N-E, Dion S, Drapeau G 1990 New selective bradykinin receptor antagonists and bradykinin B_2 receptor characterisation. Trends Pharmacol Sci 11: 156–161

Roitt I 1994 Essential Immunology, 8th edn. Blackwell Scientific Publications, Oxford

Roth J, LeRoith D et al. 1982 The evolutionary origins of hormones, neurotransmitters and other extracellular chemical messengers. N Engl J Med 306: 523–527

Rowe P M 1994 Clinical potential for TGF-β. Lancet 334: 72–73

Salmon J A, Garland L G 1991 Leukotriene antagonists and inhibitors of leukotriene biosynthesis as potential therapeutic agents. In: Jucker E (ed) Prog Drug Res 37: 10–81

Saper C B, Breder C D 1994 The neurologic basis of fever. N Engl J Med 330: 1880–1886

Samuelsson B 1983 Leukotrienes: mediators of immediate hypersensitivity reactions and inflammation. Science 220: 568–575

Snyder D W, Fleish J H 1989 Leukotriene receptor antagonists as potential therapeutic agents. Annu Rev Pharmacol Toxicol 29: 123–143

Steinman L 1993 Autoimmune disease. Scientific American 269: 74–83

Steranka L R, Farmer S G, Burch R M 1989 Antagonists of B_2 bradykinin receptors. FASEB J 3: 2019–2025

Strom T B, Kelley V R et al. 1993 Interleukin-2 receptor-directed therapies: antibody or cytokine-based targeting molecule. Annu Rev Med 44: 343–353

Thornbury N A 1994 Inflammation: key mediator takes shape. Nature 370: 251–252

Timmerman H 1990 Histamine H_3 ligands: just pharmacological tools or potential therapeutic agents? J Med Chem 33: 411

Vane J R 1971 Inhibition of prostaglandin synthesis as a mechanism of action for aspirin-like drugs. Nature New Biology 231: 232–239

Vane J, O'Grady J (eds) 1993 Therapeutic applications of prostaglandins. Edward Arnold, London

Venge P, Dahn R, Fredens K, Peterson C G B 1988 Epithelial injury by human eosinophils. Annu Rev Resp Dis 138: S54–S57

Waldman T A 1993 The IL-2/IL-2 receptor system: a target for rational immune intervention. Trends Pharmacol Sci 14: 159–163

Whicher J 1990 Control of receptor appetite. Nature 344: 584

Wigzell H 1993 The immune system as a therapeutic agent. Scientific American 269: 94–101

12 ANTI-INFLAMMATORY AND IMMUNOSUPPRESSANT DRUGS

The main *anti-inflammatory agents* are the **glucocorticoids** and the **non-steroidal anti-inflammatory drugs**. The glucocorticoids are dealt with in detail in Chapter 21 and their immunosuppressive actions are discussed briefly at the end of this chapter; the non-steroidal anti-inflammatory drugs (NSAIDs) are dealt with below. Other anti-inflammatory drugs considered in this chapter are the **antirheumatoid agents** and **drugs used to treat gout**; the **histamine H_1-receptor antagonists** are also dealt with under this heading. The main *drugs affecting the immune response* are the **immunosuppressants**; agents which increase or modify the immune response are also briefly described.

NON-STEROIDAL ANTI-INFLAMMATORY DRUGS (NSAIDs)

Non-steroidal anti-inflammatory drugs are among the most widely used of all therapeutic agents. Some important examples are listed in Table 12.1. They are frequently prescribed for 'rheumatic' musculoskeletal complaints and are often taken without prescription for minor aches and pains. There are now more than 50 different NSAIDs on the market and none of these is ideal in controlling or modifying the signs and symptoms of inflammation, particularly in the common inflammatory joint diseases. Virtually all currently available NSAIDs can have significant unwanted effects, especially in the elderly. This situation is likely to change for the better soon as a result of recent research findings.

PHARMACOLOGICAL ACTIONS

NSAIDs include a variety of different agents of different chemical classes. Most of these drugs have three major types of effect:

- *anti-inflammatory effects:* modification of the inflammatory reaction
- *analgesic effect:* reduction of certain sorts of pain
- *antipyretic effect:* lowering a raised temperature.

In general, all of these effects are related to the primary action of the drugs—inhibition of arachidonate cyclo-oxygenase and thus inhibition of the production of prostaglandins and thromboxanes—though some aspects of the action of individual drugs may occur by different mechanisms.

There are two types of cyclo-oxygenase (COX), namely COX-1 and COX-2.* COX-1 is a constitutive enzyme expressed in most tissues, including blood platelets, and is involved in cell–cell signalling and in tissue homeostasis. COX-2 is induced in inflammatory cells when they are activated and is believed to be the enzyme that produces the prostanoid mediators of inflammation. Most NSAIDs in current use are inhibitors of both isoenzymes, though they vary in the degree of inhibition of each (Meade et al. 1993, Mitchell et al. 1993). Clearly the anti-inflammatory action of the NSAIDs is related to their inhibition of COX-2 and it is probable that, when used as anti-inflammatory agents, their unwanted effects are due largely to their inhibition of

*These isoenzymes are also termed 'prostaglandin H_2 synthase (PGHS)-1 and -2'.

Table 12.1 Comparison of some commonly used NSAIDs

Drug	Plasma $t_{1/2}$ (hours)	Action			Comments
		Analg	Antipyr	Anti-infl	
Salicylic acids					
Aspirin	3–5	+	+	+	Fairly marked GIT upsets and haemorrhage. Tinnitus. Hypersensitivity reactions. Cheap and effective. A drug of first choice for mild analgesia. An encephalitis can be precipitated in children with viral infections.
Diflunisal	8–13	+	+	+	Less GIT irritation than aspirin.
Benorylate		+	+	++	Aspirin–paracetamol ester; broken down in GIT; less GIT irritation than with aspirin.
Propionic acids					All have very similar actions and side effects. Metabolised in liver. Effective and better tolerated than most other NSAIDs. Ibuprofen is a drug of first choice for inflammatory joint disease because it has the lowest incidence of unwanted effects. Fenbufen is a pro-drug, activated in the liver.
Naproxen	13	+	+	++	
Ibuprofen	2	+	+	+	
Flurbiprofen	4	+	+	+	
Fenbufen	10	+	+	–	
Ketoprofen	2	+	+	+	
Acetic acids					
Indomethacin	2	+	+	+++	One of the most potent inhibitors of cyclo-oxygenase in vitro. Clinically effective but high incidence of side effects. Headache, dizziness and GIT upsets common.
Sulindac	7(18)*	+	+	+	A pro-drug manifesting reversible activation, i.e. inter-convertible with its active sulphide metabolite; long duration of action. About half the potency of indomethacin.
Fenamates					Moderate anti-inflammatory action. GIT upsets. Diarrhoea likely. Haemolytic anaemia has been reported.
Meclofenamic acid	2	+	+	+	
Mefenamic acid	4	+	+	±	
Oxicams					
Piroxicam	45	+	+	++	GIT irritation in 20% patients. Tinnitus. Rashes. Metabolised in the liver. Is given once daily.
Tenoxicam	42–98	+	+	++	Long $t_{1/2}$ means steady state plasma concentration only after 2 weeks. Marginally less toxic than piroxicam.
Pyrazolones					
Phenylbutazone	50–100	±	+	++	Very potent. More toxic than other NSAIDs. In UK use restricted to ankylosing spondylitis.
Azapropazone	20	+	+	+	Moderate efficacy. Mild GIT irritation. Has uricosuric action.
Paracetamol	2–4	+	+	–	Safe and effective mild analgesic in therapeutic doses; less analgesic efficacy in inflammatory conditions. Chronic use can cause kidney damage. Overdose causes serious hepatotoxicity.
Tolmetin	1	+	+	+	Rapidly absorbed. Excreted in urine within 24 hours. Fairly high incidence of side effects.
Nabumetone	(24)*	+	+	++	A prodrug, converted to active metabolite in the liver. Adverse effects less marked, antipyretic effects more marked than with aspirin.

*Half-life of active metabolite
Analg = analgesic; Antipyr = antipyretic; Anti-infl = anti-inflammatory; GIT = gastrointestinal tract
See text for details of unwanted effects (p. 351)

Table 12.2 The potency of some NSAIDs on COX-1 and COX-2 (from two different studies, a and b), expressed as a ratio*: COX-2 IC_{50}/COX-1 IC_{50}

NSAID	a	b
Aspirin	166	—
Sulindac sulphide†	—	31
Indomethacin	60	22
Ibuprofen	15	1
Flurbiprofen	—	8
Piroxicam	—	10
Mefenamic acid	—	7
Diclofenac	1	—
Naproxen	1	—
Paracetamol	7‡	No effect on either enzyme
6-MNA§	—	0.14
BF389¶	0.2	—

IC_{50} = the concentration which reduces activity of the enzyme to 50% of the initial value

* The higher the figure for the ratio, the less the effect on COX-2 and the more the effect on COX-1. The figures have been rounded up.

† The active metabolite of sulindac

‡ IC_{30} value because 50% inhibition was not achieved

§ 6-Methoxy-2-naphthylacetic acid, the active metabolite of nabumetone

¶ A new compound under test

Values from: (a) Mitchell et al. (1993) — measurements of inhibition of COX-1 in intact bovine aortic endothelial cells and of COX-2 in intact macrophages stimulated with endotoxin; (b) Meade et al. (1993) — measurements in microsomal membranes from murine cells to which the cDNA of the relevant isoenzyme had been transferred by vector

COX-1. New compounds with a selective action on COX-2 are in the pipeline and could transform the approach to the treatment of inflammatory conditions. Table 12.2 gives comparisons of the inhibitory activity of some NSAIDs on COX-1 and COX-2. In summary:

- **Indomethacin**, **sulindac** and, more particularly, **aspirin**, seem to be relatively selective for COX-1; **piroxicam**, **ibuprofen**, **flurbiprofen** and **mefenamic acid** less selective.
- **Diclofenac** and **naproxen** appear to be equipotent on COX-1 and COX-2.
- BF389, a new compound, and 6-methoxy-2-napthylacetic acid, the active metabolite of the NSAID, **nabumetone**, show selective action on COX-2.

Not all NSAIDs manifest the three actions specified above to the same extent. Most are analgesic, but the degree of anti-inflammatory activity varies: some (such as **indomethacin**, **piroxicam**) are strongly anti-inflammatory, some (such as **naproxen**, **nabumetone**, **ibuprofen**) are moderately anti-inflammatory, while some (such as **paracetamol**) have essentially no anti-inflammatory activity at all.

In addition to these three categories of action, **aspirin**, in particular, has other, qualitatively different pharmacological actions (see below, p. 252).

The main pharmacological actions and the common side effects of the NSAIDs are outlined below, followed by a more detailed coverage of the salicylates and paracetamol and finally the clinical applications of the group as a whole. A comparison of some aspects of the pharmacology of some commonly used NSAIDs is given in Table 12.1.

Antipyretic effect

Normal body temperature is regulated by a centre in the hypothalamus which ensures a balance between heat loss and heat production. Fever occurs when there is a disturbance of this hypothalamic 'thermostat' that leads to the set-point of body temperature being raised. NSAIDs apparently reset the thermostat. Once there has been a return to the normal set-point, the temperature-regulating mechanisms (dilatation of superficial blood vessels, sweating, etc.) then operate to reduce temperature. Normal temperature is not affected by NSAIDs.

The mechanism of the antipyretic action of the NSAIDs is thought to be due, at least in part, to inhibition of prostaglandin production in the hypothalamus. During an inflammatory reaction, bacterial endotoxins cause the release from macrophages of a pyrogen—interleukin-1 (IL-1; Ch. 11)—and there is evidence that IL-1 stimulates the generation, in the hypothalamus, of E-type prostaglandins and that these, in turn, can cause the elevation of the set-point for temperature (reviewed by Foreman 1994). Other evidence indicates that prostaglandins are not the only mediators of fever; hence NSAIDs may have an additional antipyretic effect by mechanisms as yet unknown.

Analgesic effect

As explained in Chapter 11 and Chapter 29, several prostaglandins sensitise nociceptive afferent nerve terminals to mediators such as bradykinin. Thus, in the presence of PGE_1 or PGE_2, pain will be felt even with concentrations of inflammatory mediators, such as 5-hydroxytryptamine or bradykinin, that are too low to cause pain on their own. Recent evidence, showing that NSAIDs injected into the spinal canal can produce analgesia, suggests that inhibition of prostaglandin generation within the spinal cord may contribute to their analgesic action. NSAIDs are mainly effective against those types of pain in which prostaglandins act to sensitise nociceptors, namely pain associated with inflammation or tissue damage. Therefore, for example, they are effective in arthritis, bursitis, pain of muscular and vascular origin, toothache, dysmenorrhoea, the pain of postpartum states and the pain of cancer metastases in bone—all conditions that are associated with increased prostaglandin synthesis. In combination with opioids, they decrease postoperative pain and in some cases can reduce the requirement for opioids by as much as one-third. Their ability to relieve headache may be related to the abrogation of the vasodilator effect of prostaglandins on the cerebral vasculature.

Clinical data indicate that certain NSAIDs (e.g. **indomethacin**, **diflunisal**, **naproxen**) may also be effective in the control of some types of severe pain unrelated to inflammation (Shen 1984, Rainsford 1984).

Anti-inflammatory effects

As has been described in Chapter 11, there are many chemical mediators of the inflammatory and allergic response. Each facet of the response—vasodilatation, increased vascular permeability, cell accumulation, etc.—can be produced by several different mechanisms and, furthermore, different mediators may be of particular importance in different inflammatory and allergic conditions. Drugs such as the NSAIDs reduce mainly those components of the inflammatory and immune response in which the products of COX-2 action play a significant part, namely:

- vasodilatation
- oedema (by an indirect action; the vasodilatation facilitates and potentiates the action of mediators such as histamine which increase the permeability of postcapillary venules (p. 229)
- pain (see above).

There is conflicting evidence as to what effect NSAIDs have on *cellular accumulation* in inflammation. It has been suggested that by diverting arachidonate metabolism from the COX pathway to the 5-lipoxygenase pathway they could increase the production of the potent chemotaxin LTB_4. On the other hand, there is some evidence that many NSAIDs may *decrease* influx of leucocytes into areas of inflammation. However, such decreased influx is not a major action of NSAIDs.

Cyclo-oxygenase inhibitors, *per se*, have no effect on those processes (lysosomal enzyme release, toxic O_2 radical production) that contribute to *tissue damage* in chronic inflammatory conditions such as rheumatoid arthritis, vasculitis and nephritis. In fact, because some prostaglandins (e.g. PGE_2 and PGI_2) *decrease* lysosomal enzyme release, *reduce* the generation of toxic O_2 products and *inhibit* lymphocyte activation, NSAIDs could actually exacerbate tissue damage in the long term.* Indeed a study in 105 osteoarthritis patients indicated that the arthritis progressed more quickly in patients treated with a strong inhibitor of cyclo-oxygenase (indomethacin) than in those treated with azapropazone, a weak inhibitor (Rashad et al. 1989).

Other actions of NSAIDs

Aspirin has been reported to reduce the diarrhoea that sometimes occurs after radiation therapy for pelvic cancer and which is thought to be due to prostaglandin production in the intestinal wall. A similar production of prostaglandins may be the basis for the effect of aspirin in reducing fluid loss in experimental cholera (see Ch. 19).

One NSAID, **sulindac** (Table 12.1), is a potent inhibitor of aldose reductase in the lens of the eye. This enzyme, which reduces glucose to sorbitol, is believed to be involved in the development of cataract and peripheral neuropathy in diabetes, and sulindac is being studied for these indications.

MECHANISM OF ACTION

The main action of NSAIDs is, as stated above, *inhibition of arachidonate cyclo-oxygenase* (see Figs 11.5 and 11.8), as described originally by Vane in 1971 (p. 230).

Cyclo-oxygenase is a bifunctional enzyme, having two distinct activities—the main cyclo-oxygenase action (steps 1 and 2 in Fig. 11.8) which gives

*Certain NSAIDs can, in fact, be shown to *increase* pro-inflammatory stimuli (e.g. IL-1 generation; Bahl et al. 1994) and tissue-damaging processes (e.g. toxic oxygen radical production; Twomey & Dale 1992) by direct action on the relevant cells.

PGG_2, and a peroxidase action which converts PGG_2 to PGH_2. Different NSAIDs may inhibit the enzyme by different mechanisms, but all act at the first of the two sites, and most of the information currently available on how they affect the enzyme is derived from assays which do not distinguish between COX-1 and COX-2.

The mechanism whereby NSAIDs inhibit cyclo-oxygenase is gradually being elucidated as a result of X-ray crystallographic analysis of the enzyme and its interaction with drugs, the initial work being done on COX-1. In COX-1, the main cyclo-oxygenase site (as distinct from the peroxidase site) is a long hydrophobic channel. **Aspirin** (Fig. 12.1) causes *irreversible inactivation* of the enzyme; it acetylates the Serine 530 that is at the apex of the long channel and thereby excludes arachidonate from the channel (Picot et al. 1994). Other NSAIDs (e.g. **flurbiprofen**) bind to other sites in the channel, producing the same effect, but aspirin is the only NSAID to cause covalent, irreversible modification of the enzyme. Recovery after aspirin necessitates synthesis of new enzyme so the effect of the drug continues after the drug itself has apparently been cleared from the tissue.

Paracetamol is a weak inhibitor of both COX-1 and COX-2 (Table 12.2). This drug has analgesic and antipyretic activity but only very weak anti-inflammatory effects. It is possible that its antipyretic action is due to a selective effect on a specific COX isoenzyme in the CNS.

Other actions besides inhibition of cyclo-oxygenase may contribute to the anti-inflammatory effects of some NSAIDs. Reactive oxygen radicals produced by neutrophils and macrophages are thought to be implicated in tissue damage in some conditions, and NSAIDs that have particularly strong O_2-radical-scavenging effects as well as cyclo-oxygenase-inhibitory activity (such as **phenylbutazone** and **sulindac**) may decrease tissue damage. Furthermore, some NSAIDs may interfere with the binding of mediators (such as the chemotactic peptides derived from

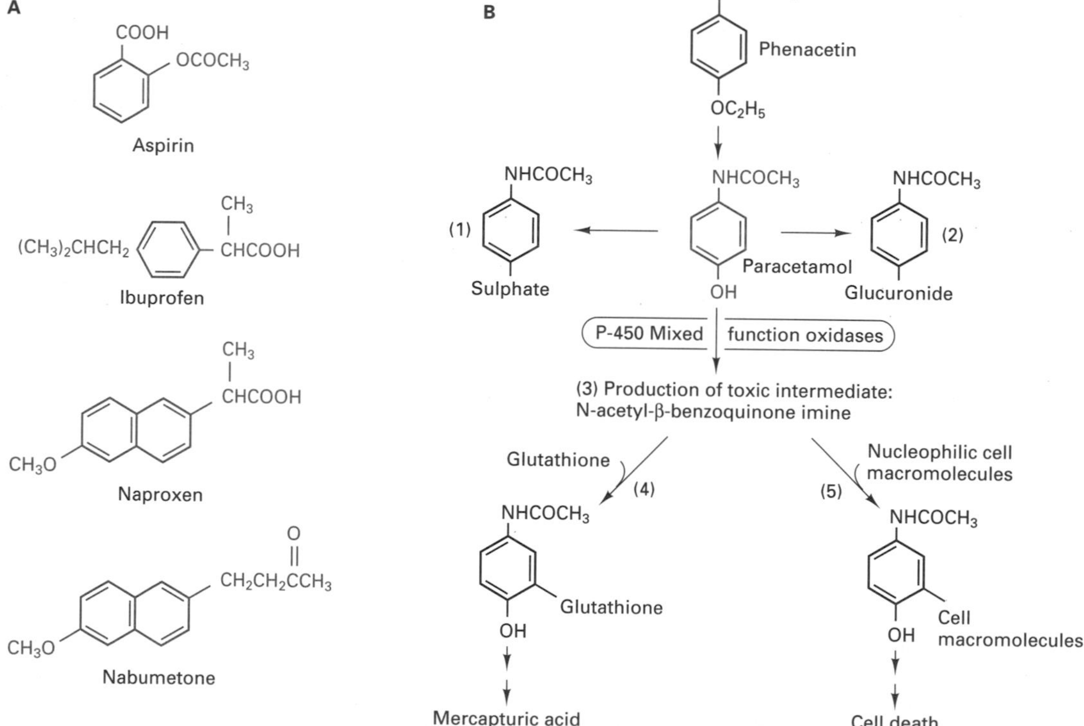

Fig. 12.1 (A) The structure of some NSAIDs; (B) the metabolism of phenacetin and paracetamol. With normal therapeutic doses paracetamol is metabolised by pathways 1 and 2, and with higher doses, by pathways 3 and 4. When glutathione is depleted, the toxic intermediate interacts with proteins and there is cell damage (reaction 5). More details on the events which can follow from reaction 5 are given in Chapter 43.

Non-steroidal anti-inflammatory drugs (NSAIDs)

NSAIDs have three major actions, all of which are due mainly to the inhibition of arachidonic acid cyclo-oxygenase in inflammatory cells (the COX-2 isoenzyme), and the resultant decrease in prostanoid synthesis.

- An anti-inflammatory action: the decrease in vasodilator prostaglandins (PGE_2, PGI_2) means less vasodilatation and, indirectly, less oedema. Accumulation of inflammatory cells is not reduced.
- An analgesic effect: decreased prostaglandin generation means less sensitisation of nociceptic nerve endings to the inflammatory mediators bradykinin and 5-hydroxytryptamine. Relief of headache is probably due to decreased prostaglandin-mediated vasodilatation.
- An antipyretic effect: this is partly due to a decrease in the mediator prostaglandin (which is generated in response to the inflammatory pyrogen, interleukin-1) that is responsible for elevating the hypothalamic set-point for temperature control in fever.

Some important examples are aspirin, ibuprofen, naproxen, indomethacin, piroxicam, paracetamol.

bacteria) to their receptors on inflammatory cells. Some of the pyrazolones have been shown to have this effect in experiments in vitro.

COMMON UNWANTED EFFECTS

Nearly a quarter of the adverse drug reactions reported officially in the UK are due to NSAIDs. These agents have also featured in the reports of drug-related deaths. Although this may be partly because NSAIDs are used extensively in the elderly, who obviously have a high mortality from natural causes, the inherent toxicity of these drugs is clearly a contributory factor. When NSAIDs are used in joint diseases (which usually necessitates fairly large doses and long-continued use) there is a high incidence of side effects—more particularly in the gastrointestinal tract but also in liver, kidney, spleen, blood and bone marrow (see Rainsford 1992). Table 12.3 outlines the risks of serious unwanted effects specific for the main NSAIDs.

Gastrointestinal disturbances

Adverse gastrointestinal events are the commonest unwanted effects of the NSAIDs, the relative risk being on average three times that in the population of non-NSAID users. Common gastrointestinal side effects are dyspepsia, diarrhoea (but sometimes constipation), nausea and vomiting. It has been estimated that one in five *chronic* users of NSAIDs will have gastric damage, which can be silent but which carries a small but definite risk of serious haemorrhage and/or perforation. Patients using **azapropazone** or **piroxicam** have the highest risk

Table 12.3 Reports of serious unwanted reactions to non-steroidal anti-inflammatory drugs*

Drug	Number of prescriptions (million)	Serious GIT reactions per million prescriptions	Other serious reactions per million prescriptions
Ibuprofen	5.47	6.6	6.6
Naproxen	4.67	32.8	8.4
Flurbiprofen	3.35	27.4	8.4
Fenbufen	1.57	35.7	33.8
Ketoprofen	3.19	33.2	5.3
Indomethacin (slow-release type)†	0.44	386.4	18.2
Sulindac	1.38	23.9	30.4
Piroxicam	9.16	58.7	9.4
Diflunisal	3.13	33.5	13.7
Azapropazone	0.91	67.0	20.9

*Taken from the CSM Update by the Committee on Safety of Medicines (1986) in Br Med J 292: 1190. The data refer to prescription-related reports on the drugs during their first five years of marketing.

†This particular formulation now withdrawn in the UK.

of gastric bleeding; there is less risk with **diclofenac** and **naproxen** and least risk with **ibuprofen** (Rodriguez & Jick 1994; Bateman 1994).

A direct irritant effect on the mucosa may contribute to the damage; it is known that tablets are more likely to cause problems than capsules, solutions or suspensions. 'Slow-release' and 'enteric-coated' preparations also cause less damage. However, NSAID-induced gastric damage is due mainly to the inhibition of the synthesis of the prostaglandins that normally inhibit acid secretion, as well as having a protective action on the mucosa and modulating its blood flow (see p. 389 and Fig. 19.2). Oral administration of prostaglandins or prostaglandin analogues such as **misoprostol** (Ch. 11, box on p. 235) can diminish gastric damage, not only in experimental animals but in man.

Skin reactions

Skin reactions are the second most common unwanted effects of NSAIDs, particularly with **mefenamic acid** (10–15% frequency) and **sulindac** (5–10% frequency). The type of skin conditions seen varies from mild rashes, urticaria, and photosensitivity reactions to more serious and potentially fatal diseases (which are fortunately rare).

Unwanted renal effects

In some patients, NSAIDs cause acute renal insufficiency. The basis of this effect is the inhibition of the biosynthesis of those prostanoids (PGE_2, PGI_2) involved in the maintenance of renal blood dynamics, and more particularly in the PGE_2-mediated compensatory vasodilatation that occurs in response to the action of noradrenaline or angiotensin II (see Ch. 18, p. 375). This syndrome, which is reversible on stopping the NSAID, does not normally occur in healthy individuals but can develop in individuals in whom there is disturbance in the noradrenergic and renin–angiotensin systems, or other kidney conditions with reduced blood flow.

Data accumulated between 1953 and 1963 indicated that *chronic* NSAID consumption could cause 'analgesic nephropathy' which comprised chronic nephritis and renal papillary necrosis. **Phenacetin** (see Fig. 12.1), now withdrawn, was regarded as the main culprit. It is rapidly metabolised to another NSAID, **paracetamol** (see Fig. 12.1), and there is now a suggestion that paracetamol (and possibly some other NSAIDs) taken regularly in high doses over a long period, could increase the risk of similar renal disease. However, the daily use of small doses of aspirin, on its own, is not reported to be hazardous for the kidney.

More detail on the toxic effects of NSAIDs on the kidney is given in Chapter 43, pages 803–804.

Other, much less common, unwanted effects of NSAIDs include bone marrow disturbances and liver disorders, the latter more likely if there is already renal impairment. Overdose of paracetamol causes liver failure (see below).

COMMONLY USED NSAIDs—THE SALICYLATES AND PARACETAMOL

The salicylates

Natural products that contain precursors of salicylic acid, such as willow bark (which contains the glycoside salicin) and oil of wintergreen (which contains methylsalicylate), have long been used for the treatment of rheumatism. Salicylic acid and acetylsalicylic acid (**aspirin**) were amongst the earliest drugs synthesised. **Sodium salicylate** is a salt of salicylic acid that has two-thirds of the potency of aspirin. Aspirin itself is relatively insoluble but its sodium and calcium salts are readily soluble. **Methylsalicylate** is used only in topical application. A newer member of this group is **diflunisal.**

Aspirin in non-inflammatory conditions

It is becoming increasingly clear that aspirin is of

General unwanted effects of NSAIDs

Unwanted effects are common, particularly in the elderly, and include:

- Dyspepsia, nausea and vomiting; also gastric damage in chronic users, with risk of haemorrhage, due to abrogation of the protective effect of PGE_2 on gastric mucosa.
- Skin reactions.
- Reversible renal insufficiency (in individuals who have noradrenergic- or angiotensin-mediated vasoconstriction) due to lack of compensatory PGE_2-mediated vasodilation.
- 'Analgesic-associated nephropathy'; this can occur following long-continued high doses of NSAIDs (more particularly paracetamol).
- Less commonly liver disorders, bone marrow depression.

benefit not only in inflammation but in several other conditions:

- It is now known that as a result of its antiplatelet action (Ch. 16, p. 344) low-dose aspirin is effective in reducing myocardial infarction, stroke and mortality in high-risk patients (see Ch. 16, p. 344).
- There is evidence that low-dose aspirin enhances the patency of coronary vessel grafts and that it may be of value in reducing the risk of venous thromboembolism.
- Epidemiological studies have suggested that regular and sustained use of aspirin reduces (virtually halves) the risk of cancer of the colon and possibly also rectal cancer (which between them cause 25 000 deaths a year in the UK).
- Meta-analysis of trials data (see Ch. 3) indicated that low-dose aspirin reduced the risk of pregnancy-induced hypertensive disease, with no adverse effects on the mother or the foetus (see Ch. 22); the most recent large clinicals trials have, however, been disappointing.
- Aspirin has been used to treat radiation-induced diarrhoea.

Pharmacokinetic aspects

As salicylates are weak acids they are largely unionised in the acid environment of the stomach and their absorption is thus facilitated. Aspirin is hydrolysed by esterases in the plasma and the tissues, yielding salicylate. With low therapeutic doses most of the salicylate in the plasma is protein-bound. With high concentrations, however, relatively less is bound and more is available for action in the tissues. Approximately 25% of the salicylate is oxidised, some is conjugated to give the glucuronide or sulphate before excretion and about 25% is excreted unchanged. The rate of urinary excretion is higher in alkaline than in acid urine since more of the unchanged salicylate will be ionised and therefore less will be reabsorbed in the tubules (see Ch. 4).

Because of partial saturation of the hepatic enzymes, the plasma half-life of aspirin will depend on the dose. With low dosage the $t_{½}$ is approximately 4 hours, and elimination follows first-order kinetics. With high doses (more than 4 g per day), elimination follows saturation kinetics (see Ch. 4) and the drug persists for more than 15 hours. (Note that the duration of action is not directly related to the plasma $t_{½}$ because of the irreversible nature of the action of the drug.)

Unwanted effects

Salicylate may produce local and systemic toxic effects.

Local effects. In the stomach, aspirin can give rise to a gastritis with focal erosions and bleeding due to inhibition of the gastric mucosal cyclo-oxygenase with consequent loss of the mucosal-protecting action of the prostaglandins (see 'Unwanted effects' above). A study of 200 individuals with normal digestive tracts, who were given aspirin, showed that most lost 2–6 ml of blood per day in the faeces; some lost a good deal more. In addition to the action on gastric mucosal cyclo-oxygenase, an inhibitory effect on platelet cyclo-oxygenase, specific to aspirin, with consequent decrease of platelet aggregation (see Ch. 16) would contribute to the bleeding.

Systemic effects. Salicylates have many of the general unwanted effects of NSAIDs outlined above (p. 251). In addition there are certain unwanted effects that occur specifically with salicylates.

Salicylism, a condition of chronic moderate toxicity, can occur with repeated ingestion of fairly large doses of salicylate. It is a syndrome consisting of tinnitus (noises in the head), dizziness, decreased hearing and sometimes also nausea and vomiting.

Other unwanted systemic effects include skin rashes and worsening of asthma in aspirin-sensitive patients. There is an association between aspirin intake and Reye's syndrome, which is a rare disorder in children. It is a combination of liver disorder and encephalopathy (CNS disturbances) that can follow an acute viral illness and it has a 20–40% mortality. It is not entirely clear to what extent aspirin is in fact implicated in its causation but the drug is best avoided in children with viral infections.

Salicylates can also cause various metabolic changes, the nature of which depends on the dose. Large therapeutic doses of salicylate *alter the acid–base balance and the electrolyte balance* and toxic doses have serious effects on these functions. The sequence of events with high doses is as follows: salicylates uncouple oxidative phosphorylation (mainly in skeletal muscle) leading to increased O_2 consumption and thus increased production of CO_2. This stimulates respiration. Salicylates also stimulate respiration by a direct action on the respiratory centre.

The resulting hyperventilation causes a respiratory alkalosis that is normally compensated for by renal mechanisms, involving increased bicarbonate excretion. This condition of *compensated respiratory alkalosis* can occur in patients receiving high therapeutic doses of salicylates. Larger doses can cause a depression of the respiratory centre, which leads eventually to retention of CO_2 and thus an increase in plasma CO_2. Since this is superimposed on a reduction in plasma bicarbonate, an *uncompensated respiratory acidosis* will occur. This may be complicated by a *metabolic acidosis*, which is due to the accumulation of metabolites of pyruvic, lactic and aceto-acetic acids (an indirect consequence of interference with carbohydrate metabolism) and the acid load associated with the salicylate itself.

Hyperpyrexia is likely to be present owing to the increased metabolic rate, and dehydration may follow from excessive vomiting.

With toxic doses of salicylates, *disturbance of haemostasis* can also occur, mainly as a result of an action on platelet aggregation. The effect of these doses on the CNS is, initially, stimulation with excitement but eventually coma and respiratory depression.

Salicylate poisoning, with the signs and symptoms outlined above, occurs more commonly, and is more serious, in children than in adults. The acid–base disturbance seen in children is usually a metabolic acidosis whereas that in adults is a respiratory alkalosis. Salicylate poisoning constitutes a medical emergency and the treatment entails correction of the acid–base disturbance, therapy for the dehydration and hyperthermia, and maintenance of kidney function. Gastric lavage and forced alkaline diuresis are used for removal of the drug (the latter procedure only if there is adequate circulatory and renal function).

Some important interactions with other drugs

Aspirin causes a potentially hazardous increase in the effect of warfarin, partly by displacing it from plasma proteins (Ch. 42) and partly because its effect on platelets interferes with haemostatic mechanisms (see Ch. 16). Sodium salicylate does not have this effect. Aspirin interferes with the effect of uricosuric agents such as **probenecid** and **sulphinpyrazone**, and since low doses of aspirin may, on their own, reduce urate excretion, aspirin should not be used in gout.

The salicylates

- Aspirin (acetylsalicylic acid), the main salicylate, causes irreversible inactivation of cyclo-oxygenase, acting mainly on the constitutive enzyme, COX-1.
- In addition to its anti-inflammatory actions, aspirin inhibits platelet aggregation and is important in the therapy of myocardial infarction.
- Salicylates are given orally and are rapidly absorbed because they are largely unionised in the acid pH of the stomach; 75% metabolised in the liver.
- Elimination follows first-order kinetics with low doses ($t_{½}$ = 4 h) and saturation kinetics with high ($t_{½}$ > 15 h).

Unwanted effects

- With therapeutic doses some gastric bleeding, usually minimal, is common.
- With large doses: dizziness, tinnitus and gastric upsets ('salicylism'). Compensated respiratory alkalosis may occur.
- With very large doses: uncompensated respiratory acidosis plus metabolic acidosis, the latter seen particularly in children.
- Aspirin can cause a hazardous increase in warfarin action (see also Table 12.1).

Paracetamol

Paracetamol (called acetaminophen in the USA) is one of the most commonly used non-narcotic analgesic–antipyretic agents. It has only weak anti-inflammatory activity. Its mechanism of action and the possible explanation of its differential actions on pain and inflammation are discussed above. In structure it is a para-aminophenol derivative (Fig. 12.1).

Pharmacokinetic aspects

Paracetamol is given orally and is well absorbed; peak plasma concentrations are reached in 30–60 minutes. A variable proportion is bound to plasma proteins and the drug is inactivated in the liver, being conjugated to give the glucuronide or sulphate (reactions 1 and 2 in Fig. 12.1). The plasma half-life of paracetamol with therapeutic doses is 2–4 hours but with toxic doses the half-life may be extended to 4–8 hours.

Unwanted effects

With therapeutic doses, side effects are few and uncommon, though allergic skin reactions sometimes

Paracetamol

- Has analgesic, antipyretic but not anti-inflammatory actions.
- It is given orally and metabolised in liver ($t_{1/2}$ = 2–4 h).
- Toxic doses cause nausea and vomiting, then, after 24–48 hours, potentially fatal liver damage by saturating normal conjugating enzymes causing the drug to be converted by mixed function oxidases to N-acetyl-p-benzoquinone imine. This, if not inactivated by conjugation with glutathione, reacts with cell proteins and kills the cell.
- Agents which increase glutathione (acetylcysteine orally or i.v.) or which increase conjugation reactions (e.g. methionine) can prevent liver damage if given early.

Clinical uses of the NSAIDs

- For analgesia in painful conditions (e.g. headache, dysmenorrhoea, backache, bony metastases of cancers, postoperative pain):
  - —the drugs of choice for short-term analgesia are **aspirin**, **paracetamol** and **ibuprofen**; more potent, longer-acting drugs (**diflunisal**, **naproxen**, **piroxicam**) are useful for chronic pain
  - —the requirement for narcotic analgesics can be markedly reduced by NSAIDs in some patients with bony metastases or postoperative pain.
- For anti-inflammatory effects in chronic or acute inflammatory conditions (e.g. rheumatoid arthritis and related connective tissue disorders, gout and soft tissue diseases). With many NSAIDs, the dosage required for chronic inflammatory disorders is considerably greater than for simple analgesia and treatment may need to be continued for long periods; thus side effects and toxic effects are likely to be seen. Treatment could be initiated with an agent known to have a low incidence of side effects, such as **ibuprofen**. If this proves unsatisfactory, more potent agents (see Table 12.1) should be used.
- To lower temperature. **Paracetamol** is preferred because it lacks gastrointestinal side effects and, unlike aspirin, has not been associated with Reye's syndrome in children.

There is substantial individual variation in clinical response to NSAIDs and considerable unpredictable patient preference for one drug rather than another.

occur. Regular intake over a long period is thought to increase the risk of kidney damage (see above, p. 252).

Toxic doses (i.e. two to three times the maximum therapeutic dose) cause a serious, potentially fatal hepatotoxicity. Renal toxicity is also reported. These toxic effects occur when the liver enzymes catalysing the normal conjugation reactions are saturated, causing the drug to be metabolised by the mixed function oxidases (reaction 3 in Fig. 12.1). The resulting toxic metabolite, N-acetyl-p-benzoquinone imine is inactivated by conjugation with glutathione (reaction 4 in Fig. 12.1), but when glutathione is depleted the toxic intermediate accumulates and reacts with nucleophilic constituents in the cell. This causes necrosis in the liver and also in the kidney tubules (reaction 5 in Fig. 12.1).

The initial symptoms of acute paracetamol poisoning are nausea and vomiting, the hepatotoxicity being a delayed manifestation that occurs 24–48 hours later. Treatment entails gastric lavage followed by oral activated charcoal. Further details of the toxic effects of paracetamol are given in Chapter 43. If the patient is seen sufficiently soon after ingestion, the liver damage can be prevented by giving the following:

- agents that increase glutathione formation in the liver (**acetylcysteine**, intravenously)
- agents that increase the conjugation reactions (**methionine**, orally).

If more than 12 hours have passed since the ingestion of a large dose, the antidotes are less likely to be useful and may cause adverse effects (e.g. nausea, allergic effects).

Benorylate is an aspirin–paracetamol ester. After metabolism in the liver it releases both active constituents. There is less gastrointestinal disturbance and blood loss than with aspirin itself and as it is more slowly absorbed than paracetamol, overdosage may not cause as much hepatotoxicity. But note that there is an increased risk of kidney damage with combinations of paracetamol and aspirin.

The clinical uses of the NSAIDs are summarised opposite.

ANTIRHEUMATOID DRUGS

Agents such as the **gold compounds**, **penicil-**

lamine, **sulphasalazine**, some 4-aminoquinoline drugs—**chloroquine** or **hydroxychloroquine**—and some immunosuppressant drugs (see below, p. 261, and Ch. 36) are believed to have a specific action in modifying the disease process in rheumatoid conditions. Some have a place in the treatment of other chronic inflammatory diseases. The agents have been termed 'disease-modifying antirheumatoid drugs' (DMARDs) to point up the comparison with the NSAIDs, which reduce symptoms but do not alleviate the underlying disease process (some may indeed make it worse). **Glucocorticoids** (see Ch. 21) are also used in these conditions.

The effects of the DMARDs are slow in onset and some (e.g. penicillamine) are not thought to have a general anti-inflammatory action. DMARDs are usually used in patients in whom the disease is progressing and causing deformities, but some authorities consider that these agents could, with benefit, be used earlier—when rheumatoid arthritis is first diagnosed. These agents improve symptoms and can reduce disease activity as measured by pain score, articular index on radiology, function, vasculitis and concentration of acute-phase proteins; however, whether they halt the long-term progress of the disease is controversial, so the term 'disease-modifying' may be inappropriate.

Gold compounds are often the drugs of first choice, with penicillamine as next choice (see Wolfe & Hughes 1988); but these two agents should not be given simultaneously because penicillamine is a metal chelator.

Gold compounds

First used in 1929 for rheumatoid arthritis, gold compounds were shown to be efficacious in double-blind clinical trials in the 1960s. The preparations used are **sodium aurothiomalate** and **auranofin**. These compounds are also used in juvenile rheumatoid arthritis.

Actions and mechanism of action

Gold compounds are relatively effective in stopping the progression of bone and joint damage in rheumatoid arthritis. The action develops slowly, the maximum effect occurring after 3–4 months. Pain and joint swelling subside and the concentration of rheumatoid factor (an IgM antibody against host IgG) falls.

The precise *mechanism of action* is not fully understood. In experimental studies, gold compounds inhibit mitogen-induced lymphocyte proliferation, reduce both the release and the activity of lysosomal enzymes, decrease the production of toxic O_2 metabolites from phagocytes, inhibit chemotaxis of neutrophils and reduce the release of mast cell mediators.* They can decrease production of IL-1. Any or all of these effects could be involved in their beneficial effects in rheumatoid disease.

Pharmacokinetic aspects

Sodium aurothiomalate is given by deep intramuscular injection; auranofin is given orally. Peak plasma concentrations of aurothiomalate are reached in 2–6 hours, most of the drug being bound to plasma protein. However, the compounds gradually become concentrated in the tissues, not only in synovial cells in joints (where the concentration is 50% of the plasma concentration) but also in macrophages throughout the body, and in liver cells, kidney tubules and the adrenal cortex. The gold complexes remain in the tissues for some time after treatment is stopped. Excretion is mostly renal, but some is excreted in the gastrointestinal tract. The $t_{1/2}$ is 7 days in the initial stages but increases with treatment, so it must be given with lengthening intervals between doses.

Unwanted effects

Unwanted effects with aurothiomalate are seen in about one-third of patients treated, and serious toxic effects in about 1 patient in 10. Unwanted effects with auranofin are less frequent and less severe.

Important unwanted effects are skin rashes (which can be severe), mouth ulcers, proteinuria and blood dyscrasias. Encephalopathy, peripheral neuropathy and hepatitis can occur. If therapy is stopped when the early symptoms appear, the incidence of serious toxic effects is relatively low.

Penicillamine

In early studies on penicillin, Abraham and his co-workers found dimethylcysteine among the substances produced by hydrolysis of penicillin and

*Aurothiomalate, though effective in vivo, is not effective in some in vitro studies (e.g. in inhibiting production of toxic oxygen metabolites) but there is evidence that it can be converted in the body to aurocyanide, which may be the active form in vivo (Graham & Dale 1990, Champion et al. 1990).

named it penicillamine. The D-isomer is used in the therapy of rheumatoid disease. It also has a role in the therapy of Wilson's disease and cystinuria (see below).

Actions and mechanism of action

About 75% of patients with rheumatoid arthritis respond to penicillamine. The effects take weeks to start and the main response is not seen for several months. The swelling of joints gradually subsides and nodules disappear. The plasma concentration of rheumatoid factor falls in most patients as does the concentration of acute-phase proteins and thus the erythrocyte sedimentation rate. The delayed hypersensitivity component of the disease process is decreased—possibly due to interference with macrophage function and thus decreased release of IL-1.

Penicillamine is also thought to modify rheumatoid disease by an effect on collagen synthesis, preventing the maturation of newly synthesised collagen. It acts at a late stage of collagen cross-linking.

The mechanism of action is still a matter of conjecture. The drug is known to have metal-chelating properties, an effect that is made use of in the treatment of hepatolenticular degeneration (Wilson's disease), in which there is copper accumulation in liver, kidneys and brain.

Penicillamine is a highly reactive thiol compound, and in addition to chelating metals, can substitute for cysteine in cysteine disulphide, the resulting complex being very much more soluble. This is the basis of its use in cystinuria—an inheritable disorder in which there is a defect in the transport of certain amino acids, associated with a very high concentration of cysteine in the urine.

Pharmacokinetic aspects

Penicillamine is given orally and only half the dose administered is absorbed. It reaches peak plasma concentrations in 1–2 hours, is 80% bound to plasma protein and excreted in the urine. Dosage is started low and increased only gradually to avoid unwanted effects.

Unwanted effects

Unwanted effects occur in about 40% of patients treated with penicillamine and may necessitate cessation of therapy. Anorexia, nausea and vomiting and disturbances of taste (the latter related to the chelation of zinc) are seen but often disappear with continued treatment. In 20% of patients proteinuria occurs. Rashes and stomatitis are the most common unwanted effects and may resolve if the dosage is lowered, as may dose-related thrombocytopenia. Other bone marrow disorders (leucopenia, aplastic anaemia) are absolute indications for stopping therapy, as are the various autoimmune conditions (e.g. thyroiditis, myasthenia gravis) that sometimes supervene.

Chloroquine

Chloroquine is a 4-aminoquinoline drug used mainly to treat malaria (Ch. 40). It has been shown to cause remission of rheumatoid arthritis but it does not retard the progression of bone damage. It is also used in both systemic and discoid lupus erythematosus.

Actions and the mechanism of action

Pharmacological effects do not come on until a month or more after the drug is started, and about half the patients treated respond. Joint swelling subsides and the concentration of rheumatoid factor is reduced.

The mechanism of action of chloroquine is not fully understood. The drug inhibits mitogen-induced lymphocyte proliferation and decreases leucocyte chemotaxis, lysosomal enzyme release and generation of toxic oxygen metabolites. It also reduces the generation of IL-1. Some of these effects may follow from the fact that it has a lysosomotrophic action, being concentrated in and raising the pH of lysosomes, particularly in phagocytic cells such as macrophages, and thus interfering with the action of the acid hydrolases.

Some effects may result from the fact that it inhibits phospholipase A_2 and therefore reduces the formation of the eicosanoids and also PAF (p. 237). It may also intercalate in the DNA and inhibit DNA and RNA synthesis, as it does in microorganisms.

Pharmacokinetic aspects and unwanted effects

The pharmocokinetic aspects and unwanted effects of chloroquine are dealt with in Chapter 40.

Sulphasalazine

Sulphasalazine was introduced for use in rheumatoid arthritis but fell into disuse for this condition and for some time now has been used mainly for chronic inflammatory bowel disease. Recent controlled trials have indicated that it is after all of value in producing remission in active rheumatoid arthritis. Only enteric-coated capsules are licensed for use in rheumatoid arthritis.

The mode of action of sulphasalazine is not clearly known but there is evidence that it can scavenge toxic oxygen metabolites produced by neutrophils.

This drug is a combination of sulphonamide (sulphapyridine) with a salicylate. It is thought to be split into its component parts in the body; both moieties may be important but 5-amino-salicylic acid is the radical scavenger. It is poorly absorbed after oral administration. Unwanted effects are usually not serious. The common side effects are gastrointestinal disturbances, malaise and headache. The absorption of folic acid is sometimes impaired; this can be countered by giving folic acid supplements. A reversible decrease in sperm count has also been reported. As with other sulphonamides, there is a possibility that blood dyscrasias and anaphylactic-type reactions will occur in a few patients.

DRUGS USED IN GOUT

Gout is a genetically determined metabolic disease in which there is over-production of purines. It is characterised by intermittent attacks of acute arthritis produced by the deposition of crystals of sodium urate (a product of purine metabolism) in the synovial tissue of joints. An inflammatory response is evoked, involving activation of the kinin, complement and plasmin systems (see Ch. 11 and Fig. 11.1), generation of lipoxygenase products such as LTB_4 (Fig. 11.9) and local accumulation of neutrophil granulocytes (Fig. 11.2). These engulf the crystals by phagocytosis, which causes generation of tissue-damaging toxic oxygen metabolites and subsequently lysis of the cells with release of proteolytic enzymes. Urate crystals also induce the production of IL-1 (Ch. 11, p. 241).

Drugs used to treat gout may act in the following ways:

- by inhibiting uric acid synthesis (**allopurinol**)
- by increasing uric acid secretion (uricosuric agents: **probenicid, sulphinpyrazone**)
- by inhibiting leucocyte migration into the joint (**colchicine**)
- by general anti-inflammatory and analgesic effects (**NSAIDs**; see p. 248).

Allopurinol

Allopurinol reduces the synthesis of uric acid by inhibiting xanthine oxidase (Fig. 12.2). It is an analogue of hypoxanthine and inhibits the enzyme mainly by substrate competition. Some degree of inhibition of de novo purine synthesis also occurs. Allopurinol is converted to alloxanthine by xanthine oxidase and this metabolite, which remains in the tissue for a considerable time, is an effective non-competitive inhibitor of the enzyme. The pharmacological action of allopurinol is largely due to alloxanthine.

The result of the action of the drug is that the concentration of the relatively insoluble urates and uric acid in tissues, plasma and urine decreases, while that of the more soluble xanthines and hypoxanthines increases. The deposition of urate crystals in tissues ('tophi') is reversed and the formation of renal stones is inhibited.

Allopurinol is the drug of choice in the long-term treatment of gout, but it is ineffective in the treatment of an acute attack and indeed makes this worse.

Pharmacokinetic aspects

Allopurinol is given orally, is well absorbed in the gastrointestinal tract, reaches peak plasma concen-

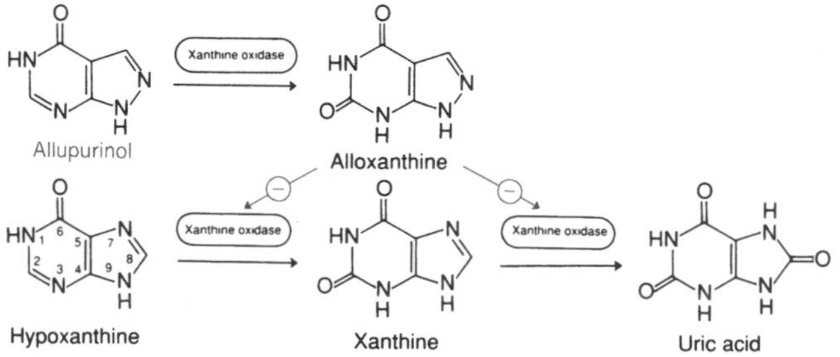

Fig. 12.2 Inhibition of uric acid synthesis by allopurinol. (See text for details.)

trations in 30–60 minutes and is distributed throughout the body water. Its half-life is 2–3 hours; it is converted to alloxanthine (Fig. 12.2) which has a half-life of 18–30 hours. Neither allopurinol nor its metabolite are bound to plasma protein. Only a small proportion of allopurinol or its metabolite is excreted as such in the urine, renal excretion being a balance between glomerular filtration and probenecid-sensitive tubular reabsorption.

Unwanted effects

Unwanted effects are few. Gastrointestinal disturbances, allergic reactions (mainly skin rashes) can occur, but disappear if the drug is stopped. Acute attacks of gout sometimes occur during the early stages of therapy.

Some important drug interactions. Allopurinol increases the effect of **mercaptopurine**, an antimetabolite that may be used in cancer chemotherapy, and also enhances the effect of another anticancer drug, **cyclophosphamide** (Ch. 36). The effect of **oral anticoagulants** is increased due to inhibition of their metabolism.

Uricosuric agents

Uricosuric agents are drugs that increase uric acid excretion by a direct action on the renal tubule. Examples are **probenecid** and **sulphinpyrazone** and the newer classes of *uricosuric diuretics* derived from ethacrynic acid (discussed in Ch. 18, p. 384).

Colchicine

Colchicine has a specific effect in gouty arthritis and can be used both to prevent and to relieve acute attacks. Its main effect is to prevent the migration of neutrophils into the joint. Its mechanism of action is thought to be by binding to *tubulin*, the protein of the microtubules, resulting in their depolymerisation. In cells such as neutrophils this effect of colchicine interferes with motility; when observed in vitro, colchicine-treated cells have a 'drunken walk'. There is some evidence that colchicine prevents the production of a putative inflammatory glycoprotein by neutrophils that have phagocytosed urate crystals.

Pharmacokinetic aspects

Colchicine is given orally, is well absorbed and reaches peak concentrations in about an hour. It is excreted partly in the gastrointestinal tract and partly in the urine.

Unwanted effects

The unwanted effects of colchicine are largely gastrointestinal—nausea, vomiting and abdominal pain. Severe diarrhoea may be a problem and with large doses may be associated with gastrointestinal haemorrhage and kidney damage. Rashes sometimes occur, also peripheral neuropathy. Long courses of treatment have occasionally resulted in blood dyscrasias.

ANTAGONISTS OF HISTAMINE

At present there are two classes of histamine antagonists: H_1- and H_2-receptor antagonists. The former group was introduced first by Bovet and his colleagues in the 1930s, at a time when the classification of the histamine receptors had not been elucidated. (Indeed the elucidation was possible only because these agents were available.) The term 'antihistamine' conventionally refers to the H_1-receptor antagonists, which affect various inflammatory and allergic mechanisms. These drugs are discussed in this section. The more recently developed H_2-receptor antagonists, the main clinical effect of which is on gastric secretion, are discussed in Chapter 19. H_3-receptor antagonists (Table 11.1b) are at present only used as investigational tools.

H_1-receptor antagonists (H_1-antihistamines)

Mepyramine and **tripelennamine** were among the first H_1-receptor antagonists produced; as a result of further research two important groups of drugs were developed—tricyclic antidepressants and the neuroleptic phenothiazines (see Chs 28 and 29). Details of some characteristic H_1-receptor antagonists are shown in Table 12.4. All are lipid soluble and all contain a substituted ethylamine moiety.

Actions

Many of the pharmacological actions of the H_1-receptor antagonists follow from the actions of histamine outlined in Chapter 11. Thus in vitro they inhibit histamine-induced contraction of the smooth muscle of the bronchi, the intestine and the uterus. They inhibit histamine-induced bronchospasm in the guinea pig in vivo but are of little value in allergic bronchospasm in man. They inhibit the increased vascular permeability caused by histamine.

Table 12.4 Some commonly used H_1-receptor antagonists

Drug	Structure*	$t_{½}$	Sedative action	Comments
Diphenhydramine	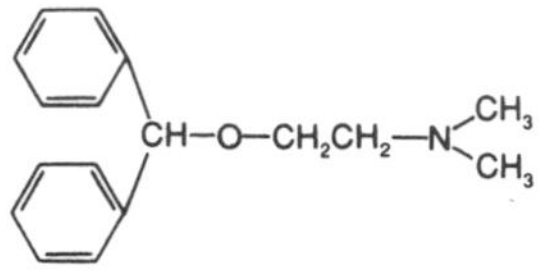	7 h	++	Some local anaesthetic action and marked muscarinic-receptor antagonism. Used in motion sickness.
Promethazine	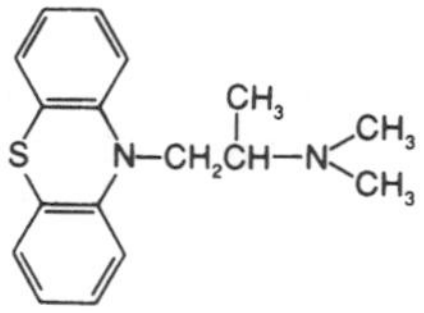	12 h	++	Some local anaesthetic action and fairly marked muscarinic-receptor antagonism. Weak α_1-receptor antagonism. Anti-emetic. Injection can be painful.
Chlorpheniramine	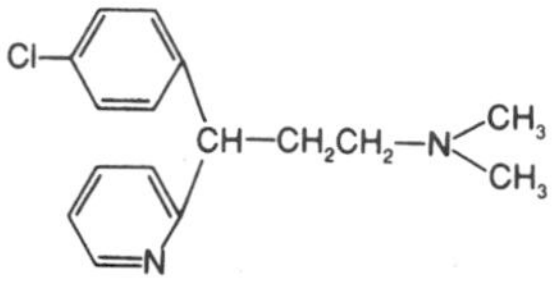	23 h	+	Potent H_1-receptor antagonism. If injected it can cause transient CNS stimulant effects.
Terfenadine	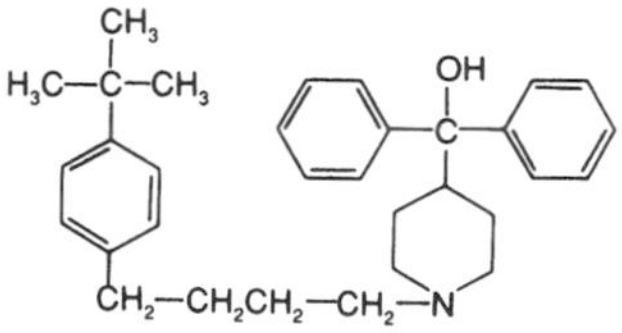	20 h	nil	Selective for H_1-receptors. No muscarinic-receptor antagonism. Peak plasma concentration within 1–2 h. Mild CNS stimulation (an 'alerting' effect) can occur.
Mequitazine	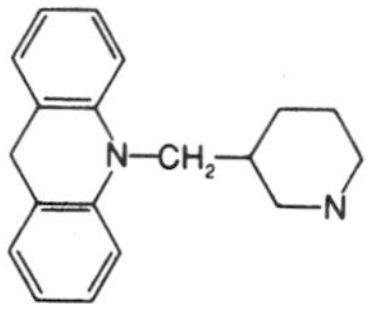	38 h	nil	Potent H_1-receptor antagonist; has minimal muscarinic-receptor antagonism. Peak plasma concentration after 6 h. High doses can impair CNS function.
Astemizole	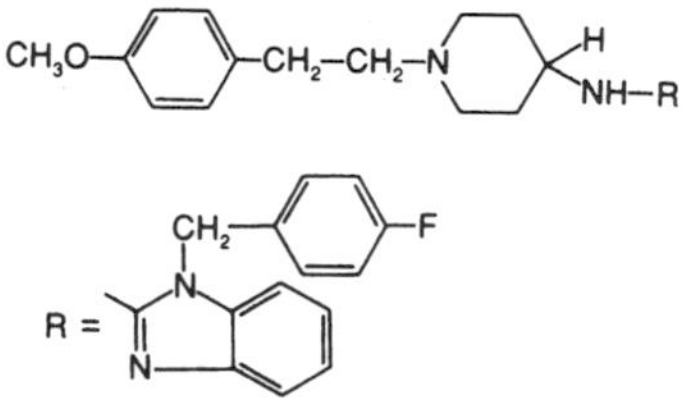	5 d (10 d)†	nil	Has minimal muscarinic-receptor antagonism. Steady state concentration not reached for several weeks; accumulation likely. Weight gain can occur. Very high doses can cause ventricular arrhythmias.

*General formula:

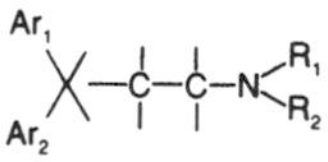

This is the general formula of the early effective H_1-receptor antagonists: Ar_1 and Ar_2 are aromatic groups. C–C represents a short chain of carbon atoms which may be saturated, branched, or part of a ring system. NR_1R_2 is generally a tertiary amino group. (See Ganellin C R 1982 In: Ganellin C R, Parsons M E (eds) Pharmacology of histamine receptors. Wright, Bristol p. 10)
† $t_{½}$ of active metabolite.

Some of the actions of these drugs do not appear to be related to blockade of H_1-receptors and may well be due to antagonist effects at other receptors such as those for 5-HT, α_1-agonists and muscarinic agonists, both peripherally and in the CNS.

Some H_1-receptor antagonists have pronounced effects in the CNS. These are usually listed as 'side effects' but they may be more clinically useful than the peripheral H_1-antagonist effects and should be recognised as such. Some are fairly strong *sedatives* and may be used for this action (e.g. **promethazine**, a phenothiazine compound; see Table 12.4). Several are *anti-emetic* and are used to prevent motion sickness (e.g. **cyclizine, dimenhydrinate, cinnarizine**; see Ch. 19, Fig. 19.8).

Many H_1-receptor antagonists (e.g. **diphenhydramine**) also show significant *antimuscarinic effects*, though their affinity is much lower for muscarinic than for histamine receptors. (As measured on the guinea-pig ileum, the pA_2 of **mepyramine**, the prototype antihistamine for the H_1-receptors, is 9.2, and for the muscarinic receptors, 5.) The combination of sedative actions with central muscarinic-receptor antagonism manifested by some agents (e.g. diphenhydramine) once led to their use in parkinsonism. But for circumstances in which selective H_1-receptor antagonism is desired, untrammelled by CNS effects, newer drugs have been developed, such as **terfenadine, astemizole** and **mequitazine** (see Table 12.4). Other, newer drugs which lack sedative action are **loratadine** and **cetirizine**.

Several H_1-receptor antagonists show weak blockade at α_1-adrenoceptors (an example is the phenothiazine, **promethazine**), and many have local anaesthetic activity (**diphenhydramine**, promethazine). **Cyproheptadine** (see Ch. 9) is a 5-HT antagonist as well as being an H_1-receptor antagonist. There are many other H_1-receptor antagonists in clinical use.

The clinical uses of H_1-receptor antagonists are summarised in the box on this page.

Clinical use of H_1-receptor antagonists

H_1-receptor antagonists can be used:

- For allergic reactions (see Ch. 11) including allergic rhinitis (hay fever), urticaria, insect bites, drug hypersensitivities. Drugs that lack sedative or muscarinic-receptor antagonist actions (e.g. **terfenadine** or **cetirizine**) are preferred.
- As anti-emetics for the prevention of motion sickness or other causes of nausea, especially those associated with vertigo (e.g. labyrinthine disorders). Muscarinic-receptor antagonist actions of some antihistamines (e.g. **cinnarizine, cyclizine**) probably contribute to efficacy but also cause side effects.
- For sedation: some H_1–receptor antagonists (e.g. **promethazine**; see Table 12.4) are fairly strong sedatives and may be used for this action.

Pharmacokinetic aspects

Most H_1-receptor antagonists are given orally, are well absorbed, reach their peak effect in 1–2 hours and are effective for 3–6 hours, though there are exceptions (see Table 12.4). Most appear to be widely distributed throughout the body, but some do not penetrate the blood–brain barrier, for example the non-sedative drugs (see Table 12.4). They are metabolised in the liver and excreted in the urine.

Unwanted effects

What is defined as 'unwanted' will depend to a certain extent on what the drugs are used for. When used for purely antihistamine actions, all the CNS effects are unwanted. When used for their sedative or anti-emetic actions, some of the CNS effects such as dizziness, tinnitus and fatigue are unwanted. Excessive doses can cause excitation and may produce convulsions in children.

The peripheral antimuscarinic actions are always unwanted. The commonest of these is dryness of the mouth, but blurred vision, constipation and retention of urine can also occur.

Unwanted effects not related to the drugs' pharmacological actions are also seen; thus gastrointestinal disturbances are fairly common while allergic dermatitis can follow topical application of these drugs.

IMMUNOSUPPRESSANT DRUGS

The drugs used for immunosuppression are **cyclosporin, glucocorticoids**, cytotoxic agents such as **azathioprine** and **cyclophosphamide**, and **anti-lymphocyte immunoglobulin**.

Cyclosporin*

Cyclosporin is a fungal peptide with powerful immunosuppressive activity, unique in that it has selective effects on lymphocytes. It was discovered by Borel and his co-workers in 1976 in the course of screening fungal products for antifungal activity. Cyclosporin was found to have only weak antifungal activity but during the concomitant toxicity testing proved to have a remarkable inhibitory effect on lymphocyte proliferation (reviewed by Borel 1994).

It is a cyclic peptide of 11 amino acids, several of which are N-methylated and one of which was previously unknown. The peptide (M_r 1203) is neutral and is unusually rich in hydrophobic amino acids; this makes it insoluble in water but soluble in lipids and other organic solvents.

Actions

Cyclosporin has revolutionised the field of organ transplantation, significantly reducing the morbidity and the incidence of rejection.

In laboratory experiments it can be shown to suppress reversibly both cell-mediated and antibody-mediated responses (Figs 11.3 and 11.4), and the therapeutic ratio for most effects is significantly greater than that of other immunosuppressive agents. It has no effect on the acute inflammatory response per se.

Cyclosporin is mainly effective in reactions in which *cell-mediated responses* play a major part, but has a marked suppressive action on some *antibody-mediated responses*, notably those which involve T helper cells, but has little effect on antibody production against antigens that stimulate B cells directly (see Ch. 11, p. 221). In general it is effective mainly at the *induction phase* of the immune response—at the phase of antigen recognition and clonal proliferation (see Figs 11.3 and 11.4) though some T cell *effector mechanisms* are also affected.

Mechanism of action

Cyclosporin has a relatively selective action on T lymphocytes. It acts at the induction stage (see Figs 11.3 and 11.4) and stops clonal proliferation of T cells by an effect at two different sites. The main effect is inhibition of the transduction pathway for the synthesis of lymphokines, particularly interleukin-2 (IL-2) (see Fig. 11.3, p. 242). It may also inhibit the expression of IL-2 receptors on the T cells that respond to IL-2. The induction of cytotoxic T lymphocytes is inhibited but not the action of already formed cytotoxic T cells. It has no effect on suppressor T cells.

Because lymphokine synthesis and secretion from activated T cells is inhibited, T-cell-dependent B cell responses will also be suppressed (Fig. 11.3).

Cyclosporin also inhibits histamine release from mast cells, and blocks the transcription of the genes for IL-3, IL-4 and LTC_4.

The inhibitory effect on interleukin-2 production is due to a relatively selective action on IL-2 gene transcription. Normally, interaction of antigen with the T_H cell receptor results in an increase of intracellular Ca^{2+} through the $InsP_3$ pathway (Ch. 2). Ca^{2+} (with calmodulin) stimulates a phosphatase, calcineurin, that activates various transcription factors; these, in turn, set in motion the transcription of interleukin-2. Cyclosporin binds with a cytosolic protein, termed 'cyclophilin'** (a member of a group now called 'immunophilins'***); the drug–immunophilin complex binds to and inhibits calcineurin and thus interferes with activation of the T_H cell and production of IL-2 and other lymphokines. The enzymic activity of cyclophilin does not appear to be involved in this mechanism.

Two other compounds have similar actions to cyclosporin. **Fujimycin**, derived from the fermentation broth of a *Streptomyces* organism, and **rapamycin**, a natural product derived from a soil microorganism, are both structurally unrelated to cyclosporin. They bind with a different immunophilin, and the complex has the same intracellular action as the cyclosporin–cyclophilin complex.

Pharmacokinetic aspects

Cyclosporin can be given orally or by intravenous infusion. The degree of absorption from the gastrointestinal tract may vary in different individuals but peak plasma concentrations are usually attained in about 3–4 hours. The plasma half-life is ~24 hours. The plasma level can be determined by radioimmunoassay. Metabolism occurs in the liver and

*Known as ciclosporine in Europe and cyclosporine in the USA.

**Recent work has shown that the immunodeficiency virus, HIV-1 (see Ch. 38), also binds to intracellular cyclophilins and it has been suggested that this may be related to the mechanism whereby the virus interferes with T_H cells.

***Immunophilins possess enzymic activity, catalysing cis-trans isomerisation of proline residues in target proteins.

most of the metabolites (of which 14 have been identified) are excreted in the bile. It accumulates in most tissues at concentrations 3–4 times that seen in the plasma. Some of the drug remains in lymphomyeloid tissue and later in fat depots for some time after administration has stopped.

Unwanted effects

Unlike most other immunosuppressive agents, cyclosporin has no depressant effects on the bone marrow. Its most serious toxic effect is on the proximal tubule of the kidney, which is reflected in increased blood urea and creatinine concentrations. This is the commonest unwanted effect and it may be a limiting factor in the use of the drug in some patients (see also Ch. 43). Hypertension can also occur. Less important unwanted effects are mild hepatotoxicity, anorexia, lethargy, hirsutism, tremor, paraesthesias (distortions of sensation), gum hypertrophy and gastrointestinal disturbances.

Glucocorticoids

The action of glucocorticoids as immunosuppressants involves both their anti-inflammatory effects and their effects on the immune response. These are described in Chapter 21 and the sites of action of the agents on cell-mediated immune reactions are indicated in Figures 11.3 and 11.4.

Cytotoxic agents

Azathioprine (Fig. 12.3) is the main cytotoxic agent used for immunosuppression and is widely used to control tissue rejection in transplant surgery. This drug is metabolised to give **mercaptopurine**, a purine analogue that inhibits DNA synthesis (see Ch. 36).

Both cell-mediated and antibody-mediated immune reactions are depressed by this drug since it inhibits clonal proliferation in the induction phase of the immune response (see Figs 11.3 and 11.4) by a cytotoxic action on dividing cells.

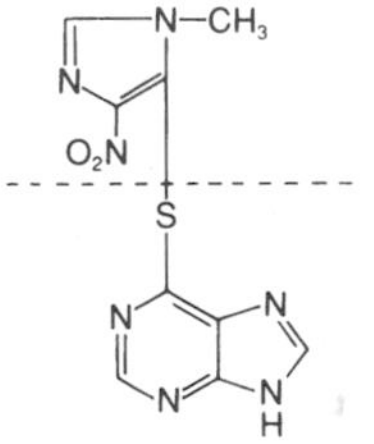

Fig. 12.3 Azathioprine. The dotted line indicates where the molecule is cleaved to release mercaptopurine.

As is the case with mercaptopurine itself, the main unwanted effect is depression of the bone marrow. Other toxic effects are nausea and vomiting, skin eruptions and a mild hepatotoxicity.

Cyclophosphamide is another cytotoxic agent with powerful immunosuppressive effects. It is an alkylating agent with a particular action on lymphocytes. Its structure is given and its mechanism of action described in Chapter 36. As an immunosuppressant it affects the clonal proliferative phase of the immune response and reduces both antibody-mediated and cell-mediated immune reactions (Figs 11.3 and 11.4).

Chlorambucil, another alkylating cytotoxic agent, is also used for immunosuppression and has effects similar to those of cyclophosphamide.

Immunoglobulins

Preparations of immunoglobulin can be derived from humans or from animals. Animal immunoglobulins can now be humanised using protein engineering techniques.

Antilymphocyte immunoglobulin is obtained by immunising horses with human lymphocytes or with foetal thymic tissue. It affects mainly T cells and cell-mediated immune reactions, leaving B cells and antibody-mediated reactions relatively unaffected. The immunoglobulin 'recognises' and binds to protein on the lymphocyte surface resulting in the exposure of the complement-binding site on the Fc portion of the immunoglobulin; this activates the complement system (Ch. 11, p. 216) leading to the lysis of the lymphocyte.

After organ transplantation it is given by intramuscular injection, initially on a daily basis but subsequently less frequently.

The *unwanted effects* are mainly those to be expected with injection of foreign protein. Antibodies against the horse immunoglobulin can be produced, anaphylactic reactions can occur (p. 224) and the complexes formed from the foreign protein with the human antibody can localise in the glomerulus of the kidney (p. 225).

Normal human immunoglobulin is derived from pooled human plasma. It is used in the treatment of some autoimmune diseases—autoimmune thrombocytopenias and haemolytic anaemias, and is being tested in a variety of other autoimmune and chronic inflammatory conditions (Dwyer 1992). It is also used as a replacement therapy in antibody deficiency states and to protect susceptible subjects

Clinical use of immunosuppressants

Immunosuppressants are used for three main purposes:

- to suppress rejection of transplanted organs and tissues (kidneys, bone marrow, heart, liver, etc.)
- to suppress graft-versus-host disease (i.e. the response of lymphocytes in the graft to host antigens) in bone marrow transplants
- to treat a variety of conditions which, while not completely understood, are believed to have an important autoimmune component in their pathogenesis. These include idiopathic thrombocytopenic purpura, some forms of haemolytic anaemia and of glomerulonephritis, myasthenia gravis, systemic lupus erythematosus, rheumatoid arthritis, psoriasis and ulcerative colitis.

Therapy for this third category involves a combination of **glucocorticoid** and **cytotoxic** agents. For transplantation of organs or bone marrow, **cyclosporin** is usually combined with a glucocorticoid, or a cytotoxic drug, or antilymphocyte immunoglobulin.

against infection with hepatitis A virus, measles or rubella (German measles).

The clinical use of immunosuppressants is summarised above.

POSSIBLE FUTURE DEVELOPMENTS

There is a great deal of research going on into anti-inflammatory immunosuppressant drugs and immunomodulatory agents, which may well result in usable drugs for clinical practice in the near future. Some of these new approaches are described below.

5-Lipoxygenase inhibitors

Several agents that inhibit 5-lipoxygenase have been developed (see Ch. 17). These compounds prevent the conversion of arachidonate to 5-HPETE (Fig. 11.12) and hence will inhibit synthesis of all the leukotrienes. Their main application is likely to be as anti-asthmatic drugs, where their reduction of the generation of LTC_4, LTD_4 and LTE_4 could be of value. It is also possible that, combined with suitable cyclo-oxygenase inhibitors, they could have many of the anti-inflammatory effects of the glucocorticoids without the toxic effects of these steroids.

Zileutin is undergoing clinical trial.

Agents that modify interleukin-1 action

Apart from the endogenous interleukin-1 antagonist (Ch. 11, p. 241), other peptides that antagonise the action of interleukin-1 or prevent its release are being developed and basic research suggests that this type of activity could be explored, with the potential of producing compounds for use in chronic inflammatory disease (Dinarello 1993).

Monoclonal antibodies

Enzymes, bacterial toxins, radionuclides, cytotoxic drugs, etc., can now be linked to monoclonal antibodies, making specific targeting of particular tissues or cell types possible. A monoclonal antibody, OKT3, has been approved for clinical use as an immunosuppressive agent in patients with transplanted kidneys. Other potential targets for immunosuppressive monoclonal antibodies are cytokines, cytokine receptors, cell adhesion molecules, and lymphocyte differentiation molecules (Hawkins et al. 1992, Russell et al. 1992, Waldman & Cobbold 1993, Winter & Harris 1993).

Immunomodulating agents

Under investigation are various synthetic compounds that might boost the host's immune response (Hadden 1993). These include stimulants such as **romuride** (developed from the adjuvant, muramyl dipeptide), **ampligen** (an interferon inducer) and various thymic peptides (**thymopentin, thymosin** α_1, **thymulin**).

REFERENCES AND FURTHER READING

Adorini L, Barnaba V et al. 1990 New perspectives on immunointervention in autoimmune diseases. Immunol Today 11: 383–386

Amos R S, Pullar T et al. 1986 Sulphasalazine for rheumatoid arthritis; toxicity in 774 patients monitored for 1 to 11 years. Br Med J 293: 420–424

Avila M H, Walker A M et al. 1988 Choice of nonsteroidal anti-inflammatory drug in persons treated for dyspepsia. Lancet 2: 556–559

Bahl A K, Dale M M, Foreman J C 1994 The effect of

non-steroidal anti-inflammatory drugs on the accumulation and release of interleukin-1-like activity by peritoneal macrophages from the mouse. Brit J Pharmacol (in press)
Bateman D N 1994 NSAIDs: Time to re-evaluate gut toxicity. Lancet 343: 1051–1052
Bennett W M, DeBroe M E 1989 Analgesic nephropathy a preventable renal disease. N Engl J Med 320: 1269–1271
Blower P R 1992 The unique pharmacological profile of nabumetone. J Rheumatol 19 (Suppl 36): 13–19
Borel J F 1994 Cyclosporine. In: Dale M M, Foreman J C, Fan T-P (eds) Textbook of immunopharmacology, 3rd edn. Blackwell Scientific Publications, Oxford, ch 29
Bray G 1993 Liver failure induced by paracetamol. Avoidable deaths still occur. Br Med J 306: 157–158
Cash J M, Klippel J M 1994 Second-line drug therapy for rheumatoid arthritis. N Engl J Med 330: 1368–1376
Champion G D, Graham G G, Ziegler J B 1990 The gold complexes. Clinical rheumatology. Baillière Tindall, vol 4
Dale M M, Foreman J C, Fan T-P 1994 Textbook of immunopharmacology, 3rd edn. Blackwell Scientific Publications, Oxford
Dinarello C A 1993 Modalities for reducing interleukin 1 activity in disease. Trends Pharmacol Sci 14: 155–158
Dwyer J M 1992 Manipulating the immune system with immune globulin. N Engl J Med 326: 107–116
Fathman C G, Myers B D 1992 Cyclosporin therapy for autoimmune disease. N Engl J Med 326: 1693–1696
Foreman J C 1994 Pyrogenesis. In: Dale M M, Foreman J C, Fan T-P (eds) Textbook of immunopharmacology, 3rd edn. Blackwell Scientific Publications, Oxford, ch 21
Friedel H A, Langtry H D, Buckley M M 1993 Nabumetone. A reappraisal of its pharmacology and therapeutic use in rheumatic diseases. Drugs 45: 132–156
Ganellin C R, Parsons M E (eds) 1982 Pharmacology of histamine receptors. Wright, Bristol
Graham G, Dale M M 1990 The activation of gold complexes by cyanide produced by polymorphonuclear leucocytes. Biochem Pharmacol 39: 1697–1702
Hadden J W 1993 Immunostimulants. Trends Pharmacol Sci 14: 169–173
Hall A J 1993 Aspirin and colorectal cancer: seems to reduce the risk. Br Med J 307: 278–279
Hawkins R E, Llewelyn M B, Russell S J 1992 Monoclonal antibodies in medicine: Adapting antibodies for clinical use. Br Med J 305: 1348–1352
Imperiale T P, Petrullis A S 1991 A meta-analysis of low-dose aspirin for prevention of pregnancy-induced hypertensive disease. J Amer Med Assoc 266: 260–264
Lands W E M 1985 Mechanisms of action of antiinflammatory drugs. Adv Drug Res 14: 147–163
Liu J 1993 FK506 and ciclosporin: molecular probes for studying intracellular signal transduction. Trends Pharmacol Sci 14: 182–188
Marshall P J, Lands W E M 1986 In vitro formation of activators for prostaglandin synthesis by neutrophils and macrophages from humans and guinea pigs. J Lab Clin Med 108: 525–534
Meade E A, Smith W L, DeWitt D L 1993 Differential inhibition of prostaglandin endoperoxide synthase (cyclo-oxygenase) isoenzymes by aspirin and other non-steroidal anti-inflammatory drugs. J Biol Chem 268: 6610–6614
Mitchell J R 1988 Acetaminophen toxicity. N Engl J Med 319: 1601–1602
Mitchell J A, Akaarasereenont P, Thierermann C, Flower R J, Vane J R 1993 Selectivity of nonsteroidal antiinflammatory drugs as inhibitors of constitutive and inducible cyclooxygenase. Proc Natl Acad Sci 90: 11693–11697
Murphy D F 1993 NSAIDs and postoperative pain. Sooner is better than later. Br Med J 306: 1493
Murray M D, Brater C B 1993 Renal toxicity of the nonsteroidal anti-inflammatory drugs. Annu Rev Pharmacol Toxicol 32: 435–465
Nicholson A N 1987 New antihistamines free of sedative side-effects. Trends Pharmacol Sci 8: 247–249
Nuki G 1983 Nonsteroidal analgesic and antiinflammatory agents. Br Med J 287: 39–43
Picot D, Lill P J, Garavito R M 1994 The X-ray crystal structure of the membrane protein prostaglandin H_2 synthase-1. Nature 367: 243–249
Rainsford K D 1984 Aspirin and the salicylates. Butterworth, London
Rainsford K D 1994 Nonsteroidal anti-inflammatory drugs. In: Dale M M, Foreman J, Fan T-P D (eds) Textbook of immunopharmacology, 3rd edn. Blackwell Scientific Publications, Oxford
Rainsford K D, Velo G P (eds) 1992 Side-effects of antiinflammatory/analgesic drugs. Kluwer Academic Publishers, Lancaster
Rashad S, Hemingway A, Rainsford K et al. 1989 Effect of nonsteroidal anti-inflammatory drugs on the course of osteoarthritis. Lancet 2: 519–522
Rodriguez L A G, Jick H 1994 Risk of gastrointestinal bleeding and perforation associated with non-steroidal anti-inflammatory drugs. Lancet 343: 769–772
Russell S J, Llewelyn M B, Hawkins R E 1992 Monoclonal antibodies in medicine: principles of antibody therapy. Br Med J 305: 1424–1429
Schreiber S L, Crabtree G R 1992 The mechanism of action of cyclosporin A and FK506. Immunol Today 13: 136–142
Sedor J R 1986 Free radicals and prostanoid synthesis. J Lab Clin Med 108: 521–522
Shen T Y 1984 The proliferation of nonsteroidal antiinflammatory drugs (NSAIDs). In: Parnham M J, Bruinvels J (eds) Discoveries in pharmacology. Vol. 2: Haemodynamics, hormones and inflammation. Elsevier, Amsterdam, p 523–553
Sibai B M, Caritis S N et al. 1993 Prevention of preeclampsia with low dose aspirin in healthy, nulliparous pregnant women. N Engl J Med 329: 1213–1218
Sigal N H, Dumont F J 1992 Cyclosporin A, FK-506, and rapamycin: pharmacologic probes of lymphocyte signal transduction. Annu Rev Immunol 10: 19–60
Simons F E R, Simons K J 1994 Drug therapy: the pharmacology and use of H_1-receptor-antagonist drugs, N Engl J Med 23: 1663–1670
Smith W L, Marnett L J 1991 Prostaglandin endoperoxide synthase: structure and catalysis. Biochim Biophys Acta 1083: 1–17
Thomson A W (ed) 1989 Cyclosporin: mode of action and clinical application. Kluwer Academic Publishers, Lancaster
Thomson A W 1989 FK-506 How much potential? Immunol Today 10: 6–9
Todd P A, Clissold S P 1990 Naproxen. A reappraisal of its pharmacology, therapeutic use in rheumatic diseases and pain states. Drugs 40: 91–137
Twomey B, Dale M M 1992 Cyclooxygenase–independent effects of non-steroidal anti-inflammatory drugs on the neutrophil respiratory burst. Biochem Pharmacol 43: 413–418

Underwood M J 1994 The aspirin papers: aspirin benefits patients with vascular disease and those undergoing revascularisation. Br Med J 308: 71–72

Vane J R 1971 Inhibition of prostaglandin synthesis as a mechanism of action for aspirin-like drugs. Nature New Biology 231: 232–239

Vane J 1994 Towards a better aspirin. Nature 367: 215–216

Vane J, Botting R 1987 Inflammation and the mechanism of action of anti-inflammatory drugs. FASEB J 1: 89–96

Waldmann H, Cobbold S 1993 the use of monoclonal antibodies to achieve immunological tolerance. Trends Pharmacol Sci 14 : 143–147

Willard J E, Lange R A, Hillis L D 1992 The use of aspirin in ischaemic heart disease. N Engl J Med 327: 175–181

Winter G, Harris W J 1993 Humanised antibodies. Trends Pharmacol Sci 14: 139–143

Wolfe C S, Hughes G V R 1988 The optimum management of arthropathies. Drugs 36: 370–381

Xie W, Robertson D L, Simmons D L 1992 Mitogen-inducible prostaglandin G/H synthase: a new target for nonsteroidal antiinflammatory drugs. Drug Development Research 25: 249–265

Zuspan F P, Samuels P 1993 Preventing preeclampsia. N Engl J Med 329: 1265–1266

DRUGS AFFECTING MAJOR ORGAN SYSTEMS

13 THE HEART

The effects of drugs on the heart will be considered under three main headings:

- effects on rate and rhythm
- effects on myocardial contraction
- effects on metabolism and blood flow.

The effects of drugs on these three aspects of cardiac function are, of course, not independent of each other. Thus, if a drug affects the electrical properties of the myocardial cell membrane, it is likely to affect both the rate and rhythm of the heart, and its contraction. Similarly, a drug that affects contraction will inevitably alter metabolism and blood flow as well. Nevertheless, from a therapeutic point of view, these three classes of effect represent distinct clinical objectives in relation to the treatment, respectively, of cardiac dysrhythmias, cardiac failure and coronary insufficiency. We will now consider certain aspects of the pathophysiology of these functions of the heart, which will provide the basis for understanding the effects of drugs upon them.

PHYSIOLOGY OF CARDIAC FUNCTION

CARDIAC RATE AND RHYTHM

Like other muscle cells, cardiac myocytes are electrically excitable, and the same underlying mechanism, namely a transient increase in membrane permeability to sodium ions in response to a depolarisation of the membrane, is responsible for this excitability in most cardiac tissues. The main differences between cardiac muscle and most other kinds of excitable cell are:

- the spontaneous, intrinsic rhythm generated by some specialised cells of the sino-atrial (SA) and atrioventricular (AV) nodes
- the long duration of the action potential and long refractory period
- the large influx of calcium ions (the 'slow inward current') during the plateau of the action potential.

The action potential of an idealised cardiac muscle cell is shown in Figure 13.1A, and is divided into four phases.

Phase 0, the rapid depolarisation, occurs when the membrane potential reaches the critical firing threshold (about −60 mV) at which point the inward current of sodium ions flowing through the voltage-dependent sodium channels becomes large enough to produce a regenerative ('all-or-nothing') depolarisation. This mechanism is the same as that responsible for action potential generation by the membrane of nerve cells (see Ch. 34). The activation of these sodium channels by membrane depolarisation is transient, and if the membrane remains depolarised for more than a few milliseconds, they close again (inactivation). They are therefore closed during the plateau of the action potential, and remain unavailable for the initiation of another action potential until the membrane repolarises.

Phase 1, the partial repolarisation, varies markedly in prominence in different parts of the heart, and occurs as the Na^+ current is inactivated. There may also be a transient voltage-sensitive outward current.

Phase 2, the plateau, results from an inward calcium current, the slow inward current. The calcium

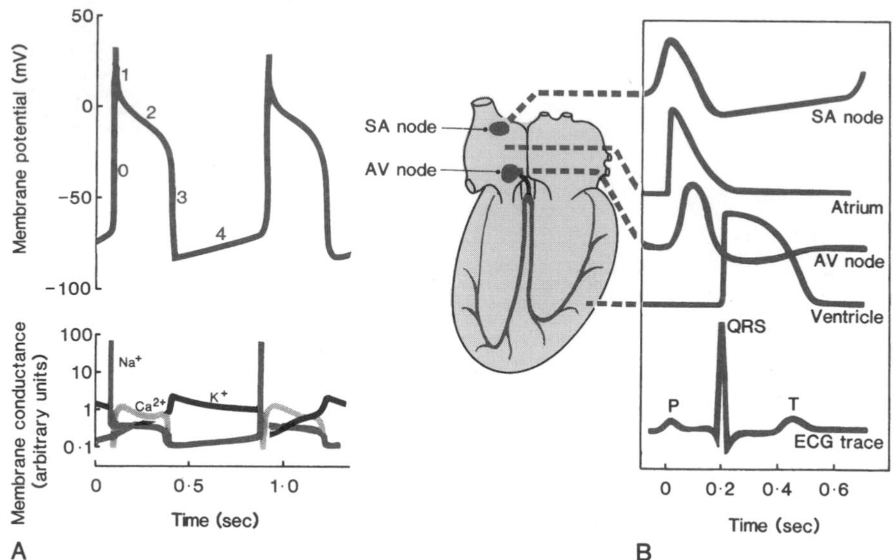

Fig. 13.1 The cardiac action potential. A. Phases of the action potential (as recorded from a cardiac Purkinje fibre): 0 = rapid depolarisation; 1 = partial repolarisation; 2 = plateau; 3 = repolarisation; 4 = pacemaker depolarisation. The lower panel shows the accompanying changes in membrane conductance for Na^+, K^+ and Ca^{2+} ions. **B.** Conduction of the impulse through the heart, with the corresponding ECG trace. Note that the longest delay occurs at the AV node, where the action potential has a characteristically slow waveform. (Adapted from: (A) Noble D 1975 The initiation of the heartbeat. Oxford University Press, Oxford)

channels show a pattern of voltage-sensitive activation and inactivation similar to the fast sodium channels, but with a much slower time-course. Activation of the contractile machinery is due partly to the increase in intracellular calcium concentration that results directly from this influx and partly from the release of calcium from the sarcoplasmic reticulum, as in skeletal muscle. In certain parts of the heart, namely the SA and AV nodes, the fast sodium current is weak or absent, and the slow inward calcium current is largely responsible for initiation and propagation of the action potential.

The plateau is assisted by a special property of the cardiac muscle membrane, known as inward-going rectification, which means that the potassium conductance falls to a low level when the membrane is depolarised. Because of this, there is little tendency for outward potassium current to restore the resting membrane potential during the plateau, so a relatively small inward calcium current suffices to maintain the plateau.

Phase 3, repolarisation, occurs as the calcium current inactivates. It happens abruptly because the inward-going rectification causes the potassium permeability to increase as soon as the membrane begins to repolarise, and the membrane potential 'flips' abruptly back to its resting level, close to the potassium equilibrium potential.

Phase 4, the pacemaker potential, is a gradual depolarisation during diastole. This has been ascribed to a slowly inactivating potassium permeability, but more recent evidence (see Noble 1985) suggests that it may be due to a gradual increase of sodium permeability. When the membrane potential reaches threshold, the fast sodium current is activated again (phase 0).

Pacemaker activity is normally found only in nodal and conducting tissue, other parts of the heart showing no inherent rhythmicity. The SA node normally discharges at a higher frequency than any other region, and so acts as pacemaker for the whole heart.

Figure 13.1B shows the action potential configuration in different parts of the heart. Phase 0 is absent in the nodal regions, where the conduction velocity is correspondingly slow (~ 5 cm/s) compared with other regions such as the Purkinje fibres (conduction velocity ~ 200 cm/s) which have the function of propagating the action potential simultaneously to the whole of the ventricular chambers. Regions that lack a fast inward current have a much longer refractory period than fast-conducting regions. This is because recovery of the slow inward current following its inactivation during the action potential takes a considerable time (a few hundred milliseconds), and the refractory period outlasts the action potential. With fast-conducting fibres, recovery from inactivation of the sodium current is quick, and the cell becomes excitable again as soon as it is repolarised.

Normally, the cardiac action potential is conducted in an orderly sequence: SA node, atrium, AV node, bundle of His, ventricle–timed by the SA node. This pattern can become disrupted either by heart disease or by the action of drugs or circulating hormones, and an important therapeutic use of drugs is to restore a normal cardiac rhythm where it has become disturbed. The commonest cause of cardiac dysrhythmia is ischaemic heart disease, and many deaths following acute myocardial infarction result from ventricular fibrillation rather than directly from contractile failure.

Disturbances of cardiac rhythm

Four basic mechanisms underlie pathological or drug-induced disturbances of cardiac rhythm:

- delayed after-depolarisation
- re-entry
- abnormal pacemaker activity
- heart block.

These will now be described in more detail.

Delayed after-depolarisation

Normal pacemaker activity, as described above, involves a spontaneous diastolic depolarisation, which initiates an action potential when it reaches threshold. Non-pacemaker cells, therefore, normally remain quiescent if not excited by the arrival of an impulse from elsewhere in the heart. Under certain circumstances, however, the phenomenon of delayed after-depolarisation occurs, which can lead to a repetitive discharge that does not depend on the arrival of an impulse from elsewhere (Fig. 13.2). The after-depolarisation immediately follows the action potential, and there is good evidence that it occurs when intracellular calcium concentration increases beyond the normal range (see January & Fozzard 1988). Thus, it is accentuated if the extracellular calcium concentration (and hence the amount of calcium entering the cell during the plateau) is increased, and also by agents such as **cardiac glycosides**, **noradrenaline** or **phosphodiesterase inhibitors** (see below) which increase intracellular calcium; it is diminished by drugs that reduce calcium entry by inhibiting the slow inward current (see below).

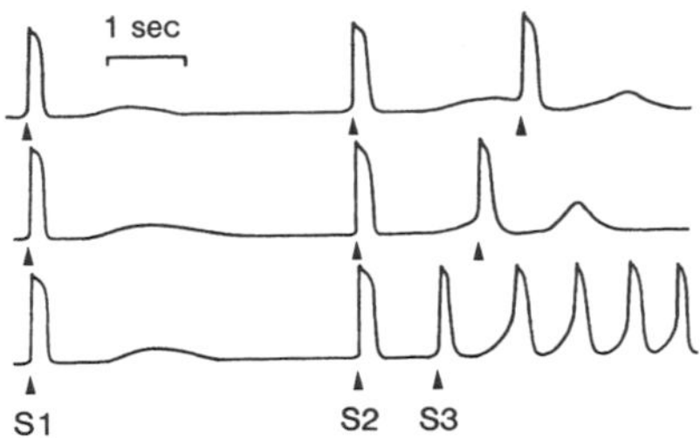

Fig. 13.2 After-depolarisation in cardiac muscle recorded from a dog coronary sinus in the presence of noradrenaline. The first stimulus (S1) causes an action potential followed by a small after-depolarisation. As the interval S2–S3 is decreased, the after-depolarisation gets larger until it triggers an indefinite train of action potentials. (Adapted from: Wit A L, Cranefield P F 1977 Circulation Res 41: 435)

After-depolarisation is the result of a net inward current (known as the *transient inward current*) that occurs when the intracellular calcium concentration $[Ca^{2+}]_i$ increases beyond its normal range. How does this rise in $[Ca^{2+}]_i$ cause an inward current? One possibility is that it results from activation of sodium–calcium exchange across the cell membrane (see Fig. 13.4). This counter-transport system acts to transfer one Ca^{2+} ion out of the cell in exchange for three Na^+ ions, resulting in a net influx of one positive charge which acts to depolarise the cell. Increasing the intracellular calcium concentration will thus produce an increase in net inward current, and therefore membrane depolarisation. Alternatively, the current may be due to a direct effect of $[Ca^{2+}]_i$ on the membrane, causing the opening of non-selective cation channels and hence entry of sodium and other ions. After-depolarisation probably underlies the 'R on T' phenomenon, the tendency of an ectopic beat falling on the T wave of the preceding QRS complex of the electrocardiogram to precipitate ventricular tachycardia. Deliberate provocation of arrhythmia in this way is utilised in invasive electrophysiological testing of patients with *life-threatening* ventricular arrhythmias to attempt to establish what drugs will be effective, an approach that continues to be hotly debated (see Ward & Camm 1993 for a recent commentary). Whatever its mechanism, the importance of the transient inward current in the genesis of dysrhythmias, and its close relation to $[Ca^{2+}]_i$, is now well established.

Re-entry

In normal cardiac rhythm, the conducted impulse dies out after it has activated the ventricles because it is surrounded by refractory tissue which it has just traversed. Re-entry describes the situation in which the impulse succeeds in re-exciting regions of the myocardium after the refractory period has subsided. A simple ring of tissue can give rise to a re-entrant rhythm if a transient or unidirectional conduction block is present (Fig. 13.3). Normally, an impulse originating at any point in the ring will propagate in both directions and die out when the two impulses meet, but if a damaged area shows either a transient block (so that one impulse is blocked but the second can get through; Fig. 13.3) or a unidirectional block, continuous circulation of the impulse can occur. This phenomenon is known as circus movement and it was first demonstrated on rings of jellyfish tissue more than 80 years ago.

The 'ring' of tissue sometimes represents an anatomically distinct anomaly such as an accessory pathway linking atria and ventricles, as in patients with Wolff–Parkinson–White syndrome. Such pathways are increasingly accessible to surgical ablation by various catheter techniques. However, more commonly the 'ring' of tissue is not anatomically distinct, but only functionally separate. If it retains a connection with the rest of the heart, it can act as a focus for high frequency re-excitation of the whole atrium or ventricle. The re-entrant rhythm will persist only if the time taken for propagation round the ring exceeds the refractory period, so it may be halted by drugs that prolong the refractory period (see below). On the other hand, myocardial damage may cause extreme slowing of action potential propagation favouring re-entry. This slowing is often associated with the attenuation or disappearance of the sodium current responsible for the fast upstroke of the action potential (Fig. 13.1). This current is reduced because the compromised cells are somewhat depolarised during diastole compared with normal cells, so the fast sodium channels remain partly or completely inactivated, leaving only the slow inward current to support propagation of the action potential.

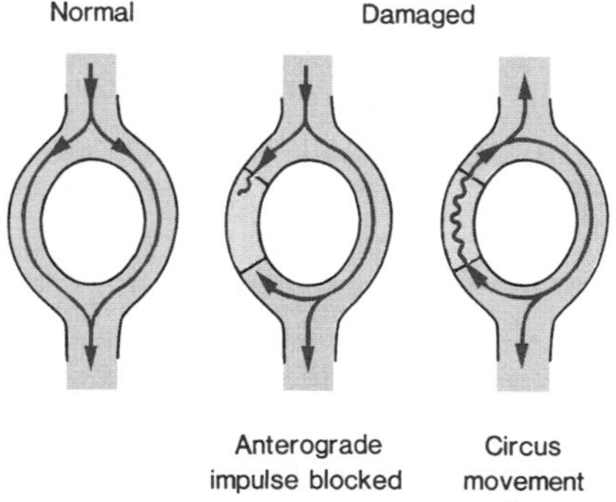

Fig. 13.3 Generation of a re-entrant rhythm by a damaged area of myocardium. The damaged area (grey) conducts in one direction only. This disturbs the normal pattern of conduction in which the impulse in the atria dies out as it converges on the AV node and permits continuous circulation of the impulse to occur.

Studies on the properties of these 'slow responses' in damaged regions of the heart have demonstrated the transient or unidirectional conduction blocks necessary to initiate a re-entrant rhythm (see Cranefield 1975).

Re-entry is thought to be the mechanism underlying many types of dysrhythmia, the pattern depending on the site of the re-entrant circuit which may be in the atria, ventricles or nodal tissue.

Abnormal pacemaker activity

Pacemaker activity in a normal heart is confined to the nodal and conducting tissues, which show slow depolarisation during phase 4. It can occur in other parts of the heart, however, particularly under pathological conditions, the main predisposing factors being:

- catecholamine action
- partial depolarisation, such as may occur in ischaemic damage.

Catecholamines, acting on β-adrenoceptors (see below), increase the rate of depolarisation during phase 4, and can cause normally quiescent parts of the heart to take on a spontaneous rhythm. Myocardial ischaemia increases sympathetic discharge to the heart, and can also cause release of adrenaline from the adrenal gland, both of which encourage the appearance of abnormal pacemakers. Partial depolarisation resulting from ischaemic damage is probably due to a decrease in the activity of the electrogenic sodium pump, and has an effect on pacemaker activity similar to that of catecholamines.

Heart block
Nodal tissue may become damaged (e.g. by infarction or fibrosis) so that it fails to conduct. If this happens to the AV node, atria and ventricles beat independently (complete AV block) at rates determined by their own pacemakers. AV block may be partial, in which case a proportion of the sinus beats are transmitted to the ventricle. This may appear in a regular pattern (e.g. 2:1 or 3:1 block) in which every second or third impulse is transmitted. The ventricular rate and cardiac output will then be low; if AV conduction fails completely in a sporadic fashion, sudden periods of unconsciousness may result (Stokes–Adams attacks).

Clinically, dysrhythmias are generally classified according to:

- the site of origin of the abnormality—atrial, junctional or ventricular
- whether the rate is increased (tachycardias) or decreased (bradycardias).

It is often unclear which of the various mechanisms discussed above are responsible. These physiological mechanisms nevertheless provide a useful starting point for understanding how antidysrhythmic drugs affect the abnormal rate and rhythm of the heart.

Cardiac dysrhythmias

- Dysrhythmias arise because of:
  - —delayed after-depolarisation, which triggers ectopic beats
  - —re-entry, resulting from partial conduction block
  - —ectopic pacemaker activity
  - —heart block.
- Delayed after-depolarisation is due to an inward current associated with abnormally raised $[Ca^{2+}]_i$.
- Re-entry is facilitated when parts of the myocardium are depolarised, conduction then depending on the Ca^{2+}-mediated 'slow response'.
- Ectopic pacemaker activity is encouraged by sympathetic activity.
- Heart block results from damage to the AV node or ventricular conducting system.
- Clinically, dysrhythmias are divided:
  - —according to their site of origin (supraventricular and ventricular)
  - —according to whether the heart rate is increased or decreased (tachycardia or bradycardia).

CARDIAC CONTRACTION

The force with which a myocardial cell contracts when invaded by an action potential depends on both intrinsic and extrinsic factors. The *intrinsic factors* include those factors that regulate the intracellular ionised calcium concentration, as well as various biochemical factors, such as availability of ATP within the myocardial cell. Together, these intrinsic factors, which are sensitive to a variety of drugs and pathological processes, regulate myocardial *contractility*. The mechanical output of the heart in situ is determined not only by contractility, but also by extrinsic circulatory factors, such as the state of the arterioles and veins, blood volume, viscosity and so on, which can also be affected by drugs and/or disease.

Myocardial contractility and viability

The contractile machinery of the myocardial cell is basically the same as that of striated muscle. The interaction between actin and myosin filaments is normally blocked by the presence of *tropomyosin* bound to the actin filament. Tropomyosin forms part of the *troponin complex*, one component of which, troponin C, has binding sites for three or four calcium ions. When calcium is bound, the conformation of the troponin complex changes, with the result that tropomyosin shifts out of the way and binding of the myosin cross-bridge to the actin filament is permitted, thus initiating the contractile process. These changes are produced when the intracellular ionised calcium concentration $[Ca^{2+}]_i$ exceeds about 10^{-7} mol/l and the system is fully activated at about 10^{-6} mol/l ionised calcium.

The main mechanisms responsible for controlling $[Ca^{2+}]_i$ are summarised in Figure 13.4. The major route of entry of calcium is the voltage-sensitive calcium channels in the surface membrane, whose activation by depolarisation gives rise to the slow inward current (see previous section). Calcium enters the cell by this route with each action potential and causes an immediate rise in $[Ca^{2+}]_i$. Depolarisation also, as in striated muscle, causes release of calcium from the sarcoplasmic reticulum which adds further to the increase in $[Ca^{2+}]_i$. Calcium entry is balanced by removal of calcium from the cell, the main agency for this being the *calcium–sodium exchange pump* (Fig. 13.4). This mechanism extrudes calcium ions in exchange for sodium ions (which are in turn extruded, in exchange for potassium ions, by the

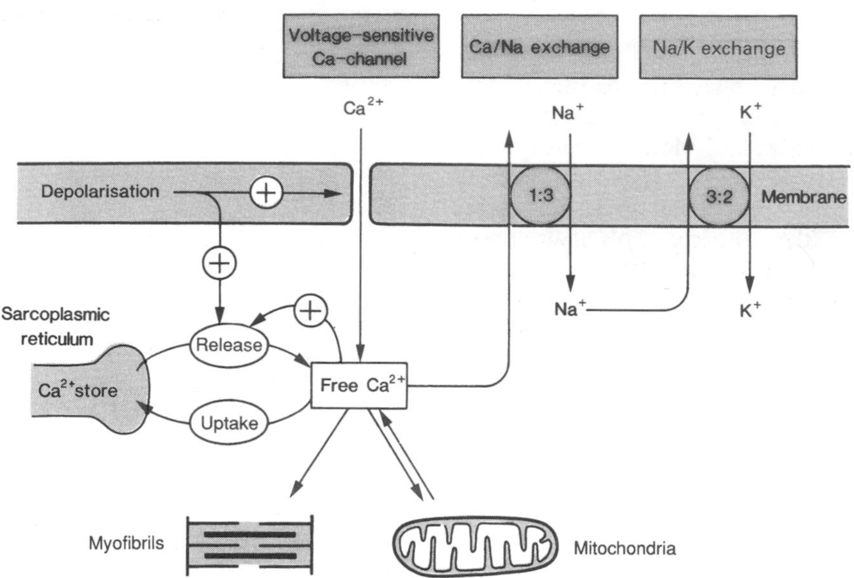

Fig. 13.4 The control of intracellular calcium in the myocardium. The phasic increase in $[Ca^{2+}]_i$ associated with the action potential results from Ca^{2+} entry through voltage-sensitive Ca^{2+} channels and the release of Ca^{2+} from sarcoplasmic reticulum (SR). The latter involves (1) depolarisation-induced release and (2) Ca^{2+}-induced Ca^{2+} release. Ca^{2+} entering the cell eventually leaves via the Ca^{2+}/Na^+ exchange system so that a steady state is maintained. This process is much slower than the exchanges between SR and free cytosolic Ca^{2+}. It functions electrogenically, because of the 1:3 coupling ratio, and is controlled by $[Na^+]_i$ as well as $[Ca^{2+}]_i$ (see also Fig. 13.12).

sodium–potassium pump). This interconnection between sodium and calcium movements across the membrane means that changes in $[Na^+]_i$, whether produced physiologically or pharmacologically, will affect $[Ca^{2+}]_i$ as well, in the same direction. Thus, inhibition of the sodium–potassium pump (e.g. by **cardiac glycosides**; see below) raises $[Na^+]_i$, slows sodium–calcium exchange, and secondarily raises $[Ca^{2+}]_i$, thus facilitating contraction. Conversely, inhibition of sodium entry (e.g. by **lignocaine**; see below) has the opposite effect.

Calcium is also exchanged between cytosol and sarcoplasmic reticulum, and between cytosol and mitochondria (Fig. 13.4). At any moment, more than 99% of the total cell calcium is sequestered by these intracellular organelles, so a small shift of calcium between these stores and the cytosol can cause a large change in $[Ca^{2+}]_i$.

Many of the effects of drugs on cardiac contractility can be explained in terms of their effects on $[Ca^{2+}]_i$, resulting from interactions with the voltage-sensitive calcium channels, the sarcoplasmic reticulum or the sodium–potassium pump. Other factors that affect the force of contraction are the availability of oxygen and glucose. Cells deprived of oxygen quickly cease to contract, though it has recently been shown by Allen and his colleagues that their electrical excitability, and the transient increase in $[Ca^{2+}]_i$ associated with the action potential, remain normal even when the contraction has disappeared. Contractile proteins are highly sensitive to intracellular pH, which drops rapidly during anaerobic glycolysis. If glycolysis is also impaired, which must happen in ischaemia because the cells are deprived of glucose as well as oxygen, the resulting fall in intracellular ATP concentration impairs the ability of the sarcoplasmic reticulum to accumulate calcium, and the mechanical failure is probably due to the loss of this store of releasable calcium within the cell, rather than to a direct effect of ATP depletion on the contractile proteins.

Such processes are probably involved in myocardial 'stunning' – contractile dysfunction that persists after ischaemia and reperfusion despite restoration of blood flow and absence of cardiac necrosis. The converse of this can also occur and is known as 'ischaemic preconditioning': this means improved ability to withstand ischaemia following previous ischaemic episodes. This clinically beneficial syndrome is demonstrable experimentally in many species and may occur in several clinical settings in man. There is some evidence that it is mediated by *adenosine* which accumulates as ATP is depleted and acts on A_1-receptors (Liu et al. 1991). This leads to activation of an inhibitory G-protein and hence inhibition of adenylate cyclase and activation of other potential effectors such as phospholipase C or the ATP-sensitive potassium channel (see Ch. 2). Exogenous adenosine or A_1-selective analogues afford a degree of protection similar to that caused by ischaemic preconditioning, and blockade of adenosine receptors prevents the protective effect of preconditioning. There is currently great therapeutic interest in developing strategies to minimise the bad effects (stunning) while maximising the good (preconditioning) for patients with angina who experience repeated brief episodes of myocardial ischaemia (see Fine & Yellon 1993 for a recent discussion).

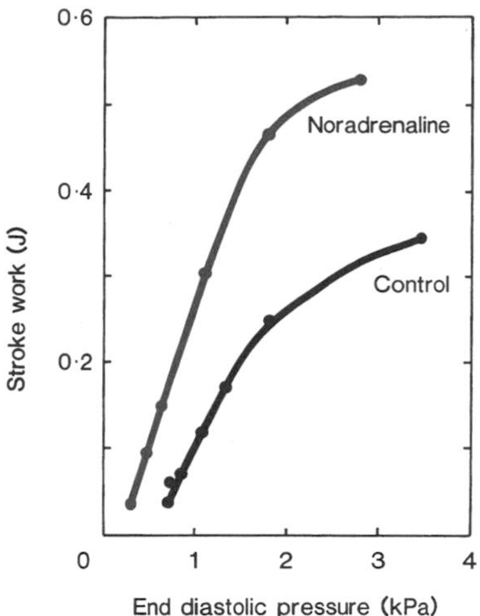

Fig. 13.5 Ventricular function curves in the dog. Intrinsic control (in this case increased myocardial contractility) is exemplified by the effect of noradrenaline infusion. Extrinsic control (the effect of external circulatory factors on the force of contraction of the heart) is shown by the relationship between stroke work and diastolic pressure. (Redrawn from: Sarnoff S J et al. 1960 Circ Res 8: 1108)

Ventricular function curves and heart failure

The force of contraction of the heart is determined partly by its intrinsic *contractility* (which, as described above, depends on the availability of intracellular calcium and ATP) and partly by extrinsic factors that affect *end-diastolic volume* and, hence, the resting length of the muscle fibres. The end-diastolic volume is determined largely by the end-diastolic pressure, and its effect on the stroke work of the heart is expressed in the Frank–Starling Law of the Heart, which reflects an inherent property of the contractile system. The Frank–Starling Law can be represented as a *ventricular function curve* (Fig. 13.5).

The *stroke work* of the ventricle is measured by the area enclosed by the pressure–volume curve during the cardiac cycle. Roughly speaking, it is given by the product of stroke volume and mean arterial pressure. As Starling showed, factors extrinsic to the heart can affect its performance in various ways, and two patterns of response are particularly important:

- An increase in central venous pressure (increased *pre-load*) without any change in peripheral resistance will increase the cardiac filling pressure, and hence the end-diastolic volume of the ventricles. This will increase the stroke volume, and thus increase both the cardiac output and the mean arterial pressure. The cardiac work and cardiac oxygen consumption both increase.
- Peripheral arteriolar vasoconstriction occurring without any change in central venous pressure constitutes an increased *after-load*. Initially, the end-diastolic volume, and hence the stroke work, will be unchanged; constancy of stroke work in the face of an increased vascular resistance means that stroke volume must decrease. As this happens, the end-diastolic volume increases which in turn increases the stroke work, until a steady state is established with an increased end-diastolic volume and the same cardiac output as before. As in the previous example, the cardiac work and cardiac oxygen consumption both increase.

The steep part of the ventricular function curve represents the normal operating range, where the central venous pressure is only a few centimetres of water above zero and a large increase in stroke work can be achieved with only a small increase in the filling pressure. In fact, under normal circumstances, the Starling mechanism seems to play little part in controlling the cardiac output, for changes in contractility, mainly due to changes in sympathetic activity, achieve the necessary regulation without any substantial change in the ventricular filling pressure (Fig. 13.5). Thus, in a normal individual, exercise causes the central venous pressure and end-diastolic volume to decrease rather than increase, because of the overriding influence of the autonomic nervous system.

In heart failure, the heart may be unable to deliver as much blood as the tissues require even when its contractility is increased by sympathetic activity. This may happen because the myocardium is damaged (e.g. by ischaemia), because narrowing or incompetence of the valves has made its pumping action inefficient or because excessive peripheral vascular resistance has increased the work required to maintain an adequate tissue blood flow (as in severe hypertension). Under these conditions the basal ventricular function curve is greatly depressed, and there is insufficient reserve, in the sense of extra contractility that can be achieved by sympathetic activity, to enable the cardiac output to be maintained without a large increase in central venous pressure occurring (Fig. 13.5). An important consequence of cardiac failure is oedema, which affects both the peripheral tissues (causing swelling of the legs) and the lungs (causing breathlessness). Oedema is caused by the increase in venous pressure, and retention of sodium (see Ch. 18), rather than by the inadequate cardiac output per se.

Myocardial contraction

- Controlling factors are:
  —intrinsic contractility
  —extrinsic circulatory factors.
- Contractility depends critically on control of intracellular Ca^{2+}, and hence on:
  —Ca^{2+} entry across the cell membrane
  —Ca^{2+} storage in the sarcoplasmic reticulum.
- The main factors controlling Ca^{2+} entry are:
  —activity of voltage-gated Ca^{2+} channels
  —$[Na^+]_i$, which affects Ca^{2+}/Na^+ exchange.
  Many things affect these two processes, including catecholamines and drugs affecting the Na^+ pump.
- Extrinsic control of cardiac contraction is due to the dependence of stroke work on the end-diastolic volume, expressed in the Frank–Starling Law.
- Cardiac work is affected independently by *after-load* (i.e. peripheral resistance) and *pre-load* (i.e. central venous pressure).
- 'Heart failure' describes the condition in which the cardiac output is insufficient to meet the circulatory needs of the body (at rest or during exercise).

MYOCARDIAL OXYGEN CONSUMPTION AND CORONARY BLOOD FLOW

In a normal human being at rest, the myocardium accounts for about 11% of total body oxygen consumption but receives only about 4% of the cardiac output as coronary blood flow, so it is, relative to its metabolic needs, one of the most poorly perfused tissues in the body. The frequency with which ischaemia occurs in the coronary circulation as a result of pathological disturbances is presumably related to this fact.

The coronary flow is, under normal circumstances, closely related to myocardial oxygen consumption, and both variables can change over a nearly 10-fold range between conditions of rest and maximal exercise.

The main physiological factors that regulate coronary flow are:

- physical factors
- vascular control by metabolites
- neural and humoral control.

Physical factors

Physical factors are mainly related to the fact that during systole the pressure exerted by the myocardium on the vessels that pass through it equals or exceeds the perfusion pressure, so that flow only occurs during diastole. Thus tachycardia, in which diastole is shortened more than systole, tends to impair coronary flow unless coronary dilatation can compensate (Fig. 13.6). During diastole, the effective perfusion pressure is equal to the difference between the aortic pressure and the ventricular pressure. Thus, if a reduction of diastolic aortic pressure occurs, or an increase in diastolic ventricular pressure, the perfusion pressure falls and so (unless other control mechanisms can compensate) does the coronary flow. Stenosis of the aortic valve is an example of a disorder that produces both of these effects, and often causes ischaemic pain ('angina') even in the absence of coronary artery disease.

Vascular control by metabolites/mediators

Vascular control by metabolites is the most impor-

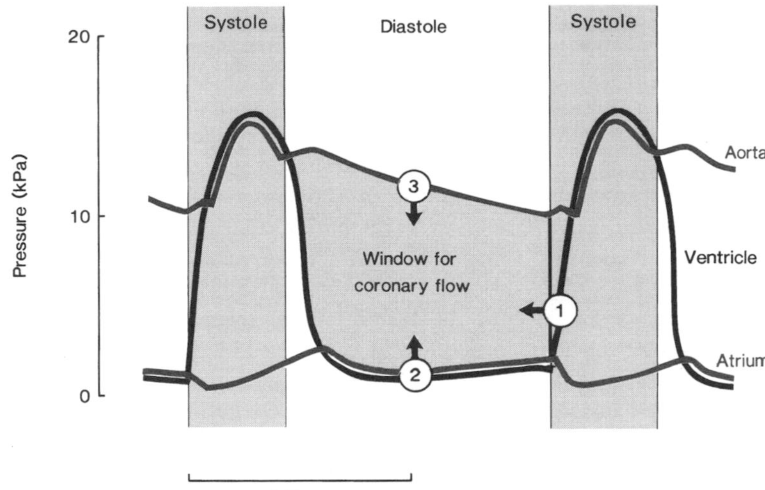

Fig. 13.6 Mechanical factors affecting coronary blood flow. The 'window' for coronary flow may be encroached upon by: (1) shortening of diastole, which occurs when the heart rate increases, (2) increased ventricular end-diastolic pressure and (3) reduced diastolic arterial pressure.

tant mechanism by which coronary flow is regulated. A reduction in arterial Po_2 causes marked vasodilatation of coronary vessels in situ, but has little effect on isolated strips of coronary artery. This suggests that it is a change in the pattern of metabolites produced by the myocardial cells, rather than the change in Po_2 per se that controls the state of the coronary vessels. *Lactic acid* is produced when the myocardium functions under hypoxic conditions, but this is relatively ineffective as a coronary dilator. A *fall in pH* also occurs, and this has some dilator effect. The most popular candidate for the dilator metabolite is *adenosine* (see Ch. 8). The rate of production of adenosine by myocardial cells increases if the tissue is hypoxic, possibly because ATP splitting under these conditions may not stop at ADP but continues all the way to adenosine.

Prostaglandins of the E series (see Ch. 11), as well as **prostacyclin,** are potent coronary dilators and are released when the heart is made ischaemic. However, inhibitors of prostaglandin synthesis have only a small effect on coronary blood flow, so it is unlikely that this system has a major physiological function.

Neural and humoral control

Coronary vessels have a dense sympathetic innervation, but the sympathetic nerves (like circulating catecholamines) exert only a small direct effect on the coronary circulation. Large coronary vessels possess α-adrenoceptors that mediate vasoconstriction, whereas smaller vessels have β_2-adrenoceptors that have a dilator effect. Normally, both effects are overshadowed by the vascular response to altered mechanical and metabolic activity, and these receptors are not of much pharmacological significance.

Coronary atherosclerosis and its consequence

Partial occlusion of coronary vessels by atheromatous deposits occurs in at least 75% of the adult population of developed countries (see Ch. 15), and the diseases that result are the major cause of illness and death in regions where starvation and the major microbial diseases have been eliminated. Important consequences of coronary obstruction are:

- anginal pain
- myocardial infarction.

Angina

Anginal pain occurs when the oxygen supply to the myocardium is insufficient for its needs. The pain has a characteristic distribution in the chest, arm and neck, and is brought on by exertion or excitement. It is a common symptom, and is unpleasant in its own right as well as providing an important diagnostic pointer to the need for investigation and treatment of coronary atheromatous disease. It is therefore an important target for therapeutic intervention (see p. 291). A similar type of pain can be produced in skeletal muscle when it is made to contract while its blood supply is interrupted, and the work of Lewis clearly showed that a chemical factor released by the ischaemic muscle is responsible for activating pain afferents. Possible candidates for this pain-producing substance include *potassium ion*, *hydrogen ion*, peptides such as *bradykinin* (Ch. 11), *adenosine*, *ADP*, and *prostaglandins*, all of which stimulate nociceptors. Since angina can occur in patients suffering from severe anaemia who have no reduction in coronary blood flow, it seems that the substance responsible must be produced in larger quantities when muscle contracts anaerobically, and it is possible that the same substance is responsible both for the regulation of coronary vessels and stimulation of pain afferents.

Three kinds of angina are recognised clinically. *Stable angina* is characterised by predictable pain on exertion. It is produced by an increased demand on the heart and is due to a fixed narrowing of the coronary vessels, almost always by atheroma. Symptomatic therapy is directed at altering cardiac work-load with **organic nitrates, β-adrenoceptor antagonists** and/or **calcium antagonists** as described below, together with treatment of the underlying atheromatous disease (Ch. 15). *Unstable angina* is characterised by pain that occurs with less and less exertion, culminating in pain at rest. The pathology is basically the same as that involved in myocardial infarction, namely a platelet–fibrin thrombus associated with a ruptured atheromatous plaque, but without complete occlusion of the vessel. The risk of infarction is substantial, and the main aim of therapy is to reduce this. **Aspirin** (Ch. 16) approximately halves the risk of myocardial infarction in this setting. *Variant angina* is much less common. It occurs at rest and is caused by coronary artery spasm, again usually in association with atheromatous disease. Therapy is with coronary artery vasodilators (e.g. **organic nitrates, calcium antagonists**).

Coronary flow, ischaemia and infarction

- The heart has a smaller blood supply in relation to its oxygen consumption than most organs.
- Normal coronary flow is controlled mainly by:
  - —physical factors, including transmural pressure during systole
  - —vasodilator metabolites.

  Autonomic innervation is less important.
- Coronary ischaemia is usually due to atherosclerosis, and causes anginal pain. Sudden ischaemia is usually due to thrombosis, and may cause cardiac infarction.
- Coronary spasm sometimes causes angina (variant angina).
- Cellular calcium overload results from ischaemia, and may be responsible for:
  - —cell death
  - —initiation of dysrhythmias.

Myocardial infarction

Death of an area of myocardium occurs when a coronary vessel is suddenly blocked by thrombosis. This is the commonest single cause of death in many parts of the world, and death usually results either from mechanical failure of the ventricle or from ventricular fibrillation. The sequence of events leading from vascular occlusion to irreversible cellular damage (see van der Vusse & Reneman 1985) is shown in Figure 13.7. An increase in $[Ca^{2+}]_i$ is the trigger for the secondary cellular damage. $[Ca^{2+}]_i$ rises initially because two ATP-dependent processes are impaired, namely uptake of calcium by the sarcoplasmic reticulum and sodium extrusion from the cell (which indirectly controls $[Ca^{2+}]_i$ because of sodium–calcium exchange). The effect of increased $[Ca^{2+}]_i$ on the tendency to dysrhythmias has already been mentioned (p. 271). Death of the cells may also be secondary to a rise in $[Ca^{2+}]_i$ through the activity of intracellular calcium-dependent proteases (see Ch. 43).

Prevention of irreversible ischaemic damage following an episode of coronary thrombosis is an important therapeutic aim, and the usefulness of drug treatment aimed at protecting myocardial cells is currently being intensively studied. The main possibilities, shown in Figure 13.7, are:

- to reduce the work-load of the heart, and thereby its metabolic needs, by the use of β-adrenoceptor antagonists or vasodilator drugs
- to inhibit calcium entry by the use of calcium antagonists (see later section).

Drug treatment aimed at preventing or reversing thrombosis is discussed in Chapter 16.

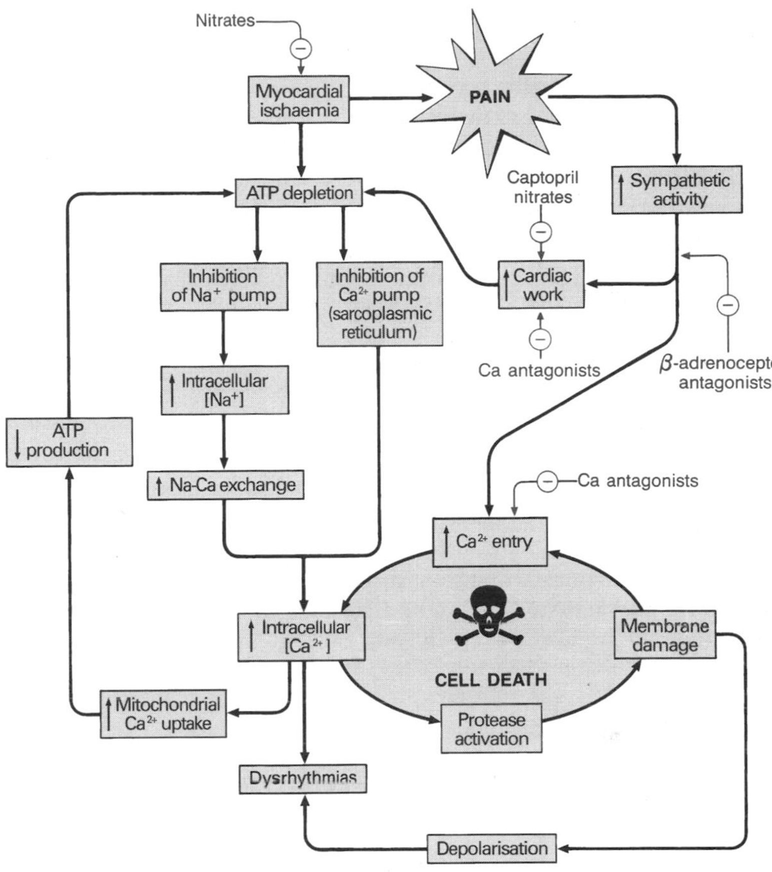

Fig. 13.7 Cellular effects of myocardial ischaemia.

ATRIAL NATRIURETIC PEPTIDE (ANP)

Atrial cells have a specialised endocrine function in relation to the cardiovascular system (see review by Ruskoaho 1992). They contain secretory granules, and store and release a 28-amino-acid peptide (ANP) which has powerful effects on the kidney and vascular system. Release of ANP occurs in response to stretching of the atria by increased central venous pressure, signalling volume overload of the circulation. Saline infusion is sufficient to evoke ANP release.

ANP is an interesting hormone. Its main effects are to increase Na^+ and water excretion by the kidney, relax vascular smooth muscle, increase vascular permeability and inhibit the release and/or actions of several hormones and mediators including aldosterone, angiotensin II, endothelin and ADH. It exerts its effects by combining with membrane receptors (which exist in at least two subtypes designated A and B) that incorporate a catalytic guanylate cyclase moiety. Binding of ANP leads to generation of cGMP within the cell. This is the same response as that produced by organic nitrates (see later) and endothelium-derived NO (Ch. 10), which, however, achieve this by interacting with soluble rather than membrane-bound guanylate cyclase. Renal glomerular afferent arterioles are dilated by ANP but efferent arterioles are constricted, so filtration pressure is increased, leading to increased glomerular filtration and enhanced Na^+ excretion. Elsewhere, ANP causes vasorelaxation especially of capacitance vessels, as do **organic nitrates**, and causes a fall in blood pressure. Binding of ANP to a third kind of binding site (designated a C 'receptor', somewhat unfortunately since it does not lead to a biological response) leads to its clearance via cellular uptake and degradation by lysosomal enzymes.

In many ways, ANP is cast as the cardiovascular hero that stands opposed to the villainous intents of vasoconstrictors such as *angiotensin*, *vasopressin* and *endothelin*, discussed in Chapter 14. Its effects could be therapeutically beneficial, for example in treating heart failure or hypertension. However, as a large peptide with a short plasma half-life, ANP itself is unsuitable as a drug, so there is considerable interest in synthetic peptide and non-peptide ANP_A agonists. There is also much interest in the alternative strategy of inhibiting its elimination, by blocking the clearance (C) 'receptors' and/or inhibiting one or more of the various ectoenzymes, notably neutral endopeptidase, that have been implicated in its degradation (see review by Roques et al. 1993). Promising results have been obtained with various neutral endopeptidase inhibitors in animal models of hypertension, and one such drug, **candoxatril**, has been used in human volunteers and in early studies of patients with heart failure in whom it increased plasma ANP, suppressed neurohumoral activity and caused haemodynamic unloading, without, however, causing diuresis.

DRUGS THAT AFFECT CARDIAC FUNCTION

Drugs that have a major action on the heart can be divided into the following groups:

- Drugs that *directly* affect myocardial cells. These include:
  - — autonomic neurotransmitters and related drugs
  - — cardiac **glycosides** and other inotropic agents
  - — antidysrhythmic drugs
  - — miscellaneous agents, including certain endogenous substances.

  The last are discussed elsewhere, for example: **methylxanthines** (see Chs 17 and 32), **adenosine derivatives** (see Ch. 14), **histamine** (see Ch. 11) and **glucagon** (see Ch. 20).
- Drugs that affect cardiac function indirectly, through actions elsewhere in the vascular system. Antianginal drugs fall into this category, as do many drugs that are used to treat heart failure.

Calcium antagonists are an important group of drugs whose main effects are on the cardiovascular system. They act both on the myocardium and on vascular smooth muscle (as well as on other cells), and are discussed as a separate group in this chapter.

AUTONOMIC TRANSMITTERS AND RELATED DRUGS

Many aspects of autonomic pharmacology have been discussed in Chapters 5, 6 and 7, so here we shall mention only aspects that particularly concern the heart.

Autonomic control of the heart

Both sympathetic and parasympathetic systems normally exert a tonic effect on the heart at rest.

Sympathetic system

The main effects that sympathetic activity produces are:

- increased heart rate (*positive chronotropic effect*; Fig. 13.8)
- increased force of contraction (*positive inotropic effect*), affecting all parts of the heart
- increased *automaticity*
- *facilitation of conduction* in the AV node
- reduced *cardiac efficiency* (i.e. O_2 consumption is increased more than cardiac work).

These effects all result from activation of β_1-receptors. There is also evidence for the existence of α-receptors, activation of which causes an increased refractory period, but this is of little significance. Coronary vessels are constricted by α-receptor activation and dilated by β-receptor activation. Sympathetic activity produces strong coronary vasodilatation and an increase in blood flow that matches the increased oxygen consumption, but this is mediated by the metabolic response of the myocardium rather than by a direct action on the coronary vessels.

The β-effects of catecholamines on the heart, though complex, are probably all due to an increase in the intracellular concentration of cAMP (see Ch. 2). The increase in heart rate results from an increase in the slope of the pacemaker potential (Figs 13.1 and 13.8). This slow diastolic depolarisation results from a voltage-sensitive inward current which is slowly switched on when the membrane potential is in the diastolic range (about –70 mV).

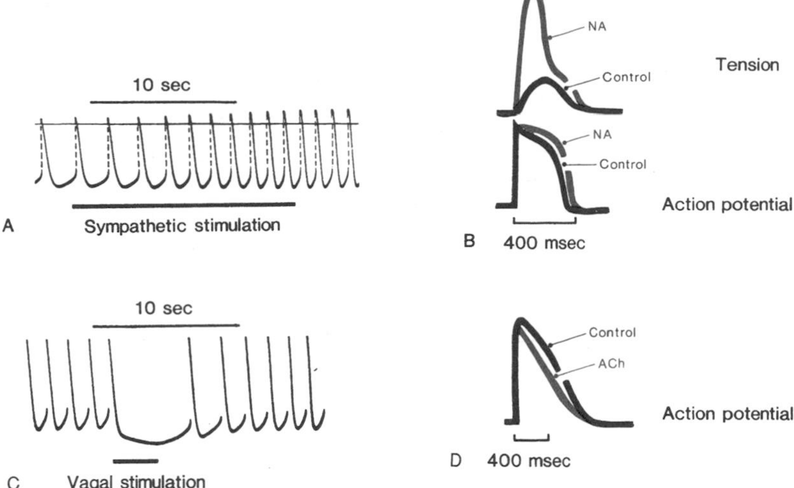

Fig. 13.8 Autonomic regulation of the heart beat. A and **B.** The effects of sympathetic stimulation and noradrenaline. **C** and **D**. The effects of parasympathetic stimulation and acetylcholine. A and C show a spontaneously beating frog sinus venosus (intracellular recording). Sympathetic stimulation increases the slope of the pacemaker potential and increases heart rate. Parasympathetic stimulation abolishes the pacemaker potential, hyperpolarises the membrane and temporarily stops the heart. B illustrates a calf ventricular muscle showing the effect of noradrenaline (NA) on action potential and tension. Prolongation of the action potential and increased tension result from an increased entry of Ca^{2+}. D shows a frog atrium in which there is a shortening of the action potential produced by acetylcholine (ACh), and a reduced tension (not shown) resulting from inhibition of Ca^{2+} entry. (From: (A and C) Hutter O F, Trautwein W 1956 J Gen Physiol 39: 715; (B) Reuter H 1974 J Physiol 242: 429; (D) Giles W R, Noble S J 1976 J Physiol 261: 103)

The effect of β-receptor activation is to shift the voltage-dependence of this process to a more depolarised potential, so that the pacemaker current is switched on earlier and faster, and reaches the firing threshold earlier.

The shape of the action potential is also changed by β-receptor activation, the plateau phase becoming more pronounced. At the same time, the contraction also becomes larger but briefer (Fig. 13.8). The accentuation of the plateau is due to an increase of the slow inward current. Patch-clamp analysis (see Ch. 2) has shown that β-receptor activation, or increased intracellular cAMP concentration, causes more calcium channels to open in response to a given depolarisation and a marked increase in the magnitude of the transient rise in $[Ca^{2+}]_i$ that accompanies the action potential (Fig. 13.9). It appears that cAMP-dependent phosphorylation of the calcium channel protein is required for the channel to function, so the number of available channels at any moment reflects the relative rates of dephosphorylation and cAMP-dependent rephosphorylation of this protein. The same mechanism

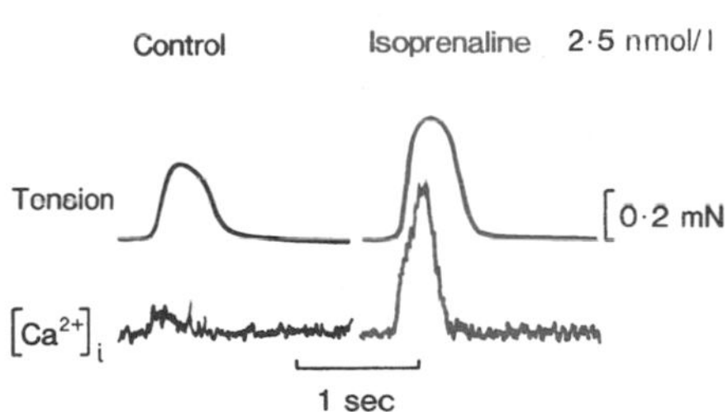

Fig. 13.9 The calcium transient in frog cardiac muscle. A group of cells was injected with the phosphorescent Ca^{2+} indicator, aequorin, which allows $[Ca^{2+}]_i$ to be monitored optically. Isoprenaline causes a large increase in the Ca^{2+} transient and in the tension produced. (From: Allen D G, Blinks J R 1978 Nature 273: 509)

probably accounts for the facilitation of AV conduction, where the sodium transient is absent, so that propagation depends on the Ca^{2+} current. Increased calcium entry may also account for increased automaticity (see p. 271) because of the effect of $[Ca^{2+}]_i$ on the transient inward current, which can result in after-discharge following a single evoked action potential (Fig. 13.2). The increased force of contraction is partly due to increased Ca^{2+} entry, but β-receptor activation also increases the Ca^{2+} sensitivity of the contractile machinery, possibly by phosphorylating troponin C; furthermore, it facilitates Ca^{2+} capture by the sarcoplasmic reticulum, thereby increasing the amount of Ca^{2+} stored intracellularly available for release by the action potential. The net result of catecholamine action is to elevate and steepen the ventricular function curve (Fig. 13.5).

β-receptor activation causes hyperpolarisation of some parts of the heart, which is particularly noticeable if the myocardium is damaged or hypoxic. This is due to stimulation of the Na^+/K^+ pump, which generates a net outward sodium current. This repolarisation may suffice to restore conduction, for example in the AV bundle, when heart block has occurred following a myocardial infarction.

The reduction of cardiac efficiency by catecholamines is important because it means that the oxygen requirement of the myocardium increases even if the work of the heart is unchanged. Myocardial infarction causes sympathetic activation, which has the undesirable effect of increasing the oxygen needs of the damaged myocardium. The mechanism of the reduction of efficiency is not certain, but one explanation is that β-receptor activation stimulates fatty acid production by promoting lipolysis (see Ch. 7), causing cardiac metabolism to shift from glucose to fatty acid utilisation which requires more oxygen per ATP molecule generated. Relatively slow adaptive and counteradaptive mechanisms involving β-receptors are brought into play during myocardial infarction: acute myocardial ischaemia leads within 15 minutes to a gradual increase in β-adrenoceptors at the cell surface. In normal hearts the increase in endogenous catecholamines is sufficient to cause desensitisation with β-receptor internalisation, but this is abolished by myocardial ischaemia leading to the balance of internalisation and externalisation of receptors being shifted toward an increase in functionally coupled cardiac β-receptors (Strasser et al. 1990).

The actions and uses of drugs that act on β-receptors are described in Chapter 7.

Parasympathetic system

Parasympathetic activity produces effects that are, in general, opposite to those of sympathetic activation, namely:

- cardiac slowing and reduced automaticity
- decreased force of contraction (mainly in atria)
- inhibition of AV conduction.

These effects result from activation of muscarinic (M_2) acetylcholine receptors, which are abundant in nodal and atrial tissue but sparse in the ventricle. These receptors are negatively coupled to adenylate cyclase, and thus reduce cAMP formation, acting to inhibit the slow calcium current, in opposition to β_1-adrenoceptors. M_2-receptors open potassium channels via G-protein coupling. The resulting increase in potassium permeability produces a hyperpolarising current that effectively opposes the inward pacemaker current; this accounts for the negative chronotropic effect and reduced automaticity (see Fig. 13.8). Cardiac slowing caused by vagal stimulation or muscarinic agonists can amount to complete cardiac standstill for many seconds, though if stimulation is maintained, a slow beat generated by ventricular conducting tissue normally reappears.

The negative inotropic effect in the atria results from inhibition of the slow inward current, and is associated with a marked shortening of the action potential (Fig. 13.8). It is very likely that both phenomena (increased K^+ permeability and reduced Ca^{2+} current) contribute to the conduction block at the AV node, where propagation is dependent on

Autonomic control of the heart

- Sympathetic activity, acting through β_1-adrenoceptors, increases heart rate, contractility and automaticity, but reduces cardiac efficiency (in relation to oxygen consumption).
- β_1-adrenoceptors act by increasing cAMP formation, which increases calcium currents.
- Parasympathetic activity, acting through M_2 muscarinic receptors, causes cardiac slowing, decreased force of contraction (atria only) and inhibition of AV conduction.
- M_2-receptors inhibit cAMP formation, and also open K^+ channels, causing hyperpolarisation.

the Ca^{2+} current. The shortening of the atrial action potential reduces the refractory period which can, paradoxically, increase the probability of re-entrant dysrhythmias in the atria. Coronary vessels lack cholinergic innervation.

As well as producing opposite effects on myocardial cells, the sympathetic and parasympathetic systems also interact at the presynaptic level. The terminals of sympathetic and parasympathetic nerves are often found close together, and there is evidence for mutual inhibition of transmitter release by the two systems.

The actions and uses of drugs that act on muscarinic receptors are described in Chapter 6.

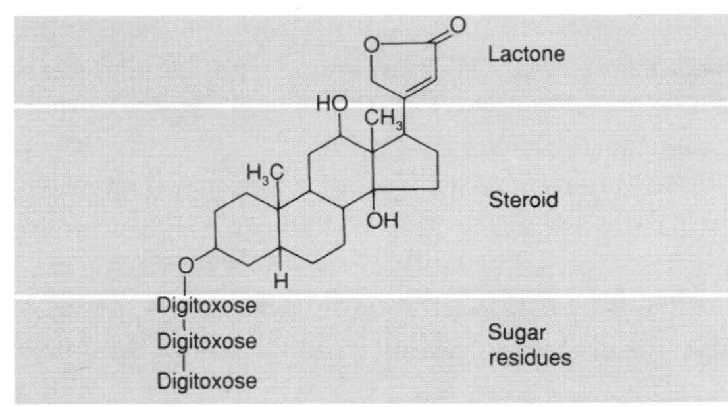

Fig. 13.10 Chemical structure of cardiac glycosides. Individual compounds vary in respect of (1) methyl and hydroxyl groups on the steroid nucleus, and (2) sugar residues.

CARDIAC GLYCOSIDES

Cardiac glycosides (reviewed by Smith 1988) come from leaves of plants of the foxglove family (*Digitalis* sp.), and have been in clinical use for many centuries. Their effectiveness in cardiac failure was described by Withering in 1775, who wrote on the use of the foxglove '. . . it has a power over the motion of the heart to a degree yet unobserved in any other medicine . . .'. Cardiac glycosides are still widely used for the treatment of cardiac failure in association with rapid atrial fibrillation, but the effectiveness of angiotensin-converting enzyme inhibitors in prolonging survival in patients with heart failure (Ch. 14) has led to decreased use of cardiac glycosides in patients in sinus rhythm although recent studies have reaffirmed their efficacy in this situation. As clinical use has declined, theoretical interest has increased, because of increasing evidence of an endogenous digitalis-like factor.

Chemistry

The leaves of the foxglove contain several cardiac glycosides with similar actions. Similar substances occur in other plants, such as squill and lily of the valley. **Digoxin** is the most therapeutically important. **Ouabain** is similar but shorter-acting; its sugar moiety (see below) consists of rhamnose, not found generally in mammals. All have the same pharmacological actions. The possibility of an endogenous digitalis-like factor in mammals (see Goto et al. 1992 for a review) has been mooted for many years, and more recently it has been established that this activity is due either to ouabain or to a closely similar substance present in plasma and synthesised in the adrenal cortex (Hamlyn et al. 1991).

The basic chemical structure (Fig. 13.10) consists of three components, a *sugar moiety*, a *steroid* and a *lactone*. The sugar moiety consists of 1–4 linked monosaccharides, some of which are not found elsewhere in nature. The lactone ring is essential for activity, and substituted lactones can retain biological activity even when the steroid moiety is removed.

Actions

The main effects of glycosides are on the heart, but some of their extra-cardiac actions are clinically important in determining toxicity. The cardiac effects are:

- cardiac slowing and reduced rate of conduction through the AV node, associated with increased vagal activity
- increased force of contraction
- disturbances of rhythm
  - — block of AV conduction
  - — increased ectopic pacemaker activity.

Useful effects include partial AV block (see below) and increased force of contraction. Unpleasant or hazardous side effects are common. One of the main drawbacks of glycosides in clinical use is the narrow margin between effectiveness and toxicity.

Mechanism of action

The cardiac glycosides exert their effects through actions both on the rate and rhythm and on the force of contraction of the heart.

Rate and rhythm. In a normal subject, glycosides *slow AV conduction* and cause cardiac slowing. This results from an increase in vagal activity due to an action on the central nervous system. AV conduction time is increased, discernible on the ECG as an increased P–R interval, due to slowing of conduction in the AV node.

Glycosides have a beneficial effect in rapid atrial fibrillation through their effects on AV conduction, and this constitutes their main therapeutic indication. If ventricular rate is excessively high, the time for diastolic filling is inadequate. Increasing the refractory period of the AV node is beneficial under these conditions, because it increases the minimum interval between impulses and reduces ventricular rate. The atrial dysrhythmia is unaffected, but the pumping efficiency of the heart improves due to improved ventricular filling. Paroxysmal supraventricular tachycardias can be terminated by cardiac glycosides by slowing AV conduction, although other drugs are usually employed for this indication (see below).

Larger doses of glycosides cause disturbances of rhythm. These may occur at plasma concentrations within, or only slightly above, the therapeutic range and are clinically important. Slowing of AV conduction can progress to AV block. In addition to depressing AV conduction, glycosides cause ectopic beats associated with increased transient inward current (see above) due to increased afterdepolarisation following the action potential. Initially this causes coupled beats (bigeminy), in which a normal ventricular beat is followed by an extra ectopic beat. This can progress to ventricular tachycardia, where there is a continuous succession of such triggered ectopic beats, and eventually to ventricular fibrillation.

Force of contraction. Glycosides cause a large increase in twitch tension in isolated preparations of cardiac muscle. Unlike catecholamines they do not accelerate relaxation (compare Figs 13.9 and 13.11). Increased tension development is due to an increased intracellular calcium transient (Fig. 13.11). The action potential is, however, only slightly affected and the slow inward current is little changed, so the increased calcium transient probably reflects a greater release of calcium from intracellular stores. The most likely mechanism for this is as follows (Fig. 13.12):

- The primary site on which glycosides act is the Na^+/K^+-ATPase of the cell membrane, which constitutes the Na^+/K^+ pump. Glycosides bind to the K^+-binding site of the enzyme, and thus inhibit the pump.

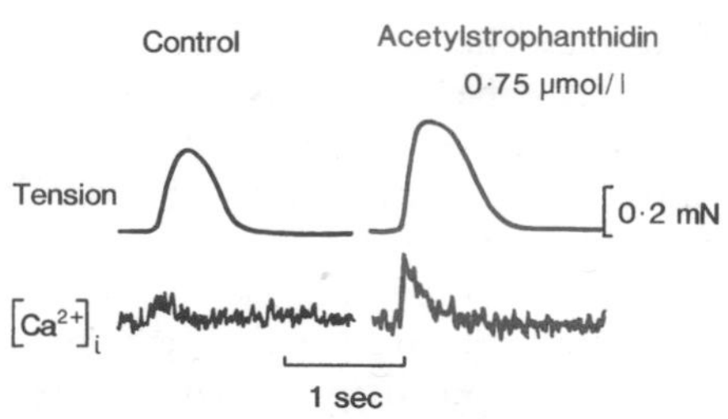

Fig. 13.11 Effect of a cardiac glycoside (acetylstrophanthidin) on the Ca^{2+} transient and tension produced by frog cardiac muscle. The effect was recorded as in Figure 13.9. (From: Allen D G, Blinks J R 1978 Nature 273: 509)

- Pump inhibition causes a rise in $[Na^+]_i$. Because Na^+/K^+ exchange is electrogenic (that is, it pumps more Na^+ ions out than K^+ ions in, and thus generates a net hyperpolarising current), inhibition causes depolarisation. This is important in producing effects on cardiac rhythm.
- Increased $[Na^+]_i$ slows extrusion of Ca^{2+}. This is because extrusion of Ca^{2+} is by a Na^+/Ca^{2+} exchange mechanism. Increasing $[Na^+]_i$ reduces the inwardly directed gradient for Na^+; the smaller this gradient the slower the extrusion of Ca^{2+} by Na^+/Ca^{2+} exchange.
- The increase in $[Ca^{2+}]_i$, though too small to activate the contractile protein directly, causes an increase in sarcoplasmic reticulum Ca^{2+} content, and thus increases the amount released by the action potential.

Interaction with extracellular potassium concentration

The effects of glycosides are increased if the plasma $[K^+]$ decreases. This is probably because of competition between the glycoside and K^+ for the Na^+/K^+-ATPase. Increased $[K^+]$ inhibits the binding of glycosides to the enzyme, and reduces their effect on sodium transport. This effect is clinically important, since **diuretics** (see Ch. 18) are often used together with glycosides in the treatment of heart failure and most of them cause a decrease in plasma $[K^+]$, thereby enhancing the tendency of the glycoside to cause unwanted dysrhythmias.

Pharmacokinetic aspects

Clinical use and unwanted effects of digoxin are summarised on page 285.

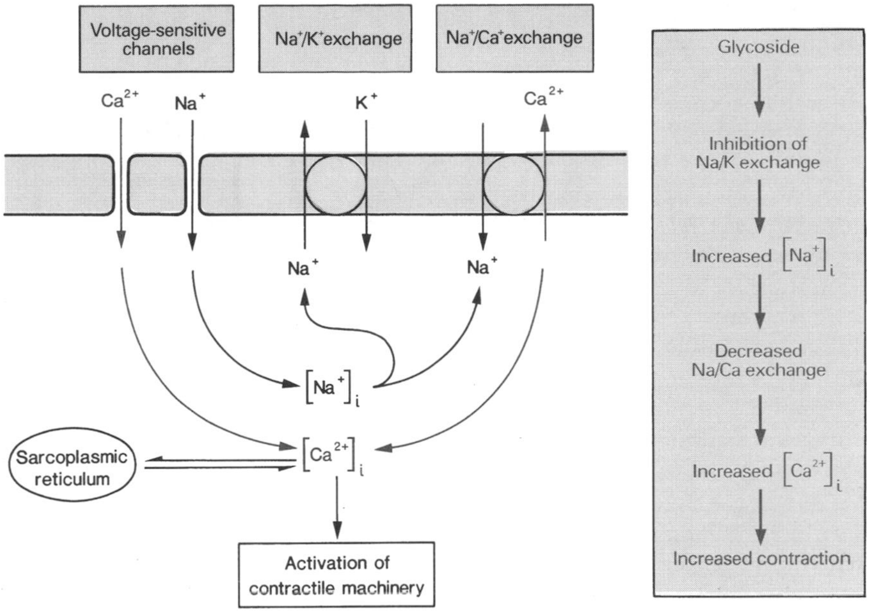

Fig. 13.12 Proposed mechanism of action of cardiac glycosides. Inhibition of Na^+/K^+ exchange indirectly inhibits Ca^{2+} extrusion from the cell, by raising $[Na^+]_i$ (see Fig. 13.4). Thus, total Ca^{2+} increases, so that more Ca^{2+} is stored in sarcoplasmic reticulum, and more is available for release in response to the action potential.

Cardiac glycosides

- Act by inhibiting Na^+/K^+ pump, thus causing increase of $[Na^+]_i$. This results in reduced Na^+/Ca^{2+} exchange, causing secondary rise in Ca^{2+} accumulation by sarcoplasmic reticulum.
- Main effect is increased force of contraction.
- Additional important effects are:
  —increase of ectopic pacemaker activity
  —impairment of AV conduction
  —increased vagal activity, causing bradycardia.
- Effects are increased by hypokalaemia.

OTHER CARDIOTONIC AGENTS

Certain β_1-adrenoceptor agonists, notably **dobutamine**, are of considerable value for treatment of acute but potentially reversible heart failure (e.g. following cardiac surgery, or in some cases of cardiogenic shock) on the basis of their positive inotropic action. Dobutamine, for reasons that are not well understood, produces less tachycardia than other β_1-agonists. It is administered intravenously. Attempts to use orally-active β-agonists to treat chronic heart failure have been disappointing. **Xamoterol,**

Digoxin

- Digoxin is the glycoside in widest clinical use.
- Uses include:
  —slowing ventricular rate in rapid atrial fibrillation
  —treatment of heart failure in patients who remain symptomatic despite optimal use of diuretics (Ch. 18) and angiotensin-converting enzyme inhibitors (Ch. 14).
- Adverse effects include nausea, vomiting, cardiac arrhythmias, confusion.
- Administration is oral or, in urgent situations, intravenous.
- Elimination is mainly by renal excretion; elimination half-time is approximately 36 hours in patients with normal renal function, considerably longer in elderly patients and those with overt renal failure in whom reduced doses are needed.
- A loading dose is used in urgent situations.
- The therapeutic range of plasma concentrations, below which digoxin is unlikely to be effective and above which the risk of toxicity increases substantially, is fairly well defined. Determination of plasma digoxin concentration is useful when lack of efficacy or toxicity is suspected.
- Clinically important interactions occur with drugs that reduce plasma K^+ (e.g. loop diuretics) or which reduce its excretion and tissue binding (e.g. amiodarone, verapamil).

a partial agonist, is partially effective in mild heart failure but deleterious in more severe disease, which makes its use problematic in a disorder whose natural history is to progress unpredictably from mild to severe.

Inhibitors of a heart-specific subtype (type III) of phosphodiesterase, the enzyme responsible for the intracellular degradation of cAMP, are positively inotropic. They increase intracellular cAMP concentration, as do β-adrenoceptor agonists, and are pro-arrhythmic for the same reason. Compounds in this group include **amrinone** and **milrinone**, which are chemically and pharmacologically very similar. Amrinone is a short-acting drug, suitable only for intravenous administration, sometimes used to treat severe acute heart failure resistant to other drugs. Milrinone is long-acting and can be used orally, but does not prolong life, perhaps because of its pro-arrhythmic action. It has been used to tide patients over who are severely symptomatic whilst awaiting some more definitive treatment such as cardiac transplantation.

ANTIDYSRHYTHMIC DRUGS

A classification of antidysrhythmic drugs in terms of their electrophysiological effects was proposed by Vaughan Williams in 1970; this provides a useful basis for discussing their mechanisms of action (see Vaughan Williams 1989), although many of the most useful drugs for treating dysrhythmias do not fit neatly into this classification (see following box).

The classes (see Table 13.1) are:

- *Class I*: drugs that block voltage-sensitive sodium channels, thus reducing the excitability of the non-nodal regions of the heart where the inward sodium current is important for propagation of the action potential. These drugs are further divided into three classes, Ia, Ib and Ic (see below).
- *Class II*: β-adrenoceptor antagonists.
- *Class III*: drugs that prolong the refractory period of the myocardium, thus tending to suppress re-entrant rhythms.
- *Class IV*: calcium antagonists, which block voltage-sensitive calcium channels and thus impair impulse propagation in nodal areas and in damaged areas of the myocardium.

Antidysrhythmic therapy

- Emergency treatment of serious arrhythmias is usually by physical means (e.g. electrical cardioversion or pacing) rather than drugs.
- Antidysrhythmic drugs can be classified by their electrophysiological effects (Vaughan Williams' classification). The main uses of drugs of different classes are summarised in Table 13.1.
- Many drugs and inorganic ions that are not classed primarily as antidysrhythmic are used clinically to treat important arrhythmias. These include:
  - —atropine (for sinus bradycardia causing haemodynamic compromise)
  - —adrenaline (in cardiac arrest due to asystole)
  - —isoprenaline (for bradycardia caused by heart block, while arranging electrical pacing)
  - —adenosine (for supraventricular tachycardia and diagnostically)
  - —calcium chloride (for ventricular tachycardia due to hyperkalaemia)
  - —magnesium chloride (for ventricular fibrillation).
- All drugs used to treat arrhythmias can themselves cause arrhythmias.
- Chronic administration of β-adrenoceptor antagonists (class II) following myocardial infarction prolongs life, but class I drugs reduce survival in patients with ventricular ectopics despite normalising the electrocardiogram. Class III agents are more effective but can cause a form of ventricular tachycardia.

The sites of action of these classes of drug are shown diagrammatically in Figure 13.13.

Many of the most useful drugs for treating arrhythmias in clinical practice do not fit into this classification. These include drugs that increase vagal activity, most notably **digoxin** (for atrial fibrillation; see above), muscarinic antagonists (e.g. **atropine** for treating sinus bradycardia), adrenoceptor agonists (e.g. **adrenaline** in asystolic cardiac arrest), **adenosine** (for supraventricular tachycardia), **calcium** salts (for ventricular arrhythmias caused by hyperkalaemia) and **magnesium** salts (for ventricular arrhythmias). Finally, it should be noted that the emergency treatment of life-threatening arrhythmias is seldom a drug in the first instance; thus *bradyarrhythmias* (e.g. heart block) may require *pacing*, and *tachyarrhythmias* often necessitate *direct current cardioversion.*

Table 13.1 Summary of antidysrhythmic drugs (Vaughan Williams' classification)

Class	Examples	Mechanism	Cardiac effects* MRD	APD	ERP	AV conduction	Contractility	Uses	Special points
Ia	Quinidine	Block of Na channels	↓↓	↑	↑	↓↓	↓		Historical interest. Atropine-like side effects
	Procainamide		↓↓	↑	↑	↓↓	↓		Historical interest. Hypersensitivity reactions
	Disopyramide		↓↓	↑	↑	↓↓	↓↓↓	Atrial and ventricular tachycardias	Strongly reduces ventricular contractility Atropine-like side effects
Ib	Lignocaine	Block of Na channels (fast dissoc.)	↓	↓	↑↑	–	–	Ventricular dysrhythmias following heart attacks	Used i.v., MRD ↓↓↓ in depol. cells
Ic	Flecainide	Block of Na channels (slow dissoc.)	↓↓↓	–	–	↓↓	↓↓	Mainly life-threatening ventricular tachycardias	May cause ventricular dysrhythmias
II	Propranolol	β-adrenoceptor antagonism	–	–	–	– or ↓	↓↓	Stress-induced tachycardias	See Ch. 7
	Metoprolol		–	–	–	–	↓↓		
III	Amiodarone	Not known	–	↑↑↑	↑↑↑	↓	–	Tachycardia in Wolff–Parkinson–White syndrome	Slow onset, long duration. Many side effects. Can cause torsades de pointes
	Sotalol		–	↑↑↑	↑↑↑	↓	↓↓	Tachyarrhythmias	In addition to class II action
IV	Verapamil	Ca-channel block	–	↓↓	–	↓↓	↓↓↓	Atrial tachyarrhythmias	Can cause severe bradycardia and hypotension. Danger if combined with β-adrenoceptor antagonists

* MRD = maximum rate of depolarisation; APD = action potential duration; ERP = effective refractory period

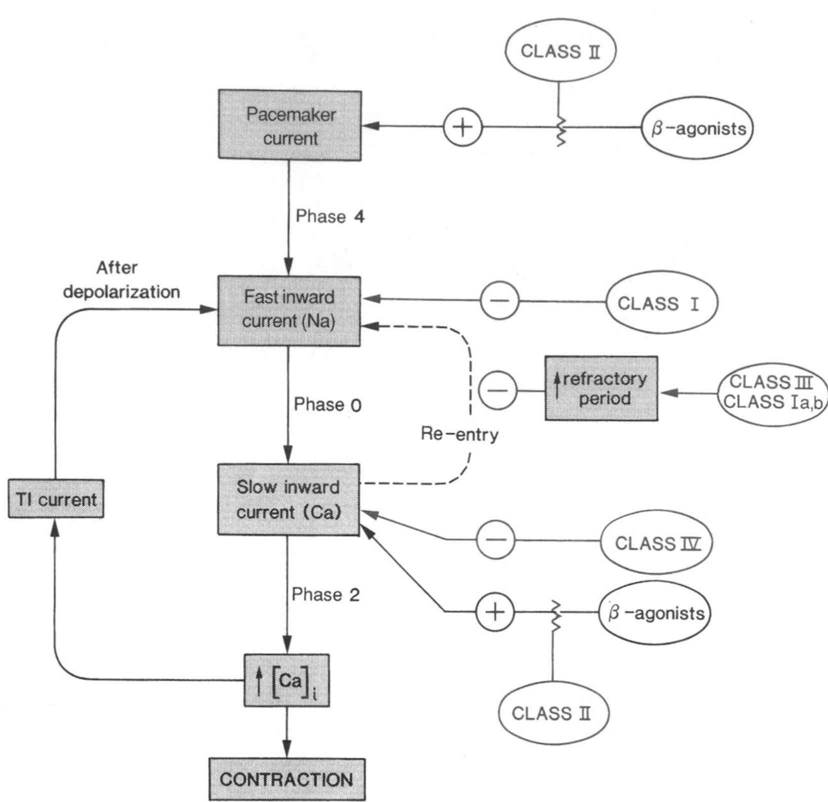

Fig. 13.13 Sites of action of antidysrhythmic drugs. (TI current = transient inward current)

Mechanisms of action

Class I drugs

Class I drugs act by *blocking sodium channels,* exactly as local anaesthetics do (see Ch. 34). Because this inhibits action potential propagation in many excitable cells, it has been referred to as 'membrane stabilising' activity, a phrase best avoided now that the ionic mechanism is well understood. Their characteristic effect on the action potential is a reduction in the rate of depolarisation during phase 0.

The reason for further subdivision of these drugs into classes Ia, Ib and Ic is that the earliest examples, **quinidine** and **procainamide** (class Ia), have different effects from many of the more recently developed agents in classes Ib and Ic, even though all share the same basic mechanism of action. A partial explanation for these functional differences comes from electrophysiological studies of the characteristics of the Na^+ channel block produced by the different types of class I drugs. The central concept is that of *use-dependent channel block.*

In general, it is the use-dependent characteristic that enables all class I drugs to block the high frequency excitation of the myocardium that occurs in dysrhythmias, without preventing the heart from beating at normal frequencies.

The work of Hille and others on the action of local anaesthetics on excitable membranes (see Ch. 34) has shown that they bind to a site within the Na^+ channel and prevent it from conducting. The channel can exist in three distinct functional states: *resting, open* and *refractory.* Channel opening occurs when it switches, in response to depolarisation, rapidly from resting to open; this is known as activation. Maintained depolarisation, as in ischaemic muscle, causes it to change more slowly from open to refractory (inactivation) and the membrane must then be repolarised for a time to restore it to the resting state.

Class I drugs bind to the channel most strongly when it is in the open or refractory state. Their action therefore shows the property of use-dependence (i.e. the more frequently the channels are activated, the greater the degree of block produced). This can be demonstrated experimentally (see Hondeghem 1989) in isolated myocardial preparations electrically stimulated at different frequencies. Normally, the rate of rise of the action potential (a measure of the number of sodium channels that are available) is affected very little by the stimulation frequency. In the presence of a class I drug, the rate of rise of the first action potential in a train is only slightly reduced, but successive action potentials become progressively more blocked. With each action potential, the opening of Na^+ channels allows further block to develop. If the preparation is then left quiescent, the lower affinity of the class I agent for the closed channels causes it gradually to dissociate, so that the block subsides. The rate at which this recovery occurs varies between different drugs and is a measure of the rate of dissociation of the drug from the channel.

Class Ib drugs, such as **lignocaine**, associate and dissociate rapidly within the time-frame of the normal heartbeat. Thus, the drug binds to the open channels during phase 0 of the action potential (affecting the rate of rise very little, but leaving many of the channels blocked by the time the action potential reaches its peak). It then dissociates in time for the next action potential, if the cardiac rhythm is normal. A premature beat, however, will be aborted because the channels will still be blocked. Furthermore, class Ib drugs bind selectively to refractory channels, and thus block preferentially when the cells are depolarised, for example in ischaemia. These properties mean that class Ib drugs are useful principally in the control of ventricular dysrhythmias following myocardial infarction.

Class Ic drugs, such as **flecainide** and **encainide**, associate and dissociate much more slowly, thus reaching a steady-state level of block that does not vary appreciably during the cardiac cycle; they also show only a marginal preference for refractory channels, so are not specific for damaged myocardium. Therefore, they cause a rather general reduction in excitability, and do not discriminate particularly against occasional premature beats, as class Ib drugs do, but will tend to suppress re-entrant rhythms which depend on unidirectional or intermittent conduction pathways operating at a low margin of safety.

Class Ia, the oldest group, lies midway in its properties between Ib and Ic.

Class II drugs

Class II drugs comprise β-adrenoceptor antagonists such as **propranolol**.

It is known that adrenaline can cause ventricular extrasystoles and even fibrillation, by its effects on the pacemaker potential and the slow inward current, carried by calcium ions, in myocardial cells (see earlier section). There is also evidence that the occurrence of ventricular dysrhythmias following myocardial infarction is partly the result of increased sympathetic activity (see Fig. 13.7), and this provides the rationale for using β-adrenoceptor-blocking drugs to reduce their occurrence. AV conduction also depends critically on sympathetic activity, and the refractory period of the AV node is increased by β-adrenoceptor-blocking drugs, which can be used in much the same way as digoxin to interfere with AV conduction in atrial tachycardias, and to slow the ventricular rate.

Class III drugs

The class III category of antidysrhythmic action was originally based on the unusual behaviour of a single drug, **amiodarone** (see below), although other drugs with similar properties (e.g. **sotalol**) have since been described. The special feature of amiodarone is its ability to prolong the cardiac action potential, though the ionic mechanism of this effect remains unclear. This prolongation is associated with an increased refractory period, which accounts for its profound ventricular and supraventricular antidysrhythmic effects. One peculiarity of the drug that makes it hard to study is that it is extensively bound in tissues and has a very long elimination half-life, so its action normally takes days or weeks to develop. For this reason, an intravenous loading dose is used in treating life-threatening arrhythmias.

Class IV drugs

Class IV agents, of which **verapamil** and **diltiazem** are the main examples, act by blocking voltage-sensitive calcium channels. As expected, they shorten the plateau phase of the action potential and reduce the force of contraction. The reduction of calcium entry has the effect of inhibiting the transient inward current (see Fig. 13.13), and thus suppressing premature ectopic beats.

Calcium antagonists also inhibit the 'slow response', a mode of conduction occurring in depolarised myocardium that may be important in sustaining re-entrant rhythms (see above).

Details of individual drugs

Table 13.1 summarises the properties of the most important antidysrhythmic drugs.

Quinidine, procainamide and disopyramide (class Ia)

Quinidine and procainamide are pharmacologically similar. Quinidine is the D-isomer of quinine, an antimalarial drug (Ch. 40). It has a venerable place in the history of antidysrhythmic drugs, but is now seldom used clinically, because safer and more effective drugs are available. (Quinidine is, however, sometimes used intravenously to treat severe falciparum malaria in patients too ill to be treated by oral quinine.) **Procainamide** is similar to **quinidine** as regards its antidysrhythmic action, but lacks atropine-like effects; its use is also currently very limited. It can produce hypersensitivity reactions, usually in the form of fever or skin rashes and blood dyscrasias, sometimes in association with autoantibodies and a systemic illness that mimics *systemic lupus erythematosus*. These reactions, though rare, can be fatal, and procainamide is now seldom used. **Disopyramide** resembles quinidine in its antidysrhythmic effects and uses, as well as its marked atropine-like effects which result in blurred vision, dry mouth, constipation and, in men, may precipitate urinary retention. It is more markedly negatively inotropic than quinidine but is less likely to cause hypersensitivity reactions.

Lignocaine (class Ib)

Lignocaine remains the most clinically important class I drug, being given by intravenous infusion to treat and prevent ventricular arrhythmias in the immediate aftermath of myocardial infarction in coronary intensive care units, although even in this setting its prophylactic use has not been proved to prolong life. It is also widely used as a local anaesthetic (Ch. 34). Its plasma half-life is about 2 hours, and it is largely removed from the portal circulation by hepatic first-pass metabolism (Ch. 4), so cannot be used orally. Its elimination is reduced if hepatic blood flow is reduced, for example by reduced cardiac output following myocardial infarction or by drugs such as **β-adrenoceptor antagonists** (which are also often used after myocardial infarction), and accumulation and toxicity may result if this is not anticipated and the rate of administration reduced accordingly.

The adverse effects of lignocaine are mainly manifestations of actions on the central nervous system, and include drowsiness, disorientation and convulsions. Because of its relatively short half-life, the plasma concentration can be adjusted fairly rapidly by varying the infusion rate.

Phenytoin (class Ib)

Phenytoin is used chiefly as an antiepileptic drug (Ch. 30), but it also has antidysrhythmic actions. The same mechanisms probably underlie its anticonvulsant and antidysrhythmic effects. It is used to counteract glycoside-induced dysrhythmias, although the basis for its efficacy in this setting is not understood.

Flecainide and encainide (class Ic)

Flecainide and encainide suppress ventricular ectopic beats. They are long-acting, and effective orally. However, they were found, in a well-controlled trial (see Ruskin 1989), actually to increase the incidence of sudden death associated with ventricular fibrillation after myocardial infarction, due to an unexpected (and unexplained) prodysrhythmic effect, so their use is now quite limited.

β-adrenoceptor antagonists (class II)

The most important β-receptor antagonists are described in Chapter 7, and several of these are used for their antidysrhythmic actions. **Propranolol**, like several other drugs of this type, has some class I action in addition to blocking β-receptors, and this may contribute to its antidysrhythmic effects, though probably not very much since the isomer with little β-antagonist activity has little antidysrhythmic activity, despite similar activity as a class I agent.

Adverse effects are described in Chapter 7, the most important ones being bronchospasm in patients with asthma or other forms of obstructive airways disease, and reduced cardiac output which can precipitate cardiac failure. It was hoped that the use of β_1-selective drugs (e.g. **metoprolol, atenolol**) would reduce the risk of bronchospasm, but the degree of selectivity of these drugs is inadequate to achieve this goal in clinical practice, although the once-a-day convenience of these drugs has led to their widespread use in patients without lung disease. Similarly, it was hoped that use of drugs with partial agonist activity (e.g. **alprenolol, pindolol**) would reduce the incidence of bronchospasm and cardiac failure, but in practice it is best to use alternative drugs in patients with lung disease or heart failure.

The main use of β-adrenoceptor antagonists as antidysrhythmic drugs is in patients recovering from myocardial infarction. They reduce mortality in the first year after a heart attack, partly at least because of their ability to prevent ventricular dysrhythmias. They are also effective for atrial dysrhythmias when these are provoked by increased sympathetic activity.

Amiodarone and sotalol (class III)
Though its mode of action is not well understood, amiodarone is a highly effective drug and is widely used. Its main action is to increase markedly the refractory period of cardiac muscle, and hence to suppress both atrial and ventricular re-entrant rhythms. Unfortunately, it has several peculiarities that complicate its use.

It has an extremely long plasma half-life (10–100 days) and accumulates extensively in the body.

Adverse effects are numerous and important; they include photosensitive skin rashes and a slate-grey/bluish discoloration of the skin, thyroid abnormalities (hypo- and hyper-, connected with its high iodine content, and rendered difficult to assess because of its effects on thyroid function tests), pulmonary fibrosis that is slow in onset but may be irreversible, corneal deposits, neurological and gastro-intestinal disturbances. Like other antidysrhythmic drugs it can have pro-arrhythmic effects: all class III drugs appear capable of causing a form of ventricular tachycardia called (somewhat whimsically) '*torsades de pointes*' (because the appearance of the ECG trace is said to be reminiscent of this ballet sequence). This occurs particularly with individuals with hereditary prolonged Q–T (Ward–Romano syndrome) and those taking other drugs that can influence Q–T, such as the H_1-receptor antagonists **astemizole** or **terfenadine** (Ch. 11) or the hypolipidaemic **probucol** (Ch. 15).

Sotalol is a β-adrenoceptor antagonist, this activity residing in the l-isomer. Unlike other β-antagonists, it prolongs the cardiac action potential and the Q–T interval due to prolongation of the slow outward potassium current. This class III activity is present in both l- and d-isomers. It appears to have similar efficacy to amiodarone in preventing chronic malignant ventricular tachyarrhythmias unassociated with acute myocardial infarction (Amiodarone vs Sotalol Study Group 1989). It shares the ability of amiodarone to cause *torsades de pointes* but lacks its other adverse effects, and is valuable in patients in whom β-receptor antagonists are not contraindicated.

Verapamil and diltiazem (class IV)
Verapamil is used to terminate and prevent paroxysmal supraventricular tachycardia (SVT), and to reduce the ventricular rate in patients with atrial fibrillation who are inadequately controlled with **digoxin**. It is not effective for ventricular dysrhythmias. It is normally given orally but can be given intravenously to terminate SVT. It has a plasma half-life of 6–8 hours, which is a problem if adverse effects follow its intravenous administration.

The main *adverse effect* is heart failure, caused by inhibition of calcium entry. This is particularly disastrous following inadvertent intravenous administration to patients with ventricular tachycardia. **Adenosine** (see below) is much safer in this setting, because of its shorter half-life. Intravenous verapamil should never be used following **β-adrenoceptor** blockade (or vice versa) because of the risk of cardiovascular collapse. Verapamil relaxes vascular smooth muscle, again by blocking calcium entry, and is sometimes used to lower blood pressure in patients with hypertension. Constipation, perhaps because of an effect on calcium entry in gastro-intestinal smooth muscle or enteric nerves, is a common and troublesome side effect of chronic therapy. If verapamil is added to **digoxin** in patients with poorly controlled atrial fibrillation the dose of digoxin should be reduced and plasma digoxin concentration checked after a few days because verapamil both displaces digoxin from tissue-binding sites and reduces its renal elimination, hence predisposing to digoxin accumulation and toxicity (see Ch. 42). **Diltiazem** is similar to verapamil, but has relatively more smooth-muscle-relaxing effect.

ANTI-ANGINAL DRUGS

Anginal pain occurs when the coronary blood flow is insufficient to meet the heart's metabolic requirements, usually because increased myocardial oxygen demand during exercise cannot be met in an area of myocardium perfused by a coronary artery with a significant fixed narrowing due to an atheromatous plaque, sometimes complicated by platelet–fibrin thrombus. It is discussed on pages 277–278. It can be counteracted by drugs that either improve perfusion of the myocardium or reduce its metabolic demand, or both. Two of the main groups of drugs that are used in angina, **organic nitrates** and **calcium antagonists**, are vasodilators and produce both of these effects. The third group are the **β-adrenoceptor antagonists**, which reduce heart rate and hence the metabolic demand. Calcium antagonists are described in a later section, and β-adrenoceptor antagonists in Chapter 7.

The box below summarises a general approach to anti-anginal drugs. A comprehensive account can be found in Abshagen (1985).

Organic nitrates (see also Ch. 10)

The ability of organic nitrates to relieve anginal pain was discovered by Lauder Brunton, a distinguished British physician, in 1867. He had found that angina could be partly relieved by bleeding, and also knew that **amyl nitrite**, which had been synthesised 10 years earlier, caused very marked flushing and tachycardia, with a fall in blood pressure, when its vapour was inhaled. He thought that the effect of bleeding resulted from hypotension, and found that amyl nitrite inhalation worked much better. It was also tried enthusiastically in many other conditions, such as cholera, without effect. Amyl nitrite, given as a vapour, was used for many years, but has now been replaced by **glyceryl trinitrate** (nitroglycerine). This substance was discovered by Nobel to be an excellent explosive, the major ingredient of dynamite. Nitroglycerine was soon discovered to cause flushing and a throbbing headache. It was realised that its action was the same as that of amyl nitrite, and it was found to be just as effective in angina. Glyceryl trinitrate is still widely used, and efforts to increase its duration of action have led to many other organic nitrates being tested, of which the most important are **isosorbide mononitrate** and **dinitrate** (Fig. 13.14). These substances all work in the same way, but differ in their duration of action.

Anti-anginal therapy

- Unstable angina is caused by platelet–fibrin thrombus on coronary artery atheroma. The most important drug is aspirin (Ch. 16) because it reduces the incidence of myocardial infarction. Glyceryl trinitrate as an intravenous infusion is very effective in relieving pain in this setting.
- Stable angina is caused by fixed coronary artery narrowing due to atheroma. Drugs and other measures to prevent progression of atheroma and cause its regression (Ch. 15) are important long-term measures.
- Duration of pain in stable angina is usually only a few minutes on stopping exercise; this can be reduced by sublingual glyceryl trinitrate.
- The frequency of anginal attacks can be reduced by regular use of:
  - —organic nitrates (e.g. isosorbide mononitrate given regularly by mouth or glyceryl trinitrate administered transdermally via a 'patch', or sublingually immediately before exertion)
  - —β-adrenoceptor antagonists (e.g. atenolol, metoprolol)
  - —calcium antagonists (e.g. diltiazem, amlodipine).
- Prinzmetal variant angina is uncommon; it is caused by coronary artery spasm often in an artery affected by atheromatous disease. The frequency and severity of attacks is reduced by coronary artery vasodilators including organic nitrates and calcium antagonists whereas β-adrenoceptor antagonists may increase vasospasm and worsen pain.

Mechanism of action

Organic nitrates act solely by relaxing smooth muscle. In common with other smooth muscle relaxants such as **sodium nitroprusside** and **atrial natriuretic peptide** (see above) they increase cGMP formation, and this is believed to be the basis of their cellular effects (see Murad et al. 1988; Fig. 13.15). The release of nitric oxide (NO) from organic nitrates involves a reaction with tissue –SH groups. NO, alone or after forming a reactive nitrosothiol intermediate, activates a soluble cytosolic form of guanylate cyclase (see Ch. 10). cGMP formation is thereby increased. Exactly how this causes

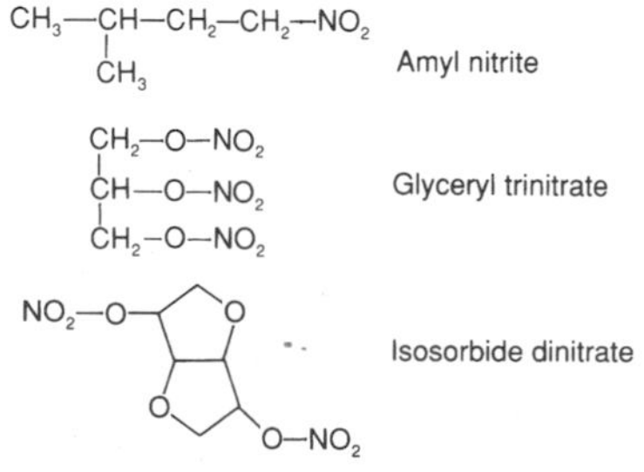

$CH_3—CH(CH_3)—CH_2—CH_2—NO_2$ Amyl nitrite

$CH_2—O—NO_2$ / $CH—O—NO_2$ / $CH_2—O—NO_2$ Glyceryl trinitrate

$NO_2—O$ … $O—NO_2$ Isosorbide dinitrate

Fig. 13.14 Structures of organic nitrates.

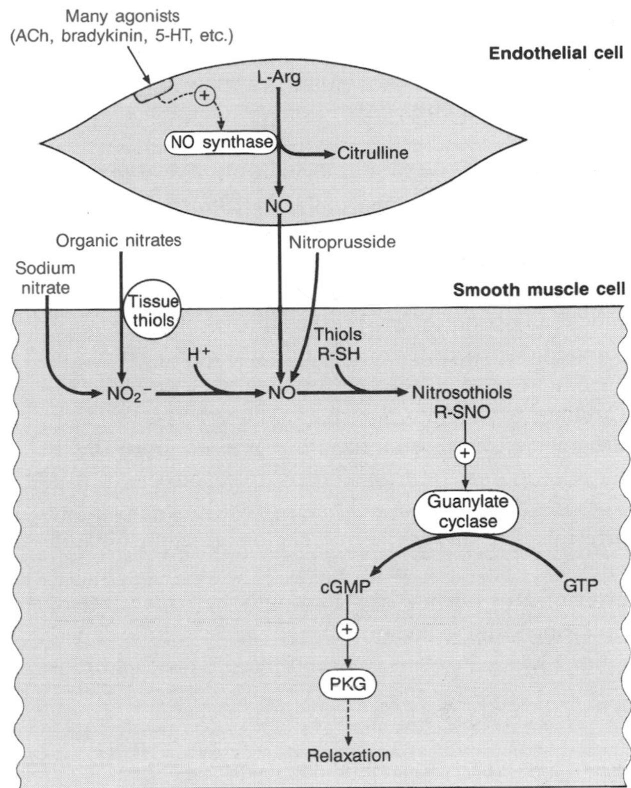

Fig. 13.15 Mode of action of nitrates.
(L-Arg = L-arginine; GTP = guanosine 5′-triphosphate; cGMP = cyclic guanosine 3′,5′ monophosphate; PKG = cGMP-dependent protein kinase)

relaxation is not yet certain, but is thought to involve (as with cAMP) activation of protein kinases, which oppose the increase in $[Ca^{2+}]_i$ caused by many contractile agonists, and/or affect the contractile proteins directly.

Pharmacological effects

Though organic nitrates relax all kinds of smooth muscle, the main effect when glyceryl trinitrate is given to normal subjects is on the cardiovascular system. There is marked dilatation of large veins, with a consequent reduction in central venous pressure (reduced pre-load), which, in the absence of heart failure, reduces cardiac output. With small doses, there is little effect on the arterioles, and the reduced stroke output is largely compensated by reflex tachycardia, so arterial pressure does not change. With larger doses, arterioles dilate, and arterial pressure falls, particularly if the subject stands up, causing dizziness. At the same time a throbbing headache is produced by dilatation of cerebral vessels.

Effects on the coronary circulation

In normal subjects, glyceryl trinitrate increases coronary flow in spite of a decrease in mean arterial pressure, implying a considerable reduction of coronary vascular resistance. Because both arterial pressure and cardiac output are decreased, myocardial oxygen consumption is reduced. This, and the increased blood flow, cause a large increase in the oxygen content of coronary sinus blood. If the coronary arteries are partially occluded by disease, however, coronary flow is not increased by nitrates. Several studies in patients who obtain relief from anginal pain with glyceryl trinitrate have shown that during an attack it either has no effect on the total coronary flow or actually reduces it, because of the fall in the arterial pressure. This might suggest that the benefit results entirely from the reduction of myocardial oxygen consumption secondary to the lowering of arterial and central venous pressure, but this view has been challenged recently by work on the regional distribution of coronary flow to different areas of the myocardium in experimental animals using the 'microsphere' technique. Very small radioactive glass beads are injected intravenously and become trapped in capillaries, the number collecting in different tissues providing a measure of local blood flow.

By this method it has been found that glyceryl trinitrate diverts blood from normal to ischaemic areas of myocardium. The mechanism appears to involve collateral vessels of fairly large calibre which are dilated by glyceryl trinitrate, enabling a partially blocked vessel to be bypassed (Fig. 13.16). It is interesting to compare this effect with that of other vasodilators (e.g. **dipyridamole**) which dilate precapillary arterioles, but not collateral vessels. This drug is as effective as nitrates, or even more so, in increasing coronary flow in normal subjects, but is not effective in angina. This is probably because the arterioles in the ischaemic region are fully dilated anyway, and the drug-induced dilatation of the arterioles in normal areas actually has the effect of diverting blood away from the ischaemic areas (Fig. 13.16). For this reason dipyridamole is administered intravenously to provide a pharmacological 'stress' in testing for arterial disease in patients who cannot exercise.

The direct relaxant action of nitrates on the coronary artery may be important in *variant angina*, where coronary spasm is pre-eminent. Other vasodilators (e.g. **dihydropyridines**) are also effective in this condition.

In summary, the anti-anginal action of nitrates involves:

- reduction of cardiac oxygen consumption, secondary to reduced arterial pressure and cardiac output
- redistribution of coronary flow towards ischaemic areas
- relief of coronary spasm in variant angina.

Tolerance and unwanted effects

Repeated administration of nitrates to smooth muscle preparations in vitro results in diminished relaxation, possibly partly because of *depletion of free*

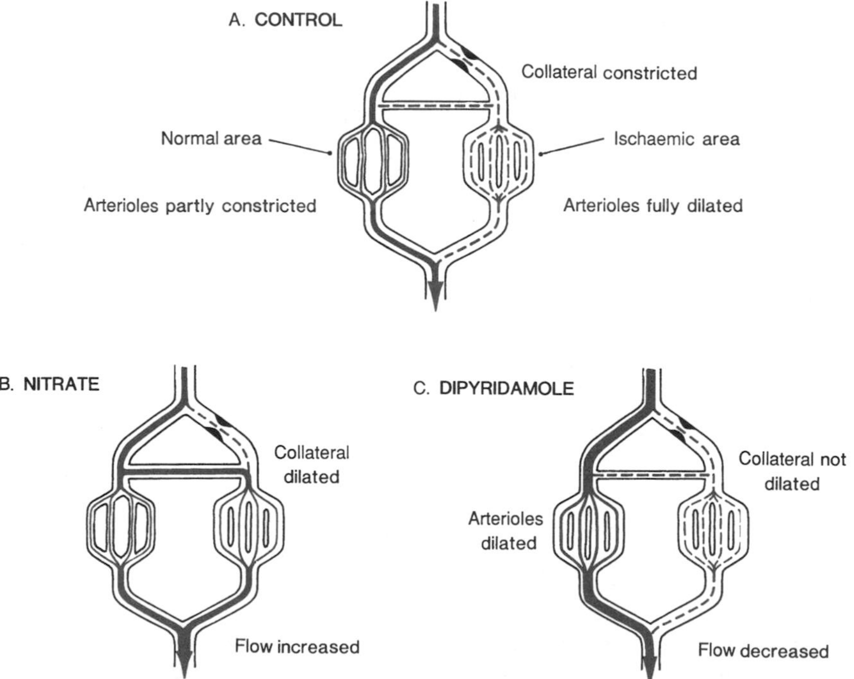

Fig. 13.16 Comparison of the effects of organic nitrates and an arteriolar vasodilator (dipyridamole) on the coronary circulation. **A.** Control. **B.** Nitrates dilate the collateral vessel, thus allowing more blood through to the under-perfused region (mostly by diversion from the adequately perfused area). **C.** Dipyridamole dilates arterioles, increasing flow through the normal area at the expense of the ischaemic area (in which the arterioles are anyway fully dilated).

–SH groups. Tolerance to the anti-anginal effect of nitrates does not occur to a clinically important extent with short-acting drugs (e.g. **glyceryl trinitrate**) unless these are administered by prolonged intravenous infusion or by frequent administration of a slow-release transdermal preparation (see below), but occurs with longer-acting drugs (e.g. **isosorbide mononitrate**).

The main *adverse effect* of nitrates is headache. This was the cause of 'Monday morning sickness' among workers in explosives factories. Tolerance to these effects develops quite quickly (which is why the symptoms appeared on Mondays and not later in the week). Formation of *methaemoglobin*, an oxidation product of haemoglobin that is ineffective as an oxygen carrier, seldom occurs when nitrates are used clinically, but can be induced deliberately with amyl nitrate in the treatment of cyanide poisoning.

Pharmacokinetic and pharmaceutic aspects

Glyceryl trinitrate is quickly metabolised by the liver to inorganic nitrite. It is quickly absorbed from the oral cavity, and is taken as a tablet which is held under the tongue, producing its effects within a few minutes. If swallowed, the drug is ineffective because of first-pass metabolism. Given sublingually, nitroglycerine is quickly converted to di- and mononitrates, which have some activity and have a half-life of about 2 hours. Its effective duration of action is only about 30 minutes. It is quite well absorbed through the skin, and a more sustained effect can be achieved by applying it as a *transdermal patch*. Once a bottle of the tablets has been opened its shelf life is quite short, because of evaporation of the volatile active substance; patients may be aware of this if their tablets no longer give them their usual headache. Patients who need only occasional treatment may benefit from a *sublingual spray* from a metered sealed container, because, although more expensive than tablets, such sprays have an indefinite shelf life.

Organic nitrates

- These are powerful vasodilators, acting mainly on capacitance vessels to reduce pre-load.
- Act by intracellular production of NO, which stimulates cGMP formation, affecting both contractile proteins and calcium regulation.
- Tolerance occurs experimentally, and is important clinically with frequent use of long-acting drugs.
- Effectiveness in angina is due partly to reduced cardiac load, partly to dilatation of collateral coronary vessels, causing more effective distribution of coronary flow. In variant angina, dilatation of constricted coronary vessels is beneficial.
- Important compounds are: glyceryl trinitrate, used sublingually for rapid anti-anginal effect; isosorbide mononitrate, used orally for prophylaxis and more sustained effect.
- No serious unwanted effects; headache and postural hypotension may occur initially. In overdose, may cause methaemoglobinaemia.

Clinical uses of organic nitrates

- Stable angina
  - —Prevention (e.g. regular isosorbide mono-nitrate; or glyceryltrinitrate sublingually immediately before exertion)
  - —Treatment (sublingual glyceryltrinitrate)
- Unstable angina: intravenous glyceryltrinitrate (as supplement to aspirin, Ch. 16)
- To reduce cardiac pre-load in patients with heart failure, expecially those unable to take angiotensin converting enzyme inhibitors (see Ch. 14)
- Uses related to relaxation of other smooth muscles (e.g. uterine, biliary) are being investigated

Long-acting organic nitrates

Isosorbide mono- and dinitrates (see Fig. 13.14) are longer-acting compounds with the same effects as nitroglycerine. Isosorbide dinitrate is rapidly metabolised in the liver to the mononitrate, which is biologically active and has a half-life of about 4 hours. Both drugs are swallowed rather than taken sublingually.

Clinical use

The clinical use of organic nitrates is summarised above.

β-adrenoceptor antagonists

β-adrenoceptor antagonists (see Ch. 7) are important in the treatment of angina. Their action depends entirely on reducing the oxygen consumption of the heart. They probably have no important effects

Table 13.2 Comparison of cardiovascular actions of antianginal drugs: nitrates, β-adrenoceptor antagonists and Ca^{2+}-channel-blocking drugs

Actions	Nitrates	β-adrenoceptor antagonists	Ca^{2+}-channel-blocking drugs		
			Nifedipine	Verapamil	Diltiazem
Blood pressure	↓	O or ↓	↓↓	↓	↓
Heart rate	↑	↓↓	↑↑	↓	↓
Cardiac output	O or ↑	↓	↑↑	↓	↓
Central venous pressure	↓↓	↑	↓	↓↓	↓
Peripheral resistance	O or ↓	↑	↓↓	↓	↓
Coronary blood flow	O	↓	↑↑	↑	↑↑

on the coronary vessels; any effect that they do produce being in the direction of constriction rather than dilatation. The overall haemodynamic effects of nitrates, β-adrenoceptor antagonists and calcium antagonists are compared in Table 13.2.

CALCIUM ANTAGONISTS

Calcium antagonists (see Nayler 1988 for a detailed account) are a chemically and pharmacologically diverse group of drugs. They include **verapamil**, several compounds of the dihydropyridine type, such as **nifedipine**, and miscellaneous other drugs including **diltiazem** (Fig. 13.17), **cinnarizine** and **prenylamine**. They affect cellular entry of calcium rather than its intracellular actions, and are referred to by some authors as 'calcium-entry blockers' to make this distinction clear. As one might expect, in view of the widespread involvement of intracellular calcium as a regulator of cell function, calcium antagonists have been shown to affect many different physiological processes, including secretion, muscle contraction, platelet function and neurotransmitter release. In practice, however, their main effects are confined to the cardiovascular system.

At first sight, one would expect a drug that blocks calcium channels to produce a collection of physiological disasters that would rapidly lead to death since so many key processes, such as muscle contraction, secretion of hormones, neurotransmitter release and so on, depend on controlled calcium entry into cells. The reasons why many calcium antagonists are useful drugs rather than lethal poisons are only partly understood. One important factor is the heterogeneity of calcium channels.

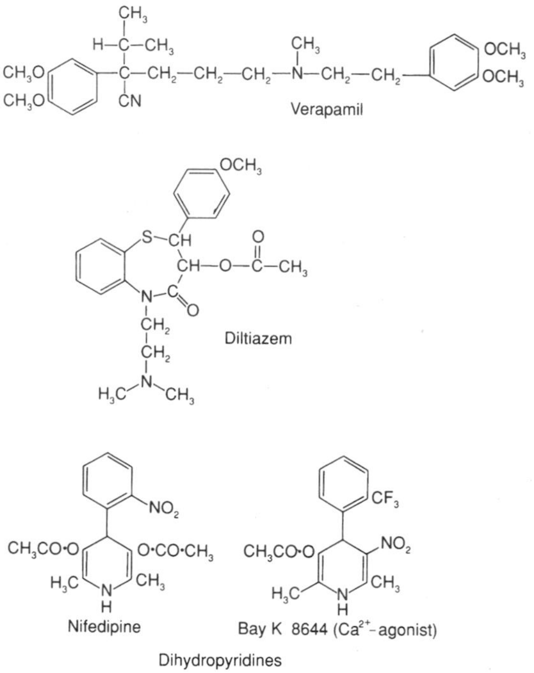

Fig. 13.17 Structures of calcium antagonists. Bay K 8644 (a calcium agonist) is included for comparison.

Types of calcium channel

The main portals of entry for calcium into cells (see Fig. 13.4) are:

- voltage-gated calcium channels, which open when the cell membrane is depolarised
- sodium–calcium exchange.

In addition, there are believed to be receptor-operated calcium channels (ROCs; see Ch. 2), which open in response to receptor ligands, such as noradrenaline acting on α_1-adrenoceptors. ROCs, however, have been very difficult to detect experimentally, and some even doubt their existence. In any event, neither ROCs nor the sodium–calcium exchange carrier appear to be targets for any of the known types of calcium antagonist, which act only on voltage-gated channels.

The properties of voltage-gated calcium channels have been studied in great detail, mainly by the use of the voltage-clamp technique applied to single cells. This technique allows the membrane potential of the cell to be held at a predetermined level, and then abruptly stepped to a new level, at the same time recording the ionic current that flows across the membrane in response to the altered membrane potential. Cell membranes contain many different kinds of voltage-gated channels (see Ch. 34); to isolate the calcium channels from the rest, it is necessary to remove the contribution of sodium currents (e.g. by omitting Na^+ from the bathing solution) and of potassium currents (by appropriate blocking agents). The calcium current can then be recorded as an inward current that flows in response to a depolarising step. The opening of single calcium channels can also be recorded by the use of the patch-clamp technique (see Ch. 2).

By these techniques, Tsien and his colleagues have found three distinct types of voltage-gated calcium channels: L, N and T. They are distinguishable on the basis of various properties, for example the voltage range over which they open, their tendency to close (inactivate) during a maintained depolarisation, their single channel conductance and their occurrence in different types of cell (see Tsien et al. 1987 for a review). Though these different types of calcium channel undoubtedly represent distinct membrane proteins, there is at present only a fragmentary understanding of their physiological functions. It is believed, however, that the channel responsible for the calcium entry that triggers neurotransmitter release may be the N channel, whereas the main channel occurring in smooth muscle is the L channel. Since most of the known calcium antagonists act preferentially or solely on the L channel, this accounts for their lack of major depressant effects on the nervous system. Another important type of calcium channel, essential to life, is that which controls the release of calcium from the sarcoplasmic reticulum of skeletal muscle. This is apparently quite distinct from the channels of the outer cell membrane, and is insensitive to the action of the blocking agents discussed here.

Another factor that leads to physiological selectivity is the characteristic of many calcium antagonists to show properties of use-dependence (i.e. they block more effectively in those cells in which the calcium channels are most active; see above discussion of class I antidysrhythmic drugs). Many also show voltage-dependent blocking actions, blocking more strongly when the membrane is depolarised. This may be partly responsible for the marked selectivity that some drugs show between different kinds of smooth muscle (e.g. vascular versus visceral), though the larger proportion of L-type channels in vascular smooth muscle also contributes to the vascular-selectivity of many calcium antagonists.

Dihydropyridines affect Ca^{2+} channel function in a complex way, not simply by a physical plug-

Calcium antagonists

- Three main types, typified by verapamil, diltiazem and dihydropyridines (e.g. nifedipine) respectively.
- Act by preventing opening of voltage-gated Ca channels (L-type).
- Mainly affect heart and smooth muscle, causing inhibition of Ca^{2+} entry associated with depolarisation.
- Selectivity between heart and smooth muscle varies: verapamil is relatively cardioselective; nifedipine is relatively smooth-muscle selective and diltiazem is intermediate.
- Vasodilator effect (mainly dihydropyridines) is mainly on resistance vessels, causing reduced after-load. Calcium antagonists also dilate coronary vessels, which is important in variant angina.
- Effects on heart (verapamil, diltiazem): antidysrhythmic action (mainly atrial tachycardias), reduced contractility and impaired AV conduction. The drugs are effective in reducing ischaemic damage in experimental animals but need to be given at time of ischaemia, so they are not of proven clinical use in reducing infarction.
- Clinical uses include: antidysrhythmic therapy (mainly verapamil, diltiazem, especially atrial tachycardias), angina (by reducing cardiac work) and hypertension.
- Unwanted effects include headache, constipation (verapamil), and ankle oedema (dihydropyridines). There is a risk of causing cardiac failure or heart block, especially with verapamil and diltiazem.

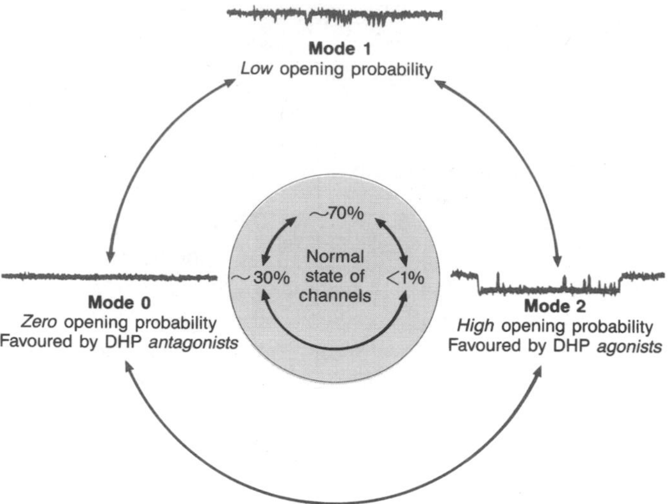

Fig. 13.18 Mode behaviour of calcium channels. The traces shown in red are patch-clamp recordings (see Ch. 2) of the opening of single Ca^{2+} channels (downward deflections) in a patch of membrane from a cardiac muscle cell. A depolarising step is imposed close to the start of each trace, causing an increase in the opening probability of the channel. When the channel is in mode 1 (top), this causes a few brief openings to occur, in mode 2 (right) the channel stays open for most of the time during the depolarising step; in mode 0 (left) it fails to open at all. Under normal conditions (centre panel) the channel spends most of its time in modes 1 and 2, and only rarely enters mode 0.

ging of the pore. This became clear when some dihydropyridines, exemplified by **Bay K 8644** (Fig. 13.17), were found to bind to the same site but to act in the converse way, that is, to promote the opening of voltage-gated calcium channels (Schramm et al 1983). Thus Bay K 8644 produces effects opposite to those of the clinically used dihydropyridines, namely an increase in the force of the cardiac contraction, and constriction of blood vessels; it is competitively antagonised by nifedipine.

Studies on the response of single calcium channels to a step depolarisation of the membrane suggest that a channel can exist in one of three distinct states (called 'modes' by Hess et al. 1984, who discovered this phenomenon; Fig. 13.18). When a channel is in mode 0 it does not open in response to depolarisation; in mode 1, depolarisation produces a low opening probability, and each opening is brief. In mode 2, depolarisation produces a very high opening probability, and single openings are prolonged. Under normal conditions, about 70% of the channels at any one moment exist in mode 1, with only 1% or less in mode 2; each channel switches randomly and quite slowly between the three modes. Dihydropyridines of the antagonist type, according to these studies, bind selectively to channels in mode 0, thus favouring this non-opening state, whereas agonists are believed to bind selectively to channels in mode 2 (see Fig. 13.18). Though cognoscenti argue heatedly about this model, it provides a useful view of how channel behaviour may be modulated in either direction from the norm. This type of two-directional modulation resembles the phenomenon seen with the GABA/benzodiazepine interaction (Ch. 27), and invites speculation about possible endogenous dihydropyridine-like mediator(s) with a regulatory effect on calcium entry.

Pharmacological effects

The main effects of calcium antagonists are confined to cardiac and smooth muscle. **Verapamil** mainly affects the heart, whereas most of the **dihydropyridines** (e.g. **nifedipine**) exert a greater effect on smooth muscle than on the heart. **Diltiazem** is intermediate in its actions.

Cardiac actions

The antidysrhythmic effects of verapamil and diltiazem have been discussed above.

All calcium antagonists can cause AV block and cardiac slowing. They also have a negative inotropic effect, which results from the inhibition of the slow inward current during the action potential plateau. In spite of this the cardiac output usually stays constant or increases, because of the reduction in peripheral resistance (Table 13.2).

Vascular smooth muscle

Calcium antagonists cause generalised arteriolar dilatation, but do not much affect the veins. They affect all vascular beds, though regional effects vary between different drugs to a considerable degree. Vasodilatation causes a fall in arterial pressure. Dihydropyridines produce marked vasodilatation without much direct effect on the heart, whereas other calcium antagonists are less selective. All of these drugs cause coronary vasodilatation in normal individuals and in patients with coronary artery spasm (variant angina), but it is not certain that this happens when coronary atherosclerosis is present (see later section).

Other types of smooth muscle (e.g. biliary tract, urinary tract and uterus) are also relaxed by calcium antagonists (especially dihydropyridines), which may be useful in treating conditions such as biliary colic.

Protection of ischaemic tissues

There are many theoretical reasons (see Nayler 1988; Fig. 13.7) why calcium antagonists might exert a cytoprotective effect in ischaemic tissues, and thus be of clinical use in treating heart attack and stroke. Reduction of calcium entry should directly limit the increase in intracellular calcium. Vasodilatation and reduction of cardiac work reduce the metabolic requirement of the cells; dysrhythmias could be reduced. Experimentally and clinically, it has been found that calcium antagonists are indeed effective, but only if given prophylactically. They do *not* appear to reduce tissue damage or mortality if they are given *after* the development of ischaemia. Paradoxically, clinical trials have suggested that they may actually be harmful if they are given shortly after the ischaemic episode, possibly because of further impairment of the already jeopardised ventricular function.

The situation appears more encouraging in relation to cerebral ischaemia (see Ch. 25), where both animal studies and clinical trials (Gelmers et al. 1988) suggest that the dihydropyridine **nimodipine** given immediately after the ischaemic episode significantly improves functional recovery and reduces mortality. It reduces the risk of cerebral vasospasm following subarachnoid haemorrhage.

Clinical uses

The main clinical uses of calcium antagonists are summarised below. Other potential uses, yet to be fully evaluated, include migraine, Raynaud's disease (Ch. 14), dysmenorrhoea and premature labour. The medical profession continues its love affair with the calcium antagonists, which are among the biggest selling drugs world-wide.

Unwanted effects

The main unwanted effects of the calcium antagonists are a direct consequence of their actions on the heart and smooth muscle. They include headache, flushing, constipation (verapamil) and ankle swelling (dihydropyridines). They can precipitate cardiac failure, and verapamil should not be used in combination with β-receptor antagonists (especially when given intravenously to patients with SVT) for this reason. In contrast, dihydropyridines are often usefully given by mouth in combination with β-adrenoceptor antagonists in treating moderately severe hypertension.

Calcium antagonists

Calcium antagonists are used mainly for the following purposes:

- As antidysrhythmic drugs (verapamil), for the treatment (intravenous) and prevention (oral) of SVT, and for atrial fibrillation inadequately controlled with digoxin.
- To treat hypertension (dihydropyridines and diltiazem): most calcium antagonists combine arteriolar vasodilatation with a negative inotropic effect, and effectively lower arterial pressure (see Ch. 14).
- To treat angina (diltiazem and dihydropyridines). Reduced cardiac oxygen consumption and coronary vasodilatation are potentially useful effects in angina, and calcium antagonists are widely used for this purpose.

REFERENCES AND FURTHER READING

Abshagen U (ed) 1985 Clinical pharmacology of antianginal drugs. Handbook of experimental pharmacology. Springer-Verlag, Berlin, vol 76

Amiodarone vs Sotalol Study Group 1989 Multicentre randomized trial of sotalol vs amiodarone for chronic malignant ventricular tachyarrhythmias. Eur Heart J 10: 685–694

Braunwald E, Mock M B, Watson J T 1982 Congestive cardiac failure: current research and clinical applications. Grune & Stratton, New York

Canvin C, Loutzenhiser R, van Breeman C 1983 Mechanism of calcium antagonist-induced vasodilatation. Annu Rev Pharmacol 23: 373–396

Cranefield P F 1975 The conduction of the cardiac impulse: the slow response and cardiac arrhythmias. Futura, New York

Fine L G, Yellon D M (chairmen) 1993 Unstable angina. Report of a meeting of physicians and scientists, University College London Medical School. Lancet 341: 1323–1327

Gadsby D C, Wit A L 1981 Electrophysiological characteristics of cardiac cells and the genesis of cardiac arrhythmias. In: Wilkerson R D (ed) Cardiac pharmacology. Academic Press, New York

Gelmers H J, Gorter K, de Weerdt C J, Wiezer H J 1988 A controlled trial of nimodipine in acute ischaemic stroke. N Engl J Med 318: 203–207

Gibbs C L 1978 Cardiac energetics. Physiol Rev 58: 174–254

Goto A, Yamada K, Yashioka M, Sugimoto T 1992 Physiology and pharmacology of endogenous digitalis-like factors. Pharmacol Rev 44: 377–399

Hamlyn J M, Blaustein M P, Bova S, Ducharme D W, Harris D W, Mandel F, Mathews W R, Ludens J H 1991 Identification and characterization of a ouabain-like compound from human plasma. Proc Natl Acad Sci USA 88: 6259–6263

Hess P, Lansmann J B, Tsien R W 1984 Different modes of Ca-channel gating behaviour favoured by dihydropyridine Ca agonists and antagonists. Nature 311: 538–544

Hondeghem L M 1989 Interaction of Class I drugs with the cardiac sodium channel. In: Vaughan Williams E M (ed) Antiarrhythmic drugs. Handbook of experimental pharmacology. Springer-Verlag, Berlin, vol 89

January C T, Fozzard H A 1988 Delayed after depolarisations in heart muscle: mechanisms and relevance. Pharmacol Rev 40: 219–227

Lee K S, Tsien R W 1983 Mechanism of calcium-channel blockade by verapamil, D 600, diltiazem and nitrendipine in single dialysed heart cells. Nature 302: 790–794

Liu G S, Thornton J, van Winkle D M, Stanly D W H, Olsson R A, Downey J M 1991 Protection against infarction afforded by preconditioning as mediated by A1 adenosine receptors in rabbit heart. Circulation 84: 350–356

Murad F, Leitman D, Waldman S, Chang C-H, Hirata M, Kohse K 1988 Effects of nitrovasodilators, endothelium-dependent vasodilators and atrial peptides on cGMP. Cold Spring Harbour Symposia on Quantitative Biology 53: 1005–1009

Nayler W G 1988 Calcium antagonists. Academic Press, London

Needleman P, Currie M G, Geller D M, Cole B R, Adams S P 1984 Atriopeptins: potential mediators of an endocrine relationship between heart and kidney. Trends Pharmacol Sci 5: 506–509

Noble D 1984 The surprising heart: a review of recent progress in cardiac electrophysiology. J Physiol 353: 1–50

Noble D 1985 Ionic mechanisms in rhythmic firing of heart and nerve. Trends Neurosci 8: 499–504

Roques B P, Noble F, Daugée V, Fournie-Zaluski M-C, Beaumont A 1993 Neutral endopeptidase 24.11: structure, inhibition and experimental and clinical pharmacology. Pharmacol Rev 45: 87–146

Ruskin J N 1989 The cardiac arrhythmia suppression trial (CAST). N Engl J Med 321: 386–388

Ruskoaho H 1992 Atrial natriuretic peptide: synthesis, release and metabolism. Pharmacol Rev 44: 479–602

Schramm M, Thomas G, Towart R, Frankowiak G 1983 Novel dihydropyridines with positive inotropic action through activation of Ca^{+}-channels. Nature 303: 535–537

Smith T W 1988 Digitalis: mechanisms of action and clinical use. N Engl J Med 518: 358–365

Strasser R H, Marquetant R, Kubler W 1990 Adrenergic receptors and sensitization of adenylyl cyclase in acute myocardial ischaemia. Circulation 82 (Suppl 3): 23–29

Tsien R W, Fox A P, Hess P, McCleskey E W, Nilius B, Nowycky M, Rosenberg R L 1987 Multiple types of calcium channel in excitable cells. Soc Gen Physiol Ser 41: 167–187

Van der Vusse G, Reneman R S 1985 Pharmacological intervention in acute myocardial ischaemia and reperfusion. Trends Pharmacol Sci 6: 76–79

Vatner S F, Hintze T H 1982 Effects of a calcium-channel antagonist on large and small coronary arteries in conscious dogs. Circulation 66: 579–588

Vaughan Williams E M 1989 Classification of antiarrhythmic actions. In: Vaughan Williams E M (ed) Antiarrhythmic drugs. Handbook of experimental pharmacology. Springer-Verlag, Berlin, vol 89

Ward D E, Camm A J 1993 Dangerous ventricular arrhythmias—can we predict drug efficacy? N Engl J Med 329: 498–499

Zsoter T T, Church J G 1983 Calcium antagonists: pharmacodynamic effects and mechanism of action. Drugs 25: 93–112 (and other articles in this volume)

14
THE CIRCULATION

This chapter is concerned mainly with the pharmacology of peripheral blood vessels. The walls of muscular arteries, arterioles, venules and veins contain smooth muscle, the activity of which is controlled by the sympathetic nervous system and various humoral factors. The parasympathetic system has no regulatory function on blood vessels, except those supplying erectile tissue. Muscular arteries and arterioles are the main resistance vessels in the circulation, while veins are capacity vessels. In terms of cardiac function, therefore, arteries and arterioles regulate the *after-load,* while veins and pulmonary vessels regulate the *pre-load* of the ventricles.

Muscular arteries control not only the resistance of the peripheral circulation, but also its compliance (i.e. the degree to which the volume of the arterial system increases as the pressure increases), an important factor in a circulatory system that is driven by an intermittent, rather than continuous, pump. Much of the blood that is ejected from the ventricle is accommodated, in the first instance, by distension of the arterial system, which absorbs the pulsations in cardiac output and delivers a relatively steady flow to the tissues. The greater the compliance of the system, the more effectively will the fluctuations be damped out, and the smaller will be the oscillations of arterial pressure with each heartbeat. This is of some importance, because cardiac work (see Ch. 13) can be reduced by introducing additional compliance into the arterial system, even if the cardiac output and mean arterial pressure are unchanged.

Several diseases affect the large and small blood vessels (e.g. atheroma and Raynaud's disease). Drug treatment of such diseases is often unsatisfactory (see p. 302). The effects of drugs on the peripheral vascular system can be broken down into:

- effects on total peripheral resistance (controlled mainly by the arterioles), which is one of the main determinants of arterial pressure and is relevant to the treatment of hypertension and shock
- effects on the resistance of individual vascular beds, which determines the local distribution of blood flow to and within different organs; such effects are relevant to the drug treatment of angina (Ch. 13), migraine (Ch. 8), Raynaud's phenomenon and circulatory shock
- effects on arterial compliance (controlled mainly by muscular arteries), which is relevant in the treatment of cardiac failure and angina
- effects on venous capacity, which determines the central venous pressure and is relevant to the treatment of cardiac failure and angina
- effects on atheroma (Ch. 15) and thrombosis (Ch. 16).

In this chapter the effects of various groups of drugs on vascular smooth muscle are first considered, and then the pharmacological approaches to the treatment of hypertension, shock and cardiac failure are discussed in more detail. The use of drugs in treating angina is discussed in Chapter 13.

VASCULAR SMOOTH MUSCLE

Like other muscle cells, vascular smooth muscle cells contract when the intracellular calcium con-

Treatment of vascular disease

Diseases of blood vessels can be classified as macrovascular or microvascular:

- *Macrovascular* disease is mainly caused by atheroma and thrombosis, treatment and prevention of which are considered in Chapters 15 and 16. When this involves peripheral arteries the commonest symptom is pain in the legs on walking ('claudication'), followed by pain at rest and, in severe cases, gangrene of the feet or legs.
- *Microvascular* disease can result from structural damage to capillary endothelium (e.g. in *diabetes mellitus*; Ch. 20) or from inappropriate vasoconstriction of arteries and arterioles. In the peripheral circulation this gives rise to *Raynaud's phenomenon* (blanching of the fingers during vasoconstriction, followed by blueness due to deoxygenation of the static blood and redness due to reactive hyperaemia following return of blood flow). This can be mild but if severe causes ulceration and gangrene of the fingers. It can occur in isolation ('Raynaud's disease') or in association with a number of other diseases including several so-called connective tissue diseases (e.g. *systemic sclerosis, systemic lupus erythematosus*).
- Treatment of peripheral atheromatous disease is often surgical (surgical reconstruction or amputation) or by angioplasty (disruption of atheroma by inflation of a balloon surrounding the tip of a catheter). Vasodilator drugs (e.g. **oxypentifylline**) are popular in some countries; they may increase blood flow at rest but controlled trials have not shown improvement in walking distance, reduction of rest pain or sustained increase in muscle blood flow during exercise.
- Treatment of Raynaud's phenomenon involves *stopping smoking* and *avoiding the cold.* Vasodilators (e.g. **nifedipine, prazosin** and **thymoxamine**) are of some benefit in severe cases.

centration rises, and vasoconstrictor substances all act by causing $[Ca^{2+}]_i$ to increase (see Bolton 1979). Vasodilator substances, many of which are clinically important, either act in an inverse manner on $[Ca^{2+}]_i$ or by interfering with the mechanisms linking $[Ca^{2+}]_i$ with the contractile machinery.

Figure 14.1 summarises the main cellular mechanisms that are thought to be involved in the control of smooth muscle contraction.

Vascular smooth muscle

- Both resistance and capacitance vessels contain smooth muscle, contraction of which is controlled by neural and humoral mechanisms.
- Smooth muscle cell contraction is initiated by a rise in $[Ca^{2+}]_i$ which activates myosin-light-chain kinase, causing phosphorylation of myosin.
- Agents causing contraction may:
  - —release intracellular Ca^{2+}, secondary to receptor-mediated $InsP_3$ formation
  - —depolarise the membrane and thus allow Ca^{2+} entry through voltage-gated Ca^{2+} channels
  - —allow Ca^{2+} entry through receptor-operated Ca^{2+} channels.
- Agents causing relaxation either:
  - —inhibit Ca^{2+} entry through voltage-gated Ca^{2+} channels either directly (e.g. nifedipine) or indirectly by hyperpolarising the membrane (K^+ activators: e.g. cromokalim)
  - —increase intracellular cAMP or cGMP concentration; cAMP causes inactivation of myosin-light-chain kinase, and may facilitate Ca^{2+} efflux; cGMP opposes agonist-induced increases in $[Ca^{2+}]_i$.

REGULATION OF $[Ca^{2+}]_i$

The regulation of $[Ca^{2+}]_i$ depends on both the entry and exit of Ca^{2+} across the plasma membrane, and on the sequestration of Ca^{2+} within the cell (see review by Gurney & Clapp 1994).

At the membrane level, calcium entry into the cell occurs as in other cells (see Ch. 13), partly through voltage-gated Ca^{2+} channels, which open when the cell is depolarised. Other mechanisms, such as Na^+/Ca^{2+} exchange (not shown in Fig. 14.1) also operate. Calcium entry is also linked to membrane receptors, though there is controversy about the details of this mechanism. It is likely, as shown in Figure 14.1, that Ca^{2+} channels of a distinct type (receptor-operated channels) are coupled to excitatory receptors either directly or via G-proteins (as in the case of K^+ channels coupled to cardiac muscarinic receptors; see Ch. 13). Thus, many vasoconstrictor agents cause both a depolarisation, associated with increased membrane permeability to cations (Na^+ and Ca^{2+}), and an increase in Ca^{2+} uptake by smooth muscle cells. This Ca^{2+} uptake is not secondary

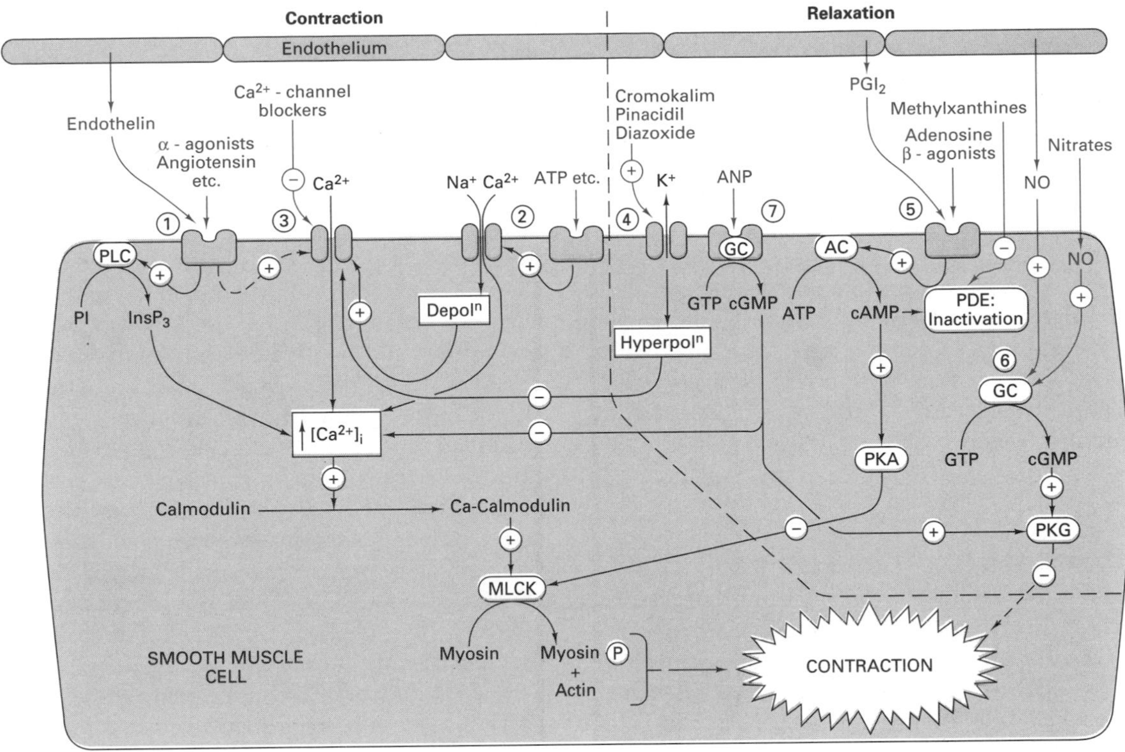

Fig. 14.1 Control of vascular smooth muscle. *Agents that elicit contraction* all do so by increasing $[Ca^{2+}]_i$, which can occur in various ways: (1) Receptors coupled to phospholipase C (PLC), which lead to inositol trisphosphate ($InsP_3$), production and the release of stored Ca^{2+}. (2) Receptor-operated channels, which allow Ca^{2+} entry and also cause depolarisation. (3) Voltage-gated Ca^{2+} channels, which open in response to depolarisation and may also be facilitated indirectly by agonists acting on α-adrenoceptors and/or cGMP.

Agents that cause relaxation may work by reducing $[Ca^{2+}]_i$, or directly on the contractile machinery: (4) K^+ channels (sensitive to intracellular ATP) are opened by drugs such as diazoxide, causing hyperpolarisation, and thus preventing voltage-gated Ca^{2+} channels from opening. (5) Receptors (e.g. for PGI_2, adenosine) coupled to adenylate cyclase, activation of which cause increased cAMP production. This acts via protein kinase A (PKA) and myosin-light chain kinase (MLCK) to inhibit contraction. cAMP also (not shown) facilitates Ca^{2+} extrusion from the cell. Inhibitors of phosphodiesterase (PDE), such as methylxanthines, protect cAMP from degradation. (6) Stimulation of soluble guanylate cyclase, by nitrovasodilators or by nitric oxide (NO) released from the endothelium, increases cGMP formation, causing relaxation opposing agonist-induced increases in $[Ca^{2+}]_i$. (7) ANP occupies a receptor that is directly coupled to membrane-bound guanylate cyclase. (Enzymes: AC = adenylate cyclase; GC = guanylate cyclase; PKA = cAMP-dependent protein kinase; PKG = cGMP-dependent protein kinase). Only the main pathways are shown in this diagram.

to the depolarisation (as it still occurs in preparations that are fully depolarised by immersion in isotonic K^+ solutions); it is also, in contrast to depolarisation-mediated Ca^{2+} uptake, unaffected by dihydropyridine-type calcium antagonists. Though the indirect evidence for receptor-operated membrane channels appears to be strong, they have so far eluded identification by numerous determined patch-clamp investigators, who like to have the last word on such matters. An alternative view is that receptor-operated channels do not exist, and that the changes in membrane permeability to Ca^{2+} are due to the effects of intracellular second messengers acting on the plasma membrane, or of a mechanism that directly links Ca^{2+} entry to the state of the intracellular Ca^{2+} stores.

Sequestration of intracellular Ca^{2+}

As in most cells, intracellular Ca^{2+} is contained mainly in the endoplasmic reticulum and in mitochondria. Many agents that contract smooth muscle do so by activating membrane-bound phospholipase C (see Ch. 2), thereby causing the intracellular formation of inositol phosphates (mainly $InsP_3$), which cause Ca^{2+} to be released from the endoplasmic reticulum. This can occur without any movement of Ca^{2+} across the plasma membrane, and provides an alternative, some say the principal, mechanism for agonist-induced contraction. Recapture of the released Ca^{2+} occurs by an ATP-driven active transport system which is subject to modulation by second messengers such as cAMP and cGMP.

Link between $[Ca^{2+}]_i$ and contraction

Smooth muscle differs from striated and cardiac muscle in that it contains no troponin, though the actin–myosin interaction functions in a similar way (see Ch. 13). In smooth muscle, Ca^{2+} regulates, through calmodulin, the activity of myosin-light-chain kinase (MLCK), an enzyme that phosphorylates one of the constituents of myosin. This enables myosin to interact with actin, thereby initiating the contractile process. This somewhat roundabout process is important, for MLCK is subject to other regulatory influences, particularly by cAMP (see Fig. 14.1). Thus many vasodilator agents increase cAMP formation; cAMP activates various protein kinases (see Ch. 2), including protein kinase A (PKA) which phosphorylates and inactivates MLCK, thus interrupting the contraction process. cAMP is also thought to enhance activity of the Ca^{2+} efflux pump. The special role of MLCK in smooth muscle explains the otherwise puzzling fact that mediators acting through an increase in cAMP inhibit smooth muscle but cause increased contraction of the heart. The greater importance of $InsP_3$-mediated Ca^{2+} release in smooth muscle is also relevant, for this process is not affected by cAMP, whereas in the heart Ca^{2+} entry through voltage-gated channels, which is strongly increased by cAMP, is more important than intracellular Ca^{2+} release. cGMP is also involved in smooth muscle relaxation through activating a kinase which has similar actions to PKA, and through sequestration of intracellular Ca^{2+}.

THE ROLE OF THE VASCULAR ENDOTHELIUM

A new chapter in our understanding of vascular control opened about 20 years ago with the realisation that the layer of endothelial cells that lines the entire vascular system acts, not just as a passive barrier keeping cells and proteins from escaping freely into the tissues, but also as a source of several substances that control the contraction of the underlying smooth muscle cells. The first was the release of *prostacyclin* (PGI_2; see Ch. 11) by endothelial cells, leading to inhibitory effects on smooth muscle and platelets, both of which act to reduce the likelihood of thrombotic occlusion (see Ch. 16). Endothelial cells from microvessels also synthesise prostaglandin (PG) E_2 which is also a vasodilator and additionally inhibits noradrenaline release from sympathetic nerve terminals while lacking the effect of PGI_2 on platelets. Prostaglandin endoperoxide intermediates (PGG_2, PGH_2) are formed in endothelial cells and act on thromboxane (TX) A_2 receptors which initiate effects opposite to those of PGI_2, providing yet another instance of the kind of two-way modulation that is familiar in the autonomic nervous system (see Chs 12 and 16). The production of *endothelium-derived relaxing factor* (EDRF)/NO (Ch. 10), and *endothelin* (see below) is another example. In moments of exasperation, one sometimes wonders whether all this makes sense or whether the designer simply could not make up

The role of the endothelium in controlling vascular smooth muscle

- Endothelial cells release various vasoactive substances, the important ones being prostacyclin (vasodilator), nitric oxide (vasodilator) and endothelin (vasoconstrictor).
- Many vasodilator substances (e.g. acetylcholine and bradykinin) act via endothelial NO production. The NO derives from arginine, and is produced when $[Ca^{2+}]_i$ increases in the endothelial cell.
- NO causes smooth muscle relaxation by increasing cGMP formation.
- Endothelin is a potent and long-acting vasoconstrictor peptide, released from endothelial cells by many chemical and physical factors. It is not confined to blood vessels, and its physiological role is not yet clear.

his mind. An important distinction appears to be whether a particular system is tonically active under basal conditions (as appears to be the case with the noradrenergic nervous system (Ch. 7) and the EDRF/NO system (Ch. 10)), or only responds to injury, inflammation, etc. as in the case of prostacyclin. Some of these latter mechanisms may prove to be functionally redundant and may represent vestiges of mechanisms that were important to our evolutionary forebears. In addition to producing an array of vasoactive mediators, the plasma membrane of endothelial cells contains several enzymes and transport mechanisms that can influence the activity of circulating substances and which are potentially important targets of drug action. An example is *angiotensin-converting enzyme* (ACE) which activates angiotensin I by converting it to the potent vasoconstrictor angiotensin II and which inactivates bradykinin and a number of other vasodilator peptides (see below).

Endothelin

Endothelin formation and secretion

Endothelin (ET), a 21-residue peptide, was discovered by Yanagisawa et al. (1988), who were able to bring the full strength of molecular biological techniques to bear to achieve the isolation, analysis and cloning of the gene for this peptide in a very short space of time. There are three distinct ET genes that encode distinct sequences (ET-1, ET-2 and ET-3) (Fig. 14.2). These three isoforms are diversely and unevenly distributed in the body (Table 14.1) suggesting that ET may have multiple functions that are not restricted to the cardiovascular system. ET-1 is the only ET present in endothelial cells and is also expressed in a wide variety of other tissues. ET-2 is much less widely distributed but is present in kidney and intestine. ET-3 is present in brain, lung, intestine and adrenal gland. ET-1 is synthesised by transcription and translation of a 212-residue precursor molecule ('prepro ET') which is processed to 'big ET-1' and finally cleaved by an endothelin-converting enzyme to ET-1. Cleavage occurs not at the usual Lys–Arg or Arg–Arg position but at a Trp–Val pair implying a very atypical endopeptidase. The best candidate for the converting enzyme is a metalloprotease which is inhibited by **phosphoramidon**. Big ET-1 is converted to ET-1 intracellularly and also on the surface of endothelial and smooth muscle cells.

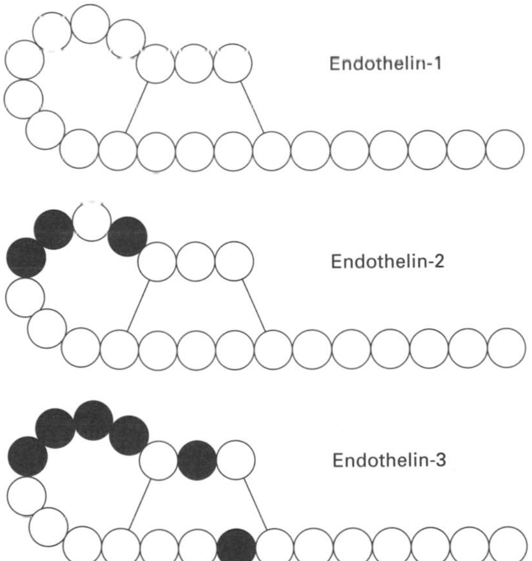

Fig. 14.2 ET-1, -2 and -3. The circles represent amino acid residues. Solid circles show differences from ET-1. The two solid lines indicate the two intramolecular disulphide linkages.

Table 14.1 Distribution of endogenous ETs and subtypes of ET receptors in various tissues

Tissues	ET-1	ET-2	ET-3	ET_A	ET_B
Vascular tissue					
Endothelium	++++				+
Smooth muscle	+			++	
Brain	+++		+	+	+++
Kidney	++	++	+	+	++
Intestines	+	+	+++	+	+++
Adrenal gland	+		+++	+	++

++++ = highest; +++ = high; ++ = moderate; and + = low levels of expression of ETs or ET-receptor mRNA and/or immunoreactive ETs
Adapted from: Masaki (1993)

Endothelial cells do not contain storage vesicles and regulation of ET production occurs at the transcription level. Stimuli include activated platelets, endotoxin, thrombin, various cytokines and growth factors, angiotensin II, arginine vasopressin, adrenaline, insulin, hypoxia and shear stress.

Endothelin receptors and responses

There are at least two types of ET-receptor, designated ET_A and ET_B (Table 14.2). ET_A-mediated

Table 14.2 Subtypes of ET receptor

Receptor	Affinity	Pharmacological response
ET_A	ET-1 = ET-2 > ET-3	Vasoconstriction Bronchoconstriction Stimulation of aldosterone secretion
ET_B	ET-1 = ET-2 = ET-3	Vasodilatation Inhibition of ex vivo platelet aggregation

From: Masaki (1993)

responses include vasoconstriction, bronchoconstriction and stimulation of aldosterone secretion. ET-1 and ET-2 are equipotent as regards these responses whereas ET-3 is less active. ET_B-initiated responses include PGI_2 release, which gives rise to transient vasodilatation following bolus intravenous injection of ET. ET_A and ET_B both belong to the superfamily of G-protein-coupled receptors (Ch. 2).

The second-messenger systems and cellular effects of ET-receptor activation are complex. ET_A-receptors are coupled to phospholipase C which initiates some of its effects. ET also stimulates Na^+/H^+ exchange, protein kinase C and mitogenesis. ET_B-receptor occupation leads to phospholipase A_2 activation, arachidonic acid mobilisation and prostaglandin or thromboxane biosynthesis depending on cell type (see Ch. 11).

Function of endothelin

Concentrations of ET-1 in circulating blood are extremely low and it does not appear to act as a hormone but rather as a paracrine or autocrine mediator. Experimental studies suggest that ET-1 is not involved in normal blood pressure regulation nor in the pathogenesis of hypertension, though it might play a part in renal and cerebral vasospasm (see Fig. 14.3). Plasma concentrations of ET-1 are raised in several pathological conditions, especially those with a component of vasospasm, including acute myocardial infarction.

In addition to vasoconstriction and fibrosis, endothelins have a number of endocrine actions. ET-1 is increased during pregnancy and is present in very high concentrations in amniotic fluid. It has been implicated in the control of uteroplacental blood flow and in the genesis of *eclampsia,* a disease of the last trimester of pregnancy characterised by

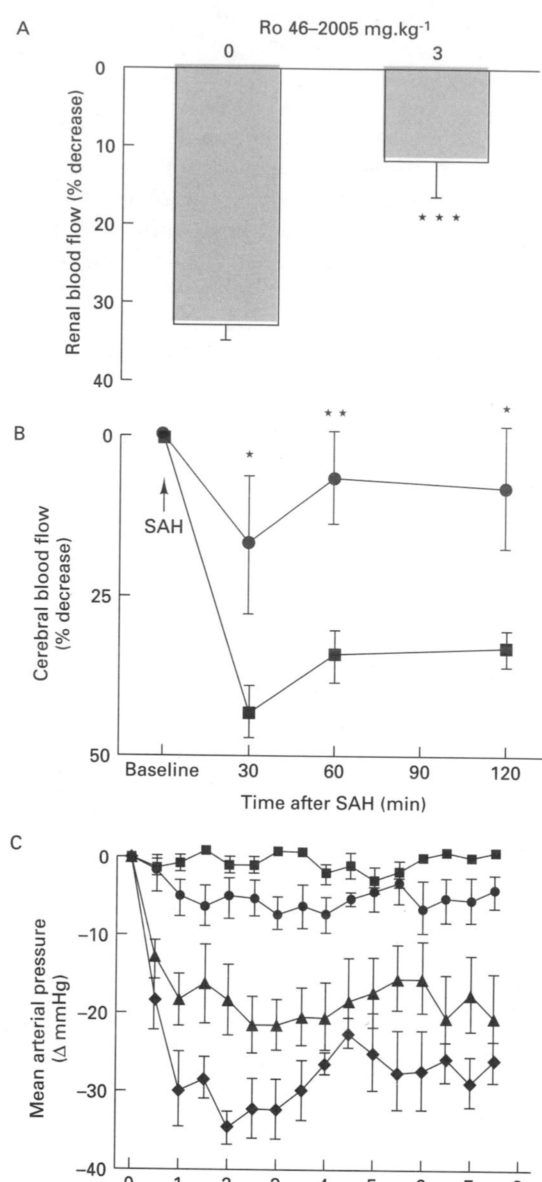

Fig. 14.3 In vivo effects of a potent non-peptide ET_A- and ET_B-receptor antagonist, Ro 46-2005 in three animal models. A. Prevention by Ro 46-2005 of post-ischaemic renal vasoconstriction in rats. **B.** Prevention by Ro 46-2005 of the decrease in cerebral blood flow after subarachnoid haemorrhage (SAH) in rats treated with placebo (squares) or with Ro 46-2005 (circles). **C.** Effect of orally administered Ro 46-2005 on mean arterial pressure in sodium-depleted squirrel monkeys treated with placebo (squares) or increasing doses of antagonist. (From: Clozel M et al. 1993 Nature 365: 759–761)

hypertension, oedema and seizures, and which is the leading cause of maternal and neonatal mortality in industrialised countries. It causes secretion of several hormones, including *atrial natriuretic peptide*, *aldosterone*, *adrenaline* and *hypothalamic* and *pituitary hormones*. The concentration of ET-1 in *thyroid follicles* is extremely high and it has been suggested that it may be involved in thyroglobulin synthesis. Recently the ET-1 gene has been disrupted in mouse embryo stem cells to produce mice deficient in ET-1. Pharyngeal arch tissues develop abnormally in mice homozygous for such gene disruption, and these animals die of respiratory failure at birth. This seems to promote ET-1 to the status of a key player in directing differentiation, a conclusion that is so unexpected as to leave one positively breathless. Heterozygotes (which produce lower amounts of ET-1 than wild-type mice) develop *elevated* blood pressures, pointing to the potential physiological importance of small amounts of ET-1, which are vasodilator and vasodepressor in intact organisms. Despite these leads, the physiological and pathological roles of endothelins are only just beginning to emerge and advice in the last edition ('watch closely') still stands.

Mechanisms of drug action on vascular smooth muscle

From the foregoing discussion, it is clear that drugs can affect vascular smooth muscle either directly, by acting on the smooth muscle cells themselves, or indirectly, by acting on endothelial cells or on

Table 14.3 Classification of vasoactive drugs that act directly on smooth muscle

Mechanism	Examples	Further details
Vasoconstrictors		
Receptor-mediated events:		
$InsP_3$ formation/Ca^{2+} release	α-adrenoceptor agonists	Ch. 7
Opening of receptor-operated channels	Vasopressin	Below; Ch. 9
Facilitation of voltage-gated Ca^{2+} channels	Angiotensin II	Below
	Endothelin	Below
	Other peptides (e.g. NPY)	Chs 5 and 9
	Dopamine*	Below; Chs 5 and 24
	5-hydroxytryptamine*	Ch. 8
	Prostaglandins*	Ch. 11
Vasodilators		
↑ cAMP: ↑ adenylate cyclase	β-adrenoceptor agonists	Ch. 7
	Adenosine	Ch. 8
	Dopamine*	
	5-hydroxytryptamine*	
	Prostaglandins*	
↓ Phosphodiesterase	Methylxanthines	Below
	Papaverine	Below
↑ cGMP	Nitrates, nitroprusside	Ch. 13
	Nitric oxide	Below; Ch. 10
	Atrial natriuretic peptide	Ch. 13
Inhibition of voltage-gated Ca^{2+} channels	Dihydropyridines	Below; Ch. 13
Opening of K^+ channels	Cromokalim, pinacidil, diazoxide, minoxidil	Below
Receptor antagonists	α_1-adrenoceptor antagonists	Ch. 7
	Angiotensin antagonists	Below
Unknown mechanisms	Hydralazine	Below
	Inhalation anaesthetics	Ch. 26
	Local anaesthetics	Ch. 34
	Various peptides (e.g. VIP, substance P, CGRP, etc.)	Ch. 9
	Many other examples	

*These agents produce mixed constrictor/dilator effects.

Table 14.4 Classification of vasoactive drugs that act indirectly

Site	Mechanism	Examples	Further details
Vasoconstrictors			
Sympathetic nerve terminals	Noradrenaline release	Amphetamine, ephedrene, tyramine	Ch. 7
	Block of NA re-uptake	Cocaine	Chs 7 and 32
Endothelium	Endothelin release from endothelial cells	Many agents, e.g.: thrombin, Ca^{2+} ionophore, TGF-β, PDGF, IL-1, TNF, angiotensin II, endotoxin, shear stress, etc.	Above
Vasodilators			
Sympathetic nerve terminals	Inhibition of NA release via presynaptic receptors	Many examples, e.g.: α_2-adrenoceptor agonists, muscarinic agonists, prostaglandins, etc.	Chs 6, 7 and 11
	Sympathetic-neurone-blocking drugs	Guanethidine, bethanidine	Ch. 7
Endothelium	Nitric oxide release	Many agents, e.g.: acetylcholine, bradykinin, substance P, Ca^{2+} ionophore, ATP, shear stress	
Central nervous system	Vasomotor inhibition	Anaesthetics	Ch. 26
		Clonidine, methyldopa	Ch. 7
Enzymes	ACE inhibition	Captopril, enalapril	Below
	Renin inhibition	Compounds in development (e.g. enalkiren)	

nerve terminals, especially those of the sympathetic nervous system. Another type of indirect action is exemplified by angiotensin-converting enzyme inhibitors (e.g. **captopril**) which block the intravascular formation of angiotensin. Tables 14.3 and 14.4 summarise the main classes of drugs that affect vascular smooth muscle, many of which are discussed in other chapters. In this chapter we present information on agents that are not covered elsewhere, and discuss the ways in which vasoactive drugs are used clinically to treat particular conditions, such as hypertension, heart failure and shock.

VASOCONSTRICTOR DRUGS

Vasoconstriction is the major effect produced by **sympathomimetic amines**, by some eicosanoids (e.g. **thromboxane A_2**; see above and Ch. 16) and by three types of peptide, namely **endothelin** (see above), **angiotensin** and **vasopressin** analogues. It also occurs with other agents, such as some **ergot alkaloids** (Ch. 8), **β-adrenoceptor antagonists** (Ch. 7) and **cardiac glycosides** (Ch. 13).

Sympathomimetic amines

Sympathomimetic amines are discussed fully in Chapter 7. Vasoconstriction is produced mainly by activation of α_1-adrenoceptors, though blood vessels also possess α_2-adrenoceptors that elicit constriction. They exert a powerful vasoconstrictor effect on the skin and mucous membranes, and on the splanchnic, hepatic and renal vascular beds, with relatively little effect on the cerebral and coronary circulations. Blood flow through skeletal muscle is not very sensitive to α-receptor agonists, but is increased by β-receptor agonists, so drugs such as **adrenaline**, which have a mixed action, effectively divert blood from the skin and splanchnic circulations to skeletal muscle.

α-adrenoceptor agonists constrict arteries, arterioles and veins. Thus, they increase peripheral resistance and reduce venous capacity, raising the central venous pressure. In the absence of any direct cardiac effect, cardiac output falls, but the reduced arterial compliance and increased arterial pressure tend to increase cardiac work.

Drugs with an almost pure α-receptor action (e.g. **phenylephrine**) cause marked bradycardia, which is a reflex response to the rise in blood pressure that is produced. The same occurs with infusions of

Vasoconstrictor substances

- The main groups are sympathomimetic amines (direct and indirect), certain eicosanoids (thromboxanes), peptides (angiotensin, vasopressin and endothelin) and a group of miscellaneous other drugs (e.g. ergot alkaloids).
- Clinical uses are limited mainly to local applications (e.g. nasal decongestion, co-administration with local anaesthetics). Usefulness in hypotensive states is not proven. Vasopressin may be used to stop bleeding from oesophageal varices in patients with portal hypertension caused by liver disease.

noradrenaline (see Fig. 7.8). Drugs with mixed α- and β-actions, which include the indirectly-acting sympathomimetic amines, such as **ephedrine**, cause marked tachycardia if administered systemically because of their β-effects on the heart. These drugs are used mainly to produce local vasoconstriction. **Adrenaline** is often added to local anaesthetic injections so as to delay removal of the local anaesthetic from the injection site, and thus prolong its action (see Ch. 34). Adrenaline must not be used with local anaesthetic injections into fingers and toes because the main digital arteries may be so constricted that necrosis occurs. Other sympathomimetic amines (e.g. **ephedrine**) may be used to cause shrinkage of congested mucous membranes, for example to cause nasal decongestion. Their effects tend to be short-lived, and chronic congestion returns worse than before so they are best restricted to short-term use.

The systemic use of sympathomimetic amines in hypotensive states is controversial (see below). It may be useful if the hypotension is due to inappropriate vasodilatation (e.g. following severe sepsis) but not in hypovolaemic states.

Dopamine

Dopamine is a precursor of noradrenaline in noradrenergic neurons (Ch. 7), and is also a transmitter in its own right in the brain (Ch. 24) and probably also in the periphery (see Ch. 5). The proposal that dopamine might serve a peripheral transmitter role came from observations that stimulation of sympathetic nerves to the kidney caused vasodilatation that was not affected by adrenoceptor-blocking agents, but was prevented by certain dopamine-receptor antagonists, such as **haloperidol** (see Ch. 24). Infusion of dopamine produced similar effects to nerve stimulation. Observations have been made on cutaneous and cerebral vascular beds, suggesting that dopaminergic vasodilatation is not restricted to renal vasculature.

Given as an intravenous infusion, dopamine produces a mixture of cardiovascular effects resulting from its agonist actions on α- and β-adrenoceptors, as well as on dopamine receptors. At low doses (e.g. 1–5 μg/kg body weight/min) dopamine is relatively selective for dopamine receptors in the renal vasculature; at higher doses effects on α- and β-adrenoceptors become progressively more evident. The main effects are:

- *vasodilatation*, particularly in the kidney but also in the mesenteric vascular bed, due to activation of dopamine receptors
- *vasoconstriction* in other vascular beds, associated with activation of α_1-adrenoceptors
- *increased force of contraction of the heart*, probably due to activation of β-adrenoceptors.

Blood pressure increases slightly, but the main effects are on the renal circulation and cardiac output.

The actions of dopamine have led to its clinical use, as an intravenous infusion, in conditions where renal failure associated with decreased renal perfusion is imminent.

Angiotensin

Angiotensin is an endogenous peptide whose physiological role and possible relevance to hypertension is discussed more fully below. The active substance, angiotensin II, is an extremely powerful vasoconstrictor, being roughly 40 times as potent as noradrenaline in raising blood pressure. Its peripheral effects resemble those of α-receptor agonists, in that it mainly affects cutaneous, splanchnic and renal blood flow, with less effect on the blood flow to brain and skeletal muscle. It does, however, reduce coronary blood flow. It lacks effects on other smooth muscle, and has less effect on the venous system than α-agonists. Outside the vascular system, its main effects are to increase the force and rate of the heart (which is due to release of noradrenaline from sympathetic nerve terminals) and to increase secretion of aldosterone from the adrenal cortex (see Ch. 21). Angiotensins also have central actions, and have been implicated in thirst and appetite for salt. Angiotensin has no routine clinical uses;

its pharmacological importance lies in the fact that other drugs (e.g. **captopril** and **losartan**; see below) affect the cardiovascular system by altering the production or action of angiotensin.

Vasopressin (antidiuretic hormone)

Vasopressin is a posterior pituitary peptide hormone (Ch. 21), important mainly for its actions on the kidney (discussed fully in Ch. 18), but it is also a powerful vasoconstrictor. There is evidence that two distinct types of receptor (V_1 and V_2) are responsible for the effects of vasopressin. The renal effect (see Ch. 18), mediated through V_2-receptors, occurs at very low concentrations of vasopressin, and involves activation of adenylate cyclase and an increase in intracellular cAMP concentration. The other effects (e.g. on smooth muscle), mediated through V_1-receptors, require much higher concentrations and involve intracellular calcium mobilisation via the phosphatidylinositol mechanism (see Ch. 2). Vasopressin causes a generalised vasoconstriction, affecting all vascular beds including the coeliac and mesenteric circulations and the coronary vessels. It is sometimes used to treat patients with bleeding oesphageal varices and portal hypertension, before more definitive treatment. It causes pallor and can precipitate cardiac ischaemia. It also affects other smooth muscle (e.g. the gastrointestinal tract and uterus) and causes abdominal cramps. For these reasons, **desmopressin**, a vasopressin analogue selective for V_2-receptors which can be administered intranasally (Ch. 21), is generally preferred for treating diabetes insipidus. An unrelated action of desmopressin is to increase circulating factor VIII and it is useful in patients with mild to moderate haemophilia or von Willebrand's disease to increase factor VIII levels before elective procedures such as tooth extraction (see Ch. 16).

VASODILATOR DRUGS

Vasodilators are a heterogeneous group of drugs, of which many are clinically important, being used in the treatment of various common and chronic conditions including hypertension, cardiac failure and angina pectoris. They may be divided for convenience into those that act directly on vascular smooth muscle and those that act indirectly by inhibiting the action of a naturally-occurring constrictor or by stimulating the production/release of an endogenous vasodilator. The main groups are listed in Tables 14.3 and 14.4. Some of them will be discussed in detail in this chapter; others are discussed elsewhere (Chs 10 and 13).

DIRECTLY-ACTING VASODILATORS

Calcium antagonists

Calcium antagonists are discussed in detail in Chapter 13. They cause a generalised vasodilatation, though there is now evidence that individual agents differ in the regional distribution of this effect. Drugs of the **dihydropyridine** type, of which many are available (see Ch. 13), act preferentially on vascular smooth muscle, whereas **verapamil** acts mainly on the heart; **diltiazem** is intermediate in specificity. The main difference that this makes is that dihydropyridines usually produce a transient reflex tachycardia as a result of their blood-pressure-lowering effect. Verapamil and diltiazem do not, because of their direct effect of slowing the heart through an action on the pacemaker.

Several calcium antagonists of the dihydropyridine type show special features:

- **nicardipine** may cause less reduction of myocardial contractility
- **amlodipine** has a much longer elimination half-life leading to less variation in plasma concentration during chronic dosing and permitting once daily dosing
- **nimodipine** has some selectivity for cerebral vasculature and is used to prevent cerebral vasospasm following subarachnoid haemorrhage.

Drugs that act on K^+ channels

Some drugs (e.g. **cromokalim**) cause smooth muscle relaxation by selectively increasing the membrane permeability to K^+, thus causing the membrane to hyperpolarise and inhibiting action potential generation. The discovery came initially from electrophysiological and ion flux studies which revealed that these drugs cause hyperpolarisation and also increase the efflux of radioactive rubidium (an ion that traverses K^+ channels). By patch-clamp recording (see Ch. 2), it was found that a specific type of high-conductance K^+ channel was opened by these agents. This discovery coincided with studies

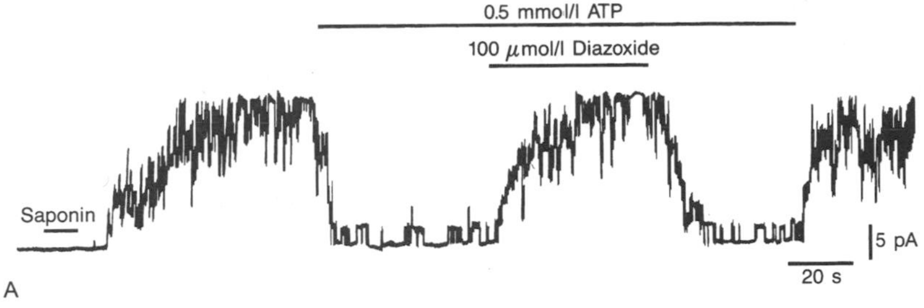

B

Cromokalim

Pinacidil

Diazoxide

Minoxidil

Fig. 14.4 Drugs that act at ATP-sensitive K^+ channels. **A.** K^+ channels opened by diazoxide. The records were obtained from insulin-secreting cells in culture by the patch-clamp technique (Ch. 2). Saponin caused permeabilisation of the cell, with loss of intracellular ATP, causing the channels to open (upward deflection) until they were inhibited by ATP. Addition of diazoxide, a vasodilator drug (which also inhibits insulin secretion; see text) causes opening of the channels. In an intact smooth muscle cell, this causes hyperpolarisation and relaxation. **B.** Structures of compounds that activate or block ATP-sensitive K^+ channels. (From: (A) Dunne et al. 1990 Br J Pharmacol 99: 169)

demonstrating the existence of ATP-sensitive K^+ channels in various different cell types. In cardiac muscle and pancreatic islet insulin-secreting cells, for example, intracellular ATP was found to close down these K^+ channels, thus causing the cell to depolarise, and this mechanism is believed to form an important link between the metabolic state of the cell and membrane function. In the case of insulin-secreting cells (see Ch. 20), a rise in plasma glucose concentration causes increased ATP production, hence K^+ channel closure and membrane depolarisation; the depolarisation results in Ca^{2+} entry and insulin secretion. Some types of antidiabetic drug (e.g. **glibenclamide**; Ch. 20; Fig. 14.4) act by mimicking the action of ATP on these channels. In the heart, ischaemia causes the intracellular ATP concentration to fall, thus opening K^+ channels, hyperpolarising the membrane and reducing excitability. This is thought to have a protective function, and similar mechanisms have now been discovered in nerve cells as well as in smooth muscle cells.

It now appears that vasodilators such as **cromokalim, pinacidil, minoxidil** and **diazoxide** work by antagonising the action of intracellular ATP on these channels (Fig. 14.4), thus opening them and causing relaxation when the ATP concentration would normally have kept them closed. Diazoxide belongs chemically to the same group as the thiazide diuretics (see Ch. 18) which also have important vasodilator properties as well as their renal actions. It causes hyperglycaemia (by inhibiting insulin secretion) which precludes its use in chronic therapy. It used to be given intravenously in the emergency treatment of hypertension, but has been superseded by other drugs (e.g. **calcium antagonists, nitroprusside**) which have fewer unwanted effects.

Minoxidil is a very potent and long-acting vasodilator, used as a drug of last resort in treating severe hypertension unresponsive to other drugs. It causes hirsutism which is unacceptable to most women, and its active metabolite is actually used as a rub-on cream to treat baldness. It causes marked salt and water retention and is usually prescribed with large doses of a loop diuretic (e.g. frusemide). It also causes marked reflex tachycardia, and a β-adrenoceptor antagonist is used to prevent this.

Pinacidil, cromokalim and its active isomer **lemakalim** are more recently developed K^+ channel activators. Drugs of this type may have other uses as smooth muscle relaxants, for example in asthma and bladder dysfunction, but have yet to establish a therapeutic niche.

Agents that act by increasing cyclic nucleotide concentration

Many drugs that relax vascular smooth muscle do so by increasing the cellular concentration of either cGMP or cAMP. Sodium nitroprusside (nitroferricyanide) is a very powerful vasodilator with little effect outside the vascular system. It breaks down spontaneously under physiological conditions to yield nitric oxide (NO) which activates soluble guanylate cyclase (Ch. 10). Unlike the organic nitrates which are enzymically converted to NO and preferentially dilate capacitance vessels, it acts equally on arterial and venous smooth muscle. Thus, both central venous pressure and arterial pressure drop, but cardiac output is not much changed, partly because of a reflex tachycardia. It is used in intensive care units for short-term treatment of hypertensive crises, to produce controlled hypotension during surgery, and for the reversible cardiac dysfunction that occurs after cardiopulmonary bypass surgery.

Although the pharmacological effects of nitroprusside are well-suited to the treatment of hypertension (see below and Ch. 13), its clinical usefulness is limited by the fact that it can only be given intravenously. In solution, particularly when exposed to light, nitroprusside is hydrolysed to cyanide. The intravenous solution has to be made up freshly from dry powder, and is protected from light by covering the container with foil. In the body, nitroprusside is rapidly converted to thiocyanate, its plasma half-life being only a few minutes, so it must be given as a continuous infusion with careful monitoring to avoid excessive hypotension. Continued use can lead to thiocyanate toxicity (weakness, nausea and inhibition of thyroid function) because thiocyanate is cleared only slowly from the bloodstream, so it is only useful for short-term treatment (usually up to 72 hours maximum).

Atrial natriuretic peptide (see Ch. 13) also causes vasodilatation by activating guanylate cyclase, but acts on the membrane-bound form of this enzyme which is directly linked with its receptor.

Many vasodilators act by increasing intracellular cAMP through activation of adenylate cyclase (see Table 14.3). Of the endogenous mediators that work in this way, β-adrenoceptor agonists are discussed in Chapter 7 and eicosanoids in Chapter 11. Purines, which also act via cAMP and have varied and widespread effects that defy simple classification, are discussed in Chapter 8. The other mechanism by which intracellular cAMP concentration may be increased is by inhibition of the enzyme, phosphodiesterase, which removes it. Drugs that act in this way include methylxanthines (e.g. theophylline) and papaverine.

Methylxanthines exert their main effects on non-vascular smooth muscle and on the central nervous system, and are discussed in Chapters 17 and 32. In addition to inhibiting phosphodiesterase, some methylxanthines are also purine-receptor antagonists, which may partly account for their smooth muscle relaxant effects. They are not used clinically as vasodilators.

Papaverine is closely related to **morphine** (see Ch. 27) and also produced by the opium poppy. Pharmacologically, it is quite unlike morphine, however, its main action being to relax smooth muscle in blood vessels and elsewhere. The mechanism of action is poorly understood, but seems to involve a combination of phosphodiesterase inhibition (as with methylxanthines) and block of calcium channels. It is used in the treatment of erectile impotence by direct injection into the corpus cavernosum of the penis (Brindley 1986). This is highly effective and, although some readers may wince, has been much appreciated by many insulin-requiring diabetics who

Types of vasodilator drugs

- ACE inhibitors (e.g. captopril, enalapril): prevent conversion of angiotensin I to angiotensin II, therefore most effective when renin production is increased.
- Organic nitrates (e.g. glyceryl trinitrate, also nitroprusside): act like endogenous NO, causing increased cGMP formation.
- Calcium antagonists (diltiazem, nifedipine and many other dihydropyridines): act by blocking Ca^{2+} entry in response to depolarisation; dilate both resistance and capacitance vessels.
- Drugs that interfere with sympathetic transmission (e.g. α_1-adrenoceptor antagonists).
- K^+-channel activators (e.g. diazoxide, cromokalim, pinacidil): open membrane K^+ channels, thus causing hyperpolarisation; thought to affect insulin-secreting cells and neurons, as well as smooth muscle, so produce various side effects.
- Angiotensin II antagonists (e.g. losartan).
- Other agents include: β_2-adrenoceptor agonists; adenosine; methylxanthines (e.g. theophylline); various diuretic agents and numerous agents that stimulate endothelial NO production.

Uses of vasodilator drugs

- Vasodilators act:
  - —to increase local tissue blood flow
  - —to reduce arterial pressure
  - —to reduce central venous pressure.
- Net effect is a reduction of cardiac pre-load (reduced filling pressure) and after-load (reduced vascular resistance), hence reduction of cardiac work.
- Main uses are:
  - —antihypertensive therapy (e.g. α_1-antagonists)
  - —treatment of angina (e.g. Ca^{2+} antagonists)
  - —treatment of cardiac failure (e.g. ACE inhibitors).

suffer from this complication of their disease and are no more needle-shy than the author of the above report whose paper describes the use of 17 drugs in one subject (himself).

Vasodilators with unknown mechanism of action

Hydralazine

Hydralazine is a vasodilator that acts mainly on arteries and arterioles, causing a fall in blood pressure accompanied by reflex tachycardia and an increased cardiac output; it has little effect on the venous system. Its mechanism of action at the cellular level has not been determined. The main use of hydralazine is as an antihypertensive drug (see below), normally administered in combination with other drugs, but its toxicity (especially an immune disorder resembling *systemic lupus erythematosus*) greatly limits its use.

Ethanol

Ethanol (see Ch. 33) exerts a strong vasodilator action in cutaneous vasculature, causing the familiar drunkard's flush.

INDIRECTLY-ACTING VASODILATOR DRUGS

The two main groups of clinically important indirectly-acting vasodilator drugs are:

- those that inhibit sympathetically-mediated vasoconstriction
- those that inhibit the renin–angiotensin system.

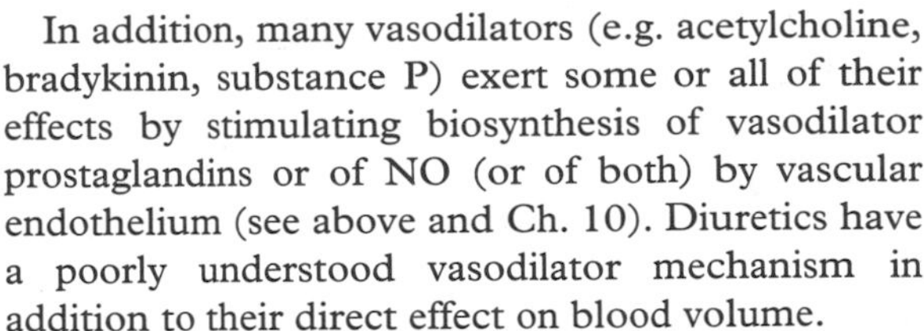

In addition, many vasodilators (e.g. acetylcholine, bradykinin, substance P) exert some or all of their effects by stimulating biosynthesis of vasodilator prostaglandins or of NO (or of both) by vascular endothelium (see above and Ch. 10). Diuretics have a poorly understood vasodilator mechanism in addition to their direct effect on blood volume.

Sympathetically-mediated vasoconstriction can be blocked at many levels, from the central nervous system down to the receptors on the smooth muscle cell; examples of such drugs are described more fully in Chapter 7.

THE RENIN–ANGIOTENSIN SYSTEM

The renin–angiotensin system is a hormonal system that interacts closely with both the sympathetic nervous system and aldosterone secretion; it plays a central role in the control of sodium excretion and body fluid volume (see review by Valloton 1987).

Renin is a proteolytic enzyme that is secreted into the circulation by cells of the *juxtaglomerular apparatus* (see Fig. 18.2), a specialised island of tissue lying at the point where the afferent arteriole, just before entering the glomerulus, comes into close apposition to a specialised part of the distal tubule (see Ch. 18). The wall of the arteriole contains a cluster of renin-containing juxtaglomerular cells, which secrete renin into the bloodstream in response to a fall in the sodium concentration of the fluid in the distal tubule. β-adrenoceptor agonists and prostacyclin also directly stimulate renin secretion. Renin acts on a plasma globulin, *angiotensinogen*, splitting off a decapeptide, *angiotensin I*, from the N-terminal end of the protein. This happens rapidly, and the renin activity in the plasma disappears within a few minutes. Angiotensin I has no appreciable activity, but is acted on by a second proteolytic enzyme, *angiotensin-converting enzyme* (ACE), that removes two more amino acids to form the highly active octapeptide, *angiotensin II* (Fig. 14.5). ACE is a membrane-bound enzyme on the surface of endothelial cells, and is particularly abundant in the lung which has a vast surface area of vascular endothelium. ACE is also present in other vascular tissues including heart, brain, striated muscle and kidney, and is not restricted to endothelial cells. Consequently, local formation of angiotensin II occurs in different vascular beds, and provides a local control independent of blood-borne angiotensin II. The gene controlling ACE is polymorphic

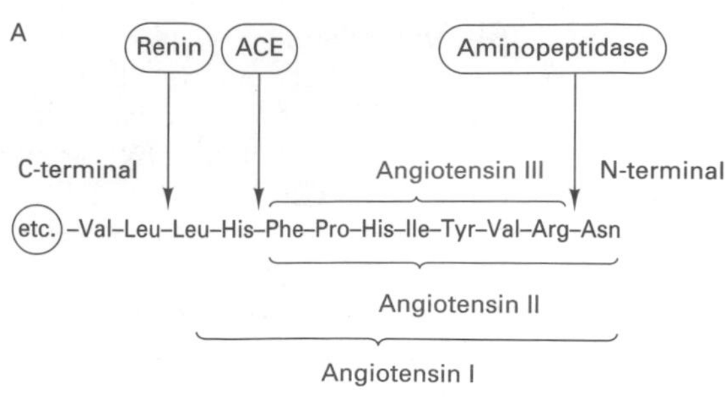

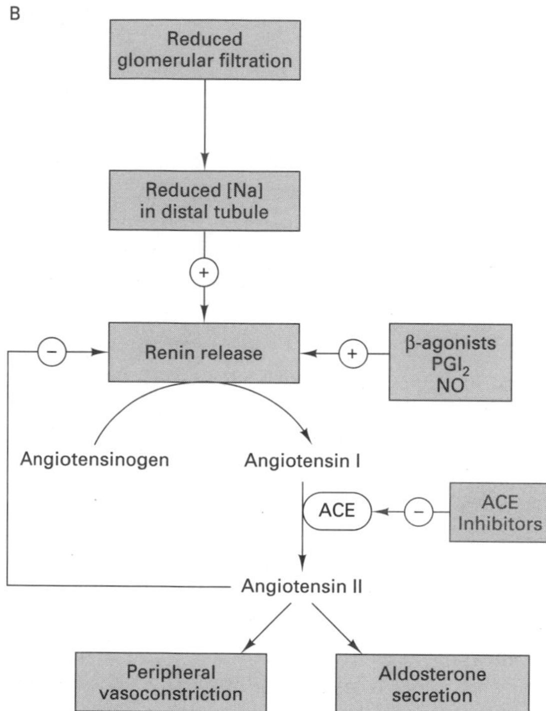

Fig. 14.5 Formation and functions of the angiotensins. **A.** Formation of angiotensin I, II and III from the N-terminal of the precursor protein, angiotensinogen. **B.** The control of angiotensin production and its main physiological effects. (ACE = angiotensin-converting enzyme)

and it has recently been found that the genotype characterised by a double deletion that gives rise to increased ACE activity is an independent risk factor for myocardial infarction (Cambien et al. 1992). If this is confirmed, it may provide a rationale for targeting ACE inhibitors (see below) toward genetically predisposed individuals. The same enzyme inactivates bradykinin (see Ch. 12) and several other vasodilator peptides. This is probably not of much physiological significance but may contribute to the pharmacological actions of ACE inhibitors. The main actions of angiotensin are:

- vasoconstriction (see above)
- secretion of aldosterone from the adrenal cortex (see Chs 18 and 21), leading to sodium and water retention.

Angiotensin II is further converted by an aminopeptidase to *angiotensin III* (Fig. 14.5) through the loss of the N-terminal Asn residue. Angiotensin III is also active, particularly in stimulating aldosterone secretion and also centrally, but its functional significance is not known.

The renin–angiotensin pathway is important in the pathogenesis of heart failure (see below) and of some kinds of hypertension, and can be influenced by drugs at four points:

- renin release
- renin activity
- ACE
- interaction of angiotensin II with vascular and/or adrenocortical receptors.

Renin release

Renin release is partly under the control of the sympathetic nervous system. It is known that stimulation of the renal sympathetic nerves causes renin release, and that this is blocked by **β-adrenoceptor antagonists**. This is one mechanism, albeit a minor one, to explain the hypotensive action of these drugs.

Renin inhibitors

Orally active renin inhibitors are currently undergoing clinical trials. These drugs (e.g. **enalkiren**, **remikiren**) reduce plasma renin activity while increasing immunoreactive renin. Plasma angiotensin II is only partially suppressed and there are only small falls in aldosterone in healthy humans. Effects on blood pressure in man (even in vigorously salt-depleted subjects) are small. The hypotensive effect of renin inhibitors may be limited by increased renin release, and because there are alternative enzymes (e.g. cathepsin G, tonin) that can generate angiotensin II in vascular tissue.

Angiotensin-converting enzyme inhibitors

Several specific ACE inhibitors have been developed, for example **captopril** (Fig. 14.6). The enzyme is a carboxypeptidase which splits off pairs of basic amino acids. Its active site contains a zinc atom. The development of captopril was one of the first examples of successful drug design based on a chemical knowledge of the target molecule. A variety of small peptides were found to be weak inhibitors of the enzyme, but these were unsuitable as drugs because of their low potency and poor oral absorption. The structure of captopril was designed to combine the steric properties of such peptide antagonists in a non-peptide molecule, which contains a sulphydryl group appropriately placed to bind to the zinc atom, coupled to a proline residue which binds to the enzyme site normally occupied by the terminal leucine of angiotensin I (Fig. 14.6).

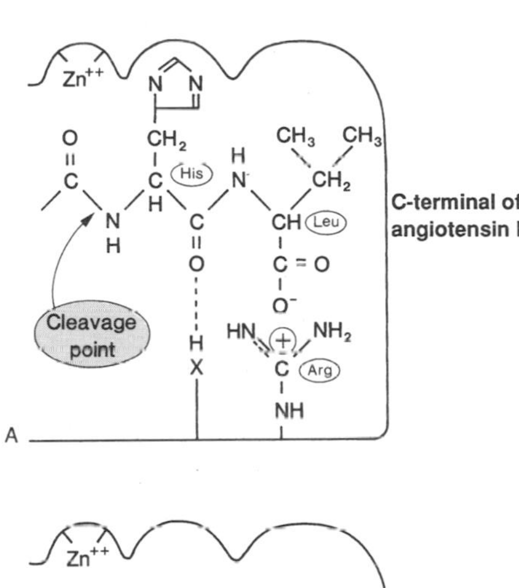

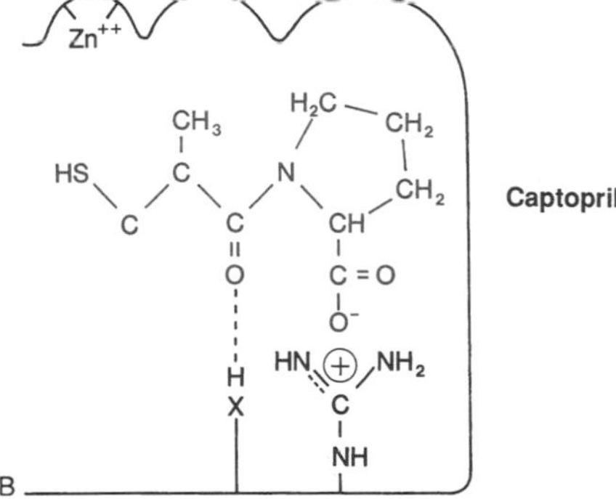

Fig. 14.6 The active site of angiotensin-converting enzyme. A. Binding of angiotensin I. **B**. Binding of the inhibitor, captopril, which is an analogue of the terminal dipeptide of angiotensin I.

Pharmacological effects

Captopril is a powerful inhibitor of the effects of angiotensin I in the whole animal. It causes a small fall in arterial pressure in normal animals or human subjects, but a much larger fall in hypertensive patients, particularly those in whom renin secretion is enhanced (e.g. in renovascular hypertension). The fall that occurs in normal, sodium-replete subjects, in whom renin secretion is small, may be partly related to inhibition of bradykinin inactivation.

ACE inhibitors affect both resistance and capacitance vessels, and thus reduce arterial pressure and cardiac load. Unlike many vasodilators, they do not affect cardiac contractility, so cardiac output normally increases. They act preferentially on angiotensin-sensitive vascular beds, which include those of the kidney, heart and brain. This selectivity may be important in sustaining adequate perfusion of these vital organs in the face of reduced perfusion pressure. Critical renal artery stenosis represents an exception to this, where ACE inhibition results in a fall of glomerular filtration rate (see below).

Several ACE inhibitors are now available, including **captopril** (duration of action approximately 8 hours), **enalapril, lisinopril** and **ramipril** (whose actions last for about 24 hours).

Clinical uses

Clinical uses of ACE inhibitors are summarised on page 316.

Unwanted effects

Captopril, the first ACE inhibitor to be introduced, was initially used in doses that, in retrospect, were excessive. In these large doses it caused rashes, taste disturbance, neutropenia, and heavy proteinuria. This pattern of adverse effects is also seen during treatment with **penicillamine** (Ch. 12) which also contains a sulphydryl group, and it has been argued that these effects are attributable to this chemical feature of the molecule rather than to ACE inhibition as such. Other ACE inhibitors that do not possess a sulphydryl group (e.g. **enalapril, ramipril**) do not cause these effects. Adverse effects that are directly related to ACE inhibition are common to all drugs of this class. These include hypotension, especially after the first dose, and especially in patients with heart failure who have been treated with loop diuretics, in whom the renin–angiotensin system is highly activated. A dry cough, which may possibly be the result of accumulation of bradykinin (Ch. 11) in the bronchial mucosa, is the commonest persistent adverse effect. Patients with bilateral renal artery stenosis predictably develop renal failure if treated with ACE inhibitors, because glomerular filtration in the face of low afferent arteriolar pressure is maintained by angiotensin-II-mediated constriction of the efferent arteriole. Such renal failure is reversible provided it is recognised promptly and the ACE inhibitor stopped. If such renal failure occurs, hyperkalaemia may be severe due to reduced aldosterone secretion, and potassium-sparing diuretics (e.g. amiloride; Ch. 18) should not be used routinely in patients treated with ACE inhibitors for this reason.

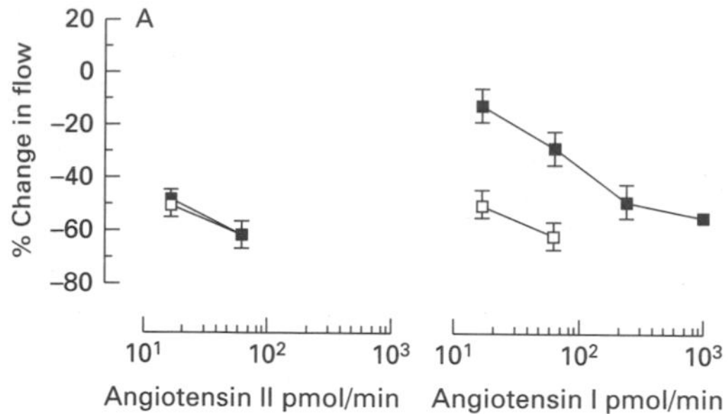

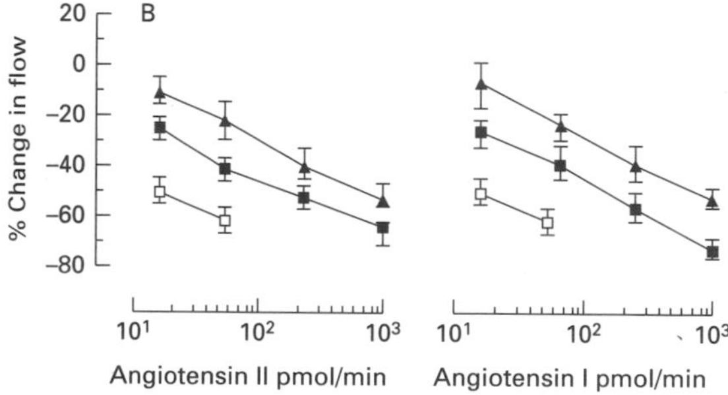

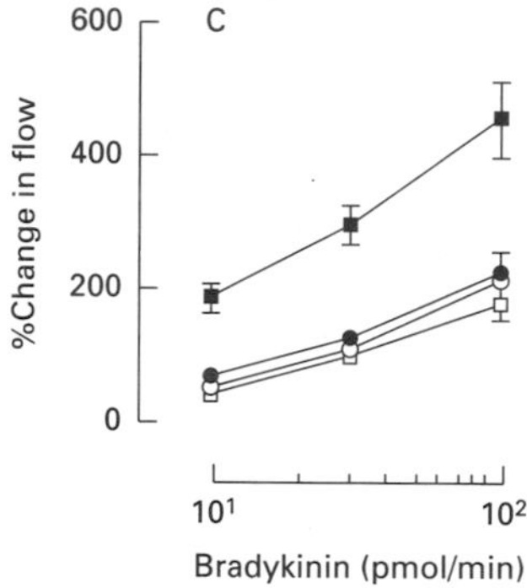

Fig. 14.7 Comparison of effects of angiotensin-converting enzyme inhibition and angiotensin-receptor blockade in the human forearm vasculature. A. Effect of brachial artery infusion of angiotensin I and angiotensin II on forearm blood flow after oral administration of placebo (open symbols) or enalapril 10 mg (solid symbols). **B.** Effect of angiotensin I and angiotensin II on forearm blood flow after oral administration of placebo (open symbols), losartan 20 mg (solid squares), or losartan 100 mg (triangles). **C.** Effect of bradykinin on forearm blood flow after placebo (open squares), enalapril 10 mg (solid squares) or losartan 20 and 100 mg. (From: Cockcroft J R et al. 1993 J Cardiovasc Pharmacol 22: 579–584)

Clinical uses of ACE inhibitors

- Hypertension
- Cardiac failure (where they improve survival)
- Following myocardial infarction (especially when there is ventricular dysfunction, even when this is mild)
- ACE inhibitors reduce proteinuria in diabetics, and are being investigated as a means of preventing renal failure in such patients

Angiotensin antagonists

Saralasin, a peptide analogue of angiotensin II, is a competitive inhibitor of the vasoconstrictor effect of angiotensin. It is a partial agonist, and must be administered parenterally so it is not used clinically any longer. More recently, attention has again focused on angiotensin-receptor antagonists with the development of a number of non-peptide, orally active pure antagonists of which **losartan** (Fig. 14.7) is the furthest advanced in development. It is hoped that such drugs will lack the adverse effects of ACE inhibitors, such as cough, that have been attributed (albeit without proof) to bradykinin accumulation. Against this is the possibility that some of the beneficial effects of ACE inhibitors (e.g. reversal of left ventricular hypertrophy) may be bradykinin/EDRF mediated (Linz & Scholkens 1992). Watch this space!

CLINICAL USES OF VASODILATOR DRUGS

It is beyond the scope of this book to provide a detailed account of the clinical uses of drugs that affect the cardiovascular system, but it is, nonetheless, useful to consider the various pharmacological approaches that are used in treating certain clinical states. The conditions that will be briefly discussed are:

- hypertension
- cardiac failure
- shock.

HYPERTENSION

Hypertension is a common and usually progressive disorder, which, if not effectively treated, results in a greatly increased probability of coronary thrombosis, strokes and renal failure. Until about 1950, there was no effective treatment, and the development of antihypertensive drugs, which greatly increase life expectancy, has been a major, but largely unsung, therapeutic success story.

There are a few recognisable and treatable causes of hypertension, such as phaeochromocytoma (Ch. 7), steroid-secreting tumours of the adrenal cortex, renal artery stenosis and so on, but the great majority of cases involve no obvious causative factor, and are grouped as essential hypertension (so called because it was originally thought that the raised blood pressure was essential to maintain adequate tissue perfusion). The underlying defect seems to be intimately related to the kidneys (as demonstrated in transplantation experiments in which kidneys are transplanted from or to animals with genetic hypertension, or from humans requiring renal transplants therapeutically: hypertension 'goes with' the kidney from a hypertensive donor and vice versa) and leads to a narrowing of the lumen of systemic arterioles. The raised peripheral vascular resistance calls into play a variety of physiological responses involving the cardiovascular system, nervous system and kidney. Certain vicious circles tend to become established, and these provide some of the targets for pharmacological attack.

Figure 14.8 summarises the major physiological control mechanisms that operate to maintain the arterial blood pressure. The two main systems involved are the sympathetic nervous system and the renin–angiotensin–aldosterone system. One of the ways in which the primary process tends to lead to progressively worsening hypertension is that renal glomerular sclerosis occurs in response to the raised pressure. The control system fails because the normal relationship between renal blood flow and arterial blood pressure is upset by the narrowing of the renal vessels. It is now well established, contrary to the earlier view that hypertension was 'essential' to sustain life, that reducing arterial blood pressure greatly improves the prognosis of patients who have diastolic pressures persistently above 95 mmHg at rest. The use of drugs to control mild hypertension (which is asymptomatic), without producing unacceptable side effects, is therefore an important clinical need, and much effort has gone into devising satisfactory therapeutic regimes.

The main points of attack for antihypertensive drugs are shown in Figure 14.8. Since these drugs usually have to be continued indefinitely, avoidance of side effects is particularly important, and the treatment of hypertension involves the staged introduction of drugs, starting with those least likely to produce side effects. The preferred regimes have changed progressively as better drugs have become available. During the 1960s, sympathetic-blocking agents (e.g. **methyldopa, guanethidine, reserpine**) were the main treatment, but these have severe side effects, respectively drowsiness, postural hypotension and depression. Diarrhoea and impotence are also common. More recently, **thiazide diuretics** or **β-adrenoceptor antagonists** have been the usual starting point, but these also have side effects, though less severe. Over the last few years **ACE inhibitors** have been increasingly used, and also **calcium antagonists**, mainly because of their relative lack of metabolic and other side effects. **α_1-adrenoceptor antagonists** have also staged something of a comeback with longer-acting drugs such as **terazosin** and **doxazosin** that are well tolerated, used once daily and have theoretically desirable effects on plasma lipids (reduced LDL/HDL ratio; see Ch. 15). Vasodilator drugs such as **nitroprusside** are used in emergencies. The harsh realities of life on antihypertensive drugs are graphically described in an article entitled '80,000 pills: a personal history of hypertension' (Mills 1989).

The main categories of antihypertensive drug are summarised in Table 14.5.

CARDIAC FAILURE

The underlying abnormality in cardiac failure (see Ch. 13) is a cardiac output that is inadequate to meet the metabolic demands of the body during exercise (and ultimately also at rest). This leads secondarily to an increased central venous pressure (increased pre-load) and to peripheral vasocon-

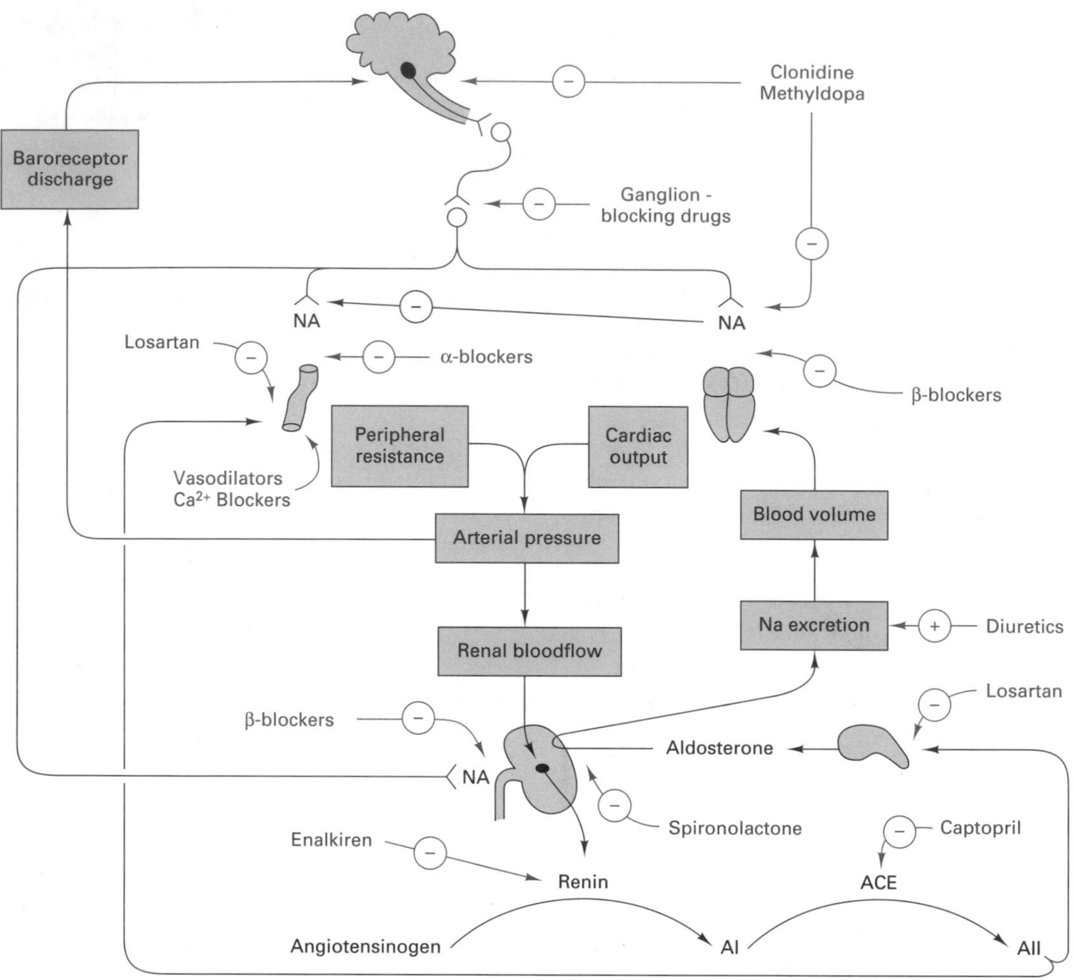

Fig. 14.8 Diagram showing the main mechanisms involved in arterial blood pressure regulation (black lines), and the sites of action of antihypertensive drugs (red lines). NA = noradrenaline, AI = angiotensin I, AII = angiotensin II, ACE = angiotensin-converting enzyme.

striction (increased after-load). It may be caused by disease of the myocardium itself (most commonly ischaemic heart disease), or by circulatory factors such as volume overload (valvular incompetence, arteriovenous shunts), etc. or pressure overload (hypertension, valvular narrowing), which require greater cardiac work to be performed to achieve a sufficient output. When the cardiac output decreases, an increase in body fluid volume occurs, partly because the increased venous pressure causes increased formation of tissue fluid, and partly because the reduced renal blood flow leads to activation of the renin–angiotensin–aldosterone system.

A highly simplified diagram of the sequence of events is shown in Figure 14.9. It can be seen that there are four main points at which drugs (see p. 320) can act:

- *Increased force of contraction.* **Cardiac glycosides** (see Ch. 13) were once the mainstay of treatment of cardiac failure, but their use is now largely restricted to patients who also have supraventricular dysrhythmias. Their adverse effects outweigh their benefits with long-term treatment in other situations. **Dobutamine** (a β_1-selective adrenoceptor agonist; see Ch. 7) is used intravenously when a rapid response is needed in the short term, for example following open heart surgery.

Table 14.5 Commonly used antihypertensive drugs

Mode of action	Drugs	Adverse effects: Postural hypotension	Adverse effects: Impotence	Other	Special features
Reduction of blood volume/indirect vasodilatation	Thiazide diuretics*	–	++	Urinary frequency, gout, glucose intolerance, hypokalaemia, hyponatraemia, thrombocytopenia	Reduce stroke in clinical trials, inexpensive
Block of β-adrenoceptors†	Propranolol Atenolol Metoprolol	–	±	Fatigue, cold peripheries	Reduce stroke in clinical trials, inexpensive, additional benefit after MI. Contraindications: asthma, heart failure, heart block, peripheral vascular disease
ACE inhibition	Captopril Enalapril	–	±	First dose hypotension, dry cough, reversible renal failure in patients with bilateral renal artery stenosis	Additional benefit in insulin-dependent diabetics with proteinuria, following MI, and in patients with heart failure; cause regression of left ventricular hypertrophy
Arteriolar vasodilatation	Ca^{2+} antagonists, e.g. nifedipine, amlodipine nicardipine	–	±	Flushing, headache, ankle oedema	
Block of α_1-adrenoceptors†	Prazosin Terazosin Doxazosin	+	±	First dose hypotension	Longer-acting drugs (e.g. terazosin, doxazosin) better tolerated than prazosin. Improve plasma lipids. Useful addition to other drugs when two drugs needed

MI = myocardial infarction, * see Ch. 18, † see Ch. 7

- *Increased fluid excretion.* **Diuretics** (see Ch. 18) are routinely used to treat cardiac failure. A diuretic may suffice on its own, but is increasingly often combined with an **ACE inhibitor**.
- *Vasodilatation.* The use of rapidly-acting vasodilators such as glyceryl trinitrate is well established for treating acute episodes of cardiac failure. The venodilator effect of these drugs is helpful in reducing venous pressure, and their effect in increasing the compliance of the arterial system is useful in reducing cardiac work. The use of arteriolar vasodilators, such as **hydralazine** or **prazosin**, for longer-term treatment has largely been replaced by ACE inhibition.
- *ACE inhibition.* **ACE inhibitors** (ACEI) are now commonly used, in combination with **diuretics**. By blocking the formation of angiotensin II they reduce both vascular resistance (thus improving tissue perfusion and reducing cardiac after-load) and the secretion of aldosterone (thus reducing Na^+ retention). They have a beneficial effect on longevity, which is greater than that provided by vasodilator therapy with a combination of organic nitrates and hydralazine. Neither digoxin nor diuretics have been shown to improve survival.

SHOCK AND HYPOTENSIVE STATES

Shock is a condition in which perfusion of vital organs is inadequate, leading to increased lactate

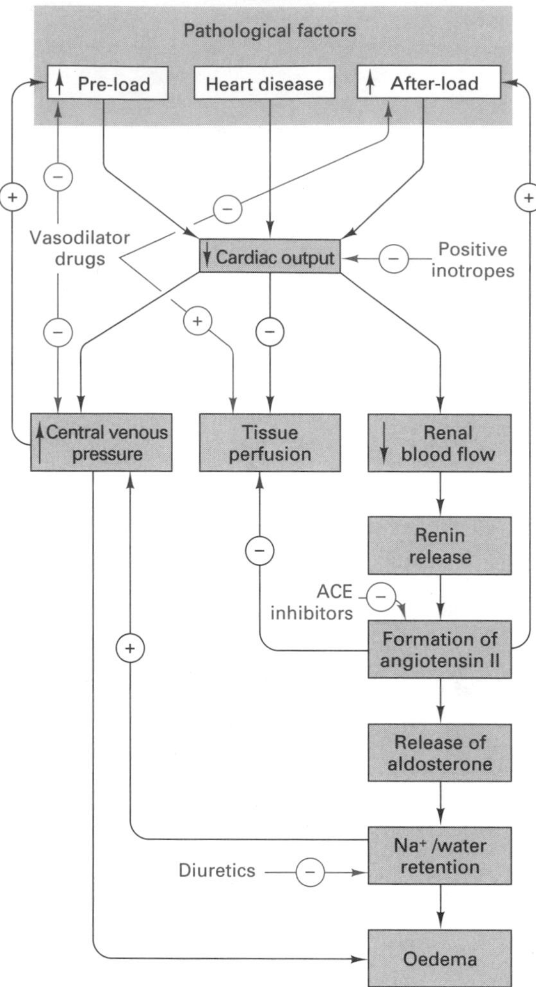

Fig. 14.9 Simplified scheme showing the pathogenesis of heart failure, and the sites of action of some of the drugs used to treat it. The symptoms of heart failure are produced by reduced tissue perfusion, oedema and increased central venous pressure.

Drugs commonly used in chronic heart failure

- *Loop diuretics* (e.g. frusemide; Ch. 18) are first-line treatment; they reduce oedema, reduce pre-load, improve symptoms caused by pulmonary oedema but increase plasma renin. They reduce plasma K^+, which may be important if they are used together with digoxin, in which case a K^+-sparing diuretic (e.g. amiloride; Ch. 18) can be added. This is often unnecessary (and may be dangerous) in patients on ACE inhibitors.
- *ACE* inhibitors (e.g. captopril, enalapril) prolong life as well as improving symptoms in patients receiving diuretics. They interrupt the renin–angiotensin system and reduce both pre-load and after-load. Captopril is shorter-acting than enalapril, which is a pro-drug. Diuretics should be withheld where possible for 24 hours (if necessary in hospital) before starting treatment, to reduce the risk of *first dose hypotension.* ACE inhibitors cause renal failure (which is reversible on stopping the drug) in patients with bilateral renal artery stenosis. They increase plasma K^+ by suppressing aldosterone; this is usually mild but may be severe in the presence of renal failure or with concurrent use of amiloride. The commonest dose-related adverse effect is dry cough.
- *Digoxin* (see Ch. 13) is of particular benefit in patients with heart failure associated with *rapid atrial fibrillation.* It is also indicated in patients who remain symptomatic despite treatment with loop diuretics and ACE inhibitors.
- *Other vasodilators.* Organic nitrates (e.g. isosorbide mononitrate) reduce pre-load, and hydralazine reduces after-load. Used in combination, these prolong life, but less effectively than ACE inhibitors. They are used when ACE inhibitors are contraindicated or not tolerated.

production, usually because of a very low arterial blood pressure. It can be caused by various insults, including haemorrhage, burns, bacterial infections and acute myocardial damage (Fig. 14.10). There may be a reduced effective circulating blood volume (hypovolaemia), caused either directly by loss of blood or by movement of fluid from the plasma to the tissues. The physiological (homeostatic) response to this is complex: vasodilatation in the vascular bed of a vital organ (e.g. brain, heart, kidney) is advantageous in favouring perfusion of that organ, but at the expense of a further reduction in blood pressure which leads to reduced perfusion of all organs. Ideally, there is a balance between vasoconstriction in non-essential vascular beds and vasodilatation in the vital organs. The dividing line between the normal physiological response to blood loss, and clinical shock is that, in the latter, tissue hypoxia produces secondary effects that tend to magnify rather than correct the primary disturbance. Thus, patients with established shock have profound and inappropriate vasodilatation in non-essential organs which is difficult to correct with

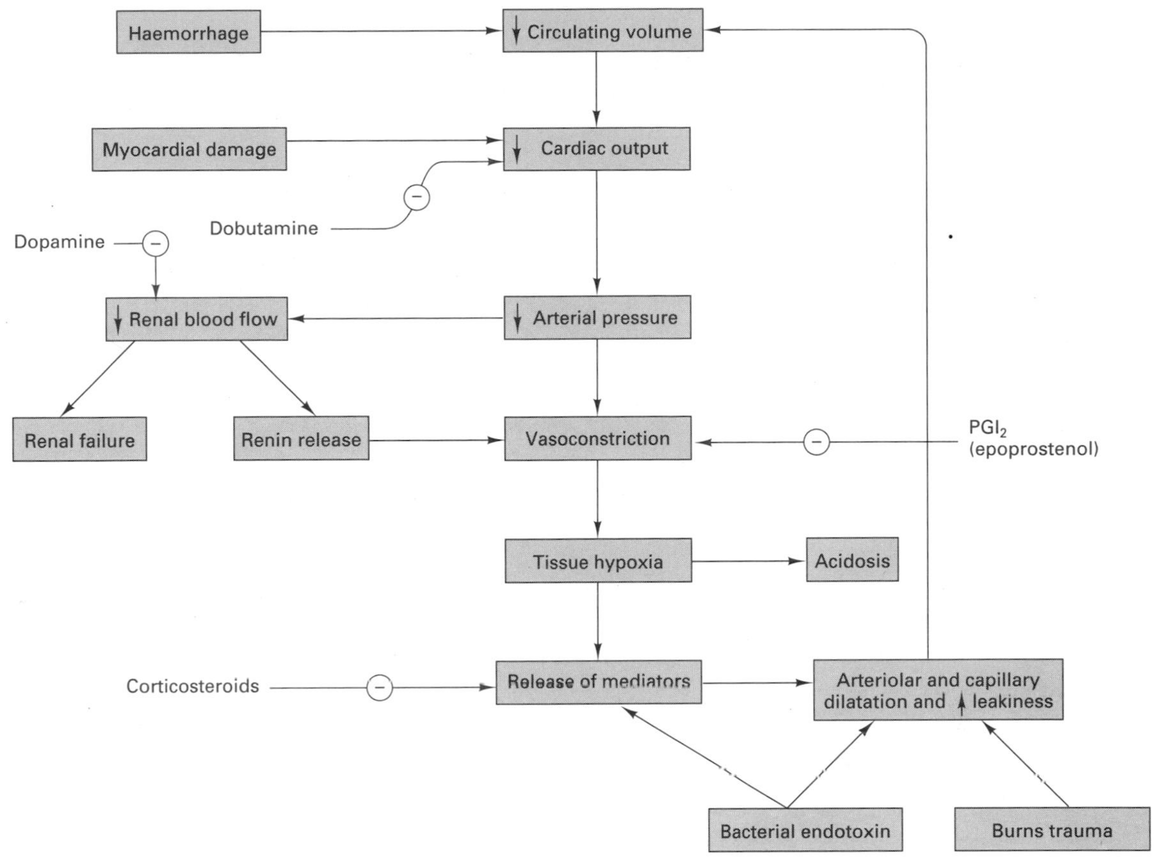

Fig. 14.10 Simplified scheme showing the pathogenesis of hypovolaemic shock, and the sites of action of two drugs (dopamine and corticosteroids) that may be used to treat it. The most important treatment is to restore circulating volume, normally by intravenous infusion.

vasoconstrictor drugs. The release of mediators (e.g. histamine, 5-hydroxytryptamine, bradykinin, prostaglandins, cytokines including interleukins and TNF, nitric oxide and, undoubtedly, a variety of yet unidentified substances) that cause capillaries to become dilated and leaky, is physiologically the opposite of what is required.

This leads in turn to multiple organ failure, and intensive therapy specialists spend much effort trying to support the circulations of such patients with cocktails of vasoactive drugs (e.g. **dobutamine, dopamine, prostacyclin**) designed to optimise flow to vital organs. In addition, there is great interest in antagonists of mediators that may be contributing to the shocked state. Clinical trials are in progress with drugs and macromolecules (including monoclonal antibodies and soluble fragments of receptors) designed to block or neutralise endotoxin, interleukins, TNF and the inducible form of NO synthase among others. So far, these efforts have not yielded fruit: experimental work strongly suggests that dose will be critical since small amounts of mediators such as NO appear to be beneficial while larger amounts are harmful (Ch. 10). Clinical trials in this setting are extremely difficult because of the unique and distinctive haemodynamic features of each patient. Volume replacement is of proven benefit if there is hypovolaemia; antibiotics are essential if there is persistent infection; corticosteroids suppress the formation of NO and of prostaglandins but are not of proven benefit once shock is established; vasoactive (dopamine, prostacyclin) and positively inotropic (adrenaline, dobutamine) drugs may help in individual patients.

REFERENCES AND FURTHER READING

Abdelrahman A M, Burrell L M, Johnston C I 1993 Blockade of the renin–angiotensin system at different sites: effect on renin, angiotensin and aldosterone. J Hypertens 11 (Suppl 3): S23–S26

Ashcroft F M 1988 Adenosine 5′-triphosphate-sensitive potassium channels. Annu Rev Neurosci 11: 97–118

Bolton T B 1979 Mechanisms of action of neurotransmitters and other substances on smooth muscle. Physiol Rev 59: 606–718

Brindley G S 1986 Pilot experiments on the actions of drugs injected into the human corpus cavernosum penis. Br J Pharmacol 87: 495–500

Cambien F, Poirier O, Lecerf L, Evans A, Cambou J-P, Arveiler D, Luc G, Bard J-M, Bara L, Ricard S, Tiret L, Amouyel P, Alhenc-Gelas F, Subrier F 1992 Deletion polymorphism in the gene for angiotensin-converting enzyme is a potent risk factor for myocardial infarction. Nature 359: 641–644

Cook N S 1988 The pharmacology of potassium channels and their therapeutic potential. Trends Pharmacol Sci 9: 21–28

Dahlof B, Pennert K, Hansson L 1992 Reversal of left ventricular hypertrophy in hypertensive patients: a metaanalysis of 109 treatment studies. Am J Hypertens 5: 95–110

Dzau V J, Sasamura H, Hein L 1993 Heterogeneity of angiotensin synthetic pathways and receptor subtypes: physiological and pharmacological implications. J Hypertens 11 (Suppl 3): S13–S18

Furchgott R F, Vanhoutte P M 1989 Endothelium-derived relaxing and contracting factors. FASEB J 3: 2007–2018

Gurney A M, Clapp L H 1994 Calcium channels and vasodilation. Adv Mol Cell Biol 8: 21–34

Jones A W 1981 Vascular smooth muscle and alterations during hypertension. In: Bülbring et al. (eds) Smooth muscle: an assessment of current knowledge. Edward Arnold, London, p 397–429

Kamm K E, Stull J T 1985 The function of myosin and myosin-light-chain kinase phosphorylation in smooth muscle. Annu Rev Pharmacol Toxicol 25: 593–620

Karihara Y, Karihara H, Suzuki H, Kodama T, Maemura K, Nagi R, Oda H, Kuwaki T, Cao W-H, Kamadan N, Jishage K, Ouchi Y, Azuma S, Toyoda Y, Ishikawa T, Kumada M, Yazaki Y 1994 Elevated blood pressure and craniofacial abnormalities in mice deficient in endothelin-1. Nature 368: 703–710

Linz W, Scholkens B A 1992 A specific β_2-bradykinin receptor antagonist HOE140 abolishes the antihypertrophic effect of ramipril. Br J Pharmacol 105: 771–772

Masaki T 1993 Endothelins: homeostatic and compensatory actions in the circulatory and endocrine systems. Endocrine Rev 14: 256–268

Mills B D 1989 80 000 pills: a personal history of hypertension. Br Med J 298: 445–448

Nayler W G 1988 Calcium antagonists. Academic Press, London

Okada K, Miyazaki Y, Takada J, Matsuyama K, Yamaki T, Yano M 1990 Conversion of big endothelin-1 by membrane-bound metalloendopeptidase in cultured bovine endothelial cells. Biochem Biophys Res Commun 171: 1192–1198

Quast U, Cook N S 1989 Moving together: K^+ channel openers and ATP-sensitive K^+ channels. Trends Pharmacol Sci 10: 431–435

Sakurai T, Yanagisawa M, Masaki T 1992 Molecular characterization of endothelin receptors. Trends Pharmacol Sci 13: 103–108

Simonson M S, Dunn J 1992 The molecular mechanisms of cardiovascular and renal regulation by endothelial peptides. J Lab Clin Med 119: 622–639

Simoons M L 1994 Myocardial infarction: ACE inhibitors for all? For ever? Lancet 344: 279–281

Timmermans P B M W M, Wong P C, Chiu A T, Herblin W F, Benfield P, Carini D J, Lee R J, Wexler R R, Saye J M, Smith R D 1993 Angiotensin II receptors and angiotensin II receptor antagonists. Pharmacol Rev 45: 205–251

Valloton M B 1987 The renin–angiotensin system. Trends Pharmacol Sci 8: 69–74

Vane J R, Anggard E E, Botting R M 1990 Regulatory functions of the vascular endothelium. N Engl J Med 323: 27–35

Vanhoutte P M 1994 Endothelin-1: A matter of life and breath. Nature 368: 693

Yanagisawa M, Kurihara H, Kimura S, Tomobe Y, Kobayashi M, Mitsui Y, Yazaki Y, Goto K, Masaki T 1988 A novel potent vasoconstrictor peptide produced by vascular endothelial cells. Nature 332: 411–415

15
CONTROL OF LIPOPROTEIN METABOLISM

LIPOPROTEINS AND ATHEROSCLEROSIS

Lipoproteins (macromolecular complexes of lipid and protein) transport lipids and cholesterol through the bloodstream. Such a transport system is essential to life, but excessive concentrations of one important class of lipoprotein known as *low density lipoprotein* (LDL; see below) increase the risk of ischaemic heart disease. Since this is the commonest cause of death and disability in industrialised societies there is great interest in drugs that reduce LDL.

Ischaemic heart disease is caused by plaques of atheroma in the coronary arteries which partially occlude one or more of these vessels and may rupture exposing subendothelial material that acts as a focus for thrombosis. Myocardial infarction is caused by such thromboses, and the role of *fibrinolytic drugs* and *antiplatelet drugs* (notably **aspirin**) in treatment and prevention of myocardial infarction is described in Chapter 16. The other approach to preventing myocardial infarction, described in the present chapter, is to attempt to reduce progression of atheroma and/or cause regression of existing atheromatous plaques. Atheroma affects other large and medium-sized arteries in addition to the coronaries and can cause *stroke*, *peripheral vascular disease* (with symptoms of pain on walking and leading in severe cases to gangrene and amputation of the leg), *renal failure* or other clinical syndromes depending on the anatomical location of lesions that are causing critical narrowings of the arterial tree.

Many large epidemiological studies, notably one based on data spanning many decades from a community called Framingham in New England, have identified a series of risk factors for atheromatous disease. Some of these cannot be altered (e.g. a family history of ischaemic heart disease) but others can (e.g. cigarette smoking, hypertension, hyperglycaemia, obesity, physical inactivity and increased plasma concentrations of total cholesterol or LDL). Pharmacological approaches to decreasing these risk factors are described in Chapters 14, 20 and 33. The present chapter describes attempts to prevent atheromatous disease by controlling lipoprotein metabolism. In addition to the common and serious problem of atherosclerosis, some unusual types of hyperlipoproteinaemia are associated with pancreatitis and other clinical disorders, and drugs that influence lipoprotein metabolism are also used for such patients.

Atherosclerosis is a *focal* disease of the intima of large and medium-sized arteries (down to approximately 3 mm external diameter). The major components of the plaque are lipid and connective tissue matrix proteins. Both extracellular and intracellular lipid are present in advanced plaques. The pathogenesis of atherosclerosis unfolds over many decades during most of which time the lesions are clinically silent, the occurrence of symptoms signalling advanced disease or supervening thrombosis. Until very recently there have been no good sub-primate models of advanced focal atherosclerotic disease, although transgenic animals deficient in specific key enzymes and receptors in lipoprotein metabolism are now rapidly transforming this scene. Nevertheless, most of our understanding of atheroma comes from human pathology and from experimental studies in primates.

The relationship between atherosclerosis and thrombosis and the LDL-cholesterol concentration in the plasma

The details of the pathogenesis of atherosclerosis are becoming clearer. The following steps are involved:

- Injury to endothelium encourages monocyte attachment, this process being markedly increased in hypercholesterolaemia. Turbulence may be responsible for the striking predilection of lesions for regions of disturbed flow such as the origin of vessels from the aorta. Injury is initially undetectable morphologically but results in endothelial cell dysfunction with altered PGI_2 (Ch. 11) and NO (Ch. 10) biosynthesis.
- Endothelial cells can also bind LDL, and, when activated (e.g. by injury), these cells and the attached monocytes/macrophages generate free radicals which oxidise the attached LDL, resulting in lipid peroxidation and destruction of the receptor needed for normal receptor-mediated clearance of LDL.
- Modified LDL is taken up by macrophages via their 'scavenger receptors'.
- Having taken up LDL, these macrophages (now *foam-cells*) migrate subendothelially. Subendothelial collections of foam-cells and T lymphocytes form the fatty streaks which presage atherosclerosis.
- Platelets, macrophages and endothelial cells release chemotaxins and growth factors. These cause proliferation of smooth muscle and deposition of connective tissue components, resulting in the formation of the atherosclerotic plaque. The excessive inflammatory fibroproliferative response leads to a dense fibrous cap of connective tissue overlying a core of lipid and necrotic debris.
- The plaque forms the substrate on which thrombosis develops subsequent to rupture (see Ch. 16, Fig. 16.10).

An additional factor, linking LDL with thrombosis, is that one species of LDL, lipoprotein(a), which is strongly associated with atherosclerosis (and is localised in atherosclerotic lesions), carries a unique apoprotein, apo(a), which is remarkably similar in structure to plasminogen. Hence lipoprotein(a) competes with and inhibits the binding of plasminogen to its receptors on the endothelial cell. Plasminogen is normally the substrate for plasminogen activator which is secreted by and bound to endothelial cells, and the interaction of the two gives rise to the fibrinolytic enzyme plasmin (see Fig. 16.10). The effect of the binding of lipoprotein(a) is that less plasmin is generated, fibrinolysis is inhibited and thrombosis promoted. LDL can also activate platelets, constituting a further thrombogenic effect of LDL.

Many steps in the atherogenic process are potential targets for pharmacological attack (e.g. by antioxidants, calcium antagonists, angiotensin-converting enzyme inhibitors or growth factor antagonists; see Cleland & Krikler 1993). These approaches have yet to prove themselves, whereas drugs that influence lipoprotein metabolism are of proven clinical efficacy and are the subject of this chapter. The pre-eminent importance of lipoproteins in the pathogenesis of atheroma is underscored by animal experiments that show that LDL cholesterol must be greater than a threshold value for early lesions (analogous to fatty streaks in humans) to develop: thus hyperlipoproteinaemia appears to be a *necessary* condition for atherogenesis. Furthermore, clinical studies have shown recently that reduction of circulating concentrations of LDL-cholesterol can cause *regression* of atherosclerotic lesions.

To understand how drugs that reduce the concentration of plasma lipids work it is necessary to know how lipids are handled in the body.

LIPOPROTEIN TRANSPORT IN THE BLOOD

Lipoproteins consist of a central core of hydrophobic lipid (triglycerides or cholesteryl esters) encased in a more hydrophilic coat of polar substances—phospholipids, free cholesterol and associated proteins (termed apolipoproteins). There are four main classes of lipoproteins, differing in the relative proportion of the core lipids and in the type of apoprotein. They also differ in size and density, and this latter property, as measured by ultracentrifugation, is the basis for their classification into:

- high density lipoproteins (HDL)
- low density lipoproteins (LDL)
- very low density lipoproteins (VLDL)
- chylomicrons.

Each of these lipoprotein classes has a specific role in lipid transport in the circulation, and there are different 'pathways' for exogenous and for endogenous lipids.

In the *exogenous pathway* (see Fig. 15.1), cholesterol and triglycerides derived from the gastrointestinal

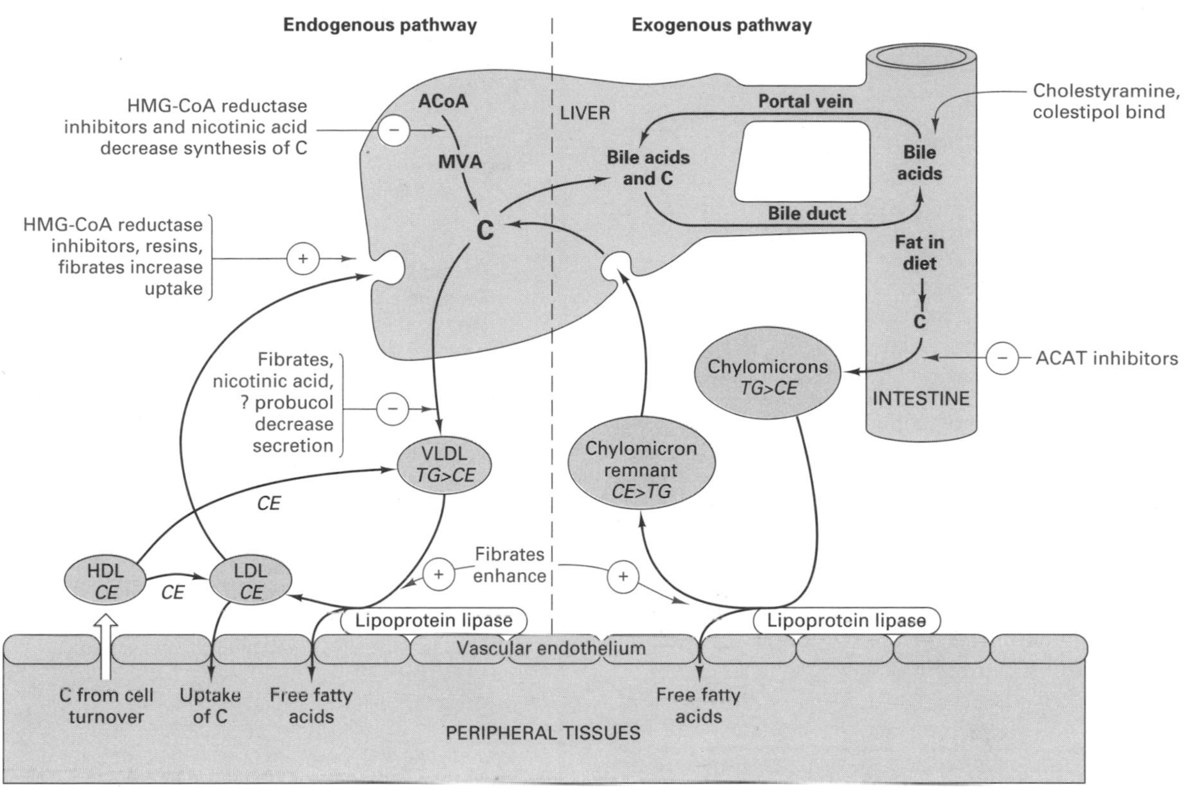

Fig. 15.1 Schematic diagram of cholesterol transport in the tissues, with the probable sites of action of the main drugs affecting lipoprotein metabolism. C = cholesterol; CE = cholesteryl ester; TG = triglyceride; MVA = mevalonate; HMG-CoA reductase = 3-hydroxy-3-methylglutaryl-CoA reductase; VLDL = very low density lipoprotein; LDL = low density lipoprotein; HDL = high density lipoprotein; ACAT = acylCoA: cholesterol acyltransferase. ACAT inhibitors are experimental.

tract are transported in the lymph and then in the plasma as *chylomicrons* (diameter 100–1000 nm) to muscle and adipose tissue. Here, on the vascular endothelial cells, the core triglycerides are hydrolysed by a surface-bound lipoprotein lipase (which requires one of the apoproteins as a co-factor) and the free fatty acids are taken up by the tissues. The chylomicron remnants (diameter 30–50 nm), still containing their full complement of cholesteryl esters, pass to the liver, bind to apolipoprotein receptors on hepatocytes, and undergo endocytosis. Cholesterol is liberated within the liver cell and may be stored, or oxidised to bile acids, or secreted in the bile unaltered. Alternatively, it may enter the endogenous pathway of lipid transport in VLDL.

In the *endogenous pathway*, cholesterol and newly synthesised triglycerides are transported as VLDL (diameter 30–80 nm) to muscle and adipose tissue where the triglycerides are hydrolysed and the fatty acids enter the tissues as described above. During this process, the lipoprotein particles become smaller (diameter 20–30 nm), but still have a full complement of cholesteryl esters and ultimately become LDL which provides the source of cholesterol for synthesis of steroids (see Chs 21 and 22), plasma membranes and bile acids (Ch. 19). Cells requiring cholesterol for these purposes synthesise receptors that recognise LDL apolipoproteins which enable them to take up LDL by receptor-mediated endocytosis. Some drugs (notably **HMG-CoA reductase inhibitors**; see below) reduce the LDL concentration in the blood by stimulating the synthesis of these receptors in hepatocytes. Cholesterol can return to plasma from the tissues in HDL particles (diameter 7–20 nm). Cholesterol is esterified with long-chain fatty acid in HDL particles, and the resulting cholesteryl esters are subsequently transferred to VLDL or LDL particles by a transfer protein present in the plasma. Epidemiological evidence shows a strong *inverse* relationship between plasma concentration of HDL and cardiovascular risk: that is the *higher* the HDL concentration the *lower* the risk.

Types of hyperlipoproteinaemia

Hyperlipoproteinaemia may be *primary* or *secondary*. The primary forms are genetically determined. Six phenotypes (Table 15.1) are recognised. These vary in the extent to which:

- the plasma cholesterol and triglyceride concentrations are raised
- particular lipoprotein classes are increased.

Secondary forms of hyperlipoproteinaemia are a consequence of other conditions such as diabetes mellitus, alcoholism, nephrotic syndrome, chronic renal failure, hypothyroidism, liver disease and administration of *drugs*, for example **β-adrenoceptor antagonists** (Ch. 7), **thiazide diuretics** (Chs 14 and 18), **oestrogens** (Ch. 22) and **isotretinoin** (an isomer of vitamin A given by mouth as well as topically in the treatment of severe acne).

LIPID-LOWERING DRUGS

Several drugs are used to decrease plasma LDL-cholesterol. Drug therapy to lower plasma lipids is only one approach to treatment and is used in addition to dietary management and correction of other modifiable cardiovascular risk factors. The selection of which patients to treat with drugs re-

Lipoprotein metabolism and hyperlipoproteinaemia

- Lipids, such as cholesterol (C) and triglycerides (T), are transported in the plasma as lipoproteins, of which there are four classes:
  - —chylomicrons which transport T and C from the GI tract to the tissues where they are split by lipoprotein lipase and the free fatty acids (FFA) are taken up. Chylomicron remnants are taken up in the liver, where C is stored, oxidised to bile acids, or released into:
  - —very low density lipoproteins (VLDL), which transport C and newly synthesised T to the tissues, where T is removed as before, leaving:
  - —low density lipoproteins (LDL) with a large component of C, some of which is taken up by the tissues and some by the liver, by endocytosis via specific LDL receptors
  - —high density lipoproteins (HDL) which adsorb cholesterol derived from cell breakdown in tissues (including arteries) and transfer it to VLDL and LDL.
- Hyperlipoproteinaemias can be primary, or secondary to some generalised disease (e.g. hypothyroidism). They are classified according to which lipoprotein particle is raised, into six phenotypes (the *Frederickson classification*). This has prognostic and therapeutic implications, but is *not* a diagnostic classification. The greatest risk of ischaemic heart disease occurs in a subset of primary type IIa hyperlipoproteinaemia due to a monogenic defect of LDL receptors called *familial hypercholesterolaemia*.

Table 15.1 Frederickson/WHO classification of hyperlipoproteinaemia

Type	Lipoprotein elevated	Chol	TG	Atherosclerosis risk	Drug treatment
I	Chylomicrons	+	+++	NE	None
IIa	LDL	++	NE	High	HMG-CoA reductase ± resins
IIb	LDL + VLDL	++	++	High	Fibrates, HMG-CoA reductase inhibitor, nicotinic acid
III	βVLDL	++	++	Moderate	Fibrates
IV	VLDL	+	++	Moderate	Fibrates (± fish oil)
V	Chylomicrons + VLDL	+	++	NE	None (± fish oil)

Chol = cholesterol; TG = triglycerides; LDL = low density lipoprotein; VLDL = very low density lipoprotein; βVDL = a qualitatively abnormal form of VLDL identified by its pattern on electrophoresis; + = increased concentration; NE = not elevated

mains controversial and is beyond the scope of this book.

The main classes of drugs used clinically are:

- bile acid binding resins
- fibrates
- HMG-CoA reductase inhibitors
- nicotinic acid.

Other drugs that are sometimes used include **probucol** and **fish oils**. D-thyroxine and neomycin are obsolete.

Bile acid binding resins

Cholestyramine (Fig. 15.2) and **colestipol** are anion exchange resins. They sequester bile acids in the intestine and prevent their reabsorption and enterohepatic recirculation (Fig. 15.1). The result is decreased absorption of exogenous cholesterol and increased metabolism of endogenous cholesterol into bile acids in the liver. This leads to increased expression of LDL receptors on liver cells and increased removal of LDL from the blood. Bile acid sequestrants are therefore mainly of use when high blood cholesterol is due to a raised LDL concentration. They aggravate hypertriglyceridaemia and should therefore not be used alone in patients with type IIb or IV hyperlipoproteinaemia.

Clinical use

Resins are used in the therapy of type IIa hyperlipidaemia (see Table 15.1). The American lipid research clinics' trial of middle-aged men with primary hypercholesterolaemia showed that addition of a resin to dietary treatment caused a mean 13% fall in plasma cholesterol and a 20–25% fall in coronary heart disease over 7 years. Cholestyramine is also effective in relieving pruritus due to accumulation of bile acids in the skin in patients with incomplete biliary obstruction.

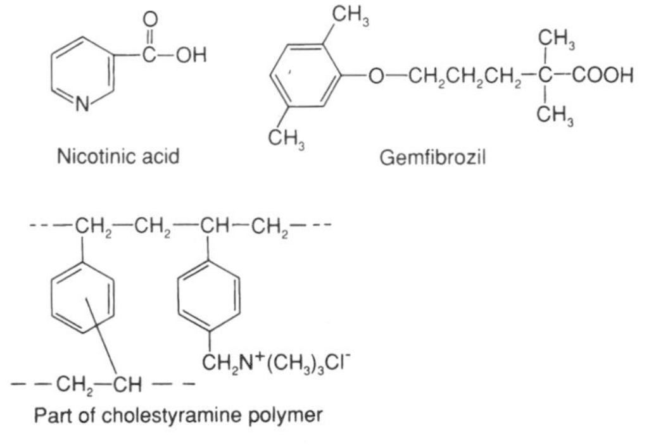

Fig. 15.2 Structures of some lipid-lowering agents.

Unwanted effects

Since resins are not absorbed, systemic toxicity is low, but gastrointestinal symptoms of nausea, abdominal bloating, constipation or diarrhoea are common and dose-related. Resins are bulky and unappetising, although this can be minimised by suspending them in fruit juice. They interfere with the absorption of fat-soluble vitamins, and of drugs such as **chlorothiazide**, **digoxin** and **warfarin**, which should therefore be taken at least 1 hour before or 4–6 hours after the resin.

Fibrates

Several fibric acid derivatives (**'fibrates'**) are used clinically including **bezafibrate, gemfibrozil, fenofibrate** and **clofibrate**. These drugs have a marked effect in lowering VLDL, and hence triglyceride, with a modest (approximately 10%) reduction in LDL and an approximately 10% increase in HDL. They are therefore used in patients with raised triglycerides as well as raised cholesterol (e.g. type IIb, type III) in preference to resins (see above). Particular care should be taken to exclude excessive **alcohol** consumption before starting treatment. Alcoholism commonly causes hypertriglyceridaemia and can cause myositis, an inflammatory disorder of striated muscle which can lead to acute renal failure in severe cases. This is also an adverse effect of fibrates (see below). **Gemfibrozil** reduces coronary heart disease by approximately one-third compared with placebo in middle-aged men with primary hyperlipoproteinaemia. **Clofibrate** predisposes to *gallstones* and its use is therefore limited to patients who have had a cholecystectomy. **Fenofibrate** has a *uricosuric* effect which may be of value in patients in whom hyperuricaemia and gout coexist with hypertriglyceridaemia.

The mechanisms of action of fibrates (see Fig. 15.2) are incompletely understood, but they stimulate lipoprotein lipase, hence increasing hydrolysis of triglyceride in chylomicron and VLDL particles as these traverse capillaries and liberating free fatty acid for storage in fat or metabolism in striated muscle. They also probably reduce hepatic VLDL production and increase hepatic LDL uptake. In addition to these effects on lipoproteins, fibrates also reduce plasma fibrinogen and improve glucose tolerance, although it is unknown if these potentially advantageous effects are clinically important. *Myositis* (see above) is unusual but can be severe. It occurs particularly in patients with renal impairment because of reduced elimination and protein binding, and fibrates should be avoided in such patients. Myositis can also be caused by **HMG-CoA reductase inhibitors** (see below) and the combined use of fibrates with this class of drugs is therefore not routine. Fibrates can cause a variety of mild gastrointestinal symptoms, but in contrast to the resins are generally convenient to take (e.g. a single dose of slow-release **bezafibrate** at bedtime) and well tolerated.

HMG-CoA reductase inhibitors

The rate-limiting enzyme in cholesterol synthesis is HMG-CoA reductase which catalyses the conversion of HMG-CoA to mevalonic acid (MVA) (see Fig. 15.1).* Several fungal metabolites are potent inhibitors of this enzyme (Fig. 15.3). **Mevastatin, lovastatin, simvastatin** and **pravastatin** have been most extensively investigated and are specific, reversible, competitive inhibitors with K_i values of approximately 1 nmol/l. Their affinity is 10 000 times greater than that of the endogenous substrate. The resulting decrease in hepatic cholesterol synthesis leads to *increased synthesis of LDL receptors* and thus *increased clearance of LDL*. In preliminary clinical trials in type IIa hyperlipidaemia, these agents have been shown to lower blood cholesterol by 33% and, when combined with **colestipol**, by 46%. The marked reduction in LDL-cholesterol could greatly reduce the risk of coronary artery disease—perhaps by as much as 50–60% (see Grundy 1988). Large-scale clinical trials to determine the effects of HMG-CoA reductase inhibitors on coronary heart disease and on overall mortality are under. The first to report shows that long-term treatment with Simvastatin substantially improves survival in patients with coronary heart disease. Meanwhile, many clinicians reserve these drugs for severely affected patients such as those with *heterozygous familial hypercholesterolaemia* or with *established atheromatous disease*—for instance following coronary artery bypass surgery—or in those with multiple risk factors for atherosclerosis.

*HMG-CoA = 3-hydroxy-3-methylglutaryl-coenzyme A

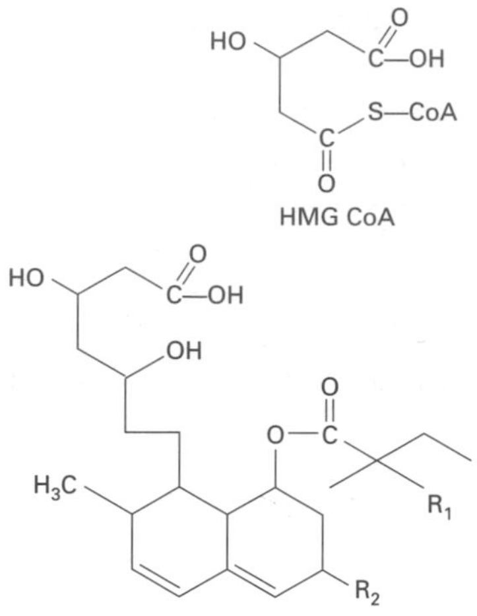

HMG CoA

	R_1	R_2
Simvastatin	CH_3	CH_3
Pravastatin	(H)	OH

(HMG CoA reductase inhibitors)

Fig. 15.3 Structure of HMG-CoA and two inhibitors of HMG-CoA reductase.

Clinical use

HMG-CoA reductase inhibitors are given by mouth. They are well absorbed and extracted by the liver, their site of action, and are subject to extensive presystemic metabolism. **Simvastatin** is an inactive lactone pro-drug which is metabolised in the liver to its active form, the corresponding β-hydroxy fatty acid. HMG-CoA reductase inhibitors are well tolerated: mild and infrequent unwanted effects include gastrointestinal disturbance, insomnia and rash. More serious adverse effects are rare but include severe myositis ('rhabdomyolysis'), hepatitis and angio-oedema. Liver function tests should be monitored and patients warned to stop the drug and report for determination of plasma creatinine kinase activity if they develop muscle aches. In contrast to their usefulness in patients with heterozygous familial hypercholesterolaemia, HMG-CoA reductase inhibitors are completely ineffective in those rare patients with the *homozygous* form of this disease who cannot make LDL receptors.

Nicotinic acid

Nicotinic acid (Fig. 15.2) is a vitamin which has been used in gram quantities as a lipid-lowering agent. **Acipimox** is a derivative of nicotinic acid which is used in lower dose and may have less marked adverse effects, although it is unclear whether the recommended dose is as effective as are standard doses of nicotinic acid. These drugs inhibit hepatic triglyceride production and VLDL secretion (see Fig. 15.1), which leads indirectly to a reduction in LDL. HDL is increased modestly. Other actions that could be advantageous in decreasing the risk of thrombosis are an increase in tissue plasminogen activator (and thus possibly increased thrombolysis) and a decrease in plasma fibrinogen (see Ch. 16).

Clinical use

Nicotinic acid is used in types II and IV hyperlipoproteinaemia. Long-term administration is associated with reduced mortality (Canner et al. 1986), but its clinical use is limited by its *unwanted effects*. These are common and include flushing, palpitations and gastrointestinal disturbances; tolerance to these effects can occur over several weeks. Flushing is associated with production of *prostaglandin* D_2 (Ch. 11) and can be limited by taking the dose half an hour after a dose of **aspirin**. High doses can cause disorders of liver function, impair glucose tolerance and increase the risk of gout.

Probucol

Probucol lowers the concentration in the plasma of both LDL and HDL. Its place in therapy has not been defined—it has distinctive properties that could be either desirable (e.g. anti-oxidant properties) or the reverse (e.g. lowering HDL and prolonging the cardiac action potential). A large clinical trial of its quantitative effects on atheroma in the femoral arteries ('PQRST') has reported recently: there was no significant change in vessel narrowing (see Walldius et al. 1994). Most of the probucol circulating in plasma is associated with LDL. Its mechanism of action is not understood. It is markedly lipophilic, and remains in the body fat for several months. Its peak effect on plasma cholesterol occurs only after 1–3 months' administration. Gastrointestinal disturbances occur in 10% of patients. Probucol should be avoided in patients with a long Q–T interval on the electrocardiogram (see Ch. 13). Drugs that prolong this interval such as **amiodarone, sotalol, astemizole** and **terfenadine** should be avoided if possible in patients who have received probucol within the past few months because of the possibility of precipitating a form of ventricular tachycardia known as 'torsades de pointes' (Ch. 13).

Drugs in hypercholesterolaemia

Drugs can:

- Sequester bile acids in the intestine and thus both reduce the absorption of exogenous cholesterol and increase the metabolism of endogenous cholesterol into bile acids, e.g. cholestyramine, colestipol.
- Inhibit de novo synthesis of cholesterol in the liver, e.g. HMG-CoA reductase inhibitors.
- Alter the relative levels of different lipoproteins: by decreasing VLDL production, by increasing the activity of lipoprotein lipase and enhancing the clearance of LDL by the liver, e.g. fibrates.

Fish oil

ω-3 marine triglycerides reduce plasma triglyceride concentrations but increase cholesterol. A purified preparation of fish oil has been used in patients with severe hypertriglyceridaemia (e.g. types IV and V) to reduce the incidence of pancreatitis. Hypertriglyceridaemia in isolation from hypercholesterolaemia is weakly if at all associated with coronary artery disease, and the use of fish oil in the hope of preventing heart disease is of unproven benefit. (In contrast, there is epidemiological evidence that eating fish regularly *does* reduce ischaemic heart disease.) The mechanism of action of fish oil on plasma triglyceride concentrations is unknown. Fish oil is rich in highly unsaturated fatty acids including *eicosapentaenoic* and *docosahexaenoic* acids and has other potentially important effects including inhibition of platelet function, prolongation of bleeding time, anti-inflammatory effects and reduction of plasma fibrinogen. Eicosapentaenoic acid substitutes for arachidonic acid in cell membranes and gives rise to 3-series prostaglandins and thromboxanes (that is, prostanoids with three double bonds in their side-chains rather than the usual two), and 5-series leukotrienes. This probably accounts for their effects on haemostasis since thromboxane A_3 is much less active as a platelet-aggregating agent than is thromboxane A_2, whereas prostaglandin I_3 is similar in potency as an inhibitor of platelet function to prostaglandin I_2 (prostacyclin). The alteration in leukotriene biosynthesis probably underlies the anti-inflammatory effects of fish oil. Fish oil is contraindicated in patients with type IIa hyperlipoproteinaemia because of the increase in LDL cholesterol that it causes.

REFERENCES AND FURTHER READING

Brett A S 1989 Treating hypercholesterolaemia. N Engl J Med 321: 676–680

Brown M S, Goldstein J L 1986 A receptor-mediated pathway for cholesterol homeostasis. Science 232: 34–47

Canner P L, Berge K G, Wenger J, Stamler J, Friedman L, Prineas R J, Fredewald W 1986 Fifteen year mortality in coronary drug project patients: long-term benefit with niacin. J Am Coll Cardiol 8: 1245–1255

Cleland J G F, Krikler D M 1993 Modification of atherosclerosis by agents that do not lower cholesterol. Br Heart J 69: S54–S62

Cobbe S M, Shepherd J 1993 Cholesterol reduction in the prevention of coronary heart disease: therapeutic rationale and guidelines. Br Heart J 69: S63–S69

Consensus Conference in Lowering Blood Cholesterol to Prevent Heart Disease 1985 JAMA 253: 2080–2086

Davies M J, Woolf N 1993 Atherosclerosis: what is it and why does it occur? Br Heart J 69: S3–S11

Durrington P N 1989 Hyperlipidaemia: diagnosis and management. Wright, London

Editorial 1988 Bile acid sequestrants and hyperlipidaemia. Lancet 1: 220–221

Elliot H 1988 The influence of clinical adrenoreceptor antagonism on plasma lipid profiles. Trends Pharmacol Sci 9: 439–442

European Atherosclerosis Society 1987 Strategies for the prevention of heart disease. Eur Heart J 8: 77–88

Frick H, Elo O, Haapa K et al. 1987 Helsinki heart study: primary prevention trial with gemfibrozil in middle-aged men with dyslipidaemia. N Engl J Med 317: 1237–1245

Goldstein J L, Brown M S 1990 Regulation of the mevalonate pathway. Nature 343: 425–430

Grundy S M 1988 HMG-CoA reductase inhibitors for treatment of hypercholesterolemia. N Engl J Med 319: 24–33

Hajjar K A, Gavish D, Breslow J L, Nachman R 1989 Lipoprotein(a) modulation of endothelial cell surface fibrinolysis and its potential role in atherosclerosis. Nature 339: 303–305

Kane J P, Malloy M J 1990 Treatment of hyperlipidemia. Annu Rev Med 41: 471–482

Lee T-J 1987 Synthesis, SARs and therapeutic potential of HMG-CoA reductase inhibitors. Trends Pharmacol Sci 8: 442–446

Lewis B 1987 Disorders of lipid transport. In: Weatherall D J, Ledingham G G, Warrel D A (eds) Oxford textbook of medicine. Oxford University Press, Oxford, p 9.108–9.123

McLean J W, Tomlinson J E, Kuang W-J et al. 1987 CDNA sequence of human apolipoprotein(a) is homologous to plasminogen. Nature 300: 132–137

Miles L A, Fless G M, Levin E G, Scann A M, Plow E F 1989 A potential basis for the thrombotic risks associated with lipoprotein(a). Nature 339: 301–303

Moncada S, Martin J F, Higgs A 1993 Symposium on regression of atherosclerosis. Eur J Clin Invest 23: 385–398

Reihner E, Rudling M et al. 1990 Influence of pravastatin, a specific inhibitor of HMG-CoA reductase, on hepatic metabolism of cholesterol. N Engl J Med 323: 224–228

Ross R 1993 The pathogenesis of atherosclerosis: a perspective for the 1990s. Nature 362: 801–809

Scandinavian Simvastatin Survival Study Group 1994 Randomised trial of cholesterol lowering in 4444 patients with coronary heart disease: the Scandinavian Simvastatin Survival Study (45). Lancet 344: 1383–1389

Scott J 1989 Lipoprotein receptors: unravelling atherosclerosis. Nature 338: 118–119

Scott J 1989 Thrombogenesis linked to atherogenesis at last? Nature 341: 22–33

Steinberg D, Parthasarathy S, Carew T E, Khoo J C, Witztum J L 1989 Beyond cholesterol: modifications of low-density lipoprotein that increase its atherogenicity. N Engl J Med 320: 915–924

Stringer M D, Gorog P G, Freeman A, Kakkar V V 1989 Lipid peroxides and atherosclerosis. Br Med J 298: 281–284

Walldius G, Erikson U, Olsson A G, Bergstrand L, Hådell K, Johansson J, Kaijser L, Lassvik C, Möldaard J, Nilsson S, Schäefer-Elinder L, Stenport G, Holme I 1994 The effect of probucol on femoral atherosclerosis: the Probucol Quantitative Regression Swedish Trial. Am J Cardiol 74: 875–883

16

HAEMOSTASIS AND THROMBOSIS

Haemostasis is the arrest of blood loss from damaged blood vessels and is essential to life. It involves three main processes:

- adhesion and activation of platelets
- fibrin formation
- vascular contraction.

The first two processes result in the formation of a haemostatic plug which blocks the breach in the vessel and stops the bleeding. The relative importance of each of the processes will depend on the size and the type of vessel (arterial, venous or capillary) which has been injured.

Thrombosis is the unwanted formation of a haemostatic plug or thrombus within the blood vessels or heart. It is a pathological condition usually associated with arterial disease or stasis of blood in the veins or atria of the heart. A *thrombus*, which forms in vivo, should be distinguished from a *blood clot*, which can form in static blood in vitro. A clot is amorphous in character, consisting of a diffuse fibrin meshwork in which all the cells of the blood are trapped. By contrast, a thrombus has a distinct structure:

- a white 'head', firm but friable, consisting mainly of platelets and leucocytes in a fibrin mesh—the leucocytes binding to specific adhesion receptors on the platelets
- a jelly-like red 'tail' which is similar in composition to a blood clot.

An *arterial thrombus*, which is usually associated with *atherosclerosis*, has a large component of platelet–leucocyte–fibrin head. Its main effect is to retard or interrupt blood flow, causing ischaemia or actual death of the tissue beyond (infarction). A *venous thrombus* usually occurs in normal veins in which the blood flow is slowed or in the chambers of the heart when the wall is damaged. It consists of a small head and a large tail which streams away in the direction of the flow. A portion of a thrombus may break away forming an *embolus* which, if it comes from the peripheral veins, may lodge in the lungs or, if it comes from the left heart, may lodge in the brain or other organs. In either case, this blocks the blood vessels, causing damage to the tissues supplied. A general outline of the events involved in arterial thrombosis is given in Figure 16.1.

Haemostasis and thrombosis

- Haemostasis is the arrest of blood loss from damaged vessels and is essential to life. The main phenomena are:
  —platelet adhesion and activation
  —blood coagulation (fibrin formation).
- Thrombosis is an unwanted pathological condition.
  —Venous thrombosis is usually associated with stasis of blood; a venous thrombus has a small platelet component and a large component of fibrin.
  —Arterial thrombosis is usually associated with atherosclerosis, and the thrombus has a large platelet component.
- A portion of a thrombus may break away, travel as an embolus and lodge in another vessel, causing ischaemia and infarction.

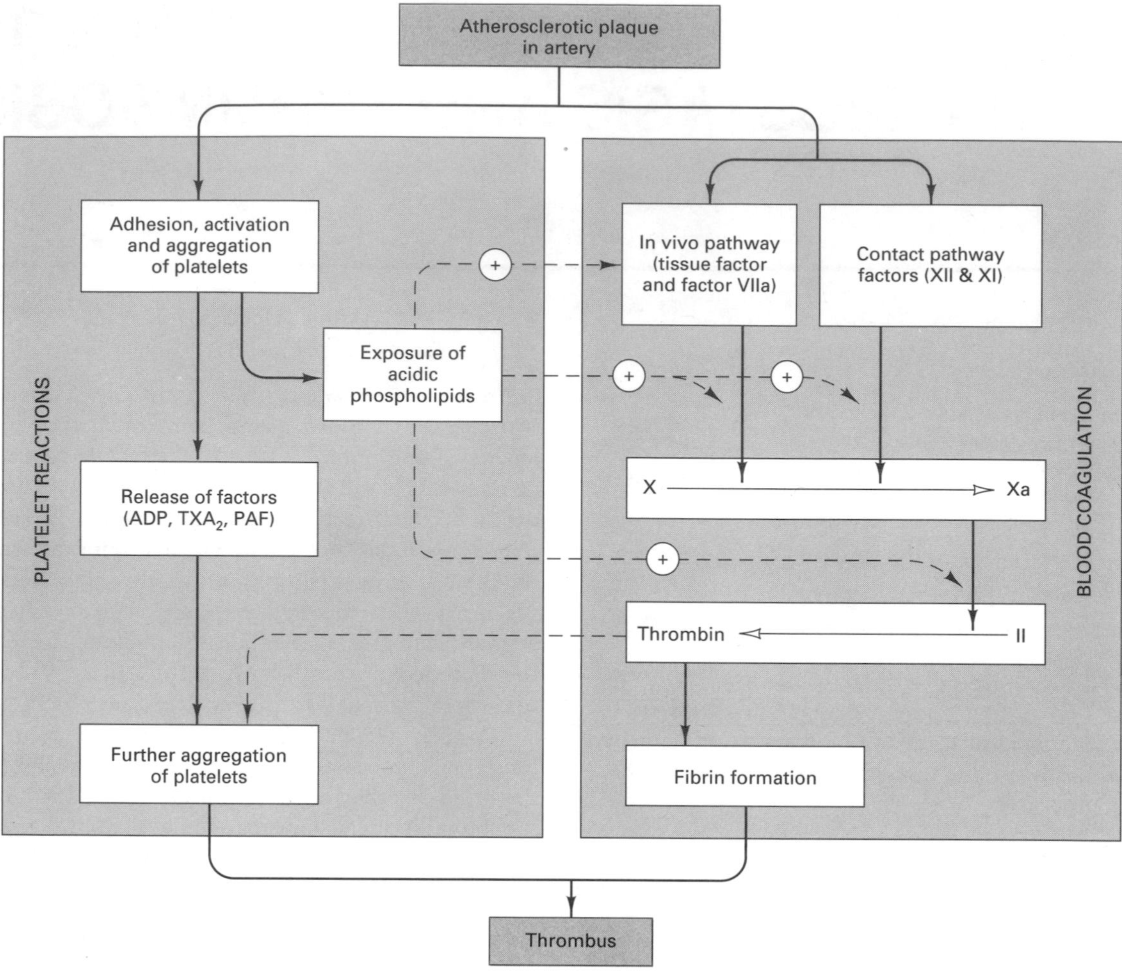

Fig. 16.1 The main events in the formation of an arterial thrombus. (A similar series of events occurs when there is vascular damage, leading to haemostasis.) The exposure of the acidic phospholipids of the platelets also provides the surface on which are localised the interactions of factors IXa and VIIa with factor X, and of factor Xa with factor II, as illustrated in more detail in Figure 16.4. Activation of factor XII also initiates the fibrinolytic pathway, which is shown in Figure 16.10.

Drug therapy to promote haemostasis is rarely necessary, being required only when this essential process is defective (e.g. in haemophilia or following excessive anticoagulant therapy). Drug therapy to modify thromboembolic diseases, on the other hand, is extensively used because these diseases are very common, being the major cause of death in the developed countries. Drugs may affect haemostasis and thrombosis in three distinct ways:

- by modifying blood coagulation (fibrin formation)
- by modifying platelet adhesion and activation
- by affecting the processes involved in fibrin removal (fibrinolysis).

BLOOD COAGULATION

Blood coagulation means the conversion of fluid blood to a solid gel or clot. The main event is the conversion of soluble fibrinogen to insoluble strands of fibrin, although fibrin itself forms only 0.15% of the total blood clot. This conversion is the last step in a complex enzyme cascade. The components (factors) are present as inactive precursors of proteolytic enzymes and cofactors, which are activated by proteolysis. Activation of a small amount of one factor catalyses the formation of larger amounts of the next factor which catalyses the formation of still larger amounts of the next, and so on, giving an amplification which results in an extremely rapid formation of fibrin.

It is usually said that there are two main pathways to fibrin formation, one termed 'intrinsic' (because all the components are present in the blood) and the other 'extrinsic' (because some components come from outside the blood). It is the so-called extrinsic pathway that is especially important in controlling blood coagulation in the body and it can accurately be called the *in vivo* pathway. The intrinsic pathway (better called the contact pathway) is activated when shed blood comes into contact with an artificial surface such as glass. The cascade is outlined in Figure 16.2 and modern ideas on the cascade are reviewed by Furie & Furie (1992).

The *in vivo* (extrinsic) *pathway* is initiated by 'tissue factor', an integral membrane protein which is expressed on the surface of tissue cells and stimulated monocytes and which may occur in atherosclerotic plaques. Tissue factor interacts with factor VIIa in the presence of calcium ions and phospholipid to convert factor X and possibly IX to

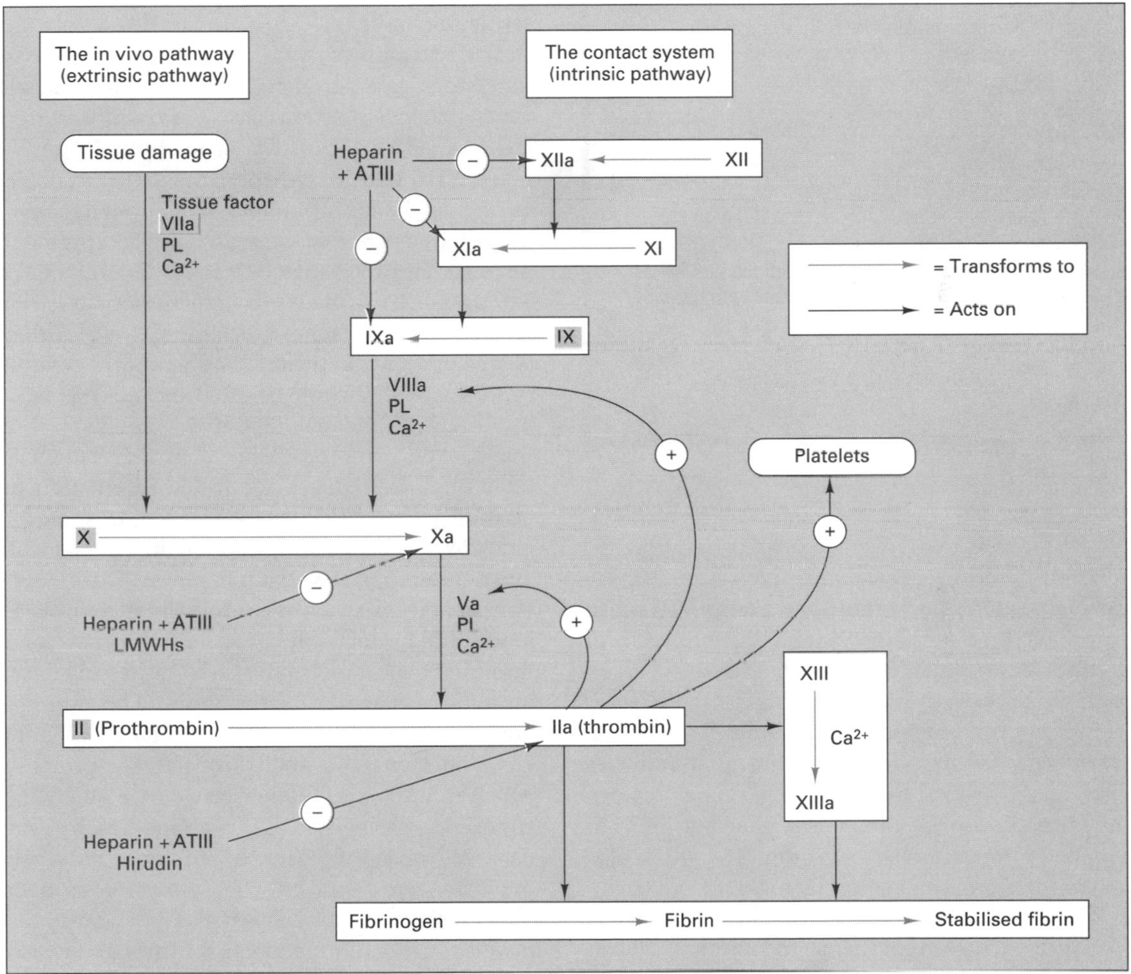

Fig. 16.2 The blood coagulation cascade with the sites of action of the anticoagulant drugs. Tissue factor also activates factor IX. Oral anticoagulants interfere with the essential post-translational γ-carboxylation of factors II, VII, IX and X (shown in light pink boxes). See Figure 16.4 for this latter action. Heparin and other antithrombin agents inactivate the enzymic forms of the coagulation factors. Coagulation of 100 ml of blood requires 0.2 mg of factor VIII, 2 mg of factor X, 15 mg of prothrombin and 250 mg of fibrinogen. (PL = a negatively charged phospholipid (supplied by activated platelets); AT III = antithrombin III; LMWHs = low-molecular-weight heparins)

Blood coagulation (fibrin formation)

The clotting system consists of a cascade of enzymes and cofactors—factors I–XIII.

- Inactive precursors are activated in series, each one giving rise to more of the next.
- The last enzyme, thrombin, derived from prothrombin (II), converts soluble fibrinogen (I) to an insoluble meshwork of fibrin in which blood cells are trapped, forming the clot.
- There are two pathways in the cascade:
  —the extrinsic pathway which operates in vivo
  —the intrinsic or contact pathway which is seen to operate in vitro.
- Both pathways result in activation of factor X, which then converts prothrombin to thrombin.
- Calcium and a negatively charged phospholipid (PL) are essential for three of the final enzyme steps, i.e. for the action of:
  —factor IX on X
  —factor VII on X
  —factor X on II.
- Binding proteins play a part, e.g. factor V in the activation of II by X.
- The negatively charged phospholipid is provided by activated platelets which have adhered to the site of damage; this localises fibrin formation.
- Blood coagulation is controlled by:
  —enzyme inhibitors, e.g. antithrombin III
  —fibrinolysis.

active enzymes which are now termed Xa and IXa. IXa, in the presence of calcium ions, a negatively charged phospholipid surface and factor VIIIa also activates factor X. Factor Xa, in the presence of calcium ions, a platelet-derived negatively charged phospholipid surface and a binding protein, factor V, activates prothrombin to give *thrombin* (IIa) the main enzyme of the cascade. Thrombin removes small fibrinopeptides from the N-terminal regions of the large fibrinogen molecules, enabling them to polymerise to form strands of fibrin. Thrombin also activates the fibrin-stabilising factor, factor XIII, to give XIIIa, a fibrinoligase, which—in the presence of calcium ions—strengthens the fibrin-to-fibrin links. In addition, thrombin acts directly on platelets to cause aggregation, generation of arachidonic acid (see below) and release of other mediators. A further function of thrombin is to activate the coagulation inhibitor, protein C.

The *contact* (intrinsic) *pathway* commences when factor XII, or 'Hageman factor', adheres to a negatively charged surface and, in the presence of high-molecular-weight kininogen and prekallikrein (see Ch. 11), becomes an active enzyme, designated XIIa. Factor XIIa activates factor XI to give XIa and factor XIa activates factor IX to IXa, after which the sequence proceeds as already described. (Patients lacking factor XII, prekallikrein, or high-molecular-weight kininogen have prolonged partial-thromboplastin time but no bleeding problems, so it appears that the proximal parts of this pathway is not crucial for blood coagulation in vivo.)

Factors XIIa, XIa, IXa, Xa, and thrombin are all serine proteases.

The two pathways described are not entirely separate and in addition there are various feedback loops which enhance reaction rates. For example, thrombin (IIa) enhances the activation of both factor V and factor VIII, and Xa enhances the activation of VII.

The acidic phospholipids mentioned above are important as *surface catalysts* and are provided by platelets and by damaged tissue. Circulating platelets do not have this procoagulant activity (which is termed 'platelet factor 3'). However, when they are aggregated and activated, the acidic phospholipids (phosphatidylinositol, phospatidic acid and, more importantly, phosphatidylserine) are expressed on the outside, thus providing a surface which facilitates the localised activation and interaction of the clotting factors. Platelets also provide some of the factor V which is important in binding, localising and accelerating the action of factor Xa.

The normal vascular endothelium actively keeps blood fluid, not only by generating several antithrombotic substances but also by expressing thrombomodulin, a receptor for thrombin. Thrombin, when bound to thrombomodulin, loses its coagulant activity and gains the ability to activate protein C—which inhibits coagulation factors Va and VIIa and stimulates fibrinolysis. Thus a clot which forms on damaged areas will not spread to intact endothelium.

Fibrinogen is not only a principal component in the coagulation pathway—it is a key component in platelet aggregation, and some fibrinogen is actually derived from platelets (see below).

As might be expected, this accelerating enzyme cascade has to be controlled and balanced by a series of inhibitors in the plasma. If it were not, all the blood in the body would solidify within minutes of the initiation of clotting. One of the most important inhibitors is an α_2-globulin, *antithrombin III,* which neutralises not only thrombin, but all the serine proteases in the cascade—Xa, IXa, XIa and XIIa. Another, heparin cofactor II, inhibits only thrombin. The endothelium of blood vessels releases *heparan sulphate* and possibly also *heparin,* both cofactors for antithrombin III (see below). Other inhibitors which play a part are α_2-macroglobulin and α_2-antitrypsin.

If the mechanisms limiting coagulation are faulty or become exhausted, a condition termed *disseminated intravascular coagulation* can occur.

Drugs are used to modify the cascade either when there is a *defect in coagulation* or when there is *unwanted coagulation.*

COAGULATION DEFECTS

Genetically determined deficiencies of clotting factors are rare. Examples are *classical haemophilia* which is due to a lack of factor VIII, and an even rarer form of haemophilia which is due to lack of factor IX (also called Christmas factor). Missing factors can be supplied by giving fresh blood or plasma or preparations of factor VIII or factor IX.

Acquired clotting defects are more common than the hereditary ones, and those most frequently seen are due to liver disease, vitamin K deficiency or the ingestion of oral anticoagulant drugs. Most acquired clotting defects require treatment with vitamin K.

Drugs affecting blood coagulation

Procoagulant drugs: vitamin K

- Reduced vitamin K acts as a cofactor in the post-translational γ-carboxylation of a cluster of glutamic acid (glu) residues in each of factors II, VII, IX and X; vitamin K is oxidised during the reaction. The γ-carboxylated glutamic acid (gla) residues are essential for the interaction of these factors with Ca^{2+} and the negatively charged phospholipid.

Oral anticoagulants, e.g. warfarin

- These act by inhibiting the reduction of vitamin K and thus inhibiting the γ-carboxylation of glu in II, VII, IX and X.
- They act only in vivo and the effect is delayed.
- Many factors modify the action; drug interactions are especially important.
- There is wide variation in patient response; the effect must be monitored by the INR.

Injectable anticoagulants, e.g. heparin, LMWHs

- These agents act by increasing the rate of action of the natural inhibitor AT III, which inactivates Xa and thrombin (and also XIIa, XIa, IXa)
- They act both in vivo and in vitro.
- Anticoagulant action is due to a unique pentasaccharide sequence with high affinity binding to AT III.
- LMWHs have the same effect on Factor X as heparin but less effect on thrombin; they have equivalent anticoagulant effect to heparin but less action on platelet function
- They are given subcutaneously or i.v. and the onset of action is rapid.

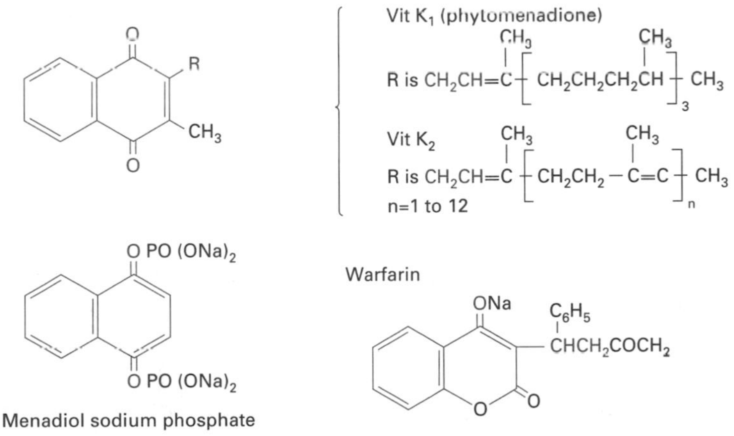

Vit K_1 (phytomenadione)

R is $CH_2CH{=}C(CH_3)[CH_2CH_2CH_2CH(CH_3)]_3CH_3$

Vit K_2

R is $CH_2CH{=}C(CH_3)[CH_2CH_2-C(CH_3){=}C]_nCH_3$

n=1 to 12

Menadiol sodium phosphate

Warfarin

Fig. 16.3 Vitamin K, its congeners and warfarin. Warfarin, a vitamin K antagonist, is used as an oral anticoagulant drug.

VITAMIN K

Vitamin K is so termed because it is the 'Koagulation' vitamin in German. It is a fat-soluble vitamin occurring in nature in two forms—as vitamin K_1 (*phytomenadione*; Fig. 16.3) in plants, and as vitamin K_2 which is synthesised by bacteria in the mammalian gastrointestinal tract. Vitamin K_2 is not a single compound but a series of substances with varying lengths of side-chains (Fig. 16.3).

Vitamin K is critically important in the formation of clotting factors II, VII, IX and X. These factors are all glycoproteins with a number of *γ-carboxy-glutamic acid* (Gla) residues clustered at the N-terminal end of the peptide chain. The γ-carboxylation occurs *after* the synthesis of the chain and the carboxylase requires vitamin K as a cofactor. The role of the vitamin can be made clear by considering the interaction of two of the clotting factors—Xa and prothrombin (factor II)—as shown in Figure 16.4. Factor Xa, on its own, is able to convert prothrombin to thrombin but it does so exceedingly slowly. In the presence of a negatively charged phospholipid surface, calcium ions and the regulatory protein, factor V, the reaction is localised to the phospholipid surface and its rate is increased about 19 000-fold. Both the phospholipid surface and factor V are supplied mainly by platelets. Calcium is necessary for the binding of factors Xa and II to the phospholipid, probably acting mainly by bridging, and this binding does not occur unless the 10 or 11 glutamic acid (glu) residues clustered at the N terminal ends of both factors II and Xa have been carboxylated (Fig. 16.4). Vitamin K in the reduced form is an essential cofactor in the carboxylation of these residues which takes place in liver cells (Fig. 16.5).

Similar considerations apply to the proteolysis of factor X by IXa and by VIIa (see Fig. 16.2).

Note that besides factors II, VII, IX and X, there are several other vitamin-K-dependent Gla-proteins in the body; examples are protein C (see above) and osteocalcin in bone. The effect of the vitamin in prevention of postmenopausal osteoporosis is under investigation.

Administration and pharmacokinetic aspects

Natural vitamin K (phytomenadione) may be given orally or by intramuscular or intravenous injection. If given by mouth, it requires bile salts for absorption and this occurs by a saturable energy-requiring process in the top part of the small intestine. A synthetic preparation, **menadiol sodium phosphate** (Fig. 16.3) is also available. It is water soluble and thus does not require bile salts for its absorption. This synthetic compound takes longer to act than

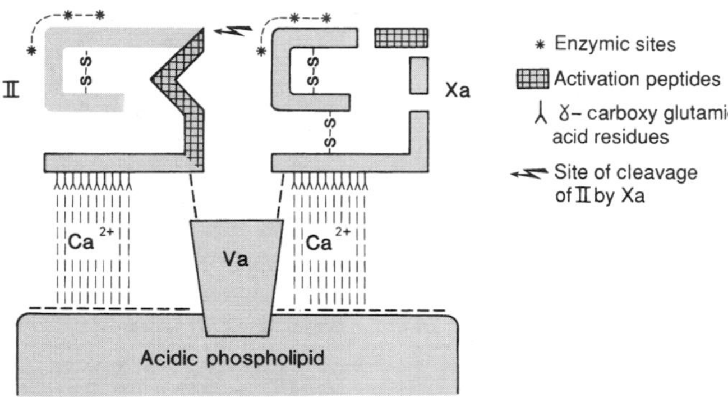

Fig. 16.4 The activation of prothrombin (factor II) by factor Xa. The peptide chains of both factors are very similar and are indicated schematically. The complex of factor Va with a negatively charged phospholipid surface (both partly supplied by aggregated platelets) forms a binding site for factor Xa and prothrombin. Platelets thus serve as a localising focus. Calcium ions are essential for the binding of the factors. When X is activated, with the removal of an activation peptide, it activates prothrombin (again with the removal of an activation peptide) liberating enzymic thrombin (shown in grey). Factor Xa is held at the surface by intrachain sulphydryl bonds, but thrombin is released. Factor V has to be converted from a non-functional to a functional binding protein (Va)—possibly by thrombin, which is thus autocatalytic. (Modified from: Jackson C M 1978 Br J Haematol 39: 1)

Clinical use of vitamin K

The treatment and/or prevention of:
- bleeding due to the oral anticoagulant drugs
- haemorrhagic disease of the newborn
- vitamin K deficiencies:
  —sprue, coeliac disease, steatorrhoea
  —lack of bile (e.g. with obstructive jaundice).

phytomenadione. There is very little storage of vitamin K in the body. It is metabolised to more polar substances which are excreted in the urine and the bile.

The clinical uses of vitamin K are summarised above.

UNWANTED COAGULATION

Unwanted coagulation occurs mainly in thrombo-embolic diseases, which are very common. (See Nachman 1992 for review of thrombogenesis and atherogenesis.) The drugs used to modify unwanted coagulation are:

- oral anticoagulants (**warfarin** and related compounds)
- injectable anticoagulants (**heparin** and newer thrombin inhibitors).

ORAL ANTICOAGULANTS

Oral anticoagulant drugs became available as an indirect result of a change in agricultural policy in North America in the 1920s. Sweet clover was substituted for corn in cattle-feed, and soon afterwards an excessive tendency to bleed after minor injury was noticed in animals so fed. This turned out to be due to the presence of *bishydroxycoumarin* in spoiled sweet clover. Congeners of this and related compounds have been developed for use in clinical medicine; all are derivatives of either coumarin or indandione. **Warfarin** (Fig. 16.3) is the most important of these; other oral anticoagulants—**nicoumalone, phenindione**—are now rarely used.

Mechanism of action

Oral anticoagulants interfere with the post-translational γ-carboxylation of glutamic acid residues in clotting factors II, VII, IX and X (see Fig. 16.5). They do this by *preventing the reduction of vitamin K* which is necessary for its action as a cofactor of the carboxylase. They will therefore act only in vivo and will not, of course, have any effect on the clotting of shed blood. Their structural similarity to vitamin K and its analogues is illustrated in Figure 16.3.

The effect of these drugs on fibrin formation takes several days to develop because of the time taken for degradation of factors already carboxylated. The onset of action of these drugs will thus depend primarily on the half-lives of the relevant factors. Factor VII, with a half-life of 6 hours, is affected first (though this does not necessarily influence coagulation very substantially), then IX, X and II with half-lives of 24, 40 and 60 hours respectively.

Administration and pharmacokinetic aspects

Warfarin is given orally and is absorbed quickly and totally from the gastrointestinal tract. It has a very small distribution volume, being strongly bound to plasma albumin (see Ch. 4). The peak concentration in the blood occurs within an hour of ingestion, but because of the mechanism of action this does not coincide with the peak pharmacological effect, which occurs about 48 hours later. The effect does not start for 12–16 hours, and lasts 4–5 days. The drugs are metabolised by the mixed function oxidases in the liver and the half-life of warfarin is about 40 hours.

Oral anticoagulants cross the placenta and they also appear in the milk during lactation. This could be important because the newborn infant is already at risk as a result of inadequate synthesis of vitamin K in the bowel.

The therapeutic use of the oral anticoagulants, particularly if long-continued, requires a careful balance between giving too little, which could leave unwanted coagulation unmodified, and giving too much, which could lead to haemorrhage. Therapy is complicated not only because the effect of a particular dose is only seen 2 days after giving it, but also because there are numerous conditions which modify the drugs' activity (see below), including a number of interactions with other drugs (see Ch. 42).

The action of an oral anticoagulant should be monitored by its effect on the *prothrombin time*, which is the time taken for clotting of citrated plasma

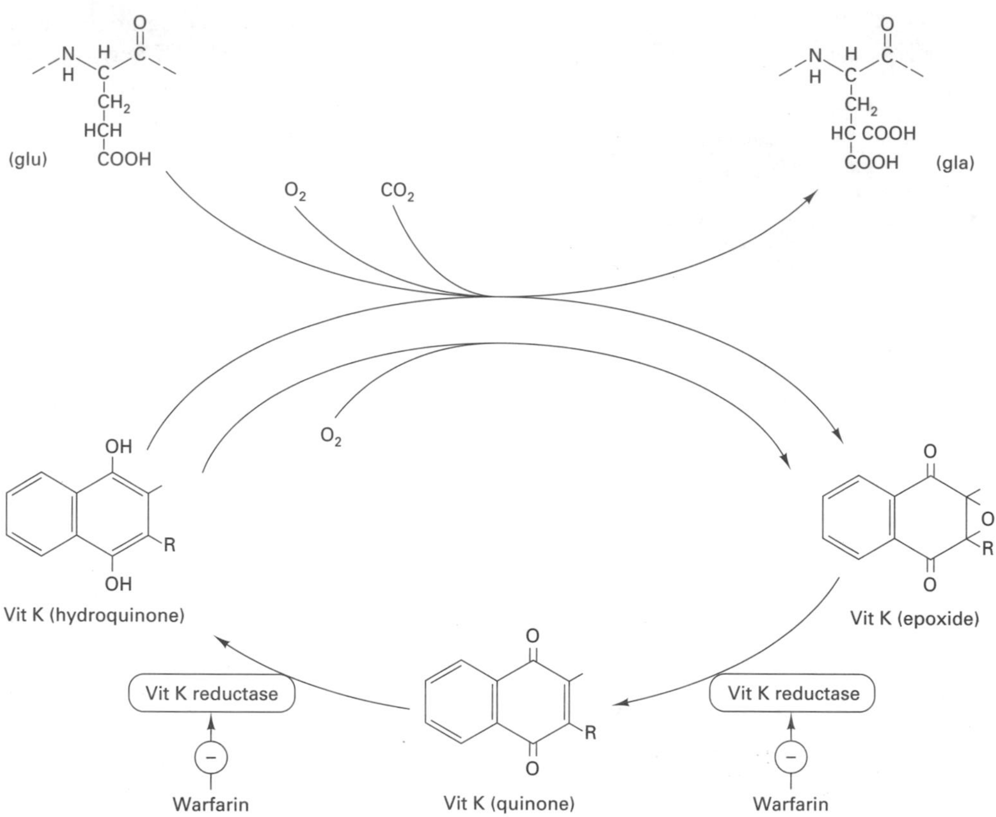

Fig. 16.5 The probable mechanism of action of vitamin K and the site of action of oral anticoagulants. After the peptide chains in clotting factors II, VII, IX and X have been synthesised, reduced vitamin K (the hydroquinone) acts as a cofactor in the conversion of glutamic acid (glu) to γ-carboxyglutamic acid (gla). During this reaction, the reduced form of vitamin K is converted to the epoxide, which in turn is reduced to the quinone and then the hydroquinone.

after the addition of calcium and standardised reference thromboplastin. The results are reported as the International Normalised Ratio (INR)—the ratio of the patient's prothrombin time to that of a control. Dosage is usually adjusted to give an INR of 2–4.

Factors increasing the pharmacological effect of the oral anticoagulants

(Note that these factors will increase the already present risk of haemorrhage.)

A decreased availability of vitamin K will obviously exacerbate the action of these drugs. Broad-spectrum antibiotics and some sulphonamides (see Ch. 37) depress the intestinal flora which normally synthesises vitamin K_2, but this does not have much effect unless there is a concurrent dietary deficiency of the vitamin.

Liver disease interferes with the synthesis of the clotting factors, and conditions in which there is a high metabolic rate, such as fever and thyrotoxicosis, increase the effect of the drugs by increasing the rate of degradation of the clotting factors.

Many drugs interact with the oral anticoagulants and increase their effect. These include:

- *Agents which inhibit the microsomal enzymes* in the liver and retard the metabolism of the oral anticoagulants. Examples include **cimetidine, salicylates, imipramine, co-trimoxazole, chloramphenicol, ciprofloxacin, metronidazole, amiodarone** and many antifungal **azoles**.
- *Agents which impair platelet aggregation and platelet function*: the **non-steroidal anti-inflammatory drugs, ticlopidine, moxalactam, carbenicillin. Aspirin** in particular can cause serious bleeding if given during warfarin therapy.

- *Agents which displace the oral anticoagulants from their binding sites* on plasma albumin result in a transient increase in their free concentration in the plasma: some **non-steroidal anti-inflammatory drugs, chloral hydrate**.
- *Agents which inhibit reduction of vitamin K*, for example **cephalosporins**.

In addition, various agents may potentiate the action of the anticoagulants by as yet unknown means.

Factors decreasing the pharmacological effect of the oral anticoagulants

There is a decreased response to these drugs during pregnancy and in some pathological conditions such as the nephrotic syndrome and anaemia.

Some drugs cause induction of the microsomal enzymes in the liver and therefore increase the degradation of warfarin (e.g. **rifampicin, carbamazepine, barbiturates, griseofulvin**). Other drugs which reduce the effect of the oral anticoagulants are **cholestyramine** (by reducing absorption), **oral contraceptives, penicillins**.

For more detail on drug interactions with warfarin see 'Guidelines on oral anticoagulation' (British Society of Haematology Committee for Standards in Haematology 1990) and Hirsh (1991b).

Unwanted effects

Haemorrhage (especially into the bowel or the brain) is the main hazard. Depending on the urgency of the situation, treatment may consist of withholding warfarin, administration of vitamin K or fresh plasma or coagulation factor concentrates. Oral anticoagulants can be teratogenic and can cause liver damage though these effects are infrequent. Necrosis of soft tissues (breast, buttock), which occurs rarely, has been attributed to inhibition of biosynthesis of endogenous vitamin-K-dependent anticoagulant substances (e.g. protein C).

The clinical use of oral anticoagulants is summarised on page 348.

INJECTABLE ANTICOAGULANTS

HEPARIN AND LOW-MOLECULAR-WEIGHT HEPARINS

Heparin was discovered in 1916 by a second-year medical student at Johns Hopkins University. During a vacation project in which he was attempting to extract thromboplastic (i.e. coagulant) substances from various tissues, he found instead, powerful anticoagulant activity. Further work made it clear that this was due to the presence of a glycosaminoglycan which was named **heparin** because it was believed to be most abundant in liver.

Strictly speaking, 'heparin' is not a single substance but a family of sulphated glycosaminoglycans (mucopolysaccharides) with a range of molecular weights from 3000 to 40 000. There is great variability among heparin molecules.

In the tissues, heparin is found in mast cells (in the form of large polymers of MW 750 000). It is also present in the plasma and in the endothelial cell layer of blood vessels. For clinical use, it is extracted from beef lung or hog intestinal mucosa, and since different preparations may differ in potency it has to be biologically assayed against an agreed international standard.

A related glycosaminoglycan, *heparan sulphate*, occurs extracellularly in many tissues, for example on the endothelium of blood vessels. This substance is, like heparin, a cofactor for antithrombin III (see below) and is physiologically important as an anticoagulant, particularly in the microcirculation. It is not used clinically.

Fragments of heparin with slightly different anticoagulant activity from the parent molecule, are now also available. The molecular weights vary from 4000 to 15 000. These preparations are referred to as **low-molecular-weight heparins** (LMWHs) to distinguish them from standard heparin.

Mechanism of action

Heparin inhibits blood clotting both in vivo and in vitro. Its main action is on *fibrin formation* but it also modifies platelet aggregation. The anticoagulant action is produced through an effect on antithrombin III. This is the naturally occurring inhibitor of the serine proteases in the coagulation cascade, acting more particularly on thrombin and factor Xa but also on factors IXa, XIa, and XIIa. Antithrombin III inhibits the action of thrombin by binding to the active serine site on the enzyme. Heparin modifies this interaction by binding to antithrombin III, changing its conformation and accelerating its rate of action so that its effect is virtually instantaneous. The binding to antithrombin III involves a unique pentasaccharide sequence (Fig. 16.6), and entails interaction between specific amino acids on anti-

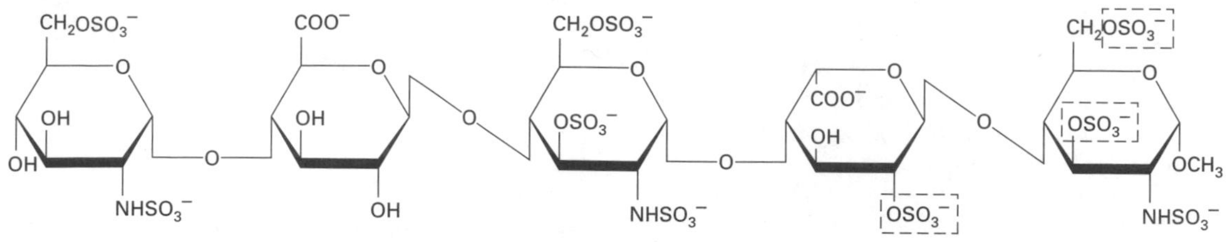

Heparin Pentasaccharide

Fig. 16.6 The pentasaccharide sequence in heparin which is the binding site for antithrombin III. The groups in solid pink boxes are critical for high affinity binding; the groups in dotted boxes increase AT III binding but are not essential for it.

thrombin III and sulphate and carboxylate groups in heparin. The distribution of the pentasaccharide sequence is random along the heparin chain.

Thrombin is considerably more sensitive to the inhibitory effect of the heparin–antithrombin III complex than factor X. To inhibit thrombin, it is necessary for heparin to bind to the enzyme as well as to antithrombin III; to inhibit factor X it is only necessary for heparin to bind to antithrombin III (see Fig. 16.7). The interaction with heparin renders the enzyme and antithrombin III inactive, but heparin is released from the complex to act on other antithrombin III molecules. With long-continued heparin therapy, there is a depletion of antithrombin III and this decreases the effect of subsequent heparin therapy.

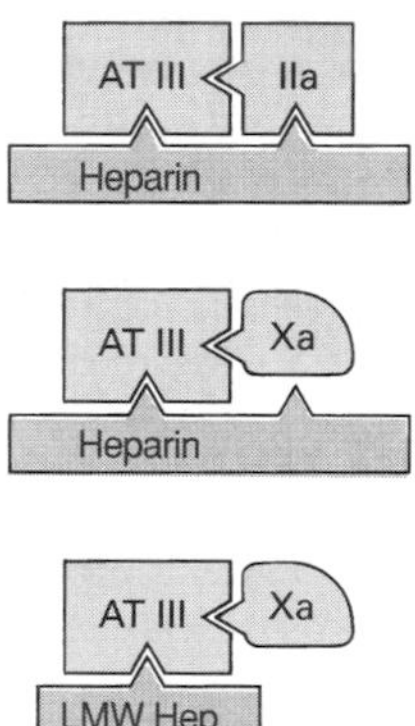

Fig. 16.7 Schematic diagram of the interaction of heparin, antithrombin III (AT III) and clotting factors. To increase the rate of inactivation of thrombin (IIa) by AT III, heparin needs to interact with both substances, but to speed up its effect on factor Xa it needs only interact with AT III. The small, low-molecular-weight heparins (LMW Hep) can increase action of AT III on factor Xa, but cannot increase the action of AT III on thrombin because they cannot bind both simultaneously. (Modified from: Hirsh & Levine 1992)

The anticoagulant action of heparin can be modified by platelets, fibrin and plasma proteins. Not only do platelets release a heparin-neutralising protein, platelet factor 4, but factor Xa, which is generated on the platelet surface (Fig. 16.4), is protected from the action of the heparin–antithrombin III complex. Thrombin when bound to fibrin is likewise protected from the action of the complex. The binding of heparin to plasma proteins (see below) decreases its bioavailability.

Low-molecular-weight heparins contain a lower proportion of the critical pentasaccharide sequence than the parent molecule. They increase the action of antithrombin III on factor Xa but not its action on thrombin, since this latter effect necessitates their binding to both enzyme and inhibitor and the molecules are in essence too small to do this (Fig. 16.7). The LMWHs exhibit less binding to plasma proteins and therefore greater bioavailability than standard heparin and furthermore are not neutralised by platelet factor 4. There is evidence that they are at least as safe and effective as unfractionated heparin. Indeed a recent meta-analysis suggested that they are more effective than regular heparin in preventing deep vein thrombosis and pulmonary embolism after orthopaedic surgery but have a similar incidence of bleeding.

Administration and pharmacokinetic aspects

Heparin is not absorbed from the gastrointestinal tract because of its charge and its large size, and it is therefore given intravenously or subcutaneously. Intramuscular injections are avoided because they result in haematoma formation. Heparin binds to a number of plasma proteins and this decreases its bioavailability. After intravenous injection there is a phase of rapid elimination followed by a more gradual disappearance thought to be due both to rapid saturable processes (involving binding to receptors on endothelial cells and macrophages) and slower first-order processes involving partly renal excretion. As a result, once the dose exceeds the saturating concentration, a greater proportion is dealt with by these slower processes and the apparent half-life increases with increasing dose. When given intravenously, the onset of action of heparin is immediate, but when given subcutaneously the onset can be delayed by up to 60 minutes. The half-life in the plasma is 40–90 minutes.

LMWHs are given subcutaneously. They have much lower affinity for heparin-binding proteins and thus have a longer half-life that is independent of dose, so the effects are more predictable and the dosing less frequent. They are excreted mainly by the kidney.

The effects of heparin can be monitored by testing the kaolin–cephalin clotting time (KCCT)* which should be increased by a factor of 1.5 to 2.5. The measurement of the ratio of the patient's activated partial-thromboplastin time (APTT) to the mean control APTT is also used. LMWHs do not prolong KCCT/APTT. An international LMWH reference preparation for monitoring the effect of LMWHs has now been established.

The clinical use of heparin and the LMWHs is summarised on page 348.

Unwanted effects

The main hazard is haemorrhage which is treated by stopping therapy and, if necessary, giving a heparin antagonist, **protamine sulphate**. This substance, a strongly basic protein which forms an inactive complex with heparin, is given intravenously as a 1% solution.

A toxic effect of heparin, reported with long-term treatment of 6 months or more, is osteoporosis with resultant spontaneous fractures. The reason for this is not known.

Hypersensitivity reactions to heparin can occur in some patients and have also been reported to occur with protamine. A transitory decrease in platelet numbers caused by heparin-induced platelet aggregation occurs within 24–36 hours in about 30% of patients and is not clinically important. A more serious thrombocytopenia occurring 2–14 days after the start of therapy is rarer. There is some evidence that LMWHs are an acceptable alternative if heparin has caused thrombocytopenia and further anticoagulation is needed.

*The KCCT is the clotting time of plasma in the presence of cephalin (a phospholipid) and kaolin, which activates the intrinsic system.

NEWER ANTITHROMBIN AGENTS

A heparinoid drug which is under investigation is **dermatan sulphate**. This acts by increasing the action of heparin cofactor II, which inhibits only thrombin; it is said to cause less bleeding than heparin.

Antithrombin-III-independent anticoagulants

Several antithrombin-III-independent inhibitors of thrombin have also recently become available, for example hirudin, hirugen, argatroban and the peptide chloromethyl ketone inhibitor, PPACK.

Hirudin, the anticoagulant substance from the medicinal leech, and the most potent known naturally occurring inhibitor of thrombin, has now been synthesised by recombinant DNA techniques and is available for clinical use. It binds to both the active catalytic site and the fibrinogen recognition site on thrombin (reviewed by Markwardt 1991). It has proved to be very effective at inhibiting experimentally produced arterial and venous thrombosis in rats. Unlike heparin, it causes little or no bleeding at clinically effective antithrombotic doses.

Given intravenously, its elimination follows first-order kinetics and its half-life is 1–2 hours. It is excreted unaltered, mainly through the kidney. After subcutaneous administration the peak plasma concentration occurs after 2–3 hours. It is a weak immunogen and the risk of allergic reactions appears to be low.

Hirugen, a synthetic dodecapeptide derived from hirudin, binds directly to thrombin and blocks access to substrates.

Argatroban is a weak competitive inhibitor of thrombin with a half-life of only a few minutes.

PPACK alkylates the active site in thrombin, inhibiting it irreversibly.

The latter three compounds can reach and inactivate thrombin which is bound to fibrin.

These newer antithrombin agents are reviewed by Weitz & Hirsh (1992) and Salzman (1992).

Ancrod

Ancrod, given intravenously, acts directly on fibrinogen to produce an unstable form of fibrin which is cleared from the blood, resulting in a depletion of fibrinogen. Ancrod has been employed for the same conditions as heparin but is not commonly used.

PLATELET ADHESION AND ACTIVATION

Platelets (or thrombocytes), though non-nucleated and, thus, strictly speaking, not entitled to be classified as cells, are capable of a complex variety of reactions which are essential for haemostasis, important for the healing of damaged blood vessels and play an as yet ill-understood part in inflammation (see Ch. 11). A low platelet count results in *thrombocytopenic purpura* in which there may be spontaneous bleeding into the skin and other tissues. In this condition the bleeding time is increased but the blood clotting time in vitro is normal.*

Platelets have an important role in arterial thromboembolism and in the response of blood vessels to injury. An important aspect of normal platelet function and of their contribution to thrombus formation is the interaction of platelets with vascular endothelium.

In a normal undamaged vessel, the endothelium plays an active part in prevention of thrombus formation. It generates and releases not only prostacyclin (see Fig. 11.8) and nitric oxide (see p. 233), both of which inhibit platelet aggregation, but also plasminogen activator (see below) and the anticoagulant substances, heparin and heparan sulphate (see p. 339). In addition, as explained above, it expresses *thrombomodulin*, a receptor/cofactor involved in the activation of the coagulation inhibitor, protein C (p. 334).

When an atherosclerotic plaque (see p. 323) is ruptured or a vessel is cut or injured, the endothelium is damaged and platelets adhere to components of the subendothelium (e.g. collagen) and become activated. Adhesion involves linking of subendothelial components to glycoprotein IIb-receptors on the platelet membrane (see below) by von Willebrand factor.** Activation involves *shape change*, which entails flattening and extension of pseudopodia; in this way, platelets can cover a small lesion in the endothelium like a sticking plaster. Shape change is followed by the *release* of several biologically active substances, some from storage granules, some synthesised de novo. Those released include ADP, fibrinogen and 5-hydroxytryptamine; those newly synthesised include platelet-activating factor and thromboxane (TX) A_2 (see Ch. 11). TXA_2 is produced in platelets from the cyclic endoperoxide, PGH_2, by thromboxane synthetase (see Fig. 11.8), the cyclic endoperoxides being produced by the action of cyclo-oxygenase on arachidonic acid (Fig. 11.8).

GPIIb/IIIa-receptors, critical for aggregation, become expressed on the platelet surface.*** Several of the substances released, in particular ADP and thromboxane A_2 (TXA_2), but also 5-hydroxytryptamine and platelet-activating factor, are potent aggregating agents, stimulating other platelets to stick to those already adhering. *Aggregation* involves links formed by fibrinogen binding to the GPIIb/IIIa-receptors on adjacent platelets. In areas of high shear the multivalent von Willebrand's factor has a similar action.

Other substances released from the platelets are factors which increase vascular permeability, factors chemotactic for white blood cells and platelet-derived growth factors which are important in repair processes but have also been implicated in atherogenesis. Platelets also release the heparin inhibitor (platelet factor 4) mentioned above. In platelets, in contrast to many other cell types, an increase in cAMP is inhibitory (see Ch. 2); thus agents which increase cAMP can inhibit some of these platelet functions.

The mass of aggregated platelets forms a plug which, together with vessel constriction, maintains haemostasis in small vessels until the platelet plug is reinforced by fibrin (see Fig. 16.1). Fibrin formation is associated with the negatively charged phospholipids which become available on the surface of activated platelets. The phospholipids act as part of the binding site for interacting coagulation factors, facilitating the localised formation of thrombin and thus fibrin (see Fig. 16.4). Thrombin has a power-

*The 'bleeding time', which is normally about 4 minutes, is measured by timing the duration of bleeding from a standard small puncture wound in the skin, the blood being blotted up every 15 seconds.

**Von Willebrand's factor is a large glycoprotein of 10^6 daltons (which is missing in von Willebrand's disease, a hereditary haemorrhagic disorder). It is synthesised by vascular endothelial cells and is also present in platelets.

***Various platelet membrane glycoproteins are receptors or binding sites for adhesive proteins.

ful action in activating and aggregating platelets. It increases the release reaction and consolidates the platelet plug, rendering the aggregation irreversible. It can be seen that many of the responses of the platelet are autocatalytic.

All these actions of the platelet are essential in haemostasis, but may be inappropriately triggered if there is pathological change in a blood vessel, such as atherosclerosis resulting in thrombosis (Figs 16.1 and 16.10). Some aspects of the role of platelets in thrombosis are discussed in Chapter 15.

ANTIPLATELET AGENTS

Platelet activation and aggregation play a critical role in thromboembolic disease and effective anti-platelet drugs are potentially of immense therapeutic

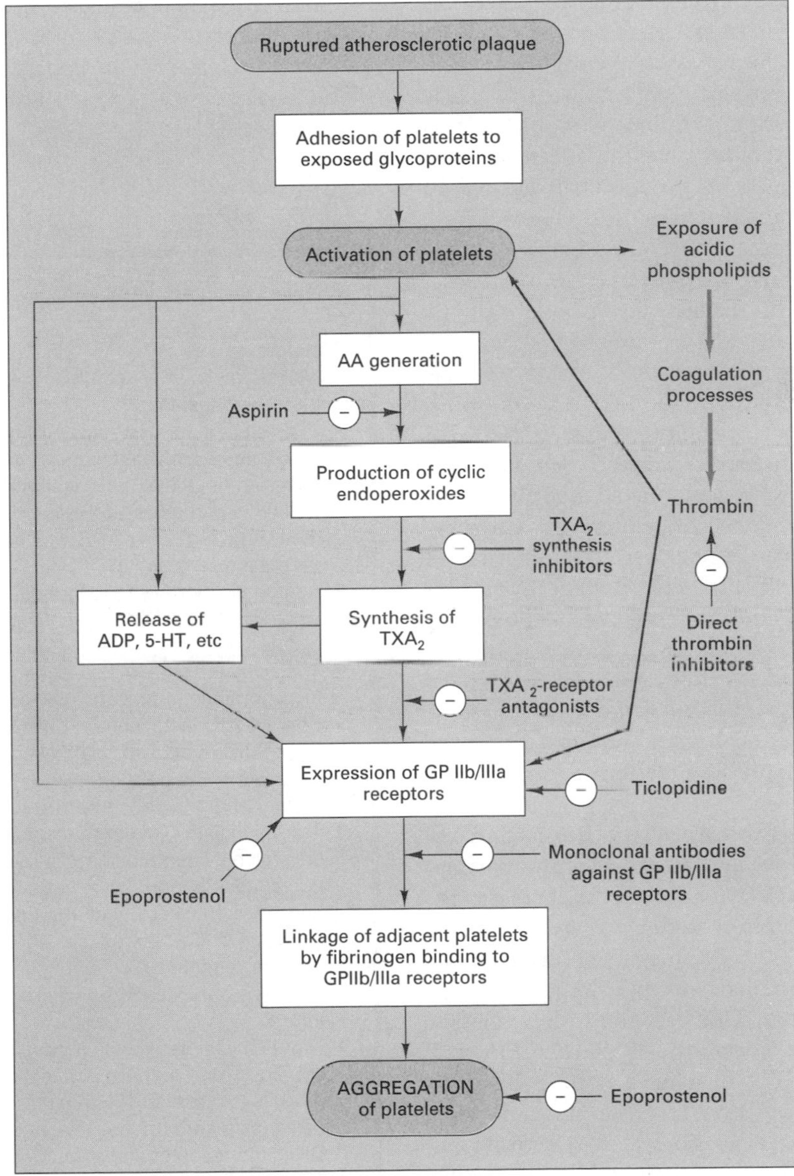

Fig. 16.8 The events involved in atherosclerotic plaque-induced activation and aggregation of platelets, with the sites of action of drugs shown. (AA = arachidonate; TXA_2 = thromboxane A_2; ADP = adenosine diphosphate)

value. Recently, advances in this area, particularly clinical trials of aspirin, have radically altered clinical practice. An outline of the main events in platelet aggregation is given in Figure 16.8—with the sites of action of antiplatelet drugs shown.

Aspirin (see Ch. 12) alters the balance between TXA_2 which promotes aggregation and prostacyclin (PGI_2) which inhibits it. Aspirin inactivates cyclo-oxygenase—acting mainly on the constitutive enzyme, COX-1 (see Vane 1994)—by irreversibly acetylating its active enzymic site. This reduces both TXA_2 synthesis in platelets and prostacyclin synthesis in endothelium. Vascular endothelial cells, however, can synthesise new enzyme whereas platelets cannot. After administration of aspirin, TXA_2 synthesis does not recover until the affected cohort of platelets is replaced—a process that takes 7–10 days. Furthermore, inhibition of the cyclo-oxygenase of the vascular endothelium requires higher concentrations of aspirin than does platelet cyclo-oxygenase. Thus low doses of aspirin given intermittently decrease the synthesis of thromboxane A_2 without drastically reducing prostacyclin synthesis, as has been shown to be the case with 3.5 mg/kg of aspirin given every 3 days to healthy volunteers. Clinical trials have now demonstrated the efficacy of aspirin in treatment regimes for acute myocardial infarction, in reducing the incidence of reinfarction following recovery and in preventing occlusive vascular disease in individuals at particular risk. Regimes for treatment of acute infarction involve fibrinolytic agents as well (see Fig. 16.9 and below).

The clinical use of aspirin is summarised on page 348.

The value of concomitant administration of **dipyridamole**—a phosphodiesterase inhibitor—remains uncertain.

TXA_2-synthesis inhibitors (e.g. **dazoxiben**, an analogue of imidazole) and **TXA_2-receptor antagonists** (e.g. **GR32191**) have been investigated. TXA_2-synthesis inhibitors actually increase prostacyclin synthesis as a consequence of diversion of endoperoxide intermediates from TXA_2 synthesis to prostacyclin synthesis. However, both these classes of drugs are weak inhibitors of platelet function in vitro. Compounds which have both TXA_2 synthetase inhibition as well as TXA_2-receptor blocking activity offer a better possibility of selectively inhibiting thromboxane synthesis while increasing prostacyclin synthesis, and drugs with this combination of activities (e.g. **ridogrel**) are in development. However, the fact that thromboxane A_2 is not the only platelet-aggregating agent might limit the therapeutic value of such drugs.

Prostacyclin is a potent inhibitor of platelet aggregation and is also able to disaggregate platelet clumps. It inhibits the transduction mechanisms for expression of the GPIIb/IIIa-receptor. It is now available, as **epoprostenol**, for clinical use but, because of its very short half-life and the need for parenteral administration, its place in therapy may be limited to such applications as cardiac bypass surgery and similar procedures and as a vasodilator and antiplatelet agent in patients in intensive care. Stable analogues of prostacyclin could extend these applications.

Platelets and antiplatelet drugs

Platelets

- Normal vascular endothelium prevents platelet adhesion.
- Platelets adhere to diseased or damaged areas and become activated, i.e. they change shape, exposing negatively charged phospholipids and GPIIb/IIIa receptors, and release various mediators, e.g TXA_2, ADP, which stimulate other platelets to aggregate.
- Aggregation entails links formed by fibrinogen binding to the GPIIb/IIIa receptors on adjacent platelets.
- The activated platelets constitute the localising focus for fibrin formation.
- Chemotactic factors and growth factors necessary for repair, but also implicated in atherogenesis, are released.

Antiplatelet drugs, e.g. aspirin

- Aspirin inhibits cyclo-oxygenase irreversibly. The balance between prostacyclin (an inhibitor of aggregation generated by vascular endothelium) and TXA_2 (a stimulant of aggregation generated by platelets) is thus altered, since the endothelium can synthesise more enzyme but platelets cannot. TXA_2 synthesis only recovers when new platelets are formed.
- Other antiplatelet agents available are: epoprostenol (synthetic prostacyclin), ticlopidine (inhibits expression of GPIIb/IIIA receptors). Drugs being tested are: monoclonal antibodies against the GPIIb/IIIa receptor and agents which either inhibit TXA_2 synthetase or block TXA_2 receptors or have both actions.

Ticlopidine inhibits the expression of the GPIIb/IIIa-receptor and its transformation into its high affinity, ligand-binding state (Fig. 16.9). Its action is slow in onset, taking 3–7 days to reach maximal effect. Its efficacy in reducing incidence of stroke is similar to that of aspirin but unwanted effects of diarrhoea, rashes, and especially leucopenia have limited its use.

Fab fragments of monoclonal antibodies against the GPIIb/IIa-receptor are being tested. They are potent inhibitors of platelet function (Fig. 16.8). In animal studies they have prevented platelet thrombus formation, decreased both the dose and the time required to achieve thrombolysis with relevant thrombolytic agents, abolished re-occlusion and decreased infarct size. In initial studies in man they have produced profound inhibition of platelet function without excessive haemorrhage, though some patients have developed reversible thrombocytopenia. Clinical trials have shown that they reduce the risk of restenosis after angioplasty, but at the expense of an increased risk of bleeding. Immunogenicity may limit the possibility of giving the agents repeatedly.

Because thrombin is a powerful stimulant of platelet activation and aggregation, drugs that inhibit its action could be regarded as antiplatelet agents and are therefore included in Figure 16.8.

FIBRINOLYSIS (THROMBOLYSIS)

When the intrinsic coagulation system is activated, the fibrinolytic or clot-dissolving system is also set in motion. This involves the action of *plasminogen*

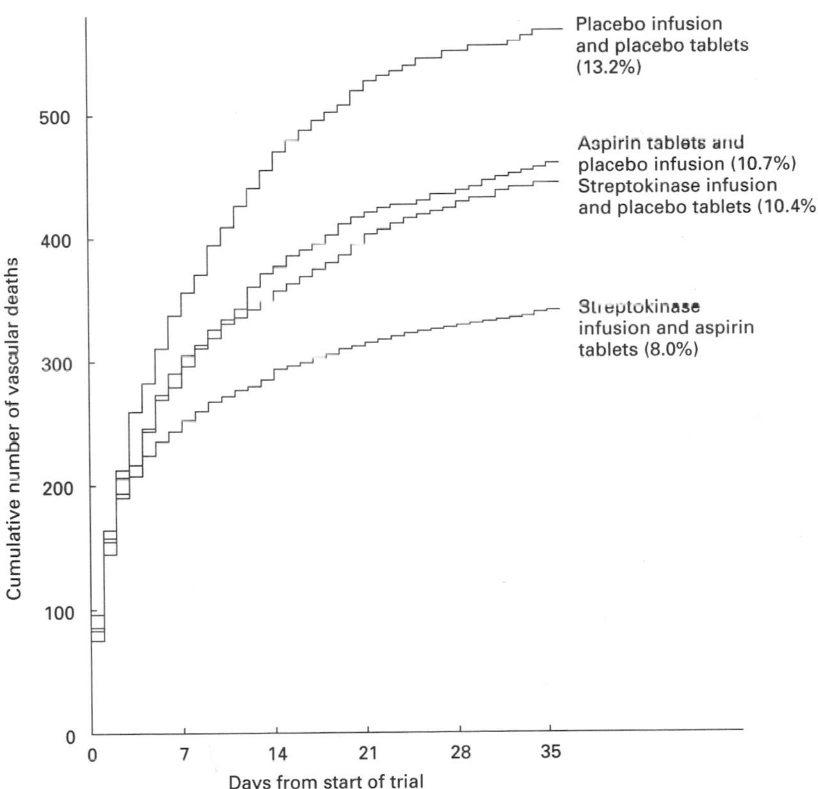

Fig. 16.9 Cumulative vascular mortality in patients with myocardial infarction treated either with placebo, aspirin alone, streptokinase alone or a combined aspirin–streptokinase regime. The figures indicate the number of deaths in the number of patients given a particular treatment, with, in brackets, the % mortality after 35 days. (ISIS-2 trial 1988 Lancet ii: 350–360)

activators. There are two endogenous plasminogen activators—tissue-type plasminogen activator (t-PA) and urokinase-type plasminogen activator (u-PA). The principal role of t-PA is in fibrinolysis whereas that of u-PA is mainly in cell migration and tissue remodelling processes.

In the blood, some plasminogen activator is derived from the endothelium of small vessels and from phagocytic cells, and some by the action of factor XII on pro-activators in plasma or tissues (Fig. 16.10). *Plasminogen*, a serum β-globulin of MW 143 000, is deposited on the fibrin strands within a thrombus. Plasminogen activators, which have a very short half-life in the circulation, are serine proteases which diffuse into the thrombus and cleave a particular Arg–Val bond in plasminogen to release the enzyme plasmin, also known as fibrinolysin (see Fig. 16.10). Plasmin is trypsin-like, acting on Arg–Lys bonds, and thus can digest not only fibrin but fibrinogen, factors II, V, and VIII and many other proteins. It is formed locally and acts on the fibrin meshwork, generating fibrin degradation products and lysing the clot. Its action is localised to the clot because the activators are effective mainly on plasminogen which is absorbed to fibrin; any plasmin which escapes into the circulation is inactivated by various plasmin inhibitors. This restriction of the locus of action is fortunate since otherwise so much plasmin would accumulate that we might run the risk of being lysed from within.

A second mechanism for stimulating fibrinolysis involves the activation of protein C by thrombin, as described above (p. 334).

Drugs may affect the fibrinolytic system by

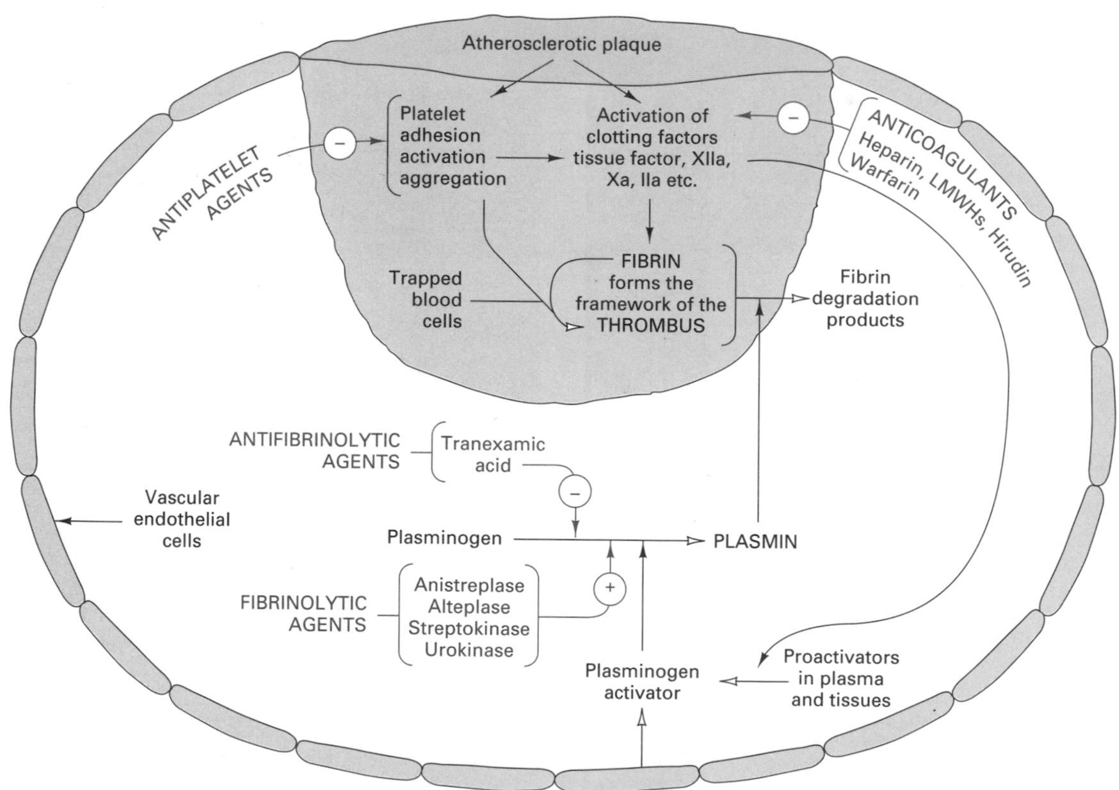

Fig. 16.10 Schematic diagram of thrombus formation showing the interaction of the fibrinolytic (thrombolytic) system with the coagulation cascade and the platelet-activation system, and the action of drugs which modify these systems. LMHs = low molecular weight heparins. For more detail of platelet activation and the coagulation cascade refer to Figures 16.1 and 16.2.

increasing the normal fibrinolytic mechanism (*fibrinolytic agents*) or by inhibiting it (*antifibrinolytic agents*).

FIBRINOLYTIC AGENTS

There are now several fibrinolytic (thrombolytic) agents available for clinical use. See Table 16.1.

Streptokinase is a non-enzymic protein with a molecular weight of 47 000 daltons. It is extracted from cultures of β-haemolytic streptococci and has to be biologically assayed and standardised. It acts indirectly, forming a stable complex with plasminogen which gains enzymic activity through a conformational change. It has proved successful in reducing mortality in suspected cases of myocardial infarction and this beneficial effect is additive with aspirin (Fig. 16.9).

It is antigenic and can cause anaphylactic reactions, albeit rarely. Furthermore its action can be reduced by antistreptococcal antibodies already present. For myocardial infarction it is infused intravenously over 60 minutes; when used for severe venous thrombosis or pulmonary embolism longer infusions (up to 72 hours) are given. One drawback is that it tends to result in a burst of plasmin formation which generates kinins (see Ch. 11) that cause hypotension.

Anistreplase (**APSAC**) is a complex of human lys-plasminogen and streptokinase which has been rendered inactive by introducing a para-anisoyl group at its catalytic centre. In the blood, the anisoyl group is removed. The half-life of removal of the p-anisoyl group to give active plasminogen–streptokinase is about 2 hours, both in the blood and in the thrombus; see Figure 16.10. Anistreplase is thus essentially a pro-drug of streptokinase. It is given as a single intravenous injection over 4–5 minutes, and fibrinolytic activity is sustained for 4–6 hours.

Alteplase (t-PA) and **duteplase** are recombinant tissue-type plasminogen activators, the first being single-chain, the second double-chain. Their enzymic activity is enhanced in the presence of fibrin to a greater extent than is that of the streptokinase–plasminogen complex, i.e. they have a higher ratio of activity for fibrin-bound plasminogen as compared with plasma plasminogen and are thus said to be 'clot selective'. t-PA is not antigenic and can be used in patients likely to have antibodies to streptokinase, such as those who have had recent streptococcal infections or who have been treated with streptokinase.

Urokinase (u-PA) is an endogenous substance

Table 16.1 Properties of fibrinolytic agents

Points of comparison	Streptokinase	Anistreplase	Urokinase*	Alteplase†
Half-life (min)	23	90	16	5–8
Activity enhanced by fibrin	+	+	++	++++
Duration of administration	i.v. infusion: loading dose for 60 min,‡ maintenance infusion for up to 72 h§	i.v. injection: 4–5 min	i.v. infusion: loading dose for 10 min, then maintenance dose over 12–24 h	i.v. injection over 1–2 min, then i.v. infusion over 3 h
Hypersensitivity reactions	Yes	Yes	No	No
Frequency of re-occlusion; estimated %	15	10	10	20
Expense	+	++	++	+++

* This is a two-chain plasminogen activator. Recombinant single-chain plasminogen activator is also available; its activity is more markedly enhanced by fibrin than is urokinase.
† This is single-chain recombinant tissue-type plasminogen activator; a double-chain preparation, duteplase, is also available.
‡ For myocardial infarction
§ For severe venous thrombosis or pulmonary embolism
Based partly on data from: Marder & Sherry 1988

Fibrinolysis and drugs modifying fibrinolysis

- A fibrinolytic cascade is initiated concomitantly with the coagulation cascade, resulting in the formation of plasmin, an enzyme which digests fibrin.
- Various agents promote the formation of plasmin from its precursor plasminogen, e.g. streptokinase, urokinase, alteplase and anistreplase (APSAC). Most have to be infused; anistreplase can be given as a single injection.
- Some drugs inhibit fibrinolysis, e.g. tranexamic acid.

which is involved in many physiological processes; a urokinase receptor is found on the surface of monocytes and many other cell types. Urokinase is secreted from cells as a single-chain pro-enzyme (scu-PA) from which the active two-chain enzymic plasminogen activator (tcu-PA) is derived by proteolysis, the two chains remaining linked by a disulphide bond. The 'urokinase' that is used clinically is tcu-PA. It is prepared from cultures of human embryonic kidney cells and has to be biologically assayed and standardised. Urokinase is enzymic and acts directly as a plasminogen activator. It is not antigenic. A loading dose is given by intravenous infusion over 10 minutes followed by a maintenance dose. It can be given repeatedly.

Recombinant single-chain urokinase plasminogen activator (**r-scuPA**) is now also available. It is converted to urokinase when it binds to fibrin.

Unwanted effects of fibrinolytic agents

The main hazard for all fibrinolytic agents is potentially serious bleeding, which may be treated by giving **tranexamic acid** (see below) and, if necessary, fresh plasma or coagulation factors. Gastrointestinal bleeding and haemorrhagic stroke can occur. Streptokinase and anistreplase can cause allergic reactions and the former is reported to produce low-grade fever in about 25% of patients treated.

Absolute contraindications to the use of these agents are active internal bleeding and cerebrovascular disease. Relative contraindications include bleeding diatheses, pregnancy, uncontrolled hypertension and any invasive procedures in which clot formation is important, such as surgery and recent serious trauma, including vigorous cardiopulmonary resuscitation.

Which fibrinolytic agent is best?

Placebo-controlled studies in patients with myocardial infarction—a major killer in the developed world—have shown that therapy with fibrinolytic agents reduces mortality (Fig. 16.9). This is an area of rapid research, development and assessment of drugs and it merits consideration. Regarding the clinically available agents, the big question is—which drug is to be preferred? To answer this one needs to turn to ISIS-3, GISSI-2, ISG and GUSTO—not sibilant names for felines but the acronyms of collaborative groups carrying out clinical trials of thrombolytic and other drugs in the therapy of myocardial infarction. Between them they have carried out some of the largest trials ever done—41 299 patients in ISIS-3 and 20 891 in GISSI-2 with its international extension, ISG. The results of these appeared to show that streptokinase (in combination therapy with aspirin; see above) was a clear winner and that the addition of heparin to the regime conferred no extra advantage (see Cobbe 1992). But the debate is not yet over because the recently announced results of the GUSTO trial (41 021 patients) indicate that tPA given rapidly intravenously combined with intravenous heparin saved more lives than streptokinase with heparin (see Horton 1993). Both regimes included oral aspirin.

Clinical use of anticoagulants, antiplatelet agents and fibrinolytic agents

- *Anticoagulants* are used in venous thromboembolism since the underlying process is predominantly coagulation (fibrin formation) with only a small component of platelet aggregation. Heparin or LMWHs are used for short-term action and warfarin for prolonged therapy.
- *Fibrinolytic agents* plus *aspirin* are used in the therapy of acute myocardial infarction; the sooner these are given after onset the better. The preferred fibrinolytic agent in the UK is streptokinase except where there has been severe streptococcal infection or previous treatment with streptokinase.
- Aspirin reduces the risk of occlusive cardiovascular disease in patients who have recovered from myocardial infarction or have unstable angina.

The debate continues and meanwhile, new fibrinolytic agents are being developed and tested—saruplase, staphylokinase, a t-PA from the saliva of the vampire bat, chimeric plasminogen activators consisting of bits of t-PA plus bits of u-PA, a recombinant fusion protein of a single-chain antifibrin antibody with truncated scu-PA. The situation is likely to change rapidly.

The clinical use of fibrinolytic agents is summarised on page 348.

ANTIFIBRINOLYTIC AND HAEMOSTATIC AGENTS

Tranexamic acid is an inhibitor of plasminogen activation and thus prevents fibrinolysis. It can be given orally or by intravenous injection. It is used to treat various conditions in which there is bleeding or risk of bleeding. It has proved valuable in the treatment of upper gastrointestinal haemorrhage, reducing mortality by 40% and decreasing the risk of rebleeding by 20–30% and the need for surgery by 30–40%. Its action in inhibiting the fibrinolytic effect of pepsin may be significant in this context.

Aprotinin inhibits proteolytic enzymes, and in addition to its use for the hyperplasminaemia which can be produced by fibrinolytic agents, it is used in patients at risk of major blood loss during cardiac surgery.

Ethamsylate reduces capillary bleeding, its main action probably being to correct impaired platelet adhesion. It is used in menorrhagia (excessive menstrual blood loss).

REFERENCES AND FURTHER READING

Antiplatelet Trialists' Collaboration 1994 Collaborative overview of randomised trials of antiplatelet therapy I, II, III. Br Med J 308: 81–105, 159–168, 235–246

Biggs R, Rizza C R 1984 Human blood coagulation, haemostasis and thrombosis, 3rd edn. Blackwell Scientific Publications, Oxford

British Society of Haematology Committee for Standards in Haematology 1990 Guidelines on oral anticoagulation: second edition. J Clin Pathol 43: 177–183

Cairns J A 1994 Oral anticoagulants or aspirin after myocardial infarction? Lancet 343: 497–498

Chesterman C N, Chong B H 1993 Uses of heparin. Br Med J 306: 871–872

Clouse L H, Comp P C 1987 The regulation of hemostasis: the protein C system. N Engl J Med 314: 1298–1304

Cobbe S M 1992 ISIS 3: The last word on thrombolysis? Streptokinase and aspirin win the vascular sweepstakes. Br Med J 304: 1454–1455

Cobbe S M 1994 Thrombolysis in myocardial infarction. The earlier the better, but how late is too late? Br Med J 308: 216–217

Collen D 1993 Towards improved thrombolytic therapy. Lancet 342: 34–36

Coller B S 1990 Platelets and thrombolytic therapy. N Eng J Med 322: 33–42

Coller B S 1992 Antiplatelet agents in the prevention and therapy of thrombosis. Annu Rev Med 43: 171–180

Collins R, Scrimgeour A, Yusuf S, Peto R 1988 Reduction in fatal pulmonary embolism and venous thrombosis by perioperative administration of subcutaneous heparin: overview of results of randomized trials. N Engl J Med 318: 1162–1173

deProst D 1986 Heparin fractions and analogues: a new therapeutic possibility for thrombosis. Trends Pharmacol Sci 12: 496–500

Doorey A J, Michelson E L, Topol E J 1992 Thrombolytic therapy of acute myocardial infarction. JAMA 268: 3108–3114

Draper G, McNinch A 1994 Vitamin K for neonates: the controversy. Br Med J 308: 867–868

Editorial 1988 Management of venous thromboembolism. Lancet 1: 275–276

Editorial 1988 Primary prevention of vascular disease by aspirin. Lancet 1: 1093–1094

Editorial 1992 Streptokinase plus aspirin does the trick: ISIS-3. Lancet 339: 780–781

Fears R 1990 Biochemical pharmacology and therapeutic aspects of thrombolytic agents. Pharmacol Rev 42: 201–224

Fennerty A, Campbell I A, Routledge P A 1988 Anticoagulants in venous thromboembolism. Br Med J 297: 1285–1286

Fibrinolytic Therapy Trialists (FTT) Collaborative Group 1994 Indications for fibrinolytic therapy in suspected acute myocardial infarction. Lancet 343: 311–322

Furie B, Furie B C 1992 Molecular and cellular biology of blood coagulation. N Eng J Med 326: 800–806

GISSI-2 (Gruppo Italiano per lo Studio Della Sopravivenza Nell'Infarto Miocardio) 1990 A factorial randomised trial of alteplase versus streptokinase and heparin versus no heparin among 12,490 patients with acute myocardial infarction. Lancet 336: 65–71

Gresele P, Deckmyn H et al. 1991 Thromboxane synthase inhibitors, thromboxane receptor antagonists and dual blockers in thrombotic disorders. Trends Pharmacol Sci 12: 158–163

Harker L A 1994 Platelets and vascular thrombosis. N Engl J Med 330: 1006–1007

Hirsh J 1991a Heparin. N Eng J Med 324: 1565–1574

Hirsh J 1991b Oral anticoagulant drugs. N Eng J Med 324: 1865–1873

Hirsh J, Levine M N 1992 Low molecular weight heparins. Blood 79: 1–17

Horton R 1993 Thrombolysis: tPA fast by GUSTO. Lancet 341: 1188

Hsia J, Hamilton W P et al. 1990 A comparison between

heparin and low-dose aspirin as adjunctive therapy with tissue plasminogen activator for acute myocardial infarction. N Engl J Med 323: 1433–1437

ISIS-2 (Second International Study of Infarct Survival) Collaborative Group 1988 Randomised trial of intravenous streptokinase, oral aspirin, both, or neither among 17,187 cases of suspected myocardial infarctions. Lancet ii: 349–360

ISIS-3 (Third International Study of Infarct Survival) Collaborative Group 1992 A randomised comparison of streptokinase vs tissue plasminogen activator vs anistreplase and of aspirin plus heparin vs aspirin alone among 41,299 patients of suspected myocardial infarction. Lancet 339: 753–770

ISG (The International Study Group) 1990 In-hospital mortality and clinical course of 20,891 patients with suspected acute myocardial infarction randomised between alteplase and streptokinase with or without heparin. Lancet 336: 71–75

Jackson R L, Busch S J, Cardin A D 1991 Glucosaminoglycans: molecular properties, protein interactions, and role in physiological processes. Physiol Rev 71: 482–530

Leizorovicz A, Simmoneau G et al. 1994 Comparison of efficacy and safety of low molecular weight heparins and unfractionated heparins in initial treatment of deep vein thrombosis: a meta-analysis. Brit Med J 309: 299–304

Longenecker G L (ed) 1985 The platelets: physiology and pharmacology. Academic Press, London

Loscalzo J, Braunwald E 1988 Tissue plasminogen activator. N Engl J Med 319: 925–931

Mann K G 1987 The assembly of blood clotting complexes in membranes. Trends Biol Sci 12: 229–233

Marder V J, Sherry S 1988 Thrombolytic therapy: current status. N Engl J Med 318: 1512–1520, 1585–1595

Markwardt F 1991 Hirudin and derivatives as anticoagulant agents. Thromb Haemost 66: 141–152

Metcalf D 1994 Thrombopoietin—at last. Nature 369: 519–520

Nachman R L 1992 Thrombosis and atherogenesis: molecular connections. Blood 79: 1897–1906

Nichols A J, Ruffolo R R et al. 1992 Development of GPIIb/IIIa antagonists as antithrombotic drugs. Trends Pharmacol Sci 13: 413–417

Ofosu F A 1989 Antithrombotic mechanisms of heparin and related compounds. In: Lane D A, Lindahl U (eds) Heparin. Edward Arnold, London, p 433–454

Patrono C 1994 Aspirin as an antiplatelet drug. N Engl J Med 330: 1287–1294

Ruggeri Z M, Ware J 1992 The structure and function of von Willebrand factor. Thromb Haem 67: 594–599

Salzman E W 1992 Low-molecular-weight heparin and other new antithrombotic drugs. N Eng J Med 326: 1017–1019

Smith P, Arnesen H, Holme I 1990 The effect of warfarin on mortality and reinfarction after myocardial infarction. N Engl J Med 323: 147–152

Suttie J W 1980 Vitamin K-dependent carboyxlation. Trends Biochem Sci 5: 302–304

Theroux P, Ouimet H et al. 1988 Aspirin, heparin or both to treat acute unstable angina. N Engl J Med 319: 1105–1111

Topol E J, Califf R M et al. 1994 Randomised trial of coronary intervention with antibody against platelet IIb/IIIa integrin for reduction of clinical restenosis: results at six months. Lancet 343: 881–889

Tuddenham E G D 1994 Thrombophilia: the new factor is old factor V. Lancet 343: 1515–1516

Underwood M J, More R S 1994 The aspirin papers. Aspirin benefits patients with vascular disease and those undergoing revascularisation. Br Med J 308: 71–72

Vane J 1994 Towards a better aspirin. Nature 367: 215–216

Vermeer C, Hamulyak K 1991 Pathophysiology of vitamin K-deficiency and oral anticoagulants. Thromb Haemost 66: 153–159

Ware J A, Heisted D D 1993 Platelet–endothelium interactions. N Eng J Med 328: 628–635

Weitz J I, Hirsh J 1992 Antithrombins: their potential as antithrombotic agents. Annu Rev Med 43: 9–16

Willard J E, Lange R A, Hillis L D 1992 The use of aspirin in ischaemic heart disease. N Engl J Med 327: 175–181

17 THE RESPIRATORY SYSTEM

The chief functions of respiration are to supply oxygen to the body and to remove carbon dioxide. In addition, the evaporation of water in the respiratory passages assists in regulating the temperature of the body.

THE REGULATION OF RESPIRATION

Respiration is controlled by spontaneous rhythmic discharges from the respiratory centre in the medulla, modulated by input from pontine and higher CNS centres and vagal afferents from the lungs. Various chemical factors affect the respiratory centre including the blood $P\text{CO}_2$ (by an action on medullary chemoreceptors) and the blood $P\text{O}_2$ (by an action on the chemoreceptors in the aortic and carotid bodies).

A moderate degree of voluntary control can be superimposed on the automatic regulation of breathing, and this implies connections between the cortex and the motor neurons innervating the muscles of respiration. Bulbar poliomyelitis and certain lesions in the brainstem result in loss of the automatic regulation of respiration without loss of voluntary regulation. This has been referred to as '*Ondine's curse*'. Ondine was a water nymph who fell in love with a mortal. When he was unfaithful to her, the king of the water nymphs put a curse on him, eliminating certain automatic functions including that of respiration. Thereafter he had to stay awake and breathe by consciously exerting voluntary control. When exhaustion finally supervened and he fell asleep, he ceased breathing.

DRUGS WHICH AFFECT RESPIRATION

Drugs may produce an effect on respiration inadvertently (e.g. the unwanted effects of some CNS depressants) or because they are intended to (e.g. respiratory stimulants).

RESPIRATORY STIMULANTS

The use of respiratory stimulants has declined in recent years, and they are now employed only in certain specific conditions (e.g. in ventilatory failure due to chronic obstructive disease of the airways) and then only under expert supervision in hospital. The main drug used is **doxapram** which stimulates both carotid chemoreceptors and the respiratory centre. It is given by continuous intravenous infusion. Unwanted effects are due mainly to the general stimulant action on the central nervous system and include tremor, dizziness and convulsions. The stimulation of the vasomotor centre is likely to cause vasoconstriction, and cardiac dysrhythmias can also occur. It should not be used in severe acute asthma (*status asthmaticus*), or in respiratory depression which is caused by drug overdose (see below) or by disease of the nervous system.

Aminophylline, in addition to its direct effect on the airways (see below, p. 358), also has a degree of central stimulant action which may contribute to the modest benefit caused by this agent in patients with emphysema.

DRUGS CAUSING RESPIRATORY DEPRESSION

Many drugs which have a depressant action on the central nervous system cause a greater or lesser degree of respiratory depression. These include the **narcotic analgesics**, **barbiturates**, many **H_1-histamine-receptor antagonists**, some **antidepressants** and **ethanol**. Most of these agents generally depress respiration only in excessive dosage, but the **opiates** cause some degree of respiratory depression in the therapeutic dose range. The respiratory depression caused by the majority of the above agents can prove fatal; however, this is less likely to occur with the benzodiazepines. These hazards are discussed in more detail in the chapters devoted to each of these agents.

Opiate analgesics and barbiturates (and possibly other CNS depressant drugs) first affect the sensitivity of respiration to increased $P\text{CO}_2$ and only later, in larger doses, do they affect the hypoxic drive.

FUNCTIONS OF THE LUNG UNRELATED TO RESPIRATION

The lung has various functions which have pharmacological and/or physiological relevance, but which have nothing to do with breathing.

Drugs which affect respiration

- Depression of respiration can be produced by excessive doses of most drugs with depressant actions on the CNS.
- Benzodiazepines cause relatively little depression (but may do so to a dangerous degree if combined with alcohol).
- Narcotic analgesics cause some degree of depression in therapeutic doses.

Angiotensin I is converted to angiotensin II (see Ch. 14) by the angiotensin-converting enzyme, which also inactivates bradykinin (p. 239). The enzyme is present on the luminal surface of the capillary endothelial cells in the lungs. Some prostaglandins are extracted from the circulation and metabolised in the lung (p. 233), as are noradrenaline and 5-hydroxytryptamine.

The lung also functions as part of the body reservoir of the blood neutrophils. Normally, at rest, only about 50% of these cells are present in the circulating blood. The remaining 50% form the 'marginated pool' which can be added to the circulation when needed, virtually doubling neutrophil numbers within seconds. Many of the marginated neutrophils are held in the blood vessels of the lungs and can be mobilised by a variety of stimuli, including exercise, infection and various pharmacological agents such as adrenaline (reviewed by McCarthy & Dale 1988).

THE REGULATION OF THE MUSCULATURE, BLOOD VESSELS AND GLANDS OF THE AIRWAYS

In the normal neurohumoral control of the airways, the *efferent pathways* are the acetylcholine-releasing parasympathetic nerves, the noradrenaline-releasing sympathetic nerves, circulating adrenaline and the non-noradrenergic, non-cholinergic (NANC) relaxant mediator. The *afferent pathways* include three different types of sensory receptor.

In pathological conditions such as asthma and bronchitis, other mediators—the inflammatory mediators (see Ch. 11) and the NANC contractile mediators—have a significant role.

The signal transduction mechanisms for the various receptors mediating contraction and relaxation of bronchiolar muscle are discussed by Dale & Hirst (1993).

The tone of the bronchial muscle affects the airways resistance, and in asthma and bronchitis the state of the mucosa and the activity of the glands also contribute. The airways resistance can be measured indirectly by instruments which record the volume or flow of forced expiration. FEV_1 is the 'forced expiratory volume in 1 second'. The 'peak expiratory flow rate' (PEFR) can also be quantitated.

Efferent pathways

Parasympathetic innervation

Parasympathetic ganglia are embedded in the walls of the bronchi and bronchioles, and the post-ganglionic fibres innervate airway smooth muscle, vascular smooth muscle and glands. There are three types of muscarinic (M) receptors present (see Ch. 6)—and at least two different theories as to how these influence parasympathetic control of smooth muscle in the airways (Barnes 1989, Goyal 1989). M_1-receptors are localised in ganglia, on the postsynaptic cells, and their stimulation facilitates neurotransmission mediated by acetylcholine acting on the nicotinic receptors.* M_2-receptors are 'autoreceptors' mediating negative feedback effects of acetylcholine on cholinergic nerves. **Pilocarpine** has relatively selective effects on M_2-receptors and, in experimental studies on human bronchi, inhibits contraction induced by electrical field stimulation of cholinergic nerves. M_3-receptors are found on bronchial smooth muscle and glands and mediate contraction of the former and secretion from the latter. Stimulation of the vagus causes broncho-constriction—mainly in the larger airways. The possible clinical relevance of the heterogenicity of muscarinic receptors in the airways is discussed on page 361.

Sympathetic innervation and catecholamines

Sympathetic nerves innervate blood vessels and glands, the released noradrenaline causing constriction of the former and inhibiting secretion by the latter. Contrary to general belief there is no sympathetic innervation of the bronchial smooth muscle; there is good experimental evidence that all 'sympathetic' effects are due to circulating catecholamines.

This statement is based on the following evidence:

- Histochemical studies show sympathetic nerves around blood vessels and submucosal glands in the bronchi, but none in the smooth muscle.
- Studies of in vitro preparations show that though airway muscle contraction following nerve stimulation can be inhibited by **atropine**, relaxation following nerve stimulation is not affected by either **β- or α-receptor antagonists** or **noradrenergic neuron blockers**; in addition, dose–response curves of relaxation with exogenous **noradrenaline** are not altered by **cocaine**. For explanation of these effects see Chapter 7. (Neuronally-induced relaxation is thought to be produced entirely by the NANC inhibitory mediators; see below.)
- In vivo studies with **tyramine**, which releases noradrenaline from sympathetic nerve terminals (see Ch. 7), indicate that though the expected cardiovascular changes occur, there is no change in FEV_1, or in peak flow in the airways. **Salbutamol**, on the other hand, a β_2-adrenoceptor agonist, *does* increase both FEV_1 and peak flow.

Autoradiography shows that β-adrenoceptors occur in the smooth muscle, the epithelium and glands, and also, in very large numbers, in the alveoli. They are also found on mast cells. In humans, virtually all the β-receptors in the airways are β_2; those in the alveoli are both β_1 and β_2. (The function of the alveolar receptors is not known.) In contrast with the muscarinic receptors, the density of β-receptors increases from trachea to bronchioles.

Stimulation of the airway β-receptors with drugs results in relaxation of smooth muscle, inhibition of mediator release from mast cells, and increased mucociliary clearance.

α-adrenoceptor agonists have no effect on normal airways but cause contraction if the airways are diseased.

Non-noradrenergic, non-cholinergic (NANC) mediators

There is experimental evidence that airway function is influenced by neuronal mediators other than acetylcholine and noradrenaline; these are referred to as NANC mediators (see Ch. 5).

The inhibitory NANC mediator is a potent bronchodilator. It can be released by electrical field stimulation (Fig. 17.1) and causes relaxation of airway smooth muscle, which is not affected by β_2-adrenoceptor antagonists, such as **propranolol,** or noradrenergic neuron blockers, such as **guanethidine**, but is prevented by **tetrodotoxin** (Ch. 34). The effect of tetrodotoxin indicates that neuronal release is involved, and the lack of effect of propranolol and guanethidine indicates that sympathetic

*There are selective antagonists at the M_1-receptor, for example **pirenzepine** (used in gastrointestinal conditions; see p. 391), **dicyclomine**, and **trihexyphenidyl** (used for parkinsonism; see Ch. 25). These drugs are not used in the respiratory system.

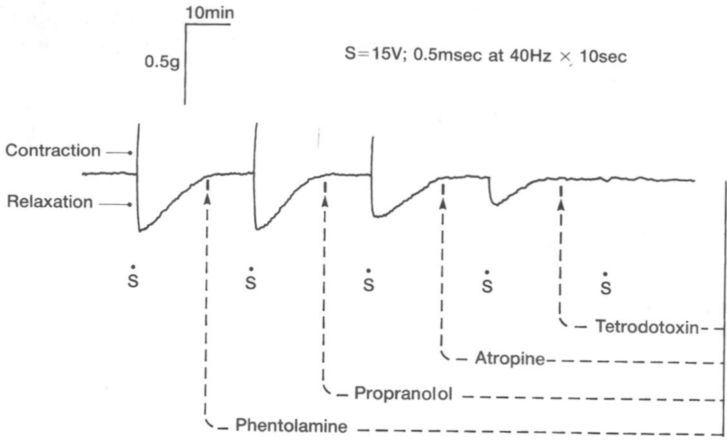

Fig. 17.1 Record of the response of a guinea-pig tracheal strip, demonstrating acetylcholine-mediated contraction and non-noradrenergic, non-cholinergic relaxation. Electrical field stimulation (S) causes a fast contraction followed by a slow relaxation. The contraction is abolished by atropine (1 μmol/l), showing that it is cholinergic. The relaxation is unaffected by the α-adrenoceptor antagonist, phentolamine (10 μm) and only marginally reduced by the β-adrenoceptor antagonist, propranolol (1 μmol/l), showing that it is not mediated through adrenoceptors. It is virtually abolished by the sodium-channel blocker, tetrodotoxin (3 μmol/l), showing that the response is neuronally mediated. (Data supplied by Dr S J Hirst. See also Coleman & Levy 1974 Br J Pharmacol 52: 167; and Richardson & Beland 1976 J Applied Physiol 41: 764)

nerves are not. This NANC inhibitory mediator is the *main* neurotransmitter relaxant in the airways, but neither its source nor its identity is known incontrovertibly. Evidence is against the involvement of purinergic nerves. One candidate, popular with experimenters, is **vasoactive intestinal peptide** (VIP); the necessary receptors can be demonstrated, and exogenous VIP causes relaxation of bronchial smooth muscle. A particularly promising candidate—with some provisional evidence in its favour—is **nitric oxide**, recently unmasked as being the endothelium-derived relaxing factor in blood vessels and subsequently shown not only to have neurotransmitter activity but also to be capable of relaxing other smooth muscle besides that in the arteries (see Ch. 10).

The stimulant NANC mediators are excitatory neuropeptides* (see Ch. 9) that can be released from sensory nerves by an axon reflex mechanism. These peptides, which are held to have a role in the delayed phase of asthma (see Fig. 17.3), include, amongst others, substance P (which increases vascular permeability and induces mucus secretion), and neurokinin A (a potent spasmogen).

The inflammatory mediators are dealt with below.

Sensory receptors

There are two categories of sensory receptor in the airways: those which affect predominantly the central control of respiration by the respiratory centre and those which have both central effects and local effects on airway resistance.

Receptors affecting the central control of the airways include the stretch receptors and the J-receptors.

Stretch receptors are slowly-adapting receptors located in the bronchial musculature; they are stimulated by distension of the airways and initiate reflexes that are important in the regulation of respiration.

J-receptors are found between the pulmonary capillaries and alveolar walls, and the related nerve fibres are unmyelinated. These receptors are thought

*These peptides are considered to be the mediators of *neurogenic inflammation*, which may also be a contributing factor in various inflammatory conditions (Ch. 11, p. 220).

by some to be 'deflation receptors' and by others to respond to congestion of the blood vessels.

Rapidly-adapting receptors, which can give rise to both central and local effects, also occur in the lung. Two other receptor types may give rise to both central and local effects (Widdicombe 1987): *irritant receptors* associated with myelinated vagal afferents, and *C-fibre receptors* associated with non-myelinated vagal fibres. Mechanical stimuli, acting mainly on irritant receptors in the upper airway, cause cough. Chemical stimuli, acting on irritant receptors and/or C-fibre receptors in the lower airways, cause bronchoconstriction and an increase in mucus secretion. Chemical stimuli producing these effects include both exogenous agents, such as ammonia, sulphur dioxide, cigarette smoke and the experimental tool, capsaicin (see Ch. 31), as well as endogenous stimuli such as the inflammatory mediators histamine, leukotrienes C_4 and D_4, and bradykinin (which can, themselves, directly cause bronchoconstriction or mucus secretion or both; see Ch. 11). In the upper airways the reflex bronchoconstriction and mucus secretion are due largely to release of acetylcholine; in the lower airways, the responses are due largely to the release of excitatory neuropeptides (see above) by axon reflexes.

These effects of neural and inflammatory mediators have relevance for the understanding of bronchial hyper-responsiveness and the delayed phase of asthma (see below and Fig. 17.2).

Regulation of airway muscle, blood vessels and glands

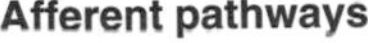

Afferent pathways

- Stretch receptors in the smooth muscle respond to marked pulmonary inflation and relay to the respiratory centre, inhibiting inspiration.
- Irritant receptors and C-fibre receptors respond to exogenous chemicals, inflammatory mediators and physical stimuli (e.g. cold air) causing bronchoconstriction and mucus secretion through acetylcholine release in the upper airway and axon reflex release of excitatory neuropeptides in the lower.

Efferent pathways

- The parasympathetic nerves mediate bronchial constriction and mucus secretion through an action on muscarinic M_3-receptors.
- Sympathetic nerves innervate blood vessels (causing constriction) and glands (inhibiting secretion), but *not* airway smooth muscle.
- Circulating adrenaline acts on β_2-receptors to relax airway smooth muscle.
- The main neurotransmitter causing relaxation of airway smooth muscle is the NANC inhibitory transmitter (identity unknown; it may be nitric oxide).
- NANC excitatory transmitters are peptides released from sensory neurons by axon reflex mechanisms.

DISORDERS OF RESPIRATORY FUNCTION

Two of the main disorders of the respiratory system are bronchial asthma and cough. Others, less susceptible to treatment, are chronic bronchitis with resultant chronic obstructive airway disease, and the adult respiratory distress syndrome.

BRONCHIAL ASTHMA

Asthma may be loosely defined as a syndrome in which there is recurrent 'reversible' obstruction of the airways in response to stimuli which are not in themselves noxious and which do not affect non-asthmatic subjects. The asthmatic subject has intermittent attacks of dyspnoea (disorder of breathing), wheezing, and cough, the dyspnoea consisting of difficulty in breathing *out*. It contrasts with the obstructive airway disease mentioned above, which is not reversible. But note that the term 'reversible' as applied to asthma needs to be qualified since it is only the acute attack of dyspnoea that is reversible; the underlying pathological change may not be reversible and indeed can progress, while in acute severe asthma (*status asthmaticus*) the airway obstruction causing the dyspnoea can take days to reverse, and in some cases is not reversible at all and proves to be fatal.

Asthma affects over 5% of the population in industrialised countries—10% in the USA according to some authorities. It is increasing in prevalence and severity and has a rising mortality (2000 p.a. in the UK at present, over 4000 in the USA) despite a substantial increase in prescribed asthma treatment (see Neville et al. 1993, Weinberger S E 1993). Some chest physicians consider that the increase in mortality may be the result of the currently available therapy not being used optimally. If this is indeed so, it may stem from the fact that recent advances in the understanding of the pathogenesis of asthma have not been universally appreciated.* Aspects relating to this are discussed by Buist (1988), Morley & Smith (1989), Burney et al. (1990), Burrows & Lebowitz (1992), Barnes & Lee (1992), Neville et al. (1993), Weinberger S E (1993).

Asthma was previously thought to be purely a type I hypersensitivity reaction (p. 224), the actual attack occurring in a sensitised individual when allergen interacted with IgE antibodies on mast cells, leading to release of histamine and other mediators, which cause a simple bronchoconstriction. That view is now known to be an over-simplification—not all asthma is due to allergy and, even in allergic asthma, elements other than the interaction of allergen with mast-cell-fixed IgE are involved. This has relevance for the use of drugs in treatment.

It is currently recognised that the characteristic features of asthma are *inflammatory changes in the airways* associated with *bronchial hyper-responsiveness*. (But note that asthma in preschool children is not associated with obvious bronchial hyper-responsiveness and chronic inflammation does not appear to be the basis of the episodic asthma associated with viral infections.) Inflammatory changes are present even in patients with very mild asthma and in some individuals these may even precede the development of overt asthma. The term bronchial hyper-responsiveness (or hyper-reactivity) refers to abnormal sensitivity to a wide range of stimuli such as irritant chemicals, cold air, stimulant drugs, etc., all of which can result in bronchoconstriction. Stimuli which cause the actual asthma attacks are many and various, and include allergens (in sensitised individuals), exercise (in which the stimulus may be cold air), respiratory infections and atmospheric pollutants such as sulphur dioxide.

The development of asthma probably involves both genetic and environmental factors, and the asthmatic attack itself consists, in many subjects, of two main phases—the immediate phase and the late (or delayed) phase. These phases can be demonstrated by tests of FEV_1 (Fig. 17.2).

This division into two phases is fairly arbitrary—

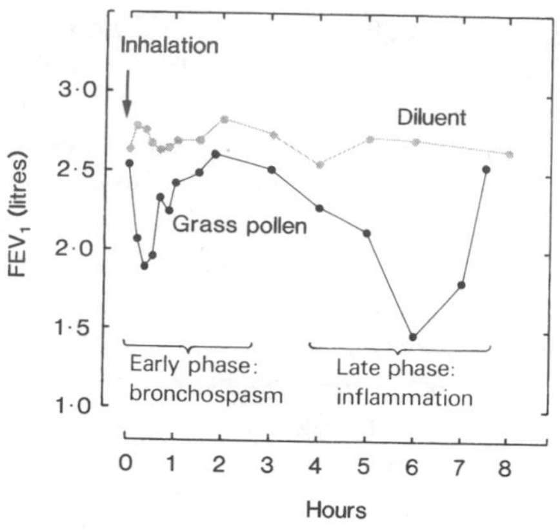

Fig. 17.2 The two phases of asthma as demonstrated by the changes in the forced expiratory volume in 1 second (FEV_1) after inhalation of grass pollen in an allergic subject. (From: Cockcroft D W 1983 Lancet 1: 253)

indeed, in some subjects, only one of the phases may be obvious—but it provides a useful basis for discussing the physiopathological changes in the bronchi as well as the locus of action and the effects of drugs used in treatment.

The full details of the complex events involved are still a matter of debate, with various authors championing their particular inflammatory cell or mediator as being the principal agent in the development of asthma. In the following paragraphs we give a simplified synthesis of the current ideas on asthma pathogenesis held by most authorities (see Holgate 1993, Weinberger S E 1993; and for a comprehensive coverage by numerous authors in 33 chapters, see Weiss & Stein 1993). We emphasise that an understanding of this topic is necessary for rational use of current (and future) drugs in the treatment of asthma.

The development of allergic asthma

In allergic asthma, exposure of genetically predisposed individuals to allergens such as pollen or proteins of the house dust mite causes sensitisation. This involves activation of a clone of T cells which then:

- generate various B-cell-activating cytokines, leading to IgE production and release
- generate various interleukins which induce expression of IgE receptors, mainly on mast cells but also on eosinophils, platelets, and macrophages.

When the IgE binds to the IgE receptors on the

*In the words of one aspiring general practitioner in 1989: 'Asthma is easy to understand and simple to treat. It's just histamine-induced bronchospasm—all you need to do is prescribe a good bronchodilator'. A detailed bibliography on recent advances therefore seems appropriate.

cells, the system becomes primed so that subsequent re-exposure to the relevant allergen will cause an asthmatic attack.

The immediate phase of the asthmatic attack

The immediate phase, i.e. the initial response, occurs abruptly and is due mainly to *spasm of the bronchial smooth muscle*. The cells involved in initiating this phase are predominantly mast cells which release histamine, but other cells—eosinophils, macrophages, platelets—could contribute, as indicated in Figure 17.3. Histamine is not the only or even the main spasmogen—LTC_4 and LTD_4 (Ch. 11, p. 235) are now known to be more important, and other mediators (e.g. neurokinin A) may also contribute. Various chemotaxins (e.g. LTB_4) and chemokines (see Ch. 11, p. 241) attract leucocytes into the area, setting the stage for the delayed phase.

It is possible that in non-allergic asthma, irritants may stimulate the irritant receptors and cause release of neuropeptide mediators from sensory nerve fibres, and that these neuropeptides then activate mast cells and other cells. Most exercise-induced asthma appears to involve mainly the phenomena of this first phase.

The late phase

The second, late phase or delayed response (see Fig. 17.2), occurs at a variable time after exposure to the eliciting stimulus and may be nocturnal. This phase is in essence a progressing *inflammatory reaction* (p. 215) initiated during the first phase. The inflammation is different from the inflammation seen, for example, in bronchitis. It has special

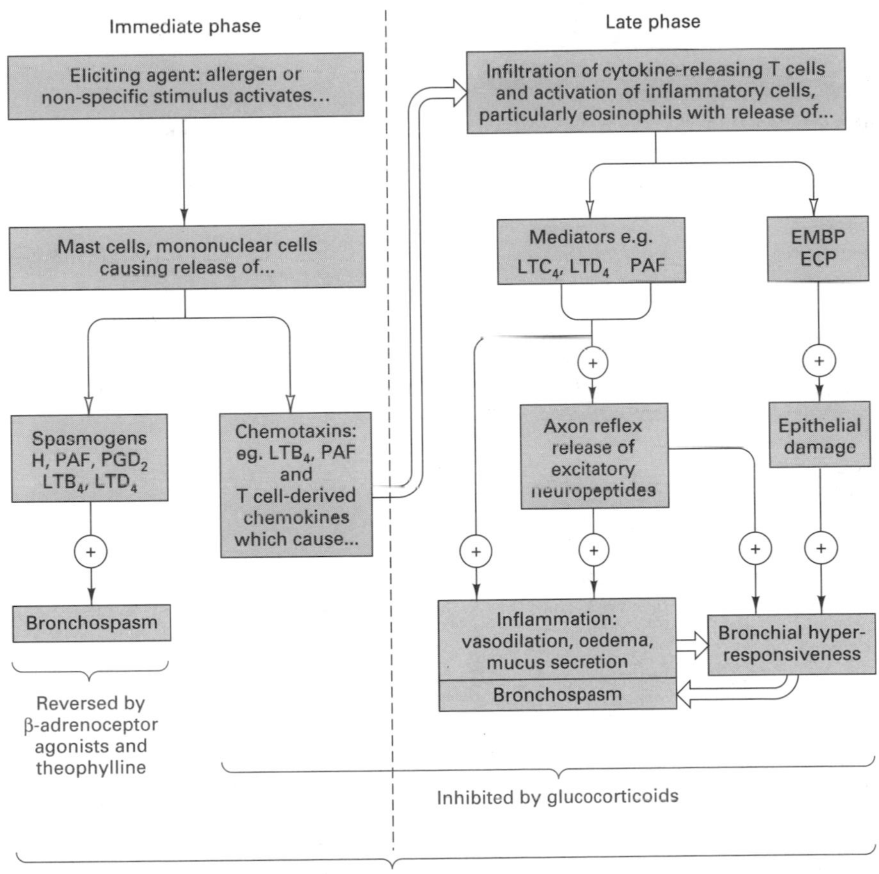

Fig. 17.3 Outline of the reactions thought to occur in asthma. (H = histamine; PAF = platelet-activating factor; LTB_4, LTC_4 and LTD_4 = leukotrienes B_4, C_4 and D_4; EMBP = eosinophil major basic protein; ECP = eosinophil cationic protein). Note that not all asthmatic subjects respond to cromoglycate or nedocromil, and that theophylline is only a second-line drug.

characteristics in that there is infiltration not only by the usual inflammatory cells (p. 217), but also, and more specifically, by activated cytokine-releasing T cells and by eosinophils, whose products cause damage and loss of epithelium—with the repercussions outlined in Figure 17.3 (reviewed by Corrigan & Kay 1992). There is also some preliminary evidence for participation of neurogenic mechanisms such as the release of the excitatory NANC peptide transmitters by axon reflex mechanisms—the relevant sensory neurons being more accessible to irritant stimuli when there is epithelial loss due to factors released from eosinophils; this is thought to be the basis of the hyper-responsiveness. Lack of the NANC relaxant could also play a part in bronchoconstriction. The relative significance of these various factors is not yet clear.

Bronchial asthma

- Asthma is defined as recurrent reversible airway obstruction. The asthmatic attack comprises wheezing, cough and difficulty in breathing out; the airways resistance is increased—manifest as a decrease in the 'forced expiratory volume in 1 sec' (FEV_1).
- Two characteristic features are:
  - —underlying inflammatory changes in the airways
  - —underlying bronchial hyper-responsiveness, i.e. abnormal sensitivity to stimuli.
- In acute severe asthma *(status asthmaticus)* the airway obstruction can be fatal.
- In many subjects the asthmatic attack consists of two phases which illustrate the pathophysiology of the condition; these are as follows:
  - —an immediate phase on exposure to eliciting agent consisting mainly of bronchospasm
  - —a later phase consisting of a special type of inflammation comprising: vasodilatation, oedema, mucus secretion and bronchospasm caused by inflammatory mediators released from eosinophils and other cells, and, possibly, neuropeptides released by axon reflexes; activated, cytokine-releasing T cells have an important role; damage to bronchial epithelium is caused by proteins released from eosinophils.
- Important mediators: histamine probably in first phase only; LTC_4, LTD_4, (and possibly Substance P, neurokinin A, and PAF) and various chemotaxins in both phases.
- Anti-asthmatic drugs include:
  - —bronchodilators
  - —anti-inflammatory agents.

There are two categories of anti-asthma drugs—**bronchodilators** and **anti-inflammatory agents**. Bronchodilators are effective in reversing the bronchospasm of the immediate phase, anti-inflammatory agents in inhibiting or preventing the inflammatory components of both phases (Fig. 17.3).

Many authorities now consider that progression of the condition, with increase in the severity of the asthmatic attacks, is due to a gradual increase in the mucosal inflammation. Over-reliance on bronchodilators, which overcome the acute attacks of bronchospasm without modifying the underlying inflammation, could well contribute to this.

The problem of how to use the above two categories of drugs in the clinical treatment of asthma is complex. A recent set of guidelines (see British Thoracic Society and Others 1993) specifies five therapeutic steps—the first involving only a short-acting β-agonist, progressing, if this type of agent is needed more than once daily, to subsequent steps involving both bronchodilators and anti-inflammatory drugs. There is now general agreement on the need to implement early anti-inflammatory treatment rather than relying on symptomatic treatment with bronchodilators alone.

DRUGS USED TO TREAT ASTHMA—BRONCHODILATORS

Drugs used as bronchodilators include the β_2-adrenoceptor agonists, the xanthines and the muscarinic-receptor antagonists.

β_2-adrenoceptor agonists

β_2-adrenoceptor agonists are dealt with in detail in Chapter 7. In asthma, their action is twofold.

Their main effect is to dilate the bronchi by a direct action on the β_2-adrenoceptors on the smooth muscle. Being physiological antagonists (see Ch. 1), they can relax the bronchial muscle despite the numerous spasmogens involved. A secondary action is to inhibit mediator release from mast cells. They may also inhibit vagal tone and increase mucus clearance by an action on cilia.

These drugs are usually given by inhalation of aerosol, powder or nebulised solution, but some may be given orally or by injection. A metered-dose inhaler is used for aerosol preparations; if patients (e.g. children, the elderly) have problems using these, 'spacer' devices can be used instead.

Two categories of β_2-adrenoceptor agonists are used in asthma:

- short-acting agents—**salbutamol** and **terbutaline**; given by inhalation, the maximum effect is within 30 minutes and the duration 4–6 hours
- longer-acting agents—**salmeterol**; given by inhalation, the duration is 12 hours.

Others are rimeterol (with shorter duration of action than salbutamol), fenoterol, pirbuterol and reprotelol. Bambuterol, a pro-drug of terbutaline, is also now available.

The unwanted effects of β_2-adrenoceptor agonists are given in Chapter 7. In the context of their use in asthma, the commonest adverse effect is tremor. It should be noted that there is increasing evidence that β-agonist tolerance can occur in asthmatic airways (see Cockroft et al. 1993, Britton 1992) and that steroids can reduce the possibility of the development of tolerance because they inhibit β-receptor down-regulation. However it is reported that, in some cases, potentially serious hypokalaemia can occur if β_2-adrenoceptor agonists are used concomitantly with the anti-asthma drugs xanthines and glucocorticoids.

Some authors have questioned the safety of β_2-adrenoceptor agonists in asthma; this is discussed and dismissed by Burrows & Lebowitz (1992); but see Britton (1992).

β_2-adrenoceptor agonists are also used to improve respiratory function in chronic obstructive lung disease.

It should be stressed that non-selective β-adrenoceptor agonists, such as adrenaline and isoprenaline, which act on both β_1- and β_2-receptors, are no longer used in asthma and that β_2-adrenoceptor *antagonists*, such as propranolol, though having no effect on airway function in normal individuals, cause wheezing in asthmatics and can precipitate a potentially serious acute asthmatic attack.

Xanthine drugs

There are three pharmacologically active, naturally occurring methylxanthines, **theophylline**, **theobromine** and **caffeine** (Fig. 17.4; see also Chs 13 and 32). The xanthine usually employed in clinical medicine is theophylline (1,3-dimethylxanthine), which can be used also as theophylline-ethylenediamine, known as **aminophylline**. Caffeine and theophylline are constituents of coffee and tea, and theobromine is a constituent of cocoa. A new compound, **enprofylline**—a propylxanthine—is under test (Fig. 17.4). It has rather different effects from the methylxanthines and may shed some light on the vexed question of the mechanism of action of these agents (see Persson 1987). Both theophylline and enprofylline have bronchodilator action, though they are rather less effective in this regard than β_2-adrenoceptor agonists.

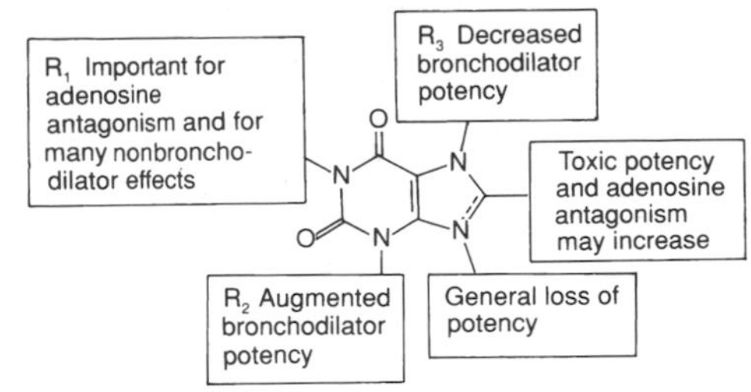

Drug	R_1	R_2	R_3
Theophylline	CH_3	CH_3	H
Caffeine	CH_3	CH_3	CH_3
Theobromine	H	CH_3	CH_3
Enprofylline	H	H	C_3H_7
Proxiphylline	CH_3	CH_3	C_3H_6OH

Fig. 17.4 The xanthine molecule, showing some pharmacological consequences of alkyl substitution. (After: Persson 1987)

Actions

Anti-asthmatic actions. Several clinical studies have shown that xanthines can be effective both in relieving the acute attack and in the treatment of 'chronic asthma'. (This latter term is used rather indiscriminately to apply to the propensity for repeated attacks and/or to a state of semi-continuous low-grade asthma.) Actions in addition to bronchodilatation seem to be involved since there is some evidence that these agents can inhibit the late phase, as shown by measurement of FEV_1 after bronchial allergen challenge (Pauwels 1989). However, they do not appear to prevent bronchial hyper-responsiveness.

Actions on the central nervous system. The methylxanthines have a stimulant effect on the CNS causing increased alertness (see Ch. 32). They can cause tremor and nervousness and can interfere with sleep. Enprofylline does not have this effect.

Actions on the cardiovascular system. All

the xanthines stimulate the heart (see Ch. 13), having positive chronotropic and inotropic actions. They cause vasodilatation in most blood vessels, though the methylxanthines can cause constriction in some vascular beds, more particularly cerebral blood vessels.

Actions on kidney. Methylxanthines have a weak diuretic effect, involving both an increased glomerular filtration rate and reduced reabsorption in the tubules. Enprofylline does not have this action.

Mechanisms of action

The way in which this group of drugs produces its effects in asthma is still unclear. One proposed mode of action is competitive antagonism of adenosine at adenosine receptors, but enprofylline, which is a more potent bronchodilator, is not an adenosine antagonist. The relaxant effect on smooth muscle has been attributed to inhibition of phosphodiesterase with resultant increase in cyclic AMP (see Fig. 14.1). An increase in cyclic AMP could also inhibit activation of inflammatory cells. However, the concentrations necessary to inhibit the isolated enzyme greatly exceed the therapeutic range. There is evidence that subtypes of the enzyme exist, which raises the possibility that inhibitors with selective action could be of value (see Nicholson & Shahid 1994). There is also evidence that the smooth muscle relaxation could be related to an effect on a cyclic *GMP* phosphodiesterase.

The methylxanthines are reported to cause release of catecholamines.

Anti-asthmatic drugs—bronchodilators

- β_2-adrenoceptor agonists (e.g. salbutamol) are first-line drugs (for details see Ch. 7).
  - —They act as physiological antagonists of the spasmogenic mediators.
  - —Salbutamol is given by inhalation; its effects start immediately and last 3–5 h.
  - —Salbutamol can also be given by intravenous infusion in status asthmaticus.
- Xanthine drugs (e.g. theophylline) are second-line drugs.
  - —The mechanism of action is uncertain but may be by inhibition of cyclic GMP- or cyclic AMP-phosphodiesterase.
  - —Theophylline has a narrow therapeutic window; unwanted effects include chronotropic and inotropic effects on the heart, CNS stimulation and gastrointestinal disturbances.
  - —It is given intravenously (by slow infusion) for status asthmaticus, or orally (as a sustained-release preparation) as a second-line treatment.
  - —It is metabolised in the liver, and liver dysfunction and viral infections increase its plasma concentration and $t_{1/2}$ (normally 12 h with sustained-release preparation).
  - —Drug interactions with theophylline are important, some (e.g. some antibiotics) increase the $t_{1/2}$, others (e.g. antiepileptic drugs) decrease it.
- Muscarinic-receptor antagonists (e.g. ipratropium bromide) are second-line drugs (see Ch. 6 for details).
  - —Ipratropium bromide binds to all muscarinic receptor subtypes (M_1, M_2 and M_3); it inhibits acetylcholine-mediated bronchospasm.
  - —It is given by aerosol inhalation.

Unwanted effects

When theophylline is used in asthma, most of its other effects, such as those on the CNS, cardiovascular system and gastrointestinal tract, are unwanted side effects. Furthermore, theophylline has a relatively low therapeutic index; the concentration range for an optimum therapeutic effect is 30–100 μmol/l, and adverse effects are likely to occur with concentrations greater than 110 μmol/l. There are various immunoassay techniques for measuring the theophylline concentration in the plasma (see Ch. 3). Gastrointestinal symptoms (anorexia, nausea and vomiting) and nervousness and tremor are sometimes seen with concentrations only slightly higher than the clinically effective levels. Serious cardiovascular and CNS effects can occur when the plasma concentration exceeds 200 μmol/l. The most serious cardiovascular effect is arrhythmia, which can be fatal. In children, seizures can occur with theophylline concentrations at or slightly above the upper limit of the therapeutic range. Seizures can be fatal in patients with respiratory compromise due to severe asthma. These CNS effects *may* be related to the decrease in cerebral blood flow reported with theophylline, and/or to adenosine antagonism. Enprofylline has neither of these latter actions but whether it does or does not cause the unwanted CNS effects has yet to be established. Unwanted effects reported with enprofylline are headache, nausea and gastrointestinal upsets.

Clinical use of theophylline

- As a second-line drug in asthma therapy, i.e. as an alternative, or in addition, to steroids and other anti-asthmatic agents in patients whose asthma does not respond adequately to β_2-adrenoceptor agonists.
- To reduce symptoms of chronic obstructive pulmonary disease.

Pharmacokinetic aspects

Xanthine drugs are given orally; it is not feasible to give them by inhalation. Rapid-release oral preparations are rarely used now because of the possibility of side effects. Sustained-release preparations have a lower incidence of side effects and furthermore result in effective plasma concentrations for as long as 12 hours. Aminophylline can also be given by *slow* intravenous injection of a loading dose followed by intravenous infusion, in the treatment of *status asthmaticus*.

Theophylline and enprofylline are both well absorbed from the gastrointestinal tract. Theophylline is metabolised in the liver and enprofylline is excreted unchanged in the urine. The plasma half-life of theophylline, based on studies with rapid-release preparations, is about 8 hours in adults but is less than half this in children, and is about 12 hours with the preferred sustained-release preparations. (But note that plasma clearance of theophylline varies widely in different subjects.) The half-life of enprofylline is 2 hours.

The half life of theophylline is *increased* in liver disease, cardiac failure, and viral infections and is *decreased* in heavy cigarette smokers and drinkers. Theophylline is implicated as a culprit in many unwanted drug interactions. Its serum concentration is increased by drugs such as **oral contraceptives**, **erythromycin**, **ciprofloxacin**, **calcium-channel blockers**, **fluconazole** and **cimetidine** (but not **ranitidine**); its serum concentration is decreased by drugs such as **rifampicin**, **phenobarbital**, **phenytoin** and **carbamazepine**. Cognisance should be taken of these factors in view of the narrowness of the range of safe and effective therapeutic concentrations.

The clinical use of theophylline is summarised on this page.

Muscarinic-receptor antagonists

Muscarinic-receptor antagonists are dealt with in detail in Chapter 6. The main compound used specifically as an anti-asthmatic is **ipratropium bromide** (see below). Oxitropium is also available. Ipratropium relaxes bronchial constriction caused by increased tone due to parasympathetic stimulation; this occurs particularly in asthma produced by irritant stimuli (see p. 354) and can occur in allergic asthma.

Ipratropium is a quaternary derivative of N-isopropylatropine. It does not discriminate between muscarinic receptor subtypes (see Ch. 6), and it is likely that its blockade of M_2-autoreceptors on the cholinergic nerves increases acetylcholine release and reduces the effectiveness of its antagonism at the M_3-receptors on the smooth muscle. It is not particularly effective against allergen challenge but it inhibits the augmentation of mucus secretion which occurs in asthma and may increase the mucociliary clearance of bronchial secretions. It has no effect on the late inflammatory phase of asthma.

It is given by aerosol inhalation. It is not well absorbed into the circulation and thus does not have much action at muscarinic receptors other than those in the bronchi. It does not cross the blood–brain barrier to any great extent. The maximum effect is not seen until after 30 minutes or so, but then lasts for 3–5 hours. It has few unwanted effects and is, in general, safe and well tolerated. It can be used with β_2-adrenoceptor agonists.

Clinical use of ipratropium bromide

- As an adjunct to β_2-adrenoceptor antagonists and steroids when these on their own do not control asthma.
- As a bronchodilator in some cases of chronic bronchitis, and in bronchospasm precipitated by β_2-adrenoceptor antagonists.

DRUGS USED TO TREAT ASTHMA—ANTI-INFLAMMATORY AGENTS

Glucocorticoids

Glucocorticoids are dealt with in detail in Chapter 21 (p. 435). They are not bronchodilators and are not effective in the treatment of the immediate response to the eliciting agent. In the management of chronic asthma, in which there is a predominant inflammatory component, their efficacy is unequivocal.

The basis of their anti-inflammatory action is discussed on page 438. Of relevance for asthma is the fact that they inhibit the generation not only of leucocyte chemotaxins such as LTB_4 and PAF (Fig. 11.5), thus reducing recruitment and activation of inflammatory cells, but also of the spasmogens, LTC_4 and LTD_4, and the vasodilators, PGE_2 and PGI_2. Bronchoalveolar lavage studies have shown that they inhibit the allergen-induced influx of eosinophils into the lung. They can up-regulate β_2-receptors, decrease microvascular permeability and reduce mediator release from eosinophils. Glucocorticoids decrease the eosinophil response to the cytokine GM-CSF and reduce the formation of various other cytokines. The reduction in the synthesis of IL-3 (the lymphokine which regulates mast cell production) may explain why *long-term* steroid treatment eventually reduces the early-phase response to allergens and prevents exercise-induced asthma.

The main compounds used are **beclomethasone**, and **budesonide**, which are given by inhalation with a metered-dose inhaler, the full effect being attained only after several days of therapy.

For chronic asthma and acute, severe or rapidly deteriorating asthma, a short course of an *oral* glucocorticoid (e.g. **prednisolone**) is indicated, combined with an inhaled steroid to reduce the oral dose required. In *status asthmaticus*, **hydrocortisone** is given intravenously followed by oral prednisolone.

Unwanted effects are uncommon with inhaled steroids. Oropharyngeal candidiasis, i.e. thrush (Ch. 39), can occur, as can dysphonia (voice problems), but these are less likely to occur if 'spacing' devices are used which decrease oropharyngeal deposition of the drug and increase airway deposition. Regular large doses can produce adrenal suppression, particularly in children, and necessitate the carrying of a 'steroid card' (see p. 442). The unwanted effects of oral glucocorticoids are given on page 441; these can sometimes occur with inhaled steroids if part of an inhaled dose is ingested. A recently introduced inhalation steroid, **fluticasone proprionate**, might overcome this problem as it has limited absorption from the gastrointestinal tract and undergoes almost complete first-pass metabolism.

Sodium cromoglycate

Sodium cromoglycate is unique in that it was first tested—and its efficacy demonstrated—in allergic asthma in man, without prior testing in animals.

Actions and mechanisms of action

Sodium cromoglycate and the related drug, **nedocromil sodium**, are not bronchodilators and they do not have any direct effects on smooth muscle, nor do they inhibit the actions of any of the known smooth muscle stimulants. If given prophylactically they can reduce both the immediate and the late-phase asthmatic responses and reduce bronchial hyper-responsiveness. They are effective in antigen-induced, exercise-induced and irritant-induced asthma, though not all asthmatic subjects respond, and it is not possible to predict which patients will benefit. It is generally said that children are more likely to respond, and these agents have become the anti-inflammatory drugs of first choice in children.

The mechanism of action is not fully understood. Cromoglycate was originally thought to act as a 'mast cell stabiliser', preventing histamine release from mast cells. However, although it has this effect it is clearly not the basis of its action in asthma because at least 20 other compounds have been produced, by various pharmaceutical companies, which are equally potent or more potent than cromoglycate at inhibiting mast cell histamine release but none have proved to have any anti-asthmatic effect at all in man.

There is evidence that cromoglycate depresses the exaggerated neuronal reflexes (including the axon reflexes involving excitatory neuropeptides) that are triggered by stimulation of the 'irritant receptors'; it suppresses the response of sensory C fibres to the irritant, capsaicin, and may inhibit the release of preformed T cell cytokines. There is some evidence that it acts as a tachykinin antagonist. A depressant effect on the interaction of PAF with eosinophils may be of significance and various other effects on the inflammatory cells and mediators involved in asthma have been described. (See review by Garland 1991.)

Pharmacokinetic aspects

Cromoglycate is extremely poorly absorbed from the gastrointestinal tract. It is given by inhalation as an aerosol, as a nebulised solution or in powder form; about 10% is absorbed into the circulation when it is given in this way. It is excreted unchanged—50% in the bile and 50% in the urine. Its half-life in the plasma is 90 minutes.

Unwanted effects

Unwanted effects are few and consist mostly of the effects of irritation in the upper respiratory tract. Hypersensitivity reactions have been reported (urticaria, anaphylaxis), but are rare.

Histamine H_1-receptor antagonists

Although mast cell mediators are thought to play a part in the immediate phase of allergic asthma (Fig. 17.2) and in some types of exercise-induced asthma, histamine H_1-receptor antagonists have had no place in therapy. Recently, well-controlled trials have shown that the newer, non-sedating antihistamines, such as **terfenadine** and **cetirizine** (see p. 261), are reasonably effective in mild atopic asthma. Other agents—**azelastine** and **ketotifen**—in which some degree of antihistamine activity has been combined with other actions, have also been assessed.

Azelastine is said to inhibit histamine release from human basophils, oxygen radical production in neutrophils, and leukotriene C_4 synthesis in guinea-pig and rat tissue. In early clinical trials it has been reported to decrease daily asthmatic attacks and reduce the level of concomitant therapy.

Ketotifen is a 5-hydroxytryptamine antagonist (Ch. 8) with some degree of H_1-receptor antagonism. It has been reported to result in some reduction in the delayed phase of airway obstruction in asthma. It is given orally and its full action is not expressed for 3–4 weeks. The main unwanted effect is drowsiness, which is less of a problem in children. The results of controlled clinical trials have been equivocal, but it may have a place in the treatment of mild childhood asthma.

Anti-asthmatic drugs—anti-inflammatory agents

Glucocorticoids (for details see Ch. 21)
- These reduce the inflammatory component in chronic asthma and are life-saving in acute severe asthma.
- They are not effective in the treatment of the immediate response to the eliciting agent.
- The mechanism of action involves decreased generation of PAF, LTC_4 and LTD_4 (see Fig. 11.5), reduced formation of cytokines and decreased activation of eosinophils and other inflammatory cells.
- They are given by inhalation (e.g. beclomethasone); systemic toxic effects are rare, but oral thrush and voice problems can occur. In deteriorating asthma, a glucocorticoid (e.g. oral prednisolone or intravenous hydrocortisone) is also given.

Sodium cromoglycate
- Given prophylactically this can prevent both phases of asthma and reduce bronchial hyper-responsiveness in many but not all patients.
- It is the anti-inflammatory drug of choice for asthma in children.
- The mechanism of action is uncertain. Depression of axon reflex release of neuropeptides, antagonism of tachykinin receptors, inhibition of cytokine release and inhibition of PAF interaction with platelets and eosinophils may be important; mast cell stabilisation is not.
- It is given by inhalation.
- Unwanted effects are minor respiratory tract irritation and (rarely) hypersensitivity.

SEVERE ACUTE ASTHMA (*STATUS ASTHMATICUS*)

Severe acute asthma is a medical emergency requiring hospitalisation. Treatment includes oxygen, inhalation of **salbutamol** in oxygen given by nebuliser, and intravenous **hydrocortisone** followed by a course of oral **prednisolone**. Additional measures include nebulised **muscarinic antagonist**, intravenous salbutamol or **aminophylline** and **antibiotics** (if bacterial infection is present).

POSSIBLE FUTURE STRATEGIES FOR ASTHMA THERAPY

Of the currently used anti-asthmatic drugs, none is ideal in that none actually 'cures' all patients of the disease. The glucocorticoids are the most active in this regard but they have potentially serious unwanted effects. Ideally what are required are new anti-inflammatory agents that are active by the oral route and that do not have the drawbacks of steroid drugs.

Several potentially useful compounds are in development.

New bronchodilators

LTD_4-receptor antagonists. Several LTD_4-receptor antagonists are in clinical trial. **Accolate** is a high affinity competitive antagonist at the LTD_4-receptor. It is given orally and has good bioavailability. It prevents antigen-induced and exercise-induced bronchospasm and relaxes the airways in mild asthma. Its bronchodilator activity is one-third that of salbutamol and its effects are additive with β_2-receptor agonists. **Pranlukast** is another LTD_4-receptor antagonist currently undergoing clinical investigation.

New anti-inflammatory drugs

5-lipoxygenase inhibitors. Several 5-lipoxygenase inhibitors are in clinical trial. These agents prevent the production of not only the spasmogenic leukotrienes LTC_4 and LTD_4, but also LTB_4, which is probably the main chemotaxin that recruits leucocytes into the bronchial mucosa and then activates them (see Ch. 11). **Zileutin** is the prototype compound. It blocks antigen- and exercise-induced bronchospasm and may inhibit or reduce late phase inflammation. It is given orally but has low potency and is short-lived, necessitating large doses three to four times daily. Other similar compounds which are more potent and longer-acting are in the pipeline. Also under investigation are agents with 5-lipoxygenase inhibitory activity by virtue of an action on FLAP, the membrane protein with which the enzyme needs to be associated in order to act on arachidonate (see Ch. 11).

New cyclic nucleotide phosphodiesterase inhibitors. Inhibitors of type IV phosphodiesterase, selective for inflammatory cells, are being developed in the hope that they will be an improvement on the currently used xanthines (see Nicholson & Shahid 1994).

PAF antagonists. So far, compounds with PAF antagonism have not been successful in clinical trials, but it may be that newer ones could prove to be useful.

DRUGS USED FOR COUGH

Cough is a protective reflex mechanism, the purpose of which is to remove foreign material and secretions from the bronchi and bronchioles. It may be inappropriately stimulated by inflammation in the respiratory tract or neoplasia. In these cases *antitussive* (or cough suppressant) drugs are sometimes used, for example for the dry painful cough associated with inflammation of the pleura or with bronchial carcinoma. It should be understood that these drugs merely suppress the symptom without influencing the underlying condition. In cough associated with bronchiectasis (suppurating bronchial inflammation) or chronic bronchitis, antitussive drugs can cause harmful sputum thickening and retention; they should not be used for the cough associated with asthma.

Antitussive drugs act by an ill-defined effect in the brainstem, depressing an even more poorly defined 'cough centre'. The **narcotic analgesics** (see Ch. 31) have effective antitussive action in doses below those required for pain relief, and various isomers of these agents, which are neither analgesic nor addictive, are also effective against cough. New opioid analogues which suppress cough by inhibiting release of excitatory neuropeptides through an action on μ-receptors (see Table 31.2) on sensory nerves in the bronchi are being assessed.

Codeine

Codeine, or methylmorphine, is one of the opium alkaloids (see Ch. 31). It has considerably less addiction liability than the main opioid analgesics and is an effective cough suppressant. However, it also decreases secretions in the bronchioles, which thickens sputum, and inhibits ciliary activity, which reduces clearance of the thickened sputum. Constipation also occurs because of the well-known action of opiates on the gastrointestinal tract (see Chs 19 and 31).

Dextromethorphan

Dextromethorphan is related to levorphanol, a synthetic narcotic analgesic. Its antitussive potency is equivalent to that of codeine and it produces only marginally less constipation and inhibition of mucociliary clearance.

Pholcodine (β-morpholinylethylmorphine), which is a non-analgesic opium alkaloid of the same chemical class as papaverine, is also used as a cough suppressant.

ADULT RESPIRATORY DISTRESS SYNDROME

The adult respiratory distress syndrome is a serious disease of the lungs which has a 60% mortality. It affects 150 000 individuals in the USA each year. It is characterised by pulmonary arterial hypertension with vasoconstriction. There is extensive injury and occlusion of the pulmonary microvasculature resulting in oedema and progressive hypoxia. Multiorgan dysfunction follows. Its causes are many and various: direct injury to the lungs (pneumonia, aspiration of gastric contents, inhalation of toxic chemicals) or systemic disorders (sepsis, drug reactions). A variety of inflammatory mediators are involved in the microvascular damage and neutrophils are known to play a significant part through the generation of toxic oxygen radicals and the release of elastase. The marginated pool of neutrophils in the lung may be of relevance here (see p. 351). Early clinical studies suggest that inhalation of **nitric oxide** is beneficial (see p. 210).

REFERENCES AND FURTHER READING

Alabaster V A, Moore B A 1993 Drug intervention in asthma: present and future. Thorax 48: 176–182

Aronson J K, Hardman M, Reynolds D J M 1992 Theophylline. Br Med J 305: 1355–1358

Banner A S 1994 Theophylline: should we discard an old friend? Lancet 343: 618–619

Barnes P J 1989 Muscarinic receptor subtypes. Thorax 44: 161–167

Barnes P J 1992 Neural mechanisms in asthma. Br Med Bull 48: 150–168

Barnes P J 1993 Anti-inflammatory therapy for asthma. Annu Rev Med 44: 229–242

Barnes P J, Lee T H 1992 Recent advances in asthma. Postgrad Med J 68: 942–953

Boggs P B 1989 The changing role of antihistamines in asthma. Ann Allergy 63: 450–451

Bone R C 1993 A new therapy for the adult respiratory distress syndrome. N Engl J Med 328: 431–432

Bosquet J, Chauez P et al. 1990 Eosinophilic inflammation in asthma. N Engl J Med 323: 1033–1039

British Thoracic Society and Others 1993 Guidelines for management of asthma: a summary. Br Med J 306: 776–782

Britton J 1992 Asthma's changing prevalence. Br Med J 304: 857–858

Bruijnzeel P L B 1989 Contribution of eosinophil-derived mediators in asthma. Int Arch Allergy Appl Immunol 90: 57–63

Buist A S 1988 Is asthma mortality increasing? Chest 93: 449–450

Burney P G J, Chinn S, Rona R J 1990 Has the prevalence of asthma increased in children? Evidence from the national study of health and growth 1973–86. Br Med J 300: 1306–1310

Burrows B, Lebowitz M D 1992 The β-agonist dilemma. N Engl J Med 326: 560–561

Chapman K R, Bryant D et al. 1989 A placebo-controlled dose–response study of enprofylline in the maintenance therapy of asthma. Am Rev Resp Dis 139: 688–693

Cockroft D W, O'Byrne P M 1993 Mechanisms of airway hyper-responsiveness. In: Weiss E B, Stein M S (eds) Bronchial asthma: mechanisms and therapeutics, 3rd edn. Little Brown, Boston, ch 4: 32–42

Cockroft D W, McParland C P et al. 1993 Regular inhaled salbutamol and airway responsiveness to allergen. Lancet 342: 833–837

Controversies in Therapeutics 1990 Theophylline in the management of airflow obstruction. (1) Addis G J: Much evidence suggests that theophylline is valuable. (2) Johnston I D A: Difficult drugs to use, few clinical indications. (3) Rubin P C: (Editorial comment) In: Br Med J 300: 928–931

Corrigan C J, Kay A B 1992 T cells and eosinophils in the pathogenesis of asthma. Immunol Today 13: 501–507

Crimi E, Brusasco V, Crimi P 1989 Effect of nedocromil sodium on the late asthmatic reaction to bronchial allergen challenge. J Allergy Clin Immunol 5: 985–990

Crossman D C, Dashwood M R et al. 1993 Sodium cromoglycate: evidence of tachykinin antagonist activity in human skin. J Appl Physiol 75: 167–172

Dale M M, Hirst S J 1993 Advances in receptor biochemistry. In: Weiss E B, Stein M S 1993 (eds) Bronchial asthma: mechanisms and therapeutics, 3rd edn. Little Brown, Boston, ch 16: 203–216

Editorial 1992 Steroids in acute severe asthma. Lancet 340: 1384–1385

Garland L G 1991 Pharmacology of prophylactic anti-asthma drugs. In: Page C P, Barnes P J (eds) Handbook of experimental pharmacology. Springer-Verlag, Berlin, vol 98, ch 9: 261–290

Garland L G, Adcock J J 1991 New drugs for asthma therapy. Agents Actions Suppl 34: 497–517

Gleich G J 1990 The eosinophil and bronchial asthma: current understanding. J Allergy Clin Immunol 85: 422–436

Goyal R K 1989 Muscarinic receptor subtypes. N Engl J Med 321: 1022–1029

Gross N J 1988 Ipratropium bromide. N Engl J Med 319: 486–494

Gross N J 1993 Anticholinergic agents. In: Weiss E B, Stein M S (eds) Bronchial asthma: mechanisms and therapeutics, 3rd edn. Little Brown, Boston, ch 64: 876–883

Holgate S 1993 Mediator and cytokine mechanisms in asthma. Thorax 48: 103–109

International Consensus Report on the Diagnosis and Management of Asthma 1992 Clin Exp Allergy 22 (Suppl): 1–72

Jenne J J, Tashkin D P 1993 Beta-adrenergic agonists. In: Weiss E B, Stein M S (eds) Bronchial asthma: mechanisms and therapeutics, 3rd edn. Little Brown, Boston, ch 55: 700–748

Kay A B 1989 Inflammatory cells in chronic asthma. Agents Actions Suppl 28: 147–161

McCarthy D A, Dale M M 1988 The leucocytosis of exercise: a review and model. Sports Med 6: 333–363

McFadden E R, Gilbert I A 1992 Asthma. N Engl J Med 327: 1928–1937

Malo J-L, Cartier A 1993 Late asthmatic reactions. In: Weiss E B, Stein M S (eds) Bronchial asthma: mechanisms and therapeutics, 3rd edn. Little Brown, Boston, ch 12: 135–146

Milgrom H, Bender B 1993 Current issues in the use of theophylline. Am Rev Resp Dis 147: 533–539

Morley J, Smith D 1989 Lung inflammation, its significance for asthma therapy. Agents Actions 26: 32–39

Neville R G, Clark R C et al. 1993 National asthma attack audit, 1991–1992. Br Med J 306: 559–562

Nicholson C D, Shahid M 1994 Inhibitors of cyclic nucleotide phosphodieterase isoenzymes—their potential utility in the therapy of asthma. Pulmonary Pharmacol 7: 1–17

Page C 1994 Sodium cromoglycate, a tachykinin antagonist? Lancet 343: 70

Page C P, Morley J 1993 Platelet-activating factor, platelets, and asthma. In: Weiss E B, Stein M S (eds) Bronchial asthma: mechanisms and therapeutics, 3rd edn. Little Brown, Boston, ch 22: 287–295

Pauwels R A 1989 New aspects of the therapeutic potential of theophylline in asthma. J Allergy Clin Immunol 83: 548–553

Persson C G A 1987 The pharmacology of anti-asthmatic xanthines and the role of adenosine. Asthma Rev 1: 61–93

Rossing T H 1989 Methylxanthines in 1989. Ann Intern Med 110: 502–504

Salmon J A, Garland L G 1991 Leukotriene antagonists and inhibitors of leukotriene biosynthesis as potential therapeutic agents. Prog Drug Res 37: 10–80

Taylor I K, Shaw R J 1993 The mechanism of action of corticosteroids in asthma. Resp Med 87: 261–277

US Department of Health and Human Services Bethesda Maryland 1991 Guidelines for the diagnosis and management of asthma. Publication No. 91-3042

Weinberger M E 1993 Methylxanthines. In: Weiss E B, Stein M S 1993 (eds) Bronchial asthma: mechanisms and therapeutics, 3rd edn. Little Brown, Boston, ch 58: 764–784

Weinberger S E 1993 Recent advances in pulmonary medicine. N Engl J Med 328: 1389–1397

Weiss E B, Stein M S 1993 (eds) Bronchial asthma: mechanisms and therapeutics, 3rd edn. Little Brown, Boston

Widdicombe J G 1987 Nervous control of airway tone. In: Nadel J A, Pauwels R, Snashall P D (eds) Bronchial hyper-responsiveness. Blackwell Scientific Publications, Oxford, p 46–67

18
THE KIDNEY

The main function of the kidney is the excretion of waste products such as urea, uric acid and creatinine. In the course of this activity it fulfils another function, crucially important in homeostasis—the regulation of the salt and electrolyte content and the volume of the extracellular fluid. It also plays a part in acid–base balance.

The kidneys receive about a quarter of the cardiac output. From the several hundred litres of plasma which flow through them each day, they filter an amount equivalent to about 15 times the extracellular fluid volume. This filtrate is similar in composition to plasma, the main difference being that it has very little protein or protein-bound substances. As it passes through the renal tubule, about 99% of it is reabsorbed while some substances are secreted, and eventually about 1.5 litres of the filtered fluid are voided as urine (Table 18.1).

The most important group of drugs employed for their effect on the kidney are the **diuretics**. In essence, these drugs increase the excretion of salt and water. They are employed mainly in the therapy of heart failure and other causes of salt and water retention (often manifested clinically as oedema, a condition in which there is an accumulation of extracellular fluid); but have another important use

Table 18.1 Reabsorption of fluid and solute in the kidney

	Filtered/day	Excreted/day	% reabsorbed
NaCl	20 000 mEq	110 mEq	99+
$NaHCO_3$	5000 mEq	2 mEq	99+
K^+	700 mEq	50 mEq	93+
H_2O	170 l	1.5 l	99+

Renal blood flow = 1200 ml/min (20–25% of cardiac output).
Renal plasma flow = 660 ml/min.
Glomerular filtration rate = 125 ml/min.

in the treatment of hypertension (see Ch. 14). Drugs may also be used to alter the pH of the urine and to modify the excretion of some organic compounds such as uric acid.

In structure, each kidney consists of an outer cortex, an inner medulla and a hollow pelvis which empties into the ureter. The functional unit is the nephron, of which there are about 1.3×10^6 in each kidney.

THE STRUCTURE AND FUNCTION OF THE NEPHRON

The nephron consists of a glomerulus, proximal convoluted tubule, loop of Henle, distal tubule and collecting duct (Fig. 18.1). The glomerulus comprises a tuft of capillaries projecting into a dilated end of the renal tubule. Most nephrons lie largely or entirely in the cortex. The remaining 12%, called the juxtamedullary nephrons, have their renal glomeruli and convoluted tubules next to the junction of the medulla and cortex, and their loops of Henle pass deep into the medulla.

The blood supply to the nephron

The nephron possesses the special characteristic of

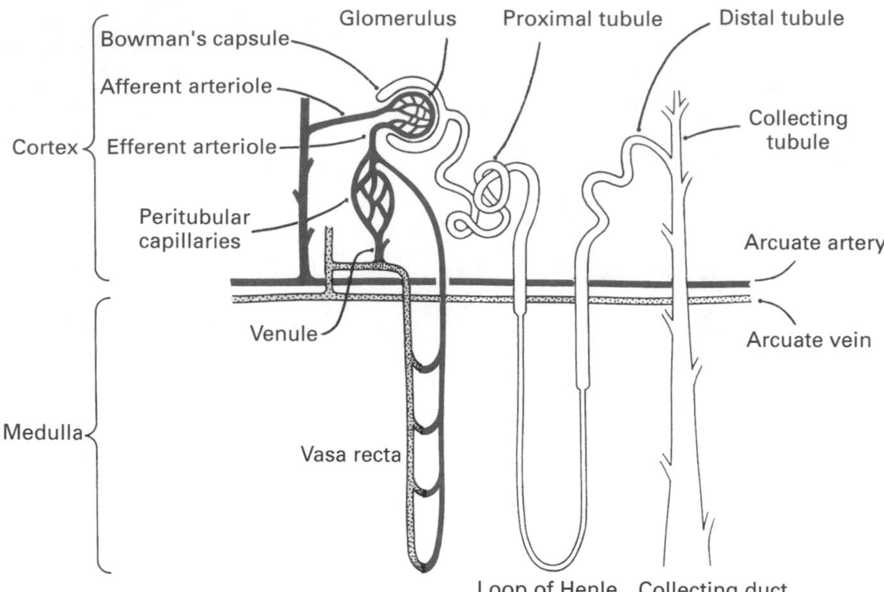

Fig. 18.1 Simplified diagram of a juxtamedullary nephron and its blood supply. The tubules and the blood vessels are shown separately for clarity. In the kidney the peritubular capillary network surrounds the convoluted tubules, and the distal convoluted tubule passes close to the glomerulus, between the afferent and efferent arterioles. (This last is shown in more detail in Fig. 18.2.)

having two capillary beds in series with each other (see Fig. 18.1). For those nephrons which lie entirely in the cortex, the afferent arterioles branch to form the capillaries of the glomerulus; these empty into the efferent arterioles which in turn branch to form a second capillary network in the cortex, around the convoluted tubules and loops of Henle of other nephrons, before emptying into the veins. In the case of the juxtamedullary nephrons, some of the branches of the afferent arterioles bypass the convoluted tubules, and instead form bundles of vessels which pass deep into the medulla with the thin loops of Henle. These loops of vessels are called *vasa recta* and they have a role in counter-current exchange (see p. 373).

The juxtaglomerular apparatus

A conjunction of afferent arteriole, efferent arteriole and distal convoluted tubule near the glomerulus comprises the *juxtaglomerular apparatus* (Fig. 18.2). At this site there are specialised cells in both the afferent arteriole and in the tubule. The latter, termed *macula densa* cells, are able to respond to changes in the rate of flow and the composition of tubule fluid, and are thought to control renin release from the specialised granular renin-containing cells

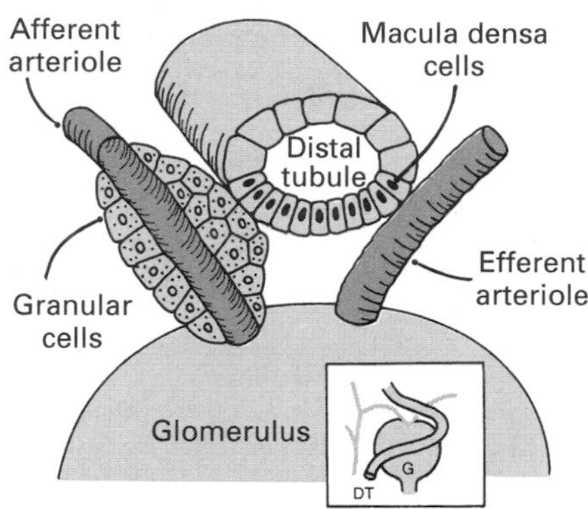

Fig. 18.2 The juxtaglomerular apparatus. The cutaway sections show the granular renin-containing cells round the afferent arteriole, and the *macula densa* cells in the distal convoluted tubule. The inset shows the general relationships between the structures. (G = glomerulus; DT = distal tubule) (Modified from: Sullivan & Grantham 1982)

in the afferent arteriole (Ch. 14). The juxtaglomerular apparatus is important in controlling the blood flow to the nephron and the glomerular filtration rate. Factors extrinsic to the kidney can influence these processes through circulating hormones and through noradrenergic sympathetic fibres which supply the afferent and efferent arterioles and the specialised cells. They will thus influence the generation of angiotensin I and II. The role of the juxtaglomerular apparatus in the control of sodium balance is dealt with below, and its role in cardiovascular dynamics is considered in Chapter 14.

Glomerular filtration

Fluid is driven from the capillaries into the tubular capsule (Bowman's capsule) by hydrodynamic force. It crosses three layers: the capillary endothelium, the basement membrane, and the epithelial cell layer of the capsule. These form a complex filter which excludes large molecules. Normally, all constituents in the plasma, except the plasma proteins, appear in the filtrate, and the blood which passes on through the efferent arteriole to the peritubular capillaries has a higher concentration of plasma proteins and thus a higher oncotic pressure than normal. (The term 'oncotic pressure' refers to osmotic pressure contributed by large molecules such as the plasma proteins.)

TUBULAR FUNCTION

In the epithelium of the tubules, as in all epithelia, the apex or luminal surface of each cell is surrounded by a *zonula occludens*, a specialised region of membrane which forms a tight junction between it and neighbouring cells, and which separates the intercellular space from the lumen (see Fig. 18.11). The movement of ions and water across the epithelium can occur both through the cells (the transcellular pathway) and between the cells through the *zonulae occludentes* (the paracellular pathway). The *zonulae* in different parts of the nephron vary in their degree of functional tightness, i.e. their relative permeability to ions. The tightness or leakiness of the epithelium of various portions of the nephron is an important factor in their function (see Taylor & Palmer 1982). Tight epithelium is found in the distal portion of the nephron, which is the site of action of the major hormones involved in the control of salt and water excretion.

Normally, 70–75% of the volume of the filtrate is absorbed back into the blood in the proximal convoluted tubule, with virtually no change in the sodium concentration or the osmotic pressure of the remaining tubular fluid. In the rest of the renal tubule the electrolyte concentrations and osmotic pressure of the filtrate vary a great deal due to differential absorption of salt and water and the effects of the antidiuretic hormone (ADH), mineralocorticoids and the counter-current system in the medulla.

A detailed account of the renal handling of sodium, chloride, water, amino acids and glucose is given by Burg (1985).

The proximal convoluted tubule

The apical or luminal surface of the cells of this part of the tubule is extensively increased by numerous microvilli, forming a brush border, and the surface area is increased by numerous ridges and folds (Fig. 18.3). The epithelium is 'leaky', i.e. the *zonula occludens* is permeable to ions and water and permits passive flows in either direction. This prevents the build-up of significant ionic or osmotic gradients; separate regulation of the movements of ions and water occurs mainly in the distal part of the tubule.

A simplified diagram of the main transport processes in the proximal tubule is given in Figure 18.4.

About 60–70% of the sodium in the filtrate is

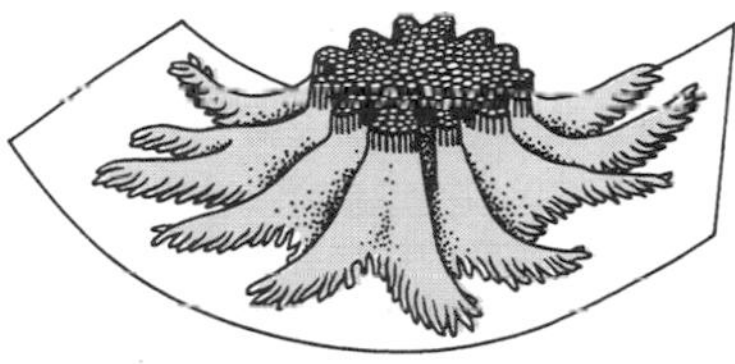

Fig. 18.3 Simplified three-dimensional reconstruction of a cell in the proximal convoluted tubule. (Modified from: Sullivan & Grantham 1982)

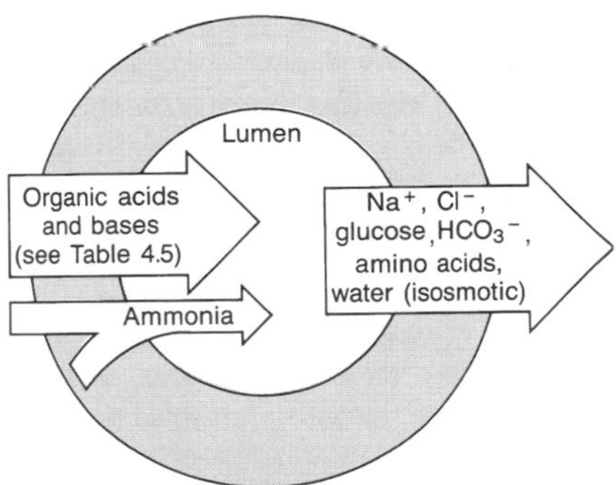

Fig. 18.4 The main transport processes in the proximal convoluted tubule. The main driving force for the absorption of solutes and water from the lumen is the Na^+/K^+-ATPase in the basolateral membrane of the tubule cells. Many drugs are secreted into the proximal tubule (see Ch. 4). (Redrawn from: Burg 1985)

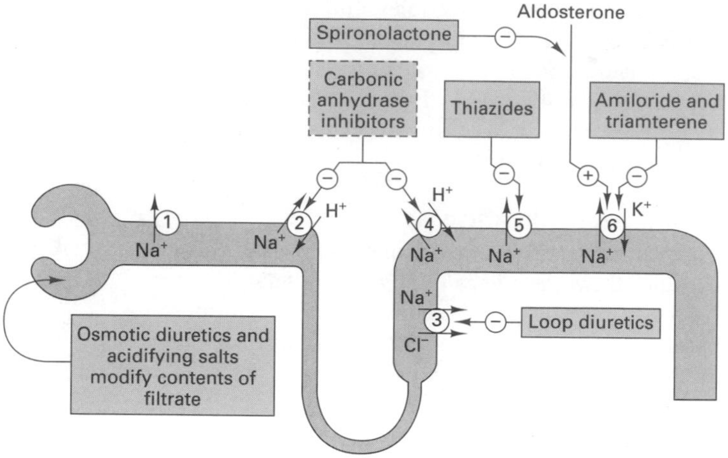

Fig. 18.5 Sodium absorption in the nephron and the main sites of action of drugs. Sites of sodium absorption: (1) Na^+ (passive Cl^- absorption); (2) Na^+/H^+ exchange; (3) Na^+ K^+ $2Cl^-$ co-transport; (4) Na^+/H^+ exchange; (5) Na^+ Cl^- co-transport, (6) Na^+/K^+ exchange. Currently used diuretics are shown in solid boxes, agents not used for their diuretic action in boxes with dotted lines.

reabsorbed in the proximal tubule. It enters the cells passively through the sodium–permeable apical membrane, and is transported out by *the primary active transport mechanism in the nephron*—the Na^+/K^+-ATPase (the sodium pump) in the baso-lateral membrane. Some sodium enters in exchange for hydrogen ions.

Water is reabsorbed as a result of the osmotic force generated by this solute reabsorption, the increased colloid osmotic pressure in the peritubular capillaries contributing to this effect.

The movement of sodium into the cell is coupled to that of other solutes by various *symport* systems.* *Glucose* enters the cell with sodium by such a symport process, the co-transport being driven by the electrochemical gradient for sodium across the apical membrane. There are similar symport processes for various *amino acids* with sodium. It is assumed that in these symport systems there is a two-site carrier in the membrane with one site for sodium and one for glucose or an amino acid. On the luminal side, where the concentration of sodium is high, sodium combines with its specific site and this increases the affinity of the other site for the other solute. Re-orientation of the binding sites to the inner side of the membrane, where the sodium concentration is low, favours dissociation of the sodium and consequently of the other solute.

*In a *symport* or co-transport system, the transport of one substance is coupled to that of another, both being transported across a membrane in the same direction, as opposed to an *antiport* system in which two substances are exchanged across a membrane.

The atrial natriuretic peptide reduces reabsorption of sodium and water in the proximal tubule.

Chloride absorption is largely passive. Some diffuses through the *zonula occludens*.

Many organic acids and bases are actively secreted into the tubule from the blood (see below, Fig. 18.4 and Ch. 4).

Bicarbonate is returned to the plasma by an indirect method involving exchange with hydrogen ions and the action of carbonic anhydrase (for detail see p. 383 and Fig. 18.15). Drugs, such as **acetazolamide**, which inhibit carbonic anhydrase, increase the volume of urine flow (i.e. are diuretic) by preventing bicarbonate reabsorption (Figs 18.5 and 18.15). They also result in a depletion of extracellular bicarbonate.

After passage through the proximal tubule, the remaining 25–30% of the filtrate, which is still isosmotic with plasma, passes on to the loop of Henle.

The loop of Henle

The loop of Henle plays an important part in regulating the osmolarity of the urine, and hence in regulating the osmotic balance of the body as a whole. Its function is summarised in Figure 18.6. The loop consists of a descending and an ascending portion (Figs 18.1 and 18.6), the ascending portion having both thick and thin segments.

The *descending* limb is highly permeable to water, which moves out passively under the influence of osmotic forces. These forces arise because the interstitial fluid of the medulla is hypertonic (see p. 373). In juxtamedullary nephrons with long loops, there

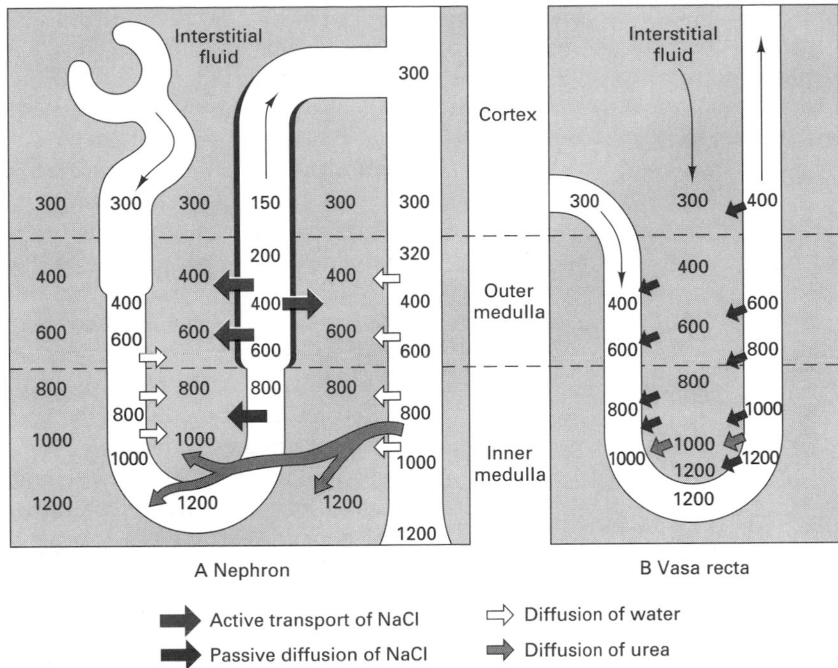

Fig. 18.6 Schematic diagram of the counter-current mechanisms for concentrating the urine. (The figures are in milliosmoles per litre.) **A.** Renal tubules. **B.** Vasa recta.

The main factors are:

- A counter-current multiplier mechanism involving the tubules and a counter-current exchange mechanism involving the vasa recta.
- A source of energy, which is supplied by the sodium pump and the active transport of sodium chloride in the ascending loop of Henle. (Loop diuretics act by inhibiting this active transport, thus interfering with the counter-current concentrating mechanism.)
- Differences in permeability between tubules carrying fluid in opposite directions. The thickened outline of the ascending limb of Henle's loop indicates decreased permeability to water in contrast to the water-permeable descending loop.
- Diffusion of salt into the vessels taking blood down into the medulla, and out of vessels passing back up to the cortex, maintaining hypertonicity in the medulla.

The absorption of water in the collecting ducts is controlled by the antidiuretic hormone. Additional active reabsorption of sodium chloride occurs in the distal tubule and is controlled by aldosterone.

is extensive movement of water out of the tubule (and also movement of urea in) so that the fluid eventually reaching the tip of the loop has a high osmolarity—up to 1500 mosmol/l under conditions of dehydration.

The *ascending* limb has very low permeability to water. In the thick segment of this limb, there is active reabsorption of sodium chloride, not accompanied by water, which reduces the osmolarity of the tubular fluid and makes the interstitial fluid of the medulla hypertonic (Figs 18.5 and 18.6). Sodium and chloride move into the cell by a co-transport system involving Na^+,K^+,$2Cl^-$, this process being driven by the electrochemical gradient for sodium produced by the Na^+/K^+-ATPase in the basolateral membrane. (Loop diuretics inhibit this process as shown in Figs 18.5 and 18.11.) Chloride then passes out of the cell into the circulation, partly by diffusion through chloride channels and partly by a symport mechanism with potassium (see Fig. 18.11). Some sodium diffuses out of the lumen through the *zonula occludens* which in this part of the nephron forms a cation-selective tight junction. Most of the potassium taken into the cell by the co-transport system cycles back to the lumen but some potassium is reabsorbed along with magnesium and calcium.

The tubular fluid, after passage through the loop of Henle, has been reduced in volume by a further 5% and, because of the absorption of salt, it is hypotonic with respect to plasma as it enters the distal convoluted tubule. The thick ascending limb of the loop of Henle is sometimes referred to as the 'diluting segment' because the absorption of salt with very little water results in this marked dilution of the filtrate.

The early distal tubule

In the early distal tubule, active salt transport, coupled with impermeability of the *zonula occludens*, continues to dilute the tubular fluid and the osmolarity falls further below that of plasma. Potassium and hydrogen ions are added to the filtrate. The transport is driven by the sodium–potassium pump in the basolateral membrane, sodium entering the cell from the lumen, accompanied by chloride by means of an electroneutral Na^+Cl^- carrier (Fig. 18.13). **Thiazide diuretics** act by inhibiting this carrier.

This part of the nephron is where calcium excretion is regulated. Parathyroid hormone and calcitriol both increase calcium reabsorption (see Ch. 21, Fig. 21.18).

The collecting tubule and the collecting duct

Several distal tubules empty into each collecting tubule and the collecting tubules join to form collecting ducts (see Fig. 18.1). The collecting tubule has two different cell types: the principal cells that reabsorb sodium and secrete potassium and the intercalated cells that are involved mainly in hydrogen ion secretion. The principal cells have sodium and potassium *channels*, not co-transporters, in the luminal membrane.

This portion of the nephron has 'tight' epithelia, i.e. the *zona occludens* has low permeability to both ions and water. Because of this property, the movement of ions and water can be dissociated and individual regulation of each can be influenced by hormones. The absorption of salt is under the control of the mineralocorticoid, **aldosterone**, and the absorption of water is under the control of the **antidiuretic hormone** (ADH), also termed **vasopressin** (see Chs 14 and 21).

Aldosterone enhances sodium reabsorption and promotes potassium excretion. It has a threefold action on sodium reabsorption. Firstly, according to recent work, it has a rapid effect through stimulation of the Na^+/H^+ exchanger by an action on membrane aldosterone receptors. Secondly, it has a delayed effect by binding to receptors within the cell (see Chs 2 and 21) and directing the synthesis of a specific mediator protein that activates sodium channels in the apical membrane which allow transcellular passage of sodium. **Amiloride** and **triamterene** inhibit these channels as shown in Figures 18.5 and 18.13. Thirdly it exerts long-term effects by increasing the number of the basolateral sodium pumps.

Aldosterone secretion is controlled indirectly by the juxtaglomerular apparatus (see Fig. 18.2) which is sensitive to the composition of the fluid in the distal tubule. A decrease in the sodium chloride concentration of the filtrate is sensed by the *macula densa* cells of the distal tubule, which stimulate renin release. This leads to the formation of angiotensin I and, subsequently, angiotensin II (see Ch. 14), which in turn stimulates the synthesis and release of aldosterone by the adrenal cortex. The renin–angiotensin–aldosterone system and the mechanism of action of aldosterone are considered in more detail in Chapters 14 (p. 313) and 21 (p. 444). **Spironolactone** exerts a diuretic effect by antagonising the action of aldosterone in this part of the nephron; shown in Figure 18.5.

Antidiuretic hormone (ADH) produces a sustained increase in the permeability to water in this part of the nephron, allowing its passive reabsorption. This hormone is secreted by the posterior pituitary gland and binds to receptors in the basolateral membrane. These receptors, which are different from those involved in vascular responses (p. 309), are termed V_2-receptors. The eventual result of stimulation of the V_2-receptors is an increase in the number of water channels in the apical membrane. Microfilaments and microtubules are important in this effect, possibly in the translocation of the vesicles.

An inhibition of the action of ADH is seen as a side effect of some drugs—**lithium carbonate** (used in psychiatric disorders; see Ch. 29), **demeclocycline** (an antibiotic; see Ch. 37) and agents which affect the microtubules such as **colchicine** (Ch. 12) and the **vinca alkaloids** (see Ch. 36).

Urea is reabsorbed from the medullary section of the collecting tubule, and passes into the interstitial tissue where it plays a part in increasing the osmolarity of this area (see Fig. 18.6). *Bicarbonate* is exchanged for hydrogen ions as in the proximal tubule, and carbonic anhydrase inhibitors act by preventing this exchange (see p. 382 and Fig. 18.5).

The main site at which the urine is concentrated is in the collecting tubule as it passes into the medulla where there is passive reabsorption of water due to the increasing osmolarity of the interstitial fluid. This absorption depends on ADH, and in its absence, the low water permeability of the collecting ducts means that the hypo-osmolarity of the distal tubular fluid is maintained as the fluid traverses the collecting ducts, and hypotonic urine is excreted.

Natriuretic peptides

Endogenous natriuretic peptides are involved in the regulation of sodium excretion in the distal nephron. The atrial natriuretic peptide, atriopeptin (see Ch. 14), is released when the atrial pressure is high. It causes solute and water diuresis, thus decreasing blood volume and therefore reducing atrial pressure. This peptide also inhibits the biosynthesis of renin, aldosterone and ADH (reviewed by Cogan 1990). Another peptide, similar to atriopeptin and termed urodilatin, is now thought to be produced in the distal tubule and is believed to promote sodium excretion and produce diuresis by action on receptors on the luminal side of the collecting duct cells.

The counter-current multiplier and exchange system in the medulla

The loops of Henle function as counter-current multipliers and the *vasa recta* as counter-current exchangers. In the ascending limb, salt is actively absorbed in the thick part and passively absorbed in the thin part. *This results in hypertonicity of the interstitial tissue.* In the descending limb, water moves out of the tubule and the fluid becomes more concentrated as it reaches the bend. There is thus an osmotic gradient in the medulla which ranges from isotonicity (300 mosmol/l) at the cortical boundary to 1200–1500 mosmol/l or more in the innermost area (see Fig. 18.6). Urea contributes to this gradient because it is more slowly reabsorbed than water throughout most of the nephron (it may be *added* to the fluid in the descending limb; Fig. 18.6) and so its concentration rises until it reaches the collecting tubules in the medulla where it diffuses out into the interstitia. It is thus 'trapped' in the inner medulla.

These differences in salt concentration are the basis of the counter-current multiplier system, the main principle being that a small horizontal osmotic gradient is multiplied vertically (see Fig. 18.6). The primary generating force is the active reabsorption of salt in the ascending limb of the loop of Henle.

The osmotic gradient would be dissipated if all the excess salt in the medulla were carried away by the blood vessels. This does not happen because the vasa recta function as counter-current exchangers in that salt diffuses passively out of the vessels which take blood to the cortex and into those which descend into the medulla (Fig. 18.6), while water diffuses out of the descending and into the ascending vessels.

Renal tubular function

- All the constituents of the plasma, other than proteins, are filtered into the tubules.
- Transport of sodium out of the tubules by the Na^+/K^+-ATPase in the basolateral membrane is the main primary active transport process throughout the tubules.
- In the proximal tubules, 75% of the filtrate is reabsorbed isosmotically and organic acids and bases are secreted into the tubular lumen.
- In the descending limb of Henle's loop, water is reabsorbed due to hypertonicity in the medulla; fluid of high osmolarity therefore reaches the thick ascending limb.
- The thick ascending limb is impermeable to water, and within it there is active, marked reabsorption of NaCl (the major factor in producing hypertonicity in the medulla). The ions are transported by a Na^+,$2Cl^-$,K^+ carrier (inhibited by loop diuretics). The filtrate is diluted.
- Counter-current mechanisms maintain hypertonicity in the medulla.
- In the distal convoluted tubule there is moderate absorption of Na^+ and Cl^- by an electroneutral carrier (inhibited by thiazides). K^+ is secreted into the tubule.
- The collecting tubules and ducts have low permeability to salts and water. Na^+ is absorbed through Na^+ channels, which are stimulated by the aldosterone mediator (and inhibited by amiloride). Aldosterone also increases the number of basolateral sodium pumps. Water absorption through water channels is stimulated by antidiuretic hormone. K^+ and H^+ are secreted into the tubule.

ACID–BASE BALANCE

The kidneys participate in the regulation of the hydrogen ion concentration of the body fluids.

Though either an acid or alkaline urine can be excreted according to need, the usual requirement is the formation of an acid urine to compensate for the tendency to a decrease in body pH consequent on the metabolic production of CO_2. The main renal mechanism is the secretion of hydrogen ions into the tubular fluid and the conservation of bicarbonate. This depends on the carbonic-anhydrase-catalysed reactions outlined on page 383 and illustrated in Figure 18.15.

POTASSIUM BALANCE

The extracellular potassium concentration is controlled rapidly and within narrow limits through regulation of potassium excretion by the kidney. This regulation is very important because small changes in extracellular [K^+] affect the function of many excitable tissues, particularly the heart, brain and skeletal muscle. Urinary potassium excretion is normally about 50–100 mEq in 24 hours, but can be as low as 5 mEq or as high as 1000 mEq. The amount which normally appears in the urine represents mainly potassium secreted into the filtrate in the collecting tubule, as much of the filtered potassium is reabsorbed in the proximal tubule and loop of Henle. Some diuretics cause significant potassium loss (see below). This may be particularly important if such potassium-losing agents are administered at the same time as cardiac glycosides (whose toxicity is increased by low plasma potassium; see Ch. 13).

In the collecting duct, potassium is transported into the cell from the blood and the interstitial fluid by the Na^+/K^+-ATPase in the basolateral membrane; it then leaks into the tubule through a selective ion channel. This potassium secretory flux is regulated by the extent to which sodium is re-absorbed, because the influx of sodium generates a lumen-negative potential difference across the cell and this increases the driving force for potassium secretion.

It follows that potassium loss will be *increased* in the following circumstances:

- When more sodium reaches the collecting duct—as occurs with the **thiazide** and **loop diuretics**, which decrease sodium absorption in early parts of the nephron and therefore increase its delivery to the collecting ducts (see pp. 378 and 377). (The high flow rate of filtrate produced by these diuretics will also favour potassium excretion by continually flushing it away, increasing the gradient from cell to lumen).
- When sodium reabsorption in the collecting ducts is markedly increased—as occurs in hyperaldosteronism. Aldosterone indirectly increases potassium excretion because of its stimulant effect on sodium uptake (see above). Aldosterone may also directly increase luminal membrane potassium permeability.

Potassium loss will be *reduced* in the following circumstances:

- When sodium reabsorption in the collecting ducts is decreased—as occurs with **amiloride** and **triamterene**, which block the sodium channel in this part of the nephron (see p. 380) and with spironolactone, which blocks the action of aldosterone (see p. 379).

Recent work suggests that the kidney has a previously unsuspected mechanism for primary, active potassium absorption in the collecting duct, possibly by a luminal membrane H^+/K^+-ATPase similar to that on gastric parietal cells.

EXCRETION OF ORGANIC MOLECULES

There are different mechanisms for the excretion of organic anions and organic cations (see Ch. 4).

Organic anions bound to plasma albumin will not appear in the glomerular filtrate, but when the blood from the glomerulus passes into the peritubular capillary plexus some of these substances (e.g. urate) are secreted into the proximal convoluted tubule (Fig. 18.4). Entry into the cell across the basolateral membrane occurs partly by passive, carrier-mediated diffusion down favourable electrical and chemical gradients and partly by active transport. Among the drugs excreted in this way are the **thiazides**, **ethacrynic acid**, **frusemide**, **salicylates** and most **penicillins** and **cephalosporins**.

Organic cations are thought to be secreted by transport processes in both the basolateral and luminal membranes. Some diuretics (**triamterene**, **amiloride**) are added to the tubular fluid in this way and many drugs are eliminated by this route, including **atropine**, **morphine** and **quinine**.

This topic is dealt with in more detail in Chapter 4 (see Table 4.5, p. 88).

ARACHIDONIC ACID METABOLITES AND RENAL FUNCTION

The metabolites of arachidonic acid, the eicosanoids, which are generated in the kidney, are now recognised as modulators of its haemodynamics and excretory functions. Details of the eicosanoids are given in Chapter 11.

Prostanoids, the products of the cyclo-oxygenase pathway, are synthesised in all parts of the kidney, the predominant products being PGE_2 in the medulla and PGI_2 in the glomeruli. Factors which stimulate their synthesis include ischaemia, mechanical trauma, circulating angiotensin II, catecholamines, antidiuretic hormone and bradykinin.

Influence on haemodynamics

Under basal conditions, prostaglandins probably do not have much effect. However, in circumstances in which vasoconstrictor agents (angiotensin II, noradrenaline) are generated and released, the vasodilator prostaglandins, PGE_2 and PGI_2, modulate the effects of these agents in the kidney by causing compensatory vasodilatation. This action is relevant to the unwanted renal effects of some NSAIDs (see Ch. 12, p. 252, and Ch. 43). Prostaglandins play a part in the control of renin release under basal conditions, and also in conditions of intravascular volume depletion.

Influence on the renal control of salt and water

The overall effect of the renal prostaglandins is to increase renal blood flow and cause natriuresis. This can, in some circumstances, be an important consideration when NSAIDs, whose action is inhibition of prostaglandin production (see Ch. 12), are used in therapy. Thus, NSAIDs can cause renal failure in several clinical conditions in which renal blood flow depends on vasodilator prostaglandins, for example cirrhosis of the liver, heart failure, nephrotic syndrome and glomerulonephritis; they exacerbate salt and water retention in patients with heart failure. See also Chapter 43.

DRUGS ACTING ON THE KIDNEY

DIURETICS

Diuretics are drugs which cause a net loss of sodium and water from the body by an action on the kidney. Their primary effect is to decrease the reabsorption of sodium and chloride from the filtrate, increased water loss being secondary to the increased excretion of salt. This can be achieved by:

- a direct action on the cells of the nephron
- indirectly modifying the content of the filtrate.

Since a very large proportion of the salt and water which passes into the tubule in the glomerulus is reabsorbed (Table 18.1), a small decrease in reabsorption can result in a marked increase in excretion. A summary diagram of the mechanisms and sites of action of various diuretics is given in Figure 18.5.

Note that the diuretics which have a direct action on the cells of the nephron (with the exception of spironolactone) act from within the tubular lumen and reach their sites of action by being secreted into the proximal tubule.

THE DEVELOPMENT OF DIURETIC DRUGS

The diuretics used prior to 1920 were **xanthines** (e.g. theophylline and caffeine) and **osmotic diuretics** (e.g. urea). The next group of compounds introduced were the **carbonic-anhydrase inhibitors**. These were developed from the sulphonamides, following on the observation that sulphanilamide (Ch. 37) caused, as a side effect, a mild diuresis.

As a result of further modifications of the original structure, **acetazolamide** (Fig. 18.7) was introduced in 1950. Further molecular modifications, in which diuretic activity was sought rather than carbonic-anhydrase inhibition, resulted in studies of meta-disulphonamides (Fig. 18.7) and gave rise eventually to **chlorothiazide** and **hydrochlorothiazide**, then **bendrofluazide**, the series showing increasing potency in promoting sodium excretion, not accompanied by equivalent potency on potassium excretion (Fig. 18.7). Numerous other similar compounds have been produced.* A by-product of

*It would be apposite to mention, in this context, that molecular modification of a derivative of sulphanilamide gave rise to the oral antidiabetic agents, the sulphonylureas, and that investigation of the goitrogenic action of sulphaguanidine led to the development of the antithyroid drugs thiouracil, propylthiouracil and methimazole (see Ch. 21).

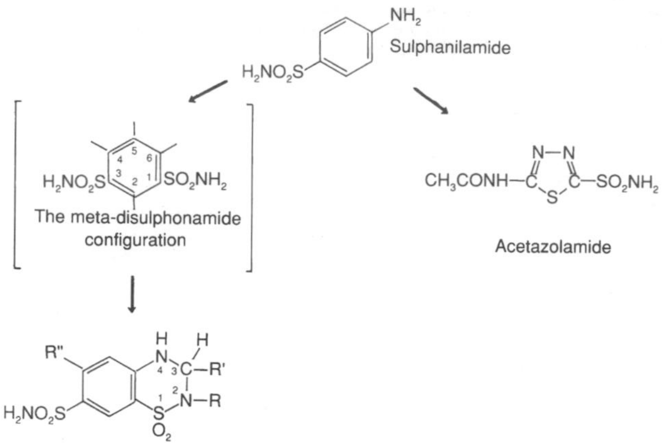

	R	R′	R″	Na	K	Cl
				μEq/min excreted†		
Chlorothiazide*	H	H	Cl	20	24	7
Hydrochlorothiazide	H	H	Cl	265	33	291
Bendrofluazide	H	CH_2–phenyl 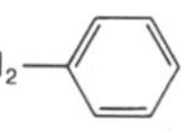	CF_3	493	61	455
Cyclopenthiazide	H	CH_2–cyclopentyl 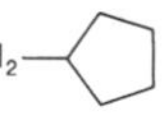	Cl	—	—	—

Fig. 18.7 Development of diuretics from sulphanilamide by molecular modification. The substituted sulphanilamide moiety is shown in red.

*This compound has a double bond between N-4 and C-3.

†The effect on excretion of ions with an intravenous dose of 0.5 mg/kg per hour.

the research on thiazides was the development of **diazoxide**, an antihypertensive agent; see Chapter 14.

Further molecular modifications led in the early 1960s to the compounds **frusemide, bumetanide** and later **piretanide** and **torasemide**. These agents, though also sulphonamide derivatives, have very few chemical features in common with the thiazides (Fig. 18.8). Their mechanism of action is also different from that of the thiazides. They are *loop diuretics* with a 'ceiling' of diuresis much higher than that of the thiazides; their action is similar to that of **ethacrynic acid** (Fig. 18.8), a compound which was developed in a quite different research programme.

Although all these compounds proved to be very effective in promoting sodium excretion, they all caused potassium loss, and this prompted the search for potassium-sparing diuretics. Aldosterone antagonists such as **spironolactone** (Fig. 18.9), introduced in 1962, partially satisfied this requirement, but they had several drawbacks. Numerous compounds were screened and eventually **amiloride** and **triamterene** emerged (Fig. 18.9). These two drugs were developed from two different research programmes, but they have rather similar sites of action.

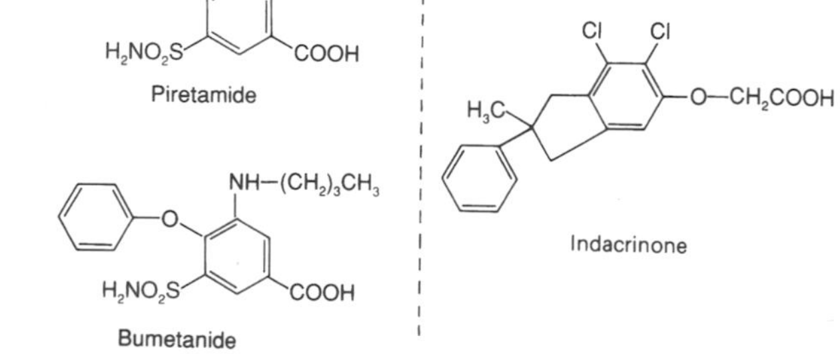

Fig. 18.8 Loop diuretics. The boxed methylene group of ethacrynic acid forms an adduct with cysteine in vivo and this adduct is thought to be the pharmacologically active form of the drug. The substituted sulphanilamide moiety is shown in red. Indacrinone has uricosuric activity.

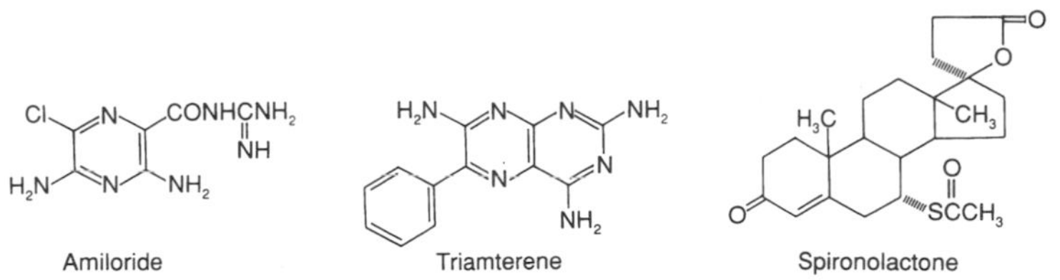

Amiloride Triamterene Spironolactone

Fig. 18.9 Potassium-sparing diuretics.

The most recent development in this area is the attempt to develop uricosuric diuretics to overcome the problem that most currently used diuretics tend to produce an increase in the plasma uric acid concentration. One such compound is **indacrinone** which is a derivative of ethacrynic acid (Fig. 18.8).

DIURETICS ACTING DIRECTLY ON THE CELLS OF THE NEPHRON

Drugs which cause a net salt loss by an action on cells must obviously affect those parts of the nephron where most of the *active* and *selective* solute reabsorption occurs:

- the ascending loop of Henle
- the early distal tubule
- the collecting tubules and ducts.

Loop diuretics

Loop diuretics are the most powerful of all diuretics, capable of causing 15–25% of the sodium in the filtrate to be excreted; thus, they are termed 'high ceiling' diuretics (see Fig. 18.10 for comparison with a thiazide). The main example is **frusemide**; others are **bumetanide, piretanide, torasemide** and **ethacrynic acid**. These drugs act primarily on the thick segment of the ascending loop of Henle, inhibiting the transport of sodium chloride out of the tubule into the interstitial tissue by inhibiting the $Na^+/K^+/2Cl^-$ carrier in the luminal membrane (see Figs 18.5 and 18.11). **Frusemide, bumetanide, torasemide** and **piretanide** have a direct inhibiting effect on the carrier, acting on the chloride-binding site. **Ethacrynic acid** forms a complex with cysteine, the complex being the active form of the drug.

As has been explained above, the reabsorption of solute at this site is the basis for the ability of the kidney to concentrate the urine by creating a hypertonic interstitial area in the medulla, which provides the osmotic force by which water is reabsorbed from the collecting tubules under the influence of the antidiuretic hormone. The action of the loop diuretics has the additional effect that more solute is delivered to the distal portions of the nephron where its osmotic pressure further reduces water reabsorption. Essentially, some of the solute which normally passes into the medullary interstitium and draws water out of the collecting ducts, now remains in the tubular fluid and holds water with it. As much as 25% of the glomerular filtrate may pass out of the nephron (compared with the normal loss of about 1%), resulting in a profuse diuresis.

Loop diuretics appear to have a venodilator action, directly and/or indirectly through the release of a renal factor. After intravenous administration to patients with acute heart failure (see Ch. 13), a therapeutically useful vascular effect is seen *before*

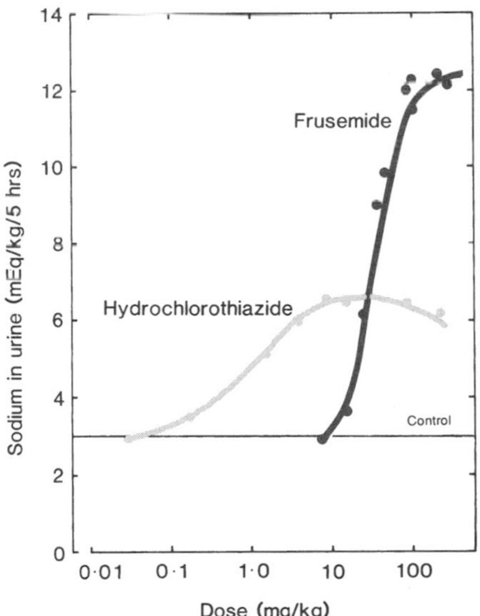

Fig. 18.10 The dose–response curves for frusemide and hydrochlorothiazide, showing differences in potency and 'ceiling'. Note that these doses are not used clinically. (Adapted from: Timmerman R J et al. 1964 Curr Ther Res 6: 88)

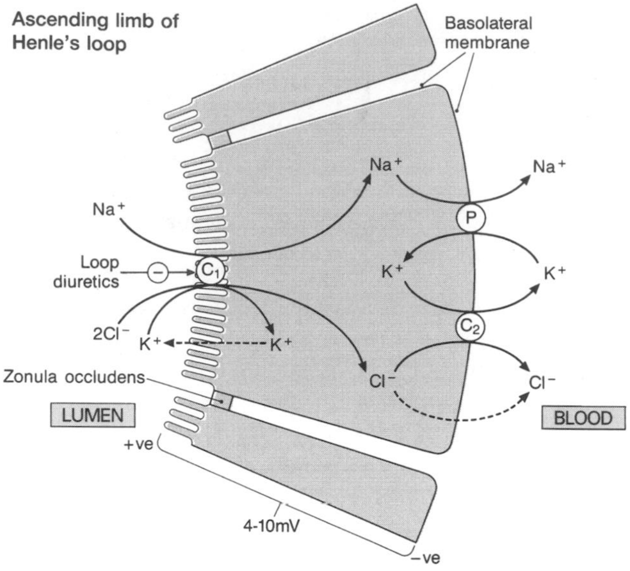

Fig. 18.11 Ion transport in the cells of the thick ascending limb of Henle's loop, showing the site of action of loop diuretics. The sodium pump (P) is the main primary active transport mechanism. Na^+, K^+ and Cl^- enter by a co-transport system (C_1). Chloride leaves the cell both by passive diffusion (dotted lines) and by an electroneutral K^+/Cl^- co-transport system (C_2). Some sodium is absorbed paracellularly, through the *zonula occludens*, and some potassium leaves the cell by passive diffusion (not shown).

the onset of the diuretic effect. **Piretanide**, in particular, has general vasodilator actions.

These drugs cause significant potassium loss (explained on p. 373). Loop diuretics may produce a metabolic alkalosis because the loss of sodium and chloride (with the resultant volume depletion), along with potassium depletion, stimulates hydrogen ion secretion and bicarbonate generation.

There is an increase in the excretion of calcium and magnesium and a decreased excretion of uric acid. The effect on calcium is made use of in the treatment of hypercalcaemia. **Torasemide*** causes less loss of potassium and calcium.

Pharmacokinetic aspects

The loop diuretics are readily absorbed from the gastrointestinal tract and may also be given by injection. They are strongly bound to plasma protein and so do not pass into the glomerular filtrate to any marked degree. They reach their site of action—the luminal membrane of the cells of the thick ascending loop—by being secreted in the proximal convoluted tubule by the organic acid transport mechanism; the fraction thus secreted will pass out in the urine. The fraction not secreted is metabolised in the liver—**bumetanide** and **torasemide** being metabolised by cytochrome P-450 pathways and **frusemide** being glucuronidated. Given orally, they

*Not used in the UK.

Diuretics

Diuretics are drugs which increase the excretion of salt (NaCl, $NaHCO_3$) and water. Normally (i.e. in the absence of diuretics), less than 1% of filtered sodium is excreted. The main diuretics are the loop diuretics and the thiazides.

- **Loop diuretics** (e.g. frusemide) cause up to 15–20% of filtered Na^+ to be excreted, with torrential urine production. They act by inhibiting the $Na^+/K^+/2Cl^-$ co-transporter in the thick ascending loop. They increase K^+ and Ca^{2+} loss. Main unwanted effects: hypokalaemia, metabolic alkalosis and hypovolaemia.
- **Thiazides** (e.g. bendrofluazide) are less potent. They act by inhibiting the Na^+/Cl^- co-transporter in the distal convoluted tubule. They increase K^+ loss and reduce Ca^{2+} loss. Main unwanted effects: hypokalaemia and metabolic alkalosis.
- **Potassium-sparing diuretics:**
  —These act in the collecting tubules and are very weak diuretics.
  —Amiloride and triamterene act by blocking the Na^+ channels controlled by aldosterone's protein mediator.
  —Spironolactone is an antagonist at the aldosterone receptor.

act within 1 hour; given intravenously, they produce a peak effect within 30 minutes. The half-lives are about 90 minutes (longer in renal failure) and the duration of action 3–6 hours, except in the case of **torasemide** which has a longer half-life and longer duration of action and can therefore be given once a day. The clinical use of loop diuretics is given below.

Unwanted effects

Some unwanted effects are common with loop diuretics, and are directly related to their renal actions. *Potassium loss* (see p. 374), resulting in low plasma potassium (hypokalaemia), and *metabolic alkalosis* due to hydrogen ion excretion are both very likely to occur. Hypokalaemia can be averted or treated by concomitant use of potassium-sparing diuretics (see below) or by potassium supplements. *Depletion of magnesium and calcium* is common, and in elderly patients, *hypovolaemia* and *hypotension*, with collapse due to sudden loss of extracellular fluid volume, can follow the profuse diuresis produced by these agents.

Unwanted effects which are not related to the renal actions of the drugs are rare. They include nausea, allergic reactions (more common in those agents related to sulphonamides) and, infrequently, deafness (compounded by concomitant use of an aminoglycoside antibiotic). Ethacrynic acid is more likely to cause GIT upsets and deafness and is consequently less widely used.

Diuretics acting on the early distal tubule

The diuretics acting at this site—sometimes referred to as the distal convoluted tubule—include the **thiazides** and related drugs.

The development of these agents is outlined above. The main thiazide is **bendrofluazide**. Others are **hydrochlorothiazide**, and **cyclopenthiazide**, but many similar drugs are available (Fig. 18.12). Of the drugs related to the thiazides and having similar actions, the main one is **chlorthalidone**, and newer ones are **indapamide**, **xipamide** and **metolazone**.

Clinical use of loop diuretics

- In patients with salt and water overload due to:
  - —acute pulmonary oedema
  - —chronic heart failure
  - —hepatic cirrhosis complicated by ascites
  - —nephrotic syndrome
  - —renal failure.
- In hypertension, especially if accompanied by renal impairment.
- In acute treatment of hypercalcaemia.

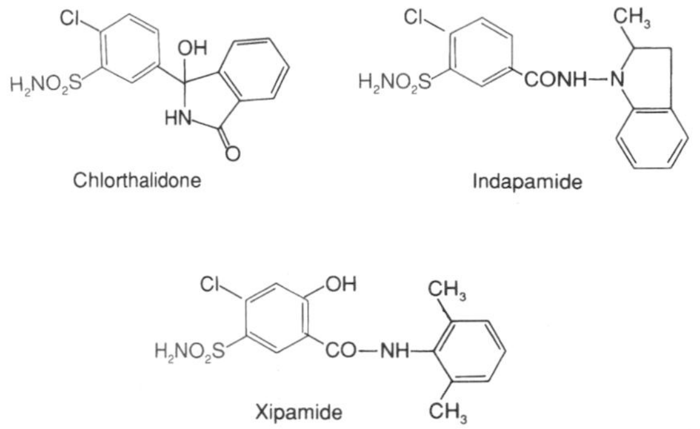

Chlorthalidone, Indapamide, Xipamide

Fig. 18.12 Some diuretics related to the thiazide compounds. The substituted sulphanilamide moiety is shown in red.

This group of drugs has a moderately powerful diuretic action (see comparison with loop diuretics in Fig. 18.10). They decrease active reabsorption of sodium and accompanying chloride by binding to the chloride site of the electroneutral Na^+/Cl^- co-transport system and inhibiting its action (Figs 18.5 and 18.13). They do not have any action on the thick ascending loop of Henle. Potassium loss with these drugs is significant (by mechanisms explained on p. 374) and can be serious. Excretion of uric acid and calcium is decreased; that of magnesium is increased.

Thiazide diuretics have a paradoxical effect in diabetes insipidus where they *reduce* the volume of urine.

Hypochloraemic alkalosis can occur.

They have some extra-renal actions—they produce vasodilatation and can cause hyperglycaemia. When used in the treatment of hypertension (Ch. 14), the initial fall in blood pressure is due to decreased blood volume resulting from diuresis, but the later phase seems to be due to a direct action on the blood vessels. Note that **diazoxide**, a non-diuretic thiazide, has powerful vasodilator effects (see Ch. 14). and also increases the blood sugar. Both actions are due to the same mechanism, namely the opening of membrane K^+ channels (see Ch. 14 and p. 310). **Indapamide** is said to lower blood pressure at sub-diuretic doses with less metabolic disturbance.

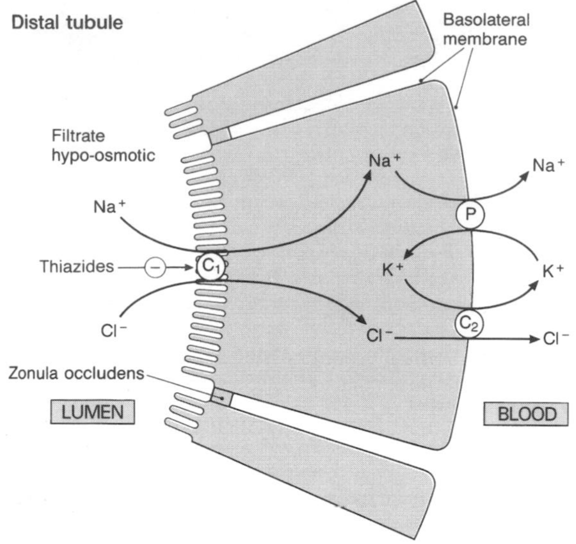

Fig. 18.13 Salt transport in the distal convoluted tubule showing the proposed site of action of thiazide diuretics. The sodium pump (P) in the basolateral membrane is the primary active transport mechanism. Na^+ and Cl^- enter by an electroneutral co-transport carrier (C_1). Some K^+ is transported out of the cell by the co-transport carrier (C_2), and some by passive diffusion (not shown). (Adapted from: Greger 1988)

Pharmacokinetic aspects

The thiazides and related drugs are all effective orally, being well absorbed from the gastrointestinal tract. All are excreted in the urine mainly by tubular secretion (see p. 373). Their tendency to increase plasma uric acid is due to competition with uric acid for tubular secretion mechanisms. With the shorter-acting drugs such as **bendrofluazide**, **hydrochlorothiazide**, **chlorothiazide** and **cyclopenthiazide**, onset of action is within 12 hours, maximum effect at about 4–6 hours and duration between 8 and 12 hours. The longer-acting drugs such as **chlorthalidone** have a similar onset but a longer duration of action and can be given on alternate days. The clinical use of thiazide diuretics is given in the following box.

Unwanted effects

These agents have a fairly large therapeutic index and serious unwanted effects are relatively rare. The main unwanted effects of thiazides are the result of some of the renal actions; a *decreased plasma potassium* is particularly significant. Others are *metabolic alkalosis*, *increased plasma uric acid* (with the possibility of gout) and *hyperglycaemia* (which could exacerbate diabetes mellitus). **Indapamide** has little obvious effect on potassium, uric acid and glucose excretion.

Unwanted effects not related to the main renal actions of the thiazides include increased plasma cholesterol (with long-term use), male impotence (reversible on stopping the drug) and, infrequently, hypersensitivity reactions (skin rashes, blood dyscrasias and, more rarely still, pancreatitis, acute pulmonary oedema). In cases of hepatic failure, thiazides can precipitate encephalopathy. An unusual but potentially serious unwanted effect is hyponatraemia.

Clinical use of thiazide diuretics

- In hypertension.
- In mild heart failure.
- In severe resistant oedema (metolazone, especially, is used, together with loop diuretics).
- To prevent recurrent stone formation in idiopathic hypercalciuria.
- In nephrogenic diabetes insipidus.

Spironolactone

Spironolactone has a limited diuretic action. It is an antagonist of aldosterone, competing for intracellular aldosterone receptors in the cells of the distal tubule (see Ch. 21). The spironolactone–receptor complex does not apparently attach to the DNA, and the subsequent processes of transcription, translation and production of mediator protein(s)—shown in Figure 18.14—do not occur. The result is an inhibition of the sodium-retaining action of aldosterone (see Fig. 18.5), and a concomitant decrease in its potassium-secreting effect. Spironolactone has subsidiary actions in decreasing hydrogen ion secretion and also uric acid excretion.

Potassium canrenoate (see below) has effects similar to spironolactone.

Pharmacokinetic aspects

Spironolactone is well absorbed from the gastrointestinal tract. Its plasma half-life is only 10 minutes but its active metabolite, canrenone, has a plasma $t_{1/2}$ of 16 hours. The action of spironolactone is

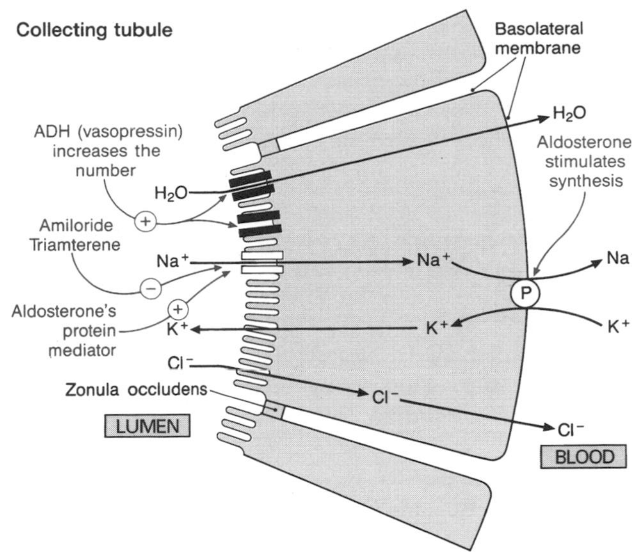

Fig. 18.14 Simplified diagram of the action of hormones and drugs on the principal cells of the collecting tubule. The cells are normally impermeable to water in the absence of antidiuretic hormone (ADH), and to sodium in the absence of aldosterone. Salt and water reabsorption in this part of the tubule are controlled physiologically by these two hormones, through their respective effects on the water channels and sodium channels. Aldosterone acts within the tubule (see p. 371). Spironolactone antagonises aldosterone action. The Na^+ pump (P) in the basolateral membrane is the main source of energy for ion movement.

believed to be largely but not entirely due to canrenone. The onset of action is very slow, taking several days to develop.

Potassium canrenoate is given parenterally. The clinical use of spironolactone is given in the box on this page.

Unwanted effects

Gastrointestinal upsets occur fairly frequently. If spironolactone is used on its own it will cause hyperkalaemia and possibly metabolic acidosis. Actions on steroid receptors in tissues other than the kidney can result in gynaecomastia, menstrual disorders and testicular atrophy. Peptic ulceration has been reported.

Triamterene and amiloride

Like spironolactone, triamterene and amiloride have a limited diuretic efficacy. They act on the collecting tubules and collecting ducts, inhibiting sodium reabsorption and decreasing potassium excretion (see Figs 18.5 and 18.14). Amiloride blocks the luminal sodium channels by which aldosterone produces its main effect, making less sodium available for transport across the basolateral membrane. Triamterene probably has a similar action. By preventing Na^+ entry they also reduce Na^+/H^+ exchange, and thus inhibit H^+ excretion, resulting in some degree of alkalinisation of the urine. Alkalinisation is less marked in the case of amiloride.

Both are mildly uricosuric, i.e. they promote the excretion of uric acid.

The main importance of these diuretics lies in their *potassium-sparing ability*. They can be given with potassium-losing diuretics like the thiazides in order to maintain potassium balance.

Pharmacokinetic aspects

Triamterene is well absorbed in the gastrointestinal tract. Its onset of action is within 2 hours and its duration of action 12–16 hours. It is partly metabolised in the liver and partly excreted unchanged in the urine. Amiloride is poorly absorbed and has a slower onset, with a peak action at 6 hours and a duration of action of about 24 hours. Most of the drug is excreted unchanged in the urine. The clinical use of triamterene and amiloride is given below.

Clinical use of the potassium-sparing diuretics

- With potassium-losing diuretics to prevent potassium loss, (spironolactone is used less frequently than amiloride or triamterene because it is poorly tolerated).
- Spironolactone is used
  - in primary hyperaldosteronism (Conn's syndrome), which is rare
  - in secondary hyperaldosteronism due to hepatic cirrhosis complicated by ascites.

Unwanted effects
The main unwanted effect is related to the pharmacological action of the drugs—hyperkalaemia, which can be dangerous. Metabolic acidosis can occur, as can skin rashes. Gastrointestinal disturbances have been reported but are infrequent.

DIURETICS WHICH ACT INDIRECTLY BY MODIFYING THE CONTENT OF THE FILTRATE

Diuretics which act by indirectly modifying the content of the filtrate do so by increasing either the osmolarity or the sodium load.

Osmotic diuretics

Osmotic diuretics are pharmacologically inert substances (e.g. **mannitol**) which are filtered in the glomerulus but incompletely reabsorbed or not reabsorbed at all by the nephron (see Fig. 18.5). They can be given in amounts sufficiently large for them to constitute an appreciable fraction of the plasma osmolarity. Within the nephron, their main effect is exerted on those parts of the nephron which are freely permeable to water—the proximal tubule, descending limb of the loop and the collecting tubules. Passive water reabsorption is reduced by the presence of the non-reabsorbable solute within the tubule; in particular a larger volume of fluid remains within the proximal tubule. This has the secondary effect of reducing sodium reabsorption, since the sodium concentration within the proximal tubule is lower than it otherwise would be, and this alters the electrochemical gradient for reabsorption.

Therefore, the main effect of osmotic diuretics is to increase the amount of water excreted, with a relatively smaller increase in sodium excretion. Hence, they are not useful in treating conditions associated with sodium retention, but have much more limited therapeutic applications. These include *acutely raised intracranial or intraocular pressure* and *prevention of acute renal failure*. In this latter condition, the glomerular filtration rate is reduced, and absorption of salt and water in the proximal tubule becomes almost complete, so that more distal parts of the nephron virtually dry up, and urine flow ceases. Retention of fluid within the proximal tubule by administration of an osmotic diuretic limits these effects.

The treatment of acutely raised intracranial pressure (cerebral oedema) and raised intraocular pressure (glaucoma) relies on the increase in plasma osmolarity by solutes that do not enter the brain or eye; this results in extraction of water from these compartments. It has nothing to do with the kidney; indeed the effect is lost as soon as the osmotic diuretic appears in the urine.

Osmotic diuretics are usually given intravenously.

Unwanted effects include transient expansion of the extracellular fluid volume and hyponatraemia due to abstraction of water from the intracellular compartment. (In patients who are totally unable to form urine, this could cause cardiac failure or pulmonary oedema or both.) Headache, nausea and vomiting can occur.

Diuretics acting on the proximal tubule

Carbonic anhydrase inhibitors (Fig. 18.15) cause increased excretion of bicarbonate with accompanying sodium, potassium and water, resulting in an increased flow of an alkaline urine and a mild metabolic acidosis. These agents, though not now used as

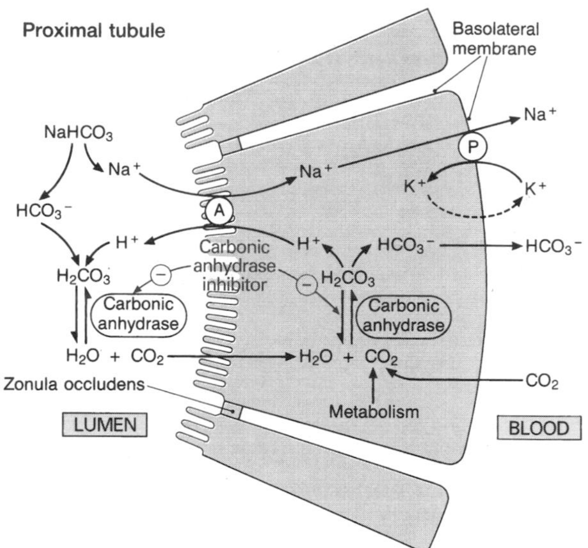

Fig. 18.15 Renal mechanisms for conserving base showing the action of carbonic anhydrase inhibitors. Sodium is absorbed and hydrogen ions secreted at the luminal surface by an antiport mechanism (A). Most bicarbonate in the filtrate is 'reabsorbed' in this way in the proximal tubule. In the distal tubule, bicarbonate is added to the plasma, and monobasic phosphate or ammonium chloride is added to the urine (not shown). The primary active transport mechanism is the sodium pump (P). Dashed lines with K^+ indicate passive diffusion. (Amiloride inhibits the Na^+/H^+ exchange or antiport, but this is not a major factor in its diuretic action.)

diuretics, may be used in the treatment of glaucoma to reduce the formation of aqueous humor, and also in some unusual types of epilepsy. Examples are **acetazolamide** (see Fig. 18.7) and **dichlorphenamide**.

Their mechanism of action is as follows. In the proximal tubule cells, carbonic anhydrase catalyses the formation of carbonic acid from CO_2 and water. The acid dissociates to form hydrogen and bicarbonate ions; the bicarbonate ion passes into the plasma and the hydrogen ion is secreted into the lumen—the secretion being balanced electrically by the opposite transport of sodium and involving an antiport system driven by the electrochemical gradient for sodium. In the lumen, the hydrogen ions combine with filtered bicarbonate ions to form carbonic acid, which dissociates to form water and carbon dioxide. This latter reaction is catalysed by carbonic anhydrase associated with the cell surface. The carbon dioxide diffuses back into the cell. The net effect of these processes is that much of the filtered bicarbonate is reabsorbed by the proximal tubule. Drugs which inhibit carbonic anhydrase increase the volume of urine flow (i.e. are diuretic) by preventing bicarbonate reabsorption (Figs 18.5 and 18.15). They also result in a depletion of extracellular bicarbonate. The effect is self-limiting as the blood bicarbonate falls.

DRUGS WHICH ALTER THE pH OF THE URINE

In various conditions it is of advantage to alter the pH of the urine, and it is possible to produce urinary pH values ranging from 5–8.5.

Agents which increase the urinary pH

Sodium or **potassium citrate** or other salts (acetate, lactate) are metabolised and the cations are excreted with bicarbonate to give an alkaline urine. This increases the action of some antibacterial drugs (**sulphonamides, streptomycin**) and may by itself have some antibacterial effects, as well as decreasing irritation or inflammation in the urinary tract. Alkalinisation is important in preventing certain drugs, such as some sulphonamides, from crystallising out in the urine; it also decreases the formation of uric acid and cystine stones.

It is possible to increase the excretion of drugs which are weak acids (e.g. **aspirin, salicylates** and some **barbiturates**) by alkalinising the urine (see Ch. 4). **Sodium bicarbonate** given intravenously is used in patients with salicylate overdose.

Note that sodium overload can be dangerous in cardiac failure, and that overload with either sodium or potassium can be harmful in renal insufficiency.

Agents which decrease urinary pH

A decrease in urinary pH can be produced with **ammonium chloride** but this is now rarely if ever used clinically except in a specialised test for renal tubular acidosis.

The ammonia is metabolised to urea in the liver, leaving chloride and hydrogen ion. The chloride displaces bicarbonate (which is dissipated by conversion to carbonic acid then to CO_2 and H_2O) so that a hyperchloraemic acidosis results. The chloride, with accompanying sodium, appears in the glomerular filtrate and passes out in the urine with an osmotic equivalent of water, causing a mild diuresis. Then the base-conserving mechanisms come into play, the tubules secrete hydrogen ions in exchange for sodium, ammonia is generated and an acid urine (containing ammonium chloride) is excreted.

DRUGS WHICH ALTER THE EXCRETION OF ORGANIC MOLECULES

The main organic molecules to be considered are uric acid and **penicillin**.

Uric acid is derived from the catabolism of the purine bases and is present in plasma mainly as ionised urate. In man it passes freely into the glomerular filtrate, and most is then reabsorbed in the proximal convoluted tubule while a small amount is simultaneously secreted into the tubule by the anion-secreting mechanisms (see p. 374). The net result is excretion of approximately 8–12% of the filtered urate. Under physiological conditions, a rise in the level of urate in the plasma results in increased secretion into the proximal tubule. This process keeps the plasma urate concentration within the normal range, but in some conditions (e.g. gout) blood levels remain high. Urate crystals are then deposited in joints, resulting in the arthritis of gout. Drugs which *increase* the elimination of urate (uricosuric agents) may be useful in such cases. (Drugs used to treat gout are dealt with in more detail in Ch. 12, p. 258.)

Some uricosuric agents *decrease* the secretion of

penicillin and may also be used for this purpose. The two main uricosuric agents are probenecid and sulphinpyrazone.

Probenecid is a lipid-soluble derivative of benzoic acid, which inhibits the reabsorption of urate in the proximal convoluted tubule and thus increases its excretion. It has the opposite effect on **penicillin**, inhibiting its secretion into the tubules and raising its plasma concentration. Given orally, probenecid is well absorbed in the gastrointestinal tract, maximal concentrations in the plasma occurring in about 3 hours. The greater proportion of the drug (90%) is bound to plasma albumin. The free drug passes into the glomerular filtrate, but more is actively secreted into the proximal tubule from whence it may diffuse back due to its high lipid solubility (see also Ch. 4).

Sulphinpyrazone is a congener of phenylbutazone (see Ch. 12) with powerful inhibitory effects on uric acid reabsorption in the proximal convoluted tubule. It is absorbed from the gastro-intestinal tract, becomes highly protein-bound in the plasma and is secreted into the proximal convoluted tubule.

Both these agents, if given in sub-therapeutic doses, actually *inhibit* secretion of urate. **Salicylates,** on the other hand, inhibit secretion in doses within their therapeutic range, producing an increase in urate levels in the blood. They may thus exacerbate gouty arthritis and will antagonise the effects of uricosuric agents.

Most diuretics tend to cause an increase in plasma uric acid. Current research is aimed at developing diuretics with uricosuric properties; **indacrinone** is onc such agent.

REFERENCES AND FURTHER READING

Barter D C 1983 Pharmacodynamic considerations in the use of diuretics. Annu Rev Pharmacol 123: 45–62

Berger B E, Warnock D G 1985 Clinical uses and mechanisms of action of diuretic agents. In: Brenner B M, Rector F C (eds) The kidney, 3rd edn. W B Saunders, Philadelphia, p 433–455

Brater D C 1991 Clinical pharmacology of loop diuretics. Drugs 41 (Suppl 3): 14–22

Breyer J, Jacobson H R 1990 Molecular mechanism of diuretic agents. Annu Rev Med 41: 265–275

Burg M B 1985 Renal handling of sodium, chloride, water, amino acids and glucose. In: Brenner B M, Rector F C (eds) The kidney, 3rd edn. W B Saunders, Philadelphia, p 145–175

Clarke R J 1991 Indapamide: a diuretic of choice for the treatment of hypertension? Am J Med Sci 301: 215–220

Cogan M G 1990 Renal effects of atrial natriuretic factor. Annu Rev Physiol 52: 699–708

Cragoe E J (ed) 1983 Diuretics: chemistry, pharmacology and medicine. John Wiley, New York

Frelin C, Vigne P, Babry P, Lazdunski M 1987 Molecular properties of amiloride action and of its Na^+ transporting targets. Kidney Int 32: 785–793

Friedel H A, Buckley M M 1991 Torasemide. A review of its pharmacological properties and therapeutic potential. Drugs 41: 81–83

Funder J W 1993 Aldosterone action. Annu Rev Physiol 55: 115–130

Goetz K L 1992 Renal natriuretic peptide (urodilatin?) and atriopeptin: evolving concepts. Am J Physiol 261: (Renal Fluid Electrolyte Physiol 30): F921–932

Greger R 1985 Ion transport mechanisms in thick ascending limb of Henle's loop of mammalian nephron. Physiol Rev 65: 760–797

Greger R 1988 Chloride transport in thick ascending limb, distal convolution and collecting duct. Annu Rev Physiol 50: 111–122

Greven J 1987 The pharmacological basis of the action of loop diuretics. In: Puschett J B, Greenberg A (eds) Diuretics II: chemistry pharmacology and clinical implications. Elsevier, Amsterdam, p 173–181

Hendry B M, Ellory J C 1988 Molecular sites for diuretic action. Trends Pharmacol Sci 9: 416–421

Houston M C 1991 Nonsteroidal anti-inflammatory drugs and antihypertensives. Am J Med 90: 42(S)–47(S)

Jamison R, Maffly R H 1976 The urinary concentrating mechanism. N Engl J Med 295: 1059–1067

Koga H, Sat H, Dan T, Aoki B 1991 Studies on uricosuric diuretics. J Med Chem 34: 2702–2708

Levenson D J, Simmons C E, Brenner B M 1982 Arachidonic acid metabolism, prostaglandins and the kidney. Am J Med 72: 354–374

Orme M 1990 Thiazides in the 1990s. Br Med J 300: 1668–1669

Reeves W B, Andreoli T E 1992 Renal epithelial chloride channels. Annu Rev Physiol 54: 29–50

Rose B D 1991 Diuretics. Kidney Int 39: 336–352

Schafer J A, Hawk C T 1992 Regulation of Na^+ channels in the cortical collecting duct by AVP and mineralocorticoids. Editorial Review, Kidney Int 41: 255–268

Schuster V L 1993 Function and regulation of collecting duct intercalated cells. Annu Rev Physiol 55: 267–288

Sullivan L P, Grantham J J 1982 The physiology of the kidney, 2nd edn. Lea & Febiger, Philadelphia

Taylor A, Palmer L G 1982 Hormonal regulation of sodium chloride and water transport in epithelia. In: Goldberger R F, Yamamoto K R (eds) Biological regulation and development. Plenum Press, New York, vol 3A: 253–298

Wasnick R, Davis J, Ross P, Vogel J 1990 Effect of thiazides on rates of bone mineral loss: a longitudinal study. Br Med J 301: 1303–1305

Wehling M, Christ M, Gerzer R 1993 Aldosterone-specific membrane receptors and related rapid, non-genomic effects. Trends Pharmacol Sci 14: 1–4

Wingo C S, Cain B D 1993 The renal ATP-ase: physiological significance and role in potassium homeostasis. Annu Rev Physiol 55: 323–347

19
THE GASTROINTESTINAL TRACT

In addition to its main function of digestion and absorption of food, the gastrointestinal tract is one of the major endocrine systems in the body. It also has its own integrative neuronal network, the enteric nervous system (see Ch. 5), which contains about the same number of neurons as the spinal cord; the topic is reviewed by Del Valle & Yamada (1990) and Wingate (1986).

THE INNERVATION AND THE HORMONES OF THE GASTROINTESTINAL TRACT

The elements under neuronal and hormonal control are the smooth muscle, the blood vessels and the glands (exocrine, endocrine and paracrine).

Neuronal control

There are two principal intramural plexuses in the tract—the *myenteric plexus* (*Auerbach's plexus*) between the outer, longitudinal and the middle, circular muscle layers, and *Meissner's plexus*, or *submucous plexus*, on the luminal side of the circular muscle layer. The plexuses are interconnected and their ganglion cells receive preganglionic *parasympathetic fibres* from the vagus which are mostly cholinergic and mostly excitatory, though some are inhibitory. Incoming *sympathetic fibres* are largely postganglionic and these, in addition to innervating blood vessels, smooth muscle and some glandular cells directly, may have endings in the plexuses where they inhibit acetylcholine secretion (see Ch. 5).

The neurons within the plexuses constitute the enteric nervous system and secrete not only acetylcholine and noradrenaline but 5-HT, purines, nitric oxide and a variety of pharmacologically active peptides. The enteric plexus contains sensory neurons which respond to mechanical and chemical stimuli.

Hormonal control

The hormones of the gastrointestinal tract include both *endocrine* secretions and *paracrine* secretions. The endocrine secretions (i.e. substances released into the bloodstream) are mainly peptides synthesised by endocrine cells in the mucosa, and the most important is **gastrin**. The paracrine secretions, or local hormones, many of them regulatory peptides, are released from special cells found throughout the wall of the tract. These hormones act on nearby cells, and in the stomach, the most important of these is **histamine**. Some of these paracrine secretions also function as neurotransmitters. Histamine, gastrin and acetylcholine are considered below in the context of the local control of acid secretion.

The *main functions* of the gastrointestinal tract which are important from a pharmacological point of view are:

- gastric secretion
- vomiting (emesis)
- the motility of the bowel and the expulsion of the faeces
- the formation and excretion of bile.

GASTRIC SECRETION

The stomach secretes about 2.5 litres of gastric juice daily. The principal exocrine secretions are pepsinogens, from the *chief* or *peptic cells*, and hydrochloric acid and intrinsic factor (see Ch. 23) from the *parietal* or *oxyntic cells*. Mucus is secreted by mucus-secreting cells found amongst the surface cells throughout the gastric mucosa. Bicarbonate ions are also secreted and are trapped in the mucus, creating a gradient of pH from 1–2 in the lumen to 6–7 at the mucosal surface. The mucus and bicarbonate form an unstirred gel-like layer protecting the mucosa from the gastric juice. Alcohol and bile can disrupt this layer. Locally produced prostaglandins stimulate the secretion of both mucus and bicarbonate. Thus, **non-steroidal anti-inflammatory drugs** (such as aspirin), which inhibit prostaglandin synthesis (see Ch. 12), will decrease the protective effect of the barrier. This partly accounts for the tendency of these agents to cause gastric ulceration and bleeding.

Disturbances in the above secretory functions are thought to be involved in the pathogenesis of peptic ulcer, and the therapy of this condition involves drugs which modify each of these factors.

THE REGULATION OF ACID SECRETION BY PARIETAL CELLS

The regulation of acid secretion by parietal cells is especially important in peptic ulcer and constitutes a particular target for drug action. The secretion of the parietal cells is an isotonic solution of HCl (150 mmol/l) with a pH less than 1, the concentration of hydrogen ion being more than a million times higher than that of the plasma.

The Cl^- is actively transported into canaliculi in the cells which communicate with the lumen of the gastric glands and thus with the lumen of the stomach. K^+ accompanies the Cl^- and is then exchanged for H^+ from within the cell by a K^+/H^+-ATPase (Fig. 19.1). H_2CO_3, formed from CO_2 and H_2O, dissociates in a reaction catalysed by carbonic anhydrase to form H^+ and HCO_3^-. The HCO_3^- exchanges across the basal membrane for Cl^-. Three main stimuli act on the parietal cells:

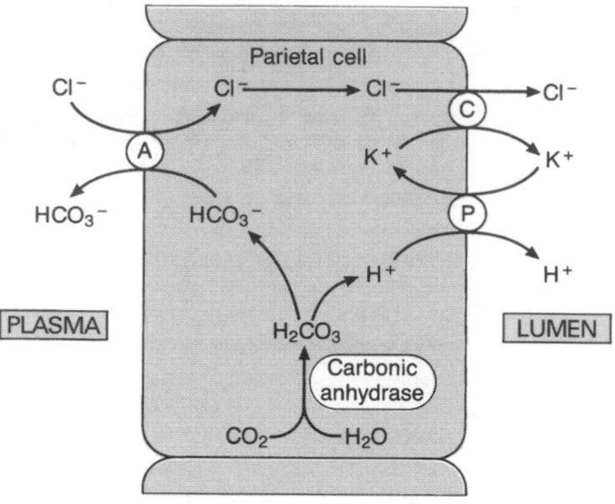

Fig. 19.1 A schematic illustration of the secretion of hydrochloric acid by the gastric parietal cell. Secretion involves a proton pump (P) which is a H^+/K^+-ATPase, a symport carrier (C) for K^+ and Cl^-, and an antiport (A) which exchanges Cl^- and HCO_3^-. A Na^+/H^+ antiport at the interface with the plasma may also have a role (not shown).

- **gastrin** (a hormone)
- **acetylcholine** (a neurotransmitter)
- **histamine** (a local hormone).

Prostaglandins E_2 and **I_2** inhibit acid secretion. Figure 19.2 summarises the actions of these chemical mediators.

Gastrin

Gastrin is a peptide hormone synthesised in endocrine cells of the mucosa of the gastric antrum and duodenum, and secreted into the portal blood. A 17-amino-acid peptide (G17) appears to be the main form of gastrin involved in the control of gastric secretion. Gastrin is closely related in its structure to cholecystokinin, which is also found in the gastrointestinal tract (and in the CNS).

Actions

The main action of gastrin is stimulation of the secretion of acid by the parietal cells. There is controversy as to the mechanism of action (discussed below). Gastrin receptors on the parietal cells have been demonstrated with radioactively labelled gastrin. Gastrin receptors are blocked by **proglumide** (Fig. 19.2), which is used only as an experimental tool.

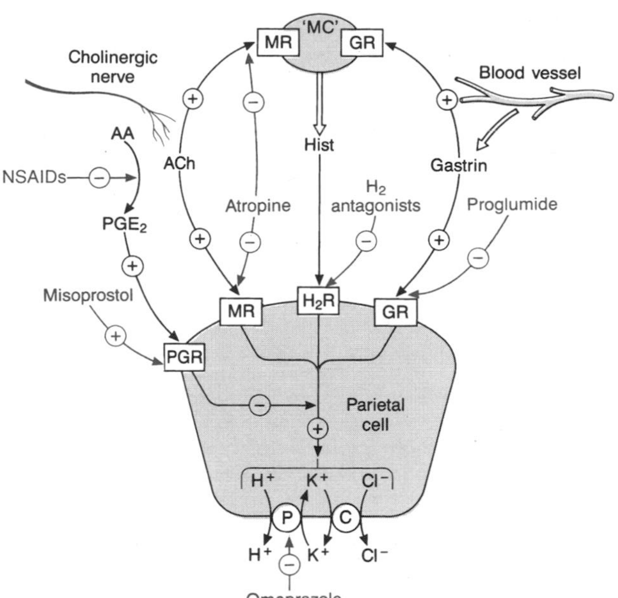

Fig. 19.2 Schematic diagram showing the one-cell and two-cell hypotheses of the action of secretagogues on the acid-secreting gastric parietal cell, giving the site of action of drugs influencing acid secretion. Acetylcholine and gastrin may act mainly directly on their receptors (the one-cell hypothesis) or partly directly, and partly by releasing histamine (the two-cell hypothesis). ('MC' = mast-cell-like, histamine-secreting cell; Hist = histamine; ACh = acetylcholine; MR = muscarinic receptor; H_2R = histamine H_2-receptor; GR = gastrin receptor; PGR = prostaglandin E_2 (PGE_2) receptor; AA = arachidonic acid; NSAIDs = non-steroidal anti-inflammatory drugs; P = proton pump (H^+/K^+-ATPase); C = symport carrier for K^+ and Cl^-).

Gastrin also indirectly increases pepsinogen secretion and stimulates blood flow and gastric motility.

Control of gastrin release

Control of gastrin release involves both neuronal mediators and blood-borne mediators, and the direct effects of the stomach contents. Within the stomach, the important stimuli are amino acids and small peptides, which act directly on the gastrin-secreting cells. Milk and solutions of calcium salts are also effective stimulants, so it is inappropriate to use calcium-containing salts as antacids.

Gastrin secretion is inhibited when the pH of the gastric contents falls to 2.5 or lower.

An excessive secretion of gastrin resulting in excessive secretion of acid is seen with rare tumours of gastrin-secreting cells—gastrinomas—the complex of signs and symptoms being called the Zollinger–Ellison syndrome.

Acetylcholine

Acetylcholine is released from neurons and stimulates specific muscarinic receptors on the surface of the parietal cells and on the surface of histamine-containing cells, as determined by studies with competitive antagonists (see Ch. 6).

Histamine

Histamine is discussed in Chapter 11. Only those aspects of its pharmacology relevant to gastric secretion will be dealt with here.

Considerable clarification of the role of histamine has followed from the development of the histamine H_2-receptor antagonists (see below). It is now known that the parietal cell has H_2-receptors and is sensitive to histamine, responding to amounts that are below the threshold concentration that acts on H_2-receptors in blood vessels. In man the histamine is derived from mast cells or histamine-containing cells similar to mast cells, which lie close to the parietal cell. There is a steady basal release

Secretion of gastric acid, mucus and bicarbonate

- Acid is secreted from gastric parietal cells by a proton-pump (K^+/H^+-ATPase).
- The three endogenous secretagogues for acid are histamine, acetylcholine and gastrin.
- PGE_2 and PGI_2 inhibit acid and stimulate mucus and bicarbonate secretion.
- Peptic ulcers are thought to be due to an imbalance between:
  —mucosal-damaging mechanisms (acid, pepsin) and
  —mucosal-protecting mechanisms (mucus, bicarbonate, local synthesis of PGE_2 and PGI_2).
- The presence of *H. pylori* may be a significant factor in duodenal ulcer genesis.

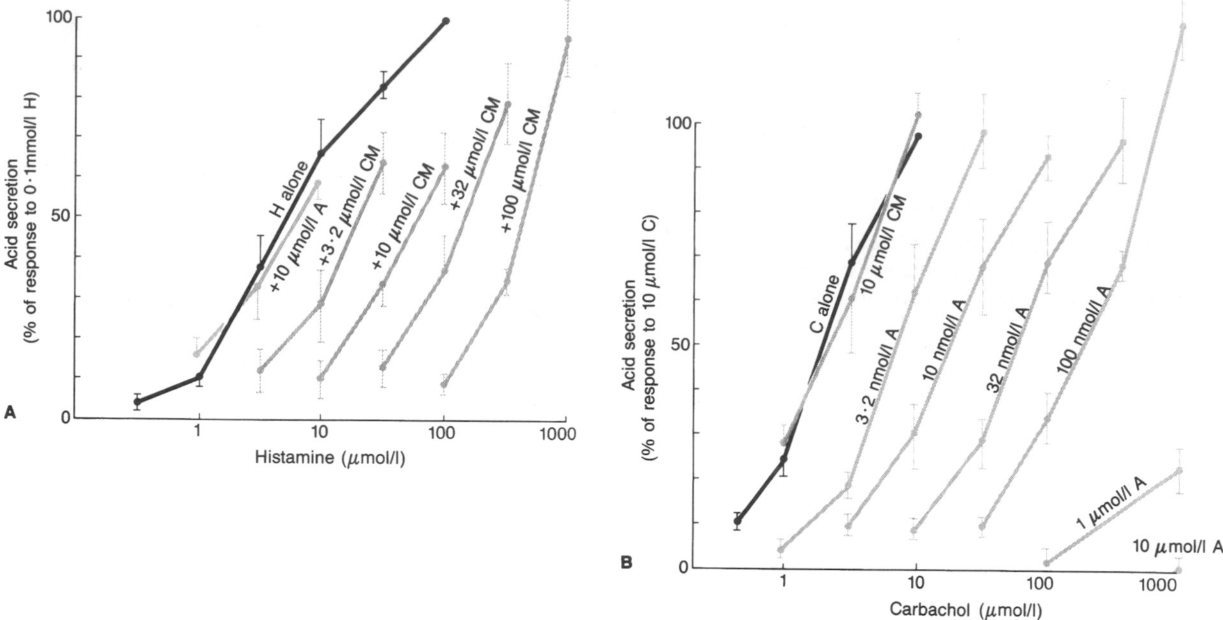

Fig. 19.3 The effect of anti-secretory agents on stimulated acid secretion in isolated canine parietal cells. Acid secretion was measured by the accumulation of a radiolabelled weak base, aminopyrine, in the secretory channels of the parietal cell. **A.** Parallel displacement of the histamine dose–response curve by cimetidine (CM) but not by atropine (A). (The pA_2 value for cimetidine calculated from such data was 6.) **B.** Parallel displacement of the carbachol dose–response curve by atropine but not cimetidine. (See Ch. 1 for discussion of parallel displacement of dose–response curves.) (Adapted from: Soll A H 1980 Am J Physiol 238: G366–375)

of histamine which can be increased by gastrin and acetylcholine.

The role of acetylcholine, histamine and gastrin in acid secretion

The exact mechanism of action of the three secretagogues on the parietal cell is not yet entirely clear. A general scheme is given in Figure 19.2 which summarises the two main theories—the *single-cell* hypothesis and the *two-cell* hypothesis.

According to the *single-cell* hypothesis, the parietal cell has H_2-receptors for histamine, muscarinic M_2-receptors for acetylcholine, and also gastrin receptors. Stimulation of the H_2-receptors increases cAMP, and stimulation of the M_2- and gastrin receptors increases cytosolic calcium; these intracellular messengers synergise to produce acid secretion. In this scheme, all three secretagogues act directly on the parietal cell. Evidence for independent action of all three secretagogues comes from experiments with isolated canine parietal cells. However, the situation in vivo is more complicated, in that cimetidine and atropine can block gastrin action. The effect on isolated parietal cells of histamine (with and without cimetidine) and carbachol (with and without atropine) is shown in Figure 19.3.

According to the *two-cell* hypothesis, gastrin and acetylcholine act either only by releasing histamine, or partly by releasing histamine and partly by direct action on their respective receptors on the parietal cell. This is discussed by Black & Shankley (1987), Soll & Berglindh (1987) and Sandvik & Waldrum (1991).

DRUGS USED TO INHIBIT OR NEUTRALISE GASTRIC ACID SECRETION

The principal pathological conditions in which it is useful to reduce acid secretion are **peptic ulceration** (both duodenal and gastric), **reflux oesophagitis** (in which gastric juice causes damage to the oesophagus) and the **Zollinger–Ellison syndrome** (a rare condition which is due to a gastrin-producing tumour).

The reason why peptic ulcers develop is not understood. It is thought that there is a shift in the balance between mucosal-damaging mechanisms (the secretion and action of acid and pepsin) and mucosal-protecting mechanisms (the secretion and action of mucus and bicarbonate). It is known that the mucosal-damaging mechanisms are increased in duodenal ulcer patients.

The mucosal-protecting mechanisms can be abrogated by NSAIDs (Ch. 12), which decrease the synthesis of prostaglandins. (Prostaglandins normally stimulate mucus and bicarbonate secretion, decrease acid secretion and cause vasodilatation, thereby increasing the elimination of acid that has diffused into the submucosa.)

A factor which might both undermine the mucosal-protecting system and also be implicated in mucosal damage, is the presence in the mucus of *Helicobacter pylori*, a Gram-negative bacillus. It is now generally agreed that this organism is a significant factor in the development of duodenal ulcers and may also be important in gastric ulcers, although its role in ulcer production is not understood. Eradication of the bacillus reduces the incidence of relapse by about 90% and some (but not as yet all*) authorities now recommend that treatment of active duodenal ulceration includes not only antisecretory therapy (to be discussed below) but colloidal bismuth (which is thought to have a toxic action on the bacillus; see below) and antibiotics, for example metronidazole plus tetracycline (see Ch. 37); Cover & Blaser 1992, Graham 1993, Forbes et al. 1994).

Antisecretory therapy of peptic ulcer is aimed at decreasing the secretion of acid with **H_2-receptor antagonists** or **proton-pump inhibitors**, and/or neutralising secreted acid with **antacids** (see Colin-Jones 1990). **Muscarinic antagonists** can be used as adjuncts to other antisecretory agents.

Histamine

Cimetidine

Ranitidine

Famotidine

Nizatidine

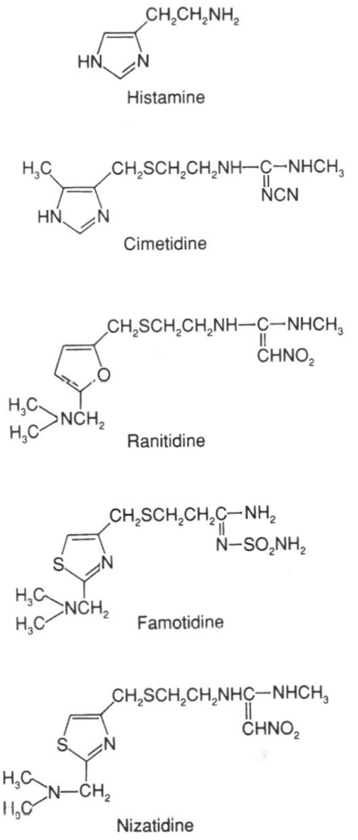

Fig. 19.4 The structure of histamine and four H_2-receptor antagonists.

H_2-RECEPTOR ANTAGONISTS

The introduction of the H_2-receptor antagonists in the mid 1970s by Sir James Black and his colleagues constituted a major breakthrough in drug treatment of peptic ulcer.

H_2-receptor antagonists competitively inhibit histamine actions at all H_2-receptors, but their main clinical use is as inhibitors of gastric acid secretion. They inhibit histamine-stimulated and gastrin-stimulated acid secretion and decrease acetylcholine-stimulated acid secretion; pepsin secretion also falls with the reduction in volume of gastric juice (Fig. 19.5). These agents not only decrease both basal and food-stimulated acid secretion by 90% or more, but promote healing of duodenal ulcers, as shown by numerous clinical trials. Relapses are likely to follow when treatment with H_2-receptor antagonists is stopped. Duodenal ulcers recur within a year in 80–90% of patients and gastric ulcers in 74%. In any event, treatment with H_2-antagonists can be given long-term with safety, to prevent relapse.

The drugs used are **cimetidine** and **ranitidine** (Fig. 19.4). Newer H_2 antagonists, such as **nizatidine** and **famotidine**, are also available. The results of experiments with cimetidine on gastric secretion in man are given in Figure 19.5. The clinical use of H_2-receptor antagonists is given in the box on page 392.

Pharmacokinetic aspects

The drugs are given orally and are well absorbed.

*The reason for the disagreement is that treatment of *H. pylori* infection is poorly tolerated and less than 100% effective.

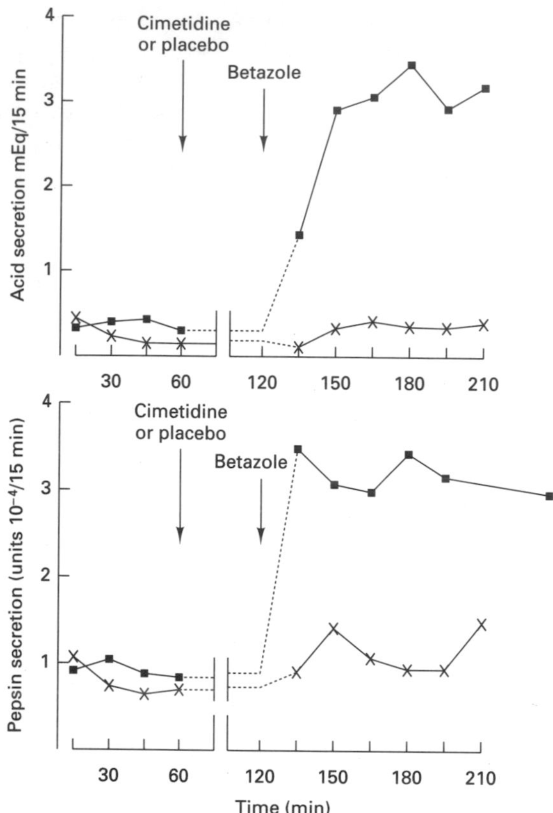

Fig. 19.5 The effect of cimetidine on betazole-stimulated gastric acid and pepsin secretion in man. Either cimetidine (×) or a placebo (■) was given orally 60 minutes prior to injecting betazole (1.5 mg/kg) subcutaneously. (Betazole, an isomer of histamine which is a relatively specific H_2-receptor agonist, stimulates gastric acid secretion.) (Modified from: Binder H J, Donaldson R M 1978 Gastroenterology 74: 371–375)

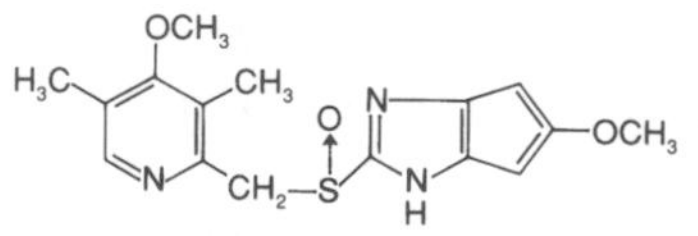

Fig. 19.6 Omeprazole.

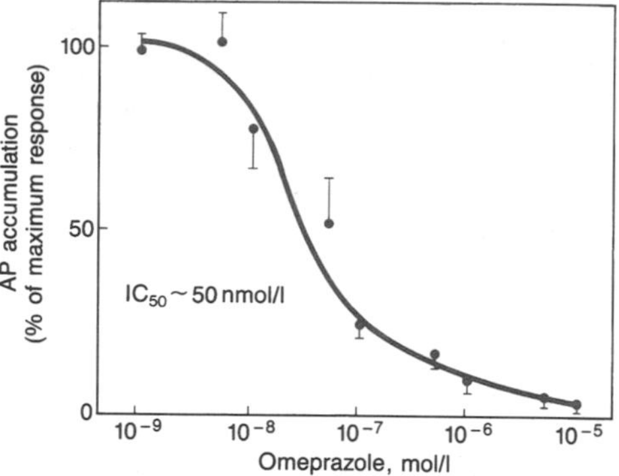

Fig. 19.7 The inhibitory action of omeprazole on acid secretion from isolated human gastric glands stimulated by 50 μmol/l histamine. Mean and standard error for tissue from eight patients. Acid secretion was measured by the accumulation of a radiolabelled weak base, aminopyrine (AP), in the secretory channels. (Adapted from: Lindberg P et al. 1987 Trends Pharmacol Sci 8: 399–402)

Preparations of cimetidine and ranitidine for intramuscular and intravenous use are also available. The half-life of cimetidine is shorter than that of ranitidine, but oral doses twice daily, even single doses nocturnally, are effective with both drugs. Famotidine and nizatidine need only be given once a day.

Unwanted effects

Unwanted effects are rare and are usually readily reversed on withdrawal of treatment. Diarrhoea, dizziness, muscle pains, transient rashes and hypergastrinaemia have been reported. Cimetidine sometimes causes gynaecomastia in men and, rarely, decrease in sexual function. This is probably due to the propensity of this agent to bind to androgen receptors, but the fact that it decreases **oestradiol** catabolism may contribute. Cimetidine also inhibits cytochrome P-450 and can retard the metabolism (and thus potentiate the action) of drugs such as the **oral anticoagulants, phenytoin, carbamazepine, quinidine, nifedipine, theophylline** and the **tricyclic antidepressants**. It can also cause confusion in the elderly. Ranitidine appears to have less effect on androgen receptors and the P-450 system. Both cimetidine and ranitidine reduce renal tubular secretion of basic drugs.

PROTON-PUMP INHIBITORS

The main agent is a substituted benzimidazole, **omeprazole,** a weak base of pKa 3.97 (Fig. 19.6). It acts by blocking irreversibly* the H^+/K^+-ATPase (the proton pump), the terminal step in the acid secretory pathway (see Figs 19.1 and 19.2). It markedly inhibits both basal and stimulated gastric

*Reversible proton-pump inhibitors are under test.

acid secretion (Fig. 19.7). It is inactive at neutral pH, but accumulates in an acid environment and is activated at a pH lower than 3, probably by protonation. It is thought to react with sulphydryl groups associated with the proton pump. The preferential accumulation of omeprazole in areas of very low pH, such as occur uniquely in the secretory canaliculi of gastric parietal cells, means that it has a specific effect on these cells. The clinical use of proton-pump inhibitors is given in the box on page 392.

Pharmacokinetic aspects

Omeprazole is given orally; but as it degrades rapidly at low pH it is administered as capsules containing enteric-coated granules to prevent inactivation in the stomach. Increased doses give disproportionately higher increases in plasma concentration (possibly because its inhibitory effect on acid secretion improves its own relative bioavailability). It is eliminated rapidly and completely by metabolism to inactive products. Although its $t_{½}$ is about 1 hour, a single daily dose affects acid secretion for 2–3 days. With daily dosage there is an increasing antisecretory effect for up to 5 days, after which a plateau is reached.

Unwanted effects

Unwanted effects are not common. They include headache, diarrhoea (both sometimes severe) and rashes. Dizziness, somnolence, mental confusion, impotence, gynaecomastia, and pain in muscles and joints have been reported.

MUSCARINIC-RECEPTOR ANTAGONISTS

Muscarinic-receptor antagonists are discussed in detail in Chapter 6. The main effects of muscarinic-receptor stimulation on the gastrointestinal tract are an increase in motility and an increase in secretory activity. The principal antagonist with clinically useful antisecretory action is **pirenzipine**. Pirenzipine is a relatively specific muscarinic M_1-receptor antagonist and is believed to act at the M_1-receptors found in parasympathetic ganglia, and possibly also on the histamine-secreting cell and the gastric parietal cell. Pirenzipine reduces basal and stimulated acid secretion at doses that have minimal effects on the heart, eye, bladder, etc. (which involve mainly M_2- or M_3-receptors). It is given orally and reported to be as effective as cimetidine in healing duodenal and gastric ulcers. However, it is more likely to produce unwanted effects, 20% of patients developing dry mouth and/or blurring of vision. The clinical use of muscarinic-receptor antagonists is given on page 392.

ANTACIDS

Antacids act by neutralising gastric acid and thus raising the gastric pH. This has the effect of inhibiting peptic activity, which practically ceases at pH 5. Given in sufficient quantity for long enough they can produce healing of duodenal ulcers but are less effective in gastric ulcers.

Based on the fact that low doses, with negligible effect on gastric acidity, have proved to have some degree of ulcer-healing potential, it has been suggested that, besides neutralising acid, they could have mucosal-protecting actions such as stimulation of bicarbonate production, enhancement of prostaglandin synthesis or reduction of *H. pylori* colonisation. There seems to be some evidence for at least the latter two of these actions (reviewed by Konturek et al. 1992).

The antacids in common use are salts of magnesium and aluminium. Magnesium salts cause diarrhoea and aluminium salts constipation, so mixtures of these two are used to preserve normal bowel function. Some preparations of these substances (e.g. magnesium trisilicate mixture and some proprietary aluminium preparations) contain high concentrations of sodium and should not be given to patients on a sodium-restricted diet.

Numerous antacid preparations are available; a few of the main ones are given below.

Magnesium hydroxide is an insoluble powder that forms magnesium chloride in the stomach. It does not produce systemic alkalosis since magnesium ion is poorly absorbed from the gut.

Magnesium trisilicate is an insoluble powder which reacts slowly with the gastric juice forming magnesium chloride and colloidal silica. This agent has a prolonged antacid effect, and it also adsorbs pepsin.

Aluminium hydroxide gel forms aluminium chloride in the stomach; when this reaches the intestine the chloride is released and is reabsorbed. Aluminium hydroxide raises the pH of the gastric juice to about 4; it also adsorbs pepsin. It acts gradually and its effect continues for several hours.

Colloidal aluminium hydroxide combines with phosphates in the gastrointestinal tract and the increased excretion of phosphate in the faeces which occurs results in decreased excretion of phosphate via the kidney. (This effect may be clinically useful for the prevention and treatment of phosphatic renal stones, the compound used being basic aluminium carbonate.)

There is a suggestion that aluminium, if absorbed, could be involved in the pathogenesis of Alzheimer's disease, though there is controversy on this point (see Ch. 25; Landsberg et al. 1992). Aluminium is said not to be absorbed to any significant extent during administration of aluminium hydroxide, but some perhaps overly cautious practitioners may prefer to use other antacids.

Sodium bicarbonate acts rapidly and is said to raise the pH of gastric juice to about 7.4. Carbon dioxide is liberated leading to the eructation of gas. This evolution of CO_2 stimulates gastrin secretion and can result in a secondary rise in acid secretion. Since some sodium bicarbonate is absorbed in the intestine, large doses or frequent administration of this antacid can cause alkalosis, the onset of which can be insidious. This agent should therefore not be prescribed for long-term treatment; nor should it be given to patients who are on a sodium-restricted diet.

Clinical use of agents affecting gastric secretion

- H_2-receptor antagonists, e.g. ranitidine:
  —peptic ulcer (drugs of choice)
  —Zollinger–Ellison syndrome (second line drugs)
  —reflux oesophagitis.
- Proton-pump inhibitors, e.g. omeprazole:
  —Zollinger–Ellison syndrome (drugs of choice)
  —peptic ulcers resistant to H_2-receptor antagonists
  —reflux oesophagitis.
- Antacids, e.g. magnesium trisilicate, aluminium hydroxide:
  —dyspepsia
  —symptomatic relief in peptic ulcer
  —adjuncts for healing of peptic ulcer?
- Bismuth chelate:
  —prevention (with antibiotics) of relapse of active duodenal ulcer.
- Muscarinic receptor antagonists, e.g. pirenzipine:
  —peptic ulcer (adjuncts to H_2-receptor antagonists).

Alginates are sometimes combined with antacids for use in reflux oesophagitis, because they are believed to increase adherence to the oesophageal mucosa. The clinical use of antacids is given on this page.

DRUGS WHICH PROTECT THE MUCOSA

Some agents, termed 'cytoprotective', are said to enhance the mucosal protection mechanisms (see above) and/or provide a physical barrier over the surface of the ulcer.

Bismuth chelate

Bismuth chelate (colloidal bismuth subcitrate, tripotassium dicitratobismuthate) is reported to be effective against *H. pylori*. Used alone it eradicates the organism in 30% of patients. A combination of bismuth chelate with **metronidazole** and **tetracyline**, given after a standard course of H_2-antagonist therapy, is reported to reduce the relapse rate with H_2-antagonist alone, as specified above, from 90% (duodenal) and 74% (gastric) to about 12%.

Bismuth chelate is believed to have other mucosal-protecting actions—coating the ulcer base, adsorbing pepsin, enhancing local prostaglandin synthesis and stimulating bicarbonate secretion.

The small amount of bismuth which is absorbed is excreted in the urine. If renal excretion is impaired, the raised plasma concentrations of bismuth can result in encephalopathy.

Unwanted effects include nausea and vomiting, and blackening of the tongue and faeces.

Sucralfate

Sucralfate is a complex of aluminium hydroxide and sulphated sucrose, which has been shown in double-blind trials to promote healing of ulcers as assessed by endoscopic examination. In the presence of acid, sucralfate releases aluminium, acquires a strong negative charge and binds to positively charged groups in proteins, glycoproteins, etc. It adheres to both damaged and normal mucosa. It can form complex gels with mucus, an action which is thought to decrease the degradation of mucus by pepsin and to limit the diffusion of hydrogen ions. In vitro studies indicate that it can inhibit the action of pepsin. It also stimulates the mucosal-protecting mechanisms—mucus and bicarbonate secretion and prostaglandin production.

It is given orally, four times daily before meals. In the acid environment of the stomach the polymerised product forms a viscous paste and about 30% is still present in the stomach 3 hours after administration. A small amount is absorbed into the systemic circulation (absorption of the released aluminium is comparable to that during administration of aluminium hydroxide as an antacid) and 1–2% of the drug given appears in the urine. It reduces the absorption of a number of other drugs, including **fluoroquinolone antibiotics**, **theophylline**, **tetracycline**, **digoxin** and **amitriptyline**. Since it requires an acid environment for activation, **antacids** given concurrently or prior to its administration will reduce its efficacy.

Unwanted effects are few, the most common being constipation which occurs in 0–15% of patients treated. Less common are dry mouth, nausea, vomiting, headache and rashes.

Misoprostol

Prostaglandins (PGs) are synthesised in large amounts by the gastric and intestinal mucosa and the E and I series can be shown to protect the deeper mucosal cells from experimental necrotic damage. A deficiency in prostaglandin production may contribute to ulcer formation. **Misoprostol** is a stable analogue of prostaglandin E_1 (PGE_1). It inhibits gastric acid secretion, both basal and that occurring in response to food, histamine, pentagastrin and caffeine by a direct action on the parietal cell (Fig. 19.2). It maintains or increases mucosal blood flow and increases the secretion of mucus and bicarbonate.

It is given orally and is used to prevent the gastric damage that can occur with chronic use of **non-steroidal anti-inflammatory drugs** (NSAIDs).

Unwanted effects are diarrhoea and abdominal cramps; uterine contractions can also occur (see Ch. 22). Prostaglandins and NSAIDs are discussed in Chapter 12.

DRUGS USED TO STIMULATE GASTRIC SECRETION

Pentagastrin consists of the 'working end' of the gastrin molecule (Trp–Met–Asp–Phe) to which a substituted β-alanine has been added. It has all the physiological actions of endogenous gastrin. It also has other, probably non-physiological effects, in that it stimulates pancreatic secretion and contracts the smooth muscle of the lower oesophageal sphincter, the gall bladder, the intestine and the colon. It inhibits gastric emptying and the absorption of glucose and electrolytes in the small intestine.

It is used diagnostically to test gastric acid secretion. It is given in a single dose of 6 μg/kg by subcutaneous or intramuscular injection. Secretion begins within 10 minutes, and the maximum response occurs within half an hour. The plasma half-life of pentagastrin is about 10 minutes. Unwanted effects are transient and include nausea and an urge to pass faeces. Flushing, increased heart rate and dizziness can also occur. Hypersensitivity reactions are occasionally seen.

VOMITING

The act of vomiting is a complicated one necessitating coordinated activity of the somatic respiratory and abdominal muscles, and the involuntary muscles of the gastrointestinal tract.

THE REFLEX MECHANISM OF VOMITING

Borison & Wang (1953) showed that the central neural regulation of vomiting is vested in two separate units in the medulla:

- *the vomiting centre*, which controls the interrelated movements of the relevant smooth muscle and striated muscle
- *the chemoreceptor trigger zone* in the *area postrema* on the floor of the fourth ventricle, close to the vagal nuclei.

The chemoreceptor trigger zone (CTZ) is sensitive to chemical stimuli and is the site of action of drugs such as **apomorphine**, **morphine** and the **cardiac glycosides**, and of emetogenic substances released by cytotoxic cancer chemotherapy drugs; these agents reach the CTZ through the bloodstream. In functional terms the CTZ lies *outside* the blood–brain barrier. An action on the CTZ is probably the mechanism by which endogenous substances produced in uraemia, radiation sickness and various clinical disorders, stimulate vomiting. The CTZ is also concerned in the mediation of motion sickness.

Motion sickness is caused by certain kinds of movement, and the origin of the stimuli is primarily

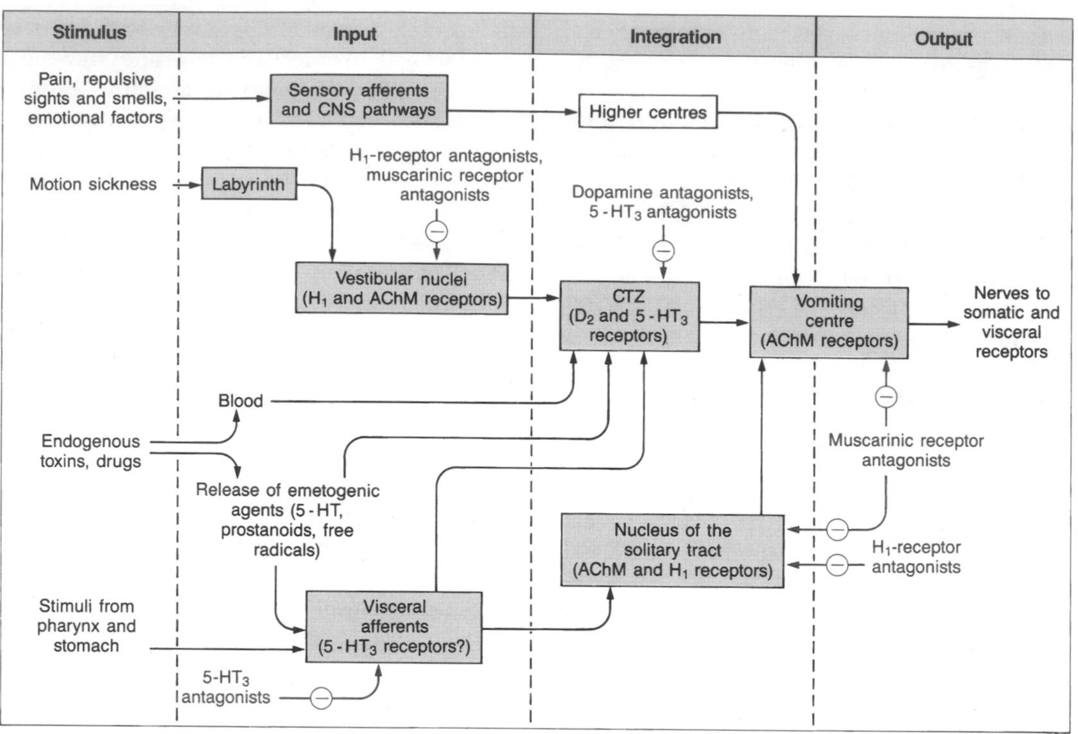

Fig. 19.8 Schematic diagram of the factors involved in the control of vomiting, with the probable sites of action of anti-emetic drugs. The cerebellum may function as a second relay or gating mechanism in the link between labyrinth and CTZ (not shown). (CTZ = chemoreceptor trigger zone; H_1 = histamine H_1; M = muscarinic; D_2 = dopamine D_2; 5-HT_3 = 5-hydroxytryptamine$_3$) (Based partly on a diagram from: Borison et al. 1981)

the vestibular apparatus. There is at least one primary afferent relay, in the vestibular nucleus, and the cerebellum may function as a secondary relay. However, it is not clear how the vestibular apparatus relays to the CTZ, since the cells of the CTZ do not appear to receive synaptic inputs, but respond only to substances in the blood and cerebrospinal fluid. A neurohumoral factor in the cerebrospinal fluid may be implicated.

Impulses from the CTZ in the *area postrema* pass to the vomiting centre. This centre is composed of those areas of the brainstem which control and integrate the visceral and somatic functions involved in vomiting. It is a physiological rather than an anatomical entity. An outline of the suggested interrelationships is given in Figure 19.8.

Vomiting can be triggered by a variety of stimuli. Some examples are given in Figure 19.8.

The main neurotransmitters considered to be involved in the control of vomiting are acetylcholine, histamine, 5-hydroxytryptamine and dopamine.* Receptors for these transmitters have been demonstrated in the relevant areas and are illustrated in Figure 19.8.

EMETIC DRUGS

In some circumstances, such as when a toxic substance has been swallowed, it may be necessary to stimulate vomiting. This should never be attempted if the patient is not fully conscious or if the substance is corrosive.

The drug usually used to produce vomiting is **ipecacuanha**, which acts locally in the stomach, its irritant action being due to the presence of two

*It has been hypothesised that enkephalins (see Ch. 9) are implicated in the mediation of vomiting, acting possibly at δ-receptors in the CTZ and at μ-receptors in the vomiting centre, and that cytotoxic drugs which cause emesis may act by inhibiting the metabolising enzymes which break down the enkephalins in the CTZ.

alkaloids *emetine* and *cephaeline*. Emetine has also been used in the treatment of amoebiasis (see Ch. 40).

For experimental studies on vomiting the drugs used are **apomorphine** which acts on the CTZ (see also p. 498) and **copper sulphate**, which acts locally in the stomach.

ANTI-EMETIC DRUGS

Different anti-emetic agents are used for different conditions, though there may be some overlap. Anti-emetic drugs are of particular importance as an adjunct to cancer chemotherapy to combat the nausea and vomiting produced by many cytotoxic drugs (see Ch. 36). These agents can cause almost unendurable nausea and vomiting. (It is reported that a young medically qualified patient being treated by combination chemotherapy for sarcoma stated that 'the severity of the nausea and vomiting at times made the thought of death seem like a welcome relief'.)

Details of the main categories of agents are given below and a summary of the main clinical uses of anti-emetic drugs is given opposite.

H_1-receptor antagonists

H_1-receptor antagonists are dealt with in Chapter 12. They have little or no activity against vomiting produced by substances acting directly on the CTZ but are effective in motion sickness and against vomiting caused by substances which act locally in the stomach. Examples are **cinnarizine, cyclizine, dimenhydrinate** and **promethazine**. It is possible that the component of antimuscarinic activity in some H_1-receptor antagonists plays a part in their effects.

In using drugs to treat the morning sickness of pregnancy, the problem of potential damage to the foetus has to be borne in mind. Promethazine is effective but, in general, all drugs should be avoided, if possible, during the first three months of pregnancy.

H_1-receptor antagonists are most effective if given before the onset of nausea and vomiting but may have some action in controlling it when established. Their peak anti-emetic effect occurs about 4 hours after ingestion and can last 24 hours.

Muscarinic-receptor antagonists

Drugs which antagonise acetylcholine at muscarinic receptors are dealt with in Chapter 6. **Hyoscine** is active against nausea and vomiting of labyrinthine origin and against vomiting due to local stimuli in the stomach but is ineffective against substances which act directly on the CTZ.

Hyoscine is the most potent agent available for the prevention of motion sickness, though it is less useful once sickness occurs. Its anti-emetic action peaks 1–2 hours after ingestion. The main unwanted actions are drowsiness and dry mouth; other side effects (e.g. blurring of vision and retention of urine) do not usually occur with the doses employed for anti-emetic effect. A transdermal preparation of hyoscine is available.

Phenothiazines

Phenothiazines are dealt with in Chapter 28; only those aspects relevant to the control of vomiting will be considered here.

Neuroleptic phenothiazines, such as **chlorpromazine, prochlorperazine** and **trifluoperazine** are effective anti-emetics, while some phenothiazines, such as **thiethylperazine**, are employed only for this purpose. They are active against agents which directly stimulate the CTZ but most are not active against emetic stimuli in the gut. They are

Clinical use of anti-emetic drugs

- H_1-receptor antagonists:
  —cyclizine: motion sickness
  —cinnarizine: motion sickness, vestibular disorders (e.g. Ménière's disease)
  —promethazine: severe morning sickness of pregnancy (but only if absolutely essential).
- Muscarinic-receptor antagonists:
  —hyoscine: motion sickness (drug of choice).
- D_2-receptor antagonists:
  —phenothiazines (e.g.thiethylperazine): vomiting caused by uraemia, radiation, viral gastroenteritis (drugs of choice); severe morning sickness of pregnancy (but only if absolutely essential)
  —metoclopramide: vomiting caused by uraemia, radiation, gastrointestinal disorders, cytotoxic drugs.
- 5-HT_3-receptor antagonists (e.g. ondansetron): vomiting caused by cytotoxic anticancer drugs (drug of choice); postoperative vomiting; radiation-induced vomiting.
- Cannabinoids (e.g. nabilone) for vomiting caused by cytotoxic anticancer drugs.

thought to act as antagonists of the dopamine D_2-receptors in the chemoreceptor trigger zone (see Fig. 19.8). However, they also have some degree of blocking action at histamine and muscarinic receptors and may have other sites of action.

Halogenation of the R_1 side-chain, as in trifluoperazine and prochlorperazine, increases anti-emetic activity and extrapyramidal effects, and decreases the occurrence of sedation and hypotension. Chlorpromazine has less prominent extrapyramidal action.

The main unwanted effects are dealt with in Chapter 28.

Phenothiazines can be given orally, rectally or parenterally, which means that unlike some anti-emetics they can be given after a patient starts to vomit.

Metoclopramide

Metoclopramide is a dopamine-receptor antagonist (Fig. 19.8) and acts in the CTZ. Like the phenothiazines, its unwanted effects are related to its blockade of other CNS dopamine receptors (see Ch. 28). Disorders of movement occur and are more common in children and young adults. Many patients feel drowsy and fatigued but some experience motor restlessness. Metoclopramide stimulates prolactin release (see Ch. 21) and can cause galactorrhoea and disorders of menstruation; diarrhoea can result from its action on gut motility (see p. 398). It is given orally, has a plasma $t_{½}$ of 4 hours and is excreted in the urine.

The anti-emetic action of high doses of metoclopramide in the nausea and vomiting caused by anticancer drugs is now thought to be due to antagonism of 5-HT_3 receptors.

Metoclopramide also has peripheral actions, increasing the motility of the stomach and intestine, which add to its anti-emetic effect and which may be used in therapy of gastrointestinal disorders (see p. 398).

5-hydroxytryptamine (5-HT) antagonists

5-hydroxytryptamine (see Ch. 8), released in either CNS or gut, is an important transmitter in emesis. Selective 5-HT_3-receptor antagonists, for example **ondansetron**, are proving to be of particular value in preventing and treating vomiting caused by cytotoxic drugs.

Ondansetron is given orally and/or by slow intravenous injection or infusion and its $t_{½}$ is 5 hours. Unwanted effects include headache and gastrointestinal upsets.

A newer 5-HT_3 antagonist, with similar actions, is **granisetron**.

Cannabinoids

A synthetic cannabinol derivative, **nabilone**, decreases vomiting due to agents which stimulate the CTZ. Its anti-emetic effect is antagonised by **naloxone** which implies that opioid receptors may be important in the action of this drug.

Nabilone is given orally, is well absorbed from the gastrointestinal tract and is metabolised in many tissues. Its plasma half-life is approximately 120 minutes, and its metabolites are excreted in the urine and faeces.

Unwanted effects are common, especially drowsiness, dizziness and dry mouth. Mood changes and postural hypotension are also fairly frequent. Some patients experience hallucinations and psychotic reactions.

Steroids

There are now several reports of the anti-emetic effect of high-dose steroids either alone or in combination with a phenothiazine. The steroids used were the glucocorticoids, **dexamethasone** and **methylprednisolone** (see Ch. 21). Their mechanism of action as anti-emetics is not known. They synergise with **ondansetron**.

Other anti-emetic agents

Other anti-emetic agents include the neuroleptic drugs **haloperidol** and **droperidol** (Ch. 28) which have given good results against strongly emetic cytotoxic drugs (e.g. cisplatin). **Domperidone**, a dopamine D_2-receptor antagonist (see Ch. 14 and below) is also used as an anti-emetic in postoperative vomiting and against moderately emetogenic anticancer drugs.

THE MOTILITY OF THE GASTROINTESTINAL TRACT

Drugs which increase movements include the *purgatives*, which accelerate the passage of food through the intestine, and *agents which increase the motility* of the gastrointestinal smooth muscle without causing purgation. The main agents decreasing movements

The reflex mechanism of vomiting

- Emetic stimuli:
  —chemicals in blood
  —neuronal input from GI tract, labyrinth and CNS.
- Impulses from chemoreceptor trigger zone, and various CNS centres relay to the vomiting centre.
- Chemical transmitters: histamine, acetylcholine, dopamine, 5-hydroxytryptamine acting on H_1, muscarinic, D_2 and 5-HT_3 receptors respectively.
- Anti-emetic drugs:
  —H_1-receptor antagonists (e.g. cyclizine)
  —muscarinic antagonists (e.g. hyoscine)
  —D_2-receptor antagonists (e.g. thiethylperazine, metoclopramide)
  —5-HT_3-receptor antagonists (e.g. ondansetron)
  —cannabinoids (e.g. nabilone).
- Main side effects of principal anti-emetics:
  —drowsiness and anti-parasympathetic effects (hyoscine, nabilone > cinnarizine)
  —dystonic reactions (thiethylperazine > metoclopramide)
  —general CNS disturbances (nabilone)
  —headache, GIT upsets (ondansetron).

are the *antidiarrhoeal* drugs and the *antispasmodics*. These four groups of agents are dealt with below.

PURGATIVES

The transit of food through the intestine may be hastened by several different methods:

- by increasing the volume of non-absorbable solid residue with *bulk laxatives*
- by increasing the water content with *osmotic laxatives*
- by altering the consistency of the faeces with *faecal softeners*
- by increasing motility and secretion (*stimulant purgatives*).

Good, comparative clinical studies of laxatives are not available; folk-lore and old wives' tales abound.

Bulk laxatives

The bulk laxatives include **methylcellulose** and certain plant gums, for example **sterculia, agar, bran** and **ispaghula husk**. These agents are polysaccharide polymers which are not broken down by the normal processes of digestion in the upper part of the gastrointestinal tract. They act by virtue of their capacity to retain water in the gut lumen and so promote peristalsis. They take several days to work but have no serious unwanted effects.

Osmotic laxatives

Osmotic laxatives consist of poorly absorbed solutes—the **saline purgatives** and **lactulose**. These maintain an increased volume of fluid in the lumen of the bowel by osmosis, which accelerates the transfer of the gut contents through the small intestine and results in an abnormally large volume entering the colon. This causes distension which leads to purgation about an hour later. Abdominal cramps can occur.

An amount of a saline purgative dissolved in sufficient water to produce an isotonic or hypotonic solution causes more rapid purgation than the same amount used as a hypertonic solution, which can cause vomiting.

The main salts in use are **magnesium sulphate** and **magnesium hydroxide**. A dose of 8 g of magnesium sulphate will retain about 120 ml of water in the lumen of the gut; this doubles the volume of the faeces. The amount of magnesium absorbed after an oral dose is usually too small to have adverse systemic effects but these salts should be avoided in small children and in patients with poor renal function, in whom they can cause heart block, neuromuscular disorders or CNS depression.

Lactulose is a semisynthetic disaccharide of fructose and galactose. In the colon, bacteria convert it to its two component sugars and, when these are fermented, the lactic and acetic acid formed function as osmotic laxatives. It takes 2–3 days to act. Unwanted effects, with high doses, are flatulence, cramps, diarrhoea and electrolyte disturbance. Tolerance can develop. After lactulose administration, the gut contents have a lower pH than normal and this decreases the activity of ammonia-producing organisms. Because of this effect, lactulose is used in the treatment of hepatic encephalopathy (a condition associated with chronic liver failure).

Faecal softeners

Docusate sodium is a surface-active compound which acts in the gastrointestinal tract in a manner similar to a detergent, and produces softer faeces. It is also a weak stimulant laxative.

Stimulant purgatives

Many agents increase peristalsis by stimulating

the mucosa of the gut (probably by initiating local reflexes), the impulses arising in the mucosa and being transmitted through the intramural plexuses to the smooth muscle of the intestine. The following are the more important purgatives in this group:

- bisacodyl
- sodium picosulphate
- preparations of senna.

These agents sometimes cause abdominal cramps; prolonged use can lead to deterioration of intestinal function, and can result in atonic colon.

Senna has laxative activity because it contains derivatives of anthracene (e.g. emodin). These substances are combined with sugars to form glycosides which must be hydrolysed before the active principles are free to act. The drug passes unchanged into the colon where bacteria hydrolyse the glycoside bond, releasing the free anthracene derivatives; these are then absorbed and have a direct stimulant effect on the myenteric plexus, resulting in smooth muscle activity and thus defaecation. Some emodin is excreted in the urine and some may appear in the milk of women who are breast feeding.

A single dose usually produces a laxative action within 8 hours, which may be accompanied by griping.

Bisacodyl stimulates sensory nerve endings in the colon. It can be given orally but is usually administered as a suppository, causing stimulation of the rectal mucosa which results in peristaltic action and defaecation in 15–30 minutes. **Sodium picosulphate** has a similar action; it is given orally.

Note that the belief that regular, daily defaecation is an absolute prerequisite for good health is embedded in folklore and tradition, but there is little to support it in modern medicine.

DRUGS WHICH INCREASE GASTROINTESTINAL MOTILITY

Some agents increase gut motility. The main groups of drugs used are:

- domperidone
- metoclopramide
- cisapride.

Domperidone

Domperidone is a dopamine-receptor antagonist acting at D_2-receptors, and is used as an anti-emetic as described above. It is also effective in increasing gastrointestinal motility. Dopamine can be shown to produce relaxation of guinea-pig gastro-oesophageal smooth muscle, but the order of potency of antagonists of this action (prazosin > phentolamine > domperidone > haloperidol) suggests that it is acting on α-adrenoceptors. Domperidone is thought to enhance motility by blocking α_1-adrenoceptors and thus decreasing their relaxant effect. Clinically, it increases lower oesophageal sphincter pressure (thus inhibiting gastro-oesophageal reflux), increases gastric emptying and enhances duodenal peristalsis. It does not stimulate gastric acid secretion. It is useful in disorders of gastric emptying and in chronic gastric reflux.

Its main unwanted effect is hyperprolactinaemia, consistent with its action on dopamine receptors (see Ch. 24).

Metoclopramide

In addition to its central effects as an anti-emetic (see above), metoclopramide exerts a significant local stimulant effect on gastric motility, causing a marked acceleration of gastric emptying with no concomitant stimulation of gastric acid secretion. It is believed to activate cholinergic neurons, but in comparison with muscarinic agonists, it appears to have less effect on the motility of the lower bowel. Metoclopramide is useful in gastro-oesophageal reflux and in disorders of gastric emptying, but is ineffective in paralytic ileus.

Cisapride

Cisapride stimulates acetylcholine release in the myenteric plexus in the upper gastrointestinal tract. This raises oesophageal sphincter pressure and increases gut motility. It is used in reflux oesophagitis and in disorders of gastric emptying. It has no anti-emetic action.

Unwanted effects, which are rare, include diarrhoea, abdominal cramps and tachycardia.

ANTIDIARRHOEAL AGENTS

Diarrhoea is the too frequent passage of faeces which are too liquid. There are numerous causes including infectious agents, toxins, anxiety, drugs, etc. The repercussions will depend not only on the cause, but also on the state of nutrition and health of the patient. They can range from discomfort and inconvenience in a healthy well-nourished adult, to a medical emergency requiring hospitalisation and parenteral fluid and electrolyte therapy. On a world-wide basis, acute diarrhoeal disease is one of the principal causes of death in malnourished infants; this is particularly important in developing countries.

Diarrhoea involves both an increase in the motility of the gastrointestinal tract and a decrease in the absorption of fluid, and thus a loss of electrolytes (particularly sodium) and water. Details of electrolyte transport in diarrhoea are given by Field et al. (1989). Cholera toxins and some other bacterial toxins produce not only loss of gut contents but a profound increase in secretion through their effect on the guanine nucleotide regulatory proteins which couple the surface receptors of the mucosal cells to adenylate cyclase (see Ch. 2).

There are three approaches to the treatment of severe acute diarrhoea:

- maintenance of fluid and electrolyte balance
- use of anti-infective agents
- use of non-antimicrobial antidiarrhoeal agents.

The maintenance of fluid and electrolyte balance by means of oral rehydration is the first priority and wider appreciation of this could save the lives of many infants in the developing world. Many cases require no other treatment. In the ileum, as in parts of the nephron, there is co-transport of sodium and glucose across the epithelial cell and, therefore, glucose enhances sodium absorption and thus water uptake; amino acids have a similar effect. Preparations of sodium chloride and glucose for oral use are available in powder form.

The use of anti-infective agents is usually not necessary in simple gastroenteritis since most infections are usually viral in origin, and those that are bacterial generally resolve without antibacterial therapy. *Campylobacter* is the commonest bacterial organism causing gastroenteritis in the UK, and severe cases may require **erythromycin** or **ciprofloxacin** (Ch. 37). Chemotherapy may be necessary in some types of enteritis (e.g. typhoid, amoebic dysentery and cholera).

General principles for the treatment of traveller's diarrhoea (frequently due to enterotoxin-producing *Esch. coli*) are detailed by DuPont & Ericsson (1993) and Gorbach (1987), who makes the pertinent remark 'travel broadens the mind and loosens the bowels'.

The use of non-antimicrobial antidiarrhoeal agents is dealt with below, and these include antimotility agents, adsorbents and agents which modify fluid and electrolyte transport.

Antimotility agents

The main pharmacological agents which decrease motility are **opiates** (details in Ch. 31) and **muscarinic-receptor antagonists** (details in Ch. 6). Agents in this latter group are seldom employed as primary therapy for diarrhoea because of their actions on other systems; but small doses of atropine are used combined with diphenoxylate (see below).

The action of **morphine**, the type-specific opiate, on the alimentary tract is complex and, furthermore, varies in different species. In man, morphine increases the tone and rhythmic contractions of the intestine but diminishes propulsive activity. Its overall effect is constipating. The pyloric, ileocolic and anal sphincters are contracted and the tone of the large intestine is markedly increased.

The main opiates used in diarrhoea are **codeine** (a morphine congener), **diphenoxylate** and **loperamide** (both pethidine congeners used only for their actions in the gut). All have unwanted effects which include nausea, vomiting, abdominal cramps, drowsiness and dizziness. Paralytic ileus can also occur. They should not be used in young children.

More than 3 000 000 people cross international borders each year. Many travel hopefully but come back ill, having encountered enterotoxin-producing *Esch. coli* or other organisms. Most infections are self-limiting and require only oral replacement of fluid and salt as detailed above, but loperamide reduces the frequency of passage of faeces and the duration of the illness.

Loperamide has a relatively selective action on the gastrointestinal tract which is related to its distribution in the body. After oral dosing in experimental animals, 85% is found in the gastrointestinal tract, and 5% in the liver. There is evidence that there is efficient enterohepatic cycling of the drug. It has low solubility in water which would discourage abuse by injection. It should not be given to patients with dysentery because it can exacerbate diarrhoea in the presence of an invasive bacterial infection.

Diphenoxylate, given once in the therapeutic dose suitable for diarrhoea, does not have morphine-like activity, though large doses (25-fold higher) produce typical opioid effects. However, its salts are, for practical purposes, insoluble in water and thus the drug does not have potential for abuse by injection. Preparations of diphenoxylate usually contain atropine as well.

Codeine and loperamide have antisecretory actions in addition to their effects on intestinal motility.

Bismuth subsalicylate, which is used for traveller's diarrhoea, is said to be safe in healthy young adults and can prevent* up to 65% of cases of diarrhoea in areas of high risk. It decreases fluid secretion in the bowel. It may work largely by virtue of its salicylate component.

Bismuth subsalicylate can cause tinnitus and blackening of the faeces and may have as yet unknown unwanted effects.

Adsorbents

Adsorbent agents are used extensively in the treatment of diarrhoea, although properly controlled trials proving adequacy have not been carried out.

The main preparations used are **kaolin, pectin, chalk, charcoal, methyl cellulose** and **activated attapulgite** (magnesium aluminium silicate).

It has been suggested that these agents may act by adsorbing microorganisms or toxins, by altering the intestinal flora or by coating and protecting the intestinal mucosa but there is no hard evidence for this.

Agents which modify fluid and electrolyte transport

Drugs which reduce secretion and/or stimulate absorption may well be of value in acute diarrhoea. **Zaldaride maleate**, a new preparation, not yet generally available, inhibits calmodulin and hence reduces secretion of water and electrolytes; it is reported to be effective in traveller's diarrhoea. Other preparations with the potential for producing these effects have been tested in the laboratory and are being investigated in man. **Non-steroidal anti-inflammatory agents** such as **aspirin** and **indomethacin** have been shown to have significant antidiarrhoeal actions both in experimental animals and in man. The effect is probably largely due to inhibition of prostaglandin synthesis (see Ch. 12) though other, as yet unknown, mechanisms may play a part.

*However, authorities recommend that drugs should not be taken prophylactically unless absolutely necessary (DuPont & Ericsson 1993).

Drugs and GI tract motility

- Purgatives:
  - —bulk laxatives, e.g. ispaghula husk (first choice for slow action)
  - —osmotic laxatives, e.g. lactulose
  - —faecal softeners, e.g. docusate sodium
  - —stimulant purgatives, e.g. senna.
- Drugs which increase motility without purgation:
  - —domperidone, used in disorders of gastric emptying.
- Drugs used to treat diarrhoea:
  - —oral rehydration with isotonic solutions of NaCl plus glucose or starch-based cereal (important in infants)
  - —antimotility agents, e.g. loperamide (unwanted effects: drowsiness and nausea)
  - —absorbents, e.g. magnesium aluminium silicate.

ANTISPASMODIC AGENTS

Drugs which reduce spasm in the gut are of value in irritable bowel syndrome and diverticular disease.

Muscarinic-receptor antagonists are dealt with in Chapter 6. They decrease spasm by inhibiting parasympathetic activity. Some of the agents available are **propantheline, mepenzolate, dicyclomine**. The last named is thought to have some additional direct relaxant action on smooth muscle. Unwanted effects—dry mouth, blurred vision, dry skin, tachycardia, difficulty with urination—are due to parasympathetic inhibition in other tissues; they are less marked and less common with dicyclomine.

Mebeverine, a derivative of reserpine, has a direct relaxant action on gastrointestinal smooth muscle. Unwanted effects are few.

DRUGS FOR CHRONIC INFLAMMATORY BOWEL DISEASE

Chronic inflammatory bowel disease comprises ulcerative colitis and Crohn's disease (a granulomatous condition affecting mainly the terminal ileum and the colon), both of uncertain aetiology. The following agents are used.

Glucocorticoids—these anti-inflammatory agents are dealt with in Chapter 21. See also Figure 11.5. Prednisolone is given locally in the bowel by suppository or enema.

Sulphasalazine is a combination of the sulphonamide, sulphapyridine, with 5-aminosalicylic acid. The latter is the active moiety; it is released in the colon and is not absorbed. Its mechanism of action is not known. It may act by scavenging free radicals, inhibiting prostaglandin and leukotriene production and/or by decreasing neutrophil chemotaxis and superoxide generation. Its unwanted effects are diarrhoea, salicylate sensitivity and interstitial nephritis. The sulphapyridine moiety is absorbed and its unwanted effects are those associated with the sulphonamides (see Ch. 37). Sulphasalazine is not useful for the actual attack of inflammatory bowel disease, but is valuable in preventing recurrence in patients who are in remission.

Newer compounds are **mesalazine** (5-aminosalicylic acid itself) and **olsalazine** (two molecules of 5-aminosalicylic acid linked by a diazo bond, which is broken by colonic bacteria).

The immunosuppressant, **azathioprine** (see Ch. 12), is used in patients with severe disease.

DRUGS AFFECTING THE BILIARY SYSTEM

Drugs used to treat cholesterol cholelithiasis

The commonest pathological condition of the biliary tract is cholesterol cholelithiasis, i.e. the formation of cholesterol gallstones. Drugs which dissolve non-calcified cholesterol gallstones are **chenodeoxycholic acid** (CDCA) and **ursodeoxycholic acid** (UDCA). CDCA is one of the two primary bile acids. UDCA, the 7 β-hydroxy epimer of CDCA, occurs in small amounts in human bile and is the main bile acid in the bear (hence 'urso'). UDCA and CDCA are interconvertible during enterohepatic cycling in man. Given orally, UDCA and CDCA are handled by the body in the same way as endogenous bile acids; both agents decrease hepatic synthesis and secretion of cholesterol. Diarrhoea is the main unwanted effect.

The clinical use of these agents is appropriate only in selected patients with gallstones as surgery is the preferred treatment in most cases.

Drugs affecting biliary spasm

The pain produced by the passage of gallstones down the bile duct (biliary colic) can be very intense, and immediate relief may be required. **Morphine** relieves the pain, owing to its central narcotic analgesic action, but locally it may have an unfavourable effect since it constricts the sphincter of Oddi and raises the pressure in the bile duct. **Buprenorphine** may be preferable. **Pethidine** has similar actions, although it relaxes other smooth muscle, for example that of the ureter. **Atropine** is commonly employed to relieve biliary spasm since it has antispasmodic action. It may be used in conjunction with morphine.

The nitrates (see Ch. 13) can produce a marked fall of intrabiliary pressure and may relieve the biliary spasm.

REFERENCES AND FURTHER READING

Innervation and hormones of the gastrointestinal tract

Del Valle J, Yamada T 1990 The gut as an endocrine organ. Annu Rev Med 41: 447–455

Walsh J H 1988 Peptides as regulators of gastric acid secretion. Annu Rev Physiol 50: 41–63

Wingate D L 1986 Neurophysiology of the gastrointestinal tract. The Gastroenterology Annual 3: 258–283

Gastric secretion

Allen A, Garnet A 1980 Mucus and bicarbonate secretion in the stomach and their possible role in mucosal protection. Gut 21: 249–262

Angus J A, Black J W 1982 The interaction of choline esters, vagal stimulation and H_2-receptor blockade on acid secretion in vitro. Eur J Pharmacol 80: 217–224

Birdsall N J M 1991 Cloning and structure function of the H_2 histamine receptor. Trends Pharmacol Sci 12: 9–10

Black J W, Shankley N P 1987 How does gastrin act to stimulate oxyntic cell secretion? Trends Pharmacol Sci 8: 486–490

Black J W, Duncan W A M, Durant C J, Ganellin C R, Parsons E M 1972 Definition and antagonism of histamine H_2-receptors. Nature 236: 385–390

Machen T E, Paradiso A M 1987 Regulation of intracellular pH in the stomach. Annu Rev Physiol 49: 19–33

Robert A 1987 Effect of drugs on gastric secretion. In: Johnson L R (ed) Physiology of the gastrointestinal tract, 2nd edn. Raven Press, New York, p 1071–1088

Sandvik A K, Waldrum H L 1991 Gastrin is a potent stimulant of the parietal cell—maybe. Am J Physiol 260: G925–G928

Soll A H, Berglindh T 1987 Physiology of isolated gastric glands and parietal cells: receptors and effectors regulating function. In: Johnson L R (ed) Physiology of the gastrointestinal tract, 2nd edn. Raven Press, New York, p 883–908

Wolfe M M, Soll A H 1988 The physiology of gastric acid secretion. N Engl J Med 319: 1707–1715

Drugs in gastric disorders

Alper J 1993 Ulcers as an infectious disease. Science 260: 159–160

Clissold S P, Campoli-Richards D M 1986 Omeprazole: a preliminary review of its pharmacodynamic and pharmacokinetic properties and therapeutic potential in peptic ulcer disease and Zollinger–Ellison syndrome. Drugs 32: 15–47

Colin-Jones D G 1990 Acid suppression: how much is needed? Br Med J 301: 564–565

Consensus Development Panel 1994 *Helicobacter pylori* in peptic ulcer disease: Consensus Development Conference statement. National Institute of Health, Bethesda, Md.

Cover T L, Blaser M J 1992 *Helicobacter pylori* and gastroduodenal disease. Annu Rev Med 43: 135–145

Feldman M, Burton M E 1990 Histamine H_2-receptor antagonists: standard therapy for acid-peptic disease. N Engl J Med 323: 1672–1680, 1749–1755

Forbes G M, Glaser M E et al. 1994 Duodenal ulcer treatment with Helicobacter eradication: seven-year follow-up. Lancet 343: 258–260

Graham D Y 1993 Treatment of peptic ulcers caused by *Helicobacter pylori.* N Engl J Med 328: 349–350

Hosking S W, Ling T K W et al. 1994 Duodenal ulcer healing by eradication of Helicobacter pylori without antacid treatment: randomised controlled trial. Lancet 343: 508–510

Isaacson P G 1994 Gastric lymphoma and *Helicobacter pylori.* N Engl J Med 330: 1310–1311

Konturek S J, Brzozowski T, et al. 1992 Antacids and mucosal protection. Eur J Gastroenterol Hepatol 4: 954–965

Landsberg J P, McDonald B, Watt F 1992 Absence of aluminium in neuritic plaque cores in Alzheimer's disease. Nature 360: 65–67

Langman M J S 1991 Omeprazole: for resistant ulcers and severe oesophageal reflux disease. Br Med J 303: 481–482

McCarthy D M 1991 Sucralfate. N Engl J Med 325: 1017–1025

Marks I N, Schmassmann A et al. 1992 Antacid therapy today. Eur J Gastroenterol Hepatol 4: 977–983

Maton P N 1991 Omeprazole. N Engl J Med 324: 965–975

Moss S, Calam J 1992 *Helicobacter pylori* and peptic ulcers: the present position. Gut 23: 289–292

Pope A J, Parsons M E 1993 Reversible inhibitors of the gastric H^+/K^+-transporting ATPase: a new class of antisecretory agent. Trends Pharmacol Sci 14: 323–325

Soll A H 1990 Pathogenesis of peptic ulcer and implications for therapy. N Engl J Med 322: 909–916

Tygat G N J, Noach L A, Rauws E A J 1992 *Helicobacter pylori.* Eur J Gastroenterol Hepatol 4: S7–S15

Walt R P 1992 Misoprostol for the treatment of peptic ulcer and anti-inflammatory-drug-induced gastroduodenal ulceration. N Engl J Med 327: 1575–1580

Weberg R 1992 Antacids and acid neutralisation. Eur J Gastroenterol Hepatol 4: 949–953

Weir D G 1988 Peptic ulceration. (Section on New Drugs) Br Med J 296: 195–200

Vomiting

Andrews P L R, Rapeport W G, Sanger G J 1988 Neuropharmacology of emesis induced by anti-cancer therapy. Trends Pharmacol Sci 9: 334–340

Borison H L, Wang S C 1953 Physiology and pharmacology of vomiting. Pharmacol Rev 5: 193–230

Borison H L, Borison R, McCarthy L E 1981 Phylogenic and neurologic aspects of the vomiting process. J Clin Pharmacol 21: 235–295

Bunce K, Tyers M, Beranek P 1991 Clinical evaluation of 5-HT_3 receptor antagonists as anti-emetics. Trends Pharmacol Sci 12: 46–48

Davis C J, Lake-Bakaar G V, Grahame-Smith D G (eds) 1986 Nausea and vomiting: mechanisms and treatment. Springer-Verlag, Berlin

Editorial 1989 Drugs acting on 5-hydroxytryptamine receptors. Lancet 2: 717–719

Editorial 1991 Ondansetron v dexamethasone for chemotherapy-induced emesis. Lancet 338: 478-479

Edwards C M 1988 Chemotherapy-induced emesis mechanisms and treatment: a review. J Roy Soc Med 81: 658–662

Lathers C M, Charles J B, Bungo M W 1989 Pharmacology in space. Part 2: Controlling motion sickness. Trends in Pharmacol Sci 10: 243–250

Smyth J F, Coleman R E et al. 1991 Does dexamethasone enhance control of cisplatin induced emesis by ondansetron? Br Med J 303: 1423–1424

Motility of the gastrointestinal tract

Avery M E, Snyder J D 1990 Oral therapy for acute diarrhoea. N Engl J Med 323: 891–894

Bateman D N, Smith J M 1989 A policy for laxatives. Br Med J 298: 1420–1421

Carpenter C C J, Greenough W B, Pierce N F 1988 Oral rehydration therapy—the role of polymeric substrates. N Engl J Med 319: 1346–1348

Costello A M de L, Bhutta T I 1992 Antidiarrhoeal drugs for acute diarrhoea in children: none work, and many may be dangerous. Br Med J 304: 1–2

DuPont H L, Ericsson C D 1993 Prevention and treatment of travellers diarrhoea. N Engl J Med 328: 1281–1287

Farthing M J G 1993 Travellers diarrhoea: mostly due to bacteria and difficult to prevent. Br Med J 306: 1425–1426

Field M, Rao M C, Chang E B 1989 Intestinal electrolyte transport and diarrhoeal disease. N Engl J Med 321: 800–806, 879–883

Gorbach S L 1987 Bacterial diarrhoea and its treatment. Lancet 2: 1378–1382

Programme for Control of Diarrhoeal Diseases: sixth programme report 1986–1987 World Health Organization WHO/CDD/88.28 p 1–119

Spiller R 1990 Management of constipation. Part 2: When fibre fails. In: Controversies in therapeutics. Br Med J 300: 1064–1065

Tedesco F J, DiPiro J T 1985 Laxative use in constipation. Am J Gastroenterol 80: 303–309

The biliary system

Bouchier I A D 1990 Gallstones. Br Med J 300: 592–597

Editorial 1992 Bile acid therapy in the 1990s. Lancet 340: 1260–1261

Johnston D E, Kaplan M M 1993 Pathogenesis and treatment of gallstones. N Engl J Med 328: 412–421

Poupon R E, Poupon R, Balkan B 1994 Ursodiol for the long-term treatment of biliary cirrhosis N Engl J Med 330: 1342–1347

Inflammatory bowel disease

Kamm M A, Senapati A 1992 Drug management of ulcerative colitis. Br Med J 305: 35–38

20

THE ENDOCRINE PANCREAS AND THE CONTROL OF BLOOD GLUCOSE

PANCREATIC ISLET HORMONES

The endocrine portion of the pancreas, namely the islets of Langerhans, contains cells that secrete **insulin, amylin, glucagon** and **somatostatin**. The glucagon-secreting cells (α_2- or A-cells) and somatostatin-secreting cells (α_1- or D-cells) are found peripherally in the islet, and the predominant, insulin-secreting cells (β- or B-cells) are found in the centre (see Fig. 20.1). These latter secrete amylin as well as insulin. Amylin opposes the action of insulin by stimulating breakdown of glycogen in striated muscle and inhibits insulin secretion, although whether these effects are biologically important remains controversial (see below). Insulin has a crucial role in the control of blood glucose, and intermediary metabolism. Diseases in which there is deficient or excessive insulin production (in diabetes mellitus or from functioning tumours of β-cells known as insulinomas respectively) are characterised by profound metabolic disturbances. Glucagon increases blood glucose; decreased glucagon secretion is not known to cause disease and excessive secretion (from functioning tumours of α_2-cells, known as glucagonomas) causes only moderate hyperglycaemia. Somatostatin has an indirect paracrine role in that it has inhibitory actions on both insulin and glucagon secretion. Somatostatin is also released from the hypothalamus and inhibits the release of growth hormone from the pituitary (p. 420).

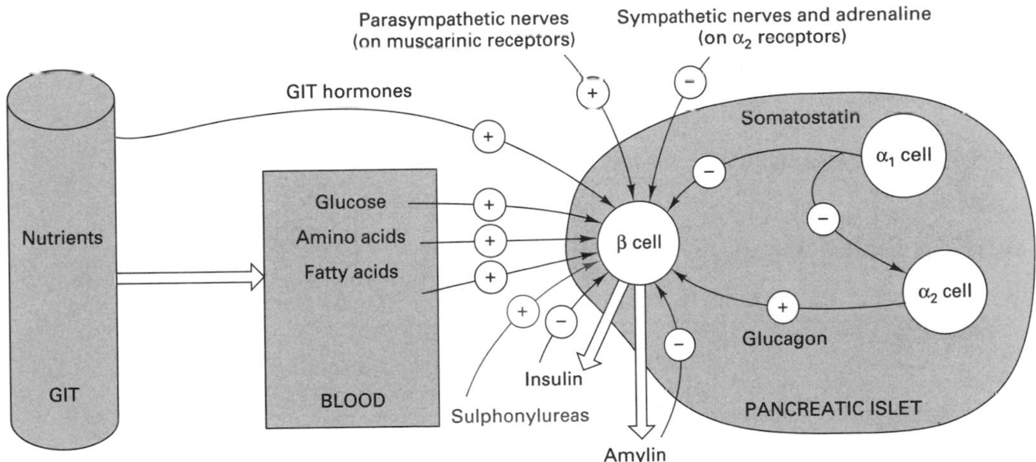

Fig. 20.1 Endogenous factors regulating insulin secretion by β-cells of the islets of Langerhans. Blood glucose is the most important factor. Drugs used to stimulate insulin secretion are shown in red. Glucagon potentiates insulin release but opposes some of its peripheral actions; see Table 20.2. (GIT = gastrointestinal tract)

INSULIN

Insulin is a polypeptide (6000 MW approx.) consisting of two peptide chains connected by two disulphide bridges. Its amino acid sequence was determined by Sanger and his co-workers in 1955. It is derived by proteolytic cleavage from a larger single-chain protein precursor (9000 MW approx.) termed proinsulin. Proteolysis removes a connecting peptide, the C-peptide, and the insulin so produced, together with the associated C-peptide, is stored in granules in the β-cells. Insulin and C-peptide are co-secreted in equimolar amounts, together with smaller and variable amounts of proinsulin.

Synthesis and secretion

The main factor controlling the synthesis and secretion of insulin is the *blood glucose* concentration (Fig. 20.1). The β-cell responds to both the *actual glucose concentration* and also to the *rate of change* of blood glucose. There is a steady basal release of insulin and also a response to a rise in blood glucose. This response has two phases—an initial rapid phase reflecting release of stored hormone, and a slower, delayed phase reflecting both release of stored hormone and new synthesis (Fig. 20.2). The response is abnormal in diabetes mellitus, as discussed later.

ATP-sensitive K^+-channels determine the resting membrane potential in β-cells. Glucose metabolism increases the intracellular concentration of ATP, which blocks these channels, causing depolarisation. This opens voltage-dependent Ca^{2+} channels, leading to Ca^{2+} influx. There is recent evidence (discussed by Turk et al. 1993) that the Ca^{2+} signal caused by D-glucose in the β-cell induces insulin secretion only in the presence of amplifying intracellular messengers including diacylglycerol (DAG), non-esterified arachidonic acid (which facilitates further Ca^{2+} entry) and 12-lipoxygenase products of arachidonic acid (mainly 12-S-HETE; see Ch. 11). Most phospholipases are activated by Ca^{2+} but it appears that free arachidonic acid is liberated in β-cells by an ATP-sensitive Ca^{2+}-insensitive ('ASCI') phospholipase A_2. Thus, both Ca^{2+} entry and arachidonic acid production are driven by ATP in the β-cell. Secretion of insulin occurs by exocytosis, in pulses every 15–30 minutes.

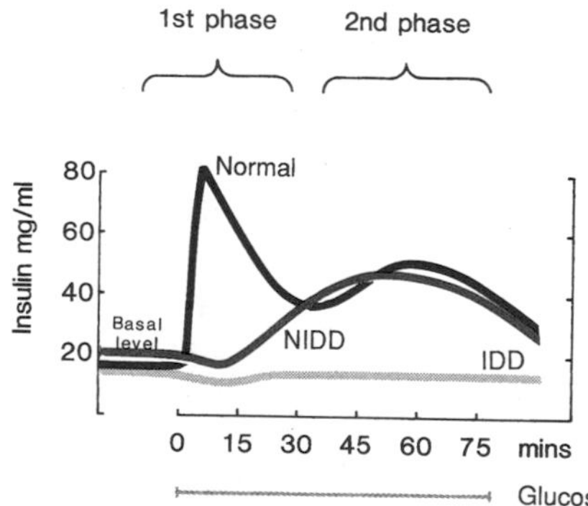

Fig. 20.2 Schematic diagram of the two-phase release of insulin which occurs with constant glucose infusion. The first phase is missing in non-insulin-dependent diabetes mellitus (NIDDM) and both are missing in insulin-dependent diabetes mellitus (IDDM). The first phase can also be produced by amino acids, sulphonylureas, glucagon and GIT hormones. (Data from: Pfeifer et al. 1981)

Stimuli to insulin release other than glucose include glucagon, amino acids (particularly arginine and leucine), fatty acids, various hormones from the gastrointestinal tract (GIT) and the **sulphonylurea drugs** (see below). These elicit only the first phase of insulin release.

GIT hormones, such as *gastrin, secretin, cholecystokinin, gastric inhibitory polypeptide* (GIP) and *enteroglucagon* are released by eating. These stimulate insulin secretion which explains why oral glucose causes a greater insulin release than intravenous glucose. Such GIT hormones (in particular GIP) provide an anticipatory signal from the GIT to the islets.

Insulin release is inhibited by somatostatin and amylin (see Fig. 20.1).

The *autonomic nervous system* has a significant inhibitory effect on insulin secretion as shown in Figure 20.1. Adrenaline increases blood glucose by inhibiting insulin release from the islets (via α_2-receptors) and by promoting glycogenolysis via β_2-receptors in striated muscle and liver. These activate adenylate cyclase, leading to conversion of glycogen phosphorylase from the inactive to the active form (see Ch. 2).

About one-fifth of the insulin store in the pancreas of the human adult is secreted daily (this is equivalent to about 5 mg) and the mean plasma concentration after an overnight fast is 20–50 pmol/l. Insulin is secreted into the portal circulation and in the fasted state its concentration in the portal vein is approximately threefold higher than in the rest of the circulation, reflecting the removal of a large amount (approximately 50%) of insulin by the liver. This differential may rise to a ratio of 10 : 1 after the islets have been stimulated by glucose.

Circulating insulin can be measured by radioimmunoassay, but this may give an overestimate because many insulin antibodies cross-react with proinsulin which can lead to errors in insulin estimation. Plasma insulin concentration is reduced in patients with insulin-dependent diabetes mellitus (see below) and markedly increased in patients with insulinomas, as is C-peptide with which it is co-released. Insulin for injection does *not* contain C-peptide, which therefore provides a means of distinguishing endogenous from exogenous insulin. This is used to distinguish insulinoma (an insulin-secreting tumour causing high circulating insulin with high C-peptide) from surreptitious injection of insulin (high insulin, normal or low C-peptide). Deliberate induction of hypoglycaemia by self-injection with insulin is a well-recognised, if unusual, manifestation of psychiatric disorder, especially in health professionals—it has also been used in murder.

Actions

Insulin is the main hormone controlling intermediary metabolism. It affects every tissue in the body but principally liver, muscle and fat (Table 20.1). Its overall effect is the conservation of body fuel supplies. Its most obvious immediate effect is to *reduce blood sugar* reflecting its general physiological function of *facilitating the uptake, utilisation and storage of glucose, amino acids and fats after a meal.* Conversely, a fall in plasma insulin causes reduced uptake of these substances into cells and increased mobilisation of endogenous fuel sources. The biochemical pathways through which insulin exerts its effects are summarised in Figure 20.3 and the molecular aspects of its mechanism are discussed below.

Carbohydrate metabolism

Insulin influences glucose metabolism in all tissues. The *liver* is especially important in this regard, the action of insulin being to decrease glycogenolysis (glycogen breakdown) and gluconeogenesis (synthesis of glucose from non-carbohydrate sources) and increase glycogen synthesis. It also increases glucose utilisation (glycolysis), but the overall effect in the liver is to increase glycogen stores.

In *muscle*, unlike liver, uptake of glucose is slow and is the rate-limiting step in carbohydrate metabolism. The main effect of insulin is to increase facilitated transport of glucose, but it also increases glycogen synthesis and glycolysis.

In *adipose tissue*, insulin increases glucose uptake by facilitating transfer of glucose transporters from an intracellular pool to the membrane. Intracellular metabolism of glucose is enhanced. One of the main end products of glucose metabolism in adipose tissue is glycerol, which is esterified with fatty acids to form triglycerides, thereby affecting fat metabolism (see below and Table 20.1).

Fat metabolism

Insulin increases fatty acid synthesis and triglyceride formation in *adipose tissue* (Table 20.1). It decreases lipolysis, partly by promoting dephosphorylation of lipases and thus inactivating them. Insulin also depresses the lipolytic action of adrenaline and growth hormone (and possibly glucagon) by opposing their stimulant action on adenylate cyclase. Insulin also causes lipogenesis in the *liver*. Indeed, when adequate amounts of insulin and carbohydrate are available there is more de novo synthesis of fatty acids in the liver than in adipose tissue.

Table 20.1 Summary of the effects of insulin on carbohydrate, fat and protein metabolism in liver, muscle and adipose tissue

Type of metabolism	Liver cells	Fat cell	Muscle
Carbohydrate metabolism	↓ gluconeogenesis ↓ glycogenolysis ↑ glycolysis ↑ glycogenesis	↑ glucose uptake ↑ glycerol synthesis ↓	↑ glucose uptake ↑ glycolysis ↑ glycogenesis
Fat metabolism	↑ lipogenesis ↓ lipolysis	↑ synthesis of triglycerides ↑ fatty acid synthesis ↓ lipolysis	–
Protein metabolism	↓ protein breakdown	–	↑ amino acid uptake ↑ protein synthesis

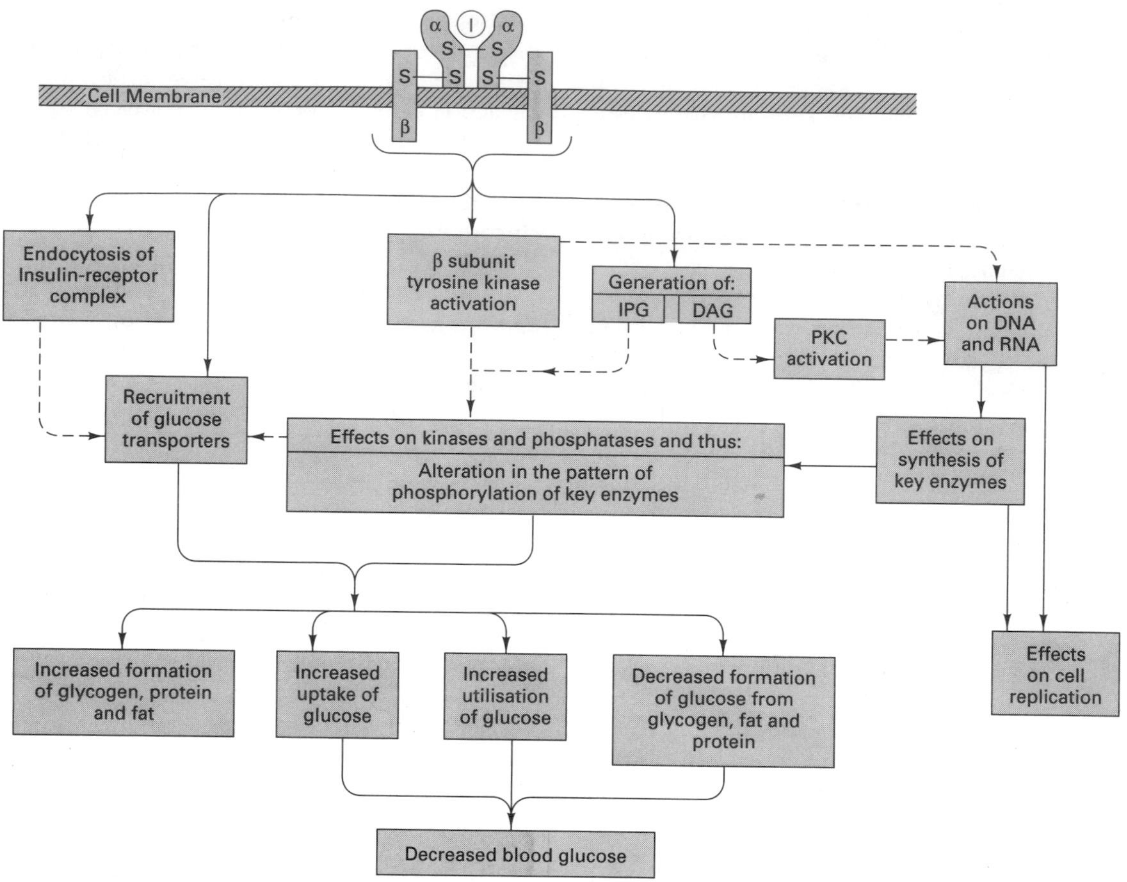

Fig. 20.3 Schematic diagram of the insulin receptor and proposed transduction events that link insulin–receptor interaction to the biological responses. (Dashed lines indicate actions for which evidence is still limited; I = insulin; IRS-1 = insulin receptor substrate 1; IPG = inositol phosphoglycan; DAG = diacylglycerol; PKC = protein kinase C)

Protein metabolism

Insulin stimulates the uptake of amino acids into *muscle* and increases protein synthesis. It also decreases protein catabolism and the oxidation of amino acids, particularly in the *liver* (see above).

Other metabolic effects

Other metabolic effects of insulin include increased transport into cells of K^+, Ca^{2+}, nucleosides and inorganic phosphate.

Long-term effects

In addition to immediate actions on metabolism, insulin has longer-term actions by increasing or decreasing the synthesis of key enzymes. Furthermore, it can stimulate cell proliferation in vitro and is implicated in growth regulation in vivo.

Mechanism of action

Insulin binds to a specific receptor on the surface of its target cells. The receptor is a glycoprotein complex (350 000 MW) consisting of two α- and two β-subunits linked by disulphide bridges (Fig. 20.3). The α-subunits are entirely extracellular and carry the insulin-binding site. The β-subunits are transmembrane proteins, and when insulin binds to the receptor these β-subunits manifest tyrosine kinase activity (see Fig. 20.3 and Ch. 2), acting upon themselves (autophosphorylation). This enhances the action of the kinase on other target proteins (see below).

At concentrations of insulin that produce maximum effects, only a small proportion (less than 10%) of receptors are occupied.

On interaction with insulin, the receptors aggregate into clusters and the insulin–receptor complexes are subsequently internalised in vesicles. The resulting loss of insulin receptors from the cell surface has been invoked to explain the insulin resistance seen in some cases of diabetes mellitus, but this remains controversial.

The transduction mechanisms for the insulin response (i.e. the events that link receptor-binding to the biological response) are still a matter of intensive research and vigorous debate. It seems likely that several pathways are involved, and it is possible that the signal transduction mechanisms for the short-term metabolic actions are different from those for the long-term effects on enzyme synthesis and cell replication. Since the immediate *metabolic actions* are mediated largely through alteration of the state of key enzymes, activation of a cascade of kinases and phosphatases must occur, initiated by tyrosine kinase on the β-subunit of the receptor.

Another hypothesis is that ligand–receptor interaction generates mediators by protease action and/or by activation of a specific phospholipase C which cleaves glycosylphosphatidylinositol to give an inositol phosphoglycan (IPG) and diacylglycerol (DAG). It is suggested that IPG modulates the activity of the kinases while DAG activates protein kinase C. There is also evidence that a guanine nucleotide protein (G-protein) has a role in regulating kinase activity. In addition, recruitment of glucose transporters is important in the metabolic action of insulin on fat cells.

The *longer-term actions* of insulin entail effects on DNA and RNA. Regulation of the rate of specific messenger RNA transcription by insulin is now well established and provides an important means of modulating enzyme activity. Both protein kinase C activation (see above) and the activation of the receptor tyrosine kinase could be implicated in the actions of insulin on cell replication. It is noteworthy that several growth factor (GF) receptors (e.g. epidermal GF and platelet-derived GF) have tyrosine kinase activity (see Ch. 2).

Endocrine pancreas and blood glucose

- Islets of Langerhans secrete insulin (and amylin) from β-cells, glucagon from α_2-cells, and somatostatin from α_1-cells.
- Many factors stimulate insulin secretion, but the main one is blood glucose.
- Insulin has essential metabolic actions as a *fuel-storage hormone,* and also affects cell growth and differentiation. It decreases blood glucose by:
  —increasing glucose uptake
  —increasing glycogen synthesis
  —decreasing gluconeogenesis
  —decreasing glycogen breakdown.
- Glucagon is a *fuel-mobilising hormone,* stimulating gluconeogenesis and glycogenolysis, also lipolysis. It increases blood sugar and also increases the force of contraction of the heart.
- Diabetes mellitus is a chronic metabolic disorder in which there is hyperglycaemia. There are two forms:
  —insulin-dependent diabetes (IDDM)
  —non-insulin-dependent diabetes (NIDDM).

GLUCAGON

Glucagon is a single chain polypeptide of 21 amino acid residues with a molecular weight of about 3000.

Synthesis and secretion

Glucagon is synthesised mainly in the α_2-cell of the islet, but also in the stomach. It has considerable structural homology with other GI tract hormones such as *secretin, vasoactive intestinal peptide* and *gastric inhibitory peptide* (see Ch. 9).

One of the main physiological stimuli to glucagon secretion is the concentration of amino acids, in particular arginine, in plasma. Thus an increase in secretion follows ingestion of a high protein meal. Secretion is stimulated by low, and inhibited by high concentrations of glucose and fatty acids in the plasma. Sympathetic nerve activity and circulating adrenaline stimulate glucagon release by an action on β-adrenoceptors. Parasympathetic nerve activity also increases secretion.

Somatostatin, from the adjacent α_1-cells in the islets, has an inhibitory action on glucagon release.

In contrast to insulin, which fluctuates with ingestion of meals, there is no very marked change in plasma glucagon concentration (measured by radioimmunoassay) throughout the day

Actions

Glucagon acts on specific receptors that are coupled by stimulatory G-proteins to adenylate cyclase, and its actions are somewhat similar to β-adrenoceptor-mediated actions of adrenaline. Unlike adrenaline, however, its metabolic effects are more pronounced than its cardiovascular actions. As regards metabolic actions, glucagon is proportionately more active on liver, and adrenaline on muscle and fat. It acts on the liver to *stimulate glycogen breakdown* and *gluconeogenesis*, and to *inhibit glycogen synthesis* and *glucose oxidation*. Consequently, it increases blood glucose, and is used to treat hypoglycaemia in unconscious patients (who cannot drink) if there is difficulty in obtaining intravenous access, and can be life-saving. It causes lipolysis in liver and fat cells, and the fatty acids so produced further increase gluconeogenesis. A prolonged rise in plasma glucagon results in *induction* of the enzymes involved in the above effects, as well as their stimulation through elevated cAMP.

Glucagon's actions on target tissues are thus the opposite of those of insulin. Paradoxically, glucagon potentiates insulin release (Figs 20.1 and 20.2).

Glucagon increases the rate and force of contraction of the heart, though less markedly than adrenaline, and is sometimes used to treat acute cardiac failure precipitated by injudicious use of β-adrenoceptor antagonists.

SOMATOSTATIN

Somatostatin is secreted by the α_1- (or D-) cells of the pancreas. It is also the growth hormone release-inhibiting factor generated in the hypothalamus (see p. 420). It provides local, paracrine, inhibitory regulation of insulin and glucagon release within the islet. **Octreotide** is a long-acting octapeptide analogue of somatostatin. It inhibits release of a number of hormones and is used clinically to relieve symptoms from several uncommon gastro-entero-pancreatic endocrine tumours, and for short-term treatment of acromegaly before surgery on the pituitary tumour (Ch. 21).

AMYLIN (ISLET AMYLOID POLYPEPTIDE)

Amyloid is deposited in the pancreas of patients with non-insulin-dependent diabetes mellitus, although it is not known if this is functionally important rather than a secondary phenomenon. In 1987 the major structural component of pancreatic amyloid was identified as a 37-amino-acid peptide now known as *islet amyloid polypeptide* or *amylin*. This is stored with insulin in secretory granules in β-cells and co-secreted with insulin in response to glucose and other stimuli. Unlike C-peptide, however, the molar ratio of secreted amyloid to insulin varies, increasing during prolonged stimulation by elevated glucose. Fasting amylin concentrations in plasma of healthy humans are around 1–10 pmol/l, post-prandial concentrations rising to 5–20 pmol/l (i.e. approximately one-tenth of plasma insulin concentrations). Pharmacological concentrations of amylin stimulate glycogen breakdown to lactate in striated muscle, with an increase in plasma lactate concentration and subsequent rise in glucose concentration that may reflect gluconeogenesis from lactate in liver. Amylin also inhibits insulin secretion (Fig. 20.1). Amylin is structurally related to *calcitonin* (see Ch. 21) and has weak calcitonin-like actions on calcium metabolism and osteoclast activity in patients with Paget's disease (a metabolic disorder of bone characterised by focal areas of increased bone turnover). It is also about 50% identical with *calcitonin gene-related peptide* (CGRP; see Ch. 9) and large intravenous doses cause vasodilatation via activation of adenylate cyclase, presumably via an action on CGRP receptors. Circulating concentrations of amylin are reduced to the detection limit of current assays in patients with insulin-dependent diabetes, and increased in patients with non-insulin-dependent diabetes. Whether amylin has a significant role in the control of glucose metabolism remains a controversial issue. Arguments favouring its endocrine role are presented by Rink et al. (1993).

CONTROL OF BLOOD GLUCOSE

The control of blood glucose (Table 20.2) must be seen in the context of the necessity of maintaining adequate fuel supplies in the face of intermittent food intake along with variable exercise and, thus, variable demand. After food intake, more fuel is available than is immediately required. Glucose is the main fuel utilised, and excess calories are stored as glycogen or fat. During fasting, these energy stores need to be mobilised in a regulated manner.

The blood glucose concentration is controlled by a feedback system between liver, muscle and fat and the pancreatic islets—the main regulatory hormone being **insulin**, the overall pattern of control of blood glucose differing in basal (i.e. fasting) and fed states.

Table 20.2 The effect of hormones on the control of blood glucose

Hormone	Main actions	Main stimulus for secretion	Main effect
Main regulatory hormone			
Insulin	↑ glucose uptake ↑ glycogen synthesis ↓ glycogenolysis ↓ gluconeogenesis	Moment-to-moment fluctuations in blood glucose	↓ blood glucose
Main counter-regulatory hormones			
Glucagon	↑ glycogenolysis ↑ gluconeogenesis	Hypoglycaemia, i.e. blood glucose less than 3 mM (e.g. with exercise, stress, high protein meals, etc.)	↑ blood glucose
Catecholamines	↑ glycogenolysis ↓ glucose uptake		
Glucocorticoids	↑ gluconeogenesis ↓ glucose uptake and utilisation		
Growth hormone	↓ glucose uptake		

DIABETES MELLITUS

Diabetes mellitus is a chronic metabolic disorder characterised by a *high blood glucose concentration* (*hyperglycaemia*) which is due to insulin deficiency and/or insulin resistance. (The normal blood glucose rarely exceeds 7 mmol/l: diabetes is diagnosed by a fasting plasma glucose ⩾ 7.8 mmol/l, or a plasma glucose ⩾ 10 mmol/l, 2 hours after a meal.) Hyperglycaemia occurs because the liver and skeletal muscle cannot store glycogen and the tissues are unable to take up and utilise glucose. When the renal threshold for glucose reabsorption is exceeded, glucose spills over into the urine (*glycosuria*) and causes an osmotic diuresis (*polyuria*) which in turn results in dehydration and increased fluid intake (*polydipsia*). Protein wasting occurs in severe diabetes due to the fact that protein metabolism is deranged and an excessive amount of protein is converted to carbohydrate. Ketosis occurs in the absence of insulin because there is increased fat breakdown to acetyl CoA. In the absence of carbohydrate metabolism, acetyl CoA is converted to aceto-acetate, β-hydroxybutyrate and acetone.

As a consequence of the metabolic derangements in diabetes, various complications develop, often over many years. Many of these are due to disease of blood vessels, either large (*macrovascular disease*) or small (*microangiopathy*). Macrovascular disease is due to accelerated atheroma which is much more common and severe in diabetic patients. Microangiopathy is a distinctive feature of diabetes mellitus and particularly affects *retina* and *kidney*. Coexistent *hypertension* is linked with progressive renal damage, and treatment of hypertension slows the progression of diabetic nephropathy. Treatment of hypertension with **angiotensin-converting enzyme inhibitors** (ACEI) appears to be more effective in this regard than treatment with other antihypertensive drugs (Ch. 14). Trials are presently in progress to determine whether ACEI are also of benefit in diabetic patients with normal blood pressures.

Diabetic *neuropathy* may involve accumulation of poorly metabolised osmotically active metabolites of glucose such as *sorbitol*, produced by the action of aldose reductase. This underpins hopes that **aldose reductase inhibitors** will be effective in preventing diabetic complications. Results to date have not been encouraging, but **tolrestat** is currently undergoing large-scale clinical trials in prevention of neuropathy, retinopathy, and nephropathy.

There are two main forms of diabetes.

- insulin-dependent diabetes mellitus (IDDM; also known as juvenile onset or Type I diabetes)
- non-insulin-dependent diabetes mellitus (NIDDM; also known as maturity onset or Type II diabetes).

In IDDM there is an absolute deficiency of insulin, and unless insulin treatment is provided the patient will die with diabetic ketoacidosis. Such patients are usually young and not obese when they first develop symptoms. There is an inherited predisposition to IDDM with a 10-fold increased incidence in first-degree relatives of an index case, and strong associations with particular histocompatibility antigens (HLA types). Studies of identical twins have shown that genetically predisposed individuals must additionally be exposed to an environmental factor such as viral infection (e.g. with Coxsackie or Echo virus). Viral infection may damage pancreatic β-cells and expose antigens that initiate a self-perpetuating autoallergic process. More than 90% of β-cells have to be destroyed before the patient becomes overtly diabetic. This natural history provides a tantalising prospect of preventing IDDM by intervening in the prediabetic stage, and a variety of strategies have been mooted including *immunosuppression* with **cyclosporin** or **azathioprine**, dietary modifications, **antioxidants**, **tumour necrosis factor** and many others. Most attention is currently being given to **nicotinamide** because of studies from New Zealand suggesting that pharmacological doses of this vitamin induce remission in patients with newly diagnosed IDDM, and delay onset of IDDM in prediabetic children with antibodies against islet cells. It is suggested that it may work by influencing DNA repair. A large controlled study is currently in progress to answer this question.

In NIDDM there is both insulin resistance (which precedes overt disease) and impaired insulin secretion. NIDDM patients are usually obese and treatment is initially dietary although supplementary oral hypoglycaemic drugs or insulin often become necessary.

The alterations in insulin secretion in the two forms of diabetes are shown schematically in Figure 20.2 and are contrasted with the normal response.

In a *normal* individual there is a basal level of insulin secretion and the response to an intravenous infusion of glucose (equivalent to what might happen after a meal) has two phases. The first phase is rapid and short-lived and the second is prolonged. In *NIDDM* there is hyperglycaemia and a normal or slightly raised basal insulin concentration. The first phase of the insulin-secretory response to glucose is virtually absent, but the delayed response is present. The response to non-glucose secretagogues (e.g. amino acids, sulphonylureas, glucagon and GI tract hormones) is nearly normal (not shown). In *IDDM* there is severe β-cell dysfunction. Basal insulin secretion is extremely low and there is virtually no response to glucose, or any other stimuli. The minimal insulin secretion is insufficient to maintain metabolic homeostasis with the result that there is hyperglycaemia, proteolysis, lipolysis and ketosis.

TREATMENT OF DIABETES MELLITUS

In IDDM, **insulin** is the main form of treatment. For many years it has been assumed, as an act of faith, that normalising plasma glucose would prevent diabetic complications. A recently published large US trial (the Diabetes Control and Complications Trial; American Diabetes Association 1993) suggests that this faith was well placed: intensively managed 13- to 39-year-old IDDM patients maintained (for 4–9 years) lower mean blood glucose concentrations (2.8 mmol/l lower) than conventionally managed patients, and had a substantial reduction in occurrence and progression of retinopathy, nephropathy and neuropathy. These benefits outweighed a threefold increase in severe hypoglycaemic attacks and modest excess weight gain. The practical implications of this study are substantial.

Realistic goals in NIDDM (especially in older obese patients) are likely to be less ambitious than in young IDDM patients. Diet is the cornerstone (albeit one with a tendency to crumble) often combined with oral agents (**metformin** and **sulphonylureas**) and/or **insulin**. Dietary management, essential in treating both forms of diabetes, is beyond the scope of this book.

INSULIN TREATMENT

The effects of insulin and its mechanism of action have been described above. It is destroyed in the gastrointestinal tract, and must be given parenterally—usually subcutaneously, but intravenously or occasionally intramuscularly in emergencies. One of the main problems in using insulin is to avoid wide fluctuations in plasma concentration and thus in blood glucose.

Insulin for clinical use was once either porcine or bovine, but is now usually human (made either by modification of porcine insulin or in microorganisms by recombinant DNA technology). Bovine insulin differs from human insulin in three amino acid residues, and porcine insulin in one.

Insulin is assayed biologically against an international standard and its dosage expressed in 'units'.

There is a confusing variety of insulins available, varying in their peak effect and duration of action. Details of some preparations are given in Table 20.3.

Early preparations were acidic, and tended to precipitate in the tissues or when mixed with other insulin formulations. To counter this, acetate-buffered neutral solutions were introduced. This type of insulin (**soluble insulin**) produces a rapid and short-lived effect, and can be given intravenously. Longer-acting preparations are made by precipitating insulin with protamine or zinc, thus forming finely divided amorphous solid or relatively insoluble crystals, which are injected as a suspension from which insulin is slowly absorbed. These include **isophane insulin**, a suspension of insulin (porcine, bovine or human) in the form of a complex with protamine; **amorphous insulin zinc suspension**, and **crystalline insulin zinc suspension** (see Table 20.3 for kinetics). Mixtures are also available.

It was hoped that improved purity of human insulin preparations would reduce the incidence of immune responses and of anti-insulin antibodies (see below) but no real advantage of human insulin has emerged during clinical trials. Manufacturing advantages have, however, led to considerable increase in the use of human insulin.

'Monocomponent' insulins are purified by anion exchange chromatography and most types of insulin are also obtainable in the purer monocomponent form. Highly purified insulins are also available.

Severe insulin resistance as a consequence of antibody formation is rare but may complicate treatment. A high titre of circulating anti-insulin antibodies is more likely to occur with bovine insulin than with porcine insulin. Note, however, that virtually all patients treated with animal insulin have antibodies against the hormone, albeit usually of low titre. 'Human' insulin is less immunogenic than animal insulin but may still evoke an antibody response, since the source of the hormone is not the only determinant of immunogenicity; insulins undergo physical changes before and after injection which can increase their potential for provoking antibodies.

Drugs in diabetes

Insulin can be extracted from porcine or bovine pancreas. 'Human' insulin is made by recombinant DNA technology or by modifying porcine insulin. It is usually given subcutaneously.

- There are three main types of insulin:
  - Fast- and short-acting soluble insulin. Peak action 2–4 hours; duration 6–8 hours. It can be given i.v.
  - Intermediate-acting, e.g. isophane insulin. Peak action 6–12 hours; duration 12–24 hours. It can be mixed with soluble insulin.
  - Long-acting, e.g. insulin zinc suspension (crystalline). Peak action 8–24 hours; duration 24–36 hours.
- The main unwanted effect is hypoglycaemia.

Oral hypoglycaemic drugs: used in NIDDM

- Biguanides (e.g. metformin):
  - act peripherally, increasing glucose uptake in striated muscle provided some insulin is present
  - assist in weight loss
  - are used with sulphonylureas when these have ceased to work adequately.
- Sulphonylureas (e.g. glipizide):
  - stimulate insulin secretion
  - can cause hypoglycaemia and weight gain
  - are only effective if β-cells are functional
  - action involves block of ATP-sensitive K^+-channels in β-cells.

Pharmacokinetic aspects

Various regimes of insulin administration may be used. A common regime for IDDM patients is to inject a combination of short- and intermediate-acting insulins twice daily, before breakfast and before the evening meal. Intensified regimes may be used to improve control of blood glucose; these involve multiple daily injections or continuous subcutaneous infusion of soluble insulin through a pump system. The most sophisticated forms of pump regulate the dose by means of a sensor which continuously measures blood glucose, but these are not routinely available.

Intravenous and intraperitoneal infusion are also used. *Intravenous* infusion of soluble insulin is used routinely in emergency treatment of *diabetic ketoacidosis*, in conjunction with large volumes of *isotonic saline* and *potassium chloride* to replace Na^+, K^+ and Cl^- depletion. *Intraperitoneal* insulin is used in IDDM patients with end-stage renal failure treated by *ambulatory peritoneal dialysis*.

Administration of insulin by the *intranasal* route

Table 20.3 Insulin preparations*

Category	Preparations	Source	With subcutaneous injection			Comments
			Onset (h)	Peak action (h)	Duration of action (h)	
Fast-action	Soluble insulin (neutral, regular)	h, p, b	0.5	2–5	5–8	Important in emergencies, e.g. ketoacidosis by i.v. infusion. If used alone, four injections are necessary daily. Can be mixed in the syringe with an intermediate insulin
Intermediate action	Isophane insulin	h, p, b	2	4–12	12–24	Used for starting twice daily injection regimes. Can be mixed with soluble insulin
	Insulin zinc suspension (amorphous)	h, p, b	2	5–10	12–16	
	Biphasic insulin	p	1	3–8	12–24	Ready mixed preparations
Long-action	Insulin zinc suspension (crystalline)	h, b	5	8–24	24–36	
	Insulin zinc suspension (mixed; amorphous + crystalline)	h, p, b	2	6–14	18–30	30% amorphous + 70% crystalline

Note: h = 'human' (prepared biosynthetically); p = porcine; b = bovine. 'Human' insulin is increasingly being used in preference to animal; many brands of animal insulin have been withdrawn.

* See also MacPherson & Feely (1990).

with adjuvants to facilitate transmucosal absorption is being investigated (though the adjuvants cause mucosal irritation).

New techniques for insulin administration being investigated are the incorporation of insulin into biodegradable polymer microspheres which can be injected, and the encapsulation of insulin with a lectin in a glucose-permeable membrane. This latter technique could be self-regulatory, because there is competitive binding of glucose and glycosylated insulin to the lectin. Once in the blood, insulin has a $t_{½}$ of about 10 minutes. It is inactivated in the liver and kidney, and 10% is excreted in the urine. Progressive renal impairment causes reduced insulin requirement.

Clinical uses of insulin

- Patients with IDDM require long-term maintenance treatment with insulin
- Many patients with NIDDM ultimately require chronic insulin treatment
- Short term treatment with insulin may be needed in patients with NIDDM during intercurrent events (e.g. infections, myocardial infarction, pregnancy, during major operations)
- An entirely separate use is in emergency treatment of hyperkalaemia, when insulin is given with glucose to lower extracellular K^+ via redistribution into cells

Unwanted effects

The main undesirable effect of insulin is *hypoglycaemia*. This is common and serious and can result in substantial morbidity and death. Regimes of intensive insulin therapy (multiple daily injections and continuous infusion) result in a threefold increase in severe hypoglycaemia. It has been suggested that patients transferred from animal to human insulin experience an alteration of the warning symptoms of hypoglycaemia from those associated with the counter-regulatory activity of the sympathetic nervous system (sweating, palpitations, tremor and so on) to those of cerebral glucose deficiency (inability to concentrate, headache, disturbances of speech and vision, culminating in loss of consciousness). Recent studies have not borne out this suspicion. The *treatment of hypoglycaemia* is to give oral **glucose** or, if the patient is unconscious or otherwise unable to drink, **intravenous glucose** (50% w/v intravenously). **Glucagon** injected intramuscularly is used if intravenous administration of glucose is not feasible.

Allergy to insulin is unusual but may take the form of local or systemic reactions.

Lipodystrophy or *fat hypertrophy* involves loss or proliferation of adipose tissue at the site of injection. It can be minimised by rotating injection sites.

Rebound hyperglycaemia (*Somogyi effect*) can follow excessive insulin administration. This results from the release of the insulin-opposing or counter-regulatory hormones in response to insulin-induced hypoglycaemia. This can cause hyperglycaemia before breakfast following an unrecognised hypoglycaemic attack during sleep in the early hours of the morning. It is essential to recognise this possibility to avoid the mistake of *increasing* (rather than reducing) the dose of insulin in this situation.

ORAL HYPOGLYCAEMIC AGENTS

The main groups of oral agents that lower blood sugar (see box on p. 415) are the **biguanides** and the **sulphonylureas** and related compounds. In addition, **acarbose** (an **α-glucosidase inhibitor**) has recently been marketed, and several other classes of drugs are in development (see below).

Biguanides

These are orally active hypoglycaemic agents that do not require functioning β-cells or affect insulin production. Their main action is probably to increase glucose uptake across the cell membrane in skeletal muscle, although they also have minor effects on glucose absorption and hepatic glucose production. **Metformin** is the only drug of this class presently available in the UK. This compound has additional metabolic actions in that it reduces plasma concentrations of low density lipoprotein and very low density lipoprotein, effects that could be useful in reducing atheroma (see Ch. 15). It has a half-life of about 3 hours, and is excreted unchanged in the urine.

Metformin does not stimulate appetite (rather the reverse!), and is consequently useful in the majority of NIDDM patients who are obese and who fail treatment with diet alone. It can be combined with sulphonylurea drugs. The main unwanted effect is transient gastrointestinal disturbance. A rare but potentially fatal toxic effect is lactic acidosis and metformin should never be given to patients with renal disease or severe pulmonary or cardiac disease. Metformin does not cause hypoglycaemia and does not result in weight gain. Long-term use may interfere with absorption of vitamin B_{12}.

Sulphonylureas

The sulphonylurea group of drugs was developed as a result of the finding that a sulphonamide derivative (used to treat typhoid) resulted in a marked lowering of blood glucose. These drugs act by stimulating insulin release (see below) and thus require functional islet cells.

There are now numerous sulphonylureas available for therapy. The first drugs of this kind used therapeutically were **tolbutamide** and **chlorpropamide**. Chlorpropamide has a long duration of action and a substantial fraction is excreted in the urine. Consequently it can cause severe hypoglycaemia in elderly patients in whom there is a progressive decline in glomerular filtration rate (Ch. 4). It causes flushing after alcohol because of a **disulfiram**-like effect (Ch. 33) and has an action like that of antidiuretic hormone on the distal nephron giving rise to hyponatraemia and water intoxication. Williams (1994) comments that 'time honoured but idiosyncratic chlorpropamide should now be laid to rest'—a sentiment with which we concur. So-called second generation sulphonylureas (see Fig. 20.4 and Table 20.4) are more potent than tolbutamide, but their maximum hypoglycaemic effect is no greater and failure of treatment to control blood sugar just as common as with the older drugs. These include **glibenclamide**, **glipizide**, and **gliclazide**. They all contain the sulphonylurea moiety, but different substitutions result in differences in potency, pharmacokinetics and duration of action (see Table 20.4). Glibenclamide is best avoided in the elderly and in patients with even

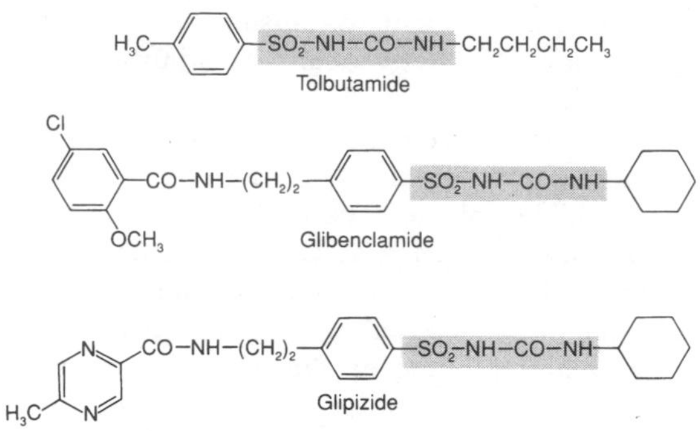

Fig. 20.4 Structures of some oral hypoglycaemic drugs. The sulphonylurea moiety is shown within the light pink box.

Table 20.4 Oral hypoglycaemic sulphonylurea drugs

Drug	Relative potency*	Duration of action and (half-life) in hours	Pharmacokinetic aspects	General comments
Tolbutamide	1	6–12 (4)	Some converted in liver to weakly active hydroxytolbutamide. Some carboxylated to inactive compound. Renal excretion	A safe drug. Least likely to cause hypoglycaemia. May decrease iodide uptake by thyroid. Contraindicated in liver failure
Glibenclamide[†]	150	18–24 (10)	Some is oxidised in the liver to moderately active products and is excreted in urine; 50% is excreted unchanged in the faeces	May cause hypoglycaemia. The active metabolite accumulates in renal failure
Glipizide	100	16–24 (7)	Peak plasma levels in 1 hour. Most is metabolised in the liver to inactive products which are excreted in urine. 12% is excreted in faeces	May cause hypoglycaemia. Has diuretic action. Only inactive products accumulate in renal failure

* Relative to tolbutamide
[†] Termed 'gliburide' in USA
All are largely protein-bound (90–95%).

mild renal impairment because of the risk of hypoglycaemia since several of its metabolites are excreted in urine and are moderately active.

Mechanism of action

The principal action of the sulphonylureas is on the β-cells of the islets (Fig. 20.1), stimulating insulin secretion (the equivalent of phase I in Fig. 20.2) and thus reducing plasma glucose concentration.

High affinity receptors for sulphonylureas are present on β-cells, and the order of potency of various sulphonylureas in binding parallels their potency in stimulating insulin release. The drugs reduce the potassium permeability of β-cells in vitro, by blocking the ATP-sensitive potassium channel (see p. 404) by which glucose regulates insulin secretion.

Basal insulin secretion and the secretory response to various stimuli are enhanced in the first few days of treatment with sulphonylurea drugs. With longer treatment, insulin secretion continues to be augmented, and there is also enhanced tissue sensitivity to insulin, the mechanism of which is not well understood.

Pharmacokinetic aspects

Sulphonylureas are well absorbed after oral administration and most reach peak plasma concentrations within 2–4 hours. The duration of action varies (Table 20.4). All bind strongly to plasma albumin, and are implicated in interactions with other drugs (e.g. salicylates and sulphonamides) that compete for these binding sites (see below and Ch. 42). Most sulphonylureas (or their active metabolites) are excreted in the urine, so their action is increased in elderly patients or in those with renal disease.

Sulphonylureas cross the placenta and stimulate foetal β-cells to release insulin; as a result, their use is contraindicated in pregnancy, and gestational diabetes is managed with diet supplemented if necessary with insulin.

Unwanted effects

The sulphonylureas are usually well tolerated. Side effects are specified in Table 20.4. In addition, as with insulin, sulphonylurea drugs *stimulate appetite* and often cause *weight gain*. This is a major concern in obese NIDDM patients. *Hypoglycaemia*, which can be severe, may occur with any of the agents. Its incidence is related to the potency and duration of action, the highest incidence occurs with chlorpropamide and glibenclamide and the lowest with tolbutamide. Such hypoglycaemia can be prolonged, and this can be serious in elderly patients and in patients with impaired renal function. About 3% of patients experience *gastrointestinal upsets. Allergic skin rashes* have been observed, and *bone marrow damage* (Ch. 43), though very rare, has been reported and is severe.

A vexed question is whether prolonged therapy with oral hypoglycaemic drugs has *adverse effects on the cardiovascular system*. A study on the treatment of NIDDM sponsored by the National Institutes of Health in the USA in 1970 found that after 4–5 years of treatment there appeared to be an *increase* in cardiovascular-related deaths in the oral-agent-treated group as compared with the groups treated with insulin or placebo. However, there was no statistically significant increase in total mortality in the sulphonylurea group as compared with the others and a reappraisal of the same data does not support the view that sulphonylurea therapy is harmful. Conversely, there is no evidence that oral hypoglycaemic drugs have beneficial cardiovascular effects.

Oral hypoglycaemic drugs

Oral hypoglycaemic drugs are only of use in the treatment of NIDDM and only as a supplement to diet. They include:

- metformin (a biguanide)
- sulphonylureas (e.g. glibenclamide)
- acarbose (an α-glucosidase inhibitor).

Drug interactions

Several compounds *augment* the hypoglycaemic effect of the sulphonylureas and several such interactions are potentially clinically important. **Non-steroidal anti-inflammatory drugs** (including **azapropazone, phenylbutazone** and **salicylates**), **coumarins**, some **uricosuric drugs** (e.g. **sulphinpyrazone**), **alcohol, monoamine oxidase inhibitors**, some **antibacterials** (including **sulphonamides, trimethoprim** and **chloramphenicol**), some **antifungal** drugs (including **miconazole** and possibly **fluconazole**) have all been reported to produce severe hypoglycaemia when given with the sulphonylureas. The probable basis of the interaction is competition for the metabolising enzymes, but interference with plasma protein binding or with excretion may play a part.

Agents that *decrease* the action of the sulphonylureas include **diuretics** (**thiazides** and **loop diuretics**) and **corticosteroids**.

α-glucosidase inhibitors

Acarbose, an inhibitor of intestinal α-glucosidase, has recently been marketed for use in NIDDM patients inadequately controlled by diet with or without other agents. It delays carbohydrate absorption, reducing the post-prandial increase in blood glucose. The commonest adverse effects are related to its main action and consist of flatulence, loose stools or diarrhoea and abdominal pain and bloating. Its precise place in treatment has still to be established, but like **metformin** it may be particularly helpful in obese NIDDM patients.

Potential new antidiabetic drugs

Several agents are currently being studied including **α_2-antagonists, inhibitors of fatty acid oxidation** and agents that *enhance the response of tissues to insulin*, notably the **thiazolidinediones**. Lipolysis in fat cells is controlled by adrenoceptors of the β_3-subtype (see Ch. 7). The possibility of using selective β_3-agonists, currently in development, in the treatment of NIDDM and obesity is being investigated.

REFERENCES AND FURTHER READING

Alberti K G M M 1993 Preventing insulin dependent diabetes mellitus. Br Med J 307: 1435–1436

American Diabetes Association 1993 Implications of the diabetes control and complications trial. Diabetes 42: 1555–1558

Bloom J D, Dutia M D, Johnson B D, Wissner A, Burns M G, Largis E E, Dolan J A, Claus T H 1992 Disodium (R,R)-5-[2-[[2-(3-chlorophenyl)-2-hydroxyethyl]-amino]propyl]-1,3-benzodioxole-2,2-dicarboxylate (CL 316,243). A potent β-adrenergic agonist virtually specific for β_3 receptors. A promising antidiabetic and antiobesity agent. J Med Chem 35: 3081–3084

Eizirik D L, Sandler S, Palmer J P 1993 Repair of pancreatic β cells. A relevant phenomenon in early IDDM? Diabetes 42: 1383–1391

Foley J E 1992 Rationale and application of fatty acid oxidation inhibitors in treatment of diabetes mellitus. Diabetes Care 15: 773–784

Frank R N 1994 Perspectives in diabetes. The aldose reductase controversy. Diabetes 43: 169–172

Gerich J E 1989 Oral hypoglycemic agents. N Engl J Med 321: 1231–1245

Hofmann C A, Colca J R 1992 New oral thiazolidinedione antidiabetic agents act as insulin sensitizers. Diabetes Care 15: 1075–1078

Klip A, Leiter L A 1990 Cellular mechanism of action of metformin. Diabetes Care 13: 696–704

MacPherson J N, Feely J 1990 Insulin. Br Med J 300: 731–736

Melander A 1987 Clinical pharmacology of sulfonylureas metabolism. Metabolism 36: 12–16

Myers M G Jr, White M F 1993 Perspectives in diabetes. The new elements of insulin signaling. Insulin receptor substrate-1 and proteins with SH2 domains. Diabetes 42: 643–650

Nuttall F Q 1993 Dietary fiber in the management of diabetes. Diabetes 42: 503–508

Pfeifer M A, Halter J B, Porte D 1981 Insulin secretion in diabetes mellitus. Am J Med 70: 579–588

Pociot F, Reimers J I, Anderson H U 1993 Nicotinamide—biological actions and therapeutic potential in diabetes prevention. Diabetologia 34: 362–365

Rink T J, Beaumont K, Koda J, Young A 1993 Structure and biology of amylin. Trends Pharmacol Sci 14: 113–118

Santiago J V 1993 Perspectives in diabetes. Lessons from the diabetes control and complications trial. Diabetes 42: 1549–1554

Suter S L, Nolan J J, Wallace P, Gumbiner B, Olefsky J M 1992 Metabolic effects of new oral hypoglycemic agent CS-045 in NIDDM subjects. Diabetes Care 15: 193–203

Turk J, Gross R W, Ramanadham S 1993 Perspectives in diabetes. Amplification of insulin secretion by lipid messengers. Diabetes 42: 367–374

Williams G 1994 Management of non-insulin-dependent diabetes mellitus. Lancet 343: 95–100

21
THE ENDOCRINE SYSTEM

The endocrine glands release **'hormones'**. This word, as introduced by Bayliss & Starling, referred to chemicals secreted without benefit of duct into the bloodstream, for action on a distant tissue. As pointed out in Chapter 11, the concept of 'hormones' as distinct from 'neurotransmitters' has become increasingly elastic. There appears to be, instead, a spectrum of agents, with substances which are predominantly neurotransmitters (e.g. acetylcholine) at one end and substances which are predominantly hormones in the classical sense (e.g. sex steroids) at the other, with a range of substances lying in between. In this chapter we consider substances which are mainly hormones in the classical Bayliss & Starling sense.*

THE PITUITARY

The pituitary gland is composed of three sections arising from two different embryological sites. The *anterior pituitary* is derived from the endoderm of the buccal cavity, as is the *intermediate lobe* (which can thus be considered for practical purposes as part of the anterior pituitary), while the *posterior pituitary* is derived from neural ectoderm. Both main parts of the gland have an intimate functional relationship with the hypothalamus, the neurons of which consist of two quite distinct systems influencing the anterior and posterior pituitary respectively.

ANTERIOR PITUITARY (ADENOHYPOPHYSIS)

The anterior pituitary secretes a number of different hormones vital for normal physiological function, some of which are involved in the regulation of other endocrine glands (Table 21.1). The cells of the anterior pituitary can be classified into corticotrophs, lactotrophs (mammotrophs), somatotrophs, thyrotrophs and gonadotrophs, according to the substances they secrete (see below).

Secretion from the anterior pituitary is largely

*However, we throw a semantic spanner into the works by citing new evidence that the action of the calcium *ion* on parathyroid cells has all the characteristics of a hormone or chemical transmitter.

Table 21.1 Hormones secreted by the hypothalamus and the anterior pituitary

Hypothalamic factor /hormone (and related drugs)	Hormone affected in anterior pituitary (and related drugs)	Main effects of anterior pituitary hormone
Corticotrophin-releasing factor (CRF)	Corticotrophin (ACTH; tetracosactrin)	Stimulates secretion of adrenal cortical hormones (mainly glucocorticoids). Maintains integrity of adrenal cortex.
Thyrotrophin-releasing hormone (TRH; protirelin)	Thyrotrophin	Stimulates synthesis and secretion of thyroid hormones, T_3 and T_4. Maintains integrity of thyroid gland.
Growth hormone-releasing factor (GHRF) Growth hormone-release inhibiting factor (GHRIF; somatostatin, octreotide)	Growth hormone (GH; somatotropin, somatropin, somatrem)	Regulates growth, partly directly, partly through evoking the release of somatomedins from the liver and elsewhere. Increases protein synthesis, increases blood glucose, stimulates lipolysis.
Gonadotrophin-releasing hormone (GnRH; somatorelin, sermorelin)	Follicle-stimulating hormone (FSH) See Chapter 22	Stimulates the growth of the ovum and the Graafian follicle in the female and gametogenesis in the male. With LH, stimulates the secretion of oestrogen throughout the menstrual cycle and progesterone in the second half.
	Luteinising hormone (LH) or interstitial-cell-stimulating hormone (ICSH) See Chapter 22	Stimulates ovulation and the development of the corpus luteum. With FSH, stimulates secretion of oestrogen throughout the menstrual cycle, and progesterone in the second half. In male, regulates testosterone secretion.
Prolactin release-inhibiting factor (PRIF). Probably dopamine. Prolactin-releasing factor (PRF)	Prolactin	Together with other hormones, prolactin promotes development of mammary tissue during pregnancy. Stimulates milk production in the post-partum period.
Melanocyte-stimulating hormone releasing factor (MSH-RF) MSH release inhibiting factor (MSH-RIF)	α-, β- and γ-melanocyte-stimulating hormones	Darken the skin in amphibia and fish. Function in man not known.

regulated by factors (hormones) derived from the hypothalamus, which reach the pituitary through the bloodstream. Blood vessels to the hypothalamus divide in its tissue to form a meshwork of capillaries—the primary plexus (Fig. 21.1), which drains into the hypophyseal portal vessels. These pass through the pituitary stalk to feed a secondary plexus of capillaries in the anterior pituitary. (Some portal veins which drain into these capillaries originate from a different primary plexus in the *posterior* pituitary.) Peptidergic neurons in the hypothalamus secrete a variety of releasing or release-inhibiting factors or hormones directly into the capillaries of the primary plexus (Table 21.1 and Fig. 21.1). These substances regulate the secretion of the following hormones from the various cells of the anterior pituitary:

- corticotrophin (ACTH) from corticotrophs
- prolactin from lactotrophs
- growth hormone from somatotrophs
- thyroid-stimulating hormone (thyrotrophin) from thyrotrophs
- gonadotrophins from gonadotrophs.

Other hormones of the anterior pituitary are the melanocyte-stimulating hormones which are secreted mainly from the intermediate lobe.

There is a balance (involving various negative feedback pathways) between the hypothalamic factors, the trophic hormones whose release they

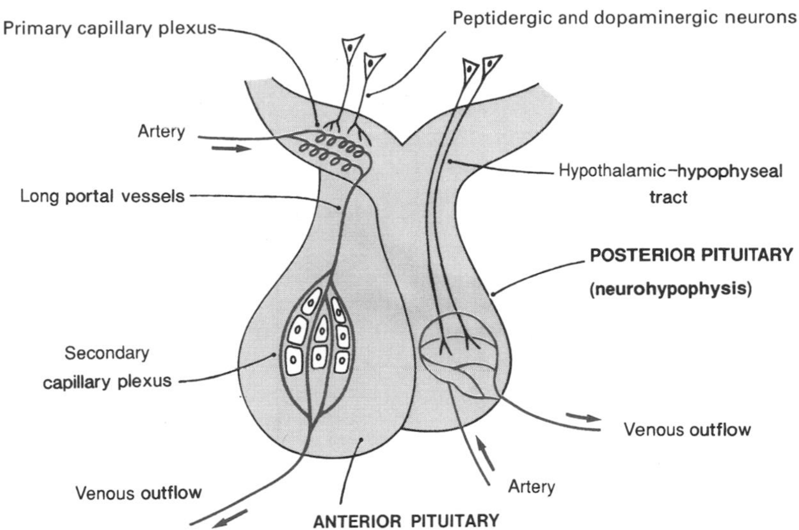

Fig. 21.1 Schematic diagram of vascular and neuronal relationships between the hypothalamus, the posterior pituitary and the anterior pituitary. The main portal vessels to the anterior pituitary lie in the pituitary stalk and arise from the primary plexus in the hypothalamus, but some (the short portal vessels) arise from the vascular bed in the posterior pituitary (not shown).

regulate and the secretions of the peripheral endocrine glands. The long negative feedback pathways, in which the mediators are the hormones which are secreted from the peripheral glands, affect both the hypothalamus and the anterior pituitary. The short negative feedback pathways involve anterior pituitary hormones acting on the hypothalamus.

The peptidergic neurons in the hypothalamus which secrete the factors that regulate the anterior pituitary are themselves influenced by higher centres in the CNS. This action is mediated through dopamine, noradrenaline, 5-hydroxytryptamine and the opioid peptides, the latter being found in very high concentration in the hypothalamus (see Ch. 9).

Another means of hypothalamic control of the anterior pituitary is exerted through the tubero-infundibular dopaminergic pathway, the neurons of which lie in close apposition to the primary capillary plexus (see Ch. 24). Dopamine can be secreted directly into the hypophyseal portal circulation and thus reach the anterior pituitary.

The anterior pituitary, in addition to being a complex endocrine gland, has some similarity to neural tissue and paracrine tissue in that some of its cells communicate with and influence each other through paracrine association (local hormone effects) and possibly also through gap junctions and electrical coupling.

HYPOTHALAMIC HORMONES

There are at least six sets of hormones (also referred to as 'factors') which originate in the hypothalamus and which regulate the secretion of anterior pituitary hormones. These are listed in Table 21.1 and are described in more detail below. Those which are available for use constitute valuable research tools as well as being of potential, and sometimes actual, clinical use in treatment and in diagnosis.

GROWTH HORMONE-RELEASING FACTOR (GHRF; SOMATORELIN)

GHRF is a peptide with 40–44 amino acid residues. It is active at a concentration of 10^{-15} mol/l. A peptide consisting of the first 29 amino acid residues has been shown to have full intrinsic activity and potency in vitro. An analogue, **sermorelin**, has been introduced as a diagnostic test for growth hormone secretion.

The main action of GHRF is summarised in

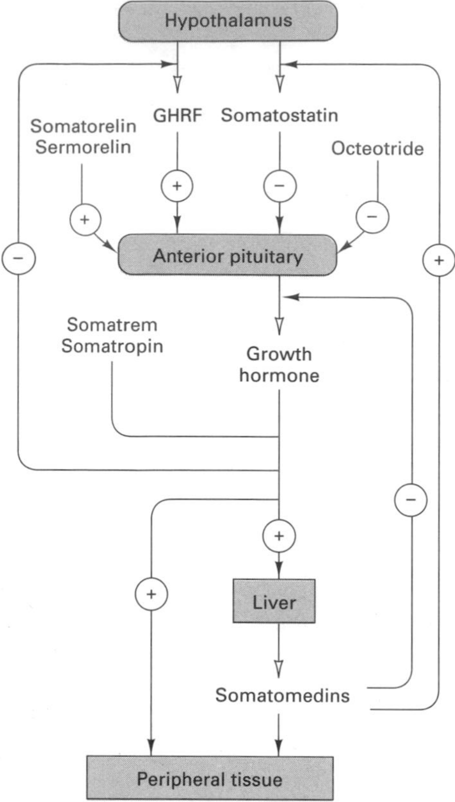

Fig. 21.2 Control of growth hormone secretion and its actions. Drugs are shown in red. (GHRF = growth hormone-releasing factor)

Figure 21.2. Its effects are potentiated by prior exposure of the secreting cells to glucocorticoids or thyroid hormone. Given intravenously, subcutaneously or intranasally, it can cause secretion of growth hormone within minutes and peak concentrations in 60 minutes. The action is selective for the somatotrophs in the anterior pituitary, no other pituitary hormones being released. Unwanted effects are rare.

SOMATOSTATIN

Somatostatin is a peptide of 14 amino acid residues and in addition to being found in the hypothalamus is present elsewhere in the CNS (where it has neuroregulatory actions) as well as in the pancreas and gastrointestinal tract. It inhibits the release of growth hormone (Fig. 21.2) and thyrotrophin from the anterior pituitary, and insulin and glucagon from the pancreas, and decreases the release of most gastrointestinal hormones. It also reduces gastric acid and pancreatic secretion.

Octreotide is a long-acting analogue of somatostatin. It is an octapeptide containing the four amino acids (Phe–Trp–Lys–Thr) known to be essential for somatostatin activity. It is used for the treatment of tumours secreting vasoactive intestinal peptide (Ch. 9), carcinoid syndrome (Ch. 8) and glucagonomas, and has a place in the therapy of Graves' ophthalmopathy, acromegaly and various other endocrine tumours. It can be of use in pancreatitis and in bleeding from oesophageal varices and gastric bleeding due to ulcer or stress gastritis.

It is given subcutaneously, the peak action is at 2 hours and the suppressant effect lasts for up to 8 hours.

Unwanted effects include pain at the injection site and gastrointestinal disturbances. Gallstones and postprandial hyperglycaemia have also been reported and acute hepatitis has occurred in a few cases.

THYROTROPHIN-RELEASING HORMONE (TRH; PROTIRELIN)

Protirelin is a tripeptide (pyroglutamyl-histidyl-proline amide), which releases thyrotrophin (and prolactin) from the anterior pituitary. It has neurotransmitter and paracrine functions as well as endocrine functions.

The response to protirelin may be inhibited by **somatostatin** and by **corticosteroids**. The prolactin-releasing action of protirelin is not influenced by plasma thyroxine levels.

It is used for the diagnosis of mild thyroid disorders. Given intravenously in normal subjects it elicits an increase in plasma thyrotrophin concentration, whereas in cases of hyperthyroidism, there is a blunted response to protirelin because the raised blood thyroxine concentration has a negative feedback effect on the anterior pituitary. The opposite occurs with hypothyroidism, in which the defect is in the thyroid itself.

CORTICOTROPHIN-RELEASING FACTOR (CRF)

CRF is a peptide which releases corticotrophin and β-endorphin from the anterior pituitary. Synthetic preparations are available. CRF acts synergistically with arginine vasopressin, and both its action and its release are inhibited by **glucocorticoids** (see Fig. 21.13).

Its main use is in diagnostic tests: to assess the ability of the pituitary to secrete corticotrophin, to assess whether a deficiency of corticotrophin is due to a pituitary or a hypothalamic defect, and to evaluate hypothalamic pituitary function after therapy for Cushing's syndrome (see p. 436 and Fig. 21.16).

GONADOTROPHIN-RELEASING HORMONE (GnRH)

Gonadotrophin-releasing hormone is a decapeptide which releases both follicle-stimulating hormone and luteinising hormone. It is also available as a preparation called **gonadorelin**. Its structure, actions and uses are described in Chapter 22.

ANTERIOR PITUITARY HORMONES

The main hormones of the anterior pituitary are listed in Table 21.1. The gonadotrophins are dealt with in Chapter 22 and thyrotrophin is considered later in this chapter (p. 428) as is corticotrophin (p. 433). The others are dealt with below.

GROWTH HORMONE (GH; SOMATOTROPIN)

Growth hormone is derived from the somatotroph cells and is found in the anterior pituitary in larger quantities than any other pituitary hormone. Secretion of growth hormone is high in the newborn, decreasing at 4 years to an intermediate level, which is then maintained until after puberty when there is a further decline.

Two preparations of growth hormone are available: **somatropin**, produced by recombinant DNA technology and identical to growth hormone, and **somatrem**, a biosynthetic compound which contains an additional methionyl residue.

Regulation of secretion

Secretion of GH is regulated by the action of hypothalamic growth hormone-releasing factor (GHRF) modulated by somatostatin or growth hormone-release-inhibiting factor (GHRIF), as described above and outlined in Figure 21.2. The neuropeptide, galanin, may also have a role in stimulating release.

One of the mediators of growth hormone action, *somatomedin C*, which is released from the liver (see below) has an inhibitory effect on growth hormone secretion by stimulating somatostatin release from the hypothalamus (Fig. 21.2).

Growth hormone release, like that of other anterior pituitary secretions, is pulsatile, and its plasma concentration fluctuates 10- to 100-fold. These surges occur repeatedly during the day and night and reflect changes in hypothalamic control. Dopamine is one of several hypothalamic neurotransmitters which are implicated in the release of growth hormone (Ch. 21), and the stimulant action of levodopa (used in treating parkinsonism; see Ch. 25) may be used in normal subjects as a test for growth hormone reserve.

Deep sleep is a potent stimulus to growth hormone secretion, particularly in children.

Actions

The main effect of growth hormone and its analogues is to stimulate normal growth, and in doing this, it affects many tissues, acting in conjunction with other hormones secreted from the thyroid, the gonads and the adrenal cortex. It stimulates the production, mainly from the liver, of several polypeptides termed *somatomedins* which are responsible for most of its anabolic actions (see Fig. 21.2). Receptors for somatomedins exist on liver cells, fat cells and cartilage cells.

Protein synthesis is stimulated by growth hormone, and the uptake of amino acids into cells is increased, especially in skeletal muscle. Somatomedins mediate many of these anabolic effects, acting on skeletal muscle and also on the cartilage at the epiphyses of long bones, thus influencing bone growth.

The effects on *carbohydrate metabolism* are complex. At high concentrations, an early 'insulin-like' effect is produced, but at physiological concentrations this does not occur.

The main action on *fat metabolism* is to act in concert with glucocorticoids to cause lipolysis.

Growth hormone also has prolactin-like effects (see below).

Disorders of production and clinical use

Deficiency of growth hormone results in pituitary dwarfism. In this condition, which can be produced by lack of GHRF or a failure of somatomedin generation or action, the normal proportions of the body are maintained.

The only established clinical use is in patients with growth hormone deficiency and in short stature due to Turner's syndrome. Satisfactory linear growth can be achieved by giving **somatropin.*** It is given subcutaneously, six to seven times per week, and therapy is most successful when started early.

The availability of the synthetic peptide has opened up the possibility of many other uses based on the anabolic and central effects; thus it could be valuable following major surgery or after extensive burns.

An excessive production of growth hormone in children results in increased growth before the epiphyses are closed and therefore gigantism. An excessive secretion of growth hormone in adults, which is usually the result of a benign pituitary tumour, results in acromegaly—a condition in which there is enlargement mainly of facial structures and of the hands and feet.** Drugs such as **levodopa** (p. 420), the dopamine agonist **bromocriptine** (see Ch. 8 and below) and **octreotide** (see p. 420) may ameliorate the condition but effective treatment consists of removal or irradiation of the tumour.

PROLACTIN

Prolactin, which is structurally related to growth hormone, is a single peptide chain (23 000 MW) consisting of 198 amino acid residues. It is secreted by mammotroph (lactotroph) cells which are abundant in the anterior pituitary and which increase in number during pregnancy, probably under the influence of oestrogen.

Regulation of secretion

Prolactin is unusual in that its secretion is under *tonic inhibitory* control by the hypothalamus (Fig. 21.3 and Table 21.1). The inhibitory influence is exerted through the dopaminergic tubero-infundibular pathway (see Ch. 24); the *prolactin release-inhibiting factor* (PRIF) secreted by the hypothalamus is generally held to be dopamine itself.

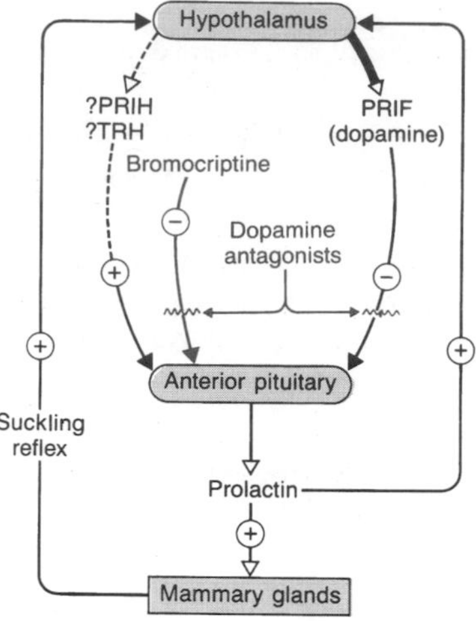

Fig. 21.3 Control of prolactin secretion and the drugs which modify it. (TRH = thyrotrophin-releasing hormone; PRF = prolactin-releasing factor; PRIF = prolactin release-inhibiting factor)

The main stimulus for prolactin release is suckling. Neural reflexes from the breast may stimulate the secretion from the hypothalamus of a *prolactin-releasing factor* (PRF) (and/or *thyrotrophin-releasing hormone* (TRH); there are receptors for TRH on the mammotrophs). Oestrogens increase both prolactin secretion and the proliferation of lactotrophs through release, from a subset of lactotrophs, of the neuropeptide, galanin.

Dopamine antagonists, for example **phenothiazines, butyrophenones** (see Ch. 28), and **domperidone**, and also *dopamine-depleting agents* such as **reserpine** (see Ch. 7) are potent stimulants of prolactin release.

Dopamine agonists such as **bromocriptine** and **apomorphine** (Ch. 30 and below) suppress prolactin release. **Levodopa**, which is decarboxylated in vivo to give dopamine (see Ch. 25), has a transient suppressant effect. Bromocriptine is also used in parkinsonism (Ch. 25); its use in relation to lactation is given on page 423.

Actions

The main function of prolactin in females is the control of milk production (one can only speculate as to what its function is in males). At parturition, when the blood level of oestrogen falls, the prolactin concentration rises and lactation is initiated. Maintenance of lactation depends on suckling, which stimulates a reflex secretion of prolactin by neural

*Growth hormone extracted from cadaver pituitaries has caused Creutzfeld–Jacob disease (see p. 754) and its use has been discontinued.

**'Acral' means distal.

Anterior pituitary and hypothalamus

- The anterior pituitary secretes hormones which regulate:
  - —the release of glucocorticoids from adrenal cortex
  - —the release of thyroid hormones
  - —ovulation in the female and spermatogenesis in the male, and the release of sex hormones (Ch. 22)
  - —growth
  - —mammary gland structure and function.
- Each anterior pituitary hormone is regulated by a specific hypothalamic releasing factor. Feedback mechanisms influence the release of these factors.
- Substances available for clinical use are:
  - —growth hormone-releasing factor (sermorelin) and analogues of growth hormone (GH, somatrem, somatropin)
  - —thyrotrophin-releasing factor (protirelin) and thyrotrophin (used to test thyroid function)
  - —octreotide, an analogue of somatostatin, which inhibits GH release
  - —corticotrophin-releasing factor, used in diagnosis
  - —gonadotrophin-releasing factor (see Ch. 22).

pathways, causing a 10–100-fold increase within 30 minutes.

Prolactin, along with other hormones, is responsible for the proliferation and differentiation of mammary tissue during pregnancy. It inhibits gonadotrophin release and/or the response of the ovaries to these trophic hormones. This is one of the reasons why ovulation does not usually occur during breast feeding, and it is believed to constitute a natural contraceptive mechanism.

According to one rather appealing hypothesis, the high postnatal concentration of prolactin reflects its biological function of 'parental' hormone. Certainly broodiness and nest-building activity can be induced in birds by prolactin injections, and equivalent 'parental' behaviour can be induced in mice and rabbits. It is rather attractive to think that it might have a similar action in humans, but this is conjectural.

Modification of prolactin secretion

Prolactin itself is not used clinically; in the context of prolactin physiology, the main clinical need is to *decrease* its secretion, and the agent used for this purpose is **bromocriptine**.

Bromocriptine is well absorbed orally, and peak concentrations occur after 2 hours. It is metabolised in the liver and excreted in the bile. Unwanted reactions include nausea and vomiting, which may be ameliorated by taking the drug with meals. Dizziness, constipation and postural hypotension may also occur.

CORTICOTROPHIN

Corticotrophin (also termed adrenocorticotrophic hormone or ACTH) is the adenohypophyseal endocrine secretion which controls the synthesis and release of the glucocorticoids of the adrenal cortex. It is dealt with later in this chapter (p. 443).

MELANOCYTE-STIMULATING HORMONES (MSH)

There are three melanocyte-stimulating hormones, α-, β- and γ-MSH. They are derived from pro-opiomelanocortin (see Fig. 9.3) and are released mainly from the cells of the intermediate lobe under the influence of two hypothalamic hormones—a releasing factor (MSHRF) and a release-inhibiting factor (MSHRIF)—see Table 21.1. In fish and amphibians, MSH has a skin-darkening effect by virtue of its action in dispersing the pigment granules of melanocytes. Its action in man is not clearly understood, but there is experimental evidence that α-MSH may have a role in temperature regulation.

The clinical use of bromocriptine

- To prevent lactation without causing pain or engorgement of the breast, as well as to suppress established lactation; it is more effective than oestrogens in this latter action.
- To treat galactorrhoea, i.e. non-puerperal lactation due to excessive prolactin secretion (hyperprolactinaemia*).
- To treat prolactin-secreting pituitary tumours (prolactinomas).
- In the treatment of parkinsonism (Ch. 25) and of acromegaly.

* Hyperprolactinaemia, an increased concentration of prolactin in the blood, can also occur as a side effect of neuroleptic drugs (Ch. 28) or oral contraceptives.

POSTERIOR PITUITARY (NEUROHYPOPHYSIS)

The posterior pituitary gland consists largely of the axons of nerve cells which lie in the supraoptic and paraventricular nuclei of the hypothalamus. These axons form the hypothalamic–hypophyseal tract, and the fibres terminate in dilated nerve endings in close association with capillaries in the posterior pituitary gland (Fig. 21.1). Peptides, synthesised in the hypothalamic nuclei, pass down the axons into the posterior pituitary where they are stored and eventually secreted into the bloodstream.

The two main hormones of the posterior pituitary are **oxytocin** (which contracts the smooth muscle of the uterus; see Ch. 22) and the **antidiuretic hormone** (ADH) (Fig. 21.4). The latter hormone is also called **vasopressin** (see Chs 14 and 18).

The structure of the posterior pituitary hormones was determined by du Vigneaud and his co-workers in the 1950s. This same group synthesised the peptides and worked out the main structure/activity relationships. Natural ADH is a nonapeptide, with a sulphydryl bridge connecting residues 1 and 6 which is necessary for physiological activity. Residue 8 is arginine in all mammalian species except pigs, in which it is lysine. Oxytocin differs from ADH in having leucine at position 8 and isoleucine at position 3 (Fig. 21.4).

Several peptides have been synthesised which vary in their antidiuretic, vasopressor and oxytocic (uterine stimulant) properties.

ANTIDIURETIC HORMONE (ADH; VASOPRESSIN)

Regulation of secretion and physiological role

ADH released from the posterior pituitary has a crucial role in the control of the water content of the body through its action on the cells of the distal part of the nephron and the collecting tubules in the kidney (see Ch. 18). Specific nuclei in the hypothalamus which control water metabolism lie close to the nuclei which synthesise and secrete ADH.

Posterior pituitary

- The posterior pituitary secretes:
  - —oxytocin (see Ch. 22)
  - —the antidiuretic hormone (vasopressin) which acts on V_2-receptors in the distal kidney tubule to increase water reabsorption, and, in higher concentrations, on V_1-receptors to cause vasoconstriction. (It also increases factor VIII concentration and participates in the control of ACTH secretion.)
- Substances available for clinical use are vasopressin, and the analogues, desmopressin, lypressin, terlipressin.

One of the main stimuli to ADH release is an *increase in plasma osmolality*. The normal plasma osmolality is 282 mosm/kg, ADH release being stimulated in response to stimulation of 'osmoreceptors' if this rises to 287 mosm/kg or above. A *decrease in circulating blood volume* is another major factor causing secretion of ADH, the stimulus being an increase in renin and angiotensin production (see Ch. 18). Angiotensin also releases ADH. All these factors produce a sensation of thirst.

The main disorder of ADH secretion is *diabetes insipidus*, a condition in which there is continuous production of copious amounts of hypotonic urine. It results from either reduced circulating ADH, termed *neurohypophyseal diabetes insipidus*, or an impaired response of the nephron to normal ADH levels, termed *nephrogenic diabetes insipidus*. This latter is due in many cases to defective V_2-receptors (see below).

The receptors for ADH

There are two classes of receptors for ADH (vasopressin)—V_1 and V_2. The V_2-receptors are coupled to adenylate cyclase, and the V_1-receptors, of which there are two types—V_{1a} and V_{1b}—are coupled to inositol phosphate production.

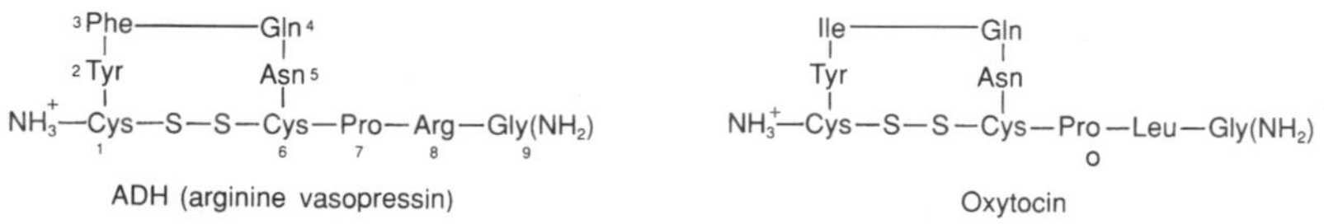

3 Phe—Gln 4
2 Tyr | Asn 5
NH_3^+—Cys—S—S—Cys—Pro—Arg—Gly(NH_2)
1 6 7 8 9
ADH (arginine vasopressin)

Ile—Gln
Tyr | Asn
NH_3^+—Cys—S—S—Cys—Pro—Leu—Gly(NH_2)
Oxytocin

Fig. 21.4 The structures of the two posterior pituitary peptides.

Actions

Renal actions

ADH binds to V_2-receptors in the basolateral membrane of the cells of the distal tubule and collecting ducts of the nephron. Its main effect is to increase the permeability of the luminal membrane to water. (Details of this action are given on p. 371.) It also transiently increases sodium absorption.

Numerous pharmacological agents interact with ADH in its action on the kidney. **Chlorpropamide** and **carbamazepine** enhance sensitivity to ADH. ADH action is counteracted by the general anaesthetic **methoxyflurane** (see Ch. 26), by **lithium carbonate** (see Ch. 29) and by the antibiotic **demeclocycline**. This last agent is used to treat patients with excessive water retention due to excessive secretion of ADH. Since microtubules are involved in the action of ADH, agents which modify these organelles, such as **colchicine** (see Ch. 11) and the **vinca alkaloids** (see Ch. 36), will also reduce ADH effects.

Non-renal actions

ADH causes contraction of *smooth muscle*, particularly in the cardiovascular system, by acting on V_{1a}-receptors (see Ch. 14). The affinity of these receptors for ADH is lower than that of the V_2-receptors, and smooth muscle effects are only seen with doses larger than those affecting the kidney.

In addition to its actions on the kidney and on smooth muscle, ADH has actions on a variety of other tissues:

- It stimulates aggregation and degranulation of platelets by an action on V_1-receptors and increases the concentration of factor VIII of the blood coagulation cascade by an action on V_2-receptors.
- Released into the pituitary 'portal' circulation, it promotes the release of corticotrophin from the anterior pituitary by an action on V_{1b}-receptors (see Fig. 21.13).
- It promotes hydrocortisone release by a direct action on V_1-receptors on adrenocortical cells.
- Within the central nervous system it acts as a neuromodulator and neurotransmitter.
- It has antipyretic activity; released endogenously, it may function as a modulator of fever.
- It accelerates glycogen breakdown in liver cells.

Preparations used and pharmacokinetic aspects

The preparations of antidiuretic peptides available for clinical use are **vasopressin** (which is ADH itself), **lypressin** (Lys[8]-vasopressin) and **desmopressin** (1-deamino-DArg[8]-vasopressin). These have, respectively, 0.8 times and 12 times the anti-diuretic potency of vasopressin but 60% and 0.4% of its vasopressor potency. **Terlipressin** (triglyceryl-lysine vasopressin) has low but protracted vasopressor action and minimal antidiuretic properties. **Felypressin** (Phe[2]-Lys[8]-vasopressin) is predominantly vasoconstrictor in action.

Vasopressin is given by subcutaneous or intramuscular injection, or by intravenous infusion. Lypressin and desmopressin are usually given intranasally as snuff or spray, though preparations of desmopressin for injection are available. Terlipressin is given intravenously.

Vasopressin and lypressin are rapidly eliminated, both having a plasma half-life of 10 minutes and a short duration of action. Metabolism is by tissue peptidases, and 33% of vasopressin is removed by the kidney. Desmopressin is less subject to degradation by peptidases, and its plasma half-life is 75 minutes.

Clinical use of vasopressin and analogues

- Treatment of neurohypophyseal *diabetes insipidus:* lypressin, desmopressin. (Chlorpropamide (a sulphonylurea used in diabetes; see Ch. 20) and carbamazepine (an antiepileptic drug; see Ch. 30) potentiate the action of endogenous and exogenous ADH and may also be used in the therapy of *diabetes insipidus.* Drugs which may be effective also in *nephrogenic diabetes insipidus*, are, paradoxically, the thiazide diuretics (p. 378) and the related compound chlorthalidone.
- The initial treatment of bleeding oesophageal varices: vasopressin, terlipressin, lypressin. (Octreotide is also used but sclerotherapy is the main treatment.)
- As prophylactic therapy in haemophilia: vasopressin, desmopressin (by increasing the concentration of factor VIII; somatostatin is also effective).
- Felypressin is used as a vasoconstrictor with local anaesthetics (see Chs 14 and 33).
- Desmopressin is used in older children and adults with persistent enuresis.

Various synthetic peptide and non-peptide agonists and antagonists of vasopressin have been synthesised and are used as experimental tools.

The clinical use of vasopressin and analogues is given on page 425.

Unwanted effects

There are few unwanted effects if the antidiuretic peptides are used intranasally in therapeutic doses. Nausea and abdominal cramps, and hypersensitivity reactions have been reported. Intravenous vasopressin may cause spasm of the coronary arteries with resultant angina, and it frequently causes abdominal and uterine cramps.

OXYTOCIN

Oxytocin is discussed in Chapter 22.

THE THYROID

The thyroid is essential for many physiological processes. It secretes three main hormones: **thyroxine** (**T_4**), **triiodothyronine** (**T_3**) and **calcitonin**. T_4 was isolated from thyroid tissue in crystalline form by Kendall in 1914 and subsequently synthesised by Harington & Barger in 1927. The presence in the thyroid of T_3, which is three- to fivefold more active than thyroxine, was shown by Gross & Pitt-Rivers in 1952.

T_4 and T_3 are critically important for normal growth and development and for energy metabolism. Calcitonin is involved in the control of plasma calcium and is dealt with later in this chapter (p. 451). The term 'thyroid hormone' will be used here to refer to T_4 and T_3.

Synthesis, storage and secretion of thyroid hormone

The functional unit of the thyroid is the follicle or acinus. Each follicle consists of a single layer of epithelial cells around a cavity, the follicle lumen, which is filled with a thick colloid containing principally *thyroglobulin*. Thyroglobulin is a large glycoprotein, each molecule of which contains about 115 tyrosine residues. It is synthesised, glycosylated and then secreted into the lumen of the follicle where iodination of the tyrosine residues occurs. Surrounding the follicles is a rich capillary network, and the rate of blood flow through the gland is very high in comparison with other tissues. The main steps in the synthesis, storage and secretion of thyroid hormone (Fig. 21.5), are as follows:

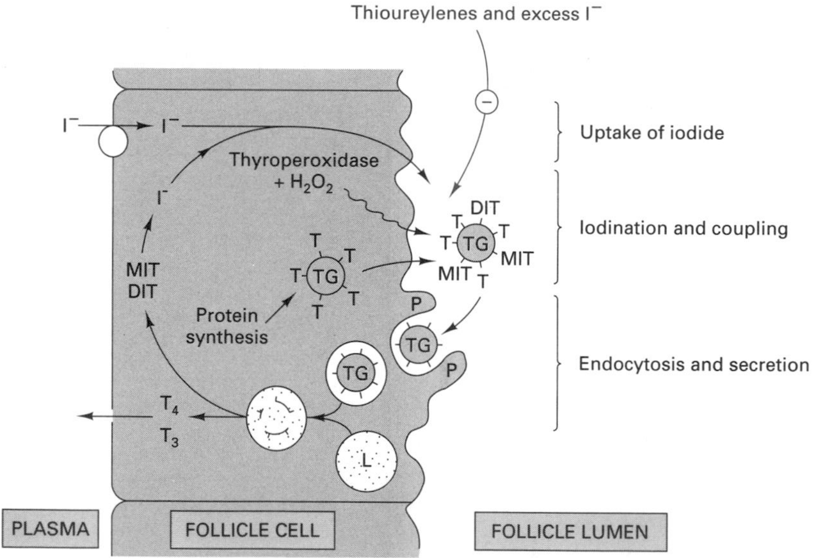

Fig. 21.5 Diagram of thyroid hormone synthesis and secretion with the sites of action of drugs which modify it. See text for details. (TG = thyroglobulin; T = tyrosine; MIT = monoiodotyrosine; DIT = diiodotyrosine; T_4 = thyroxine; T_3 = triiodothyronine; L = lysosome; P = pseudopod)

- uptake of plasma iodide by the follicle cells
- oxidation of iodide and iodination of tyrosine residues in the thyroglobulin of the colloid
- secretion of thyroid hormone.

Uptake of plasma iodide by the follicle cells
This is an energy-dependent transport process occurring against a gradient, which is normally about 25 : 1. It is inhibited by **thiocyanate** and **perchlorate**.

Oxidation of iodide and iodination of tyrosine residues in the thyroglobulin of the colloid
This process is brought about by an enzyme, thyroperoxidase, at the inner, apical surface of the cell at the interface with the colloid. It is very rapid—labelled iodide (^{125}I) can be found in the lumen within 40 seconds of intravenous injection—and requires H_2O_2 as an oxidising agent. Iodination (referred to as 'organification' of iodine) occurs *after* the tyrosine has been incorporated into thyroglobulin. The process believed to occur is shown in Figure 21.6.

Tyrosine is iodinated first at position 3 on the ring and then, in some molecules, on position 5 as well, forming *monoiodotyrosine* (MIT) in the first case, and *diiodotyrosine* (DIT) in the second. Two of these molecules are then coupled—either MIT with a DIT to form T_3 or two DIT molecules to form T_4 (Fig. 21.7). The mechanism for coupling is not fully known but is believed to involve a peroxidase system similar to that involved in iodination. About one-fifth of the tyrosine residues in thyroglobulin are iodinated.

The iodinated thyroglobulin of the thyroid forms a large store of thyroid hormone and, as is explained below, there is a relatively slow turnover of hormone in the tissues. This is in contrast to other endocrine secretions, such as growth hormone secreted by the anterior pituitary or the hormones of the adrenal cortex, which are synthesised on demand.

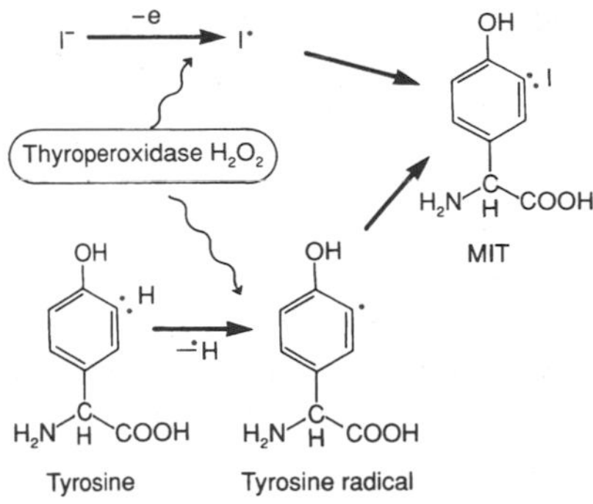

Fig. 21.6 Iodination of tyrosyl by the thyroperoxidase–H_2O_2 complex. This probably involves two sites on the enzyme, one of which removes an electron from iodide to give the free radical, I•, and another removes a monohydrogen (monoelectron) from tyrosine to give the tyrosine radical (shown by the red dot). Formation of monoiodotyrosine (MIT) results from addition of the two radicals.

Secretion of thyroid hormone
Although T_4 and T_3 comprise only a small proportion of the thyroglobulin, the whole molecule is broken down when the hormones are secreted. The process involves the endocytosis of thyroglobulin by the follicle cells (see Fig. 21.5). This starts with the formation of pseudopods which

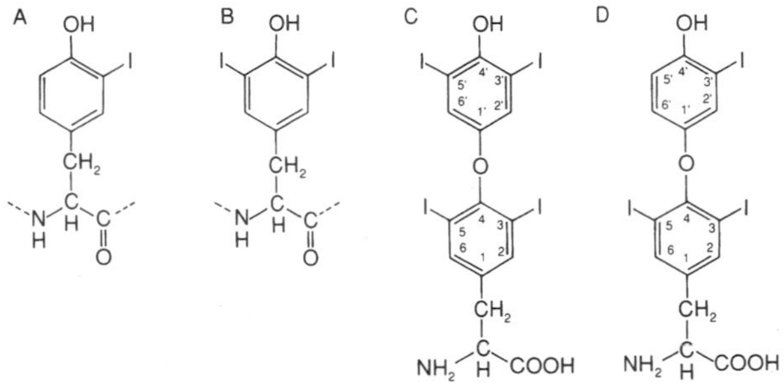

Fig. 21.7 Iodinated tyrosine residues.
A. 3-monoiodotyrosine. **B.** 3,5-diiodotyrosine. Both are shown in peptide linkage, as in thyroglobulin. **C.** Thyroxine (T_4). **D.** 3,5,3′-triiodothyronine (T_3). When T_4 is used as a drug it is given as the salt of the amino acid.

engulf some of the colloid in the lumen. The endocytic vesicles then fuse with lysosomes, proteolytic enzymes act on thyroglobulin, and T_4 and T_3 are released and secreted into the plasma. The MIT and DIT which are released at the same time are normally metabolised within the cell, the iodide being removed enzymically and re-used.

Regulation of thyroid function

The main controlling mechanism (see Fig. 21.8) is through thyrotrophin (thyroid-stimulating hormone, TSH), a glycoprotein released from the thyrotroph cells of the anterior pituitary under the influence of the hypothalamic hormone, TRH (see p. 420). Another hypothalamic secretion which affects thyrotrophin release is somatostatin (see p. 420) which reduces basal thyrotrophin release.

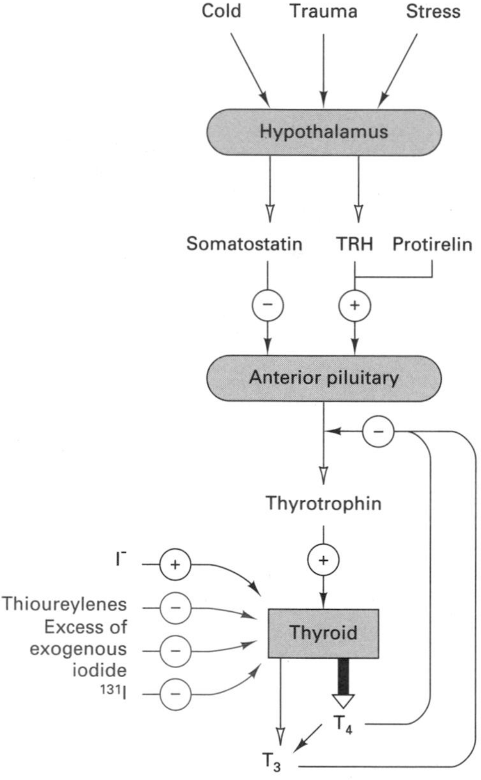

Fig. 21.8 Regulation of thyroid hormone secretion. Agents used clinically are shown in red. For the endogenous substances (shown in black) the thickness of the lines indicates the relative importance of each factor. Iodide (I^-) is essential for thyroid hormone synthesis, but excess of exogenous iodide (30 × the daily requirement of iodine) inhibits the increased thyroid hormone production which occurs in thyrotoxicosis. (TRH = thyrotrophin-releasing hormone)

The production of thyrotrophin is also influenced by a negative feedback effect of thyroid hormones, T_3 being more active than T_4. The extent of conversion of T_4 to T_3 and its degradation in the tissues (see below) will affect the plasma concentration and thus influence the negative feedback effect on thyrotrophin release.

The control of the secretion of thyrotrophin thus depends on a balance between the actions of T_4 and TRH, and probably also somatostatin, on the pituitary, but even high concentrations of thyroid hormone do not *completely* inhibit thyrotrophin secretion.

Thyrotrophin acts on receptors on the membrane of thyroid follicle cells and its main second messenger is cAMP. It has a half-life of about 50 minutes in the circulation. It controls all aspects of thyroid hormone synthesis:

- the uptake of iodide by follicle cells, by an action on the synthesis of the transport proteins; *this is the main mechanism by which it regulates thyroid function*
- the synthesis and secretion of thyroglobulin
- the generation of hydrogen peroxide and the iodination of tyrosine
- endocytosis and proteolysis of thyroglobulin
- secretion of T_3 and T_4
- the blood flow through the gland
- the transcription of the thyroperoxidase and thyroglobulin genes, thus having a trophic action on the thyroid cells.

The other main factor influencing thyroid function is the plasma iodide concentration. About 100 nmol of T_4 is synthesised daily, necessitating the gland taking up approximately 500 nmol of iodide each day (equivalent to about 70 μg of iodine). A reduced iodine intake with reduced plasma iodide concentration will result in a decrease of hormone production and an increase in thyrotrophin secretion. An increased plasma iodide has the opposite effect, though this may be modified by other factors (see below). The overall feedback mechanism responds to changes of iodide only slowly—over fairly long periods, days or weeks. There is a large reserve capacity for the binding and uptake of iodide in the thyroid which can thus be increased fivefold. The size and vascularity of the thyroid are reduced by an increase in plasma iodide. A prolonged decrease of iodine in the diet results in a continuous excessive secretion of thyrotrophin and eventually in an increase in vascularity, and hypertrophy of the gland.

Actions of the thyroid hormones

The physiological actions of the thyroid hormones fall into two categories:

- those affecting metabolism
- those affecting growth and development.

Effects on metabolism

The hormones are regulators of metabolism in most tissues, T_3 being three to five times more active than T_4 (Fig. 21.9). They produce a general increase in the metabolism of carbohydrates, fats and proteins. Most of these effects involve modulation of the actions of other hormones such as insulin, glucagon, the glucocorticoids and the catecholamines, although the thyroid hormones also control, directly, the activity of some of the enzymes of carbohydrate metabolism. There is an increase in O_2 consumption and heat production which is manifested as an increase in basal metabolic rate. This reflects action on some tissues, such as heart, kidney, liver and muscle, but not others, such as the gonads, brain and spleen. The calorigenic action is important as part of the response to a cold environment. Administration of thyroid hormone results in augmented cardiac rate and output and increased tendency to dysrhythmias such as atrial fibrillation.

Effects on growth and development

The thyroid hormones have a critical effect on growth, partly by a direct action on cells and partly indirectly by influencing growth hormone production and potentiating its effects. The hormones are important for a normal response to parathormone and calcitonin, and for skeletal development; they are particularly necessary for normal growth and maturation of the CNS.

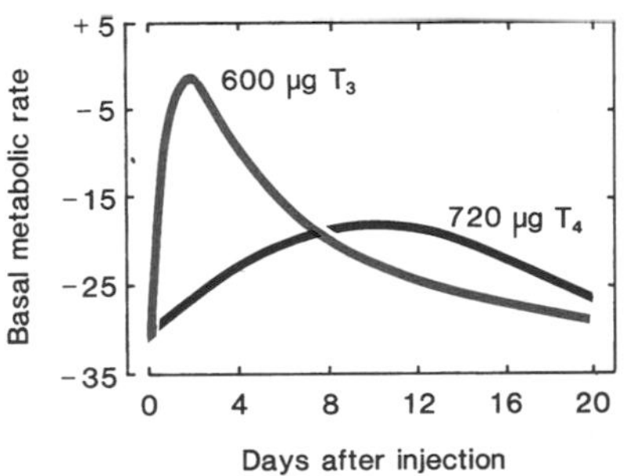

Fig. 21.9 Schematic diagram of the effect of single equimolar doses of T_3 and T_4 on basal metabolic rate in a hypothyroid subject. Note that this figure is meant only to illustrate differences in potency; thyroxine is not given clinically in a single bolus dose but in regular daily doses so that the effect builds up to a plateau. (From: Blackburn C M et al. 1954 J Clin Invest 33: 819)

Mechanism of action

The hormones act by a mechanism rather similar to that of the steroids (p. 439 and Fig. 21.15). After they enter the cell, T_4 is converted to T_3 which binds with high affinity to a specific receptor protein associated with DNA in the nucleus (see Ch. 2). The binding induces a conformational change in the receptor protein and this leads to the synthesis of specific messenger RNA and protein, the effects produced depending on the cell type.

The affinity of the receptors for T_4 is less by a factor of 4–10, and only small amounts of T_4 are bound. Thus T_4 can be regarded mainly as a *prohormone*.

Transport and metabolism

The normal plasma concentrations of the hormones, which can be measured by radioimmunoassay (Ch. 3), are 10^{-7} M for T_4 and 2×10^{-9} M for T_3. Virtually all of the T_4 and T_3 in the circulation is bound to plasma protein, the main protein being thyroxine-binding globulin (TBG). Small amounts of the hormones are bound to albumin.

In the tissues, T_4 is mono-deiodinated; one-third is converted to T_3 which is the main hormone regulating energy metabolism, while about 40% is converted to the inactive 3,3′,5′-triiodothyronine (also termed reverse T_3 or rT_3), which may inhibit the calorigenic actions of T_3. The generation of T_3 remains fairly constant over a wide range of T_4 concentrations.

The thyroid hormones are eventually degraded by de-iodination, deamination and conjugation with glucuronic and sulphuric acids. This occurs mainly in the liver, and the free and conjugated forms are excreted partly in the bile and partly in the urine. The metabolic clearance of T_3 is 20 times faster than that of T_4 (which is about 6 days).

In summary:

- There is a large pool of T_4 in the body; it has a low turnover rate and is found mainly in the circulation.
- There is a small pool of T_3 in the body; it has a fast turnover rate and is found mainly intracellularly.

ABNORMALITIES OF THYROID FUNCTION

Hyperthyroidism (thyrotoxicosis)

In thyrotoxicosis there is excessive activity of the thyroid hormones with a high metabolic rate, an increase in temperature and sweating and a marked sensitivity to heat. Nervousness, tremor, tachycardia, fatigability and increased appetite associated with loss of weight occur. There are several types of hyperthyroidism but only two are common: *diffuse toxic goitre* (also called Graves' disease or exophthalmic goitre) and *toxic nodular goitre*.

Diffuse toxic goitre is an organ-specific autoimmune disease caused by thyroid-stimulating immunoglobulins directed at the thyrotrophin receptor. As is indicated by the name, patients with exophthalmic goitre have protrusion of the eyeballs. The pathogenesis of this condition is not understood, but it is thought to have an immunological basis. There is also increased sensitivity to catecholamines.

Toxic nodular goitre is due to a benign neoplasm or adenoma and may develop in patients with long-standing simple goitre (see below). This condition does not usually have concomitant exophthalmos.

The antidysrhythmic drug, **amiodarone** (Ch. 13), has a propensity to cause hyperthyroidism.

Thyroid

- Thyroid hormones are synthesised by iodination of tyrosine residues on thyroglobulin within the lumen of the thyroid follicle.
- The thyroglobulin is endocytosed and thyroxine (T_4) and triiodothyronine (T_3) are secreted.
- Synthesis and secretion of T_3 and T_4 are regulated by thyrotrophin, and influenced by plasma iodide.
- T_3 and T_4 actions are:
  - —to stimulate metabolism generally, causing increased O_2 consumption and increased metabolic rate
  - —to influence growth and development.
- Within cells, the T_4 is converted to T_3 which interacts with a receptor causing DNA-directed mRNA and protein synthesis.
- There is a large pool of T_4 in the body; it has a low turnover rate and is found mainly in the circulation.
- There is a small pool of T_3 in the body; it has a fast turnover rate and is found mainly intracellularly.
- Abnormalities of thyroid function include:
  - —hyperthyroidism (thyrotoxicosis), either diffuse toxic goitre or toxic nodular goitre
  - —hypothyroidism; in adults this causes myxoedema, in infants, cretinism
  - —simple non-toxic goitre, due to dietary iodine deficiency.

Hypothyroidism

A decreased activity of the thyroid results in hypothyroidism, one form of which is termed *myxoedema*. It is immunological in origin and the manifestations are low metabolic rate, slow speech, deep hoarse voice, lethargy, bradycardia, sensitivity to cold and mental impairment. Patients also develop a characteristic thickening of the skin which gives the condition its name. *Hashimoto's thyroiditis*, a chronic autoimmune disease in which there is an immune reaction against thyroglobulin or some other component of thyroid tissue, can lead to hypothyroidism and myxoedema. Therapy of thyroid tumours with **radioiodine** (see below) is another cause of hypothyroidism.

Thyroid deficiency during development, caused by congenital absence or incomplete development of the thyroid, causes *cretinism* which is characterised by gross retardation of growth and mental deficiency.

Amiodarone, described above as causing hyperthyroidism, can also result in hypothyroidism. **Lithium** (Ch. 29) inhibits thyroid hormone release, and it is used in some countries for the treatment of hyperthyroidism.

A dietary deficiency of iodine, if prolonged, causes a rise in plasma thyrotrophic hormone and eventually an increase in the size of the gland. This condition is known as *simple* or *non-toxic goitre*. Another cause is ingestion of goitrogens (e.g. from cassava root). The enlarged thyroid usually manages to produce normal amounts of thyroid hormone, though if the iodine deficiency is very severe, hypothyroidism may supervene.

DRUGS USED IN DISEASES OF THE THYROID

Drugs are used in:

- hyperthyroidism
- hypothyroidism.

DRUGS USED IN HYPERTHYROIDISM

Hyperthyroidism may be treated surgically or

Thiourea   Carbimazole   Methimazole   Propylthiouracil

Fig. 21.10 Antithyroid drugs.

pharmacologically. In general, surgery is preferred only where there are mechanical problems due to compression of the trachea.

Although the condition of hyperthyroidism can be controlled with drugs, the disease is not 'cured' since the drugs do not alter the underlying autoimmune mechanisms. Furthermore, there is little evidence that therapy of any kind affects the course of the eye disease associated with Graves' disease.

Thioureylenes

Thioureylenes are the most important antithyroid agents and the main compounds are **carbimazole, methimazole** and **propylthiouracil** (Fig. 21.10). They are related to thiourea, the thiocarbamide group (S–C–N) being essential for antithyroid activity.

Action

Thioureylenes decrease the output of thyroid hormones from the gland and cause a gradual reduction in the signs and symptoms of thyrotoxicosis, the basal metabolic rate and pulse rate returning to normal over a period of 3–4 weeks. Their mode of action is not completely understood, but there is evidence that they inhibit the iodination of tyrosyl residues in thyroglobulin (see Figs 21.5, 21.6 and 21.11). It is thought that they inhibit the thyroperoxidase-catalysed oxidation reactions by acting as substrates for the postulated peroxidase–iodinium complex, thus competitively inhibiting the interaction with tyrosine. Propylthiouracil has the additional effect of reducing the de-iodination of T_4 to T_3 in peripheral tissues.

Pharmacokinetic aspects

Thioureylenes are given orally. Carbimazole is rapidly converted to methimazole, and it is this which has pharmacological activity in vivo. Methimazole is distributed throughout the body water and has a plasma half-life of 6–15 hours. An average dose of carbimazole produces more than 90% inhibition of thyroid organification of iodine within 12 hours. The clinical response to this and other antithyroid drugs, however, may take several weeks (Fig. 21.12). This is not only because thyroxine has a long half-life but also because the thyroid may have large stores of hormone which need to be depleted before the drug's action can be manifest. Propylthiouracil may act somewhat more rapidly because of its effect in inhibiting peripheral conversion of T_4 to T_3.

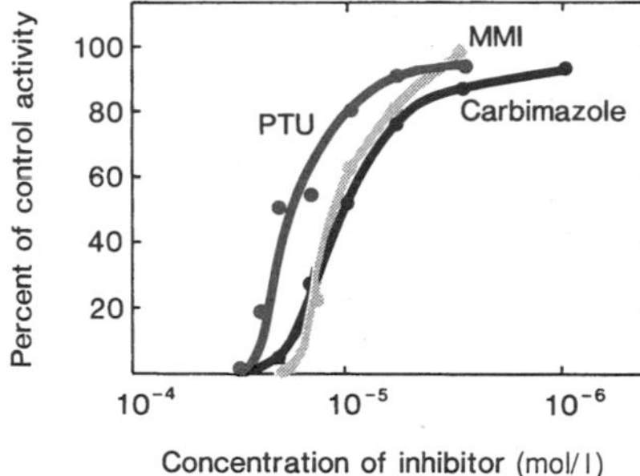

Fig. 21.11 Dose–response curves for inhibition of thyroperoxidase-catalysed iodination of thyroglobulin. The IC_{50} for carbimazole: 10.5 μmol/l; for methimazole (MMI): 11.5 μmol/l; and for propylthiouracil (PTU): 18.5 μmol/l. (Modified from: Taurog A 1976 Endocrinology 98: 1031)

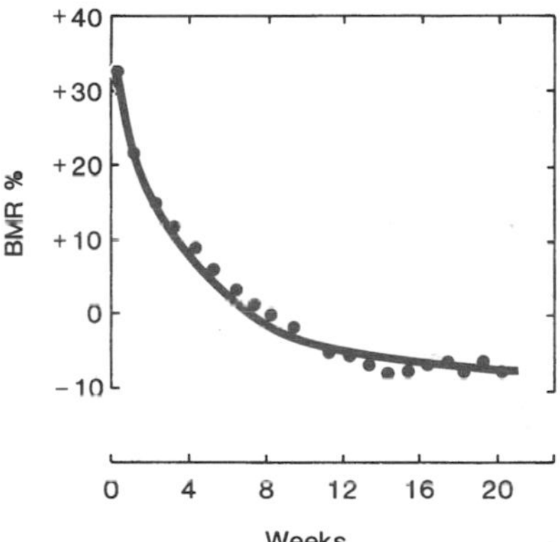

Fig. 21.12 Average time-course of fall of BMR during treatment with an antithyroid drug, carbimazole. The curve is exponential, corresponding to a daily decrease in BMR of 3.4%. (From: Furth E O et al. 1963 J Clin Endocrinol Metab 23: 1130)

Both methimazole and propylthiouracil cross the placenta and also appear in the milk, but this effect is less pronounced with propylthiouracil because it is more strongly bound to plasma protein. After degradation, the metabolites are excreted in the urine, propylthiouracil being excreted more rapidly than methimazole. The thioureylenes are not concentrated in the thyroid.

Unwanted effects

The most important unwanted effect is granulocytopenia (see Ch. 43), which, fortunately, is relatively rare, having an incidence of 0.1–1.2% and being reversible if the drug is stopped. Rashes are more common (2–25%), and other symptoms such as headaches, nausea, jaundice and pain in the joints occasionally occur.

Radioiodine

The isotope used is ^{131}I. Given orally, it is taken up and processed by the thyroid in the same way as the stable form of iodide, eventually becoming incorporated into thyroglobulin. It emits both β-particles and γ-rays. The γ-rays pass through the tissue, but the β-radiation has a very short range and exerts a cytotoxic action virtually restricted to the cells of the thyroid follicles. ^{131}I has a half-life of 8 days; by 2 months its radioactivity has effectively disappeared. It is used in one single dose, but its cytotoxic effect on the gland is delayed for 1–2 months and does not reach its maximum for a further 2 months.

The uptake of ^{131}I and other isotopes of iodine may be used as a test of thyroid function. A tracer dose of the isotope is given orally or intravenously and the amount accumulated by the thyroid is measured by a gamma scintillation counter placed over the gland.

Hypothyroidism will eventually occur after treatment with radioiodine, particularly in patients with Graves' disease, but is easily managed by replacement therapy with thyroxine. The risk of development of carcinoma of the thyroid, once considered to be a hazard, is now known to be negligible, as is the risk of infertility. However, radioiodine is best avoided in children and also in pregnant patients because of potential damage to the foetus.

Iodine/iodide

Iodine was the original agent used to treat thyrotoxicosis, but its effect is unreliable when it is used as a sole agent in therapy. It is converted in vivo to iodide (I^-).

When high doses of iodine are given to thyrotoxic patients, the symptoms subside within 1–2 days. There is inhibition of the secretion of thyroid hormones and, over a period of 10–14 days, a marked reduction in vascularity of the gland, which becomes smaller and firmer. Iodine solution in potassium iodide ('Lugol's iodine') is given orally. With continuous administration its effect reaches maximum within 10–15 days and then decreases.

The mechanism of action is not entirely clear; it may inhibit iodination of thyroglobulin, possibly by inhibiting the H_2O_2 generation which is necessary for this process.

The main uses are for the preparation of hyperthyroid subjects for surgery and as part of the treatment of severe thyrotoxic crisis (thyroid storm).

Allergic reactions can occur—these include angio-oedema, rashes, drug fever, lacrimation, conjunctivitis, pain in the salivary glands and a coryza-like syndrome.

Perchlorate and other anions

A number of inorganic anions (perchlorate and thiocyanate) compete with iodide for the iodide

Drugs in thyroid disease

Drugs for hyperthyroidism:

- **Thioureylenes** (e.g. propylthiouracil) decrease the synthesis of thyroid hormones; the mechanism is through inhibition of thyroperoxidase thus reducing iodination of thyroglobulin. Given orally.
- **Radioiodine**, given orally, is selectively taken up by thyroid and damages cells; it emits short range β-radiation which affects only thyroid follicle cells. Hypothyroidism will eventually occur.
- **Iodine**, given orally in high doses, transiently reduces thyroid hormone secretion and decreases vascularity of the gland.

Drugs for hypothyroidism:

- **Thyroxine** has all the actions of endogenous T_4, (see box on p. 430); given orally
- **Liothyronine** (T_3) has all the actions of endogenous T_3 (see box on p. 430); given intravenously.

transport system in the membrane of the follicle cell. They also cause loss of inorganic iodide which has already been taken up. They are of experimental and historical interest.

Propranolol

β-adrenoceptor antagonists, for example propranolol (Ch. 7), are not in fact antithyroid agents, but they are useful for decreasing many of the signs and symptoms of hyperthyroidism—the tachycardia, dysrhythmias, tremor and agitation. They are used in preparation for surgery, for the initial treatment of most hyperthyroid patients while the **thioureylenes** or **radioiodine** are taking effect, and as part of the treatment of thyroid storm.

Guanethidine, a noradrenergic blocking agent (Ch. 7), is used in eye drops to ameliorate the exophthalmos of hyperthyroidism (which is not relieved by antithyroid drugs); it acts by relaxing the sympathetically innervated smooth muscle that causes eyelid retraction. Glucocorticoids and surgical decompression are also sometimes needed for ophthalmic Graves' disease.

> **Clinical use of drugs acting on the thyroid**
>
> **The thioureylenes are used:**
> - for hyperthyroidism (diffuse toxic goitre), at least 1 year of treatment being necessary; recurrence occurs eventually in over half the patients but can be managed by a repeat course of treatment
> - as a preliminary to surgery for toxic goitre
> - as part of the treatment of thyroid storm (very severe hyperthyroidism); propylthiouracil is preferred because of its action in decreasing the conversion of T_4 to T_3 in the tissues.
>
> **Radioiodine is used:**
> - as first-line treatment for hyperthyroidism (particularly in the USA); recurrence is rare provided the dose is adequate
> - for treatment of relapse of hyperthyroidism after thioureylene therapy or surgery
> - in some thyroid tumours—to ablate residual tumour tissue after surgery.
>
> **Thyroid hormones**
> - **Thyroxine** is the standard replacement therapy for hypothyroidism.
> - **Liothyronine** is the treatment of choice for myxoedema coma.

DRUGS USED IN HYPOTHYROIDISM

There are no drugs that specifically augment the synthesis or release of thyroid hormones. The only effective treatment of hypothyroidism, unless it is due to iodine deficiency (which is treated with iodide; see above), is to administer the thyroid hormones themselves—used as replacement therapy. **Thyroxine** and **triiodothyronine** (**liothyronine**) are available and are given orally. Thyroxine is the drug of choice, liothyronine being reserved for the rare condition of myxoedema coma when its more rapid action is required for emergency treatment.

The actions and mechanisms of action of T_4 and T_3 are detailed on page 429.

Unwanted effects may occur with overdose, and in addition to the signs and symptoms of hyperthyroidism there is a risk of precipitating angina pectoris, cardiac dysrhythmias or cardiac failure.

The clinical use of drugs acting on the thyroid is given on this page.

CORTICOTROPHIN AND ADRENAL STEROIDS

The steroids secreted by the adrenal cortex have two main actions:

- those seen primarily in the resting state and which are 'permissive' in nature, i.e. they permit or facilitate the actions of other hormones
- those which occur in response to a threatening environment.

These latter actions are crucial for survival, an animal deprived of its adrenal cortex being able to survive only in rigorously controlled conditions.

The principal adrenal steroids are those with *mineralocorticoid* and *glucocorticoid* activity, but some *sex steroids*—mainly androgens—are also secreted. The mineralocorticoids affect water and electrolyte balance and the main endogenous hormone is **aldosterone**. The glucocorticoids affect carbohydrate and protein metabolism and the main endogenous hormones are **hydrocortisone** and **corticosterone**. The two actions are not completely separated in naturally occurring steroids, some glucocorticoids having quite substantial effects on water and electrolyte balance. In addition to their metabolic effects, glucocorticoids also have anti-inflammatory and immunosuppressive activity, and it is for these actions that they are most commonly used therapeutically. When they are used as anti-inflammatory and immunosuppressive agents, all of their other actions are unwanted side effects. Synthetic steroids have been developed in which it has been possible to separate the glucocorticoid from the mineralocorticoid actions (see Table 21.2), but it has not been possible to separate the anti-inflammatory actions from the other actions of the glucocorticoids.

A deficiency in corticosteroid production, *Addison's disease*, is characterised by muscular weakness, low blood pressure, depression, anorexia, loss of weight and hypoglycaemia. Addison's disease may have an autoimmune aetiology, or may be due to destruction

Table 21.2 Comparison of the main corticosteroid agents (using hydrocortisone as a standard)

Compound	Relative affinity for glucocorticoid receptors*	Approx. relative potency in clinical use: Anti-inflam.	Approx. relative potency in clinical use: Sodium-retaining	Duration of action after oral dose	Comments
Hydrocortisone (cortisol)	1	1	1	S	Drug of choice for replacement and emergencies
Cortisone	0.01	0.8	0.8	S	Cheap. Inactive until converted to hydrocortisone. Not used as anti-inflammatory because of mineralocorticoid effects
Corticosterone	0.85	0.3	15	S	–
Prednisolone	2.2	4	0.8	I	Drug of choice for systemic anti-inflammatory and immunosuppressive effects
Prednisone	0.05	4	0.8	I	Inactive until converted to prednisolone. Anti-inflammatory and immunosuppressive
Methylprednisolone	11.9	5	minimal	I	Anti-inflammatory and immunosuppressive
Triamcinolone	1.9	5	none	I	Relatively more toxic than others. Anti-inflammatory and immunosuppressive
Dexamethasone	7.1	30	minimal	L	Anti-inflammatory and immunosuppressive, used especially where water retention is undesirable, e.g. cerebral oedema. Drug of choice for suppression of ACTH production
Betamethasone	5.4	30	negligible	L	Anti-inflammatory and immunosuppressive, used especially where water retention is undesirable. Used for suppression of ACTH production
Beclomethasone		+	–	–	Anti-inflammatory and immunosuppressive. Used topically and as an aerosol
Budesonide		+	–	–	(as above)
Deoxycortone	0.19	neg.	50	–	
Fludrocortisone	3.5	15	150	S	Drug of choice for mineralocorticoid effects
Aldosterone	0.38	none	500	–	Endogenous mineralocorticoid

*Human foetal lung cells

Duration of action: S : $t_{1/2}$ = 8 – 12 ; I : $t_{1/2}$ = 12 – 36 h; L : $t_{1/2}$ = 36 – 72 h

Data for relative affinity obtained from: Baxter & Rousseau, 1979

of the gland by chronic inflammatory conditions such as tuberculosis. A decreased production of *endogenous* corticoids also occurs when glucocorticoids are given therapeutically for prolonged periods; this can result in deficiency eventually, when treatment is discontinued.

When corticosteroids are produced in excess, the clinical picture depends on which of the steroids predominate. Excessive glucocorticoid activity results in *Cushing's syndrome*, the manifestations of which are outlined in Figure 21.16. This can be caused by hypersecretion from the adrenal glands or by prolonged administration of glucocorticoids. An excessive production of mineralocorticoids results in disturbances of sodium and potassium balance. This may occur with hyperactivity of the adrenals or tumours of the glands (*primary hyperaldosteronism*, or Conn's syndrome, an uncommon but important cause of hypertension; see Ch. 14), or with excessive renin–angiotensin action such as occurs in kidney disease, cirrhosis of the liver or congestive cardiac failure (*secondary hyperaldosteronism*). Excessive production of adrenal androgens results in *adrenal virilism*.

The glucocorticoids are dealt with below and the mineralocorticoids on page 444.

GLUCOCORTICOIDS

Synthesis and release

Adrenal steroids are not stored preformed; they are synthesised and released as needed, and the main physiological stimulus for synthesis and release of the glucocorticoids is *corticotrophin* (adrenocorticotrophic hormone or ACTH) secreted from the anterior pituitary gland (see p. 423). Corticotrophin secretion is regulated partly by *corticotrophin-releasing factor* (CRF) derived from the hypothalamus (see Table 21.1) and partly by the level of glucocorticoids in the blood. (Antidiuretic hormone, which may reach the pituitary through short portal vessels from the posterior pituitary, may also have a role.) The release of CRF in turn is controlled by the level of glucocorticoids and, to a lesser extent, of corticotrophin in the blood, and is influenced by input from the central nervous system. There is a basal release of glucocorticoids. Opioid peptides normally exercise a tonic inhibitory control on the secretion of CRF. Psychological factors can affect the release of CRF, as can stimuli such as excessive heat or cold, injury or infections; this is the mechanism, in fact, by which the pituitary adrenal system is activated in response to a threatening environment. The interrelationship of these factors is outlined in Figure 21.13.*

There is normally a diurnal variation in the concentration of endogenous corticosteroids in the blood, between approximately 450 nmol/l at 8 a.m. and 110 nmol/l at 4 p.m.

The starting substance for synthesis of glucocorticoids is *cholesterol* which is obtained mostly from the plasma and is present in the lipid granules of the cells of the middle layer of the adrenal cortex. The steps involved in synthesis are outlined in Figure 21.14. The first step, the conversion of cholesterol to *pregnenolone* is the rate-limiting step and is regulated by ACTH. Some of the reactions in the synthesis can be inhibited by drugs.

Metyrapone prevents the β-hydroxylation at C_{11} and thus the formation of hydrocortisone and corticosterone (Fig. 21.14). Synthesis is stopped at the 11-deoxycorticosteroid stage and, as these substances have no negative feedback effects on the hypothalamus and pituitary, there is a marked increase in ACTH in the blood. Metyrapone can therefore be used to test ACTH production and may also be used in some cases of Cushing's syndrome. **Trilostane** blocks an earlier step in the pathway—the 3β-dehydrogenase.

Corticotrophin and the adrenal steroids

- Corticotrophin (ACTH) stimulates synthesis and release of **glucocorticoids** (e.g. hydrocortisone) from adrenal cortex (also some androgens).
- Corticotrophin-releasing factor (CRF) from the hypothalamus regulates corticotrophin release and is in turn regulated by neural factors and negative-feedback effects of plasma glucocorticoids.
- Mineralocorticoid (e.g. aldosterone) release from the adrenal cortex is controlled by the renin–angiotensin system.

*When released, the corticosteroids pass first through the adrenal medulla because both the medulla and cortex of the adrenal gland have a common blood supply. Glucocorticoids play a part in controlling the conversion of noradrenaline to adrenaline, through a stimulant action on the relevant methyltransferase (see Ch. 7).

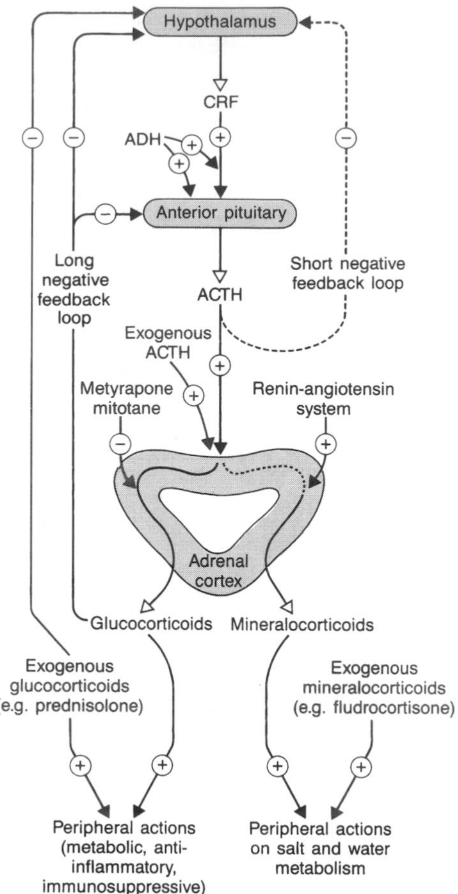

Fig. 21.13 Regulation of synthesis and secretion of adrenal corticosteroids. The long negative feedback loop is more important than the short one (dashed line). ACTH has only a minimal effect on mineralocorticoid production (indicated by dotted line).
(ACTH = adrenocorticotrophic hormone (corticotrophin); ADH = antidiuretic hormone (vasopressin); CRF = corticotrophin-releasing factor)

Aminoglutethimide inhibits an earlier stage in the synthetic pathway and has the same effect as metyrapone. **Amphenone B**, mainly an experimental tool, blocks the 21β-, the 17α- and the 11β-hydroxylase reactions.

Mitotane, a derivative of DDT, decreases corticosteroid synthesis mainly by a cytotoxic action on the cells and is used only in inoperable tumours of the adrenal cortex. It has a selective action on the adrenal cortex, but its precise mechanism of action is not known.

Actions

The pharmacological actions of the glucocorticoids may be considered under three main headings:

- general effects on metabolism, water and electrolyte balance and organ systems
- negative-feedback effects on the anterior pituitary and hypothalamus
- anti-inflammatory and immunosuppressive effects.

General metabolic and systemic effects

The main metabolic effects are on carbohydrate and protein metabolism. The hormones cause both a decrease in the uptake and utilisation of glucose and an increase in gluconeogenesis, resulting in a tendency to hyperglycaemia (see Ch. 20). There is a concomitant increase in glycogen storage which may be due to insulin secretion in response to the increase in blood sugar. There is decreased protein synthesis and increased protein breakdown, particularly in muscle. Glucocorticoids have a 'permissive' effect on the lipolytic response to catecholamines and other hormones, which act by increasing intracellular cAMP concentration (see Ch. 2). Such hormones cause lipase activation through a cAMP-dependent kinase, the synthesis of which requires the presence of glucocorticoids (see below). Large doses of glucocorticoids given over a long period result in the redistribution of fat characteristic of Cushing's syndrome (see Fig. 21.16).

The glucocorticoids, in non-physiological concentrations, have some mineralocorticoid actions (see below), causing sodium retention and potassium loss—probably by occupying mineralocorticoid receptors.

Glucocorticoids tend to produce a negative calcium balance by decreasing calcium absorption in the gastrointestinal tract and increasing its excretion by the kidney. This can result in osteoporosis (see below).

Negative feedback effects on the anterior pituitary and hypothalamus

Both endogenous and exogenous glucocorticoids have a negative feedback effect on the secretion of CRF and ACTH (see Fig. 21.13). Administration of exogenous glucocorticoids depresses the secretion of CRF and ACTH thus inhibiting the secretion of endogenous glucocorticoids and causing atrophy of the adrenal cortex. If therapy is prolonged, it may

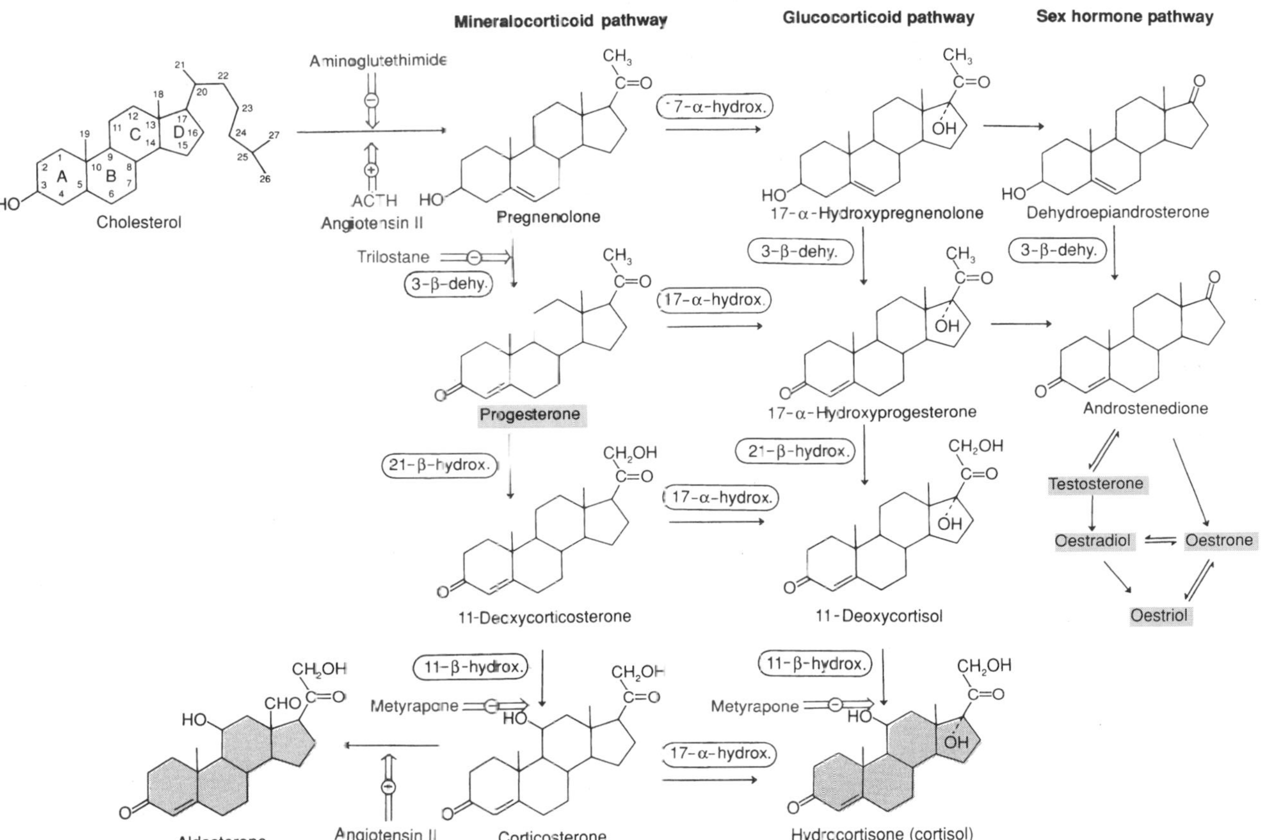

Fig. 21.14 Main pathways in the biosynthesis of corticosteroids and adrenal androgens with sites of action of drugs indicated. Note that the drugs have selective actions on different cortical cell types. Glucocorticoids are produced by cells of the zona fasciculata and their synthesis is stimulated by ACTH; aldosterone is produced by cells of the zona glomerulosa and its synthesis is stimulated by angiotensin II. Metyrapone inhibits glucocorticoid synthesis, aminoglutethimide inhibits both glucocorticoid and sex hormone synthesis, and trilostane blocks synthesis of all three types of adrenal steroid. (Further details of sex steroid biosynthesis are given in Fig. 22.3.) (3-β-dhy. = 3-β-dehydrogenase; 17-α-hydrox. = 17-α-hydroxylase; 21-β-hydrox. = 21-β-hydroxylase; 11-β-hydrox. = 11-β-hydroxylase)

take many months to return to normal function when the drugs are stopped.

Anti-inflammatory and immunosuppressive effects

When given therapeutically, glucocorticoids have powerful anti-inflammatory and immunosuppressive effects. They inhibit both the early and the late manifestations of inflammation, i.e. not only the initial redness, heat, pain and swelling (p. 216), but also the later stages of wound healing and repair and the proliferative reactions seen in chronic inflammation (p. 225). They affect *all* types of inflammatory reactions whether caused by invading pathogens, by chemical or physical stimuli or by inappropriately deployed immune responses such as are seen in hypersensitivity or autoimmune disease (p. 224).

The anti-inflammatory effects of the glucocorticoids are due to actions on blood vessels, inflammatory cells and inflammatory mediators.

Actions on blood vessels and inflammatory cells:

- Decreased vasodilatation and fluid exudation, associated with a direct vasoconstrictor action on small blood vessels.
- Decreased action of T helper cells and reduced clonal proliferation of T cells, mainly through decreased production of IL-2 (see Ch. 11, Figs 11.3 and 11.4). When used clinically to suppress graft rejection, glucocorticoids suppress the initiation and generation of a 'new' immune response more efficiently than a response that is already established and in which clonal proliferation has already occurred.
- Decreased accumulation of leucocytes in the area of inflammation, associated with a decrease in the release of monocytes and an increase in the release of neutrophils from the bone marrow.
- Reduced generation and release of tissue-damaging toxic oxygen radicals from neutrophils and macrophages.
- Reduced efficacy of cytokine-activated macrophages in dealing with intracellular microorganisms.
- Decreased fibroblast function and therefore less production of collagen and glycosaminoglycans; the contribution of these events to chronic inflammation is reduced but so also is healing and repair.
- Reduced function of osteoblasts (which lay down bone matrix) and increased activity of osteoclasts (which digest bone matrix), and thus a tendency to develop osteoporosis. The effect on osteoclasts is indirect—through decreasing the intestinal absorption of calcium, resulting in increased parathormone secretion, which in turn stimulates these cells.

Action on the mediators of the inflammatory and immune responses:

- Decreased production of prostanoids and leukotrienes (see Fig. 11.5).

Glucocorticoids

Drugs used: hydrocortisone, prednisolone and dexamethasone.

Metabolic actions

- On carbohydrates: decreased uptake and utilisation of glucose, and increased gluconeogenesis; this causes a tendency to hyperglycaemia.
- On proteins: increased catabolism, reduced anabolism.
- On fat, there is a permissive effect on lipolytic hormones, and a redistribution of fat, as in Cushing's syndrome.

Regulatory actions

- On hypothalamus and anterior pituitary: a negative-feedback action resulting in decrease of endogenous glucocorticoids.

Anti-inflammatory and immunosuppressive actions

- On vascular events: reduced vasodilatation, decreased fluid exudation.
- On cellular events:
  - —in areas of acute inflammation: decreased number and activity of leucocytes
  - —in areas of chronic inflammation: decreased activity of mononuclear cells, decreased proliferation of blood vessels, less fibrosis
  - —in lymphoid areas: decreased clonal expansion of T and B cells and decreased action of cytokine-secreting T cells.
- On inflammatory and immune mediators:
  - —decreased production and action of many cytokines (IL-1, IL-2, IL-3, IL-4, IL-5, IL-6, IL-8, TNFγ and GM-CSF)
  - —reduced generation of eicosanoids and platelet-activating factor
  - —decrease in complement components in the blood.
- Overall effects: reduction in chronic inflammation and autoimmune reactions but also decreased healing and diminution in the protective aspects of the inflammatory response.

- Decreased generation of cytokines, for example IL-1, IL-2, IL-3, IL-4, IL-5, IL-6, IL-8, TNF-γ (see Table 11.2) and GM-CSF (see Ch. 23, p. 485).
- Reduction in the concentration of complement components in the plasma (see p. 216).
- Decreased histamine release from basophils.

These anti-inflammatory and immunosuppressive actions of the glucocorticoids have generally been considered to be 'pharmacological' actions only, i.e. to be qualitatively different from the metabolic and regulatory actions of endogenously produced glucocorticoids—which were thought to be 'physiological' effects. In 1984, Munck and co-workers put forward a hypothesis which makes more sense. They suggested that the anti-inflammatory and immunosuppressive actions *do* have a physiological role in that they prevent 'overshoot' of the body's immensely powerful defence reactions, which might otherwise themselves threaten homeostasis. The fact that the magnitude and duration of inflammation is greatly increased in adrenalectomised as compared with sham-operated rats provides experimental support for this hypothesis.

The consequence of these powerful actions of the glucocorticoids is that they can be of immense value when used to treat certain conditions in which there is hypersensitivity and unwanted inflammation, but they carry the hazard that they can suppress the necessary protective responses to infection and can decrease essential healing processes.

Mechanism of action

Glucocorticoid effects involve interactions between the steroids and intracellular receptors that belong to the superfamily of nuclear receptors. This superfamily also includes the receptors for mineralocorticoids, the sex steroids, thyroid hormones, vitamin D_3 and retinoic acid—all agents that interact with DNA and modify gene transcription (see Ch. 2). There are believed to be 10 to 100 steroid-responsive genes in each cell.

The glucocorticoids, after entering cells, bind to specific receptors in the nucleus (Fig. 21.15A). These receptors, which have a high affinity for glucocorticoids are found in virtually all tissues—about 3000 to 10 000 per cell, the number varying in different tissues. After interaction with the steroid, the receptor becomes 'activated', i.e. it undergoes a conformational change which exposes a DNA-binding domain (see Figs 21.15B, 2.3 and 2.4). The steroid–receptor complex then binds to the DNA, and either induces (i.e. initiates transcription of) or represses (prevents transcription of) particular genes. The former involves the formation of specific messenger RNAs, which direct the synthesis of specific proteins; in the latter this is prevented and the production of certain proteins is inhibited. Some of the effects of the glucocorticoids on gene transcription are brought about through interaction of the steroid–receptor complex with a *transcription factor activator protein** termed 'AP-1'; this is a heterodimer of Fos and Jun proteins which are the products of Fos and Jun proto-oncogenes.** (For simple outlines of this topic, see Barnes & Adcock 1993, King 1992; for a more detailed review, see Landers & Spelsberg 1992).

AP-1 is involved in the induction of several genes, for example for collagenase, IL-2, the IL-2 receptor and the inducible cyclo-oxygenase (COX-2). The glucocorticoid–receptor complex can bind to, and inhibit the function of, AP-1.

The results of glucocorticoid modification of gene transcription

The detailed mechanisms whereby the nuclear events outlined above result in the known actions of glucocorticoids are not yet fully understood. However, some information which is relevant for the anti-inflammatory effects of the glucocorticoids is available.

Glucocorticoids and eicosanoid generation:

- It has been established that the glucocorticoids decrease prostanoid generation. It is now clear that the enzyme which gives rise to those prostanoids that are involved in inflammation is an inducible cyclo-oxygenase, termed COX-2—induced in inflammatory cells (monocytes, macrophages, synoviocytes, endothelial cells, fibroblasts) by inflammatory stimuli (cytokines, endotoxin, etc.; see Fig. 11.5). Exogenous glucocorticoids inhibit expression of COX-2 by inhibiting transcription of the relevant gene (either directly or by interfering with the function of AP-1) and thus

*These activator proteins bind to the DNA upstream from the start site of transcription and act as enhancers of transcription.

**See Chapter 36, page 698, for more information on oncogenes.

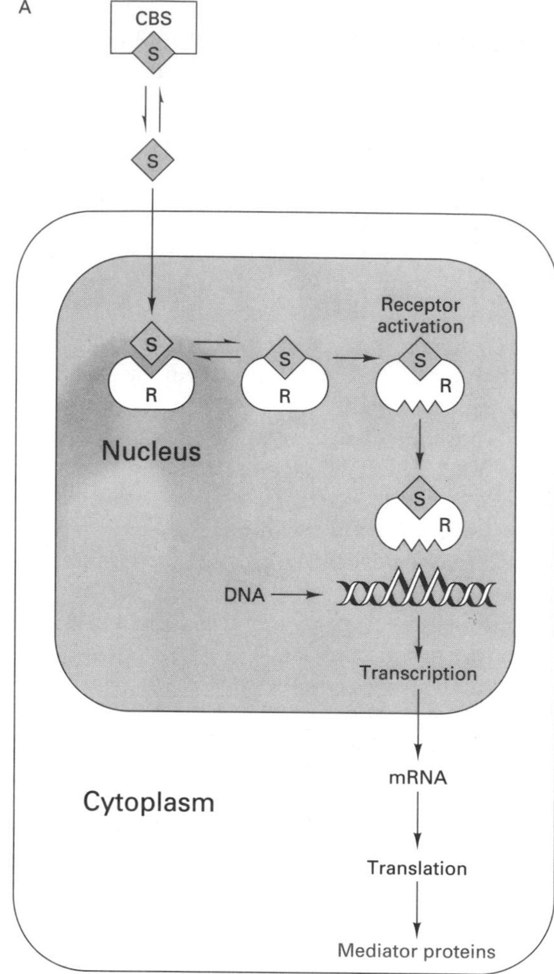

B
H2N
Zn++
Zn++
COOH
(i)
(ii)
(iii)
(iv)

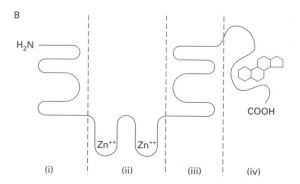

Fig. 21.15 Mechanism of action of glucocorticoids at the cellular level and the functional domains of the glucocorticoid receptor. A. Diagram showing glucocorticoid-mediated induction, i.e. the initiation of transcription. Note that the glucocorticoids can also repress induction. (S = steroid; R = receptor; CBG = corticosteroid-binding globulin) After the binding of steroid to receptor and before interaction with DNA, there is dimer formation, i.e. the linking of two steroid–receptor complexes (not shown). **B.** Diagram of the glucocorticoid receptor domains with the main functions associated with each domain. Note that three domains are involved in transcription and three in dimer formation. (i) Regulatory domain: activates gene-specific transcription, and can bind other protein factors. (ii) The DNA-binding domain: determines which genes will be influenced by the receptor (it contains two 'zinc fingers' which wrap around the DNA helix), controls transcriptional activation (i.e. positive as opposed to negative genomic events) and is involved in dimer formation. (iii) Hinge domain: is involved in nuclear localisation, transcription and dimer formation. (iv) Steroid-binding domain: binds steroid and is involved in nuclear localisation and dimer formation. (Modified from: Landers & Spelsberg 1992)

reduce prostanoid generation in inflammatory cells, but have little or no effect on the constitutive enzyme, COX-1. Endogenous glucocorticoids maintain a tonic inhibition of COX-2 expression.

- There is preliminary evidence that glucocorticoids *inhibit transcription of the gene* for phospholipase A_2 (PLA_2), the enzyme which gives rise not only to the prostanoids but also to platelet-activating factor and the leukotrienes (see Fig. 11.5). There is also evidence that glucocorticoids *induce the formation of an anti-inflammatory protein mediator*—lipocortin-1—which acts by inhibiting the activity of PLA_2. Lipocortins are members of a family of calcium-regulated, phospholipid-binding proteins termed 'annexins'. There is controversy about the mechanism whereby lipocortin-1 inhibits PLA_2; it may sequester the phospholipid substrate and/or directly inhibit the enzyme. Either mechanism could contribute to the decrease in the production of both platelet-activating factor and the eicosanoids observed in the presence of glucocorticoids. Recent data indicate that lipocortin-1 may also inhibit the IL-1-induced migration of leucocytes and that recombinant lipocortin-1 has anti-inflammatory action in vivo.*

Glucocorticoid effects on bone. It has long been known that glucocorticoids influence bone

*There is controversy as to whether lipocortins are primary mediators of the anti-inflammatory effects of the glucocorticoids. This is discussed by Davidson & Dennis (1989).

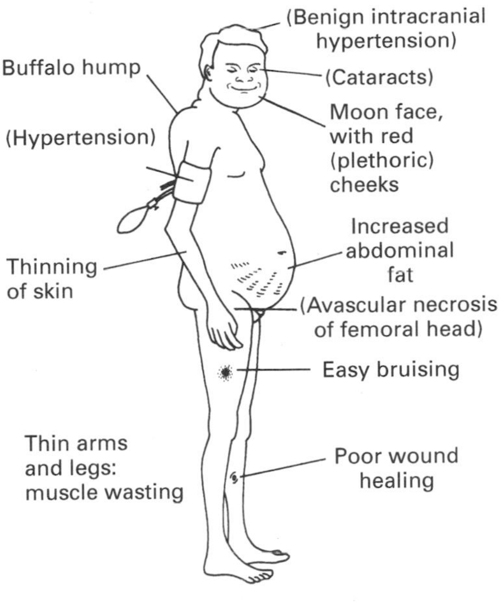

Fig. 21.16 Effects of prolonged glucocorticoid excess: iatrogenic Cushing's syndrome. Italicised effects are particularly common. Less frequent effects, related to dose and duration of therapy, are shown in brackets. (Adapted from: Baxter & Rousseau 1979)

by regulation of calcium and phosphate metabolism and through effects on collagen synthesis by osteoblasts and collagen degradation by collagenase, and that one of the main unwanted effects of these agents is osteoporosis (see Fig. 21.16). Recent evidence indicates that glucocorticoids accomplish these effects, at least in part, by the following actions:

- modification of the basal and induced transcription of the collagenase gene by interfering with the function of AP-1—the major enhancer factor in collagenase gene transcription
- blocking of vitamin-D_3 induction of the osteocalcin gene (see p. 450) in osteoblasts.

The glucocorticoid-induced decrease of *other inflammatory mediators*, such as the cytokines and complement components, could be due to direct inhibition of transcription or interference with intracellular transduction events.

Mechanism of action of the glucocorticoids

Glucocorticoids interact with intracellular receptors; the resulting steroid–receptor complex then interacts with DNA to modify gene transcription—inducing synthesis of some proteins and inhibiting synthesis of others.

- For metabolic actions, most mediator proteins are enzymes, e.g. cAMP-dependent kinase, but not all actions on genes are known.
- For anti-inflammatory and immunosuppressive actions, some actions at the level of the genes are known:
  - —inhibition of transcription of the gene for COX-2 (which is normally induced by inflammatory mediators and gives rise to inflammatory prostanoids)
  - —block of vitamin D_3-mediated induction of the osteocalcin gene in osteoblasts and modification of transcription of the collagenase gene
  - —possibly increased synthesis of an anti-inflammatory mediator protein, lipocortin 1, which inhibits phospholipase A_2 and blocks production of platelet-activating factor and all the eicosanoids.

As far as the *metabolic actions* of glucocorticoids are concerned, several relevant enzymes can be shown, in vitro, to be induced by glucocorticoids (e.g. the cAMP-dependent kinase mentioned above on p. 436), but these do not as yet explain all of the metabolic actions seen in vivo.

Unwanted effects

Unwanted effects are more likely to occur with large doses or prolonged administration and should not occur with replacement therapy. These effects are inherent in the three categories of pharmacological actions associated with the drugs:

- *Suppression of the response to infection or injury.* An intercurrent infection can be potentially very serious unless recognised and treated with antimicrobial agents along with an increase in the dose of steroid. Wound healing may be impaired, but peptic ulceration is probably not the problem it has been considered to be in the past, the incidence being only slightly higher in patients treated with steroids than in controls. However, patients on concurrent high doses of **aspirin** (e.g. in rheumatoid arthritis) would be more at hazard from peptic ulceration.

- *Suppression of the patients' capacity to synthesise corticosteroids.* Sudden withdrawal of the drugs after prolonged therapy may result in acute adrenal insufficiency.* Careful procedures for phased withdrawal should be followed, the rate of withdrawal depending mainly on duration of therapy. Recovery of full adrenal function usually takes about 2 months, though in some cases it may take 18 months or more.
- *Metabolic effects.* When the drugs are used in anti-inflammatory and immunosuppressive therapy, the metabolic actions and the effects on water and electrolyte balance and organ systems are unwanted side effects, and iatrogenic Cushing's syndrome may occur (see Fig. 21.16). The osteoporosis previously mentioned (see above, p. 441), with the attendant hazard of fractures, is probably one of the main limitations to long-term glucocorticoid therapy. Another limitation is the development of muscle wasting and weakness. The tendency to hyperglycaemia which occurs with exogenous glucocorticoids may develop into actual diabetes. In children, the metabolic effects (particularly those on protein metabolism) may result in inhibition of growth, even with fairly low doses, though this is not likely to occur unless treatment is continued for more than 6 months. A depressant effect on DNA synthesis and cell division in some tissues may also be implicated in this effect, though this antiproliferative action is not as general as that produced by antimitotic drugs.

There is often euphoria, but some patients may become depressed or develop psychotic symptoms. An effect on the blood supply to bone can result in avascular necrosis of the head of the femur.

The incidence of cataracts is higher after prolonged administration of the glucocorticoids in patients with rheumatoid arthritis, and cataracts have occurred in children as well.

Other toxic effects which have been reported are glaucoma, raised intracranial pressure, hypercoagulability of the blood, fever and disorders of menstruation. Oral thrush (a fungal infection, see Ch. 38) frequently occurs when glucocorticoids are taken by inhalation.

Pharmacokinetics and unwanted actions of the glucocorticoids

- Administration: oral, topical and parenteral; the drugs are bound to corticosteroid-binding globulin in the blood and enter cells by diffusion; metabolised in the liver.
- Unwanted effects are seen mainly with prolonged systemic use as anti-inflammatory or immunosuppressive agents (in which case all the metabolic actions are unwanted), but not usually with replacement therapy. The most important are:
  - —suppression of response to infection
  - —suppression of endogenous glucocorticoid synthesis
  - —metabolic actions (see above)
  - —osteoporosis
  - —iatrogenic Cushing's syndrome (see Fig. 21.16).

Pharmacokinetic aspects

Glucocorticoids may be given by a variety of routes. Most are active when given orally. All can be given systemically, either intramuscularly or intravenously. They may also be given topically—injected intra-articularly, given by aerosol into the respiratory tract, administered as drops into the eye or the nose, or applied in creams or ointments to the skin. There is much less likelihood of systemic toxic effects after topical administration, though such effects can occur if large quantities are used. When prolonged use of systemic glucocorticoids is necessary, alternate-day therapy may decrease the unwanted effects.

The endogenous glucocorticoids are carried in the plasma bound to corticosteroid-binding globulin (CBG) and to albumin. CBG has one hydrocortisone-binding site per molecule and has a high affinity for naturally occurring glucocorticoids. It is present in plasma in very low concentration and accounts for about 77% of hydrocortisone bound. CBG does not bind synthetic steroids. Albumin has a lower

*It is advisable that a patient on long-continued glucocorticoid therapy should carry a card stating: 'I am on STEROID TREATMENT which should not be stopped abruptly, and in the case of intercurrent illness may need to be increased'. This is because the exogenous glucocorticoids will have suppressed the necessary general hypothalamo–pituitary–adrenal response to the stress of illness or trauma.

Clinical use of glucocorticoids

- Replacement therapy for patients with adrenal failure (e.g. Addison's disease). All the actions of the corticosteroids are required, and a mineralocorticoid will need to be given along with a glucocorticoid.
- Anti-inflammatory/immunosuppressive therapy (see also Ch. 12):
  - —in asthma (by inhalation or, in severe cases, systemically; see Ch. 17)
  - —topically in various inflammatory conditions of skin, eye, ear or nose (e.g. eczema, allergic conjunctivitis or rhinitis)
  - —in hypersensitivity states (e.g. severe allergic reactions to drugs or insect venom)
  - —in miscellaneous diseases with autoimmune and inflammatory components (e.g. rheumatoid arthritis and other 'connective tissue' diseases, inflammatory bowel diseases, some forms of haemolytic anaemia, idiopathic thrombocytopenic purpura)
  - —to prevent graft-versus-host disease following organ or bone marrow transplantation.
- In neoplastic disease (see also Ch. 35):
  - —in combination with cytotoxic drugs in treatment of specific malignancies (e.g. Hodgkin's disease, acute lymphocytic leukaemia)
  - —to reduce cerebral oedema in patients with metastatic or primary brain tumours (dexamethasone is the drug used)
  - —as a component of anti-emetic treatment in conjunction with chemotherapy (see Ch. 19).

When they are used as anti-inflammatory and immunosuppressive agents, all of their metabolic actions are unwanted side effects.

affinity for hydrocortisone, but its plasma concentration is very much higher; it binds both natural and synthetic steroids. Both CBG-bound and albumin-bound steroids are biologically inactive.

Steroids, being small lipophilic molecules, enter their target cells by simple diffusion.

Hydrocortisone has a plasma half-life of 90 minutes, though its main biological effects occur only after 2–8 hours. The main step in inactivation is the reduction of the double bond between C_4 and C_5. This occurs in liver cells and elsewhere. The ketone at C_3 is reduced in the liver, and most compounds are then linked enzymically to sulphate or glucuronic acid at the C_3 hydroxyl, and finally excreted in the urine. Hydrocortisone may undergo an oxidation at C_{17} to give a 17-ketosteroid along with a two-carbon fragment. Virtually all of the metabolites are excreted within 72 hours. Metabolism is slowed if there is a double bond between carbon atoms 1 and 2 (methylprednisolone and prednisolone) and if there is a fluorine atom at C_9 (dexamethasone, betamethasone). Cortisone and prednisone are inactive until converted in vivo to hydrocortisone and prednisolone respectively.

The clinical use of the glucocorticoids is given on this page.

Dexamethasone can also be used to test hypothalamic–pituitary–adrenocortical function in the 'dexamethasone suppression test'. A low dose, usually given at night, should suppress the hypothalamus and pituitary, and result in reduced corticotrophin secretion and hydrocortisone output, the hydrocortisone being measured in the plasma about 9 hours later. Failure of suppression implies hypersecretion of corticotrophin or of glucocorticoids (Cushing's syndrome).

GLUCOCORTICOID ANTAGONISTS

Mifepristone (RU486), first described as a progesterone antagonist and potential abortifacient (see p. 461 and Fig. 21.4), also has a high affinity for the glucocorticoid receptor. It antagonises glucocorticoid effects in several cellular systems in vitro. Given orally in man, it has been shown to inhibit the effect of dexamethasone on the hypothalamo–pituitary–adrenal axis. In preliminary clinical studies, it has proved to be relatively effective in Cushing's syndrome.

CORTICOTROPHIN

Corticotrophin (ACTH; see Table 21.1 and p. 423) is a polypeptide hormone with 39 amino acid residues. A peptide consisting of the first 20 residues from the N-terminal end retains the full biological activity of the whole molecule, but removal of even one residue from the N-terminal end inactivates the hormone completely. Corticotrophin itself is rarely used in therapy because it provokes antibody formation. **Tetracosactrin**, a synthetic polypeptide that consists of the first 24 N-terminal amino acids, is used instead; it is less immunogenic than corticotrophin because the immunogenicity resides mainly in the 15 amino acids at the C-terminal end.

Regulation of secretion

The physiological release of corticotrophin is controlled by a balance between stimulatory and inhibitory factors (see Fig. 21.13). Its release is *stimulated* by corticotrophin-releasing factor (CRF; see Table 21.1). CRF release from the hypothalamus is under neural control, particularly from the limbic system. Stimuli which cause CRF to be released are, as explained above, various stressful physical and emotional conditions and factors which interfere with the body's ability to maintain homeostasis—heat, cold, infections, toxins, injury and so on. Other hormones which can stimulate corticotrophin release are the catecholamines and the posterior pituitary hormone, ADH (vasopressin; p. 424). This last also potentiates the action of CRF (Fig. 21.13).

Corticotrophin release is *inhibited* by corticosteroids, acting partly on the anterior pituitary directly, and partly on the secretion of CRF. The effect of the steroids on the hypothalamus is referred to as the 'long negative feedback loop'. Corticotrophin concentration in the blood also influences CRF release (the 'short negative feedback loop'), but this is less important.

The concentration of corticotrophin in the blood can be assessed by the dexamethasone suppression test (see p. 443).

Actions

Corticotrophin and tetracosactrin have two actions on the adrenal cortex:

- Stimulation of the synthesis and release of glucocorticoids from the adrenal cortex. (There is also a slight release of aldosterone and weakly androgenic steroids.) The main effect is to increase the concentration of the starting substrate for steroid synthesis, cholesterol (Fig. 21.14). The action is very rapid—a release of glucocorticoids occurs within minutes of injection and the main biological actions are those of the steroids released.
- A trophic action on adrenal cortical cells, and regulation of the levels of key mitochondrial steroidogenic enzymes.

Pharmacokinetic aspects and clinical use

Corticotrophin and tetracosactrin are broken down in the gastrointestinal tract and therefore have to be given parenterally.

The main use of tetracosactrin is in the diagnosis of adrenal cortical insufficiency. The drug is given intramuscularly, and then the concentration of hydrocortisone in the plasma is measured by radioimmunoassay (see Ch. 3).

MINERALOCORTICOIDS

The main endogenous mineralocorticoid is **aldosterone**, which is produced in the outermost of the three zones of the adrenal medulla, the *zona glomerulosa*. Its main action is to increase sodium reabsorption by an action on the distal tubules in the kidney, with concomitant increased excretion of potassium and hydrogen ions (see Ch. 18). An excessive secretion of mineralocorticoids, as in Conn's syndrome, causes marked sodium and water retention with resultant increase in the volume of extracellular fluid, hypokalaemia, alkalosis and hypertension. A decreased secretion, as in Addison's disease, causes increased sodium loss which is relatively more pronounced than water loss. The osmotic pressure of the extracellular fluid is thus reduced, resulting in a shift of fluid into the intracellular compartment and a marked decrease in extracellular fluid volume. There is a concomitant decrease in the excretion of potassium ions resulting in hyperkalaemia, and also a moderate decrease in plasma bicarbonate.

Regulation of aldosterone synthesis and release

The control of the synthesis and release of aldosterone is complex. Control depends mainly on the electrolyte composition of the plasma and on the angiotensin II system (Fig. 21.13 and Chs 14 and 18). Low plasma sodium or high plasma potassium concentrations affect the *zona glomerulosa* cells of the adrenal directly, stimulating aldosterone release. A depletion in body sodium also activates the *renin–angiotensin system* (see Fig. 14.5). One of the effects of angiotensin II is to increase the synthesis and release of aldosterone.

Mechanism of action

Aldosterone, like other steroids, binds to specific intracellular receptors. Unlike the glucocorticoid-binding receptors which occur in most tissues, aldosterone receptors occur in only a few target tissues such as the kidney, and in the transporting epithelia of the colon and bladder. Cells containing mineralocorticoid receptors also contain 11-β–hydroxysteroid dehydrogenase. This enzyme converts glucocorticoids to metabolites that have only low affinity for the mineralocorticoid receptors, thus ensuring that the cells are affected only by bona fide mineralocorticoids.

As with the glucocorticoids, the interaction of ligand with receptor initiates DNA transcription, initiating transcription of specific proteins resulting in:

- an early increase in the number of sodium channels in the apical membrane of the cell, mainly by the activation of previously quiescent channels; the protein mediator that activates these channels has not been identified
- a later phase of increase in the number of Na^+/K^+-ATPase molecules in the basolateral membrane (see Ch. 18, Fig. 18.4).

There is also evidence for a rapid non-genomic effect of aldosterone on Na^+ influx, through an action on the Na^+/H^+ exchanger in the apical membrane.

Increased K^+ secretion into the tubule results from the influx of K^+ into the cell through the action of the basal Na^+/K^+-ATPase, coupled with an increased efflux of K^+ through apical K^+ channels. (For reviews, see Wehling et al. 1993, Bastl & Hayslett 1992.)

Spironolactone is a competitive antagonist of aldosterone, and it also prevents the mineralocorticoid effects of other adrenal steroids on the renal tubule (p. 380).

Clinical use

The main clinical use of mineralocorticoids is in replacement therapy (Table 21.2). The most commonly used drug is **fludrocortisone** (Table 21.2 and Fig. 21.13) which can be taken orally.

> **Mineralocorticoids**
>
> - Fludrocortisone is given orally to produce a mineralocorticoid effect. This agent:
>   - —increases Na^+ reabsorption in distal tubules and increases K^+ and H^+ efflux into the tubules
>   - —acts, like most steroids, on intracellular receptors that modulate DNA transcription causing synthesis of protein mediators
>   - —is used with a glucocorticoid in replacement therapy.

PARATHYROID HORMONE, VITAMIN D, AND BONE MINERAL HOMEOSTASIS

Calcium and phosphate both have intracellular and extracellular functions in the body. The intracellular role of calcium is as a second messenger, regulating the activity of a variety of enzymes. Phosphate is an integral component of nucleic acids, nucleotides, phospholipids and many proteins; it is important in the 'energy-currency' of the cell, and phosphorylation/dephosphorylation reactions control the state of activity of many, if not most, enzymes. Extracellularly, calcium and phosphate are critically important constituents of bone. Extracellular calcium concentration also affects the electrical excitability of nerve and muscle cells—a reduction of plasma calcium concentration causes spontaneous muscle contraction (tetany).

Calcium and phosphate homeostasis is controlled by parathyroid hormone and a family of hormones derived from vitamin D.

The structure of bone

The cells involved in bone formation are osteoblasts, which synthesise and secrete the organic matrix of bone (the osteoid), and osteoclasts, which resorb it. The principal component of bone matrix is collagen, but there are also other components such as osteocalcin (a vitamin-K-dependent protein that binds calcium by virtue of γ-carboxyglutamic acid residues; cf. Ch. 16, p. 336) and various phosphoproteins, one of which, osteonectin, binds to both calcium and collagen and thus links these two major constituents of bone matrix. Calcium phosphate crystals in the form of hydroxyapatite $[Ca_{10}(PO_4)_6(OH)_2]$ are deposited in the osteoid, converting it into hard bone matrix. Bone is continuously being remodelled, a process whereby the synthesis of bone matrix and the deposition of mineral salts is balanced by bone resorption. The latter process—bone resorption, the work of osteoclasts—is stimulated mainly by parathyroid hormone and calcitriol, a hormone derived from vitamin D (see below). The production of new bone is largely controlled by newly discovered morphogenic factors termed *bone morphogenic proteins* (BMPs)—known by some as *osteogenic proteins* (OPs). At least seven bone morphogenic proteins have been identified and for several the genes have been cloned. The proteins appear to belong to the transforming growth factor-β family of regulatory proteins. They are thought to stimulate local undifferentiated mesenchymal cells to differentiate into chondrocytes (which secrete collagen) and osteoblasts. Bone itself contains OPs and the main production site of one of these, OP-1, is the kidney—which also generates the only other known morphogen, erythropoietin (see Ch. 23). In early clinical trials, preparations of these morphogens, applied locally, have successfully promoted healing of bone defects. They will soon be available for clinical use and should prove valuable in facilitating union of fractures and in arthrodesis. (See Lancet Editorial 1992, Alper 1994.)

A significant pathological condition affecting bone is *osteoporosis*, occurring particularly in elderly women as a result of age-related alteration in bone homeostasis; it can also result from glucocorticoid administration. The use of drugs to prevent and/or treat osteoporosis is considered by Riggs & Melton (1992). Other diseases of bone requiring drug therapy are *rickets** and *osteomalacia*, in which there are defects in bone mineralisation—a common cause being vitamin D deficiency—and *Paget's disease* in which there is distortion of the processes of bone resorption and remodelling.

Calcium

More than 90% of the calcium in the body is in the skeleton, mostly as crystalline hydroxyapatite (see above) but some as non-crystalline phosphates and carbonates. Together, these make up half the bone mass. The daily turnover of the minerals in bone involves about 700 mg of calcium, as the bone is continuously remodelled.

Intracellular calcium constitutes only a small proportion of body calcium, but it has a major role in cellular function (see Ch. 2). An influx of calcium with increase of calcium in the cytosol is part of the transduction mechanism of many cells, thus the concentration of calcium in the extracellular fluid and the plasma needs to be controlled with great precision. The concentration of calcium in the cytoplasm of cells is about 100 nmol/l, whereas in the plasma it is about 2.5 mmol/l. About 40% of plasma calcium is bound to plasma proteins, and 10% is in the form of complexes with various anions. The remaining 50% is present as free ionised calcium.

*The term rickets is used when the defect occurs in growing bone.

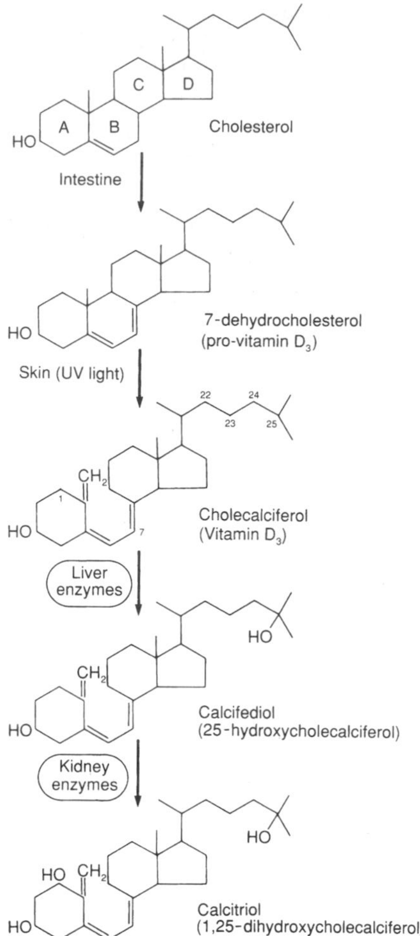

Fig. 21.17 The basic structures of the members of the vitamin D_3 system. The B ring of the precursor 7-dehydrocholesterol is cleaved by UV irradiation. Both vitamin D_2 (calciferol) and its precursor, ergosterol (neither shown here), have a double bond between C22 and C23 and a methyl group at C24. Hydroxylation at various sites results in the active vitamin D metabolites.

The normal plasma calcium concentration is regulated by complex interactions between **parathormone** and various forms of **vitamin D** (Figs 21.17, 21.18 and 21.19). **Calcitonin** also plays a part.

Calcium absorption in the intestine involves a calcium-binding protein whose synthesis is regulated by calcitriol (see Fig. 21.18 and below). It is probable that the overall calcium content of the body is regulated largely by this absorption mechanism. Normally, urinary calcium excretion remains more or less constant. However, with high blood calcium concentrations, urinary excretion increases, and with

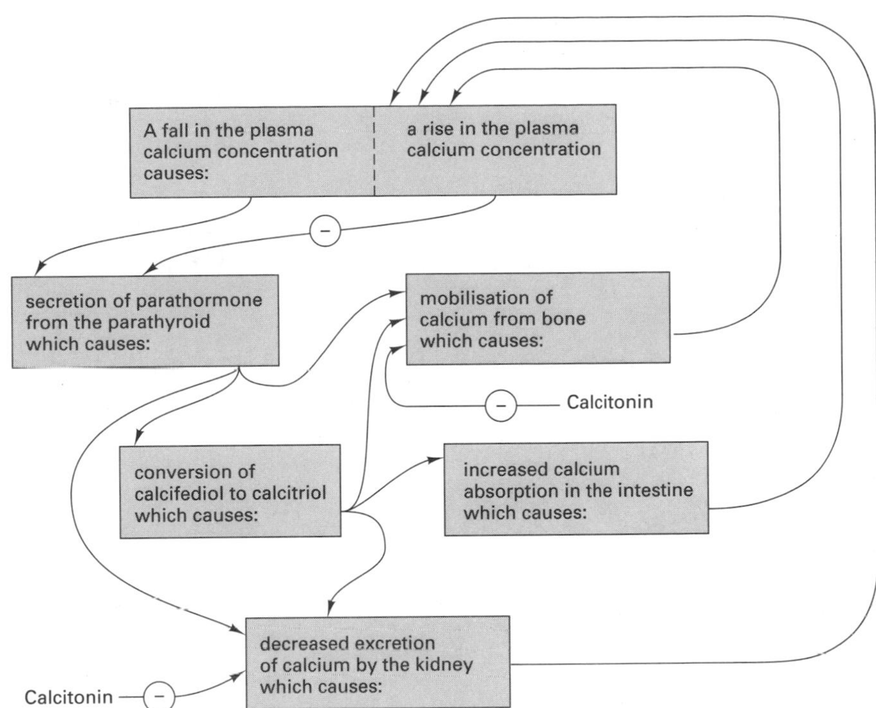

Fig. 21.18 The main factors involved in maintaining the concentration of calcium in the plasma. Calcifediol and calcitriol are metabolites of vitamin D_3 and constitute the 'hormones' 25-hydroxy vitamin D_3 and 1,25-dihydroxy vitamin D_3 respectively. (Calcitonin, secreted by the thyroid, inhibits calcium mobilisation from bone and decreases its resorption in the kidney, thus reducing blood calcium.)

low blood concentrations, urinary excretion can be reduced by parathormone and calcitriol, both of which enhance calcium reabsorption in the renal tubules (Fig. 21.18).

The main causes of hypocalcaemia are hypoparathyroidism, vitamin D deficiencies, congenital rickets and some kidney diseases. The main causes of hypercalcaemia are hyperparathyroidism and malignancies.

Calcium salts used therapeutically include **calcium gluconate** and **calcium lactate**, given orally. Calcium gluconate is also used for intravenous injection; intramuscular injection is not used because of the danger of local necrosis. An oral preparation of **hydroxyapatite** is available.

Clinical use of calcium salts

- In dietary deficiencies and for chronic hypocalcaemia due to hypoparathyroidism or malabsorption (given orally).
- Hypocalcaemic tetany (given i.v.).
- Osteoporosis:
  —with oestrogen and calcitonin in postmenopausal osteoporosis; regimes involving calcium with vitamin D preparations and/or etidronate and/or calcitriol are also being tested (see below)
  —with calcitriol and calcitonin for corticosteroid-induced osteoporosis (see below).
- Cardiac dysrhythmias caused by severe hyperkalaemia (given i.v).

The clinical use of the calcium salts is given in the following box.

Unwanted effects

Oral calcium salts can cause gastrointestinal disturbance. Intravenous administration requires care and is contraindicated in patients on cardiac glycosides (see Ch. 13).

Phosphate

Phosphates are critically important in the structure and function of the cells of the body. They play a

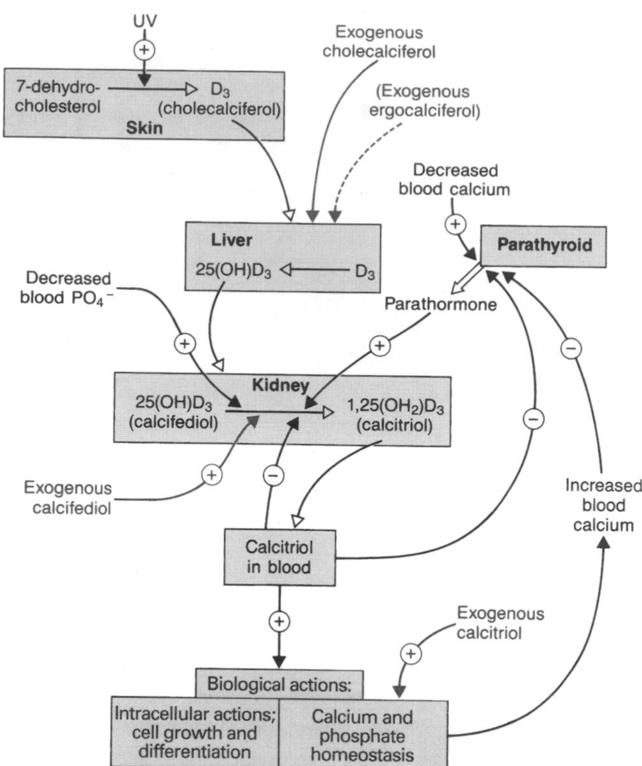

Fig. 21.19 Summary of the actions of the vitamin D endocrine system. Drugs which affect the system are shown in red. Exogenous ergocalciferol, vitamin D_2 (shown in brackets), is converted to the corresponding D_2 metabolites in liver and kidney, as is the D_2 analogue, dihydrotachysterol. Alfacalcidol (1α-hydroxycholecalciferol) is 25-hydroxylated to calcitriol in the liver.

significant part in enzymic reactions in the cell; they have roles as intracellular buffers and in the excretion of hydrogen ions in the kidney. They are a major component of bone and constitute one of the factors which modify the calcium concentration in tissues, in part by an effect on the synthesis of calcitriol (Fig. 21.19).

Phosphate absorption is an energy-requiring process regulated by calcitriol (see below). Phosphate deposition in bone, as hydroxyapatite, depends on the plasma concentration of parathormone, which, with calcitriol, tends to mobilise both calcium and phosphate from the bone matrix. Phosphate is excreted by the kidney. About 90% is filtered in the glomerulus, and most of this is reabsorbed in the proximal tubule. Parathormone inhibits reabsorption and thus increases excretion.

Phosphate deficiency and hypophosphataemia can occur in nutritional deficiency states (e.g. in alcoholics and patients receiving parenteral nutrition) and may require oral or, exceptionally, intravenous replacement. Hyperphosphataemia is a common problem in patients with renal failure, and is treated with calcium- or aluminium-containing antacids (Ch. 19) that bind phosphate and prevent its absorption from the gut.

PARATHYROID HORMONE (PARATHORMONE)

Parathormone is a single chain polypeptide of 84 amino acids, the essential activity of which is contained in residues 1–34 of the N-terminal part of the molecule. It is an important regulator of calcium metabolism. Parathormone increases the plasma calcium concentration by mobilising calcium from bone, by promoting its reabsorption by the kidney and, in particular, by stimulating the synthesis of calcitriol which in turn increases calcium absorption from the intestine and synergises with parathormone in mobilising bone calcium (Figs 21.18 and 21.19). Parathormone promotes phosphate excretion, and thus its net effect is to increase the concentration of calcium in the plasma and lower that of phosphate.

The mobilisation of calcium from bone by parathormone is mediated, at least in part, by stimulation of osteoclast activity, and the effect on these cells and on the cells of the kidney tubules involves

Table 21.3 Vitamin D and its main derivatives

Compound	Alternative name	Notes
Vitamin D_3	Cholecalciferol*	Formed in skin from dehydrocholesterol by u.v. irradiation
Vitamin D_2	Ergocalciferol* (calciferol*)	Formed in plants by u.v. irradiation of ergosterol
25-hydroxy-vitamin D_3	Calcifediol	Formed in liver from cholecalciferol or ergocalciferol. Main 'storage' form of vitamin D. Thought to be important in reabsorbing calcium in the renal tubules and regulating calcium flux in muscle
1,25-dihydroxy vitamin D_3	Calcitriol*	Formed from calcifediol in kidney. Most potent metabolite in regulating plasma [Ca^{2+}]
Analogue of vitamin D_2	Dihydrotachysterol*	A crystalline compound prepared by reduction of vitamin D_2. Activated by 25-hydroxylation of the liver
1α-hydroxy-cholecalciferol	Alfacalcidol*	A synthetic 1α-hydroxylated derivative of vitamin D_3. Undergoes hepatic 25-hydroxylation to calcitriol

* Compounds available for clinical use

activation of adenylate cyclase (see Ch. 2). Osteoblast activity is also inhibited, thus decreasing calcium deposition by decreasing the amount of matrix available for mineralisation.

Parathormone is synthesised in the cells of the parathyroid glands and stored in vesicles. The principal factor controlling secretion is the concentration of ionised calcium in the plasma, low plasma calcium stimulating secretion. The parathyroid cell has a calcium sensor in its membrane, consisting of seven serpentine membrane-spanning segments and two large extracellular lobes. Calcium binding causes the two lobes to bend towards each other over the calcium ion in the manner of a Venus fly-trap; the conformational change activates a G-protein which in turn activates phospholipase C (see Ch. 2) leading to inhibition of parathormone secretion.* The plasma phosphate concentration has no effect on the secretion of the hormone.

There is little or no clinical use for parathormone as such. Hypoparathyroidism is best treated by vitamin D—acute hypoparathyroidism necessitating the use of intravenous calcium and injectable vitamin D preparations.

VITAMIN D

Vitamin D is a prehormone which is converted in the body into a number of biologically active metabolites. These function as true hormones, circulating in the blood and regulating the activities of various cell types (see Reichel et al. 1989). The main action is the maintenance of plasma calcium by increasing calcium absorption in the intestine, mobilising calcium from bone and decreasing its renal excretion (see Fig. 21.18). Vitamin D itself is really a family of sterol derivatives. In humans, there are two sources of vitamin D:

- dietary ergocalciferol (D_2), derived from ergosterol in plants
- cholecalciferol (D_3) generated in the skin from 7-dehydrocholesterol by the action of ultraviolet irradiation, the 7-dehydrocholesterol having been formed from cholesterol in the wall of the intestine (Table 21.3).

Cholecalciferol is a secosteroid—i.e. a steroid in which one of the rings has undergone fission, in this case ring B. The basic structure is outlined in Figure 21.17. Vitamin D_3 is converted to 25,hydroxyvitamin D_3 (**calcifediol**) in the liver, and this is converted to a series of other metabolites of varying activity in the kidney, the most potent of which is 1,25,dihydroxyvitamin D_3 (**calcitriol**) (see Figs 21.17 and 21.19).

Calcifediol is the main metabolite found in the circulation and may constitute a storage form of the hormone. The synthesis of calcitriol from calcifediol is regulated by parathyroid hormone, and is also influenced by the phosphate concentration in the plasma and by the calcitriol concentration itself through a negative feedback mechanism (Fig. 21.19). Receptors for calcitriol have been identified in vir-

*Now that calcium is known to have its own cellular receptor complete with signal transduction mechanism, the erstwhile definition of 'hormone/chemical transmitter' has become confusingly blurred.

Parathyroid, vitamin D and bone mineral homeostasis

- The vitamin D family are true hormones.
- There is conversion from precursors to calcifediol in the liver, then to the main hormone, calcitriol, in kidney.
- Calcitriol increases plasma calcium by mobilising it from bone, increasing its absorption in the intestine and decreasing its excretion by the kidney.
- Parathyroid hormone increases blood calcium by increasing calcitriol synthesis, mobilising calcium from bone and reducing renal calcium excretion.
- Calcitonin (secreted from the thyroid) reduces calcium resorption from bone by inhibiting osteoclast activity.
- Drugs affecting this system are:
  - —the vitamin D preparations: ergocalciferol, calcitriol; given orally
  - —disodium etidronate, which reduces bone turnover in Paget's disease; given orally or by i.v. infusion
  - —salcatonin (synthetic salmon calcitonin); given s.c. or i.m.

tually every tissue except liver and it is now considered that calcitriol may be important in the functioning of many cell types, possibly participating in the regulation of intracellular calcium and in the control of cell differentiation and growth—particularly in bone marrow. (Reviewed by Reichel et al. 1989.)

The main actions of calcitriol are the stimulation of absorption of calcium and phosphate in the intestine and the mobilisation of calcium from bone, but it also increases calcium reabsorption in the kidney tubules (Fig. 21.18).

Clinical use of vitamin D preparations

- To prevent and to treat various forms of rickets, osteomalacia and vitamin D deficiency due to malabsorption and liver disease (ergocalciferol).
- To treat the hypocalcaemia associated with hypoparathyroidism (ergocalciferol).
- To treat the osteodystrophy of chronic renal failure, which is due to decreased calcitriol generation (calcitriol or alphacalcidol).

Plasma calcium levels should be routinely monitored (usually weekly) during therapy with vitamin D.

Its effect on bone probably involves synergism with parathormone (Fig. 21.18). It decreases collagen synthesis by osteoblasts, and its effect on these cells is believed to be by the classical steroid pathway, involving intracellular receptors and an effect on the DNA. It promotes maturation of osteoclasts and indirectly stimulates their activity. However, the effect on bone is complex; and is clearly not confined to mobilising calcium, since in clinical vitamin D deficiency (see below), in which the mineralisation of bone is impaired, administration of vitamin D restores bone formation. One explanation may lie in the fact that calcitriol has been shown to stimulate synthesis of osteocalcin, the vitamin-K-dependent, calcium-binding protein of bone matrix.

The main vitamin D preparation used clinically is **ergocalciferol**; also available for clinical use are **alfacalcidol** and **calcitriol** (Table 21.3). These latter preparations are more expensive than ergocalciferol and for most purposes offer little advantage over it. The exception is in patients with severe renal failure who are unable to 1-hydroxylate vitamin D in the kidney and therefore require alfacalcidol or calcitriol for treatment of renal rickets. All can be given orally and are well absorbed from the intestine. Vitamin D preparations are fat soluble and bile salts are necessary for absorption. Injectable forms of calciferol are available.

Pharmacokinetic aspects

All forms of vitamin D are given orally. Vitamin D is bound to a specific α-globulin in the blood, and the plasma half-life is about 22 hours. However, it can be found in the fat for many months. Enterohepatic recirculation of the vitamin occurs, and the main route of elimination is in the faeces.

The clinical use of vitamin D preparations is given on this page.

Unwanted effects

Excessive intake of vitamin D causes hypercalcaemia, the manifestations of which are gastrointestinal disturbances, physical weakness and fatigue. Renal effects include a reduced ability to concentrate the urine, resulting in polyuria and polydipsia. If hypercalcaemia persists, calcium salts are deposited in the kidney causing renal failure.

Some anticonvulsant drugs (e.g. phenytoin; see Ch. 30) can increase requirement for vitamin D. Vitamin D given to a nursing mother is secreted into the milk; high doses should be avoided because of the theoretical risk of hypercalcaemia in the infant.

CALCITONIN

Calcitonin is a hormone secreted by the specialised 'C' cells found in the thyroid follicles.

Actions

The main action of calcitonin is on bone; it inhibits calcium resorption by binding to a specific receptor on osteoclasts inhibiting their action. In the kidney it decreases the reabsorption of both calcium and phosphate in the proximal tubules. Its overall effect is to decrease the plasma calcium concentration.

Regulation of secretion

Secretion is determined mainly by the plasma calcium concentration. Pentagastrin stimulates its secretion and, conversely, exogenous calcitonin reduces gastrin secretion.

Administration, pharmacokinetics and unwanted effects

The preparations available for clinical use (see below) are porcine (natural) **calcitonin** and **salcatonin** (synthetic salmon calcitonin). Synthetic human calcitonin is now also available. Porcine calcitonin may contain traces of thyroid hormones and can lead to the production of antibodies. Calcitonin is given by subcutaneous or intramuscular injection, and there may be a local inflammatory action at the injection site. It can also be given intranasally. The plasma half-life of calcitonin is 4–12 minutes.

Nausea and vomiting may occur, as may facial flushing, an unpleasant taste in the mouth and a tingling sensation in the hands.

Clinical use of calcitonin/salcatonin

- To lower the plasma calcium in hypercalcaemia—for example that associated with neoplasia.
- To treat Paget's disease of bone (it not only relieves the pain but may reduce some of the neurological complications).
- As part of the therapy of postmenopausal and corticosteroid-induced osteoporosis.

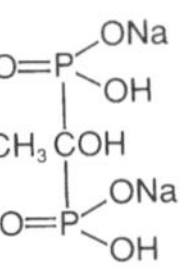

Fig. 21.20 Disodium etidronate.

OTHER AGENTS USED IN DISORDERS OF CALCIUM AND PHOSPHATE METABOLISM

Several other substances may be of value in conditions of disturbed calcium and phosphate homeostasis. These include:

- bisphosphonates
- plicamycin
- glucocorticoids
- oestrogens.

Bisphosphonates

Bisphosphonates (also termed diphosphonates), are enzyme-resistant analogues of pyrophosphate, the naturally occurring inhibitor of mineralisation in bone, the P–O–P structure of pyrophosphate being replaced by P–C–P. They impede the bone-resorbing activity of osteoclasts in a dose-dependent manner and thus reduce the turnover of bone.

The main diphosphonate at present available for clinical use is **disodium etidronate** (Fig. 21.20). Others are disodium pamidronate and sodium clodronate.

Disodium etidronate is given orally, about 10% is absorbed, and 50% of the absorbed drug accumulates in bone, the rest being excreted unchanged by the kidney. That portion of the drug which is taken up by bone remains for several weeks.

It is used for up to 6 months for Paget's disease of bone, malignant hypercalcaemia and osteoporosis (in which it improves spinal bone mass and is thought to prevent vertebral fractures). Bisphosphonates are being tested for the treatment of cancer metastases to bone.

Disodium etidronate has a narrow therapeutic margin and, if given for too long, can *increase* the risk of fractures due to reduced calcification of bone.

Glucocorticoids

It has been pointed out earlier in this chapter that one of the unwanted effects of glucocorticoid therapy is osteoporosis. This is due partly to decreased intestinal absorption of calcium and phosphate associated with increased renal excretion, and partly to an inhibition of bone formation. This latter action is thought to be partly due to an indirect inhibition of osteoclast activity (see p. 438). These effects can be made use of in the therapy of some types of hypercalcaemia, particularly that associated with sarcoidosis.

Plicamycin

Plicamycin (mithramycin), an antibiotic once used in cancer chemotherapy, inhibits resorption of bone. It is an inhibitor of RNA synthesis in osteoclasts and thus blocks calcium mobilisation from bone. Given intravenously, it is used in refractory hypercalcaemia caused by malignancy. Hepatic and renal toxicity and thrombocytopenia limit its use.

Gallium nitrate

Gallium nitrate inhibits bone resorption; it is thought that it adsorbs to and decreases the solubility of hydroxyapatite crystals. Given by continuous intravenous infusion, it is being tested as therapy for hypercalcaemia. It is nephrotoxic and is reported to cause hypophosphataemia.

Oestrogens

Oestrogens have an important place in the prevention of post-menopausal osteoporosis (see Ch. 22). They are thought to act by opposing the calcium-mobilising, bone-resorbing effect of parathormone.

REFERENCES AND FURTHER READING

The hypothalamus and pituitary

Daughaday W H 1990 Clinical applications of corticotrophin releasing hormone. Mayo Clin Proc 5: 1026–1027

Davies R R, Johnston D G 1987 Growth hormone releasing factors. J Roy Soc Med 80: 3–5

Editorial 1990 All aboard for octreotide. Lancet 2: 909–911

Jørgensen J O L 1991 Human growth hormone replacement therapy: pharmacological and clinical aspects. Endocr Rev 12: 189–205

Jørgensen J O L, Christiansen J S 1993 Growth hormone therapy. Lancet 341: 1247–1248

László F A, László F, De Wied D 1991 Pharmacology and clinical perspectives of vasopressin antagonists. Pharmacol Rev 43: 73–104

Leong D A, Frawley S, Neill J D 1983 Neuroendocrine control of prolactin secretion. Annu Rev Physiol 45: 109–127

Lightman S L 1993 Molecular insights into diabetes insipidus. N Engl J Med 328: 1562–1563

Manger J A 1990 Thyroid-stimulating hormone: biosynthesis, cell biology, and bioactivity. Endocr Rev 11: 354–385

Owens M J, Nemeroff C B 1991 Physiology and pharmacology of corticotropin-releasing factor. Pharmacol Rev 43: 425–464

Page R B 1982 Pituitary blood flow. Am J Physiol 243: E427–442

Reichlin S 1983 Somatostatin. N Engl J Med 309: 1495–1501, 1556–1563

Ryan R J, Charlesworth C M, McCormich D J et al. 1988 The glycoprotein hormones: recent studies of structure–function relationships. FASEB 2: 2661–2669

Ruvkun G 1992 A molecular growth industry. Nature 360: 711–712

Sung J J Y, Chung S C S et al. 1993 Octreotide infusion or emergency sclerotherapy for variceal hemorrhage. Lancet 342: 637–641

Vance M L 1994 Hypopituitarism. N Engl J Med 330: 1651–1662

Wass J A H 1993 Acromegaly: treatment after 100 years. Br Med J 307: 1505–1506

Wynick D, Hammond P J et al. 1993 Galanin regulates basal and oestrogen-stimulated lactotroph function. Nature 364: 529–532

The thyroid

Berry M J, Larsen P R 1992 The role of selenium in thyroid hormone action. Endocr Rev 13: 207–220

Feldt-Rasmussen U, Glinoer D, Orgiazzi J 1993 Reassessment of antithyroid drug therapy of Graves' disease. Annu Rev Med 44: 323–334

Franklin J F, Sheppard M 1992 Radioiodine for hyperthyroidism: perhaps the best option. Br Med J 305: 728–729

Larkins R 1993 Treatment of Graves' ophthalmopathy. Lancet 342: 941–942

Ludgate M 1992 Structure–function relationships in the thyrotropin (TSH) receptor. In: Edwards C R W, Lincoln D W (eds) Recent advances in endocrinology and metabolism. Churchill Livingstone, Edinburgh, ch 3

Nygaard B, Hegedüs 1993 Radioiodine treatment of multinodular non-toxic goitre. Br Med J 307: 828–832

Oppenheimer J H, Schwartz H L et al. 1987 Advances in our understanding of thyroid hormone action at the cellular level. Endocr Rev 8: 288–308

Pitt-Rivers R, VanderLaan W P 1984 The therapy of thyroid diseases. In: Parnham M J, Bruinvels J (eds) Discoveries in pharmacology. Vol. 2: Haemodynamics, hormones and inflammation. Elsevier Science Publishers, Amsterdam, ch 7

Toft A D 1994 Thyroxine therapy. N Engl J Med 331: 174–180

Utiger R D 1992 Vanishing hypothyroidism. N Engl J Med 326: 561–563

Volpe R 1987 Immunoregulation in autoimmune thyroid disease. N Engl J Med 316: 44–45

ACTH and the adrenal corticosteroids

Barnes P J, Adcock I 1993 Anti-inflammatory actions of

steroids: molecular mechanisms. Trends Pharmacol Sci 14: 436–441
Bastl C, Hayslett J P 1992 The cellular action of aldosterone in target epithelia. Kidney Internat 42: 250–264
Baxter J D, Rousseau G G (eds) 1979 Glucocorticoid hormone action. Monographs on endocrinology. Springer-Verlag, Berlin, vol 12
Beato M 1989 Gene regulation by steroid hormones. Cell 56: 335–344
Davidson F F, Dennis E A 1989 Biological relevance of lipocortins and related proteins as inhibitors of phospholipase A_2. Biochem Pharmacol 38: 3645–3651
DeWitt D L, Meade E A 1993 Serum and glucocorticoid regulation of gene transcription and expression of the prostaglandin H synthase-1 and prostaglandin H synthase-2 isoenzymes. Arch Biochem Biophys 306: 94–102
Fisher L A 1989 Corticotrophin-releasing factor: endocrine and autonomic integration of responses to stress. Trends Pharmacol Sci 10: 189–193
Flower R J 1988 Lipocortin and the mechanism of action of the glucocorticoids. Br J Pharmacol 94: 987–1015
Flower R J, Dale M M 1994 The anti-inflammatory effects of corticosteroids. In: Dale M M, Foreman J C, Fan T-P (eds) Textbook of immunopharmacology, 3rd edn. Blackwell Scientific Publications, London
Flower R J, Rothwell N J 1994 Lipocortin-1: cellular mechanisms and clinical relevance. Trends Pharmacol Sci 15: 71–76
Geisow M J, Walker J H et al. 1987 Annexins: new family of Ca^{2+}-regulated phospholipid binding proteins. Biosci Rep 7: 289–297
Goulding N J, Godolphin J L et al. 1990 Anti-inflammatory lipocortin I production by peripheral blood leucocytes in response to hydrocortisone. Lancet 1: 1416–1418
Guslandi M, Tittobello A 1992 Steroid ulcers: a myth revisited. Br Med J 304: 655–656
King R J B 1992 Effects of steroid hormones and related compounds on gene transcription. Clin Endocrinol 36: 1–14
Krane S M 1993 Some molecular mechanisms of glucocorticoid action. Br J Rheumatol 32: 3–5
Landers J P, Spelsberg T C 1992 New concepts in steroid hormone action: transcription factors, proto-oncogenes, and the cascade model of gene expression. Crit Rev Eukaryotic Gene Expression 2: 19–63
Munck A, Guyre P M, Holbrook N J 1984 Physiological functions of glucocorticoids in stress and their relation to pharmacological actions. Endocr Rev 5: 25–44
Quinn S J, Williams G H 1988 Regulation of aldosterone secretion. Annu Rev Physiol 50: 409–426
Schleimer R P, Claman H N, Oronsky A 1989 (eds) Anti-inflammatory steroid action: basic and clinical aspects. Academic Press, San Diego, p 1–543
Spitz I M, Bardin C W 1993 Mifepristone (RU 486)—a modulator of progestin and glucocorticoid action. N Engl Med J 329: 404–410
Sternberg et al. 1992 The stress response and the regulation of inflammatory disease. Ann Intern Med 117: 854–866
Taylor A L, Fishman L M 1988 Corticotrophin-releasing hormone. N Engl J Med 319: 213–222
Taylor I K, Shaw R J 1993 The mechanism of action of corticosteroids in asthma. Respir Med 87: 261–277
Wehling M, Christ M, Gaezer R 1993 Aldosterone-specific membrane receptors and related rapid, non-genomic effects. Trends Pharmacol Sci 14: 1–4

Parathyroid hormone, vitamin D, and bone mineral homeostasis

Adamson B B, Gallacher S J 1993 Mineralisation defects with pamidronate for Paget's disease. Lancet 342: 1459–1460
Alper J 1994 Boning up: newly isolated proteins heal bad breaks. Science 263: 323–324
Barnes D 1987 Close encounters with an osteoclast. Science 236: 914–916
Bilezikian J P 1992 Management of acute hypercalcemia. N Engl J Med 326: 1196–1203
Brown E M 1991 Extracellular Ca^{2+} sensing, regulation of parathyroid cell function, and role of Ca^{2+} and other ions as extracellular (first) messengers. Physiol Rev 71: 371–711
Brown E M, Gamba G et al. 1993 Cloning and characterization of an extracellular Ca^{2+}-sensing receptor from bovine parathyroid. Nature 366: 575–580
Carano A et al. 1990 Biphosphates directly inhibit the bone reabsorption activity of isolated avian osteoclasts in vitro. J Clin Invest 85: 456–461
Chestnut C H 1992 Osteoporosis and its treatment. N Engl J Med 326: 406–408
Conklin B R, Bourne H R 1994 Homeostatic signals: marriage of the flytrap and the serpent. Nature 367: 22
Editorial 1989 Low-dose vitamin D analogues for renal osteodystrophy. Lancet (i): 1364–1365
Editorial 1992 New bone? Lancet 339: 463–464
Fleisch H 1987 Biphosphonates—history and experimental basis. Bone 8: S23–S28
Glorieux F H 1991 Rickets, the continuing challenge. N Engl J Med 325: 1875–1877
Heaney R P 1993 Thinking straight about calcium. N Engl J Med 328: 503–505
Kraut J A, Coburn J W 1994 Bone, acid, and osteoporosis. N Engl J Med 330: 1821–1822
Mitlak B H, Nussbaum S R 1993 Diagnosis and treatment of osteoporosis. Ann Rev Med 44: 265–277
Mundy G R 1994 Osteoporosis: boning up on genes. Nature 367: 216–217
Norman A W, Litwack G 1987 The calcium-regulating hormones: vitamin D, parathyroid hormone, calcitonin. In: Hormones. Academic Press, San Diego, p 355–395
Overgaard K, Hansen M et al. 1992 Effect of salcatonin given intranasally on bone mass and fracture rates in established osteoporosis: a dose–response study. Br Med J 305: 556–561
Reichel H, Koeftler H P, Norman A W 1989 The role of the vitamin D endocrine system in health and disease. N Engl J Med 320: 980–991
Riggs B L, Melton L J 1992 The prevention and treatment of osteoporosis. N Engl J Med 327: 620–627
Sambrook P, Birmingham J et al. 1993 Prevention of corticosteroid osteoporosis: a comparison of calcium, calcitriol, and calcitonin. N Engl J Med 328: 1747–1752
Subramaniam M, Colvard D et al. 1992 Glucocorticoid regulation of alkaline phosphatase, osteocalcin, and proto-oncogenes in normal human osteoblast-like cells. J Cellular Biochem 50: 411–424

General reading

Evans R M 1988 The steroid and thyroid hormone superfamily. Science 240: 889–895
Moore D D 1989 Promiscuous behaviour in the steroid hormone superfamily. Trends Neurosci 12: 165–168

22
THE REPRODUCTIVE SYSTEM

ENDOCRINE ASPECTS

Hormonal control of the reproductive system in both the male and female involves *sex steroids* from the gonads, the *hypothalamic peptides* and the *glycoprotein gonadotrophins* from the anterior pituitary.

HORMONAL CONTROL OF THE FEMALE REPRODUCTIVE SYSTEM

At puberty an increased output of the hormones of the hypothalamus and anterior pituitary stimulates secretion of oestrogenic sex steroids. These are responsible for the maturation of the reproductive organs and the development of the secondary sexual characteristics, and also for a phase of accelerated growth followed by closure of the epiphyses of the long bones. Sex steroids are thereafter involved in the regulation of the cyclic changes expressed in the menstrual cycle and are important in pregnancy. A simplified outline of the interrelationship of these substances in the physiological control of the menstrual cycle is given in Figures 22.1 and 22.2.

The menstrual cycle is taken as beginning with the start of menstruation. This lasts for 3–6 days, during which the superficial layer of the endometrium of the uterus is shed. When the menstrual flow stops, the endometrium regenerates.

A releasing factor, the gonadotrophin-releasing hormone (**GnRH**), is secreted in a pulsatile fashion from peptidergic neurons in the hypothalamus; it stimulates the anterior pituitary to release gonado-

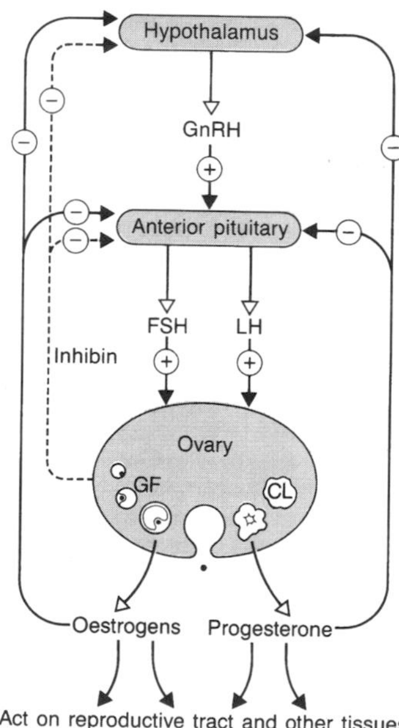

Fig. 22.1 Hormonal interrelationship in the control of the female reproductive system. (GF = Graafian follicle; CL = corpus luteum; LH = luteinising hormone; FSH = follicle-stimulating hormone; GnRH = gonadotrophin-releasing hormone)

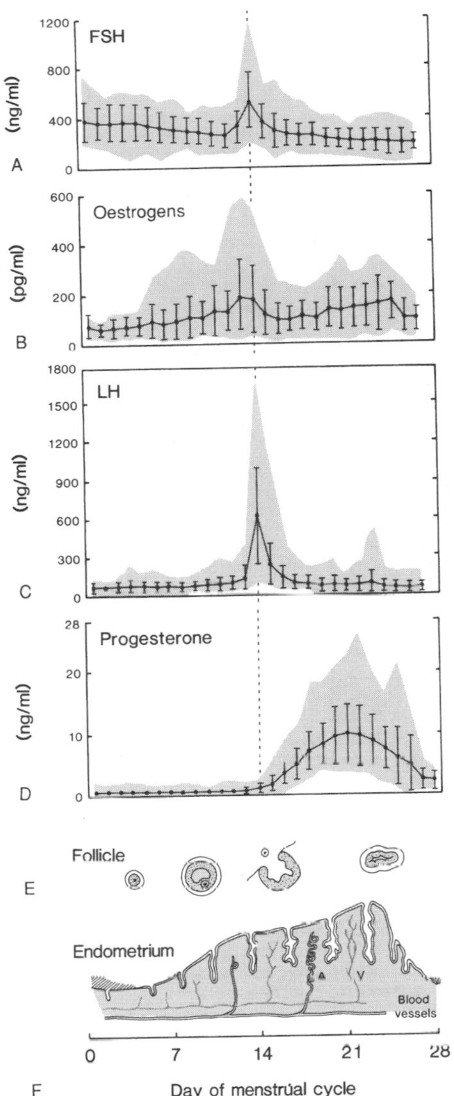

Fig. 22.2 Plasma concentrations of ovarian hormones and gonadotrophins in women during normal menstrual cycles. Values are the mean ± standard deviation of 40 women. The shaded areas indicate the entire range of observations. Day 1 is the onset of menstruation. **E** and **F** show diagrammatically the changes in the ovarian follicle and the endometrium during the cycle. Ovulation on day 14 of the menstrual cycle occurs with the midcycle peak of LH, represented by the dashed line. (After: Van de Wiele R L, Dyrenfurth I 1974 Pharmacol Rev 25: 189–217)

trophic hormones (Fig. 22.1)—the follicle-stimulating hormone (**FSH**) and the luteinising hormone (**LH**). In the first phase of the cycle, FSH is the main gonadotrophin released (Fig. 22.2A). It acts on the ovaries, promoting the development of small groups of follicles, each of which contains an ovum. One of these develops faster than the others and forms the *Graafian follicle* (Figs 22.1 and 22.2E), and the rest degenerate.

The ripening Graafian follicle has a fluid-filled centre surrounded by granulosa cells within which lies the ovum, and surrounding these is a layer of thecal cells. **Oestrogens** are produced by the granulosa cells stimulated by FSH, from androgen precursor molecules derived from thecal cells stimulated by LH. The oestrogens (Fig. 22.2B), are responsible for the *early, proliferative* phase of endometrial regeneration which occurs from day 5 or 6 until midcycle (see Fig. 22.2F). During this phase the endometrium increases in thickness and vascularity, and at the peak of oestrogen secretion there is a prolific cervical secretion of mucus of pH 8–9, rich in protein and carbohydrate, which is thought to make the passage of the spermatozoa easier. The secreted oestrogens have a negative feedback effect on both the anterior pituitary and the hypothalamus, decreasing FSH and GnRH release (Fig. 22.1). The high oestrogen secretion just before midcycle sensitises LH-releasing cells of the pituitary to the action of the GnRH and thus is instrumental in determining the midcycle surge of LH secretion (Fig. 22.2C), which causes rapid swelling and rupture of the main follicle, resulting in ovulation (Fig. 22.2E). Oestrogen may also influence the LH surge by a direct effect on the hypothalamic release of GnRH. If fertilisation occurs, the fertilised ovum passes down the fallopian tubes to the uterus, starting to divide as it goes.

An important action of the oestrogens is to promote the formation of progesterone receptors in target tissues. They also have mild anabolic effects and tend to increase retention of salt and water.

There is some evidence that, in addition to its effect on oestrogen secretion, FSH stimulates the Graafian follicle to secrete **inhibin**, a 31-kDa glycoprotein, which also has a negative feedback effect on FSH but not LH production.

Under the influence of LH, the cells of the ruptured follicle proliferate and the follicle develops into the *corpus luteum* which secretes **progesterone** (Fig. 22.2C, D and E). During the second part of the menstrual cycle, this hormone acts on the oestrogen-primed endometrium, stimulating the *secretory* phase of its regeneration which renders the endometrium suitable for the implantation of a fertilised ovum (Fig. 22.2F). At this stage the cervical mucus becomes more viscid, less alkaline, less copious and in general less welcoming for the sperm. Progesterone has a negative feedback effect on the hypothalamus and pituitary, decreasing the release of LH. It also has a *thermogenic* effect, causing a rise in body temperature of about 0.5°C which commences at ovulation and is maintained until the end of the cycle. If implantation of the ovum has not occurred, progesterone secretion stops, and its sudden cessation is the main cause of the onset of menstruation.

If implantation does occur and pregnancy results, the *corpus luteum* continues to secrete progesterone, which, by its effect on hypothalamus and anterior pituitary, prevents further ovulation. During pregnancy, the corpus luteum also secretes *relaxin*—a peptide hormone that inhibits spontaneous uterine contractions, softens the cervix and lengthens the interpubic ligament in preparation for parturition; relaxin also has modulatory actions on the cardiovascular system.

As pregnancy proceeds, the placenta develops hormonal functions and secretes **gonadotrophins**, **progesterone** and **oestrogens**. Progesterone secreted during pregnancy controls the development of the secretory alveoli in the mammary gland, while oestrogen stimulates the lactiferous ducts. After parturition, oestrogens, along with **prolactin** (see Ch. 21, p. 422), are responsible for stimulating and maintaining lactation, though high doses of exogenous oestrogen will inhibit it.

Hormonal control of the female reproductive system

- The menstrual cycle starts with menstruation.
- Hypothalamic GnRH acts on the anterior pituitary to release FSH and LH, which act on the ovary.
- FSH stimulates follicle development and is the main hormone controlling oestrogen secretion. LH stimulates ovulation at midcycle and is the main hormone controlling subsequent progesterone secretion from the corpus luteum.
- Oestrogen controls the proliferative phase of the endometrium, progesterone the later secretory phase; both have negative feedback effects on the hypothalamus and anterior pituitary.
- If a fertilised ovum is implanted, the corpus luteum continues to secrete progesterone during the pregnancy.

Oestrogens are dealt with below, progestogens (progesterone-like drugs) on page 460, androgens on page 463, and the gonadotrophins on page 466.

THE BEHAVIOURAL EFFECTS OF SEX HORMONES

As well as exerting a cyclical control over the menstrual cycle, sex steroids affect sexual behaviour. Two types of control are recognised, namely *organisational* and *activational*. The former refers to the fact that sexual differentiation of the brain can be permanently altered by the presence or absence of sex steroids at a key stage in development. In rats, administration of androgens to females within a few days of birth modifies their development, resulting in virilisation of behaviour. Conversely, neonatal castration of male rats causes them to develop behaviourally as females. It is believed that brain development in the absence of sex steroids follows female lines, but that it can be switched to the male pattern by exposure of the hypothalamic cells to androgen at a key stage of development. In rats, this sensitive phase extends for a few days either side of birth, but in guinea pigs it occurs during foetal development.

In primates, similar but less complete behavioural virilisation of female offspring has been demonstrated following androgen administration or hypersecretion in pregnant mothers. This probably happens in humans also, if pregnant women secrete, or are treated with, androgens.

The *activational* effect of sex steroids refers to their ability to modify sexual behaviour after brain development is complete. In general, oestrogens and androgens increase sexual activity in the appropriate sex.

OESTROGENS

Oestrogens are synthesised mainly by the ovary but also in fairly large amounts by the placenta, and in small amounts by the testis in males and by the adrenal cortex in both sexes. Some other tissues, such as liver, muscle, fat and hair follicles, can also convert steroid precursors into oestrogens.

The starting substance for oestrogen synthesis is cholesterol (see Fig. 21.14). The immediate precursors to the oestrogens are androgenic substances—androstenedione or testosterone (Fig. 22.3).

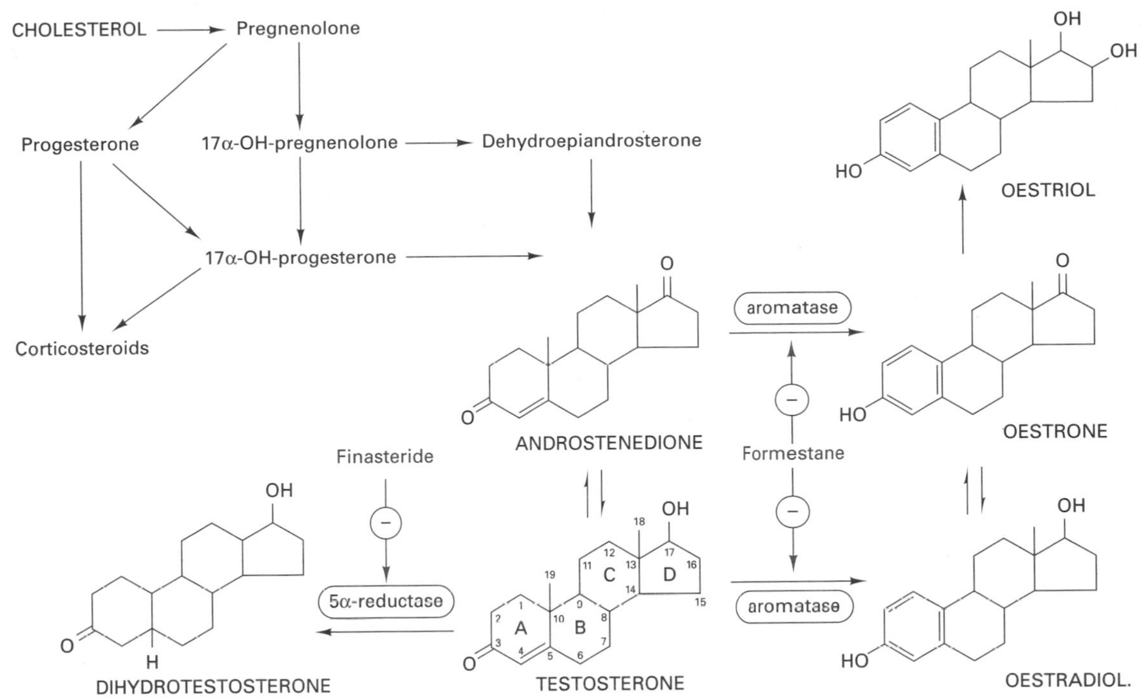

Fig. 22.3 The biosynthetic pathway for the androgens and oestrogens with sites of drug action. (See also Fig. 21.14.) Finasteride is used in benign prostatic hyperplasia and formestane to treat breast cancer in postmenopausal women.

There are three main endogenous oestrogens in humans—**oestradiol**, **oestrone** and **oestriol** (Fig. 22.3). Oestradiol is the most potent and is the principal oestrogen secreted by the ovary. At the beginning of the menstrual cycle, the plasma concentration is 0.2 nmol/l rising to ~ 2.2 nmol/l in midcycle (see Fig. 22.2). In the liver, oestradiol is converted to oestrone which may be converted to oestriol (Fig. 22.3). Oestradiol and oestrone are the two main endogenous oestrogens and are readily interconvertible. Oestrone may be sulphated in the liver and the oestrone sulphate so formed can be converted back to oestrone by sulphatases. Because oestrone is in equilibrium with oestradiol, it has been suggested that it constitutes a storage form of the hormones.

Oestriol is sometimes referred to as an 'impeded' oestrogen. It is regarded as a partial agonist, i.e. an oestrogen of low efficacy. More probably it is short-acting since, if its concentration in the plasma is maintained (as under physiological conditions), it is as potent as oestradiol.

Actions

The effects of oestrogens given as drugs depend on the age at which they are administered. Given at age 11–13 (with progestogens) for primary hypogonadism, oestrogens stimulate the development of the secondary sexual characteristics and the phase of accelerated growth. In the adult with primary amenorrhoea, oestrogens, given cyclically with a progestogen, will induce an artificial cycle. Their main use in adult women, however, is for oral contraception and in postmenopausal hormone replacement therapy (HRT), and their pharmacological actions when thus used are described on pages 467 and 461 respectively.

Oestrogens have several metabolic actions which may become manifest when they are used as drugs. They cause some degree of retention of salt and water (as occurs with endogenous oestrogens in the latter half of the menstrual cycle) and they have mild anabolic actions. The concentration of serum triglycerides and of high density lipoproteins is raised, whereas that of low density lipoproteins is decreased (these effects may contribute to the relatively low risk of atheromatous disease in premenopausal women; see Ch. 15). An impairment in glucose tolerance can occur in some individuals.

Oestrogens increase the coagulability of the blood.

Table 22.1 Oestrogens

Drug	Comment
Oestradiol	A natural oestrogen. Usually given i.m. Long-acting preparations are available. Oestradiol valerate is active by mouth. Patch preparations for transdermal use have proved effective.
Oestriol	A natural oestrogen. Can be given orally.
Oestrone	Given orally as piperazine oestrone sulphate. Oestrone sulphate is the main ingredient of an oral preparation of equine oestrogens.
Ethinyloestradiol	Semi-synthetic. Given orally. Effective and cheap. The drug of choice. Used in many oral contraceptive preparations.
Mestranol	Synthetic. Converted to ethinyloestradiol in the body.
Dienoestrol	Used topically in the vagina.
Chlorotrianisene	A synthetic non-steroidal agent. Given orally. Taken up in fat depots from which it is slowly released. Converted into a more active compound in the body.

There is some increase in the plasma concentration of various clotting factors (X, II), an increase in platelet aggregation, a decrease in the antithrombin III concentration, an increase in plasminogen and changes in the fibrinolytic system. The increase in coagulability is the basis for the increased risk of thromboembolism which occurred with contraceptive pills containing a high oestrogen content. The low doses of oestrogens now used in contraceptive pills and in HRT produce little change in clotting mechanisms.

Mechanism of action

As with other steroids, the action of oestrogen involves binding to intracellular receptors, the interaction of the resultant complexes with nuclear sites and subsequent genomic effects—either gene transcription (i.e. DNA-directed RNA and protein synthesis) or gene repression (inhibition of transcription). More details are given in Chapters 2 and 21; see especially Figure 21.15.

Oestrogen receptors occur mainly in the cells of its principal target tissues: the reproductive system (uterus, vagina, mammary glands) and the anterior pituitary and hypothalamus. These tissues contain about 15 000 to 21 000 high-affinity oestrogen-binding sites per cell but smaller numbers of sites also occur in the liver, kidney, adrenal and ovary. One of the principal effects of the oestrogens on DNA is the induction of synthesis of progesterone receptors in target tissues such as uterus, vagina, anterior pituitary and hypothalamus.

Progesterone decreases oestrogen receptor expression in the reproductive tract even in the presence of continuously high plasma oestrogen concentrations, by interfering with the de novo synthesis of the receptors. **Prolactin** increases the numbers of oestrogen receptors in the mammary gland and liver but has no effect on those in the uterus.

Preparations

Many preparations of oestrogens are available.* Some of the more commonly used ones are listed in Table 22.1 and some chemical structures are given in Figs 22.3 and 22.4.

The clinical use of oestrogens is given on page 459.

Pharmacokinetic aspects

Both the natural and synthetic oestrogens used in therapy are well absorbed in the gastrointestinal tract, but after absorption, the natural oestrogens are rapidly metabolised in the liver, whereas the synthetic oestrogens and non-steroidal oestrogen-like compounds are less rapidly degraded. There is a variable amount of enterohepatic cycling. Most oestrogens are readily absorbed from skin and mucous membranes and can be given by transdermal patches. They may be given topically in the vagina as creams or pessaries for local effect. In the plasma, natural oestrogens are bound to albumin

*Note that very different doses of oestrogens are used for different conditions, for example ethinyloestradiol is used in a dose of 10–20 μg/day for postmenopausal hormone replacement therapy, 20–50 μg/day in the combined contraceptive pill, 1–3 mg/day for breast cancer.

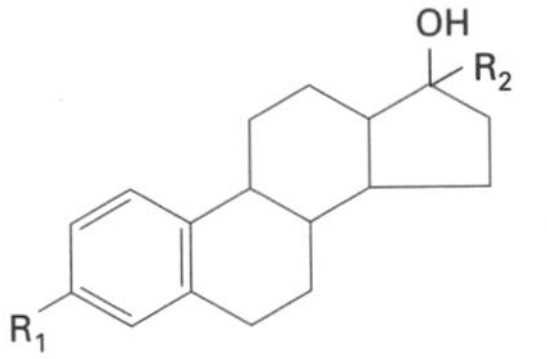

Synthetic oestrogens**	R_1	R_2
Ethinyloestradiol	OH	C≡CH
Mestranol	CH_3O	C≡CH

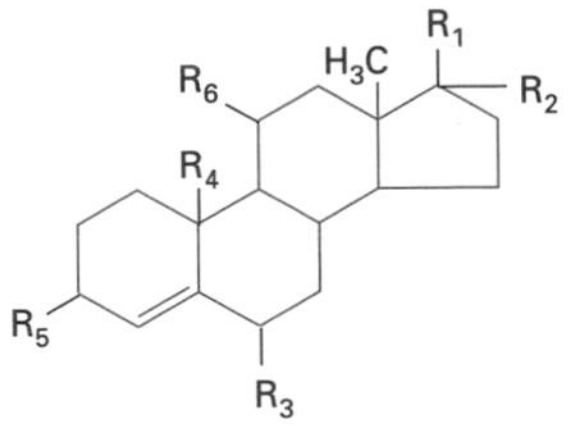

Synthetic progestogens†

	R_1	R_2	R_3	R_4	R_5	R_6
Norethisterone	OH	C≡CH	H_2	H	=0	H_2
Levonorgestrel	OH	C≡CH	H_2	H	=0	H_2
Desogestrel	OH	C≡CH	H_2	H	H_2	CH_2
Norgestimate	$OCOCH_3$	C≡CH	H_2	H	=NOH	H_2
Medroxyprogesterone acetate	$COCH_3$	O·acetate	CH_3	‡	=O	H_2

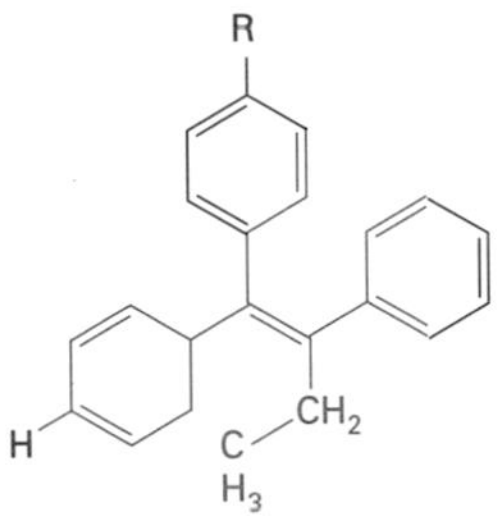

Anti-oestrogen	R
Tamoxifen*	**-O-$CH_2CH_2N(C_2H_5)_2$**

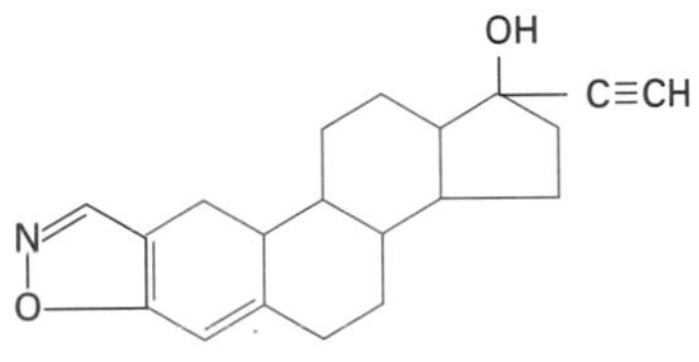

Danazol
(weak progestogen; inhibitor of gonadotrophin secretion)

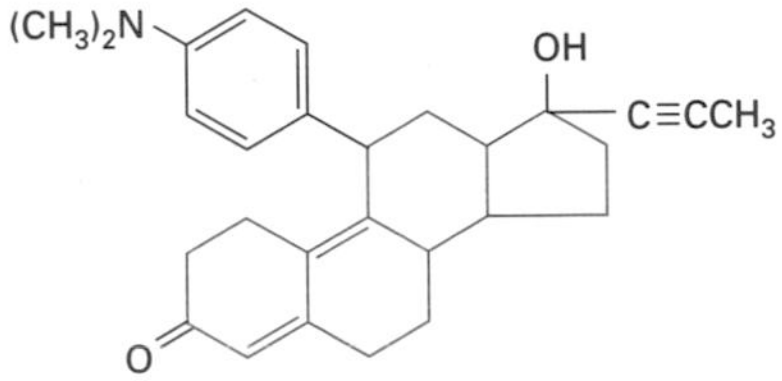

Mifepristone
(anti-progestogen)

Fig. 22.4 Synthetic compounds with oestrogenic, anti-oestrogenic, progestogenic and anti-progestogenic actions. (‡ = CH_3(C5 = C6))
† Compare with progesterone in Figure 21.14.
* See Wiseman (1994), Figure 3.
** Compare with oestrogen in Figure 22.3.

Clinical use of oestrogens

- Replacement therapy, as in hypo-ovarian conditions.
- Treatment of menopausal symptoms or for postmenopausal replacement therapy.
- Contraception.
- Vaginitis (topical oestrogen preparations are used).
- Therapy of prostatic cancer and for some cases of breast cancer (these uses have largely been superseded by other hormonal manipulations; see Ch. 36).

Very different doses are used for these different indications; see footnote on page 458.

and to a sex-steroid-binding globulin. Natural oestrogens are excreted in the urine as glucuronides and sulphates.

Unwanted effects

In general, the unwanted effects of oestrogens are tenderness in the breasts, nausea, vomiting, anorexia, retention of salt and water with resultant oedema, and increased risk of thromboembolism and of alteration of carbohydrate metabolism (see below). More details of the unwanted effects which can occur with oral contraceptives are given on page 467.

Used for postmenopausal replacement therapy, oestrogens frequently cause menstruation-like bleeding, and can produce endometrial hyperplasia unless given cyclically with a progestogen. When administered to males, oestrogens result in feminisation.

Oestrogens should not be given to pregnant women, especially during the first few months of pregnancy when development of the reproductive organs of the foetus is occurring. There is evidence that carcinoma of the vagina and the cervix is more common in young women whose mothers were given the synthetic oestrogen preparation, stilboestrol, in early pregnancy (see Ch. 43). Whether this particular effect occurs with other oestrogen preparations is not known, but an increased incidence of genital abnormalities in both male and female progeny has been reported.

ANTI-OESTROGENS

Anti-oestrogens (Fig. 22.4) are inactive or weakly active themselves, but compete with natural oestrogens for binding sites in target organs.

Tamoxifen is an anti-oestrogen which is used mainly in the treatment of oestrogen-dependent breast cancer. It produces the same side effects as the oestrogens themselves, but they are less marked. This drug binds to the oestrogen receptor in the nucleus, but there is little or no stimulation of transcription, possibly because the complex binds to a different nuclear acceptor site. Moreover, the complex does not readily dissociate, so there is interference with the recycling of receptors. Tamoxifen is discussed in more detail in Chapter 36.

Oestrogens and anti-oestrogens

- The endogenous oestrogens are oestradiol (the most potent), oestrone and oestriol; there are numerous exogenous oestrogens, e.g. ethinyloestradiol, mestranol.
- Mechanism of action: interaction with intranuclear receptors in target tissues, binding of the steroid–receptor complex to DNA resulting in modification of gene transcription.
- The pharmacological effects depend on the age of the recipient:
  - —At age 11–13 they stimulate development of the secondary sexual characteristics in hypo-ovarian conditions.
  - —Given cyclically in the adult female they induce an artificial menstrual cycle.
- Anti-oestrogens compete with oestrogens for the nuclear receptor. Tamoxifen is used in oestrogen-dependent breast cancer. Clomiphene induces ovulation by inhibiting the negative feedback effects on the hypothalamus and anterior pituitary.

Clomiphene (see Fig. 22.6) and **cyclofenil** inhibit oestrogen binding in the hypothalamus and anterior pituitary, so preventing the normal modulation by negative feedback and causing increased secretion of GnRH and gonadotrophins. This results in a marked stimulation and enlargement of the ovaries and increased oestrogen secretion. The main effect of their anti-oestrogen action is that they *induce ovulation*. These compounds are used in treating infertility due to lack of ovulation. Multiple pregnancies can occur.

PROGESTOGENS

The natural progestational hormone or progestogen is *progesterone* (see Figs 21.14 and 22.3) which is secreted mainly by the *corpus luteum* in the second part of the menstrual cycle. Small amounts are also secreted by the testis in the male and the adrenal cortex in both sexes, and large amounts are secreted by the placenta.

Mechanism of action

Progestogens act by the same mechanism as other steroids (see Ch. 21, p. 439 and Fig. 21.15). The presence of adequate numbers of progesterone receptors depends on the prior action of oestrogens (see p. 455).

Preparations

There are two main groups of progestogens:

- *The naturally-occurring hormone and its derivatives* (see Fig. 21.14). **Progesterone** itself is virtually inactive orally because after absorption it is metabolised in the liver. Preparations are available for intramuscular injection and for topical use in the vagina and rectum. Hydroxyprogesterone is an intermediate in the pathway of synthesis of hydrocortisone and testosterone (see Fig. 21.14), and has progesterone-like activity. It is given by intramuscular injection as **hydroxyprogesterone hexanoate**—the esterification at C_{17} inhibiting its further enzymic conversion. **Medroxyprogesterone** can be given orally or by injection. **Dydrogesterone**, which is given orally, has only the peripheral actions of progesterone and does not have an inhibitory action on gonadotrophin release.

- *Testosterone derivatives*. **Ethisterone, norethisterone** (see Fig. 22.4), **norgestrel, ethynodiol**, and **allyloestrenol** are all derivatives of testosterone with progesterone-like activity, and all can be given orally. The first two have some androgenic activity and are metabolised to give oestrogenic products. Newer progestogens used in contraception are given on page 467.

Actions

The pharmacological actions of the progestogens are in essence the same as the physiological actions described above. Specific effects relevant to contraception are detailed on page 467.

Pharmacokinetic aspects

Injected progesterone is bound to albumin, not to the sex-steroid-binding globulin. Some is stored in adipose tissue. It is metabolised in the liver, and the products, **pregnanolone** and **pregnanediol**, are conjugated with glucuronic acid and excreted in the urine.

The main *clinical use* of progestogens is in contraception (see below). They have an ill-defined place in the therapy of various gynaecological conditions such as menstrual disorders, endometriosis and dysmenorrhoea. They are also used in the treatment of endometrial carcinoma, and, in conjunction with oestrogen, for hormone replacement therapy.

Unwanted effects include weak androgenic actions of some of the progestogens derived from testosterone. Other unwanted effects are considered under 'Drugs used for contraception'.

ANTI-PROGESTOGENS

Mifepristone (Fig. 22.4) is a partial agonist at progesterone receptors; thus it has some inherent progestogen agonist properties but inhibits progesterone action. It sensitises the uterus to the action of prostaglandins. It is given orally and has a plasma half-life of 21 hours.

Mifepristone is used as a medical alternative to surgical termination of pregnancy. Given within 49 days of the last menstrual period, mifepristone, in a single oral dose, followed 48 hours later by the prostaglandin analogue, **gemeprost**, given as an intravaginal pessary (see p. 473), results in complete abortion in 95% of cases. There is evidence that mifepristone combined with oral **misoprostol*** is also effective.

If given in the late follicular phase of the menstrual cycle, mifepristone inhibits ovulation and hence has potential as a postcoital contraceptive agent. It is also being assessed as a treatment for breast cancer.

Mifepristone also has a significant antagonist action at the glucocorticoid receptor, though in higher concentration.

Progestogens and anti-progestogens

- The endogenous hormone is progesterone. Examples of exogenous hormones are the progesterone derivative, medroxyprogesterone, and the testosterone derivatives, norethisterone and norgestrel.
- Mechanism of action: as for oestrogens. Prior oestrogen action is required for the synthesis of progesterone receptors.
- Main pharmacological use: in oral contraception regimes.
- The anti-progestogen, mifepristone, in combination with prostaglandin analogues, is an effective medical alternative to surgical termination of early pregnancy.

POSTMENOPAUSAL HORMONE REPLACEMENT THERAPY (HRT)

Oestrogens, the main hormones used for HRT in postmenopausal women, have clear-cut beneficial effects:

- Reduction in the menopausal symptoms associated with the decline in oestrogen production, namely the hot flushes, inappropriate sweating, paraesthesias, palpitations, atrophic vaginitis, mood changes, etc.
- Reduction in the incidence of coronary heart disease (the commonest cause of death in postmenopausal women). Unopposed oestrogen (i.e. with no accompanying progestogen) reverses the postmenopausal 'atherogenic' lipid profile and is epidemiologically associated with a 45% reduc-

*For use in protection against NSAID-induced gastric damage, see page 393.

tion in the risk of ischaemic heart disease; this reduction of risk may be partially reversed by the addition of progestogens to the HRT regime, which is necessary for women with an intact uterus.

- Reduction of osteoporotic change and the concomitant risk of fracture. Postmenopausal osteoporosis may be partly due to the loss of the physiological effect of oestrogen which normally antagonises parathormone and hence decreases bone resorption (see Ch. 21). Oestrogens given in HRT increase calcium absorption and decrease its excretion, decrease bone resorption and prevent bone loss. Progestogens, given with oestrogens, may have a slight synergistic effect in preventing osteoporosis. Withdrawal of oestrogens is followed by rapid bone loss.

The use of oestrogen in HRT has some drawbacks, as follows:

- An increase in the risk of endometrial cancer. This risk can be reduced if progestogens are given for 10 days each month.
- A possible slight increase in the risk of breast cancer. Meta-analyses of five studies indicate that 10 years of treatment with unopposed oestrogen increases the risk by 1.1–1.3 fold.
- Uterine bleeding; this occurs if cyclical progestogens are included in the HRT regime.
- Minor gastrointestinal symptoms and mood changes (the latter mainly due to the progestogen component).

For an overall review of HRT see Jacobs & Loeffler (1992), Belchetz (1994).

Oestrogens used in HRT can be given orally (conjugated equine oestrogens, oestradiol, oestriol), vaginally (oestriol), by transepidermal patch (oestradiol) or by subcutaneous implant (oestradiol). A steroid marketed specifically for the treatment of postmenopausal vasomotor and vaginal symptoms is **tibolone**, which has weak oestrogenic, progestogenic and androgenic properties; it need not be given with a progestogen so bleeding is not a problem.

As regards the question of duration of use, it has been suggested (Belchetz 1994) that:

- In women with a uterus, HRT with combined oestrogen and progestogen could, with benefit, be continued indefinitely for postmenopausal symptoms or to prevent osteoporosis.
- In women without a uterus, HRT with unopposed oestrogen could, with benefit, be continued indefinitely for the above reasons and also to prevent cardiovascular disease.

There is still some controversy about the use of HRT in that some authorities state that HRT should be given only to women who have a high risk of coronary heart disease or who have had a hysterectomy (Grady et al. 1992), but most consider that the benefits far outweigh the risks (Whitcroft & Stevenson 1992); it has even been said that HRT 'is probably the most important advance in preventative medicine in the Western world in the last half century' (Studd 1992).

HORMONAL CONTROL OF THE MALE REPRODUCTIVE SYSTEM

As in the female, endocrine secretions from the hypothalamus, anterior pituitary and gonads control the male reproductive system. A simplified outline of the interrelationship of these factors is given in Figure 22.5. The gonadotrophin-releasing hormone (**GnRH**) controls the secretion of gonadotrophins by the anterior pituitary. This secretion is not cyclical as in the female but constant, though in both sexes it is pulsatile (see below). **FSH** is responsible for the integrity of the seminiferous tubules and, after puberty, is important in gametogenesis through an action on the Sertoli cells which nourish and support the developing spermatozoa. **LH**, which in the male is also called *interstitial cell stimulating hormone* (**ICSH**), stimulates the interstitial cells (Leydig cells) to secrete androgens—in particular **testosterone**. The secretion of LH begins at puberty, and the testosterone secreted is responsible for the maturation of the reproductive organs and the development of the secondary sexual characteristics. Thereafter, the primary function of testosterone is the maintenance of spermatogenesis and hence fertility—an action mediated by the Sertoli cells. This steroid is also important in the maturation of the spermatozoa as they pass through the epididymis and vas deferens. A further action is a feedback effect on the anterior pituitary, modulating its sensitivity to GnRH and thus influencing the concentration of ICSH in the circulation. In addition it has marked anabolic effects in puberty causing

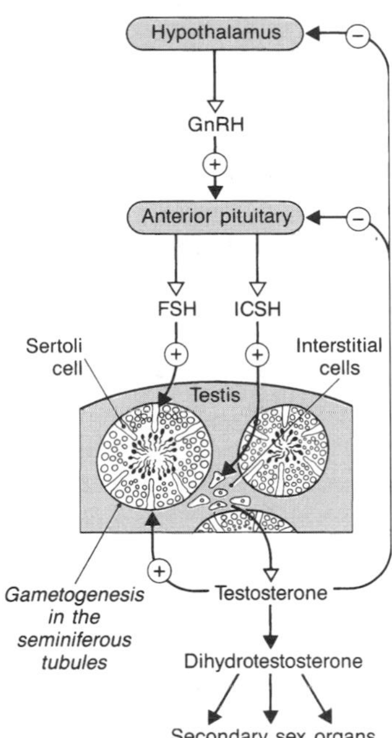

Fig. 22.5 Hormonal interrelationships in the control of the male reproductive system. (GnRH = gonadotrophin-releasing hormone; FSH = follicle-stimulating hormone; ICSH = interstitial-cell-stimulating hormone (equivalent to luteinising hormone in the female))

development of the musculature and increased bone growth resulting in a rapid increase in height. This is followed by closure of the epiphyses of the long bones.

Though the secretion of testosterone is controlled largely by ICSH, FSH may also play a part, possibly by inducing the release from the Sertoli cells (which are its primary target) of a factor similar to GnRH. The interstitial cells which synthesise testosterone also have receptors for **prolactin**, and this substance may influence testosterone production by increasing the number of receptors for ICSH.

ANDROGENS

Testosterone is the main natural androgen, and it is synthesised not only by the interstitial cells of the testis in males, but in small amounts by the ovary in females and the adrenal cortex in both sexes. Adrenal production of androgens is under the control of corticotrophin. Cholesterol is the starting substance (see Figs 21.14 and 22.3), and precursor substances are dehydroepiandrosterone and androstenedione, which may be released from the gonads and the adrenal cortex in both sexes and subsequently converted to testosterone in the liver (see Fig. 22.3).

Actions

In general the effects of exogenous androgens are the same as those of the endogenous hormones and will depend on the age of the patient to whom they are given.

If administered to males at the age of puberty, there is rapid development of the secondary sexual characteristics, maturation of the reproductive organs and a marked increase in muscular strength. Height increases more gradually. The anabolic effects can be accompanied by retention of salt and water. The skin becomes thickened and sometimes darkens, and the sebaceous glands become more active (which can result in acne). There is growth of hair on the pubic and axillary regions and on the face. The vocal cords hypertrophy resulting in a lower pitch to the voice. Androgens cause a feeling of well-being and an increase in physical vigour and may increase libido. Whether they are responsible for sexual behaviour as such is controversial, as is their contribution to aggressive behaviour.

If given to prepubertal males, the individuals concerned do not reach their full height because of premature closure of the epiphyses of the long bones.

Administration to women results in masculinisation changes similar to those seen in the pubertal male. The initial effects are on the skin (acne and growth of facial hair) and the voice. These are reversible. If treatment is continued, there is development of the musculature and of the male pattern of baldness, hypertrophy of the clitoris and further deepening of the pitch of the voice. With long-continued administration many of the effects are irreversible.

Mechanism of action

Testosterone is converted to dihydrotestosterone in most target cells by a 5α-reductase, though it is testosterone itself which is involved in virilisation of the genital tract in the male embryo and in the regulation of ICSH production. Both testosterone and dihydrotestosterone modify gene transcription

Androgens and the hormonal control of the male reproductive system

- GnRH from the hypothalamus acts on the anterior pituitary to release both FSH, which stimulates gametogenesis, and LH (also called interstitial-cell-stimulating hormone) which stimulates androgen secretion.
- The endogenous hormone is testosterone; an exogenous preparation is mesterolone.
- Mechanism of action: as for oestrogens.
- Main uses of androgens: for replacement therapy, as anabolic agents and to treat mammary cancer in women.

by the same mechanisms as other steroids (see p. 439).

Preparations

Testosterone itself can be given by subcutaneous implantation. **Testosterone enanthate** and **testosterone proprionate** are given by intramuscular depot injection. **Testosterone undecanoate** and **mesterolone** can be given orally.

The clinical use of androgens is given in the box above.

Pharmacokinetic aspects

Testosterone is rapidly metabolised in the liver if given orally, though this does not happen if it is absorbed from the buccal mucosa or from rectal suppositories. Virtually all testosterone in the circulation is bound to plasma protein—mainly to the sex-steroid-binding globulin. The half-life of free testosterone is 10–21 minutes. It is inactivated in the liver by conversion to androstenedione (see Fig. 22.3) which has weak androgenic activity, and 90% of its metabolites are excreted in the urine. Synthetic androgens are less rapidly metabolised and some are excreted in the urine unchanged.

Clinical use of androgens

- For replacement therapy in testicular failure. This condition is associated with hypogonadism or hypopituitarism. In the latter condition, growth hormone therapy is used until puberty, when androgens may be added to the treatment regime.
- As anabolic agents (see below).
- For treatment of mammary carcinoma in women. When receptors for oestrogens or progestogens are present in the cancer cells, the modification of the hormonal environment by the use of androgens can result in regression of the tumour.
- For treatment of osteoporosis, sometimes together with an oestrogen.

Unwanted effects

Unwanted effects of treatment with testosterone include eventual decrease of gonadotrophin release with resultant infertility, and salt and water retention leading to oedema. Adenocarcinoma of the liver has been reported. In children, the androgens cause disturbances in growth and in females, acne and masculinisation (see p. 463).

ANABOLIC STEROIDS

It is possible to modify the structure of androgens so as to enhance the anabolic effects and decrease other effects. Many have been produced; examples are **nandrolone**, **ethyloestrenol**, **oxymetholone** and **stanozolol**. They are believed to increase protein synthesis and enhance muscle development, resulting in weight gain. These agents are used to decrease the itching of chronic biliary obstruction and in the therapy of some aplastic anaemias. They may have a place in the treatment of debilitating and wasting conditions and in terminal disease, in which they can improve appetite and promote a welcome feeling of well-being. They are used in some cases of hormone-dependent metastatic mammary cancer.

Unwanted effects can occur, in particular cholestatic jaundice.

Anabolic steroids are used, surreptitiously, by some athletes in the expectation that they will increase strength and athletic performance. Carefully controlled studies have shown that the drugs do not necessarily have this effect in healthy individuals, whereas they do carry a definite risk of the serious side effects (see Hallagan et al. 1989). As anabolic steroid abusers may take up to 26 times the therapeutic dose, the unwanted effects are not only those specified above under 'androgens', but numerous others including testicular atrophy, sterility and gynaecomastia in men, and inhibition of ovulation, hirsutism, deepening of the voice, alopecia and acne in women. In both sexes there is increased risk of coronary heart disease, and there have been instances of sudden death in young athletes in which there was a strong suspicion that anabolic steroid use had been contributory.

ANTI-ANDROGENS

Drugs can have anti-androgen action by inhibiting the enzymes which give rise to the active steroids or by competing with endogenous androgens for their receptors.

Finasteride inhibits the enzyme 5α-reductase that converts testosterone to dihydrotestosterone (Fig. 22.3) which has greater affinity for androgen receptors. Finasteride does not itself bind to androgen receptors or have any hormonal actions, nor does it inhibit the formation of any other steroids. It is well absorbed after oral administration, has a half-life of about 7 hours and is excreted in the urine and faeces.

It is used to treat benign prostatic hyperplasia and, in women, may have a role in treating male-pattern baldness, hirsutism and possibly acne.

Both oestrogens and progestogens have anti-androgen activity, oestrogens mainly by inhibiting gonadotrophin secretion and progestogens by competing with androgens in target organs. **Cyproterone** is a derivative of progesterone and has weak progestational activity. It is a partial agonist at androgen receptors, competing with dihydrotestosterone for receptors in androgen-sensitive target tissues. Through its effect in the hypothalamus it depresses the synthesis of gonadotrophins. It is used mainly to treat prostatic cancer during initiation of GnRH treatment. It is also used in the therapy of precocious puberty in males, and of masculinisation and acne in women. It seems also to have an effect in the central nervous system, decreasing libido. It has been proposed for use in the treatment of severe hypersexuality in male sexual offenders.*

*As with the oestrogens, very different doses are used for these different conditions, for example 2 mg/day for acne, 100 mg/day for hypersexuality, 300 mg/day for prostatic cancer.

GONADOTROPHIN-RELEASING HORMONE: AGONISTS AND ANTAGONISTS

Gonadotrophin-releasing hormone (GnRH) controls the secretion by the anterior pituitary of both FSH and LH.

The secretion of GnRH is controlled by neural input from other parts of the brain and, in the female particularly, through negative feedback by the sex steroids (Figs 22.1 and 22.6). Exogenous **androgens**, **oestrogens** and **progestogens** all inhibit the secretion of the peptide, but only the progestogens, when given on their own, seem to have this effect without having marked hormonal actions on peripheral tissues. This is presumably because in the absence of oestrogen there is less induction of progesterone receptors in the reproductive tract.

Synthetic GnRH is termed **gonadorelin** and its amino-acid sequence is Pyroglu–His–Trp–Ser–Tyr–Gly–Leu–Arg–Pro–Gly–NH_2.

Numerous analogues of GnRH, both agonists and antagonists, have been synthesised. Analogues with agonist activity are **leuprolin**, **goserelin** **buserelin** and **nafarelin**, the last being 200 times more potent than endogenous GnRH.

An agent which inhibits the release of both GnRH and the gonadotrophins is **danazol** (see below).

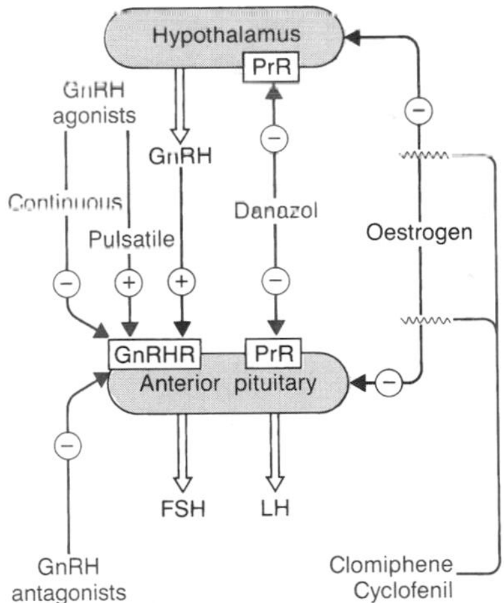

Fig. 22.6 The regulation of gonadotrophin release from the anterior pituitary by endogenous gonadotrophin-releasing hormone (GnRH) and drugs. (GnRHR = GnRH receptor; PrR = progestogen receptor; FSH = follicle-stimulating hormone; LH = luteinising hormone)

Clomiphene and **cyclofenil** stimulate gonadotrophin release by inhibiting the negative feedback effects of endogenous oestrogen (see above and Fig. 22.6).

Administration of the antagonists results in a decrease not in total FSH per se but in biologically active FSH, because greater amounts of the deglycosylated FSH isoforms with antagonist action are released (see below).

Pharmacokinetics and clinical use

GnRH antagonists were synthesised because it was thought they might constitute a new non-steroidal method of contraception. This approach has so far been less rewarding than expected, but is still being explored.

GnRH agonists, given subcutaneously in pulsatile fashion by a miniaturised pump, can stimulate gonadotrophin release (Fig. 22.6) and have been used successfully to induce ovulation. Continuous use has, paradoxically, the opposite effect—desensitising the pituitary and *inhibiting gonadotrophin generation* (Fig. 22.6). For this inhibitory action on gonadotrophin production, GnRH analogues are given by subcutaneous injection, by nasal spray or as depot preparations. GnRH analogues given in this fashion are used in various conditions in which gonadal suppression is desirable, such as endometriosis (an excessive production of endometrial tissue), precocious puberty, sex-hormone-dependent cancers (particularly advanced prostatic cancer), and hirsutism due to the polycystic ovary syndrome. Continuous, non-pulsatile administration will also lead to inhibition of spermatogenesis and ovulation. This latter effect has been used to permit timed follicular recruitment by exogenous FSH for the harvesting of oocytes for in vitro fertilisation, and intranasal administration is being considered for use in contraception (see below, p. 469).

The *unwanted effects* of the GnRH agonists are hypo-oestrogenism, which is associated with hot flushes, decreased libido and headache. With prolonged use, osteoporosis may be a problem. GnRH and its analogues are reviewed by Conn & Crowley (1991).

DANAZOL

Danazol inhibits the output of gonadotrophins (Fig. 22.6), affecting particularly the midcycle surge in the female and inhibiting steroid synthesis in the ovary. It is also active in males, reducing androgen synthesis and spermatogenesis. It has weak androgenic activity.

It is used in various conditions in which decreased sex hormone production would be beneficial, more particularly endometriosis, but also gynaecomastia in men, menorrhagia (excessive menstruation) and other menstrual disorders. Unwanted effects are common and include gastrointestinal disturbances, weight gain, fluid retention, dizziness, muscle cramps and headache. It has a virilising action in females.

Gestrinone has similar actions to danazol and is also used in endometriosis.

GONADOTROPHINS AND ANALOGUES

Follicle-stimulating hormone (FSH) and luteinising hormone (LH) are produced in moderate amounts by the anterior pituitary (see Ch. 21 and Table 21.1) in both males and females, and in large amounts by the placenta during pregnancy in the female. These hormones are glycoproteins with two different subunits, designated α and β; biological specificity depends on the β-subunit.

Preparations

Substances with gonadotrophin activity are extracted from biological material. **Chorionic gonadotrophin** is prepared from the urine of pregnant women; it has mainly LH activity. Preparations extracted from the urine of postmenopausal women

Gonadotrophin-releasing hormone (GnRH) and gonadotrophins

- GnRH is a decapeptide; gonadorelin is the synthetic form. Nafarelin is a potent analogue.
- Given in pulsatile fashion they stimulate gonadotrophin release, given continuously they inhibit it.
- The gonadotrophins, FSH and LH, are glycoproteins.
- Preparations of gonadotrophins (e.g. menotrophin extracted from postmenopausal urine), are used to treat infertility due to lack of ovulation.
- Danazol is a modified progestogen which inhibits gonadotrophin production by an action on the hypothalamus and anterior pituitary.

include **human menopausal gonadotrophins** and **menotrophin**, which contain both FSH and LH, and **urofollitrophin** which contains only FSH. A preparation of recombinant FSH is also now available.

The gonadotrophin preparations have to be given by injection. They are used primarily to treat infertility due to lack of ovulation.

DRUGS USED FOR CONTRACEPTION

ORAL CONTRACEPTIVES

There are two main types of oral* contraceptives:

- combinations of an oestrogen with a progestogen (the combined pill)
- progestogen alone (the progestogen-only pill).

(For review, see Baird & Glasier 1993.)

The combined pill

The oestrogen in most combined preparations is **ethinyloestradiol**, though a few preparations contain **mestranol** instead. The progestogen may be **norethisterone**, **levonorgestrel**, **ethynodiol**, or the newer compounds **desogestrel**, **gestodene** and **norgestimate** which are more potent, have less androgenic action and cause less change in lipoprotein metabolism. The oestrogen content of the pill should be no more than 30–35 μg of ethinyloestradiol or its equivalent,** and the progestogen content should also be low. This combined pill is taken for 21 consecutive days followed by 7 pill-free days. The mode of action is thought to be as follows:

- The oestrogen inhibits the release of FSH and thus suppresses the development of the ovarian follicle.
- The progestogen inhibits the release of LH and thus prevents ovulation, and it also makes the cervical mucus less suitable for the passage of sperm.
- Together they alter the endometrium in such a way as to discourage implantation.

They may also interfere with the coordinated contractions of cervix, uterus and fallopian tubes which are thought to be necessary for successful fertilisation and implantation. When administration ceases after 21 days, it is the withdrawal of the progestogen which precipitates menstruation.

The progestogen-only pill

The drugs used are **norethisterone**, **norgestrel**, **megestrol**, **levonorgestrel** or **ethynodiol**. The pill is taken daily without interruption. The mode of action is primarily on the cervical mucus which is made inhospitable to sperm. The progestogen probably also hinders implantation through its effect on the endometrium and on the motility and secretions of the fallopian tubes (described above).

Potential unwanted and beneficial effects of the combined pill

The experience of the last 25 years indicates that the combined pill constitutes a safe and effective method of contraception. There are distinct health benefits from taking the pill (see below) and serious adverse effects are rare. However, minor unwanted effects constitute possible drawbacks to its use and several important questions need to be considered.

Possible drawbacks

- There can be a gain in weight, due to fluid retention or an anabolic effect or both.
- General symptoms, such as nausea, flushing, dizziness, depression or irritability occur in some individuals.
- Skin changes, such as acne and/or an increase in pigmentation are occasionally reported.
- Amenorrhoea of variable duration on cessation of taking the pill is sometimes seen. Permanent loss of fertility is rare and normal cycles of menstruation usually commence fairly soon.

Questions that need to be considered

Is there an increased risk of cardiovascular disease? The combined pill, if containing high doses of oestrogen, increases blood coagulability (see p. 456 and footnote on p. 467). With low oestrogen dosage, the risk is small and is confined

*For oral contraceptives to be effective, they must of course be absorbed. Gastrointestinal disturbances with vomiting and diarrhoea may impair absorption. A bout of traveller's diarrhoea, for example, could have unexpected consequences.

**Pills containing more than 50 μg oestrogen were shown, in the 1970s, to be associated with increased coagulability of the blood and an increased risk of deep vein thrombosis and, in some cases, pulmonary embolism.

to specific subgroups in whom other factors contribute, such as smoking (which can increase the risk substantially) and long-continued use of the pill, especially in women over 35 years old. On the other hand, oestrogens are thought to reduce the risk of cardiovascular disease by protecting the arterial walls against atheromatous change. Furthermore, pills containing the newer progestogens increase the levels of high density lipoproteins, which also has a protective effect.

The consensus seems to be that low doses of oestrogen do not increase the risk of cardiovascular disease in women who have no pre-existing disease of the circulatory system. (But note that there are some dissenting voices, e.g. Lidegaard 1993.)

Is there an increase in the risk of breast cancer? Some meta-analyses show a 1.3- to 1.8-fold increase in risk; some show no increase at all. The question of whether there is an association between the combined pill and breast cancer appears to be unresolved.

Does the pill increase the risk of hypertension? Some degree of hypertension occurs in about 4–5% of women who take the combined pill, and pre-existing hypertension can be increased. The effect is usually reversible.

Does the pill increase the risk of cervical cancer? One study reported a small increase in the relative risk (1.3–1.8) in women who had taken the pill for more than 5 years. It appears that oral contraceptives could promote,* rather than initiate, cervical neoplasia (which correlates highly with sexual activity). When this and other factors are taken into account, it appears that there is no increase in risk.

Is there an impairment in glucose tolerance? Older progestogen preparations could impair glucose tolerance; the newer compounds are thought not to have this effect.

Does the pill increase the risk of liver cancer? Liver cancer is rare in most parts of the world, but there is evidence that the risk is increased in women who have taken the pill for 8 or more years.

Beneficial effects

The use of the combined pill markedly decreases the incidence of amenorrhoea, irregular periods and intermenstrual bleeding. The incidence of iron deficiency anaemia and of premenstrual tension is reduced, as is the incidence of benign breast disease, uterine fibroids and functional cysts of the ovaries. There is less risk of thyroid disease and of cancer of the ovaries. Two studies have shown a reduction in the occurrence of rheumatoid arthritis and two have not. Amongst the beneficial effects should be included the fact that unwanted pregnancy has been avoided, in the light of the further fact that pregnancy carries an overall maternal mortality ranging from 1 in 10 000 in developed countries to 1 in 150 in Africa.

In general, as stated by Baird & Glasier (1993), 'the evidence suggests that after risk factors (e.g. smoking, hypertension, and obesity) have been identified, combined oral contraceptives are safe for most women for most of their reproductive lives'.

Potential beneficial and unwanted effects of the progesterone-only pill

Inhibition of ovulation is variable and inconsistent. The contraceptive effect is less reliable than that of the combination pill, and missing a dose may result in conception. Disturbances of menstruation

Oral contraceptives

The combined pill
- The combined pill contains an oestrogen and a progestogen. It is taken for 21 consecutive days out of 28.
- Mode of action: the oestrogen inhibits FSH release and therefore follicle development; the progestogen inhibits LH release and therefore ovulation, and makes cervical mucus inhospitable for sperm; together they render the endometrium unsuitable for implantation.
- Drawbacks: weight gain, nausea, mood changes and skin pigmentation can occur.
- Serious unwanted effects are rare. A small proportion of women develop reversible hypertension; there is evidence both for and against an increased risk of breast cancer.
- There are several beneficial effects.

The progestogen-only pill
- The progestogen-only pill is taken continuously. It differs from the combined pill in that the contraceptive effect is less reliable and is mainly due to the alteration of cervical mucus. Irregular bleeding is likely to occur. It does not interfere with lactation.

*See Chapter 43 for explanation of 'promotion'.

are common; in particular there is liable to be irregular bleeding. Only a small proportion of women use this form of contraception and information on the long-term risks is not available.

An advantage is that the progesterone-only pill can be taken after parturition as, unlike oestrogen-containing pills, it does not interfere with lactation.

OTHER DRUG REGIMES USED FOR CONTRACEPTION

Postcoital oral contraceptives

An effective postcoital method of contraception could be very useful under some circumstances. To be effective it would have to be instituted within about 72 hours of unprotected intercourse.

A single dose of **mifepristone** is reported to be efficacious.

Oestrogen alone in a high dose (25 mg) daily for 5 days, or in a low dose (100 μg) combined with a **progestogen** twice a day for 12 days is reported to be successful. Nausea and vomiting are likely to occur (and the pills may then be lost).

Contraception with depot progestogen

Medroxyprogesterone can be given intramuscularly as a contraceptive. This is effective and safe. However, menstrual irregularities are common, and infertility may persist for many months after cessation of treatment.

Progestogen implants

Routes of administration which bypass the liver, thus avoiding first-pass metabolism, have been developed. **Levonorgestrel** implanted subcutaneously in six non-biodegradable capsules is being used by ~3 million women world-wide. The tubes slowly release their progestogen content over 5 years. Common unwanted effects are irregular bleeding and headache.

Hormone-impregnated vaginal rings

Vaginal rings impregnated with **levonorgestrel** or **ethynyloestradiol** plus **desorgestrel** are available. The former is left in place for 3 months at a time; it has the same disadvantages and advantages as the progestogen-only pill. The latter is worn for 21 days out of 28. The long-term effects are not known.

A **progestogen-impregnated intrauterine device** is proving to be a useful contraceptive in older women with menstrual problems.

Contraceptives for males

Oral contraceptives for males are still in the experimental stage.

Possible future development

New approaches to the use of drugs for contraception include:

- intrasnasal administration of a gonadotrophin-releasing hormone agonist (see p. 466); this would down-regulate the receptors for FSH and LH
- progesterone antagonists (e.g. **mifepristone**); preliminary trials suggest that, given in the follicular phase of the cycle, mifepristone may be an effective once-a-month contraceptive.

THE UTERUS

The physiological and pharmacological responses of the uterus vary in different species, and at different stages of pregnancy.

The motility of the uterus

Uterine muscle contracts rhythmically both in vitro and in vivo. These contractions originate in the muscle itself and are not abolished by interference with the nerve supply. There is no intrinsic nerve plexus which controls the muscle, such as occurs in the gastrointestinal tract.

Both the force and the frequency of contractions of uterine muscle vary greatly during the menstrual cycle, the variation being due to the effect of the complex hormonal changes which occur during the cycle.

The non-pregnant human uterus shows weak spontaneous contractions during the first part of the cycle. At about the 14th day, larger and more prolonged contractions can be recorded, and during menstruation, strong coordinated contractions can occur.

In early pregnancy, uterine movements are depressed, but towards the end of the 9-month period, contractions start to occur; these increase in force and become fully coordinated during parturition. Myometrial cells in the fundus act as pacemakers and give rise to conducted action potentials, the electrophysiological activity of these pacemaker cells being regulated by the sex hormones.

Administration of **oestrogen** hyperpolarises myometrial cells, suppressing spontaneous activity, and subsequent administration of **progesterone** increases this effect. During pregnancy, a condition of electrical and mechanical quiescence and relative inexcitability is produced by endogenous progesterone acting locally at the site of implantation of the foetus.

Innervation of the uterus and the action of sympathomimetic amines

The nerve supply to the uterus includes both excitatory and inhibitory sympathetic fibres. The uterus also receives some parasympathetic fibres from the sacral outflow, but these nerves have no role in the control of uterine motility.

Sympathetic stimulation causes mixed stimulatory and inhibitory actions on the uterus, the predominant effect varying with the species and with the hormonal condition of the uterus.

Noradrenaline stimulates the uterus in both pregnant and non-pregnant women, by action on α-adrenoceptors. **Adrenaline** inhibits the uterus in both pregnant and non-pregnant women by an action on β-adrenoceptors. Selective β_2-adrenoceptor agonists, such as **salbutamol**, **terbutaline**, and **ritodrine**, inhibit both the spontaneous and oxytocin-induced contractions of the pregnant uterus and have a limited place in obstetric practice. These uterine relaxants—termed tocolytic agents—are used in selected patients to prevent premature labour and also to prevent foetal asphyxia when myometrial stimulants have resulted in hypertonus and excessive uterine contractions. See Chapter 7 for details of mechanism of action and unwanted effects.

Ritodrine was in fact developed specifically for obstetric use but there is conflicting evidence as to the efficacy and safety of this and other β_2-adrenoceptor agonists when used to prevent preterm labour. The results of some (but not all) studies have indicated that these agents not only do not reduce perinatal infant morbidity or mortality but can produce potentially fatal maternal pulmonary oedema by causing sodium and water retention and therefore volume overload (see Leveno & Cunningham 1992).

Adrenoceptor antagonists are without effect on the motility of the human uterus.

Calcium antagonists may have a role in obstetrics. Preliminary studies have found **nifedipine** (see Ch. 13) to be an effective uterine relaxant (tocolytic agent). Very recently it has been reported that glyceryl trinitrate, applied as a patch to the skin, is highly effective in delaying pre-term labour.

Posterior pituitary hormones and uterine function

As explained in Chapter 21, the neurohypophyseal hormones are important in the regulation of myometrial activity. **Oxytocin** release can be stimulated by certain peripheral stimuli such as suckling. Cervical dilatation can also cause its release. The non-pregnant human uterus and the uterus in early pregnancy have greater sensitivity to **vasopressin** than to oxytocin.

DRUGS CAUSING CONTRACTION OF THE UTERUS

Agents which stimulate the pregnant uterus and are of importance in obstetrics are:

- oxytocics: oxytocin and ergometrine
- E and F type prostaglandins.

Oxytocin

Oxytocin for clinical use is prepared synthetically. Its chemical structure is given in Figure 21.4. The S–S bond of cystine is crucial for its activity, the biological action being completely lost if it is reduced.

Actions

On the uterus. Oxytocin contracts the uterus. There is an oestrogen-mediated increase in oxytocin receptors in the myometrium during pregnancy, which reaches maximum during labour, and the uterus develops a high degree of sensitivity to oxytocin at parturition. Oxytocin, given by slow intravenous infusion at term, causes regular coordinated contractions which travel from fundus to cervix, and both the amplitude and the frequency of the contractions are related to dose, the uterus relaxing completely between contractions. (There may be a slight transient increase in tone when the infusion is started.)

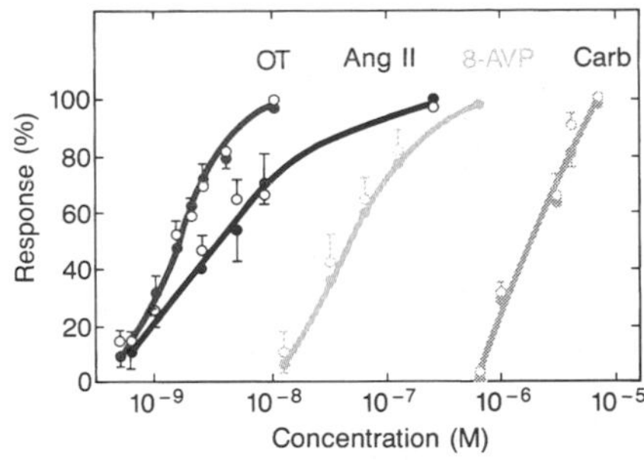

Fig. 22.7 Dose–response curves for uterine contraction. Uterine tissue was obtained from rats pre-treated (24 h) with stilboestrol. Two different strains of rats were used as indicated by the two types of symbol. (OT = oxytocin; Ang II = angiotensin II; 8-AVP = vasopressin; Carb = carbachol) (Adapted from: Hollenberg M D et al. 1983 Trends Pharmacol Sci 4: 310)

Figure 22.7 illustrates the effect of oxytocin and other spasmogens on the rat uterus.

Large doses cause an increase in the frequency of the contractions such that there is incomplete relaxation between them. Very high doses cause sustained contractions which interfere with blood flow through the placenta and lead to foetal distress or death.

On the mammary gland. Oxytocin causes contraction of the myo-epithelial cells of the mammary gland, which leads to 'milk let-down'—the expression of milk from the alveoli and ducts. Oxytocin given by intranasal spray facilitates milk let-down and results in significantly enhanced milk collection when a breast pump is used (Fig. 22.8).

Other actions. Oxytocin has a vasodilator action, when given by intravenous injection, and a weak vasopressin-like antidiuretic action which can result in water intoxication if large doses are infused. This may constitute an unwanted effect if oxytocin is used in patients with cardiac or renal disease, or pre-eclampsia.*

The clinical use of oxytocin is given in the box on page 473.

Pharmacokinetic aspects

Oxytocin can be given by intravenous injection or intramuscularly, but is most often given by intravenous infusion. It is inactivated in the liver and kidneys and by circulating placental oxytocinase.

Unwanted effects with large doses include transient but serious hypotension with associated tachycardia. If oxytocin is given by rapid intravenous injection, ECG abnormalities can occur, as can water intoxication in both mother and foetus (see above).

An analogue of oxytocin that competitively inhibits the effect of oxytocin and could suppress preterm labour is being investigated.

Ergometrine

Ergot (*Claviceps purpurea*) is a fungus which grows on rye and on certain grasses and contains an extraordinary variety of pharmacologically active substances (see Ch. 8). Ergot poisoning, which occurred frequently in Europe in the past, was often associated with abortion and it was clear that ergot contained an active principle which had powerful effects on the uterus. In 1935, **ergometrine** was isolated and was recognised as the oxytocic principle in ergot.

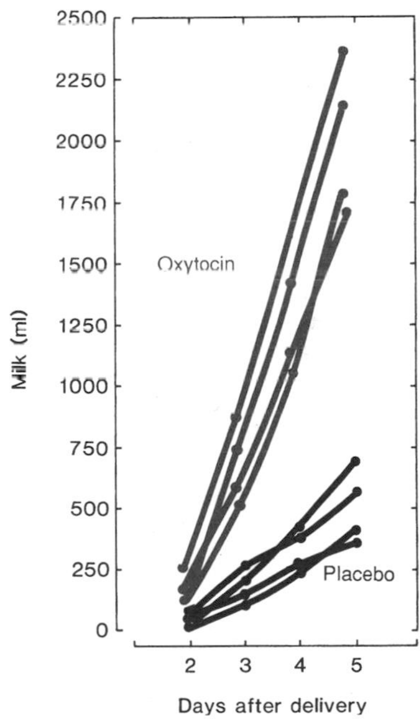

Fig. 22.8 Cumulative amount of milk obtained during second to fifth days after delivery by using breast pump on four occasions each day in primiparous women. The subjects were given either oxytocin or a placebo by nasal spray. (Data from: Ruis H et al. 1981 Br Med J 283: 341)

*Eclampsia is a pathological condition (involving, among other things, high blood pressure) which can occur in pregnant women.

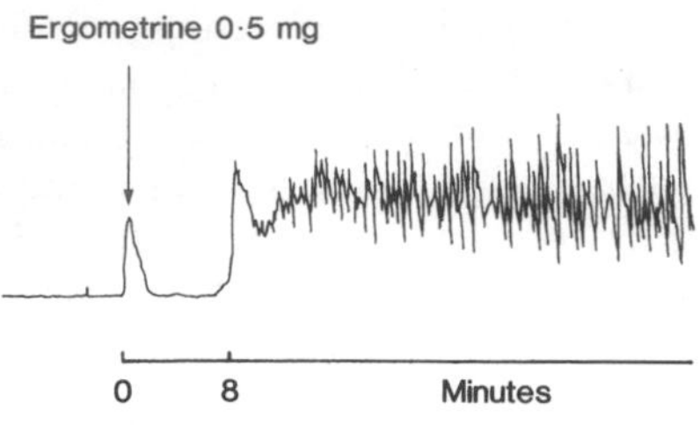

Fig. 22.9 Contractions of the human uterus at the end of the first week of puerperium recorded by intrauterine balloon. Ergometrine, 0.5 mg by mouth, gave a series of rapid uterine contractions after 8 minutes. (After: Moir C 1935; see Br Med J 1964 2: 102)

Actions

Ergometrine has a rapid stimulant effect on the postpartum human uterus in vivo. Its action depends partly on the state of the organ, thus on a normally contracting uterus, ergometrine has little effect, but if the uterus is quiescent, it initiates a prolonged series of strong contractions (Fig. 22.9).

Ergometrine has a moderate degree of vasoconstrictor action.

The mechanism of action of ergometrine on smooth muscle is not understood. It is possible that it acts on α-adrenoceptors, like the related alkaloid ergotamine, which is a partial agonist on these receptors (see Ch. 7), though it may produce effects through stimulation of 5-HT receptors.

The clinical use of ergometrine is given in the box on page 473.

Pharmacokinetic aspects and unwanted effects

Ergometrine can be given orally, intramuscularly or intravenously. It has a very rapid onset of action and its effect lasts for 3–6 hours.

Ergometrine can produce vomiting, probably by an effect on dopamine D_2-receptors in the chemoreceptor trigger zone (see Fig. 19.8). Vasoconstriction with an increase in blood pressure associated with nausea, blurred vision and headache can occur, as can vasospasm of the coronary arteries resulting in anginal pain.

> **Drugs acting on the uterus**
>
> - Oxytocin causes regular coordinated uterine contractions, each followed by relaxation.
> - Ergometrine, an ergot alkaloid, causes uterine contractions with an increase in basal tone.
> - Prostaglandin analogues, e.g. dinoprostone (PGE_2) and dinoprost ($PGF_{2\alpha}$), cause increased tone and contractions of the body of the pregnant uterus but relaxation of the cervix.
> - β_2-adrenoceptor analogues (e.g. ritodrine) inhibit both spontaneous and oxytocin-induced contractions of the pregnant uterus.

Prostaglandins

Endogenous prostaglandins

The endometrium and the myometrium of the uterus have significant prostaglandin-synthesising capacity, particularly in the second, proliferative phase of the menstrual cycle. The vasoconstrictor prostaglandin, $\mathbf{PGF_{2\alpha}}$, is generated in particularly large amounts and is thought to be implicated in the ischaemic necrosis of the endometrium which precedes menstruation. The vasodilator prostaglandins, $\mathbf{PGE_2}$ and **prostacyclin**, are also generated by the uterus. (Prostaglandins are discussed in detail in Ch. 11.)

In addition to their vasoactive properties, the E and F type prostaglandins cause contractions of both the non-pregnant and the pregnant uterus. The sensitivity of the uterine muscle to prostaglandins increases during gestation.

Prostaglandins play a significant role in two of the main disorders of menstruation, **dysmenorrhoea** (painful menstruation) and **menorrhagia** (excessive blood loss).

Menorrhagia, in the absence of uterine pathology, appears to be due to a combination of increased vasodilatation and reduced haemostasis, the increased vasodilatation being associated with an increased production of PGE_2 and PGI_2 as compared with $PGF_{2\alpha}$. Haemostasis depends on both platelet aggregation and fibrin formation, the former providing a surface for the latter (Fig. 16.1). There are fewer platelets in menstrual blood than in normal blood, and they have a reduced capacity to aggregate and to synthesise thromboxane A_2. Increased generation by the uterus of prostacyclin (which inhibits platelet aggregation) will clearly impair haemostasis as well as causing vasodilatation.

Dysmenorrhoea of the spasmodic type is now known to be associated with increased production of the spasmogenic prostaglandins, PGE_2 and $PGF_{2\alpha}$.

Non-steroidal anti-inflammatory drugs (see

Ch. 12) can be used with success to treat spasmodic dysmenorrhoea. Taken for a few days immediately before and during the marked blood loss, they can also be of value in menorrhagia, though 20% of patients with this condition do not respond at all.

Exogenous prostaglandins

On the pregnant uterus, prostaglandins of the E and F series promote a series of coordinated contractions of the body of the organ, along with relaxation of the cervix; they also, in contrast to oxytocin, tend to increase uterine tone. In early and middle pregnancy, oxytocin generally cannot cause expulsion of the uterine contents (since, at this time, the myometrial cells are not very sensitive to its action), whereas the prostaglandins can, and are therefore abortifacient.

The prostaglandins used in obstetrics are **dinoprostone** (PGE_2), **carboprost** (15-methyl $PGF_{2\alpha}$) and **gemeprost** (a PGE_1 analogue). **Misoprostol** (a PGE_1 analogue), introduced for use in the gastrointestinal tract (see Ch. 11), has been used with success in obstetric practice.

Dinoprostone can be given intravaginally as a gel or as tablets or by the extra-amniotic route as a solution. Carboprost is given by deep intramuscular injection. Gemeprost is given intravaginally by pessary.

Clinical uses of drugs acting on the uterus

Stimulants
- Oxytocin is used to induce or augment labour when the uterine muscle is not functioning adequately. It can also be used to treat postpartum haemorrhage and to promote lactation.
- Ergometrine can be used to treat postpartum haemorrhage.
- A preparation containing both oxytocin and ergometrine is used for the management of the third stage of labour; the two agents together can also be used, prior to surgery, to control bleeding due to incomplete abortion.
- Dinoprostone given by the extra-amniotic route is used for late (second trimester) therapeutic abortion; given as vaginal gel, it is used for cervical ripening and induction of labour.
- Gemeprost, given as vaginal pessary, following mifepristone, is used as a medical alternative to surgical termination of pregnancy (up to 63 days' gestation).
- Carboprost can be used to treat postpartum haemorrhage in patients who do not respond to oxytocin or ergometrine.

Myometrial relaxants (tocolytics)
- β-adrenoceptor agonists (e.g. ritodrine) are used to prevent preterm labour.
- Glyceryl trinitrate also has promise.

The clinical use of prostaglandin analogues is given on this page.

Unwanted effects include uterine pain, nausea and vomiting, which are reported to occur in about 50% of patients when the drugs are used as abortifacients. Dinoprost may cause cardiovascular collapse if it escapes into the circulation after intra-amniotic injection. Phlebitis at the site of intravenous infusion has occurred. Systemic side effects are also likely to occur when prostaglandins are given as abortifacients, by intravaginal pessary. When combined with the progestogen antagonist **mifepristone** (see p. 461), which sensitises the uterus to prostaglandins, lower doses of the prostaglandins can be used for termination of pregnancy, and the incidence and severity of side effects are correspondingly reduced.

REFERENCES AND FURTHER READING

Endocrine aspects

Baird D T, Glasier A F 1993 Hormonal contraception. N Engl Med J 328: 1543–1549
Belchetz 1994 Hormonal treatment of postmenopausal women. N Engl J Med 330: 1062–1071
Beller F K, Ebert C 1985 Effect of oral contraceptives on blood coagulation: a review. Obstet Gynecol Surv 40: 425–436
Chaudhury R R 1981 Pharmacology of estrogens. International encyclopaedia of pharmacology & therapeutics, section 106. Pergamon Press, Oxford
Chetkowski R, Meldrum D R et al. 1986 Biologic effects of transdermal estradiol. N Engl J Med 314: 1615–1621
Chez R A 1989 Clinical aspects of three new progestogens: desogestrel, gestodene and norgestimate. Am J Obstet Gynecol 160: 1296–1300
Conn P M, Crowley W F 1991 Gonadotrophin-releasing hormone and its analogues. N Engl J Med 324: 93–103
Drife J O 1989 The benefits of combined oral contraceptives. Br J Obstet Gynaecol 96: 1255–1260
Drife J O 1989 New developments in contraception. Prog Obstet Gynaecol 7: 249–261

Editorial 1987 LHRH analogues for contraception. Lancet 1: 1179–1181
Editorial 1992 New gonadotrophins for old? Lancet 340: 1442–1443
Editorial 1993 OCs o-t-c ('Oral contraceptives over-the-counter'). Lancet 342: 565–566
Filshie M, Guilleband J 1989 Contraception: science and practice. Butterworths, London
Fotherby K 1989 Oral contraceptives and lipids. Br Med J 298: 1049–1050
Fraser H M, Waxman J 1989 Gonadotrophin-releasing hormone analogues for gynaecological disorders and infertility: a real advance. Br Med J 298: 475–476
Glasier A, Thong K J et al. 1992 Mifepristone (RU 486) compared with high-dose estrogen and progestogen for emergency postcoital contraception. N Engl J Med 327: 1041–1044
Grady D, Rubin S M et al. 1992 Hormone therapy to prevent disease and prolong life in postmenopausal women. Ann Int Med 117: 1016–1037
Hallagan J B, Hallagan L F, Snyder M 1989 Anabolic androgenic steroid use by athletes. N Engl J Med 321: 1042–1046
Henrich J B 1992 The postmenopausal estrogen/breast cancer controversy. J Am Med Assoc 268: 1900–1902
Hodgen G D 1989 General application of GNRH agonists in gynecology: past, present and future. Obstet Gynecol Surv 44: 293–296
Jacobs H S, Loeffler F E 1992 Postmenopausal hormone replacement therapy. Br Med J 305: 1403–1408
Kedar R P, Bourne T H et al. 1994 Effects of tamoxifen on uterus and ovaries of postmenopausal women in a randomised breast cancer prevention trial. Lancet 343: 1318–1321
Landers J P, Spelsberg T C 1992 New concepts in steroid hormone expression: Transcription factors, proto-oncogenes, and the cascade model for steroid regulation of gene expression. Crit Rev Eukaryotic Gene Expression 2: 19–63
Larsson K, Beyer C 1981 In: Hrdina P D, Singhal R L (eds) Neuroendocrine regulation and altered behaviour. Croom Helm, London, p 95–118
Leveno K J, Cunninghan F G 1992 β-adrenergic agonists for preterm labor. N Engl J Med 327: 349–352; see also letters p 1758–1760
Lidegaard O 1993 Oral contraception and risk of a cerebral thromboembolic attack: results of a case control study. Br Med J 306: 956–963
Lukas S E 1993 Current perspectives in anabolic-androgenic steroid abuse. Trends Pharmacol Sci 14: 61–68
Martin K A, Freeman M W 1993 Postmenopausal hormone replacement therapy. N Engl J Med 328: 1115–1117
Mascarenhas L 1994 Long-acting methods of contraception. Br Med J 308: 991–992
Mooradian A D, Morley J E, Korenman S G 1987 Biological actions of androgens. Endocrinol Rev 8: 1–28
Nablusi A A, Folsom A R 1993 Association of hormone-replacement therapy with various cardiovascular risk factors in postmenopausal women. N Engl J Med 328: 1069–1076
Peyron R, Aubény E et al. 1993 Early termination of pregnancy with mifepristone (RU 486) and the orally active prostaglandin misoprostol. N Engl J Med 328: 1510–1513
Rittmaster R S 1994 Finasteride. N Engl J Med 330: 120–125
Ross R K, Paganini-Hill A, Mack T M, Henderson B E 1989 Cardiovascular benefits of estrogen replacement therapy. Am J Obstet Gynecol 160: 1301–1306
Spitz I M, Bardin C W 1993 Mifepristone (RU 486)—modulator of progestogen and glucocorticoid action. N Engl J Med 329: 404–410
Studd J 1992 Complications of hormone replacement therapy in post-menopausal women. J R Soc Med 85: 376–378
Whitcroft S I J, Estevenson J C 1992 Hormone replacement therapy: risks and benefits. Clin Endocrinol 36: 15–20
Wiseman H 1994 Tamoxifen: new membrane-mediated mechanisms of action and therapeutic advances. Trends Pharmacol Sci 15: 83–89

Uterus

Berde B, Schild H O (eds) 1978 Ergot alkaloids. Handbook of experimental pharmacology. Springer-Verlag, Berlin, vol 49
Carsten M E, Miller J D 1987 A new look at uterine muscle contraction. Am J Obstet Gynecol 157: 1303–1315
Dawood M Y 1989 Evolving concepts of oxytocin for induction of labor. Amer J Perinatol 6: 167–172
Elder M G 1983 Prostaglandins and menstrual disorders. Br Med J 287: 703–704
El-Refaey H, Calder L et al. 1994 Cervical priming with prostaglandin E_1 analogues, misoprostol and gemeprost. Lancet 343: 1207–1209
Huzar G, Roberts J M 1982 Biochemistry and pharmacology of the myometrium and labor: regulation at the cellular and molecular levels. Am J Obstet Gynecol 142: 225–236
Jenkins J S, Nussey S S 1991 The role of oxytocin: present concepts. Clin Endocrinol 34: 515–525
Spielman F J, Herbert W N P 1988 Maternal cardiovascular effects of drugs that alter uterine activity. Obstet Gynecol Surv 43: 516–522
Wray S 1993 Uterine contraction and physiological mechanisms of modulation. Am J Physiol 264 (Cell Physiol 33): C1–C18

23
THE HAEMOPOIETIC SYSTEM

The main components of the haemopoietic system are the bone marrow and the blood, with the spleen and the liver as important accessory organs. The spleen constitutes a blood store and also acts as a graveyard for time-expired red blood cells. The liver stores **vitamin B_{12}**, which is essential for erythrocyte generation, synthesises many of the principal constituents of the plasma, and is involved in the process of breakdown of the haemoglobin liberated when the red blood cells are destroyed. In addition, the kidney manufactures a factor, '**erythropoietin**', which stimulates red cell production, and various other cells synthesise and release haemopoietic growth factors—termed **colony-stimulating factors**—which regulate the production of leucocytes and platelets. The function of platelets is discussed in Chapter 16 and that of leucocytes in Chapter 11.

The term 'erythron' is used to describe the circulating red blood cells and their precursors. In a healthy adult the erythron is in a steady state, cell loss being precisely balanced by new production of cells.

The main function of the red cells is to carry oxygen, and their oxygen-carrying power depends on their haemoglobin content. About 3.3 mg of iron is contained in 1 g of haemoglobin, and the production of haemoglobin depends on the supply of iron. Anaemia results when the red cells are too few in number or do not contain the normal amount of haemoglobin, or are abnormal in other respects.

Types of anaemia

Severe haemorrhage will produce an acute anaemia, but a normal healthy person has a remarkable power to regenerate erythrocytes, and even after sudden substantial blood loss, the haemoglobin content of the blood can be restored to normal within a relatively short time. Chronic anaemia results from chronic minor blood loss, from dietary deficiency or from the disorder of an organ (e.g. stomach, liver) concerned in the manufacture of the factors essential for the formation of red blood cells.

The symptoms of anaemia are mainly a result of anoxia and are usually more severe if the anaemia develops rapidly.

The following is a convenient classification of anaemias according to the causes:

- *Deficiency of factors necessary for erythropoiesis*, such as:
  - iron (microcytic hypochromic anaemia)
  - folic acid and vitamin B_{12} (megaloblastic anaemia)
  - vitamin C, thyroxine.
- *Depression of the bone marrow.* This may affect the formation and development of the red cells, leucocytes or platelets. In complete aplastic anaemia, the formation of all these blood cells is deficient. Aplastic anaemia affecting only red cells or only platelets is rare. However, agranulocytosis—a condition in which leucocytes and other cells of the myeloid series are absent—occurs somewhat more frequently as a result of severe infection or the administration of certain drugs (Ch. 43), or exposure to radioactive substances.
- *Excessive destruction of red blood cells.* These are termed 'haemolytic' anaemias and are due either to the breakdown of red corpuscles which are defective, to autoimmune reactions (see Ch. 11, p. 225) or to the effects of poisons or infections.

The principal agents used in the treatment of

anaemia are **iron, vitamin B_{12}** and **folic acid**, and this chapter will deal mainly with these agents. Vitamin C will only be mentioned briefly.

The use of agents which stimulate the proliferation and maturation of the red and white blood cells will also be covered.

IRON

Iron is a transition metal with two important properties relevant to its biological role:

- the ability to exist in several oxidation states
- the tendency to form stable coordination complexes.

The body of a 70-kg man contains about 4 g of iron, 65% of which circulates in the blood as the oxygen-transporting molecule, haemoglobin. About one-half of the remainder is stored in the liver, spleen and bone marrow, chiefly as *ferritin* and *haemosiderin*. The iron in these molecules is available for fresh haemoglobin synthesis. The rest, which is not available for haemoglobin synthesis, is present in myoglobin, cytochromes and various other enzymes.

The distribution of iron in an average normal adult male is shown in Table 23.1. The values for an average female would be about 55% of these. Since most of the iron in the body is either part of—or destined to be part of—the haemoglobin in red cells, the most obvious clinical result of iron deficiency is anaemia, and the only *pharmacological* action of iron is to provide material for haemoglobin synthesis.

Table 23.1 The distribution of iron in the body of a normal 70-kg male

Protein	Tissue	Iron content (mg)
Haemoglobin	Erythrocytes	2600
Myoglobin	Muscle	400
Enzymes (cytochromes, catalase, etc.)	Liver and other tissues	25
Transferrin	Plasma and extracellular fluid	8
Ferritin and haemosiderin	Liver	410
	Spleen	48
	Bone marrow	300

Data from: Jacobs & Worwood: in Hardisty & Weatherall (1982)

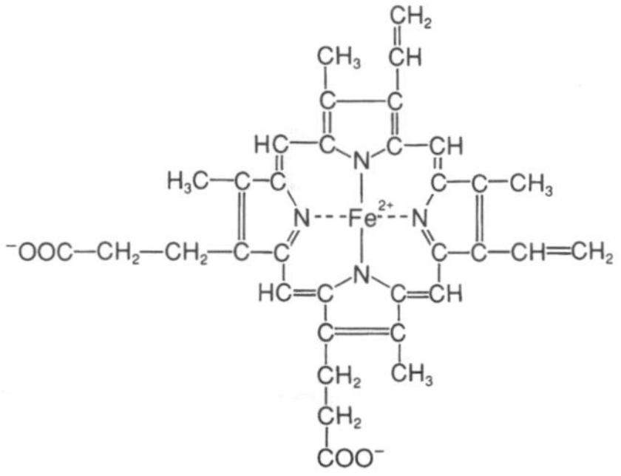

Fig. 23.1 The structure of haem.

Haemoglobin is made up of four protein chain subunits (globins), each of which contains one *haem* moiety. Haem consists of a tetrapyrrole porphyrin ring containing ferrous (Fe^{2+}) iron (Fig. 23.1). Each haem group can carry one O_2 molecule, which is bound reversibly to the Fe^{2+} and to a histidine residue in the particular globin chain to which the haem is linked. This reversible binding is the basis of O_2 transport.

Iron turnover and balance

Both the normal physiological turnover of iron and *pharmacokinetic factors* affecting iron when it is given therapeutically will be dealt with here.

The normal daily requirement for iron is approximately 5 mg for men, and 15 mg for growing children and for women during the reproductive period. A pregnant woman needs between two and ten times this amount because of the demands of the foetus and the increased requirements of the mother.* The average diet in Western Europe provides 15–20 mg of iron daily, mostly in meat. Iron in meat is generally present as haem and about 20–40% of haem iron is available for absorption; this is not altered by other factors in the diet. The human body appears to be specifically adapted to absorb iron in the form of haem. It is thought that one reason why modern man has problems in maintaining iron balance (there are an estimated 500 million people with iron deficiency in the world)

*Each pregnancy 'costs' the mother 680 mg of iron, equivalent to 1300 ml of blood, due to the demands of the foetus, plus an extra 450 mg to meet the requirements of the expanded blood volume.

is that the change from hunting to grain cultivation 10 000 years ago led to cereals, which have a relatively small amount of utilisable iron, constituting a significant proportion of the diet.

Non-haem iron in food is mainly in the ferric state and this needs to be converted to ferrous iron for absorption. Ferric iron, and to a lesser extent ferrous iron, has low solubility at the neutral pH of the intestine, but in the stomach, iron dissolves and binds to mucoprotein which functions as a carrier, transporting the iron to the intestine. In the presence of ascorbic acid, fructose and various amino acids, iron is detached from the carrier, forming soluble low molecular weight complexes which enable it to remain in soluble form in the intestine. Ascorbic acid stimulates iron absorption partly by forming soluble iron–ascorbate chelates and partly by reducing ferric iron to the more soluble ferrous form.

Phosphates and phytates inhibit iron absorption by forming insoluble iron complexes. **Tetracycline** forms an insoluble iron chelate resulting in impaired uptake of both substances; tannates (e.g. in tea) also interfere with iron absorption.

The amount of iron in the diet and the various factors affecting its availability are thus important determinants in absorption, but the *regulation* of iron absorption is a function of the intestinal mucosa, influenced by the body's iron stores. In fact, the absorptive mechanism holds a central role in iron balance since it is the sole mechanism by which body iron can be controlled.

The site of iron absorption is the duodenum and upper jejunum, and absorption is a two-stage process involving firstly a rapid uptake across the brush border and then transfer from the interior of the cell into the plasma (Fig. 23.2). The second stage, which is rate-limiting, is known to be energy dependent. Haem iron, as explained above, is absorbed as intact haem and the iron is released in the mucosal cell by the action of haem oxidase. Non-haem iron is absorbed in the ferrous state. Within the cell, ferrous iron is oxidised to ferric iron which is bound to an intracellular carrier, a transferrin-like protein; the iron is then either held in storage in the mucosal cell as *ferritin* (if body stores of iron are high) or passed on to the plasma (if iron stores are low).

Iron is carried in the plasma bound to *transferrin*—a β-globulin with two binding sites for ferric iron—which is normally only 30% saturated. Plasma contains 4 mg of iron at any one time, but the daily turnover is about 30 mg (Fig. 23.3). Most of the iron which enters the plasma is derived from the mononuclear phagocyte system, following the degradation of time-expired erythrocytes. Intestinal absorption and mobilisation of iron from storage depots contribute only small amounts. Most of the iron which leaves the plasma daily is used for haemoglobin synthesis by red cell precursors. These cells have receptors which bind transferrin molecules, releasing them after the iron has been taken up.

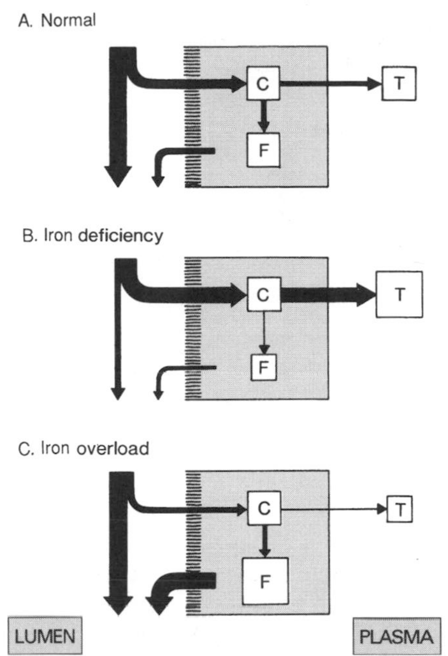

Fig. 23.2 Schematic illustration of one of the main theories of iron absorption (and thus the regulation of iron balance) by intestinal mucosal cells. Iron in the food is absorbed into the mucosal cells and bound to a transferrin-like carrier molecule (C), from where it is transferred to either transferrin (T) in the plasma or ferritin (F) within the cell. The amount transferred is influenced by the degree of iron-saturation of plasma transferrin. The iron in the ferritin is lost when the cell is sloughed off. The thickness of the arrows indicates the amount of iron transferred. (Modified from: Ganong W F 1987 Review of medical physiology, 13th edn. Appleton & Lange, San Mateo, California)

Iron is stored in two forms—soluble ferritin and insoluble haemosiderin. *Ferritin* is found in all cells, the mononuclear phagocytes of liver, spleen and bone marrow containing especially high concentrations. It is also present in plasma. The precursor of ferritin, apoferritin, is a large protein of molecular

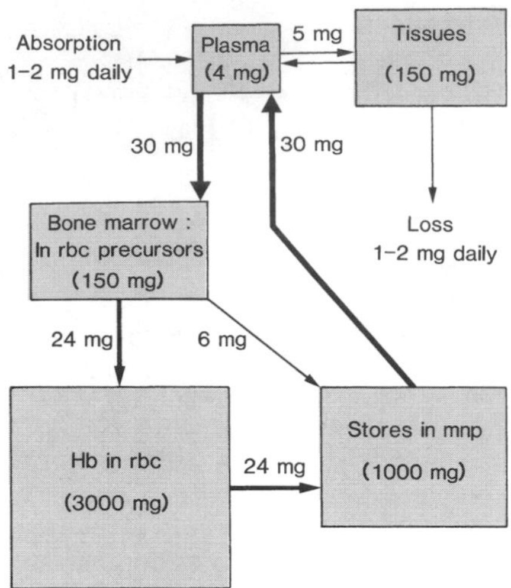

Fig. 23.3 Schematic illustration of the distribution of iron in the body, with an indication of the daily intake, movement between compartments, and loss.
(Hb = haemoglobin; rbc = red blood cells; mnp = mononuclear phagocytes) (Data from: Jacobs & Worwood, in Hardisty & Weatherall 1982)

weight 450 000, composed of 24 identical polypeptide subunits which enclose a cavity in which up to 4500 iron molecules can be stored. Apoferritin takes up ferrous iron, oxidises it and deposits the ferric iron in its core. In this form it constitutes ferritin, the primary storage form of iron, from which the iron is most readily available. The life span of this iron-laden protein is only a few days. *Haemosiderin* is a degraded form of ferritin in which the iron cores of several ferritin molecules have aggregated, following partial disintegration of the outer protein shells.

The ferritin in plasma has virtually no iron associated with it. It is in equilibrium with the storage ferritin in cells and its concentration in the plasma provides an estimate of total body iron stores.

The body has no means of actively excreting iron. Small amounts leave the body through the peeling off of mucosal cells containing ferritin, and even smaller amounts leave in the bile, the sweat and the urine. A total of about 1 mg is lost daily. The iron balance is therefore critically dependent on the active absorption mechanism in the intestinal mucosa. This absorption is influenced by the iron stores in the body, but the precise mechanism of this control is still a matter of debate. It is suggested that the amount of ferritin in the intestinal mucosa may be important in regulating absorption, as may the balance between ferritin and the transferrin-like carrier molecule in these cells. The daily movement of iron in the body is illustrated in Figure 23.3, and one of the main theories of the regulation of iron absorption and iron balance is illustrated schematically in Figure 23.2.

The clinical use of iron is given on page 479.

Administration

Iron is usually given orally but may be given parenterally in special circumstances.

Several different preparations of ferrous iron salts are available for oral administration. The main one is **ferrous sulphate**, which has an elemental iron content of 200 µg per mg. Others are ferrous succinate, ferrous gluconate, and ferrous fumarate, with elemental iron concentrations of 350 µg, 120 µg and 330 µg per mg respectively. These are all absorbed to a comparable extent.

Parenteral iron is rarely given but may be necessary in individuals who are not able to absorb oral iron due to malabsorption syndromes or as a result of surgical procedures or inflammatory conditions

Iron

- Iron is important for the synthesis of haemoglobin; it is also present in myoglobin, and in the cytochromes and other enzymes.
- Ferric iron (Fe^{3+}) must be converted to ferrous iron (Fe^{2+}) for absorption in the GIT.
- Absorption involves active transport into mucosal cells, whence it can be transported into the plasma and/or stored intracellularly as ferritin; in iron deficiency, the former route predominates.
- Iron loss occurs mainly by sloughing of ferritin-containing mucosal cells; iron is not excreted in the urine.
- Iron in plasma is bound to transferrin, and most is used for erythropoiesis. Some is stored as ferritin in other tissues. Iron from time-expired erythrocytes enters the plasma for re-use.
- Preparation: ferrous sulphate.
- Unwanted effects: GI tract disturbances. Severe toxic effects occur if large doses are ingested; these can be countered by desferrioxamine, an iron chelator.

> **Clinical use of iron**
>
> Iron deficiency anaemia, which can be due to:
> - chronic blood loss (e.g. with menorrhagia)
> - increased demand (e.g. in pregnancy and early infancy)
> - inadequate dietary intake or absorption (uncommon in developed countries).

involving the gastrointestinal tract. The preparations used are **iron-dextran** or **iron-sorbitol**, both given by deep intramuscular injection. Iron-dextran (but not iron-sorbitol) can be given by slow intravenous infusion, but this method of administration should only be used if absolutely necessary because of the risk of anaphylactoid reactions.

Unwanted effects

The unwanted effects of oral iron administration are dose-related and include nausea, abdominal cramps and diarrhoea.

Acute iron toxicity, usually seen in young children who have swallowed attractively coloured iron tablets in mistake for sweets, occurs after ingestion of large quantities of iron salts. This can result in severe necrotising gastritis with vomiting, haemorrhage and diarrhoea, followed by circulatory collapse.

Chronic iron toxicity or iron overload is virtually always due to causes other than ingestion of iron salts, the commonest being the giving of repeated blood transfusions to treat haemolytic anaemias, notably the thalassaemias. Patients on chronic transfusion programmes need regular therapy with desferrioxamine (see below).

The treatment of acute and chronic iron toxicity involves the use of iron chelators. The agent in common use is **desferrioxamine**, which is given both intragastrically (to bind iron in the bowel lumen and prevent its absorption following acute overdose) and intramuscularly and, if necessary, intravenously. In severe poisoning it is given by slow intravenous infusion. Desferrioxamine forms a complex with ferric iron which is excreted in the urine.

A new, oral iron chelator, L1, is under test. It forms neutral iron complexes and is able to remove iron from transferrin, ferritin and haemosiderin—acting mainly in the liver. L1 is partly metabolised in the liver and excreted in the urine. The plasma $t_{½}$ is approximately 90 minutes. Unwanted effects, mainly gastrointestinal disturbances, are relatively infrequent, but transient agranulocytosis has been reported as has a single case of a fatal lupus-like syndrome.

FOLIC ACID AND VITAMIN B_{12}

Vitamin B_{12} and folic acid are necessary constituents of man's diet, the active forms of these agents being essential for DNA synthesis and cell proliferation. Deficiency of either vitamin B_{12} or folate will have effects principally in those tissues in which there is rapid cell turnover—bone marrow and the gastrointestinal tract—though dividing cells in other tissues are also likely to be affected. The main manifestation of such deficiency is *megaloblastic haemopoiesis* in which there is a marked disorder of erythroblast (pronormoblast) proliferation and defective erythropoiesis. There are increased numbers of large abnormal erythrocyte precursors in the bone marrow due to the fact that during the cell cycle of the proliferating cells (see Fig. 36.1) absence of these substances results in decreased DNA synthesis. The nucleated red blood cell precursors consequently have a high RNA : DNA ratio, and many do not go on to form erythrocytes. Those erythrocytes which are produced are large cells (macrocytes) with normal cytoplasm and haemoglobin but with an increased susceptibility to destruction. Many, instead of being neat biconcave discs, are distorted in shape. Some degree of leucopenia and thrombocytopenia usually accompanies the anaemia.

The principal cause of vitamin B_{12} deficiency is decreased absorption of the vitamin due either to a lack of **intrinsic factor** (see below) or to conditions which interfere with its absorption in the ileum.

Intrinsic factor is secreted by the stomach and is essential for B_{12} absorption. It is lacking in patients with *pernicious anaemia* and in individuals who have had gastrectomies. Pernicious anaemia is a condition in which there is atrophic gastritis, thought to be due, in most cases, to a genetically-determined, local autoimmune reaction. There is often a concurrent neurological disorder—*subacute combined degeneration of the spinal cord.* The anaemia was originally termed 'pernicious' because it seemed to be untreatable, but in 1926 Minot & Murphy showed that there was a remarkable response to the feeding of raw liver. Castle and his associates subsequently established that liver contained an **extrinsic factor** (later defined as **vitamin B_{12}**), and that this, together with an 'intrinsic factor' present in normal gastric juice, was necessary for normal maturation of red cells.

Other conditions resulting in B_{12} deficiency include disorders of the terminal ileum (e.g. Crohn's disease, surgical resection), long-continued nitrous oxide anaesthesia (which inactivates the vitamin), various inflammatory conditions of the bowel and fish tapeworm infestations. (The effect of the last is ascribed to sequestration of the vitamin by the worm and occurs in Finland where raw fish is a delicacy.)

Part of the reason that Minot & Murphy obtained a response with raw liver in pernicious anaemia was the presence in this tissue of **folic acid**. Wills suggested in the 1930s that the vegetable extract 'Marmite' contained a similar anti-anaemia factor, and established that it could correct nutritional anaemia in monkeys. This factor (transiently called vitamin M—the Marmite factor) was also eventually shown to be folic acid.

FOLIC ACID

Folic acid (pteroylglutamic acid) consists of a pteridine ring, para-aminobenzoic acid and glutamic acid (Fig. 23.4). It probably does not occur in nature as such, but can be regarded as the parent compound of a group of naturally occurring folates.

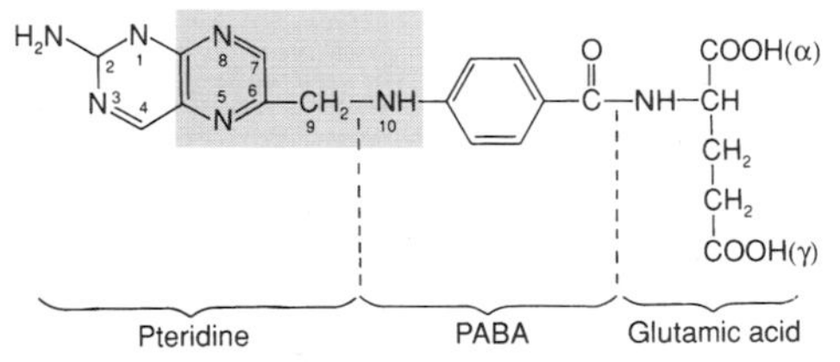

Fig. 23.4 Folic acid (pteroylglutamic acid). Folates may also contain: (1) extra hydrogens at positions 7 and 8 (dihydrofolate) or at 5, 6, 7 and 8 (tetrahydrofolate); (2) one-carbon units such as a methyl group ($-CH_3$) at N^5, a formyl group (–CHO) at N^5 or N^{10}, a methylene ($-CH_2-$) or a methenyl (=CH–) group between N^5 and N^{10}; (3) additional glutamic acid residues attached to the γ-carboxyl of the glutamate moiety. The area in the light pink box is the part of the molecule involved in one-carbon transfers in purine and pyrimidine synthesis.

These differ from folic acid in several respects. Different states of reduction of the pteridine ring may occur, several one-carbon units may be attached to N^5 or N^{10} or both, and additional glutamic acid residues may be attached to the glutamate moiety by unusual γ-peptide bonds, giving folate polyglutamates. (Some aspects of folate structure and metabolism are dealt with in Ch. 36.)

Folates are found in liver, green vegetables, yeast, nuts, cereals, fruit, etc., and the average daily diet in Western Europe contains about 600 μg, of which about 100 μg is absorbed. The folates in food are in the form of polyglutamates. They are converted to the monoglutamate—5,methyltetrahydrofolate—before absorption, and are transported in the blood in this form, most bound loosely to α_2-macroglobulin but some tightly bound to a specific folate-binding protein. The folates in tissues are mostly polyglutamates.

Actions

Folates are essential for DNA synthesis in that they are cofactors in the synthesis of purines and pyrimidines. They are also necessary for reactions involved in amino acid metabolism. In all reactions, *the polyglutamates are considerably more active than the monoglutamates*. For activity, folate must be in the tetrahydro form, in which it is maintained by the enzyme dihydrofolate reductase. This enzyme reduces dietary folic acid to tetrahydrofolate (FH_4) in a two-step reaction, and also reduces the dihydrofolate (FH_2) produced from FH_4 during thymidylate synthesis (see Figs 23.5 and 36.8). Folate antagonists act by inhibiting dihydrofolate reductase (see also Chs 35, 36 and 40).

The de novo synthesis of purines requires two folate-dependent, one-carbon transfer reactions for the insertion of carbon atoms at position 2 and position 8 (Fig. 23.6).

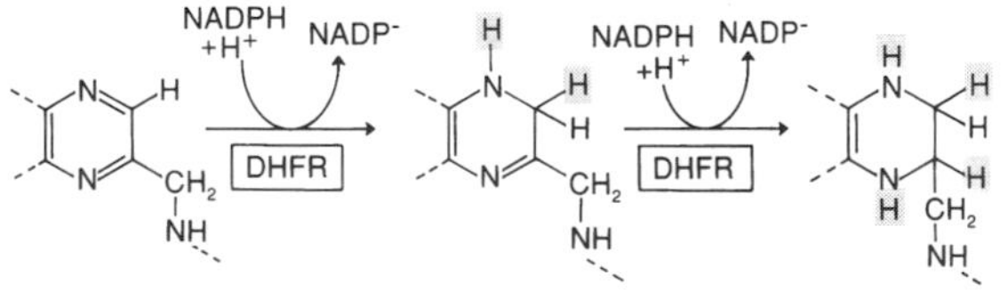

Fig. 23.5 The reduction of folic acid to dihydrofolate then to tetrahydrofolate by the enzyme dihydrofolate reductase (DHFR). Only a portion of the pteridine moiety of the folate molecule is included (that portion shown in the light pink box in Fig. 23.4).

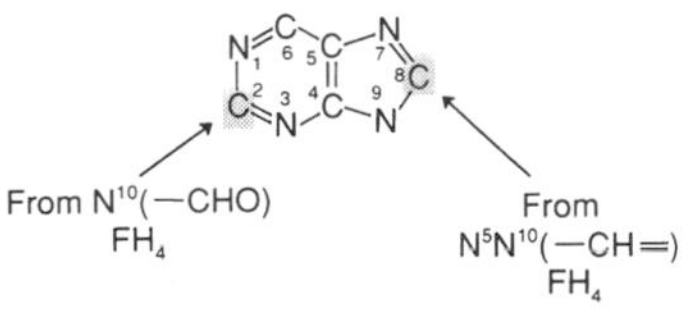

From $N^{10}(-CHO)$ FH_4

From $N^5N^{10}(-CH=)$ FH_4

Fig. 23.6 The purine ring. Carbon atoms 2 and 8 are derived from one-carbon transfers from N^{10} formyl-tetrahydrofolate [$N^{10}(-CHO)FH_4$] and N^5N^{10} methenyl-tetrahydrofolate [$N^5N^{10}(-CH=)FH_4$] respectively.

Folates are especially important for the conversion of deoxyuridylate monophosphate (DUMP) to deoxythymidylate monophosphate (DTMP) which is catalysed by the enzyme, thymidylate synthetase. This is a methylation reaction in which a folate acts as a $-CH_3$ donor (Fig. 23.7). During this reaction, tetrahydrofolate (FH_4) is oxidised to dihydrofolate (FH_2) (see Figs 23.7 and 36.8) and must therefore be reduced before it can act again. The thymidylate synthetase reaction is rate-limiting in mammalian DNA synthesis.

Folates are also important in various amino acid interconversion reactions but these are of less relevance for the role of folates in haemopoiesis than those specified above.

The clinical use of folic acid is given on page 483.

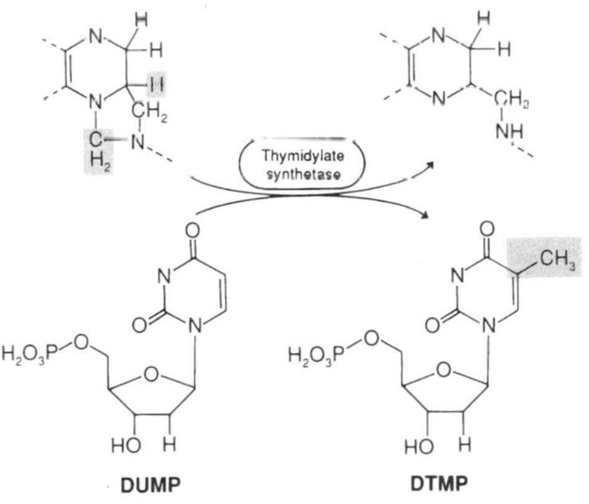

Fig. 23.7 The synthesis of 2-deoxythymidylate (DTMP). DTMP is synthesised by the transfer of a methyl group from N^5N^{10}-methylene tetrahydrofolate (FH_4) to 2-deoxyuridylate (DUMP), the FH_4 being oxidised to dihydrofolate (FH_2) in the process. Only a portion of the pteridine moiety of the folates is included in the diagram — that portion shown in the pink box in Figure 23.4.

Pharmacokinetic aspects

Folic acid is usually given orally, but preparations for parenteral use are available. In the intestine, folic acid is transferred across the mucosa unchanged. Folates are taken up into the liver and into bone marrow cells by active transport, there being separate carrier mechanisms for folic acid, reduced folates and methotrexate (see also Ch. 36). The carrier-mediated uptake of reduced folate is considerably more effective than that of folic acid. Within the cells, folic acid is reduced and methylated or formylated before being converted by polyglutamate synthetase to the polyglutamate form through sequential addition of two to five glutamate moieties. **Folinic acid**, a synthetic tetrahydrofolic acid, is converted much more rapidly to the polyglutamate form. Recent studies suggest that methyltetrahydrofolate is a poor substrate for polyglutamate formation, unlike dihydrofolate, tetrahydrofolate and formyltetrahydrofolate. (This has relevance for the effect of vitamin B_{12} deficiency on folate metabolism, as is explained below.)

Unwanted effects

Unwanted effects do not occur even with large doses of folic acid.

It is important to determine whether a megaloblastic anaemia is due to a folate or a vitamin B_{12} deficiency, since, if vitamin B_{12} deficiency is treated with folic acid, the blood picture may improve and give the appearance of cure while the neurological lesions get worse.

VITAMIN B_{12}

Vitamin B_{12} is a complex cobalamin compound. Some authors use the term 'vitamin B_{12}' specifically for *cyanocobalamin*, but it is often used (and will be used here) to include other pharmacologically active cobalamins.

Vitamin B_{12} is sometimes referred to as 'extrinsic factor' to differentiate it from the 'intrinsic factor' which is produced by the parietal cells of the gastric mucosa and is necessary for the absorption of B_{12}. In nature, B_{12} occurs mainly as *methyl-cobalamin* (methyl-B_{12}) and *5′-deoxyadenosylcobalamin* (ado-B_{12}). These are active forms of the vitamin, but they are unstable and convert spontaneously to *hydroxocobalamin* on exposure to light.

The vitamin B_{12} used medically is hydroxocobalamin. In the diet, the principal sources of vitamin B_{12} are meat (particularly liver), eggs and dairy products. All cobalamins, dietary and therapeutic, must be converted to the methyl and ado forms for activity in the body.

The average daily diet in Western Europe contains 5–25 μg of B_{12} and the daily requirement is 2–3 μg. Absorption requires intrinsic factor (p. 479)—a glycoprotein of 45 000 MW which is a secretory product of the parietal cells of the stomach. One molecule of intrinsic factor binds tightly one molecule of B_{12}. In the complex so formed, the surface peptide bonds of intrinsic factor that are susceptible to the action of proteolytic enzymes are protected by infolding. The stomach secretes a huge excess of intrinsic factor—what limits absorption is the amount the ileum is capable of absorbing. B_{12} is transferred across the cell in an energy-requiring step, intrinsic factor being removed by lysosomal enzymes on the way.

B_{12} is transported in the plasma by B_{12}-binding proteins called *transcobalamins* (TCs). The most important is TCI—an α_1-globulin of 57 000 MW secreted mainly by granulocyte precursors—which carries virtually all the B_{12} present in serum and is normally about 60% saturated. It takes up B_{12} from the liver and gives it up only very slowly to tissues. The complex of TCI–B_{12} has a plasma half-life of about 10 days, and it is thought that it may constitute a storage form of the vitamin.

The vitamin is stored in the body, 80% in the liver and the rest in the kidney, adrenal, pancreas and other organs, the total body store being about 4 mg.

The daily requirement is so low that, if B_{12} absorption is stopped suddenly—as after a total gastrectomy—it takes 2–4 years for evidence of deficiency to become manifest.

Actions

Vitamin B_{12} is required for two main biochemical reactions in man:

- the conversion of methyl-FH_4 to FH_4
- isomerisation of methylmalonyl-CoA to succinyl-CoA.

The conversion of methyl-FH_4 to FH_4

The reaction involves both conversion of 5-methyltetrahydrofolate (methyl-FH_4) to FH_4 and homocysteine to methionine, and the enzyme which accomplishes this is homocysteine–methionine methyl-transferase; the reaction requires B_{12} as cofactor and 5-methyltetrahydrofolate as the methyl donor. It is thought that the 5-methyltetrahydrofolate donates the methyl group to B_{12}, the cofactor. The methyl group is then transferred to homocysteine to form methionine (Fig. 23.8). This vitamin-B_{12}-dependent reaction thus has a significant role in the generation of the tetrahydrofolate from methyltetrahydrofolate.

Methyltetrahydrofolate (the form in which folates are usually carried in blood and in which they enter cells) is a functionally inactive form of folate. Vitamin B_{12} deficiency results in the 'trapping' of folate in the inactive methyltetrahydrofolate form and the consequent depletion of all intracellular folate polyglutamate coenzymes (which are necessary for early stages of DNA synthesis), since methyltetrahydrofolate is not converted to the polyglutamate form, which is the active form of the coenzyme (see above, p. 480).

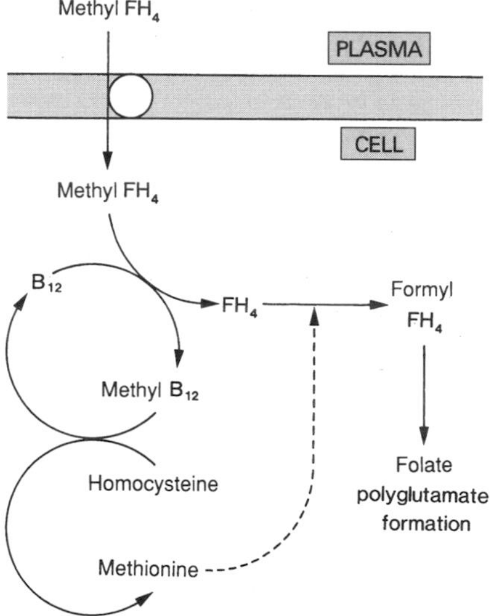

Fig. 23.8 The role of vitamin B_{12} in the synthesis of folate polyglutamate co-enzymes. 5-methyltetrahydrofolate monoglutamate (methyl-FH_4) enters the cells by active transport. The methyl group is transferred to homocysteine to form methionine via vitamin B_{12}, which is bound to the apoenzyme, homocysteine–methionine methyltransferase. (Vitamin B_{12} is shown as 'B_{12}' and as 'methyl B_{12}', but the enzyme is not shown.) Methionine is important in the donation of formate (shown by dashed line) for the conversion of tetrahydrofolate (FH_4) to formyl tetrahydrofolate (formyl-FH_4) which is the preferred substrate for the formation of folate polyglutamates.

Vitamin B_{12} and folic acid

Both vitamin B_{12} and folic acid are needed for DNA synthesis. Deficiencies affect mainly erythropoiesis.

Folic acid

- Folic acid consists of a pteridine ring, p-aminobenzoic acid and a glutamate residue.
- There is active uptake into cells and reduction to tetrahydrofolate (FH_4) by dihydrofolate reductase; extra glutamates are then added.
- Folate polyglutamate is a cofactor (a carrier of one-carbon units) in the synthesis of purines and pyrimidines (especially thymidylate).

Vitamin B_{12} (hydroxocobalamin)

- B_{12} needs an 'intrinsic factor' (a glycoprotein) secreted by gastric parietal cells for absorption.
- It is required for:
  - —conversion of methyl-FH_4 (inactive form of FH_4) to active formyl-FH_4, which, after polyglutamation, is a cofactor in the synthesis of purines and pyrimidines (see above)
  - —isomerisation of methylmalonyl-CoA to succinyl-CoA.
- B_{12} is given by injection.

B_{12}-dependent methionine synthesis may also affect the synthesis of folate polyglutamate co-enzymes by an additional mechanism. There is evidence that the preferred substrate for poly-glutamate synthesis is formyltetrahydrofolate, and the conversion of tetrahydrofolate to formyltetra-hydrofolate requires a formate donor such as methionine.

The proposed role of vitamin B_{12} in folate coenzyme synthesis is indicated in Figure 23.8.

It is through the events described above and shown in Figure 23.9 that the metabolic processes in which vitamin B_{12} and folic acid are involved, are linked and are implicated in the synthesis of DNA.

Isomerisation of methylmalonyl-CoA to succinyl-CoA

The isomerisation reaction is part of a route by which propionate is converted to succinate. Through this pathway, cholesterol, odd-chain fatty acids, some amino acids and thymine may be used for energy production via the tricarboxylic acid cycle, or for gluconeogenesis. Vitamin B_{12}, in the form of deoxyadenosyl cobalamin (ado-B_{12}) is a cofactor in the reaction (Fig. 23.9). In vitamin B_{12} deficiency

L-methylmalonyl-CoA —(Mutase)→ Succinyl-CoA

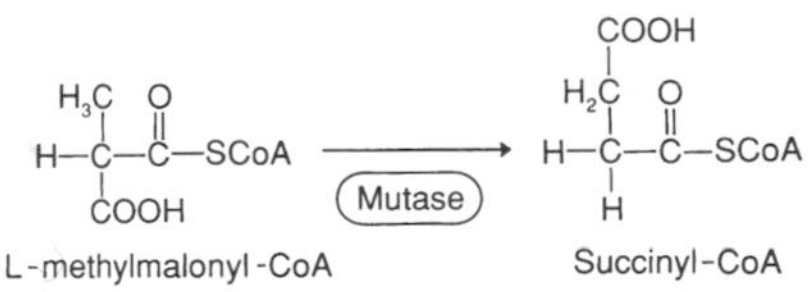

Fig. 23.9 The conversion of L-methylmalonyl-CoA to succinyl-CoA by methylmalonyl-CoA mutase. 5′-deoxyadenosyl B_{12} (ado-B_{12}) acts as a co-enzyme.

states, the reaction cannot occur and methylmalonyl-CoA accumulates. It has been postulated that this causes fatty acid synthesis in neural tissue to be distorted, and that this is the basis of the neuropathy which occurs in these states. The results of other studies suggest that the neurological lesions may be due to a block of methionine synthesis (see above) and thus of S-adenosylmethionine formation and hence defective methylation reactions in lipid (e.g. phosphatidylcholine) synthesis.

The clinical use of vitamin B_{12} is summarised in the following box.

Administration and pharmacokinetic aspects

When vitamin B_{12} is used as a drug, it is almost

Clinical use of folic acid and hydroxocobalamin

Folic acid is used:

- to treat megaloblastic anaemia due to folate deficiency which can be caused by:
  - —poor diet (commonly in alcoholics)
  - —malabsorption syndromes
  - —the use of some drugs (rare), e.g. the folate antagonist, methotrexate, or antiepileptics
- prophylactically in individuals at hazard from developing folate deficiency, for example:
  - —pregnant women (especially if there is a risk of birth defects)
  - —premature infants
  - —patients with severe chronic haemolytic anaemias, including haemoglobinopathies (e.g. sickle cell anaemia).

Hydroxocobalamin is used:

- to treat pernicious anaemia and other causes of vitamin B_{12} deficiency
- prophylactically after surgical operations which remove the site of production of intrinsic factor (e.g. total gastrectomy).

always given by intramuscular injection, since B_{12} deficiency is virtually always due to malabsorption of the vitamin. Plasma transport and distribution of therapeutically administered B_{12} are similar to that of vitamin B_{12} absorbed from the diet (see above).

At the beginning of treatment of pernicious anaemia, six or more injections are given at 2- or 3-day intervals, to saturate body stores; thereafter maintenance therapy is required. Most patients require lifelong therapy. Unwanted effects do not occur.

VITAMIN C

Vitamin C is ascorbic acid. Deficiency of this vitamin leads to *scurvy*, in which there is tenderness and swelling of the joints, tenderness of the gums with loosening of the teeth and, frequently, anaemia. Ascorbic acid is important in the maintenance of the integrity of the intercellular material of skin, cartilage periosteum and bone, and for the integrity of the capillary endothelium. It may have a role in the synthesis of collagen. It may also have a role in folate metabolism, but its exact role in erythropoiesis is not known. The anaemia of scurvy responds to small doses of vitamin C, as do the other manifestations of the scorbutic state.

HAEMOPOIETIC GROWTH FACTORS

Every 60 seconds, a human being must generate about 120 million granulocytes and 150 million erythrocytes, as well as numerous mononuclear cells and platelets. The cells responsible for this remarkable productivity are derived from a relatively small number of self-renewing, pluripotent stem cells laid down during embryogenesis. Maintenance of haemopoiesis necessitates a careful balance between self-renewal on the one hand, and differentiation into the various types of blood cell on the other. The factors involved in controlling this balance are the *haemopoietic growth factors* which direct the division and maturation of the progeny of these cells down eight possible lines of development (Fig. 23.10). These cytokine growth factors are glycoproteins with high biological activity, acting at concentrations of 10^{-12}–10^{-10} mol/l. They are normally present at very low concentrations in the plasma, but the levels can increase very rapidly by 1000-fold within hours—in response to stimulation. **Erythropoietin** is the factor which regulates the red cell line and the signal for its production is blood loss and/or low tissue O_2 tension. The **colony-stimulating factors** regulate the myeloid divisions of the white cell line and also the platelet line, and the main stimulus for their production is infection. See also Table 11.2.

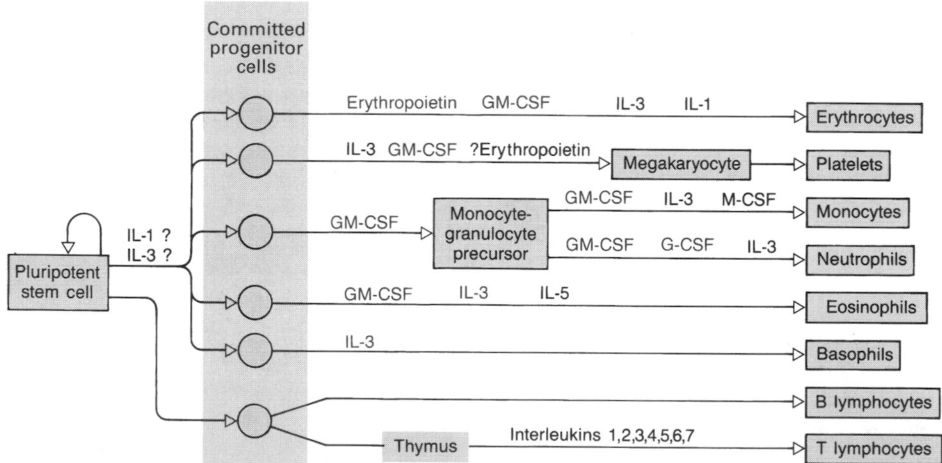

Fig. 23.10 Simplified diagram of the role of haemopoietic growth factors in blood cell differentiation. The factors shown in red are in clinical use. Thrombopoietin, recently described, directs differentiation down the megakaryocyte/platelet line (not shown). (CSF = colony-stimulating factor; GM-CSF = granulocyte-macrophage-CSF; G-CSF = granulocyte-CSF; M-CSF = macrophage-CSF; IL-3 = interleukin-3, or multi-CSF; IL-1 = interleukin-1) (Adapted from: Clark S C, Kamen R 1987 Science 236: 1229) (See also Figs 11.3 and 11.4 and Table 11.2.)

The genes for three of the haemopoietic factors have been cloned and recombinant erythropoietin, recombinant granulocyte-colony-stimulating factor and recombinant granulocyte-macrophage-colony-stimulating factor are being used clinically. Recombinant thrombopoietin has recently been produced. Some of the other haemopoietic growth factors (e.g. interleukin-1, interleukin-2 and various cytokines) are covered in Chapter 11.

EPOIETIN

The growth factor erythropoietin was discovered in 1906. It is produced in juxtatubular cells in the kidney and also in macrophages, and its action is to stimulate committed erythroid progenitor cells to proliferate and generate erythrocytes (Fig. 23.10). The gene has been cloned and two forms of recombinant human erythropoietin, **epoietin alpha** and **epoietin beta** are now available. These are clinically indistinguishable and will be referred to here as simply as 'epoietin'.

The clinical use of epoietin is given below.

Pharmacokinetic aspects

Epoietin can be given intravenously, subcutaneously and intraperitoneally, the response being greatest after subcutaneous injection and fastest after intravenous injection.

Unwanted effects

Flu-like symptoms, which are transient, are likely to occur. Hypertension is common and can cause encephalopathy with headache, disorientation and sometimes convulsions. Iron deficiency can be induced because more iron is required for the enhanced erythropoiesis and there can be an increase in blood viscosity since the plasma volume does not increase commensurately with the increase in red cell mass.

The risk of thrombosis during dialysis is increased.

Clinical use of epoietin

- The main use is for the anaemia of chronic renal failure; in this condition there is a decrease in erythrocytes due to the decrease in the production of erythropoietin by the diseased kidney, and also to the blood loss associated with dialysis.
- Other *potential* future uses are: the anaemia of AIDS (which is exacerbated by zidovudine treatment); the anaemia of chronic inflammatory conditions such as rheumatoid arthritis; the anaemia of cancer; the anaemia which occurs in premature infants.

COLONY-STIMULATING FACTORS (CSFs)

The colony-stimulating factors (CSFs) are so called because they were found to stimulate the formation of maturing colonies of leucocytes in semi-solid medium in vitro. CSFs not only stimulate particular committed progenitor cells to proliferate (Fig. 23.10), but cause irreversible differentiation. The responding precursor cells have membrane receptors to CSFs and may express receptors for more than one factor, thus permitting collaborative interactions between factors.

Granulocyte-macrophage-colony-stimulating factor (GM-CSF) is produced by many cell types and is important in the control of at least five of the eight lines of blood cell development. Granulocyte-colony-stimulating factor (G-CSF) is produced mainly by monocytes, fibroblasts and endothelial cells, and controls primarily the development of neutrophils. Recombinant forms of two of these CSFs are now in clinical use: Granulocyte-CSF (**G-CSF**) is available as **filgrastim** and **lenograstim**, and granulocyte-macrophage-CSF (GM-CSF) as **molgramostim**, and **sargramostim**. Unlike their naturally occurring counterparts, these CSFs are not glycosylated.

Actions

GM-CSF stimulates the development of the progenitors of neutrophils, monocytes, eosinophils, and (under some circumstances) megakaryocytes and erythrocytes (Fig. 23.10). It also enhances the functional activity of the mature cells—the superoxide production, phagocytosis, lysosomal enzyme secretion of granulocytes, and the tumouricidal and microbicidal action of monocytes. In addition, it prolongs the survival of neutrophils and eosinophils. Stimulated neutrophils manifest some decrease in motility. GM-CSF may increase the production of other cytokines.

G-CSF acts only on the neutrophil line (Fig. 23.10)

Clinical uses of the CSFs

CSFs are used in specialist cancer chemotherapy centres:

- To reduce the severity and duration of the neutropenia induced by cytotoxic drugs during:
  - —conventional anticancer chemotherapy
  - —intensive courses of chemotherapy which damage the haemopoietic tissue necessitating autologous bone marrow rescue.

(Note that the CSFs are not given simultaneously with cytotoxic drugs.)

- To stimulate release into the circulation of progenitor cells which can then be harvested and given with, or instead of, bone marrow cells after high-dose, intensive chemotherapy.

Other possible roles: in aplastic anaemia; for myelodysplasia; for the anaemia which occurs in AIDS and is exacerbated by zidovudine.

—increasing the proliferation and maturation of neutrophils, stimulating their release from bone marrow storage pools and enhancing their chemotactic and phagocytic functions.

A possible new development in this field is **romuride**, a synthetic immunostimulant related to muramyldipeptide (see Ch. 11), which has been shown experimentally and in early clinical trials to restore leucocyte and platelet numbers in patients who have had anticancer chemotherapy.

The clinical use of colony-stimulating factors is given on this page.

Pharmacokinetic aspects

Both GM-CSF and G-CSF can be given either subcutaneously or by intravenous infusion. With both agents, a subcutaneous injection of 5–10 μg/kg gives a peak serum concentration within 4 hours, and the subsequent serum concentration (10 ng/ml or more) is maintained for 8–24 hours.

Unwanted effects

Both CSFs are well tolerated. Bone pain occurs in 10–20% of patients.

GM-CSF frequently produces fever and can cause skin rashes, muscle pain and lethargy. There may be pain and reddening at the site of the injection. With intravenous infusion, a syndrome of flushing, hypotension, tachycardia, breathlessness, nausea and vomiting and arterial oxygen desaturation has occurred; this is reversed by giving oxygen and intravenous fluids. At high doses (>20 μg/kg per day) pleural and pericardial effusions, venous thrombosis and pulmonary embolism, have been reported.

G-CSF has produced mild dysuria (rare) and reversible abnormalities in liver function tests. Vasculitis has been reported with long-term use.

Simultaneous administration of these CSFs (which cause stimulation of haemopoietic progenitor cells) with myelotoxic anticancer drugs should be avoided because of the possibility of serious bone marrow depression.

REFERENCES AND FURTHER READING

Adamson J W, Eschbach J W 1990 Treatment of the anemia of chronic renal failure with recombinant human erythropoietin. Annu Rev Med 41: 349–360

Azuma I 1992 Development of the cytokine inducer romuride: experimental studies and clinical application. Trends Pharmacol Sci 13: 425–428

Beck W S 1988 Cobalamin and the nervous system. N Engl J Med 318: 1752–1754

Chanarin I et al. 1981 How vitamin B_{12} acts. Br J Haematol 47: 487–491

Cotes P M 1988 Erythropoietin: the developing story. Br Med J 296: 805–806

Csieff C A 1990 Biology and clinical aspects of hemopoietic growth factors. Annu Rev Med 41: 483–496

Dexter T M, White H 1990 Growth without inflation. Nature 344: 380–381

Erslev A J 1991 Erythropoietin. N Engl J Med 324: 1339–1344

Finch C A, Hueber S H 1982 Perspectives in iron metabolism. N Engl J Med 306: 1520–1528

Hambley H, Mufti G J 1990 Erythropoietin: an old friend revisited. Br Med J 300: 621–622

Hardisty R M, Weatherall D J (eds) 1982 Blood and its disorders. Blackwell Scientific Publications, Oxford
Jacobs A, Worwood M: Iron metabolism, deficiency and overload. ch 5: 149–197
Hoffbrand A V: Vitamin B_{12} and folate metabolism. ch 9: 199–263

Khwaja A, Goldstone A H 1991 Haemopoietic growth factors. Br Med J 302: 1164–1165

Kontoghiorghes G J 1991 Oral iron chelation is here. Br Med J 303: 1279–1280

Levine M 1986 New concepts in the biology and biochemistry of ascorbic acid. N Engl J Med 314: 892–902

Lieschke G J, Burges A W 1992 Granulocyte colony-stimulating factor and granulocyte-macrophage colony-stimulating factor. N Engl J Med 327: 1–35, 99–106

Metcalf D 1989 Haemopoietic growth factors. Lancet 1: 825–827, 885–887
Metcalf D 1994 Thrombopoietin—at last. Nature 369: 519–520
Oski F A 1993 Iron deficiency in infancy and childhood. N Engl J Med 329: 190–193
Shadduck R K et al 1992 Clinical applications of granulocyte-macrophage colony-stimulating factor. Seminars in Haematology 1992 (Whole issue on GM-CSF) 29(4) (Suppl 3): 1–42
Sieff C A 1990 Biology and clinical aspects of haematopoietic growth factors. Annu Rev Med 41: 483–496
Spivak J L 1993 Recombinant erythropoietin. Annu Rev Med 44: 243–253
Steinberg S E 1984 Mechanisms of folate homeostasis. Amer J Physiol 246: G319–324
Steward W P 1993 Granulocyte and granulocyte-macrophage colony-stimulating factors. Lancet 342: 153–160
Wald N J, Bower C 1994 Folic acid, pernicious anaemia, and prevention of neural tube defects. Lancet 343: 307
Whetton A D 1990 The biology and clinical potential of growth factors that regulate myeloid cell production. Trends Pharmacol Sci 11: 285–289

THE CENTRAL NERVOUS SYSTEM

24

CHEMICAL TRANSMISSION AND DRUG ACTION IN THE CENTRAL NERVOUS SYSTEM

There are two reasons why understanding the action of drugs on the CNS presents a particularly challenging problem. The first is that centrally acting drugs are of special significance to mankind. Not only are they of major clinical and therapeutic importance,* but they are also the drugs that humans most commonly administer to themselves without the intervention of the medical profession (e.g. alcohol, tea and coffee, cannabis, nicotine, opiates, amphetamines and so on). The second reason is that the CNS is functionally far more complex than any other system in the body, and this makes the understanding of drug effects very much more difficult. Thus, the relationship between the behaviour of individual cells and that of the organ as a whole is far less direct in the brain than, for example, in the heart or kidney. In these latter organs, a detailed understanding of how a drug affects the cells gives us a fairly clear idea of what effect it will produce on the organ (and on the animal) as a whole. In the brain, this is simply not true. Thus, we may know that a drug mimics the action of 5-HT in its effect on nerve cells, and we know empirically that this type of action is often associated with drugs that cause hallucinations, but the link between these two events remains wholly mysterious. In recent years, investigation of the cellular and biochemical effects produced by centrally acting drugs has progressed rapidly, but the gulf between the description of drug action at this level and the description of drug action at the functional and behavioural level remains, for the most part, very wide. Attempts to bridge it seem, at times, like throwing candy floss into the Grand Canyon.

A few bridgeheads have none the less been established, some more firmly than others. Thus the relationship between dopaminergic pathways in the extrapyramidal system and the effects of drugs in alleviating or exacerbating the symptoms of parkinsonism (see Ch. 25) is clear-cut. Less well established are the postulated connections between hyperactivity in dopaminergic pathways and schizophrenia (see Ch. 28), and between the functions of noradrenaline and 5-HT in certain parts of the brain and the symptoms of depression (see Ch. 29). At the other end of the spectrum, attempts to relate the condition of epilepsy to an identifiable cellular disturbance (see Ch. 30) have been very disappointing, even though the abnormal neuronal discharge pattern in epilepsy seems, on the face of it, a much simpler kind of disturbance than, for example, the abnormal perception and behaviour of a schizophrenic patient.

The aim of this chapter is to describe briefly the present state of knowledge about some of the main transmitter systems that are important in the brain, concentrating on those systems which form the basis of reasonably coherent explanations of the effects of centrally acting drugs. We also discuss the functions of excitatory amino acids, whose possible role in neurodegenerative disorders is considered further in Chapter 25. The unexpected role of nitric oxide as a mediator in the brain, which has caused a flurry

*A 1977 study of general practitioners prescribing in the UK showed that one person in six was given a prescription for a centrally acting drug in 1 year. In women aged 45–59 years, the figure was one in three.

of excitement among neurobiologists, is also discussed (see also Ch. 10). More detailed accounts will be found in textbooks such as Webster & Jordan (1989), Cooper, Bloom & Roth (1991), Ashton (1992). At the end of this chapter a simple classification of the main groups of psychotropic drugs is given.

In the last 10–15 years, ideas about transmitter action in the CNS have changed quite radically, particularly in two respects.

Firstly, the number of putative transmitters has jumped from about 10 'classical' transmitters (mainly small monoamines and amino acids) to 40 or more, with the discovery of a host of neuropeptides (see Ch. 9). At the same time, the number of distinct receptor types for many of the known transmitter agents has increased, mainly through the work of molecular biologists. For all of the main non-peptide transmitters, there appear to be three or four (or more) separate receptor subtypes, often with very distinct patterns of distribution within the brain.

Secondly, the concept of what is meant by a neurotransmitter has broadened considerably. The original concept envisaged a substance released by one neuron and acting rapidly, briefly, and at short range on the membrane of an adjacent neuron, producing a change in conductance which either increased or decreased the excitability of the postsynaptic cell. It is now clear that chemical mediators within the brain can produce slow and long-lasting effects (over minutes or hours); that they can act rather diffusely, at a considerable distance from their site of release; and they can produce diverse effects, for example on transmitter synthesis and on the expression of neurotransmitter receptors, in addition to affecting the ionic conductance of the postsynaptic cells. The term '*neuromodulator*' ('*neuroregulator*' in some texts) has been coined to denote a neuronally released mediator, the actions of which do not conform to the conventional (if unwritten) view of how a neurotransmitter should act (see also Ch. 5). The term 'neuromodulator' is hard to define, and is in danger of being used indiscriminately to describe any chemical mediator the actions of which are ill understood. It covers not only the neuropeptide mediators, which often act slowly and remotely from where they are released, but also mediators such as nitric oxide and arachidonic acid metabolites, which are not stored and released like conventional neurotransmitters, and may come from non-neuronal cells as well as neurons. In general, neuromodulation (see Ch. 5) describes the control of *synaptic plasticity*, including short-term events, such as the regulation of presynaptic transmitter release or postsynaptic excitability, and longer-term events such as neuronal gene regulation.

The impact of these conceptual developments on the interpretation of how centrally acting drugs exert their effects is yet to come. The increasing number of putative chemical mediators and receptors, and the diversity of the effects ascribed to them have increased enormously the range of potential points of attack for centrally acting drugs, compared with the situation existing a few years ago. On the one hand, this frustrates the efforts of authors like ourselves to present the subject simply, but on the other hand, it opens up new therapeutic possibilities in the form of drugs that selectively activate or block the various receptor subtypes. Examples from the dopamine and 5-HT fields are discussed briefly.

INDIVIDUAL NEUROTRANSMITTERS

The following chemical mediators are discussed in this chapter:

- noradrenaline
- dopamine
- 5-HT
- acetylcholine
- excitatory amino acids
- inhibitory amino acids: γ-aminobutyric acid (GABA) and glycine
- histamine
- nitric oxide.

NORADRENALINE

Many aspects of noradrenergic transmission have been discussed in Chapter 7. The basic processes responsible for the synthesis, storage, release and re-uptake of noradrenaline are the same in the brain as in the periphery, and the same types of noradrenergic receptor are also found in pre- and postsynaptic locations in the brain. Here we will consider anatomical and functional aspects of central noradrenergic pathways and their possible involvement in different types of mental disorder.

Central noradrenergic pathways

Though the existence of noradrenaline in the brain was demonstrated biochemically in the 1950s and its transmitter role was suspected, detailed analysis of its neuronal distribution only became possible when the fluorescence technique, based on the formation of a fluorescent derivative of catecholamines when tissues are exposed to formaldehyde, was devised by Falck & Hillarp. This technique enabled detailed maps of the pathways of noradrenergic, dopaminergic and 5-HT-containing neurons to be produced. Very detailed information is available for laboratory animals, such as the rat, but the same basic features have also been found in more limited studies of human brains. The cell bodies of noradrenergic neurons are found exclusively in the pons and medulla, where they form a number of discrete clusters. These rather small clumps of neurons send extensively branching axons to many other parts of the brain (Fig. 24.1) including the cerebral cortex, limbic system, hypothalamus, cerebellum and spinal cord. The most prominent cluster of noradrenergic neurons is the *locus ceruleus*, which is found in the grey matter of the pons. Although it contains, in the rat, only 1000–2000 neurons, axons from these cells, running in a discrete *dorsal noradrenergic bundle*, give rise to many millions of noradrenergic nerve terminals throughout the cortex, hippocampus and cerebellum. It is an extremely diffuse system, and the nerve terminals do not form close, discrete, synaptic contacts, but appear to release transmitter at some distance from the target cell. These characteristics have caused the noradrenergic system to be likened to a neural aerosol—a touch on the *locus ceruleus* push-button and large areas of the brain are diffusely sprayed with noradrenaline.

Other noradrenergic neurons lie close to the locus ceruleus in the pons and medulla. Axons from these cells run via the *ventral noradrenergic bundle*, and provide a similarly diffuse innervation to the hypothalamus, hippocampus and other parts of the forebrain. These cells also project to the cerebellum and spinal cord, and here, too, the terminals form a diffuse network rather than discrete synaptic contacts.

Functional aspects

If noradrenaline is applied by micro-ionophoresis to individual cells in the brain, the effect most often seen is inhibitory, and in most cases it is produced by activation of β-adrenoceptors. Activation of adenylate cyclase, with resulting accumulation of cAMP, has been unequivocally demonstrated as the mechanism of action in several types of CNS neuron. In some situations, however, noradrenaline has an excitatory effect, which is mediated by either

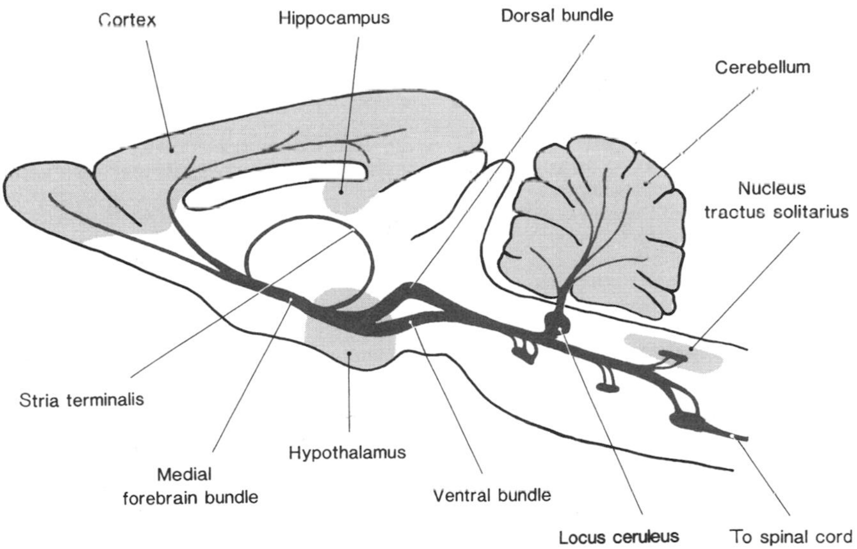

Fig. 24.1 Noradrenergic pathways in the rat brain. The location of the main groups of cell bodies and fibre tracts are shown in red. Light pink areas show the location of noradrenergic terminals.

α- or β-adrenoceptors. There is still, as mentioned above, a wide gulf between these fairly well characterised neuronal mechanisms and an understanding of the behavioural and physiological responses in which noradrenergic neurons are believed, on the basis of lesioning studies and drug effects, to participate. The most important of these behavioural and physiological functions are:

- reward system and mood
- state of arousal
- blood pressure and neuroendocrine regulation.

Reward system and mood

If electrodes are implanted in the region of the noradrenergic projection from the *locus ceruleus* to the limbic system and cortex of experimental animals, and the electrodes are connected to a switch that the animal can learn to operate, the animals quickly adopt a high rate of self-stimulation. This response is inhibited by drugs that prevent noradrenergic transmission. Studies of this kind have led to the suggestion (see Ashton 1992) that the noradrenergic, as well as dopaminergic, pathways constitute a 'reward' system, though the relationship of this psychological construct to subjective feelings in man is uncertain. Consistent with this view, some drugs of abuse, such as cocaine and amphetamine (see Ch. 33) act biochemically to enhance noradrenergic and dopaminergic transmission, possibly representing the human version of the self-stimulation paradigm.

The catecholamine hypothesis of affective disorders, originally formulated by Schildkraut (1965) suggests that *depression* results from a functional deficiency of noradrenaline in certain parts of the brain, while mania results from an excess. The evidence is discussed in Chapter 29.

Arousal

Various lines of evidence suggest that activation of noradrenergic pathways can produce behavioural arousal. One is that amphetamine-like drugs, which are known to act by releasing catecholamines in the brain, increase wakefulness, alertness and exploratory activity. Another is that the electrical activity of locus ceruleus neurons in conscious animals is highly responsive to sensory stimuli. Stimuli of an unfamiliar or threatening kind excite these noradrenergic neurons much more effectively than familiar stimuli. Furthermore, there is a close relationship between mood and state of arousal. Depressed patients are usually lethargic and unresponsive to external stimuli; also **reserpine**, which inhibits noradrenergic transmission, causes both depression and sedation. This association of symptoms may reflect the dual role of noradrenergic neurons in controlling both mood and arousal.

Blood pressure regulation

The realisation that central, as well as peripheral, noradrenergic synapses play a role in blood pressure regulation comes mainly from investigation of the mechanisms of action of hypotensive drugs such as **clonidine** and **methyldopa** (see Chs 7 and 14), both of which were shown to decrease the discharge of sympathetic nerves emerging from the central nervous system. It was then shown that they cause marked hypotension when injected locally into the vasomotor centres or into the fourth ventricle, in much smaller amounts than are required when the drugs are given systemically. Noradrenaline, injected locally into the region of the vasomotor centres, has a similar effect. Pharmacological studies with agonists and antagonists show that these responses are due to activation of α_2-adrenoceptors, which, on the basis of lesion studies, appear to be located postsynaptically (in contrast to most peripheral α_2-adrenoceptors, which are presynaptic). Noradrenergic synapses in the medulla probably form part of the baroreceptor reflex pathway, since stimulation or antagonism of α_2-adrenoceptors in this part of the brain has a powerful effect on the activity of baroreceptor reflexes. Thus, clonidine markedly increases the bradycardia and hypotension that occur in response to mechanical distension of the carotid sinus, and **α-adrenoceptor-blocking drugs** have the opposite effect.

Other noradrenergic neurons, apart from those in the baroreceptor reflex arc, are important as well. Ascending fibres run to the hypothalamus, and descending fibres run to the lateral horn region of the spinal cord, acting to increase sympathetic discharge in the periphery. Noradrenergic transmission does not actually form an essential link in the baroreceptor reflex pathway, but regulatory noradrenergic neurons greatly influence the activity of the reflex. These regulatory neurons probably originate in the pons and medulla; a similar type of regulation also occurs in the spinal cord. It has been suggested that these regulatory neurons may release adrenaline, rather than noradrenaline. Some

Noradrenaline in the CNS

- Mechanisms for synthesis, storage, release and re-uptake of noradrenaline in the CNS are essentially the same as in the periphery, as are the receptors (Ch. 7).
- Noradrenergic cell bodies occur in discrete clusters, mainly in the pons and medulla, one important such cell group being the locus ceruleus.
- Noradrenergic pathways, running mainly in the ventral and dorsal noradrenergic bundles, terminate diffusely in the cortex, hippocampus, hypothalamus, cerebellum and spinal cord.
- The actions of noradrenaline are mainly inhibitory (β-receptors), but some are excitatory (α- or β-receptors).
- Noradrenergic transmission is believed to be important in: control of mood (functional deficiency resulting in depression), and function of 'reward system'; 'arousal' system, controlling wakefulness and alertness; blood pressure regulation.
- Psychotropic drugs that act partly or mainly on noradrenergic transmission in the CNS include: antidepressants, cocaine, amphetamine. Some antihypertensive drugs (e.g. clonidine, methyldopa) act mainly on noradrenergic transmission in the CNS.

catecholamine-containing cells in the brainstem contain PNMT (the enzyme that converts noradrenaline to adrenaline; see Ch. 7) and inhibition of this enzyme appears to prevent the normal regulation of the baroreceptor reflex.

DOPAMINE

Appreciation of the role of dopamine in the brain, as a transmitter in its own right and not merely as a precursor of noradrenaline, came in the mid-1960s, during a remarkable decade of progress—the 'monoamine years'—when a combination of neurochemistry and neuropharmacology led to many important discoveries about the role of CNS transmitters, and about the ability of drugs to influence these systems. It was found that the distribution of dopamine in the brain is highly non-uniform, and more restricted than the distribution of noradrenaline. A large proportion of the dopamine content of the brain is found in the *corpus striatum*, a part of the extrapyramidal motor system concerned with the coordination of movement (see Ch. 25), and there is also a high concentration in certain parts of the *limbic system*.

The synthesis of dopamine follows the same route as that of noradrenaline (see Ch. 7), namely conversion of tyrosine to dopa (the rate-limiting step, catalysed by tyrosine hydroxylase) followed by decarboxylation (catalysed by dopa decarboxylase). Dopaminergic neurons lack dopamine β-hydroxylase, and thus do not produce noradrenaline.

Dopamine is largely recaptured, following its release from nerve terminals, by a specific dopamine transporter, similar to that for other monoamines (see Giros & Caron 1993) and is metabolised by MAO and COMT, the pathways being exactly analogous to those for noradrenaline (Fig. 24.2). The main products are *dihydroxyphenylacetic acid* (DOPAC), which is formed by oxidative deamination (MAO) followed by enzymic oxidation of the resulting aldehyde, and *homovanillic acid* (HVA), the methoxy-derivative of DOPAC, formed by the action of COMT. These substances are present in the brain, and the content of HVA is often used as an index of dopamine turnover. Drugs that cause the release of dopamine increase HVA concentration, often without changing the concentration of dopamine. DOPAC and HVA, and their sulphate conjugates, are excreted in the urine, which provides another index of dopamine release that can be used in human subjects.

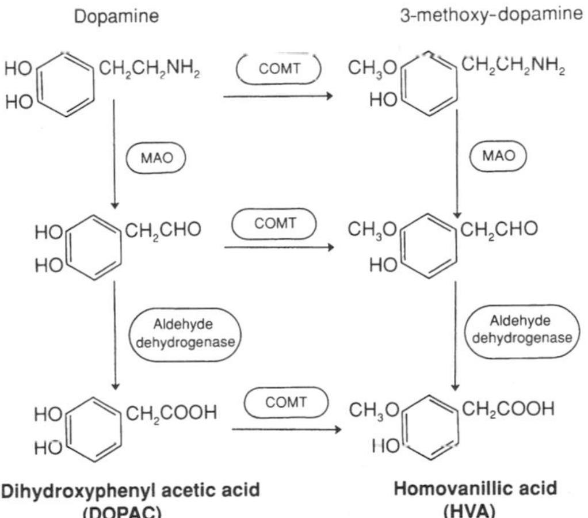

Fig. 24.2 The main pathways for dopamine metabolism in the brain. (MAO = monoamine oxidase; COMT = catechol-O-methyl transferase)

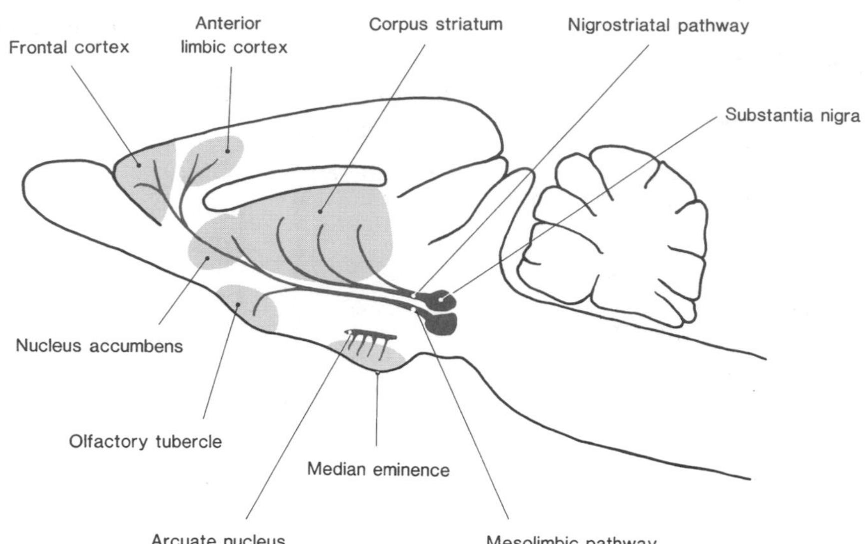

Fig. 24.3 Dopaminergic pathways in the rat brain, drawn as in Figure 24.1.

Dopamine pathways in the CNS

The mapping studies of Dahlstrom & Fuxe in 1965, based on fluorescence staining, showed that dopaminergic neurons form three main systems (Fig. 24.3). The first of these, accounting for about 75% of the dopamine in the brain, is the *nigrostriatal pathway*, the cell bodies of which lie in the *substantia nigra* (forming the A9 cell group) and the axons of which terminate in the *corpus striatum*. These fibres run in the medial forebrain bundle along with many noradrenaline- and 5-HT-containing fibres. The second important system is the *mesolimbic pathway*, the cell bodies of which lie in various groups in the midbrain (mainly the A10 cell group) and the fibres of which project, also via the medial forebrain bundle, to parts of the limbic system, especially the *nucleus accumbens*. Finally, the *tubero-infundibular system* is a group of short neurons running from the arcuate nucleus of the hypothalamus to the median eminence and pituitary gland, the secretions of which they regulate. There are also many local dopaminergic interneurons in the olfactory cortex, and in the retina. The abundance of dopamine-containing neurons in the human striatum can be appreciated from the image shown in Figure 24.4, which was obtained by injecting a dopa derivative containing radioactive fluorine, and scanning with a computerised detection system (*positron emission tomography* or *PET scanning*; see Barrio et al. 1988) to display the distribution of radioactivity in the brain 3 hours later.

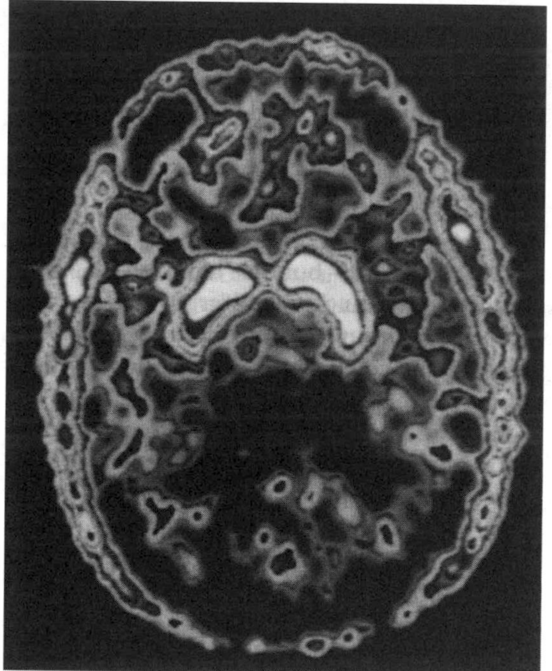

Fig. 24.4 Dopamine in the basal ganglia of a human subject. The subject was injected with 5-fluoro-dopa, labelled with the positron-emitting isotope ^{18}F, which was localised 3 hours later by the technique of positron emission tomography. The isotope is accumulated (white areas) by the dopa-uptake system of the neurons of the basal ganglia, and to a smaller extent in the frontal cortex. It is also seen in the scalp and temporalis muscles. (From: Garnett E S et al. 1983 Nature 305: 137)

Dopamine may also function as a transmitter in the periphery (see Ch. 5).

Dopamine receptors

Two types of receptor, D_1 and D_2, were distinguished on pharmacological and biochemical grounds; they are linked, respectively, to activation and inhibition of adenylate cyclase. Gene cloning studies have split these into further subgroups (see Sibley & Monsma 1993, Civelli et al. 1993). The D_1 family now includes D_1 and D_5, while the D_2 family, which is pharmacologically more important in the CNS, has been split into D_2, D_3 and D_4 (see Table 24.1). All of them, as expected, belong to the family of G-protein-coupled transmembrane receptors described in Chapter 2. They are expressed in the brain in distinct but overlapping areas. The dopamine receptors relevant to the actions of antipsychotic drugs (Ch. 28) mainly belong to the D_2 family, but the cellular mechanisms remain unclear, because the cells are difficult to study in isolation. In pituitary lactotroph cells, where D_2-receptors cause inhibition of prolactin secretion (see Ch. 21), the cellular mechanism is evidently complex (see Vallar & Meldolesi 1989), involving not only adenylate cyclase inhibition, but also inhibition of calcium mobilisation and opening of potassium channels, the general picture being similar to the cardiac inhibitory effects of muscarinic agonists (Ch. 13). Elegant studies on retinal cells (see Rogawski 1987) suggest other functions of D_1- and D_2-receptors. Thus D_1-receptors, which are localised to the horizontal cells, have been found to control the activity of intercellular gap junctions (sites of high electrical conductance that link adjacent cells, and thus couple them electrically), whereas D_2-receptors regulate the physical extension of processes by other retinal cells. Whether such events occur in the CNS is not known.

The D_4-receptor, which may be implicated in

Table 24.1 Dopamine receptors

	Receptor family	
	D_1 (subtypes: D_1, D_5)	D_2 (subtypes: D_2, D_3, D_4)
Agonists		
Dopamine	+ (low potency)	+ (high potency)
Apomorphine	PA (low potency)	+ (high potency)
Bromocriptine	PA (low potency)	+ (high potency)
Antagonists		
Phenothiazines	+ (low potency)	+ (high potency, non-selective)
Butyrophenones	+ (low potency)	+ (high potency, D_2-selective)
Spiperone	–	+ (high potency, non-selective)
Sulpiride	–	+ (high potency, non-selective)
Clozapine	+ (medium potency)	+ (high potency, D_4-selective)
Second messengers	Increase cAMP	Decrease cAMP Increase K^+-conductance
Location and function		
CNS	Mainly postsynaptic inhibition	Presynaptic and postsynaptic inhibition
Limbic system (mood & emotional stability; stereotypy)	Mainly D_1	D_2, D_3, D_4
Corpus striatum (motor control)	D_1	D_2 (not D_4)
Hypothalamus (autonomic control)	Mainly D_5	Mainly D_3
Pituitary (inhibition of hormone secretion)		D_2
Blood vessels (dilatation)	Mainly D_5	
Heart (increased force)	Mainly D_5	
Sympathetic nerve terminals (inhibition of release)		D_2

Note: PA = partial agonist; low potency implies activity in the micromolar range; high potency implies activity in the nanomolar range.

the pathogenesis of schizophrenia (see Ch. 28), has recently been shown to display an unexpected polymorphism in humans (Van Tol et al. 1992), with a varying number of repeat sequences being expressed in one of the intracellular loops. It is possible that this is associated with mental disorders such as schizophrenia, but this has not been established.

Dopamine, like many other transmitters and modulators, acts presynaptically as well as postsynaptically. Presynaptic D_3-receptors occur mainly on dopaminergic neurons, for example those in the striatum and limbic system, where they act to inhibit dopamine synthesis and release. Dopamine antagonists, by blocking these receptors, increase dopamine synthesis and release, and cause accumulation of dopamine metabolites in these parts of the brain. They also cause an increase in the rate of firing of dopaminergic neurons (see Cooper et al. 1991), probably by blocking a neuronal feedback pathway.

Dopamine receptors also mediate various effects in the periphery (mediated by D_1-receptors), notably renal vasodilatation and increased myocardial contractility, and dopamine itself is used clinically in the treatment of circulatory shock (see Ch. 14).

Functional aspects

The functions of dopaminergic pathways are rather better understood than those of pathways involving other transmitters. This is partly because selective agonists and antagonists are available for dopamine receptors (Table 24.1), and partly because dopaminergic neurons can be selectively destroyed by local injection of 6-hydroxydopamine (see Ch. 7) into small areas of the brain. The functions divide broadly into:

- motor control (nigrostriatal system)
- behavioural effects (mesolimbic and mesocortical systems)
- endocrine control (tubero-infundibular system).

Dopamine and motor systems

Ungerstedt showed, in 1968, that bilateral destruction of the *substantia nigra* in rats, which destroys the nigrostriatal neurons, causes profound catalepsy, the animals becoming so inactive that they die of starvation unless artificially fed. Unilateral lesions produced by 6-hydroxydopamine injection caused the animal to turn in circles *towards* the lesioned side. There is evidence that this abnormal locomotion results from an imbalance of dopamine action in the *corpus striatum* between the two sides of the brain. Thus, unilateral injection of **apomorphine** (a dopamine-like agonist) into the striatum causes circling away from the injected side. If apomorphine is given systemically to normal rats it causes, as one would expect, no asymmetrical pattern of locomotion, but if given systemically to animals with unilateral lesions of the substantia nigra made days or weeks earlier, apomorphine causes circling *away* from the lesioned side. This is thought to be due to denervation supersensitivity (see Ch. 5), which arises because the destruction of dopaminergic terminals on one side causes a proliferation of dopamine receptors, and hence supersensitivity to apomorphine, of the cells on that side of the striatum. In these animals, administration of drugs that act by releasing dopamine (e.g. **amphetamine**) cause turning *towards* the lesioned side, since the dopaminergic nerve terminals are only present on the normal side. This 'turning model' has been extremely useful in investigating the action of drugs on dopaminergic neurons and dopamine receptors (see Ungerstedt 1971).

Parkinson's disease (discussed in more detail in Ch. 25) is a progressive motor disturbance that occurs mainly in elderly patients, whose main symptoms are rigidity and tremor, together with extreme slowness in initiating voluntary movements (hypokinesia). It is known to be associated with a deficiency of dopamine in the nigrostriatal pathway.

Many antipsychotic drugs (see Ch. 28) are D_2-receptor antagonists, whose major side effect is to cause movement disorders, probably associated with block of D_2-receptors in the nigrostriatal pathway.

Behavioural effects

Administration of **amphetamine** to rats, which releases both dopamine and noradrenaline, causes a cessation of normal 'ratty' behaviour (exploration and grooming) and the appearance of repeated 'stereotyped' behaviour (rearing, gnawing and so on) unrelated to external stimuli. These effects are prevented by **dopamine antagonists**, and by destruction of dopamine-containing cell bodies in the midbrain, but not by drugs that inhibit the noradrenergic system. These amphetamine-induced motor disturbances in rats probably reflect hyperactivity in the nigrostriatal dopaminergic system (A9 cell group; see Fig. 24.3) since they are abolished by lesions in this area.

Amphetamine also causes a general increase in motor activity, which can be measured, for example, by counting electronically the frequency at which a rat crosses from one part of its enclosure to another. This effect, in contrast to stereotypy, appears to be related to the mesolimbic dopaminergic pathway originating from the A10 cell group (see Fig. 24.3). There is evidence (see Ch. 28) that schizophrenia in man is associated with dopaminergic hyperactivity, and many attempts have been made to detect behavioural effects of dopamine in animals that might be related to the symptoms of human schizophrenia. It has been found that chronic administration of amphetamine to a few rats in a large colony produces various types of abnormal social interaction, including withdrawal and aggressive behaviour, but it is extremely difficult to quantify such effects or to establish their relationship to schizophrenia in man.

Neuroendocrine function

The tubero-infundibular dopaminergic pathway (see Fig. 24.3) is involved in the control of *prolactin* secretion. The hypothalamus secretes various mediators (mostly small peptides; see Ch. 21), which control the secretion of different hormones from the pituitary gland. One of these, which has an inhibitory effect on prolactin release, is dopamine. This system is of considerable clinical importance. It was observed many years ago that ergot derivatives (see Ch. 8) suppress lactation, whereas antipsychotic drugs (see Ch. 28) have the opposite effect, even to the point of causing breast development and lactation in males. These effects were subsequently found to be due to changes in prolactin secretion, and studies on isolated pituitary glands confirmed that dopamine and related agonists strongly inhibit prolactin secretion, an effect that is abolished by many antipsychotic drugs, which block dopamine receptors. One dopamine receptor agonist, **bromocriptine**, derived from ergot, is used clinically to suppress prolactin secretion by tumours of the pituitary gland.

Another hormone whose secretion is regulated by dopamine is growth hormone. In normal subjects dopamine receptor activation increases growth hormone secretion, but, paradoxically, it inhibits the excessive secretion responsible for acromegaly, a condition in which bromocriptine has a useful therapeutic effect, provided it is given before excessive growth has taken place (see Ch. 21).

Vomiting

Pharmacological evidence strongly suggests that dopaminergic neurons have a role in the production of nausea and vomiting. Thus, nearly all dopamine-receptor agonists (e.g. bromocriptine) and other drugs that increase dopamine release in the brain (e.g. levodopa; Ch. 25) cause nausea and vomiting as side effects, while many dopamine antagonists (e.g. phenothiazines, Ch. 28; metoclopramide, Ch. 19) have anti-emetic activity. D_2-receptors occur in the area of the medulla (*chemoreceptor trigger zone*) associated with the initiation of vomiting (Ch. 19), and are assumed to mediate this effect.

Dopamine in the CNS

- Dopamine is a neurotransmitter as well as being the precursor for noradrenaline. It is degraded in a similar fashion to noradrenaline, giving rise mainly to DOPAC and HVA, which are excreted in the urine.
- There are three main dopaminergic pathways:
  - —nigrostriatal pathway, important in motor control
  - —mesolimbic pathways, running from groups of cells in the midbrain to parts of the limbic system, especially the nucleus accumbens
  - —tubero-infundibular neurons running from the hypothalamus to the pituitary gland, whose secretions they regulate.
- There are two main families of dopamine receptor, D_1 and D_2, linked, respectively, to stimulation and inhibition of adenylate cyclase. They are further divided into subtypes. Most of the known functions of dopamine appear to be mediated by receptors of the D_2 family.
- One member of the D_2 family, the D_4 receptor, shows marked polymorphism in humans, and may be implicated in schizophrenia.
- Parkinson's disease is associated with a deficiency of nigrostriatal dopaminergic neurons.
- Behavioural effects of an excess of dopamine activity consist of stereotyped behaviour patterns, and can be produced by dopamine-releasing agents (e.g. amphetamine) and dopamine agonists (e.g. apomorphine).
- Excessive dopamine activity has been implicated in schizophrenia, but the evidence is equivocal.
- Hormone release from the anterior pituitary gland is regulated by dopamine, especially prolactin release (inhibited) and growth hormone release (stimulated).
- Dopamine acts on the chemoreceptor trigger zone to cause nausea and vomiting.

5-HYDROXYTRYPTAMINE

The occurrence and functions of 5-HT in the periphery are described in Chapter 9. Interest in 5-HT as a possible CNS transmitter dates from 1953, when Gaddum found that *lysergic acid diethylamide* (LSD), a drug known to be a powerful hallucinogen, acted as a 5-HT antagonist on peripheral tissues, and suggested that its central effects might also be related to this action. The presence of 5-HT in the brain was demonstrated a few years later. Even though brain accounts for only about 1% of the total body content, 5-HT occupies a central position in the neurochemical hegemony (see Green 1985).

The formation, storage and release of 5-HT (see Fig. 8.1) are very similar to those of noradrenaline. The precursor substance is tryptophan, an amino acid derived from dietary protein, the plasma content of which varies considerably according to food intake and time of day. Tryptophan is taken up into neurons by an active transport process, converted by tryptophan hydroxylase to *5-hydroxytryptophan* and then decarboxylated by a non-specific amino acid decarboxylase to 5-HT. Tryptophan hydroxylase can be selectively and irreversibly inhibited by *p-chlorophenylalanine* (PCPA). Availability of tryptophan, and the activity of tryptophan hydroxylase are thought to be the main processes that regulate 5-HT synthesis. The decarboxylase is very similar, if not identical, to DOPA decarboxylase, and does not seem to play any role in regulating 5-HT synthesis. Following release, 5-HT is largely recovered by neuronal uptake, this mechanism being inhibited by many of the same drugs (e.g. **tricyclic antidepressants**) that inhibit catecholamine uptake. The carrier is not identical, however, and inhibitors show some specificity between the two systems (see Ch. 29). 5-HT is degraded almost entirely by MAO (Fig. 8.1), which converts it to 5-hydroxyindole acetaldehyde, most of which is dehydrogenated to form 5-hydroxyindoleacetic acid (5-HIAA), which is excreted in the urine.

Central 5-HT pathways

Mapping of neurons containing 5-HT has been carried out by techniques similar to those used for noradrenergic neurons, namely fluorescence histochemistry, immunofluorescent labelling of specific enzymes (tryptophan hydroxylase) and the observation of specific markers that are taken up by nerve terminals or cell bodies and transported to other parts of the neuron. The distribution of neurons containing 5-HT is very similar to that of noradrenergic neurons, and quite different from that of dopamine-containing neurons (Fig. 24.5). The cells occur in several large clusters in the pons and upper medulla, which lie close to the midline (raphe) and are often referred to as *raphe nuclei*. The rostrally situated nuclei project, via the median forebrain bundle, which also contains many noradrenergic fibres, in a diffuse way to many parts of the cortex, hippocampus, limbic system and hypothalamus, the whole arrangement being very similar to that of the noradrenergic system. The caudally situated cells project to the medulla and spinal cord.

Functional aspects

Many studies on the effects of 5-HT and related compounds on individual neurons have shown that it can interact with several types of receptor (see Ch. 8, Table 8.1; Peroutka 1988) and elicit various kinds of cellular response (Table 24.2).

The precise localisation of 5-HT neurons in the brainstem has allowed their electrical activity to be studied in detail, and correlated with behavioural and other effects produced by drugs thought to affect 5-HT-mediated transmission. 5-HT cells show an unusual, highly regular slow discharge pattern, and are strongly inhibited by 5-HT_1-receptor agonists, suggesting a local inhibitory feedback mechanism.

In vertebrates, certain physiological and behavioural functions relate particularly to 5-HT pathways, namely:

- hallucinations and behavioural changes
- sleep, wakefulness and mood
- control of sensory transmission.

Hallucinatory effects

Many centrally acting 5-HT analogues (e.g. LSD) are hallucinogenic (see Ch. 32; Green 1985), and depress the firing of 5-HT neurons. These neurons exert an inhibitory influence on cortical neurons, and it is suggested that the loss of cortical inhibition resulting from suppression of activity in these neurons underlies the hallucinogenic effect, as well as certain behavioural effects in experimental animals, such as the 'wet-dog shakes' that occur in rats when the 5-HT precursor, 5-HTP, is administered (see Green 1985).

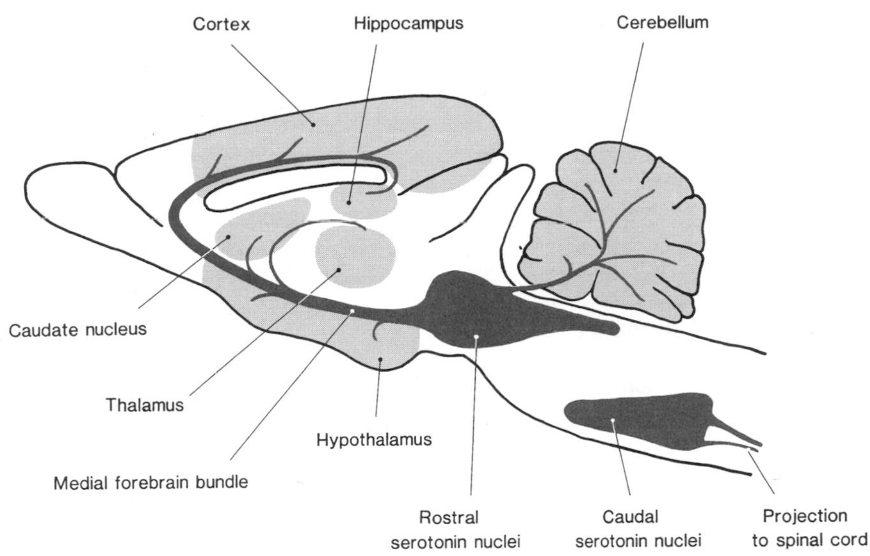

Fig. 24.5 5-HT pathways in the rat brain, drawn as in Figure 24.1.

Table 24.2 Main locations and functions of 5-HT receptors in the brain

	Receptor				
	5-HT_{1A}	5-HT_{1C}	5-HT_{1D}	5-HT_2	5-HT_3
Location	Limbic system Hypothalamus Cortex Dorsal horn	Choroid plexus Basal ganglia	Cortex Striatum Dorsal horn	Neocortex (esp. motor) Limbic system	Limbic system Area postrema
Function					
Synaptic	Postsynaptic inhibition	Postsynaptic excitation (slow)	Presynaptic inhibition	Postsynaptic excitation (slow)	Postsynaptic excitation (fast)
Behavioural	Mood/emotion Nociception	CSF secretion Motor function	Motor function	Stereotyped behaviour Mood/emotion Hallucinations	Anxiety Emesis

Sleep, wakefulness and mood

Lesions of the raphe nuclei, or depletion of 5-HT by PCPA administration abolish sleep in experimental animals, whereas micro-injection of 5-HT at specific points in the brainstem induces sleep. Attempts to cure insomnia in man by giving 5-HT precursors (tryptophan or 5-hydroxytryptophan) have, however, proved unsuccessful. There is evidence that 5-HT, as well as noradrenaline, may be involved in the control of mood (see Ch. 29), and the use of tryptophan to enhance 5-HT synthesis has been tried in depression, with equivocal results.

Sensory transmission

After lesions of the raphe nuclei or administration of PCPA, animals show exaggerated responses to many forms of sensory stimulus. They are startled much more easily, and also quickly develop avoidance responses to stimuli that would not normally produce this effect. It appears that the normal ability to disregard irrelevant forms of sensory input requires intact 5-HT pathways. The 'sensory enhancement' produced by hallucinogenic drugs may be partly due to antagonism of 5-HT. 5-HT also exerts an inhibitory effect on transmission in the pain pathway, both in the spinal cord and in the brain, and there is a synergistic effect between 5-HT and analgesics such as morphine (see Ch. 31). Thus depletion of 5-HT by PCPA, or selective lesions to the descending 5-HT-containing neurons that run to the dorsal horn, antagonise the analgesic effect of morphine, while inhibitors of 5-HT uptake have the opposite effect. 5-HT is also thought to be an inhibitory transmitter in the retina. These effects, on nociception and retinal function, may be aspects of the more general inhibitory effect of 5-HT on sensory input (see above). The correlation of these behavioural phenomena with specific receptor subtypes is not yet clear; Table 24.2, though oversimplified, summarises current views.

Other functions in which 5-HT has been implicated include the control of food intake and various autonomic and endocrine functions, such as the regulation of body temperature, blood pressure, and sexual function. Further information can be found in Green (1985) and Marsden & Heal (1992), and the putative role of 5-HT in psychiatric disorders is discussed by Siever et al. (1991).

It will be realised that 5-HT is involved in many very important physiological processes, and there is clearly scope for new drugs that influence 5-HTergic transmission in a selective way. Such drugs are now becoming available: for example, antidepressants that act by blocking 5-HT re-uptake (Ch. 29); **buspirone**, a 5-HT_{1A}-receptor agonist (Ch. 8), is effective in treating anxiety (Ch. 27); 5-HT_3-receptor antagonists, such as **ondansetron** (Ch. 8), which are used principally as anti-emetic agents (see Ch. 19), are active in animal models of anxiety, and may prove to be clinically useful in this context.

5-hydroxytryptamine in the CNS

- The processes of synthesis, storage, release, re-uptake and degradation of 5-HT in the brain are very similar to events in the periphery (Ch. 8).
- Availability of tryptophan is the main factor regulating synthesis.
- Urinary excretion of 5-HIAA provides a measure of 5-HT turnover.
- 5-HT neurons are concentrated in the midline raphe nuclei in the pons and medulla, projecting diffusely to the cortex, limbic system, hypothalamus and spinal cord, similarly to the noradrenergic projections.
- Functions associated with 5-HT pathways include:
  - —various behavioural responses (e.g. hallucinatory behaviour, 'wet-dog shakes')
  - —feeding behaviour
  - —control of mood and emotion
  - —control of sleep/wakefulness
  - —control of sensory pathways, including nociception
  - —control of body temperature
  - —vomiting.
- 5-HT can exert inhibitory or excitatory effects on individual neurons, acting either presynaptically or postsynaptically.
- The main receptor subtypes (see Table 24.2) in the CNS are: 5-HT_{1A}, 5-HT_{1B}, 5-HT_{1D}, 5-HT_2, 5-HT_3. Associations of behavioural and physiological functions with these receptors have been partly worked out.

ACETYLCHOLINE

There are numerous cholinergic neurons in the central nervous system, and the basic processes by which acetylcholine is synthesised, stored and released are the same as in the periphery (see Ch. 6). Various biochemical markers have been used to locate cholinergic neurons in the brain, the most useful being choline acetyltransferase (CAT), the enzyme responsible for acetylcholine synthesis, which can be labelled by immunofluorescence. Acetylcholine itself cannot be made visible by histochemical techniques. The location of acetylcholinesterase, which can readily be stained, is sometimes used to indicate the presence of acetylcholine, but its distribution is widespread and not specific to cholinergic pathways. Biochemical studies on acetylcholine precursors and metabolites are generally more difficult than corresponding studies on other amine transmitters, because the relevant substances, choline and acetate, are less distinctive biochemically, and involved in many processes other than acetylcholine metabolism.

Central cholinergic pathways

Acetylcholine is very widely distributed in the brain, occurring in all parts of the forebrain (including the cortex), midbrain and brainstem, though there is rather little in the cerebellum. Some of the main cholinergic pathways in the brain are shown in

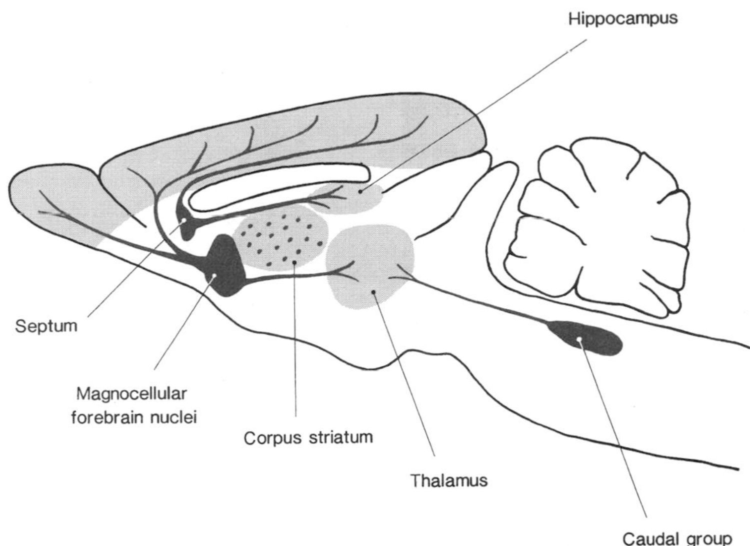

Fig. 24.6 Cholinergic pathways in the rat brain, drawn as in Figure 24.1.

Figure 24.6 (see Woolf 1991). The anterior horns and roots of the spinal cord, and the motor nuclei of the cranial nerves contain about five times as much acetylcholine as other parts of the CNS, reflecting the presence of cholinergic motoneurons supplying skeletal muscle. There is a diffuse cholinergic innervation supplying all areas of the forebrain, and the cell bodies of these cholinergic neurons lie in a small area of the basal forebrain, forming the magnocellular forebrain nuclei (so called because the cell bodies are conspicuously large). Other groups of cholinergic neurons occur in the septum, from which the septohippocampal projection arises, and in the pons, from which fibres run to the thalamus and cortex (see Fig. 24.6).

Short cholinergic interneurons are also found in the striatum and in the nucleus accumbens (two areas where dopaminergic neurons are important). The role of the striatal cholinergic neurons in connection with parkinsonism and Huntington's chorea is discussed in Chapter 25.

Acetylcholine receptors in the brain

The effect of acetylcholine on individual neurons is usually excitatory, and may be mediated by either nicotinic or muscarinic receptors, of which several subtypes occur in the brain (see Ch. 6). Some neurons show an inhibitory response, mediated by muscarinic receptors.

The muscarinic receptors in the brain are very similar in their pharmacological properties to those elsewhere (see Ch. 6), and it is believed that the central actions of **muscarinic antagonists** and anticholinesterases depend on block and stimulation of these receptors, respectively. Muscarinic receptors act presynaptically to inhibit acetylcholine release from cholinergic neurons, and muscarinic antagonists, by blocking this inhibition, markedly increase acetylcholine release. Most of the behavioural effects associated with cholinergic pathways seem to be produced by acetylcholine acting on muscarinic, rather than nicotinic receptors.

Nicotinic receptors are much sparser in the brain than muscarinic receptors, and little is known about their function. They resemble peripheral nicotinic receptors in their molecular structure (see Ch. 2), but many different subtypes exist (see Role 1992). In a few cases, specific agonists and antagonists have been identified, which should help to clarify their functional role. Surprisingly, there is only one example (the Renshaw synapse; see below) where nicotinic ACh receptors are known to participate in excitatory transmission; elsewhere this does not seem to be their role. These receptors probably mediate the effects of nicotine itself (see Ch. 33).

Many of the drugs that block nicotinic receptors (e.g. **tubocurarine**; see Ch. 6) do not cross the blood–brain barrier, and even those that do (e.g. **mecamylamine**) produce no major CNS side effects.

Functional aspects

The first cholinergic synapse to be investigated in the CNS was that of the Renshaw cell in the ventral horn of the spinal cord. These small interneurons receive an excitatory cholinergic innervation from a branch of the axon of the motoneuron. This synapse works through nicotinic receptors, and its pharmacological properties are very similar to those of the neuromuscular junction (Ch. 6). The Renshaw cell in turn activates interneurons that form inhibitory synaptic connections with motoneurons.

Other functional characteristics of cholinergic pathways have been deduced mainly from studies of the action of drugs that mimic, accentuate or block the actions of acetylcholine on muscarinic receptors, so the evidence tends to be indirect and circumstantial.

The main functions ascribed to cholinergic pathways are related to arousal and learning, and motor control. Electroencephalographic (EEG) recording has often been used to monitor the state of arousal in man or in experimental animals. A drowsy, inattentive state is associated with a large amplitude, low frequency EEG record, which switches to a low amplitude, high frequency pattern on arousal by any sensory stimulus (Fig. 24.7). Administration of **physostigmine** (an anticholinesterase that crosses the blood–brain barrier) produces EEG arousal, whereas **atropine** has the opposite effect. It is presumed that the cholinergic projection from the ventral forebrain to the cortex mediates this response. The relationship of this response to behaviour is confusing, however, for the EEG changes produced by physostigmine are the same as those produced by **amphetamine**, whereas the behavioural effects are not. Thus physostigmine in man causes a state of lethargy and anxiety, and in rats it depresses exploratory activity, whereas amphetamine has the opposite effects. Furthermore, atropine causes excitement and agitation, and increases exploratory activity in rats.

There is much evidence that cholinergic pathways, in particular the septohippocampal pathway, are involved in learning and short-term memory (see Hagan & Morris 1988). For example (Fig. 24.8), mice may be trained to execute a maze-running manoeuvre in response to a buzzer, and many will remember the correct response when re-tested 7 days later. If they are given an intracerebral injection of a muscarinic agonist, **arecoline,** immediately after the training session, the percentage forgetting

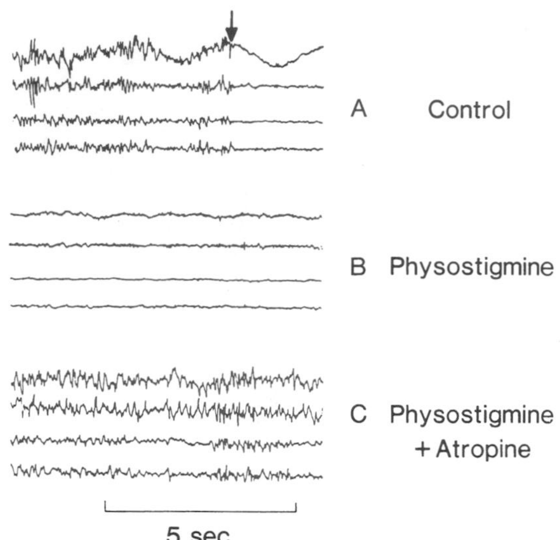

Fig. 24.7 The effect of physostigmine and atropine on EEG activity in a conscious cat. A. Normal resting EEG, with a sudden cessation of slow wave activity (the arousal response) following a sharp sound (arrow). **B.** After physostigmine, showing arousal pattern throughout. **C.** After atropine, which antagonises the effect of physostigmine, re-establishing the resting EEG pattern. (From: Bradley P B, Elkes J 1957 Brain 80: 77)

the correct response 7 days later is reduced, whereas an injection of the muscarinic antagonist, **hyoscine** (scopolamine) has the opposite effect. In the experiment shown in Figure 24.8 a deliberate bias was introduced, in that the mice selected for the arecoline test were particularly dim (the fast-learners having been excluded), and the training was brief, so that the forgetting rate in the control group was about 70%; an optimal dose of arecoline reduced this to about 15%. The hyoscine test was done on the cleverest mice (the no-hopers being excluded), and the training was more thorough, so the forgetting rate in the control group was only about 20%; the highest dose of hyoscine increased this to 70%. Though discordant results have also been reported, there is now general agreement, based on pharmacological and lesioning techniques, that the septohippocampal cholinergic pathway, acting through muscarinic receptors, is important in learning and short-term memory. Hyoscine also impairs memory in human subjects (Sahakian 1988), and amnesia is a well-documented effect of hyoscine used as pre-anaesthetic medication in clinical practice. It is notable that most of these positive results have been

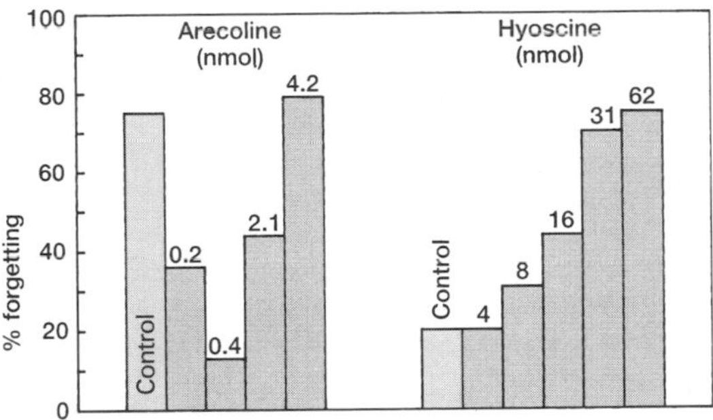

Fig. 24.8 Effect of arecoline and hyoscine on learning. Mice were trained to perform a behavioural feat in order to avoid an electric shock, and tested for their ability to remember it 7 days later. The group that performed least well (left) were given the cholinergic agonist **arecoline** by intracerebroventricular injection; at low doses, their performance improved markedly, but at higher doses, their performance declined. The group that performed best in the initial test were given the muscarinic-receptor antagonist **hyoscine**, which caused a deterioration of their performance. (From: Flood et al. 1981 Brain Res 215: 177–185)

obtained with hyoscine, and that atropine in similar studies has often been found to have no effect.

Some studies have also shown improvement of learning by anticholinesterase drugs or muscarinic agonists, such as arecoline, which enter the brain, but this finding has not been universal (see Sahakian 1988), and in several studies in man it has been found that the state of lethargy, nausea and general misery produced by physostigmine adversely affects learning.

The involvement of cholinergic neurons in neurodegenerative conditions such as dementia and Parkinson's disease is discussed in Chapter 25.

Acetylcholine in the CNS

- Synthesis, storage and release of acetylcholine in the CNS are essentially the same as in the periphery (Ch. 6).
- ACh is widely distributed in the CNS, important pathways being:
  - —basal forebrain (magnocellular) nuclei, which send a diffuse projection to most forebrain structures
  - —septohippocampal projection
  - —short interneurons in the striatum and nucleus accumbens
  - —recurrent inhibitory pathway from spinal motoneurons.
- Certain neurodegenerative diseases, especially dementia and parkinsonism (see Ch. 25) are associated with abnormalities in cholinergic pathways.
- Both nicotinic and muscarinic ACh receptors occur in the CNS. The former mediate the central effects of nicotine. The recurrent motoneuron inhibitory (Renshaw) pathway is the only known example of transmission mediated by nicotinic receptors.
- Muscarinic receptors appear to mediate the main behavioural effects associated with ACh, namely effects on arousal, and on learning and short-term memory.
- Centrally acting anticholinesterase drugs (e.g. physostigmine) and muscarinic agonists (e.g. arecoline) are reported to improve performance in short-term memory, though their clinical usefulness is unproven.
- Muscarinic antagonists (e.g. hyoscine) cause amnesia.
- Acetylcholinesterase released from neurons may have functional effects distinct from cholinergic transmission.

Secreted acetylcholinesterase

In addition to its well-established role as a membrane enzyme responsible for the rapid hydrolysis of acetylcholine (see Ch. 6), there is evidence that acetylcholinesterase may itself be released by neuronal activity and be capable of modulating neuronal excitability (see Appleyard 1992). This view, somewhat heretical, is supported by evidence suggesting that injection of purified AChE into regions of the brain devoid of cholinergic synapses can cause various behavioural effects. One possibility is that AChE possesses some protease activity, and that its effects are secondary to the production of peptide fragments from local protein substrates. Whatever the mechanism, the concept of an enzyme functioning as a released neural mediator is a novel one, whose implications remain to be explored.

EXCITATORY AMINO ACIDS

Excitatory amino acids (EAA) as CNS transmitters

Amino acids, particularly glutamate and aspartate, and possibly homocysteate (Fig. 24.9) are the principal and ubiquitous transmitters mediating fast excitatory synaptic responses in the central nervous

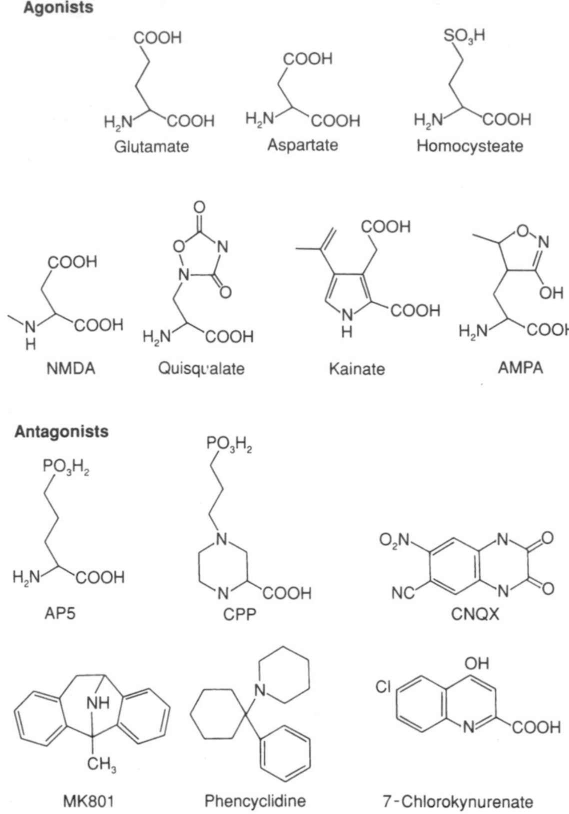

Fig. 24.9 Structures of excitatory amino acid (EAA)-receptor agonists and antagonists.

system. The realisation of their importance has come slowly, starting in the 1950s. At this time, work on the peripheral nervous system had highlighted the transmitter roles of acetylcholine and catecholamines, and as the brain also contained these substances, there seemed little reason to look further. To the hurrying paparazzi writing the EAA news of the 1990s this is, in Krnjevic's phrase, the era of Prehistory. The presence of γ-aminobutyric acid (GABA; see below) in the brain, and its powerful inhibitory effect on neurons, were discovered in the 1950s, and its transmitter role was postulated. At the same time, work by Curtis' group in Canberra showed that glutamate and various other acidic amino acids produced a strong excitatory effect, but it seemed inconceivable that such workaday metabolites could actually be transmitters. There then followed the Dark Ages of the 1960s, when neither GABA nor EAAs were thought to be more than pharmacological curiosities, even by their discoverers. The Renaissance came in the 1970s, when the role of another amino acid, glycine, was established as an inhibitory transmitter in the spinal cord, giving the lie to the idea that the transmitters had to be specialised or ornate molecules, too beautiful to do anything but sink into the arms of a receptor. Once glycine had been accepted, acceptance of GABA quickly followed. A great deal of pharmacological effort went into finding antagonists for EAA effects, particularly by Watkins, working in Bristol. From this work came the realisation that there are several types of EAA receptor, and it was the finding that antagonists for one of these receptors can block synaptic transmission in the CNS that finally established the theory.

In the last 15 years, there has been an exuberant proliferation of EAA research, referred to by Krnjevic as the Baroque era. To do full justice to what has been discovered is beyond the range of this book, but the interested reader can find his or her way by consulting review articles, for example Lodge & Collingridge (1990), Hicks et al. (1987), Monaghan et al. (1989), Kemp & Leeson (1993), Schoep & Conn (1993), Seeburg (1993). Here we will concentrate on those aspects that have important pharmacological implications. So far, no drugs have been introduced on the basis of EAA mechanisms, but activity in this area is intense, and the future therapeutic prospects look very encouraging.

Metabolism and release of amino acids

Glutamate, like GABA, is widely and fairly uniformly distributed in the CNS. It has an important metabolic role, being involved in both carbohydrate and nitrogen metabolism, the metabolic and neurotransmitter pools being linked by transaminase enzymes that catalyse the interconversion of glutamate and α-oxoglutarate (Fig. 24.10). The main sources of glutamate and aspartate are the Krebs cycle intermediates, though glutamine also serves as a source. These intermediates and reactions occur in virtually all cells, so they have not been particularly useful in understanding the transmitter function of EAAs. The close relationship between the pathways for the synthesis of EAAs and inhibitory amino acids (GABA and glycine), shown in Figure 24.10, also makes it difficult to use experimental manipulations of transmitter synthesis to study the functional role of individual amino acids.

Though the evidence was slow in coming, it is now well established that glutamate is stored in

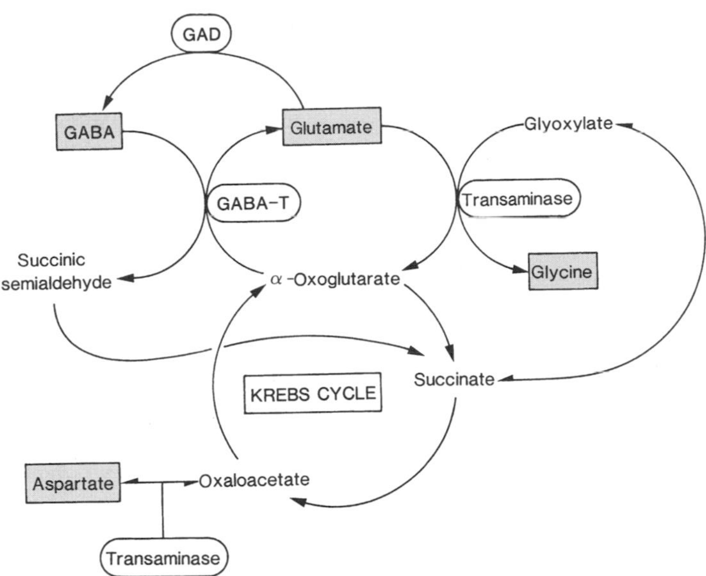

Fig. 24.10 Metabolism of transmitter amino acids in the brain. (GABA = gamma-aminobutyric acid; GAD = glutamic acid decarboxylase; GABA-T = GABA transaminase) Transmitter substances are marked with light pink boxes.

synaptic vesicles and released by calcium-dependent exocytosis. Furthermore, the use of receptor antagonists (see below) has confirmed its importance as a transmitter at many central synapses.

The action of glutamate is terminated mainly by carrier-mediated re-uptake into the nerve terminals and neighbouring glial cells. This transport can, under some circumstances (e.g. depolarisation by increased extracellular potassium), operate in reverse and constitute a source of glutamate release (see Attwell et al. 1993); a process which may occur under pathological conditions such as brain ischaemia (see Ch. 25).

EAA receptors

On the basis of studies with selective agonists and antagonists, three main subtypes of EAA receptors can be distinguished, namely *NMDA*, *AMPA* and *metabotropic* receptors (Table 24.3), all of which have been cloned and studied in great detail (see Seeburg 1993, Schoep & Conn 1993). NMDA (N-methyl-D-aspartate) and AMPA (α-amino-3-hydroxy-5-methyl-isoxazole) receptors are named on the basis of the selective agonists that have been discovered. Both types are directly coupled to cation channels (ionotropic receptors), though their conductance and ion selectivities are different. The metabotropic receptor falls into the class of G-protein-coupled receptors, and acts mainly to release inositol phosphates and diacylglycerol as intracellular second messengers (see Ch. 2); in some situations, metabotropic receptors appear to act through cAMP or arachidonic acid. Cloning studies, you will not be surprised to learn, have revealed a plethora of subtypes of both the ionotropic and metabotropic glutamate receptors. Ionotropic receptors of the AMPA type consist, at the last count, of nine distinct subunits, and there are five known types of NMDA-receptor subunit (Seeburg 1993). Like many other ligand-gated ion channels, the receptors are oligomeric, with individual subunits combining in bewildering 'mix-and-match' combinations to form functional ion channels. The metabotropic receptor, like other G-protein-coupled receptors, is a monomer with seven transmembrane helical domains (see Ch. 2), but it too comes in five or six distinct varieties which appear to activate distinct second messenger systems (Schoep & Conn 1993). Expression of the different subunits shows clear topographic patterns in the brain, but we have hardly begun to understand the significance of this extreme organisational complexity.

AMPA receptors are often divided into two pharmacological subtypes (AMPA and kainate).

Their distribution in the brain is different, but their functions appear to be very similar: both types are thought to participate in fast excitatory transmission.

Specific antagonists for NMDA receptors have been developed by Watkins and his colleagues (see Watkins et al. 1990) by modifying the structure of NMDA. The longer-chain phosphonate analogues, AP5 and AP7 (Fig. 24.9) have been used in many studies; more potent analogues such as CPP and CGS 19755 have been introduced more recently. Though potent, none of these compounds readily crosses the blood–brain barrier, and none so far are suitable for clinical use. Selective receptor antagonists for other types of EAA receptor are shown in Table 24.3.

Studies on the effects of EAA antagonists on synaptic transmission in the CNS suggest that AMPA receptors are responsible for fast excitatory transmission, and operate at many, probably most, CNS synapses. NMDA receptors, on the other hand, are involved in slower excitatory synaptic responses, and in certain types of synaptic plasticity (Fig. 24.12), as discussed below. The metabotropic receptors appear to have a more complex neuromodulatory function, and probably play a part in phenomena such as synaptic plasticity and excitotoxicity (Ch. 25).

The receptors can be selectively labelled, and regional binding studies show that most EAA receptors occur in the cortex, basal ganglia and sensory pathways. NMDA and AMPA receptors are co-localised, but kainate receptors have a somewhat different distribution.

Special features of NMDA receptors

NMDA receptors and their associated channels have been studied in more detail than the other types, especially by Ascher and his colleagues, working in Paris. They show several unusual properties, principally the following:

- They are highly permeable to Ca^{2+}.
- They are readily blocked by Mg^{2+} ions, and this

Table 24.3 Excitatory amino acid receptors

	NMDA		AMPA/kainate	Metabotropic
	Receptor site	Modulatory site		
Endogenous agonist	Glutamate ? Aspartate	Glycine	Glutamate	Glutamate
Other agonists	NMDA	D-serine	AMPA Quisqualate Kainate Domoate	Quisqualate Ibotenate ACPD
Antagonists	D-AP5 CPP CGS 19755	Kynurenate Dichlorokynurenate	CNQX	—
Channel blockers	Dizocilpine (MK 801) Phencyclidine Ketamine Mg^{2+}		—	Not applicable
Effector mechanism	Ligand-gated channel (Slow kinetics) (High Ca^{2+}-permeability)		Ligand-gated channel (Fast kinetics) (Low Ca^{2+}-permeability)	G-protein-coupled (Activation of phospholipase C, causing Ca^{2+} release and PLC activation)
Location	Postsynaptic		Postsynaptic ? Presynaptic (kainate type)	Postsynaptic Presynaptic
Functional role	Slow EPSP Synaptic plasticity (e.g. LTP) Excitotoxicity		Fast EPSP ? Presynaptic inhibition	Modulation (many mechanisms) Excitotoxicity

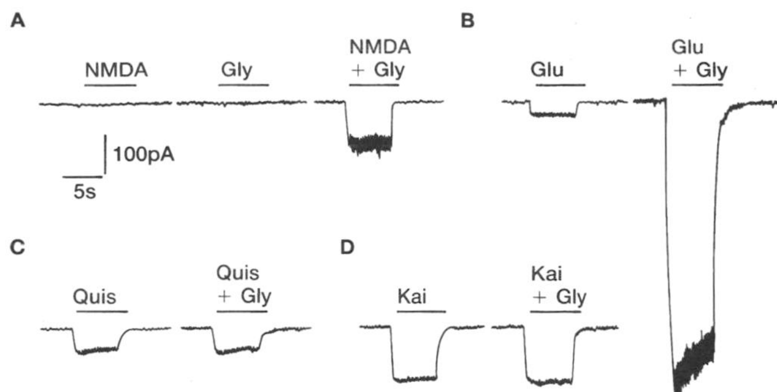

Fig. 24.11 Facilitation of N-methyl-D-aspartate (NMDA)-receptor activation by glycine. Recordings from mouse brain neurons in culture (whole cell patch-clamp technique). Downward deflections represent inward current through EAA-activated ion channels. **A.** NMDA (10 μmol/l) or glycine (1 μmol/l) applied separately had little or no effect, but together produced a response. **B.** The response to glutamate (10 μmol/l, Glu) was strongly potentiated by glycine (1 μmol/l, Gly). **C** and **D.** Responses of AMPA receptors to quisqualate (Quis) and kainate (Kai) were unaffected by glycine. (From: Johnson & Ascher 1987)

block shows marked voltage dependence (i.e. it occurs when the cell is normally polarised, but disappears if the cell is depolarised).

- Channel opening requires *glycine* as well as glutamate (Fig. 24.11; see Thomson 1989); there appears to be a distinct binding site for glycine (the modulatory site; see Table 24.3), separate from the glutamate-binding site, and both have to be occupied for the channel to open. This discovery, made by Johnson & Ascher (1987), caused a stir, because glycine had long been recognised as an inhibitory transmitter, so to find it facilitating excitation ran counter to the prevailing doctrine. EAA specialists are quick on their feet, however, and now refer to glycine as an *EAA-co-agonist* without so much as a blink.
- Certain well-known anaesthetic and psychotomimetic agents, such as **ketamine** (Ch. 26) and **phencyclidine** (Ch. 32), are selective blocking agents for NMDA-operated channels. A newer compound, **dizocilpine**, shares this property.

Functional aspects of NMDA receptors

Recent evidence suggests that, whereas AMPA and kainate receptors are mainly responsible for fast excitatory synaptic transmission in the CNS, NMDA receptors (which often coexist with AMPA/kainate receptors and make a small contribution to excitatory transmission under normal conditions) may have more subtle functions. Three such roles which are now generally accepted are:

- *long-term potentiation*
- *excitotoxicity* (discussed in Ch. 25)
- the *pathogenesis of epilepsy* (discussed in Ch. 28).

Long-term potentiation (LTP). LTP (see Anwyl 1989, Bliss & Collingridge 1993) is the term used to describe a remarkably long-lasting (hours in vitro, days or weeks in vivo) enhancement of synaptic transmission that occurs at various CNS synapses following a short (conditioning) burst of presynaptic stimulation, typically at about 100 Hz for 1 second. It has been studied in great detail in the hippocampus (Fig. 24.12), and its importance lies in its probable relevance to learning and memory, processes in which the hippocampus is known to play a central role. It has been argued that 'learning', in the synaptic sense, can occur if synaptic strength is somehow enhanced after a period of *simultaneous* activity in both pre- and postsynaptic neurons. LTP shows this characteristic; it does not occur if presynaptic activity fails to excite the postsynaptic neuron, or if the latter is activated independently, for instance by different presynaptic input. Thus LTP involves both the presynaptic and postsynaptic components of EAA synapses. The facilitatory process also appears to involve both pre- and postsynaptic elements; the release of glutamate is increased, and so is the sensitivity of the postsynaptic membrane to glutamate. The following experimental results have led to the model shown in Figure 24.13.

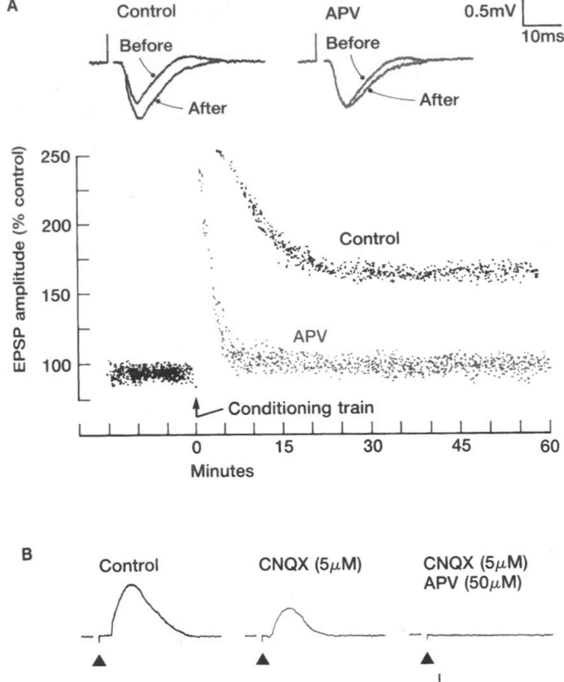

Fig. 24.12 Effects of EAA-receptor antagonists on synaptic transmission. A. APV (NMDA antagonist) prevents long-term potentiation (LTP) in the rat hippocampus without affecting the fast EPSP. Top records show the extracellularly recorded fast EPSP (downward deflection) before, and 50 minutes after, a conditioning train of stimuli (100 Hz for 2 s). The presence of LTP in the control preparation is indicated by the increase in EPSP amplitude. In the presence of APV (50 μmol/l), the normal EPSP is unchanged, but LTP does not occur. Lower trace shows EPSP amplitude as a function of time. The conditioning train produces a short-lasting increase in EPSP amplitude which still occurs in the presence of APV, but the long-lasting effect is prevented. **B.** Block of fast and slow components of EPSP by CNQX (AMPA-receptor antagonist) and APV (NMDA-receptor antagonist). EPSP (upward deflection) in hippocampal neuron recorded with intracellular electrode is partly blocked by CNQX (5 μmol/l), leaving behind a slow component, which is blocked by APV (50 μmol/l). (From: (A) Malinow R, Madison D V, Tsien R W 1988 Nature 335: 821; (B) Andreasen M, Lambert J D, Jensen M S 1989 J Physiol 414: 317-336)

- LTP requires the activation of NMDA receptors, for NMDA antagonists prevent it, without affecting normal, non-potentiated transmission (which depends on AMPA/kainate receptors).
- LTP occurs only if the postsynaptic cell is depolarised at the time when the conditioning burst of stimulation is delivered.
- Calcium entry into the postsynaptic cell is required, and there is evidence that activation of protein kinase C (see Ch. 2) is involved in the mechanism of potentiation.
- LTP is reduced by agents which block the synthesis or effects of nitric oxide or carbon monoxide (see below). One or both of these mediators may be the hitherto elusive 'retrograde messenger' through which events in the postsynaptic cell are able to influence the presynaptic nerve terminal.

It is believed that two special properties of the NMDA receptor and channel underlie its involvement in LTP, namely voltage-dependent channel block by Mg^{2+} and its high Ca^{2+} permeability. At normal membrane potentials the NMDA channel is blocked by Mg^{2+}; a sustained postsynaptic depolarisation produced by glutamate acting repeatedly on AMPA/kainate receptors, however, removes the Mg^{2+} block, and NMDA receptor activation then allows Ca^{2+} to enter the cell. This rise in $[Ca^{2+}]_i$ in the postsynaptic cell is believed to activate protein kinases, and thereby (by mechanisms that are not fully elucidated) to enhance the sensitivity of the AMPA/kainate receptors that mediate the normal transmission process (Fig. 24.13). The metabotropic EAA receptor may also be involved. Activation of this receptor results in the formation of $InsP_3$ and diacylglycerol (see Ch. 2) in the postsynaptic cell, thus contributing to the increase in $[Ca^{2+}]_i$ and also activating protein kinase C, which is known to play a part in maintaining LTP (Anwyl 1989).

Though LTP is now quite well understood as a synaptic phenomenon, its relationship to learning and memory remains very controversial. Some evidence is suggestive: for example, NMDA-receptor antagonists applied to the hippocampus impair learning in rats; also, 'saturation' of LTP by electrical stimulation of the hippocampus has been found to impair the ability of rats to learn a maze. On the other hand, LTP-like changes have not been detected after learning has taken place. Nevertheless, pharmacologists are actively seeking drugs capable of enhancing LTP in the hope that they will improve learning and memory.

LTP is now emerging as just one manifestation of the general phenomenon of *synaptic plasticity* through which neuronal connections respond to

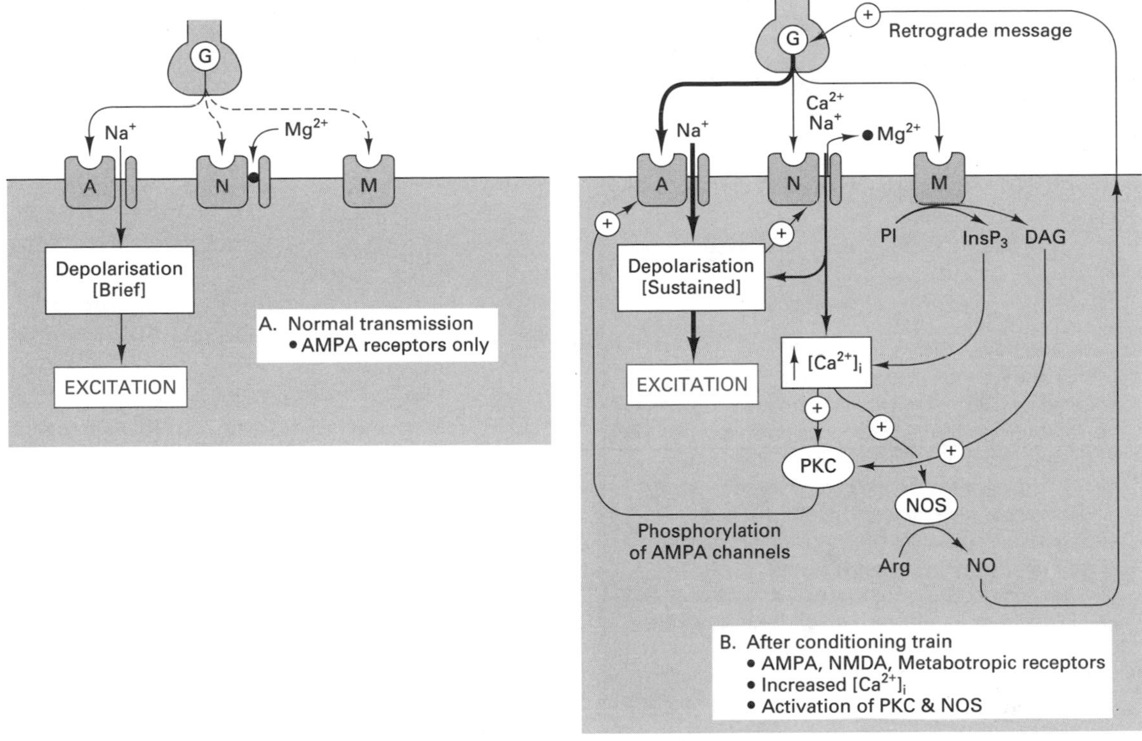

Fig. 24.13 Mechanisms of long-term potentiation (LTP). A. With infrequent synaptic activity, glutamate activates mainly AMPA receptors. There is insufficient glutamate to activate metabotropic receptors, and NMDA-receptor channels are blocked by Mg^{2+}. **B.** After a conditioning train of stimuli, enough glutamate is released to activate metabotropic receptors, and NMDA channels are unblocked by the sustained depolarisation. The resulting increase in $[Ca^{2+}]_i$ activates PKC and NOS. PKC phosphorylates various proteins, including AMPA receptors (causing facilitation of transmitter action) and other signal transduction molecules controlling gene transcription (not shown) in the postsynaptic cell. Release of NO facilitates glutamate release (retrograde signalling, otherwise known as *NO turning back*). (G = glutamate; A = AMPA receptor; N = NMDA receptor; M = metabotropic receptor; PI = phosphatidylinositol; $InsP_3$ = (1,4,5) inositol triphosphate; DAG = diacylglycerol; PKC = protein kinase C; NOS = nitric oxide synthase)

changes in the activity of the nervous system. *Short-term potentiation* and *long-term depression* also occur as quite distinct processes, and are also thought to involve EAA receptors (see Malenka & Nicoll 1993).

EAA antagonists

Much effort, particularly by Watkins and his colleagues, has gone into the search for selective EAA antagonists, partly to provide tools for better understanding the physiological roles of the different types of EAA receptor, and partly as potential therapeutic agents with which to treat, for example, epilepsy and neurodegenerative disorders.

The main types of EAA antagonists are shown in Table 24.3 and Figure 24.9.

At the receptor level, selective antagonists exist for NMDA, and other recent agents (e.g. **CNQX**; Fig. 24.9) show a degree of selectivity for AMPA/kainate receptors. In contrast to the NMDA-receptor antagonist **AP-5**, CNQX is able to block the fast excitatory response to synaptically released glutamate (Fig. 24.12). So far, most of these compounds, though very useful as experimental tools in vitro, are unable to penetrate the blood–brain barrier, so they are not effective when given systemically.

NMDA receptors, as discussed above, require glycine as well as NMDA to activate them, so blocking of the glycine site is an alternative way to produce antagonism. **Kynurenic acid**, and the more potent chloro-analogue, act in this way. Another site of block is the channel itself, where various substances act, for example **ketamine**, **phencyclidine** and

Excitatory amino acids

- EAAs, namely glutamate, aspartate, and possibly homocysteate, are the main fast excitatory transmitters in the CNS.
- Glutamate is formed mainly from the Krebs cycle intermediate, α-oxoglutarate, by the action of GABA-aminotransferase.
- There are three main EAA receptor subtypes (Table 24.3):
  —NMDA
  —AMPA/kainate
  —metabotropic.
- NMDA and AMPA/kainate receptors are directly coupled to cation channels; metabotropic receptors act through intracellular second messengers.
- The channels controlled by NMDA receptors are highly permeant to Ca^{2+} and are blocked by Mg^{2+}.
- AMPA/kainate receptors are involved in fast excitatory transmission; NMDA receptors mediate slower excitatory responses and, through their effect in controlling Ca^{2+} entry, play a more complex role in controlling synaptic plasticity (e.g. long-term potentiation).
- Competitive NMDA-receptor antagonists include AP5, and CPP; the NMDA-operated ion channel is blocked by dizocilpine, as well as by the psychotomimetic drugs, ketamine and phencyclidine.
- CNQX is an antagonist with some selectivity for the AMPA/kainate-receptor antagonist.
- NMDA receptors require glycine as a co-agonist, in addition to glutamate; 7-chlorokynurenate blocks this action of glycine.
- Excessive entry of Ca^{2+} produced by NMDA-receptor activation can result in cell death—excitotoxicity (see Ch. 25).
- EAA-receptor antagonists have yet to be developed for clinical use, but expectations are high.

dizocilpine (see Lodge & Johnson 1990). These agents are lipid soluble, and thus able to cross the blood–brain barrier.

The potential therapeutic interest in NMDA antagonists lies mainly in the reduction of brain damage following strokes (Ch. 25) and in the treatment of epilepsy (Ch. 30). The major drawback of these agents is their tendency to cause hallucinatory and other disturbances (also a feature of phencyclidine; Ch. 32), so their usefulness remains to be assessed (see Lipton 1993).

GAMMA-AMINOBUTYRIC ACID (GABA)

Synthesis, storage and function

GABA occurs in brain tissue, but not in other mammalian tissues, except in trace amounts. In the brain it is particularly abundant (about 10 μmol/g tissue) in the nigrostriatal system, but occurs at lower concentrations (2–5 μmol/g) throughout the grey matter.

GABA is formed from glutamate (Fig. 24.10) by the action of *glutamic acid decarboxylase* (GAD), an enzyme that has been used, with immunohistochemical labelling, to map the distribution of GABA-synthesising neurons in the brain. GABA is destroyed by a transamination reaction, in which the amino group is transferred to α-oxoglutaric acid (to yield glutamate), with the production of succinic semialdehyde, and then succinic acid. This reaction is catalysed by *GABA-transaminase* (GABA-T), a widespread enzyme believed to be located in mitochondria. GABA-ergic neurons have an active GABA uptake system, and it is this, rather than GABA-T, which removes the GABA after it has been released.

GABA is thought to function as an inhibitory transmitter in many different CNS pathways. The most detailed studies have been carried out on the cerebellum, cerebral cortex, hippocampus and striatum. In most situations GABA is found in short interneurons, the only long GABA-ergic tracts being those running to the cerebellum and striatum. The widespread distribution of GABA, and the fact that virtually all neurons are sensitive to its inhibitory effect, suggest that its function is ubiquitous in the brain. It has been estimated that GABA serves as a transmitter at about 30% of all the synapses in the CNS.

GABA receptors

When the importance of GABA as an inhibitory transmitter was recognised, it was thought likely that a GABA-like substance might prove to be effective in controlling epilepsy and other convulsive states; since GABA itself fails to penetrate the blood–brain barrier, a search was begun for more lipophilic GABA analogues. One such substance is the p-chlorophenyl derivative of GABA (**baclofen**; see Bowery 1982) which was introduced in 1972. However, differences between the actions of GABA and baclofen soon became evident. Baclofen, like GABA, inhibits the release of transmitter from many types of nerve terminal, but, unlike GABA, has little postsynaptic inhibitory effect. Furthermore, the postsynaptic inhibitory effect of GABA is blocked competitively by the convulsant drug, **bicuculline**, but the actions of baclofen are not antagonised. Other GABA-like substances (e.g. **muscimol**) produce the postsynaptic bicuculline-sensitive effects of GABA, but not the presynaptic, bicuculline-resistant effects. Pharmacologists love nothing more than spotting a new receptor, so the former effects were assigned to $GABA_A$ receptors, and the latter to $GABA_B$ receptors (Table 24.4; see reviews by Simmonds 1983, Bowery 1993).

Electrophysiological studies of the action of GABA on CNS neurons (see review by Bormann 1988) have shown that its postsynaptic inhibitory effect is mediated mainly by $GABA_A$ receptors, which are coupled directly to anion channels, and thus cause an increase in chloride permeability of the postsynaptic membrane; this has the effect of reducing the depolarisation produced by excitatory transmitter action. $GABA_B$ receptors, on the other hand, are located mainly on presynaptic terminals, belong to the family of G-protein-coupled receptors (Ch. 2), and act via intracellular second messengers. The details are not yet known, but the end results are an increased K^+ conductance (causing membrane hyperpolarisation) and inhibition of voltage-sensitive Ca^{2+} channels, leading to inhibition of transmitter release.

GABA exerts this type of inhibitory effect on presynaptic nerve terminals at many sites in the brain and peripheral nervous system (e.g. dopamine-releasing terminals of the striatum and peripheral sympathetic terminals).

Cloning of $GABA_A$ receptors has shown that, as expected, they belong to the class of ligand-gated ion channels, similar in their general architecture to nicotinic ACh receptors and ionotropic glutamate receptors. They also show similar molecular complexity in the form of multiple subunits, which are differentially expressed in different brain regions, and which confer different pharmacological properties (see Burt & Kamatchi 1991, Luddens & Wisden 1991).

Drugs affecting GABA-mediated transmission

Various selective agonists for $GABA_A$ and $GABA_B$ receptors are known (Table 24.4), the principal examples being **muscimol** ($GABA_A$ selective) and **baclofen** ($GABA_B$ selective). Selective antagonists exist for both $GABA_A$ receptors (e.g. **bicuculline**) and for $GABA_B$ receptors (e.g. **phaclofen**). These agents have been very useful in experimental studies, but are not used therapeutically.

The convulsant effect of **picrotoxin** (Ch. 32) is due to its ability to block the chloride channel associated with the $GABA_A$ receptor, thus blocking the postsynaptic inhibitory effect of GABA.

A remarkable relationship exists between $GABA_A$ receptors and the actions of the **benzodiazepine** group of drugs, which have powerful sedative and anxiolytic effects (see Ch. 27). These drugs selectively potentiate the effects of GABA on $GABA_A$ receptors, and there is evidence that they bind with high affinity to an accessory site on the $GABA_A$ receptor, in such a way that the binding of GABA is facilitated and its pharmacological activity is enhanced. It is interesting that $GABA_A$ receptors occur in a variety of peripheral neurons (e.g. autonomic ganglion cells) where GABA has no transmitter role; at these sites, however, there is no potentiating effect of benzodiazepines. Certain barbiturates (see Ch. 27) also potentiate $GABA_A$ effects, but they are much less selective than benzodiazepines, and the relevance of this phenomenon to their overall depressant actions on the nervous system is uncertain (see Ch. 26).

Table 24.4 Classification of GABA receptors

	Receptor type	
	$GABA_A$	$GABA_B$
Effects	Postsynaptic inhibition ↑ Cl^- conductance	Presynaptic inhibition ↓ Ca^{2+} conductance ↑ K^+ conductance
Agonists		
GABA	+	+
Baclofen	–	+
Muscimol	+	–
Antagonists		
Bicuculline	Competitive	–
Picrotoxin	Non-competitive	–
Phaclofen	–	+
Potentiators		
Benzodiazepines	+	–
Barbiturates	+	–

Reconstitution studies with cloned $GABA_A$ receptors show that sensitivity to benzodiazepines depends critically on one of the five receptor subunits. It was recently found (Korpi et al. 1993) that a mutant rat that is particularly susceptible to the behavioural effects of benzodiazepines has a single point mutation in this particular subunit.

GLYCINE

The amino acid glycine is present in particularly high concentration (5 µmol/g) in the grey matter of the spinal cord. Applied ionophoretically to motoneurons or interneurons it produces an inhibitory hyperpolarisation that is indistinguishable from the inhibitory synaptic response. Most significantly, **strychnine** (see Ch. 32), a convulsant drug that acts mainly on the spinal cord, blocks both the synaptic inhibitory response and the response to glycine. This, together with direct measurements of glycine release in response to nerve stimulation, provides strong evidence for its physiological transmitter role. β-alanine has pharmacological effects and a pattern of distribution very similar to glycine, but its action is not blocked by strychnine.

The role of glycine in facilitating excitatory responses mediated by NMDA has been mentioned above (p. 509). This effect is quite distinct from its inhibitory functions; for example the action of glycine at NMDA receptors is blocked by 7-chlorokynurenate, but not by strychnine. So far there is much speculation, but not much evidence, about the physiological role of glycine's action at NMDA receptors. The very low concentrations of glycine required for this effect, in relation to the concentration normally present in the brain, suggest that it may serve as a constant enabling factor for NMDA-receptor-mediated effects of glutamate, rather than as a regulatory mechanism. Don't bet on it, though.

Inhibitory amino acids: GABA and glycine

- GABA is the main inhibitory transmitter in the brain.
- It is present fairly uniformly throughout the brain; there is very little in peripheral tissues.
- GABA is formed from glutamate, by the action of GAD (glutamic acid decarboxylase). It is removed mainly by re-uptake, but also by deamination, catalysed by GABA-transaminase.
- There are two types of GABA receptor, $GABA_A$ and $GABA_B$.
- $GABA_A$ receptors, which occur mainly postsynaptically, are directly coupled to chloride channels, opening of which reduces membrane excitability. Muscimol is a specific $GABA_A$ agonist, and the convulsant, bicuculline, is an antagonist.
- Other drugs that interact with $GABA_A$ receptors and channels include (i) benzodiazepine tranquillisers, which act at an accessory binding site to facilitate the action of GABA, and (ii) convulsants such as picrotoxin, which block the anion channel.
- $GABA_B$ receptors are mainly responsible for presynaptic inhibition, and act via second messengers. Baclofen is a $GABA_B$-receptor agonist, and phaclofen is an antagonist.
- Glycine is an inhibitory transmitter mainly in the spinal cord, acting on its own receptor, which functionally resembles the $GABA_A$ receptor.
- The convulsant drug, strychnine, is a competitive glycine antagonist. Tetanus toxin acts mainly by interfering with glycine release.

HISTAMINE

Histamine has been discussed as a possible neurotransmitter for many years, and the evidence supporting this is now strong (see Schwartz et al. 1991). It is present in the brain in much smaller amounts than in other tissues, such as skin and lung, and much of the brain content of histamine is due to mast cells rather than neurons. If the mast cells are depleted, however, some histamine remains, and this is associated with the nerve-ending fraction of the brain homogenate. Vesicular storage of histamine in neurons, and calcium-dependent release evoked by electrical stimulation, have been demonstrated. Histamine receptors are widely distributed in the brain.

The biosynthetic enzyme, histidine decarboxylase, is present mainly in neurons, and is probably a better marker than histamine itself, since mast cells, whose histamine store turns over much more slowly than that of neurons, have relatively little histidine decarboxylase.

Anatomically, histamine-containing neurons originate mainly from a small region of the hypothalamus, and their axons run in the medial forebrain bundle (which carries a variety of monoamine-containing projections) to large areas of the cortex and midbrain. Stimulation of the medial forebrain produces an inhibitory response in cortical and hippocampal neurons, which is partly blocked by metiamide, an H_2-receptor antagonist.

Applied ionophoretically to central neurons, histamine produces either excitatory or inhibitory effects. In most cases the excitatory effects are blocked by H_1 antagonists and the inhibitory effects by H_2 antagonists. H_1-receptors are biochemically coupled to phospholipase C and phospholipid hydrolysis, whereas H_2-receptors act through adenylate cyclase and cAMP generation. A third type of receptor, H_3, is much less well understood, but may function mainly as a presynaptic inhibitory receptor.

Although many selective agonists and antagonists of the various histamine receptor subtypes are known (see Ch. 11), the effects of these agents on central nervous system function are generally modest. Though suggestions as to its function abound (see Schwartz et al. 1991), histamine remains a minor player on the neurotransmitter stage.

NITRIC OXIDE

Nitric oxide as a peripheral mediator is discussed in Chapter 10. Its significance as an important chemical mediator in the nervous system has become apparent only since 1988, and demands a considerable readjustment of our views about neurotransmission and neuromodulation. The main defining criteria for transmitter substances—namely that neurons should possess machinery for synthesising and storing the substance, that it should be released from neurons by exocytosis, that it should interact with specific membrane receptors, and that there should be mechanisms for its inactivation—do not apply to nitric oxide. Moreover, it is an inorganic toxic gas, not at all like the kind of molecule we are used to. Recent evidence, however, clearly assigns to nitric oxide, and probably also to **carbon monoxide**, an important mediator function (see Bredt & Snyder 1992, Vincent & Hope 1992, Verma et al. 1993).

The evidence for nitric oxide as a mediator comes mainly from: (a) the widespread distribution in neurons of nitric oxide synthase (NOS), the enzyme which produces NO from arginine, and the correspondence of this distribution with that of soluble guanylate cyclase, the target enzyme on which NO acts (see Ch. 10); (b) studies showing that inhibition of NOS has marked effects on various types of synaptic plasticity. Much less is known so far about carbon monoxide, but the parallels seem to be close (Table 24.5). The distribution of the CO-generating enzyme, haem oxygenase, differs from that of NOS, but also corresponds closely with that of guanylate cyclase.

The constitutive form of NOS is mainly confined to two kinds of cells, namely vascular endothelial cells and neurons—both peripheral and central. Within the brain, it is particularly abundant in the cerebellum and hippocampus. Activation of NOS occurs in response to a rise in intracellular calcium concentration, through the mediation of the calcium-

Table 24.5 Nitric oxide and carbon monoxide as mediators

	Nitric oxide (NO)	Carbon monoxide (CO)
Formation		
Precursor	Arginine	Haem
Enzyme	NO synthase (NOS)	Haem oxygenase
Inhibited by	L-NMMA L-NAME	Zn protoporphyrin
Activated by	Intracellular Ca^{2+}	Not known
Effect	Activates soluble guanylate cyclase Increases cGMP	Activates soluble guanylate cyclase Increases cGMP
Inactivated by	Haemoglobin	Haemoglobin
Implicated in	Vasodilatation (Ch. 10) Smooth muscle relaxation (Ch. 10) LTP/LTD (this chapter) Neuroprotection/neurotoxicity (Ch. 25)	? LTP (this chapter)

binding protein, calmodulin (see Ch. 2). NO is produced within seconds and escapes rapidly from the neuron by diffusion. There is no storage or specialised release mechanism. It can act either within the neuron or on neighbouring neurons or glial cells.

A flurry of work is in progress to elucidate the functional role of NO in the nervous system. There is good evidence that it is involved in various types of synaptic plasticity, especially long-term potentiation (LTP) and long-term depression (LTD), which are discussed above. It also has complex effects on neuronal survival in pathological conditions such as cerebral ischaemia (see Ch. 25).

The role of carbon monoxide (CO, better known as a poisonous gas present in vehicle exhaust, which binds strongly to haemoglobin, producing death by tissue anoxia) as a CNS mediator is less well established, but the synthetic enzyme, haem oxygenase, is widely distributed. CO, like NO, stimulates soluble guanylate cyclase, and may well have a physiological role.

Undoubtedly, further functions of NO and CO in the brain will soon be identified, and novel therapeutic approaches are expected to come from targeting the different steps in the synthetic and signal transduction pathways for these surprising mediators. We may have to endure the ponderous whimsy of many 'NO' puns, but it should be worth it.

THE CLASSIFICATION OF PSYCHOTROPIC DRUGS

Psychotropic drugs are defined as those that affect mood and behaviour. Because these are extremely complex functions, arriving at a satisfactory classification of drug effects is far from straightforward, and no single basis for classification has been found to be satisfactory. Thus, classification on a chemical basis, which produces categories such as **benzodiazepines, butyrophenones**, etc. does not give much guide to pharmacological effects. A pharmacological or biochemical classification, on the other hand, is appealing for drugs whose mechanism of action is reasonably well understood (e.g. **monoamine-oxidase inhibitors, catecholamine uptake blockers**, etc.), but there are still many instances (e.g. **hallucinogens**) where the mechanism of action is too poorly understood to form the basis of a reliable classification. Another possibility is to adopt an empirical classification based on clinical use, and divide drugs into categories such as **antidepressants, antipsychotic agents**, etc. but this has the weakness that some important psychotropic drugs have no clinical use, or their use may have changed or been superseded according to clinical fashion. **Amphetamine**, for example, a drug with well-characterised effects on mood and behaviour, has had an extremely chequered clinical history and would have been dismissed, revived and reclassified many times if a purely clinical classification had been adopted.

Because no single basis for classifying psychotropic drugs is satisfactory, different authorities tend to offer a variety of hybrid, and often incompatible schemes, and the scene is undoubtedly one of some confusion.

The following classification (see Tyrer 1982) is based on that suggested in 1967 by the World Health Organization; although not watertight it provides a useful basis for the material presented later (Chs 27–29 and 32).

- **Anxiolytic sedatives**
  Synonyms: hypnotics, sedatives, minor tranquillisers
  Definition: drugs that cause sleep and reduce anxiety
  Examples: barbiturates, benzodiazepines and ethanol
  See Chapters 27 and 33
- **Antipsychotic drugs**
  Synonyms: neuroleptic* drugs, antischizophrenic drugs, major tranquillisers
  Definition: drugs that are effective in relieving the symptoms of schizophrenic illness
  Examples: phenothiazines and butyrophenones
  See Chapter 28
- **Antidepressant drugs**
  Synonym: thymoleptics*

---

*These strange terms are the remnants of a classification proposed by Javet in 1903, who distinguished psycholeptics (depressants of mental function), psychoanaleptics (stimulants of mental function), and psychodysleptics (drugs that produce disturbed mental function). The term neuroleptic (literally 'nerve-seizing') was coined 50 years later to describe chlorpromazine-like drugs (see Ch. 28). It gained favour, presumably by virtue of its brevity rather than its literal meaning.

Definition: drugs that alleviate the symptoms of depressive illness
Examples: monoamine oxidase inhibitors and tricyclic antidepressants
See Chapter 29

- **Psychomotor stimulants**
Synonym: psychostimulants
Definition: drugs that cause wakefulness and euphoria
Examples: amphetamine, cocaine and caffeine
See Chapter 32
- **Hallucinogenic drugs**
Synonyms: psychodysleptic drugs (see footnote on p. 516), psychotomimetic agents
Definition: drugs that cause disturbance of perception (particularly visual hallucinations) and of behaviour in ways that cannot be simply characterised as sedative or stimulant effects
Examples: lysergic acid diethylamide (LSD), mescaline and phencyclidine
See Chapter 32.

Some drugs defy classification in this scheme; for example, **lithium** (see Ch. 29), which is used in the treatment of manic-depressive psychosis, and **ketamine** (see Ch. 26), which is classed as a dissociative anaesthetic, but produces psychotropic effects rather similar to those produced by phencyclidine.

Another category that has come into vogue is *nootropic drugs*, meaning drugs that enhance mental performance (see Ch. 25). It was coined to define drugs resembling **piracetam**, which were reported to improve mental function in various tests by an unknown mechanism. Clinical trials of such drugs in dementia have shown them to be largely ineffective, and the term appears to reflect the wish of the discoverers of piracetam to give the drug a status that it does not obviously deserve.

CLINICAL USE OF PSYCHOTROPIC DRUGS

The term *psychosis* refers to a group of mental disorders (e.g. schizophrenia, manic-depressive psychosis; see Chs 28 and 29), which are considered to be endogenous in origin (i.e. they represent some inherent malfunction of the brain), as distinct from *neurosis*, typified by anxiety states, phobias, and so on, which is regarded as an abnormal reaction to external circumstances (see Ch. 27). Though still useful, this distinction is not clear-cut. Thus, many, if not most, patients complaining of excessive anxiety also show features of depression, and schizophrenic patients frequently appear depressed or anxious in addition to showing the characteristics of schizophrenia. Correspondingly, the use of drugs in psychiatric illness often ignores the conventional demarcations into specific therapeutic categories such as anxiolytic agents, antipsychotic drugs, antidepressant drugs, etc. which are listed above. The simple-minded pharmacologist, confronted with the realities of clinical practice, may find this confusing. Here we will adhere to the conventional pharmacological categories, but it needs to be emphasised that in clinical use these distinctions may be less clear-cut.

REFERENCES AND FURTHER READING

Aghajanian G K 1993 Central 5-HT receptor subtypes: physiological responses and signal transduction mechanisms. In: Marsden C A, Heal D J (eds) Central serotonin receptors and psychotropic drugs. Blackwell, Oxford

Anwyl R 1989 Protein kinase C and long-term potentiation in the hippocampus. Trends Pharmacol Sci 10: 236–239

Appleyard M E 1992 Secreted acetylcholinesterase: non-classical aspects of a classical enzyme. Trends Neurosci 15: 485–490

Ashton H 1992 Brain function and psychotropic drugs. Oxford University Press, Oxford

Attwell D, Barbour B, Szatkowski M 1993 Nonvesicular release of neurotransmitter. Neuron 11: 401–407

Barrio J R, Huang S, Phelps M E 1988 In vivo assessment of neurotransmitter biochemistry in humans. Annu Rev Pharmacol Toxicol 28: 213–230

Bliss T V P, Collingridge G L 1993 A synaptic model of memory: long-term potentiation in the hippocampus. Nature 361: 31–38

Bormann J 1988 Electrophysiology of $GABA_A$ and $GABA_B$ receptor subtypes. Trends Neurosci 11: 112–116

Bowery N G 1982 Baclofen: 10 years on. Trends Pharmacol Sci 3: 400–403

Bowery N G 1993 $GABA_B$ receptor pharmacology. Annu Rev Pharmacol Toxicol 33: 109–147

Bredt D S, Snyder S H 1992 Nitric oxide, a novel neuronal messenger. Neuron 8: 3–11

Burt D R, Kamatchi G L (1991) $GABA_A$ receptor subtypes: from pharmacology to molecular biology. FASEB J 5: 2916–2923

Civelli O, Bunzow J R, Grandy D K 1993 Molecular diversity of the dopamine receptors. Annu Rev Pharmacol Toxicol 32: 281–307

Cooper J R, Bloom F E, Roth R H 1991 Biochemical basis of neuropharmacology. Oxford University Press, New York
Giros B, Caron M 1993 Molecular characterization of the dopamine transporter. Trends Pharmacol Sci 14: 43–49
Green A R (ed) 1985 Neuropharmacology of serotonin. Oxford University Press, Oxford
Hagan J J, Morris R G M 1988 The cholinergic hypothesis of memory: a review of animal experiments. In: Iversen L L, Iversen S, Snyder S H (eds) Handbook of psychopharmacology. Plenum Press, New York, vol 20: 237–323
Hicks T P, Lodge D, McLennan H (eds) 1987 Excitatory amino acid transmission. Liss, New York
Johnson J W, Ascher P 1987 Glycine potentiates the NMDA response in cultured mouse brain neurons. Nature 325: 529–531
Kemp J A, Leeson P D 1993 The glycine site of the NMDA receptor—five years on. Trends Pharmacol Sci 14: 20–25
Korpi E R, Kleingoor C, Kettermann H, Seeburg P H 1993 Benzodiazepine-induced motor impairment linked to point mutation in cerebellar $GABA_A$ receptor. Nature 361: 356–359
Lipton S A 1993 Prospects for clinically tolerated NMDA antagonists: open-channel blockers and alternative redox states of nitric oxide. Trends Neurosci 16: 527–532
Lodge D, Collingridge G 1990 Les agents provocateurs: a series on the pharmacology of excitatory amino acids. Trends Pharmacol Sci 11: 22–24 (series of reviews in this journal published in 1990)
Lodge D, Johnson K M 1990 Noncompetitive excitatory amino acid receptor antagonists. Trends Pharmacol Sci 11: 81–86
Luddens H, Wisden W 1991 Function and pharmacology of multiple $GABA_A$ receptor subunits. Trends Pharmacol Sci 12: 49–51
Malenka R C, Nicoll R A 1993 NMDA-receptor-dependent synaptic plasticity: multiple forms and mechanisms. Trends Neurosci 16: 521–527
Marsden C A, Heal D J (eds) 1992 Central serotonin receptors and psychotropic drugs. Blackwell, Oxford
Monaghan D T, Bridges R J, Cotman C W 1989 The excitatory amino acid receptors: their classes, pharmacology, and distinct properties in the function of the nervous system. Annu Rev Pharmacol Toxicol 29: 365–402
Peroutka S J 1988 5-Hydroxytryptamine receptor subtypes: molecular, biochemical and physiological characterization. Trends Neurosci 11: 496–500
Rogawski M A 1987 New directions in neurotransmitter action: dopamine provides some important clues. Trends Neurosci 10: 200–205
Role L W 1992 Diversity in primary structure and function of nicotinic acetylcholine receptor channels. Curr Opin Neurobiol 2: 254–262
Sahakian B J 1988 Cholinergic drugs and human cognitive performance. In: Iversen L L, Iversen S, Snyder S H (eds) Handbook of psychopharmacology. Plenum Press, New York, vol 20: 373–425
Schildkraut J J 1965 The catecholamine hypothesis of affective disorders: a review of supporting evidence. Am J Psychiatry 122: 509–522
Schoep D D, Conn P J 1993 Metabotropic glutamate receptors in brain function and pathology. Trends Pharmacol Sci 14: 13–20
Schwartz J-C, Arrang J-M, Garbarg M, Pollard H, Ruat M 1991 Histaminergic transmission in the mammalian brain. Physiol Rev 71: 1–51
Seeburg P H 1993 The molecular biology of mammalian glutamate receptor channels. Trends Neurosci 16: 359–365
Sibley D R, Monsma F J 1992 Molecular biology of dopamine receptors. Trends Pharmacol Sci 13: 61–69
Siever L J, Kahn R S, Lawlor B A, Trestman R L, Lawrence T L, Coccaro E F 1991 Critical issues in defining the role of serotonin in psychiatric disorders. Pharm Rev 43: 509–525
Simmonds M A 1983 Multiple GABA receptors and associated regulatory sites. Trends Neurosci 6: 279–281
Thomson A 1989 Glycine modulation of the NMDA receptor/channel complex. Trends Neurosci 12: 349–353
Tyrer P J 1982 Drugs in psychiatric practice. Butterworth, London
Ungerstedt U 1971 On the anatomy, pharmacology and function of the nigrostriatal dopamine system. Acta Physiol Scand Suppl 367
Vallar L, Meldolesi J 1989 Mechanisms of signal transduction at the dopamine D_2 receptor. Trends Pharmacol Sci 10: 74–77
Van Tol H M M, Wu C M, Guan H C, Ohara K, Bunzow J R 1992 Multiple dopamine D_4 receptor variants in the human population. Nature 358: 149–152
Verma A, Hirsch D J, Glatt C E, Ronnett G V, Snyder S H 1993 Carbon monoxide: a putative neural messenger. Science 259: 381–384
Vincent S R, Hope B T 1992 Neurons that say NO. Trends Neurosci 15: 108–113
Watkins J C, Krogsgaard-Larsen P, Honore T 1990 Structure–activity relationships in the development of excitatory amino acid receptor agonists and competitive antagonists. Trends Pharmacol Sci 11: 25–33
Webster R A, Jordan C C (eds) 1989 Neurotransmitters, drugs and disease. Blackwell, Oxford
Woolf N J 1991 Cholinergic systems in mammalian brain and spinal cord. Prog Neurobiol 37: 475–524

25
NEURODEGENERATIVE DISORDERS

MECHANISMS OF NEURODEGENERATION

With few exceptions, CNS neurons cannot divide, nor can they regenerate when their axons are interrupted. Thus, any pathological process causing neuronal loss generally has irreversible consequences. At first sight, this appears to be very unpromising territory for pharmacological intervention, and indeed drug therapy currently has rather little to offer, except in the particular case of Parkinson's disease (see below). Nevertheless, the high incidence and social impact of neurodegenerative brain disorders has resulted in a massive research effort in recent years, and considerable advances have been made, which may be translated into therapeutic progress in the not-too-distant future. In this chapter, we discuss:

- mechanisms responsible for neuronal death, especially **excitotoxicity** and **oxidative stress**
- pharmacological approaches (so far hypothetical) to preventing neuronal loss
- pharmacological approaches to compensation for neuronal loss.

The discussion focuses mainly on three common neurodegenerative conditions, namely dementia (Alzheimer's disease), ischaemic brain damage (stroke) and Parkinson's disease. The hurried reader may safely skip straight to page 527 without missing anything of current therapeutic importance.

EXCITOTOXICITY

Though it seems surprising, in view of their established role as neurotransmitters, EAAs are able to cause neuronal death (see Choi 1988). A low concentration of glutamate applied to neurons in culture kills a large proportion of the cells, and local injection of a glutamate analogue, such as kainic acid, has been widely used as a method for destroying neurons in vivo. This effect of kainic acid is not direct, but depends on the excitation of local glutamate-releasing neurons, and it is the release of glutamate that leads to neuronal death. It is known that these cytotoxic actions are mediated through NMDA receptors, for they are blocked by NMDA antagonists, and that calcium entry is a necessary step. The sequence of events (referred to as excitotoxicity; see Olney 1990, Beal 1992) resulting in cell death (Fig. 25.1) is similar to what happens in cardiac muscle cells (Ch. 13) during cardiac ischaemia. There are many possible ways in which Ca^{2+} overload may kill cells, including activation of intracellular proteases and lipases, impaired mitochondrial function as the mitochondria take up Ca^{2+} from the cytosol, generation of free radicals, etc. (see Ch. 43). Two additional mechanisms triggered by the rise in Ca^{2+} may also contribute to excitotoxicity. First, NO synthesis (see Chs 10 and 24) appears to be important, since inhibitors of NO synthase are able to protect against glutamate-induced neurotoxicity (Dawson et al. 1991); the mechanism is not well understood, but may be related to free

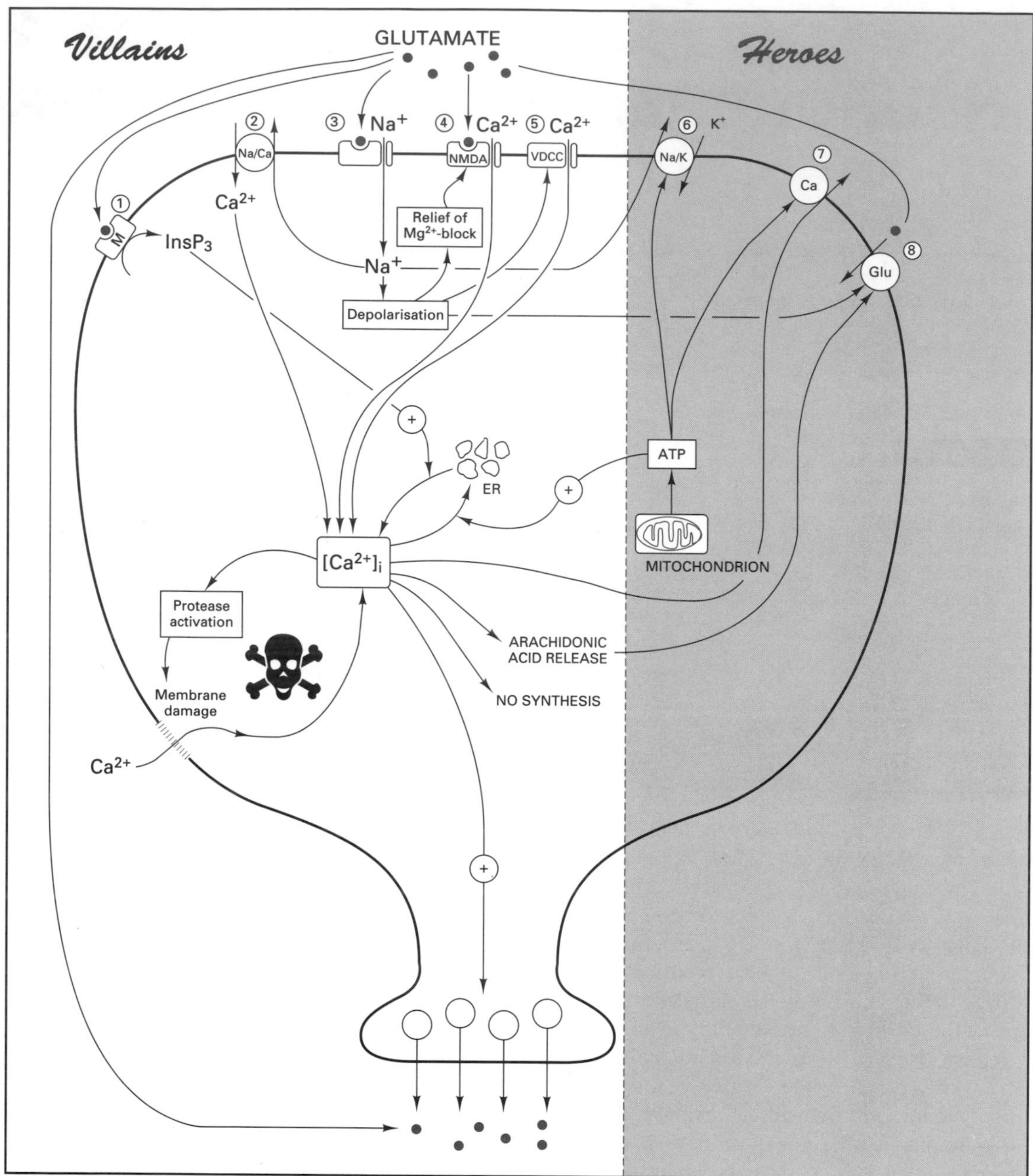

Fig. 25.1 Mechanisms of excitotoxicity. ER = endoplasmic reticulum.

radical production (see below). Secondly, production of arachidonic acid may inhibit the glutamate uptake carrier, thus causing the action of glutamate to be enhanced.

Defence against glutamate neurotoxicity is clearly an important issue if our brains are to stay alive. Mitochondrial energy metabolism provides a main line of defence (see Beal et al. 1993). Mitochondrial ATP production fuels both the sodium/potassium pump (thereby sustaining the membrane potential) and calcium uptake by the endoplasmic reticulum, both of which provide protection against excitotoxicity. It may be that impaired ATP production is a common precipitating factor in various neurodegenerative conditions, and that it works by rendering neurons vulnerable to excitotoxic damage.

Though there is much speculation about excitotoxicity in relation to neurodegenerative disease (see review by Lipton & Rosenberg 1994), the only clear experimental data showing its involvement in brain pathology is in ischaemic brain damage (see below). Excitotoxicity is believed to occur in severe epilepsy (see Ch. 30) in which appreciable neuronal degeneration, leading eventually to progressive dementia, accompanies the bursts of neuronal activity that occur during epileptic attacks. It is also postulated as a major factor in Parkinson's disease and Huntington's disease (see below; Beal 1992, Lipton & Rosenberg 1994).*

In addition, there are several examples of neurodegenerative conditions caused by environmental toxins, acting as agonists on glutamate receptors (see Olney 1990). Domoic acid is a glutamate analogue produced by mussels, which was identified as the cause of an epidemic of severe mental and neurological deterioration in a group of Newfoundlanders in 1987. On the island of Guam, a syndrome combining the features of dementia, paralysis and Parkinson's disease has been tracked down to an excitotoxic amino acid, β-methylamino-alanine, present in the seeds of a local cycad. Discouraging the consumption of these seeds is now reducing the incidence of the disease. At a more down-to-earth level, the copious addition of monosodium glutamate to food as a 'flavour enhancer' raises the question of possible neurotoxicity. The 'Chinese restaurant syndrome'—an acute attack of neck stiffness and chest pain—is known to result from excessive glutamate, but so far the possibility of more serious neurotoxicity is only hypothetical.

Possible therapies based on the excitotoxicity concept include the development of glutamate-receptor (especially NMDA-receptor) antagonists (see Ch. 24), calcium-channel-blocking drugs (Ch. 14), and inhibitors of calcium-activated proteases. None have yet been developed and proven as therapies, but activity in this area is intense (see Lipton & Rosenberg 1994).

*A recent clinical trial (Bensimon et al. 1994) has suggested that treatment with an inhibitor of EAA transmission, **riluzole**, is of some benefit to patients with *amyotrophic lateral sclerosis*, a fatal paralytic disease resulting from progressive degeneration of motoneurons. Riluzole appears to inhibit both the release and the postsynaptic action of glutamate.

OXIDATIVE STRESS

The brain derives nearly all its energy from mitochondrial oxidative phosphorylation, which generates ATP at the same time as reducing molecular O_2 to H_2O. Under certain conditions, highly reactive species, for example $\bullet O_2^-$, $\bullet OH$ free radicals, and H_2O_2 may be generated as side products of this process (see Coyle & Puttfarken 1993). Oxidative stress is the result of excessive production of these reactive species. They can also be produced as a by-product of other biochemical pathways, including NO synthesis and arachidonic acid metabolism (which are implicated in excitotoxicity; see above and Fig. 10.3), as well as the mixed function oxidase system (see Ch. 4). Unchecked, reactive oxygen radicals attack many key molecules, including

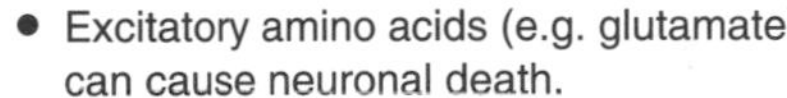

Excitotoxicity and oxidative stress

- Excitatory amino acids (e.g. glutamate) can cause neuronal death.
- Excitotoxicity is associated mainly with activation of NMDA receptors, but other types of EAA receptors also contribute.
- Excitotoxicity results from a sustained rise in intracellular calcium concentration (calcium overload).
- Excitotoxicity can occur under pathological conditions (e.g. cerebral ischaemia) in which excessive glutamate release occurs. It can also occur when chemicals such as kainic acid are administered.
- Raised intracellular calcium causes cell death by various mechanisms, including activation of proteases, formation of free radicals, and lipid peroxidation. Formation of NO and arachidonic acid are also involved.
- Various mechanisms act normally to protect neurons against excitotoxicity, the main ones being calcium transport systems, mitochondrial function and the production of free radical scavengers.
- Oxidative stress refers to conditions (e.g. hypoxia) in which the protective mechanisms are compromised, and neurons become more susceptible to excitotoxic damage.
- Excitotoxicity due to environmental chemicals may contribute to some neurodegenerative disorders.
- Measures designed to reduce excitotoxicity include the use of glutamate antagonists, calcium-channel-blocking drugs and free radical scavengers; none are yet proven for clinical use.

enzymes, membrane lipids and DNA. Not surprisingly, defence mechanisms are provided, in the form of enzymes such as superoxide dismutase (SOD) and catalase, as well as antioxidants, such as ascorbic acid, glutathione and α-tocopherol (vitamin E), which act normally to keep these reactive species in check. It is possible that accumulated or inherited mutations in enzymes such as those of the mitochondrial respiratory chain lead to a congenital or age-related increase in susceptibility to oxidative stress, which is manifest in different kinds of inherited neurodegenerative disorders (such as Huntington's disease), and in age-related neurodegeneration (see Beal et al. 1993).

Therapeutic interventions based on the oxidative stress concept have yet to be proven, but theoretical possibilities include the use of free radical scavengers and antioxidants, as well as the inhibition of NO synthase and arachidonic acid production.

ISCHAEMIC BRAIN DAMAGE

Ischaemic brain damage, along with Parkinson's disease (see below), is one of the few neurodegenerative disorders that can be studied in animals, and much is known about the mechanisms involved. After heart disease and cancer, strokes are the commonest cause of death in Europe and North America, and they cause major handicap in about 1% of the population. It is clear that the loss of neurons following interruption of blood supply to the brain is not simply due to the cells dying for lack of oxygen. A complex cascade of events takes place, including movements of ions, pH changes, generation of mediators such as NO and arachidonic acid, production of free radicals, and the development of cerebral oedema (see Kogure et al. 1993). Following acute ischaemia, these processes can take many hours to develop, so there is potential for reversing or ameliorating the process in its early stages.

There is strong evidence that glutamate excitotoxicity delivers the final neuronal death blow in ischaemic brain damage (Rothman & Olney 1986, McCulloch 1992). Thus, it is known that ischaemia causes depolarisation of neurons, and the release of large amounts of glutamate. Ca^{2+} can be shown to enter the cells, mainly as a result of glutamate acting on NMDA receptors, for both Ca^{2+} entry and cell death following cerebral ischaemia are inhibited by NMDA-receptor- or channel-blocking drugs (see Ch. 24).

Attempts to develop drugs to improve the outcome after strokes have so far been disappointing. **Nimodipine** (a calcium-channel antagonist; see Ch. 14), which was expected to improve cell survival by reducing calcium entry following depolarisation, was ineffective in clinical trials; it actually increased the risk of cerebral haemorrhage, possibly by causing vasodilatation. NMDA antagonists, such as **dizocilpine**, and other glutamate-receptor antagonists, are effective in animal models, but have not yet been tested thoroughly in man. It appears that most NMDA antagonists produce unpleasant psychological symptoms in man, which will certainly be a disadvantage, though it may not preclude their use in emergency situations. The use of **adenosine analogues**, which act presynaptically to inhibit glutamate release, is another therapeutic possibility, not yet proven. A critical factor in any therapy for stroke will be the time 'window' available between the vascular event and irreversible neuronal loss.

DEMENTIA AND ALZHEIMER'S DISEASE

Loss of intellectual ability with age is considered to be a normal process, and the definition of pathological dementia is quite vague. Alzheimer's disease was originally defined as *presenile* dementia, but it now appears that the same pathology underlies the dementia irrespective of the age of onset. The term *dementia of the Alzheimer type* (DAT) thus denotes all dementias that do not have an obvious organic cause, such as stroke, brain damage or alcohol. Its prevalence rises sharply from the age of about 60 years, and reaches 90% or more by the age of 95. Until recently, age-related dementia was considered to result from the steady and unavoidable loss of neurons that goes on throughout life, possibly accelerated by a failing blood supply associated with atherosclerosis. It is now clear that DAT is associated with quite specific biochemical abnormalities, which raises the hope—not yet realised—of being able to inhibit the neurodegenerative process by drug treatment. The biochemical mechanisms are well reviewed by Selkoe (1991, 1993), Gottfries (1992), Mullan & Crawford (1993); approaches to therapy are discussed by Davis et al. (1993).

PATHOLOGICAL CHANGES

DAT is associated with a general shrinkage of brain tissue, but with relatively little loss of cortical neurons. Two microscopic features are characteristic of the disease, namely *amyloid plaques*, consisting of amorphous extracellular deposits of β-amyloid protein, and *neurofibrillary tangles*, comprising filaments of a phosphorylated form of a protein normally associated with intraneuronal microtubules. These appear also in normal brains, though in smaller numbers, and their physical occurrence may predate the onset of dementia by many years. There is considerable evidence, albeit indirect, to relate Alzheimer's disease with abnormalities in the constitution or processing of these two proteins, though other mechanisms, such as slow virus infection, or aluminium toxicity, may also be involved.

Amyloid deposits consist of a 40- to 42-residue protein, Aβ (sometimes called β/A4; Fig. 25.2), which is believed to be the main culprit responsible for neurodegeneration. Aβ is produced by proteolytic cleavage of a much larger *amyloid precursor protein* (APP), which is a membrane protein normally expressed by many CNS neurons. The cleavage of APP is a complex process; normally the large extracellular domain is snipped off and released as soluble APP, which may exert various regulatory functions (see Mattson et al. 1993). Formation of Aβ requires extracellular cleavage at a different point, and an additional cleavage in the intramembrane domain of APP (Fig. 25.2). It is believed that this special pattern of cleavage occurs either as a result of mutations in the APP gene (which have been demonstrated in a rare form of inherited early-onset DAT), or because of abnormal types of

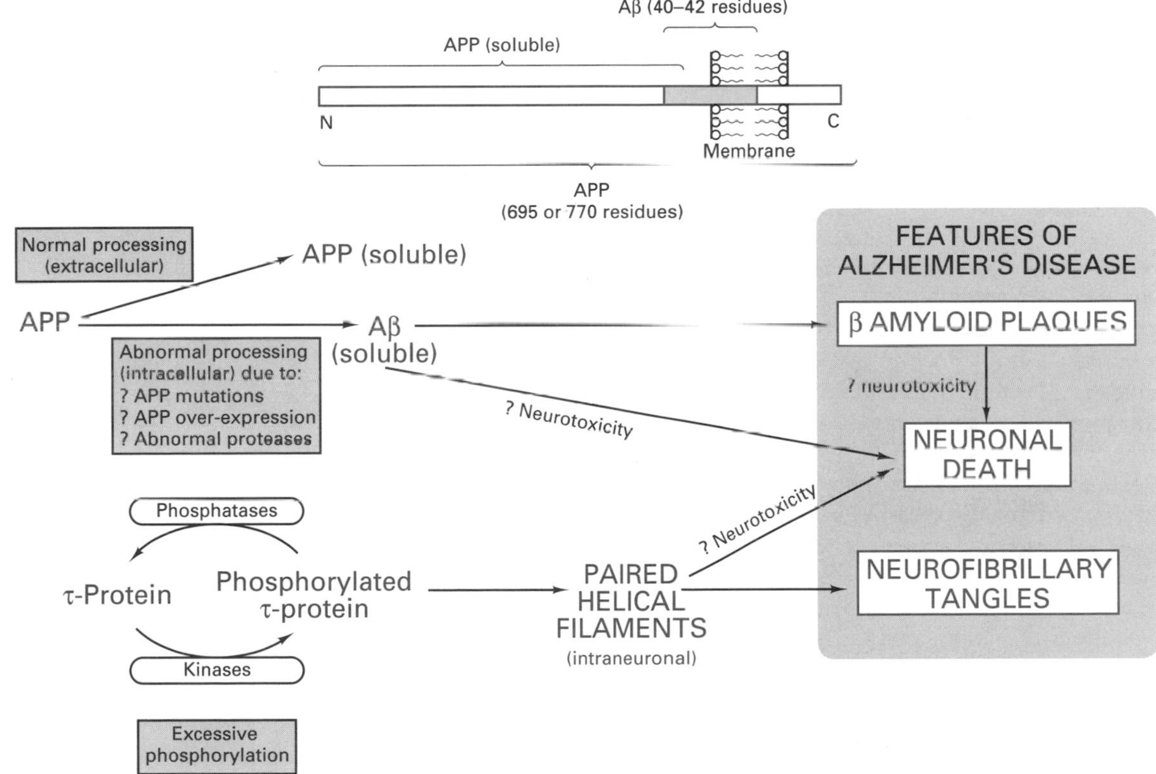

Fig. 25.2 Pathogenesis of Alzheimer's disease. The amyloid precursor protein (APP) is normally processed by extracellular cleavage to produce the secreted (soluble) form of the protein, which is not associated with neuronal damage. Abnormal processing by cleavage at different sites, results in formation of the soluble Aβ fragment, which causes neurodegeneration and the deposition *of amyloid plaques.* The microtubule-associated τ-protein is excessively phosphorylated in Alzheimer's disease, and aggregates as intracellular *paired helical filaments*, which may be toxic to the cell, later giving rise to extracellular *neurofibrillary tangles.*

protease activity. In fact, Aβ formation occurs at a low level in normal cells, so DAT may represent only a small quantitative shift in the pathway. How Aβ production is linked to neurodegeneration remains controversial, and some authors regard it as bystander rather than assassin. There is, however, increasing evidence that Aβ is inherently neurotoxic (see Mattson et al. 1993) and can also enhance the effect of other neurotoxins, including glutamate (see above). The other main player on the biochemical stage is the protein of which the neurofibrillary tangles are composed, the *τ-protein* (Fig. 25.2), though its exact role in the pathogenesis is unclear. This protein is a normal constituent of neurons, being associated with intracellular microtubules. In DAT it becomes abnormally phosphorylated, and is deposited intracellularly as *paired helical filaments* with a characteristic microscopic appearance. When the cells die, these filaments aggregate as extracellular neurofibrillary tangles. Whether intracellular deposition of the filaments harms the cell is not certain, but inhibiting the phosphorylation reaction is one of the biochemical strategies being explored in the hope of finding a way to inhibit progress of the disease.

Though changes in many transmitter systems have been demonstrated in DAT brains, mainly from measurements on post-mortem brain tissue, a relatively selective loss of cholinergic neurons in the basal forebrain nuclei is characteristic. This discovery, made in 1976, implied that pharmacological approaches to restoring cholinergic function might be feasible. Lesions of the nucleus basalis produce cognitive and learning deficits in experimental animals.

Choline acetyl transferase (CAT) activity in the cortex and hippocampus is reduced considerably (30–70%) in DAT but not in other psychological disorders, such as depression or schizophrenia, and acetylcholinesterase activity is also greatly reduced. The number of muscarinic receptors, determined by binding studies, is not affected, but the number of nicotinic receptors, particularly in the cortex, is reduced.

So far, there are no animal models for DAT which adequately reproduce the underlying neurodegenerative process, which occurs spontaneously only in higher primates. Transgenic mice incorporating the APP gene mutation discovered in families with inherited early-onset DAT have been produced, but appear not to show characteristic DAT pathology. This lack of good animal models makes the testing of potential DAT therapies very difficult.

Dementia and Alzheimer's disease

- Progressive dementia (dementia of Alzheimer type; DAT) is a normal accompaniment of advancing age, distinct from vascular dementia associated with brain infarction.
- The main pathological features of DAT comprise amyloid plaques, neurofibrillary tangles, and a loss of neurons (particularly cholinergic neurons of the basal forebrain).
- Amyloid plaques consist of the Aβ fragment of amyloid precursor protein (APP), a normal neuronal membrane protein. The causes of excessive Aβ formation are not known, but may include: mutations affecting APP; excessive phosphorylation of APP; abnormal APP proteases. There is some evidence that Aβ is neurotoxic.
- Neurofibrillary tangles comprise aggregates of a highly phosphorylated form of a normal neuronal protein. The relationship of these structures to neurodegeneration is not known.
- Loss of cholinergic neurons is believed to account for much of the learning and memory deficit in DAT.
- Currently available therapies for DAT are only marginally effective at best; most have shown little or no benefit in controlled trials. The most widely used are putative vasodilators (dihydroergotamine), muscarinic agonists (arecoline, pilocarpine) and anticholinesterases (physostigmine, tacrine).

THERAPEUTIC APPROACHES

In spite of the recent advances in understanding the mechanism of neurodegeneration in DAT, there are still no effective therapies. The main approaches are summarised in Table 25.1 (see also Davis et al. 1993). The cholinesterase inhibitor, **tacrine**, was recently introduced, on the basis that enhancement of cholinergic transmission might compensate for the cholinergic deficit that occurs in DAT. Trials have given equivocal results, and any improvement in cognitive performance among DAT patients is likely to be limited at best (Davis et al. 1992).

PARKINSON'S DISEASE

NATURE OF PARKINSON'S DISEASE

Parkinson's disease is a progressive disorder of movement that occurs most commonly in the elderly. The main symptoms are:

- tremor at rest, usually starting in the hands and resulting in 'pill-rolling' movements, which tend to diminish during voluntary activity
- muscle rigidity, which is detectable as an increased resistance to passive limb movement
- decrease in the frequency of voluntary movements (hypokinesia), which is partly the result of muscle rigidity, but partly due to an inherent inertia of the motor system, which means that motor activity is difficult to stop as well as to initiate.

Parkinsonian patients show a characteristic shuffling gait with short paces, which takes some effort for them to begin, and once in progress they cannot quickly stop or change direction. Parkinson's disease is commonly associated with dementia, though this is probably a reflection of the same degenerative process affecting other parts of the brain, rather than a direct consequence of the damage to the basal ganglia that is responsible for the motor symptoms.

Parkinson's disease often occurs with no obvious underlying cause, but it may be the result of viral encephalitis or other types of pathological damage. It can also be drug-induced, the main drugs that cause it being those that reduce the amount of dopamine in the brain (e.g. **reserpine**; see Ch. 7), or block dopamine receptors (e.g. neuroleptic drugs, such as **chlorpromazine**; see Ch. 28). In contrast to schizophrenia and many other neurological and behavioural disorders, Parkinson's disease shows no hereditary tendency, and an environmental cause seems more likely (see below).

Table 25.1 Therapeutic approaches in dementia

Approach	Mechanism	Drugs and therapies	Status
Available or in development			
Improved blood flow/ psychostimulation	Vasodilatation Effects on monoamine receptors	Dihydroergotoxine Pentoxyfylline	Many trials of vasodilators, psychostimulants, antidepressants, etc. Efficacy not proven
Nootropic agents*	Not known	Piracetam	Improved learning and memory in animal models Efficacy not proven
Cholinergic replacement therapy	Cholinesterase inhibitors	Physostigmine Tacrine	Modest efficacy claimed in some trials Hepatotoxicity reported with tacrine
	Muscarinic agonists	Arecoline Pilocarpine New compounds in development	Some efficacy in animal models Peripheral side effects Not yet tested
Hypothetical			
Improved neuronal survival	Neurotrophic factors	Nerve growth factor (NGF) and other growth factors	Improved forebrain cholinergic function in animal models Special delivery systems needed for human use
Halting disease process	Inhibition of amyloid formation	APP protease inhibitors Inhibitors of APP phosphorylation	Not yet developed
	Inhibition of τ-protein deposition	Inhibitors of phosphorylation	Not yet developed
	Inhibition of excitotoxicity	Glutamate antagonists Ca-channel blockers Protease inhibitors, etc.	Being developed mainly in other indications (e.g. stroke)

*Drugs which enhance mental performance. Their existence is controversial (see p. 517).

NEUROCHEMICAL CHANGES

Parkinson's disease has been known for many years to be due to a disorder of the basal ganglia, but its neurochemical origin was discovered by Hornykiewicz in 1960 (see review by Hornykiewicz & Kish 1986), who showed that the dopamine content of the substantia nigra and corpus striatum (see Ch. 24) in post-mortem brains of Parkinson's disease patients was extremely low (usually less than 10% of normal), and this was later correlated with a loss of the cell bodies of dopaminergic neurons from the substantia nigra and degeneration of nerve terminals in the striatum. Noradrenaline and 5-HT contents were also low in these patients, but much less affected than dopamine, and other evidence showed that cells containing these amines were still alive and functioning, whereas the dopamine cells were largely absent. Further studies have shown that symptoms of Parkinson's disease appear when the striatal dopamine content is reduced to 20–40% of normal (see review by Schultz 1982). Lesions of the nigrostriatal tract or chemically induced depletion of dopamine in experimental animals also produce symptoms of Parkinson's disease. The symptom that is most clearly related to dopamine deficiency is hypokinesia, which occurs immediately and invariably in lesioned animals. Rigidity and tremor involve more complex neurochemical disturbances of other transmitters (particularly acetylcholine, noradrenaline, 5-HT and GABA) as well as dopamine. In experimental lesions, two secondary consequences follow damage to the nigrostriatal tract, namely a hyperactivity of the remaining dopaminergic neurons, which show an increased rate of transmitter turnover, and an increase in the number of dopamine receptors, which produces a state of denervation hypersensitivity (see Ch. 5). These compensatory mechanisms presumably act to preserve transmission in the face of a declining number of neurons, and are important in relation to the therapeutic effectiveness of levodopa (see below). Positron emission tomography (PET) scanning of living patients, and post-mortem brain studies also suggest that D_1-receptors proliferate in Parkinson's disease, and are down-regulated during treatment with levodopa (see Guttman & Seeman 1986).

ACTION OF MPTP

New light was thrown on the possible aetiology of Parkinson's disease by a chance event. In 1982, a group of young drug addicts in California suddenly developed an exceptionally severe form of the disease (known as the 'frozen addict' syndrome), and the cause was traced to the compound 1-methyl-4-phenyl-1,2,3,6-tetrahydropyridine (MPTP), which was a contaminant in a preparation intended as a heroin substitute (see Langston 1985). MPTP has been found to cause irreversible destruction of nigrostriatal dopaminergic neurons in various species, and to produce a Parkinson's disease-like state in primates. MPTP acts by being converted to a toxic metabolite, MPP^+, by the enzyme monoamine oxidase (specifically by the MAO-B subtype; see Ch. 29). MPP^+ is taken up by the dopamine transport system, and thus acts selectively on dopaminergic neurons; it inhibits mitochondrial oxidation reactions, and thus increases oxidative stress (see above; Tipton & Singer 1993). MPTP appears to be selective in destroying nigrostriatal neurons, and does not affect dopaminergic neurons elsewhere—the reason for this is unknown. **Selegiline**, a selective MAO-B inhibitor (Ch. 29), prevents MPTP-induced neurotoxicity. It is also used in treating Parkinson's disease (see below), on the basis of its ability to inhibit dopamine breakdown, and the possibility now arises that it might also be working by blocking the metabolic activation of a putative naturally occurring, or environmental, MPTP-like substance, which is involved in the causation of Parkinson's disease. Speculation that MPTP-like neurotoxicity may account for Parkinson's disease is supported by evidence that a very similar defect of mitochondrial function has been detected in brain regions affected by the disease. Whether or not this speculation proves to have any substance, MPTP is proving to be a very useful experimental tool for studying the causes and treatment of the disease.

Parkinson's disease

- Degenerative disease of the basal ganglia causing tremor at rest, muscle rigidity and hypokinesia, often with dementia.
- Often idiopathic, but may follow virus infection. Can be drug induced (neuroleptic drugs).
- Associated with marked loss of dopamine from basal ganglia.
- Can be induced by MPTP, a neurotoxin affecting dopamine neurons in the corpus striatum.

The intrinsic cholinergic neurons of the corpus striatum (which has the highest content of ACh, CAT and AChE in the brain) are also involved in Parkinson's disease (as well as Huntington's disease; see below). ACh release from the striatum is strongly inhibited by dopamine, and it is suggested that hyperactivity of these cholinergic neurons (associated with a lack of dopamine) leads to hypokinesia, rigidity and tremor (characteristic of Parkinson's disease) whereas hypoactivity (associated with a surfeit of dopamine, secondary to a deficiency of GABA) results in hyperkinetic movements and hypotonia (characteristic of Huntington's disease; see Fig. 25.3). The use of muscarinic antagonists in the treatment of Parkinson's disease, and of anticholinesterase drugs in the treatment of Huntington's disease fits in with this general scheme. Up to a point, redressing the balance between the dopaminergic and cholinergic neurons appears to be able to compensate for an overall deficit or surfeit of dopaminergic function.

DRUG TREATMENT OF PARKINSON'S DISEASE

The corpus striatum is exceptionally rich in acetylcholine as well as dopamine. Acetylcholine has excitatory effects, whereas dopamine is mainly inhibitory, and it has been suggested that the symptoms of Parkinson's disease (and Huntington's disease; see below) result from an imbalance between these two systems (Fig. 25.3). Accordingly, drug treatment is aimed at restoring this balance.

The drugs that are effective in the treatment of Parkinson's disease fall into the following categories (see Calne 1993, Kopin 1993):

- drugs that replace dopamine (e.g. **levodopa,** often used concomitantly with peripherally acting dopa decarboxylase inhibitors, e.g. **carbidopa, benserazide**)
- drugs that mimic the action of dopamine (e.g. **bromocriptine, pergolide, lisuride**)
- drugs that enhance dopamine release, and may be neuroprotective
- MAO-B inhibitors (e.g. **selegiline**)
- drugs that release dopamine (e.g. **amantadine**)
- acetylcholine antagonists (e.g. **benztropine**).

Implantation of dopamine-rich fragments of brain or adrenal tissue into the striatum of patients with Parkinson's disease, following the demonstration in rats that behavioural changes associated with a loss of dopaminergic neurons could be partly restored in this way, has so far given disappointing results. Initial clinical trials of this procedure (see Bjorklund 1992, Baker & Ridley 1992) have attracted great publicity, but the long-term benefit is not clear. Another approach, which looks promising in experimental animals (Jiao et al. 1993), but has not yet been tested in man, is the use of gene therapy to transfect the tyrosine hydroxylase gene into cerebral tissues, and thus increase dopamine production.

Levodopa

Levodopa (with a dopa-decarboxylase inhibitor, see below) is now the first-line treatment for Parkinson's disease. It is well absorbed from the small intestine, a process which relies on active transport, though much of it is inactivated by monoamine oxidase in

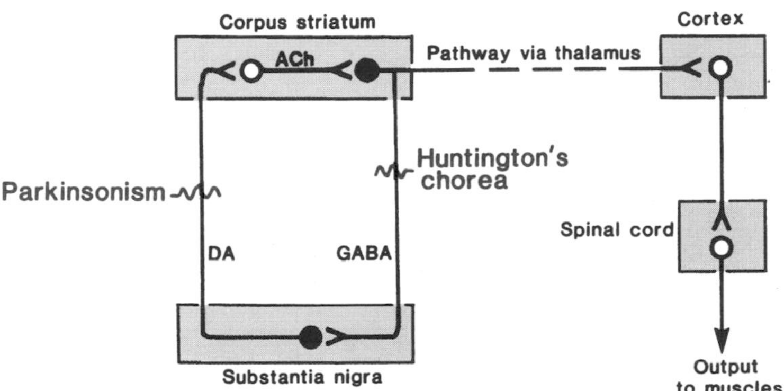

Fig. 25.3 Simplified diagram of the organisation of the extrapyramidal motor system, and the lesions that are believed to occur in Parkinson's disease and Huntington's disease.

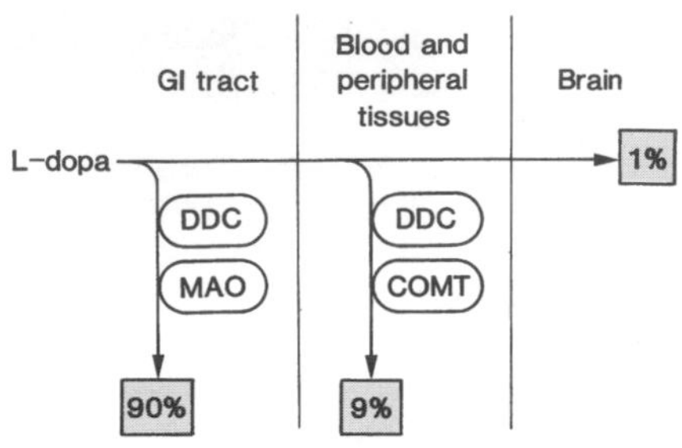

Fig. 25.4 The fate of levodopa (L-dopa) after oral administration. (DDC = dopa decarboxylase; MAO = monoamine oxidase; COMT = catechol-O-methyl transferase)

the wall of the intestine (Fig. 25.4). The plasma half-life is short (about 2 hours), and about 95% of the drug is converted to dopamine in peripheral tissues, where dopa decarboxylase is widespread. Less than 1% enters the brain. Decarboxylation occurs rapidly within the brain, since dopa decarboxylase is by no means confined to neurons. It is known that the anti-Parkinson effect of levodopa depends on dopamine formation in the brain because the effect is prevented by decarboxylase inhibitors that enter the brain but not by those, such as **carbidopa** (see below), that do not. It is not certain whether the effect depends on an increased release of dopamine from the few surviving dopaminergic neurons or to a 'flooding' of the synapse with exogenous dopamine. Animal studies suggest that levodopa can act even when no dopaminergic nerve terminals are present. On the other hand, the therapeutic effectiveness of levodopa decreases as the disease advances, so part of its action may rely on the presence of functional dopaminergic neurons.

Therapeutic effectiveness of levodopa

At the beginning of treatment with levodopa, with the dose gradually built up to achieve the optimal effect, many trials have shown that about 80% of patients show improvement, particularly of rigidity and hypokinesia, and about 20% are restored virtually to normal motor function. As time progresses, the effectiveness of levodopa gradually declines (Fig. 25.5). In a typical study, Sweet & McDowell (1975) found that, out of 100 patients treated with levodopa for 5 years, only 34 were better than they had been at the beginning of the trial, 32 patients having died and 21 having withdrawn from the trial. It is likely that the loss of effectiveness of levodopa mainly reflects the natural progression of the disease, for there is no evidence that drug treatment can affect the underlying pathological process. Levodopa was found in the above clinical trial to improve the life expectancy of Parkinson patients, though it remained shorter than that of controls of the same age. This is probably the result of improved motor function rather than an effect on the disease process.

Unwanted effects of levodopa

There are two main types of unwanted effect:

- The development of *involuntary choreiform movements*, which happens in the majority of patients within 2 years of starting levodopa therapy. These movements usually affect the face and limbs, and can become very severe. They disappear if the dose of levodopa is reduced, but this causes rigidity to return. It is not known why the margin between the beneficial and the unwanted effect becomes progressively narrower, but it appears to be related to the duration of levodopa treatment rather than to the underlying disease.
- Rapid fluctuations in clinical state, where hypokinesia and rigidity may suddenly worsen for anything from a few minutes to a few hours, and then improve again. This '*on–off effect*' is not seen in untreated Parkinson's disease patients or with other anti-Parkinson drugs. It can produce such a sudden loss of mobility that the patient stops while walking and feels rooted to the spot, or is unable to rise from a chair in which he had sat down normally a few moments earlier. The mechanism of this remarkable effect is not understood. In some patients, rigidity and hypokinesia occur as the plasma dopa concentration falls after a dose, but often the attacks are unrelated to levodopa dosage.

In addition to these slowly developing side effects, levodopa produces several acute effects, which are experienced by most patients at first but tend to disappear after a few weeks. The main ones are:

- *Nausea and anorexia.* Domperidone, a peripherally acting dopamine antagonist, may be useful in preventing this effect (see below).
- *Hypotension.* This is usually of minor importance, but may cause postural hypotension in patients on antihypertensive drugs.
- *Psychological effects.* Levodopa, by increasing

dopamine activity in the brain, can produce a schizophrenia-like syndrome (see Ch. 28) with delusions and hallucinations. A more common effect, seen in about 20% of patients, is the occurrence of confusion, disorientation, insomnia or nightmares.

Optimisation of levodopa treatment

Three strategies have been devised to enhance the central effects of levodopa and minimise its peripheral effects:

- inhibition of dopa decarboxylase in the periphery by **carbidopa** or **benserazide**
- inhibition of dopamine degradation in the central nervous system by the monoamine oxidase inhibitor, **selegiline**
- block of dopamine receptors in the periphery by **domperidone**.

Carbidopa inhibits dopa decarboxylase but does not penetrate the blood–brain barrier. It therefore inhibits the formation of dopamine from levodopa peripherally but not in the brain. Combined with levodopa it enables the dose of levodopa to be reduced four- to eightfold and greatly reduces the peripheral side effects. The central side effects are not, of course, reduced, but it has been claimed that the proportion of patients showing clinical benefit is increased. A combination of carbidopa and levodopa is now used routinely in treating Parkinson's disease. Benserazide is similar.

Selegiline is a monoamine oxidase (MAO) inhibitor that is selective for MAO-B, which predominates in dopamine-containing regions of the central nervous system. It therefore lacks the unwanted peripheral effects of non-selective MAO inhibitors, and, in contrast to them, does not provoke the 'cheese reaction' or interact so frequently with other drugs (see Ch. 29). Selegiline is often combined with levodopa, but can be used on its own in early cases of Parkinson's disease; it clearly retards the progression of symptoms by a few months (Parkinson Study Group 1993). Whether it actually retards the neurodegenerative process is unproven. A recent large-scale trial (Fig. 25.5) showed no difference when selegiline was added to levodopa/benserazide treatment.

Domperidone is a dopamine antagonist related to **haloperidol** (see Ch. 28), which does not penetrate the blood–brain barrier. Its usefulness as a means of reducing the side effects of levodopa is being assessed.

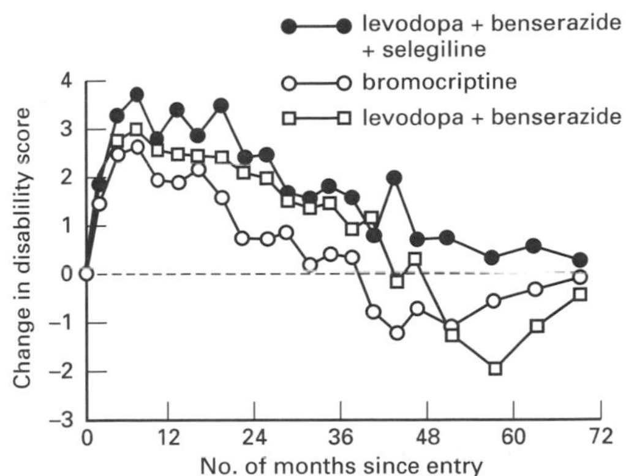

Fig. 25.5 Comparison of levodopa/benserazide, levodopa/benserazide/selegiline and bromocriptine on progression of Parkinson's disease symptoms. Patients (249–271 in each treatment group) were assessed on a standard disability rating score. Before treatment, the average rate of decline was 0.7 units/year. All three treatments produced improvement over the initial rating for 2–3 years, but the effect declined, either because of refractoriness to the drugs, or to disease progression. Bromocriptine appeared slightly less effective than levodopa regimes, and there was a higher drop-out rate due to side effects in this group. (Parkinson's Disease Research Group 1993)

Other drugs used in Parkinson's disease

Bromocriptine

Bromocriptine, derived from the ergot alkaloids (see Ch. 8), is a potent agonist at dopamine (D_1) receptors in the central nervous system. It has an inhibitory effect on the anterior pituitary gland, and was first introduced for the treatment of galactorrhoea and gynaecomastia (Ch. 21), but is effective also in Parkinson's disease. A large-scale trial (Fig. 25.5) showed its effect to be similar to that of levodopa. Its duration of action is longer (plasma half-life 6–8 hours) so that it does not need to be given so frequently. It was hoped that bromocriptine might be effective in patients who had become refractory to levodopa because of a progressive loss of dopaminergic neurons from the corpus striatum, but this has not been clearly established. Other dopamine-receptor agonists, such as **lisuride** and **pergolide**, have been developed and are undergoing trial. **Apomorphine**, given by self injection, is being evaluated in patients with severe on-off effect.

Amantadine

Amantadine was introduced as an antiviral drug, and discovered by accident in 1969 to be beneficial in Parkinson's disease. Many possible mechanisms for its action have been suggested, based on neurochemical evidence of increased dopamine release, inhibition of amine uptake or a direct action on dopamine receptors. Most authors now suggest, although not with much conviction, that increased dopamine release is primarily responsible for the clinical effects.

Amantadine is less effective than levodopa or bromocriptine, and its action declines with time. Its side effects are considerably less severe, though qualitatively similar to those of levodopa.

Acetylcholine antagonists

Atropine and related drugs have been used for many years in treating Parkinson's disease, and were the main form of treatment before levodopa was discovered. Muscarinic acetylcholine receptors exert an excitatory effect, opposite to that of dopamine, on striatal neurons (see Fig. 25.3) and also exert a presynaptic inhibitory effect on dopaminergic nerve terminals. Suppression of these effects thus makes up, in part, for a lack of dopamine. The action of muscarinic antagonists is more limited than that of levodopa, and they diminish tremor more than rigidity or hypokinesia (which are more disabling in their effects). Furthermore, their side effects—dry mouth, constipation, impaired vision, urinary retention—are often troublesome; they are used mainly to treat Parkinson's disease in patients receiving neuroleptic drugs (which are dopamine antagonists and thus nullify the effect of L-dopa; see Ch. 28). The drugs used for this purpose (e.g. **benztropine**) have less peripheral effect in relation to their central effect than does atropine. Drowsiness and confusion are the main unwanted effects. Patients suffering from Parkinson's disease very often show some degree of dementia, and acetylcholine antagonists would be expected to exacerbate this (see above).

The clinical use of drugs in Parkinson's disease is summarised in the following box.

> **Drugs used in Parkinson's disease**
>
> - Drugs act by counteracting deficiency of dopamine in basal ganglia or by blocking muscarinic receptors.
> - The most effective drug is levodopa, a dopamine precursor which passes the blood–brain barrier.
> - Other useful drugs include: bromocriptine (dopamine agonist), selegiline (MAO-B inhibitor), amantadine (? enhances dopamine release) and benztropine (muscarinic-receptor antagonist).
> - Levodopa is effective in most patients initially, but often loses efficacy after about 2 years.
> - Levodopa does not affect underlying disease process; selegiline may do so, but direct evidence is lacking.
> - Main unwanted effects of levodopa are: involuntary movements, which occur in most patients within 2 years; unpredictable 'on–off effect'. Others are: nausea, hypotension and occasionally psychotic symptoms.
> - Efficacy of levodopa may be improved by:
>   —combination with peripheral decarboxylase inhibitor (carbidopa) to reduce side effects and increase efficacy
>   —combination with selegiline
>   —combination with peripheral dopamine antagonist (domperidone).

HUNTINGTON'S DISEASE

Huntington's disease is an inherited (autosomal dominant) disorder resulting in progressive brain degeneration, which usually becomes manifest in the middle of life. It leads to progressive dementia and severe involuntary sudden jerky (choreiform) movements, which make speech and feeding progressively more difficult. The nature of the primary biochemical defect remains undetermined. The disease causes a widespread loss of cortical cells, which is presumably responsible for producing dementia, and also loss of cells from the corpus striatum, which causes the motor disturbance. Glutamate-mediated excitotoxicity involving striatal and cortical neurons has been postulated. Bird & Iversen (1974), in a study of post-mortem brains from patients with Huntington's disease, found that the dopamine content of the striatum was normal or slightly increased, while there was a 75% reduction in the activity of glutamic acid decarboxylase, and a smaller and more variable reduction in the activity of choline acetyltransferase. It is believed that the loss of GABA-mediated inhibition in the striatum produces a hyperactivity of dopaminergic synapses. There is also an under-activity of cholinergic transmission, so the syndrome is in some senses a mirror image of Parkinson's disease (Fig. 25.3). The effects of drugs that influence dopaminergic transmission are correspondingly the opposite of those that are observed in Parkinson's disease, dopamine antagonists being effective in reducing the involuntary movements, while drugs such as levodopa and bromocriptine make them worse. Drugs do not affect the underlying cause of the disease.

REFERENCES AND FURTHER READING

Baker H F, Ridley R M 1992 Neural transplantation in primates: towards brain repair in humans. Rev Neurosci 3: 175–190

Beal M F 1992 Role of excitotoxicity in human neurological disease. Curr Opin Neurobiol 2: 657–662

Beal M F, Hyman B T, Koroshetz W 1993 Do defects in mitochondrial energy metabolism underlie the pathology of neurodegenerative diseases? Trends Neurosci 16: 125–131

Bensimon G, Lacomblez L, Meininger V 1994 A controlled trial of riluzole in amyotrophic lateral sclerosis. N Engl J Med 330: 585–591

Bird E J, Iversen L L 1974 Huntington's chorea. Postmortem acetyltransferase and dopamine in basal ganglia. Brain 97: 457–472

Bjorklund A 1992 Dopaminergic transplants in experimental parkinsonism: cellular mechanisms of graft-induced functional recovery. Curr Opin Neurobiol 2: 683–689

Calne D B 1993 Treatment of Parkinson's disease. N Engl J Med 329: 1021–1027

Choi D W 1988 Calcium-mediated neurotoxicity: relationship to specific channel types and role in ischaemic damage. Trends Neurosci 11: 465–469

Coyle J T, Puttfarken P 1993 Oxidative stress, glutamate and neurodegenerative disorders. Science 262: 689–695

Davis K L et al. 1992 A double-blind placebo-controlled multicenter study of tacrine for Alzheimer's disease. N Engl J Med 327: 1253–1259

Davis R E, Emmerling M R, Jaen J H, Moos W H, Spiegel K 1993 Therapeutic intervention in dementia. Crit Rev Neurobiol 7: 41–83

Dawson V L, Dawson T M, London E D, Bredt D S, Snyder S H 1991 Nitric oxide mediates glutamate neurotoxicity in primary cortical cultures. Proc Natl Acad Sci USA 88: 6368–6371

Gottfreis C G 1992 Clinical and neurochemical aspects of diseases with cognitive impairment. Rev Neurosci 3: 191–205

Guttman M, Seeman P 1986 Dopamine D_1 receptor density in Parkinsonian brain is constant for duration of disease, age, and duration of L-DOPA therapy. Adv Neurol 45: 51–57

Hornykiewicz O, Kish S J 1986 Biochemical pathology of Parkinson's disease. Adv Neurol 45: 19–34, 183–190

Jiao S, Gurevich V, Wolff J A 1993 Long-term correction of rat model of Parkinson's disease by gene therapy. Nature 362: 450–453

Kogure K, Hossmann K-A, Siesjo B K (eds) 1993 Neurobiology of ischaemic brain damage. Elsevier, Amsterdam

Kopin I 1993 The pharmacology of Parkinson's disease therapy: an update. Ann Rev Pharmacol Toxicol 32: 467–495

Langston W J 1985 MPTP and Parkinson's disease. Trends Neurosci 8: 79–83

Lipton S A 1993 Prospects for clinically tolerated NMDA antagonists: open-channel blockers and alternative redox states of nitric oxide. Trends Neurosci 16: 527–532

Lipton S A, Rosenberg P A 1994 Excitatory amino acids as a final common pathway for neurologic disorders. N Engl J Med 330: 613–622

McCulloch J 1992 Excitatory amino acid antagonists and their potential for treatment of ischaemic brain damage in man. Br J Clin Pharmacol 34: 106–114

Mattson M P, Barger S W, Cheng B, Liederburg I, Smith-Swintoky V L, Rydel R E 1993 β-amyloid precursor protein metabolites and loss of neuronal Ca^{2+} homeostasis in Alzheimer's disease. Trends Neurosci 16: 409–415

Mullan M, Crawford C 1993 Genetic and molecular advances in Alzheimer's disease. Trends Neurosci 16: 398–403

Olney J W 1990 Excitotoxic amino acids and neuropsychiatric disorders. Annu Rev Pharmacol Toxicol 30: 47–71

Parkinson's Disease Research Group 1993 Comparisons of therapeutic effects of levodopa, levodopa and selegiline, and bromocriptine in patients with early, mild Parkinson's disease: three year interim report. Br Med J 307: 469–472

Parkinson Study Group 1993 Effects of tocopherol and deprenyl on the progression of disability in early Parkinson's disease. N Engl J Med 328: 176–183

Rothman S M, Olney J W 1986 Glutamate and the pathophysiology of hypoxic–ischaemic brain damage. Ann Neurol 119: 105–111

Schultz W 1982 Depletion of dopamine in the striatum as an experimental model of Parkinsonism: direct effects and adaptive mechanisms. Prog Neurobiol 18: 121–166

Selkoe D J 1991 Amyloid protein and Alzheimer disease. Scientific American, Nov: 40–47

Selkoe D J 1993 Physiological production of the β-amyloid protein and the mechanism of Alzheimer's disease. Trends Neurosci 16: 403–409

Sweet R D, McDowell F H 1975 Five years' treatment of Parkinson's disease with levodopa. Therapeutic results and survival of 100 patients. Ann Intern Med 83: 456–463

Tipton K F, Singer T P 1993 Advances in our understanding of the mechanisms of neurotoxicity of MPTP and related compounds. J Neurochem 61: 1191–1206

26 GENERAL ANAESTHETIC AGENTS

General anaesthetics are used as an adjunct to surgical procedures in order to render the patient unaware of, and unresponsive to, painful stimulation. They are given systemically, and exert their main effects on the central nervous system, in contrast to local anaesthetics (see Ch. 34) which work by producing a local block of conduction of sensory nerve impulses from the periphery to the central nervous system. Though we now take them for granted, general anaesthetics are the drugs that paved the way for much of modern surgery.

Many drugs, including, for example, **ethanol** and **morphine**, can produce a state of insensibility and obliviousness to pain, but are not used as anaesthetics. For a drug to be useful as an anaesthetic it must be readily controllable, so that induction and recovery are rapid, allowing the level of anaesthesia to be adjusted as required during the course of the operation. For this reason it was only when inhalation anaesthetics were first discovered, in 1846, that surgical operations under controlled anaesthesia became a practical possibility. Until that time surgical skill consisted largely of being able to operate at lightning speed, and most operations were amputations. Inhalation is still the most useful route of administration for anaesthetics, though there are also some drugs that are sufficiently rapidly metabolised or redistributed in the body to be given as anaesthetics by the intravenous route.

The use of **nitrous oxide** to relieve the pain of surgery was suggested by Humphrey Davy in 1800. He was the first person to make nitrous oxide and he tested its effects on several people, including himself and the Prime Minister, noting that it caused euphoria, analgesia and loss of consciousness. The use of nitrous oxide, billed as 'laughing gas', became a popular fairground entertainment, and came to the notice of an American dentist, Horace Wells, who had a tooth extracted under its influence, while he himself squeezed the inhalation bag. **Ether** also first gained publicity in a disreputable way, through the spread of 'ether frolics' at which it was used to produce euphoria among the guests (explosions, too, one might have thought). William Morton, also a dentist and a student at Harvard Medical School, used it successfully to extract a tooth in 1846 and then suggested to Warren, the chief surgeon at Massachusetts General Hospital, that he should administer it for one of Warren's operations. Warren grudgingly agreed, and on 16 October 1846 a large audience was gathered in the main operating theatre; after some preliminary fumbling, Morton's demonstration was a spectacular success. 'Gentlemen, this is no humbug' was the most gracious comment that Warren could bring himself to make to the assembled audience. A more wordy appreciation came later from Oliver Wendell Holmes (1847), the neurologist–poet–philosopher who first coined the word 'anaesthesia'. 'The knife is searching for disease, the pulleys are dragging back dislocated limbs—Nature herself is working out the primal curse which doomed the tenderest of her creatures to the sharpest of her trials, but the fierce extremity of suffering has been steeped in the waters of forgetfulness, and the deepest furrow in the knotted brow of agony has been smoothed forever'. Morton subsequently sank into an endless and bitter dispute with one of his collaborators over the patent rights, and contributed nothing more to medical science. In the same year James Simpson, professor of obstetrics in Glasgow, used **chloroform** to relieve the pain of childbirth, bringing on himself fierce denunciation from the clergy, one of whom wrote: 'Chloroform is a decoy of Satan, apparently offering itself to bless women; but in the end it will harden society and rob God of the deep, earnest cries which arise in time of trouble, for help'. Opposition was effectively silenced in 1853 when Queen Victoria gave birth to her seventh child under the influence of chloroform, and the procedure became known as 'anaesthésie à la reine'.

PHYSICOCHEMICAL THEORIES OF ANAESTHESIA

Unlike most drugs, inhalation anaesthetics, which include a diverse group of substances such as **halothane**, **nitrous oxide** and **xenon**, belong to no recognisable chemical class. The shape and electronic configuration of the molecule is evidently unimportant, and the pharmacological action requires only that the molecule has certain physicochemical properties. The lack of chemical specificity argues against there being any distinctive 'receptor' for anaesthetics (see Ch. 1); instead we need to consider in which 'phase' of the cell the drugs are acting. Anaesthetics appear to act principally on the cell membrane (see below), and theories of anaesthesia focus on interactions with the two main components of the membrane, namely lipids and proteins.

- *Lipid.* It is suggested that by dissolving in the membrane lipid, anaesthetic drugs affect its physical state in such a way as to alter the function of the membrane.
- *Protein.* The interaction of anaesthetic molecules with hydrophobic domains of membrane proteins (ion channels, receptors, etc.) may affect their function in such a way as to disrupt the normal mechanisms by which the ion permeability of the membrane is controlled.

Accounts of the different theories of anaesthesia are given by Franks & Lieb (1987, 1994), Wann & Macdonald (1988), Halsey (1989).

LIPID THEORY

The lipid theory derives from the extensive work of Overton & Meyer, published between 1899 and 1901, who showed a close correlation between *anaesthetic potency* (measured in terms of the concentration needed to produce reversible immobilisation of swimming tadpoles) and *lipid solubility* (measured as the olive-oil : water partition coefficient) in a diverse group of simple and unreactive organic compounds. This led to the theory, formulated by Meyer in 1937: 'Narcosis commences when any chemically indifferent substance has attained a certain molar concentration in the lipids of the cell. This concentration depends on the nature of the animal or cell but is independent of the narcotic.'

The relationship between anaesthetic activity and lipid solubility has been repeatedly confirmed. Figure 26.1 shows results obtained in man where the *minimal alveolar concentration* (MAC) required to produce a lack of response to painful stimulation is plotted against lipid solubility, for various inhalation anaesthetics whose oil : water partition coefficient varies over a 10 000-fold range. MAC is inversely proportional to the potency of an anaesthetic. The Overton–Meyer studies did not suggest any particular mechanism, but revealed an impressive correlation which any theory of anaesthesia needs to take into account. Experiments with various hydrophobic solvents showed that the correlation with anaesthetic potency was closest for olive oil or octanol, which have physicochemical properties similar to those of membrane lipids; thus most theories postulate that anaesthesia is caused by an alteration of membrane function.

How might the introduction of inert foreign molecules into the cell membrane cause a functional disturbance? One theory proposes that *volume expansion* is the underlying mechanism. A phenomenon that has been held to support this view is that of *pressure reversal* of anaesthesia. If animals, such as newts, are immobilised by addition of anaesthetic to the water in which they swim, application of

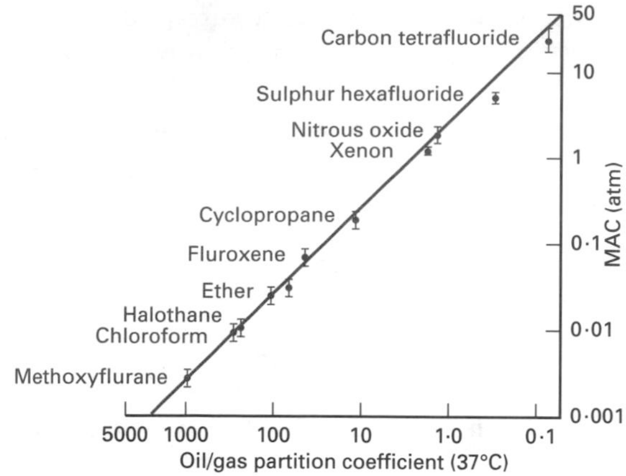

Fig. 26.1 Correlation of anaesthetic potency with oil : gas partition coefficient. Anaesthetic potency in man is expressed as minimum alveolar partial pressure (MAC) required to produce surgical anaesthesia. There is a close correlation with lipid solubility, expressed as the oil : gas partition coefficient. (From: Halsey 1989)

hydrostatic pressure to about 100 atmospheres immediately restores their mobility, and anaesthesia returns as soon as the pressure is lowered (Miller et al. 1973). Quantitative analysis of this phenomenon suggests that hydrostatic compression of the lipid phase of the membrane is responsible, and the results are compatible with the suggestion that anaesthesia occurs when the volume of the lipid phase is expanded by about 0.4% as a result of the intrusion of anaesthetic molecules. Pressure is thought to act simply by opposing this volume expansion. There is independent evidence that anaesthetics do indeed cause membranes to expand (e.g. in the red cell) slightly, but there are quantitative discrepancies between these results and those of pressure reversal experiments, so the interpretation is not clear at present (see Wann & Macdonald 1988). It is interesting that pressure reversal has also been observed when anaesthesia is produced by intravenous agents such as barbiturates, and with local anaesthetics, though there are discrepancies which mean that lipid volume expansion cannot explain all of the actions of these drugs.

Another theory involves an *increase in membrane fluidity* (i.e. a disordering of the regular packing of the hydrophobic tails of membrane phospholipids) as the mechanism by which the intrusion of anaesthetic molecules affects membrane function. Membrane fluidity can be measured by the technique of electron spin resonance (ESR) spectroscopy, in both natural membranes and artificial lipid bilayers. Many studies have shown that anaesthetics increase fluidity. This effect correlates, in general, with anaesthetic activity, though relatively high concentrations are needed. The effect of clinical concentrations would correspond only to a minute increase in fluidity, such as might occur if the temperature was increased by less than 1°C, so the relevance of this phenomenon to the pharmacological actions of anaesthetics is not clear. Actually, raising the temperature *reduces* the potency of anaesthetic agents, the opposite of what the fluidity theory predicts.

PROTEIN THEORY

Though there is good evidence that anaesthetics can bind to protein molecules, well-documented for haemoglobin and myoglobin as well as for various enzymes, there is little direct evidence to suggest that this can account for anaesthesia. In most cases, the concentration of anaesthetic agents needed to affect protein conformation or enzyme activity are much greater than those needed for anaesthesia. On the other hand, extensive studies on *luciferase* (the enzyme responsible for the luminescent reaction of fireflies and certain bacteria) have shown a striking parallel with anaesthesia (see Franks & Lieb 1987). This enzyme is a pure soluble protein, so effects of anaesthetics acting indirectly on associated lipids are ruled out. There turns out to be a close correlation between anaesthetic potency and potency in inhibiting this enzyme for a wide range of compounds, suggesting that anaesthetics may bind to a hydrophobic domain of the protein. Similar interactions with functional membrane proteins such as receptors or ion channels are postulated to underlie the phenomenon of anaesthesia.

The protein theory may also account for a general feature of anaesthetic action, namely *the cut-off phenomenon*, which is hard to explain on the basis of lipid interactions. In many homologous series anaesthetic potency increases steadily, along with lipid solubility, as the length of the hydrocarbon chain is increased. Beyond a certain point, however, potency suddenly drops even though lipid solubility continues to increase. This may mean that anaesthetics do, after all, bind to a site of predetermined size, which is more likely to correspond to a particular domain of a protein molecule than to interaction with an essentially fluid lipid phase (see Franks & Lieb 1987). There is also evidence, from ESR studies of rat brain in vivo, that halothane molecules in the brain during anaesthesia bind to saturable sites, and are immobilised when bound. These results are in keeping with a protein rather than a lipid environment, since association of halothane with membrane lipids shows neither saturability nor immobilisation.

In summary, it seems clear from the correlation of potency with lipid solubility that the interaction of anaesthetic molecules with one or more hydrophobic regions of the cell membrane underlies their effects. Whether the primary association is with the lipid bilayer or with one or more distinct proteins, or at the interface between the two, is still uncertain, but recent evidence tends to argue in favour of a protein site. The receptor crusade, it seems, is threatening even the last bastion of resistance, the Overton–Meyer theory of narcosis.

Theories of anaesthesia

- Many simple, unreactive compounds produce narcotic effects.
- Anaesthetic potency is closely correlated with lipid solubility (Overton–Meyer correlation), not with chemical structure, suggesting that anaesthesia involves interaction with a hydrophobic domain of the cell.
- The two main theories of anaesthesia postulate interaction with the lipid membrane bilayer or with hydrophobic binding sites on protein molecules.
- Theories involving the lipid bilayer involve two possible mechanisms:
  —volume expansion
  —membrane fluidisation.
  The phenomenon of pressure reversal of anaesthesia is consistent with the volume expansion mechanism, but can be explained in other ways. The relatively weak effects of temperature changes are difficult to reconcile with the membrane fluidisation hypothesis.
- The phenomenon of cut-off (loss of biological activity beyond a certain point in an homologous series of compounds, even though lipid solubility continues to increase) is difficult to explain in terms of lipid theories.
- There is increasing evidence that anaesthetics may act by binding to discrete hydrophobic domains of protein molecules, though the nature of the protein(s) that are involved in anaesthesia has not been settled.

THE EFFECTS OF ANAESTHETICS ON THE NERVOUS SYSTEM

At the cellular level, anaesthetics inhibit the conduction of action potentials and also inhibit transmission at synapses. The effect on axonal conduction, however, requires considerably higher concentrations than the effect on synaptic transmission, and is probably unimportant in practice. During surgical anaesthesia transmission along peripheral nerves is unaffected, and experiments on transmission within the central nervous system in experimental animals have revealed that excitatory synaptic transmission is much more susceptible to anaesthetic action than is axonal conduction (see Pocock & Richards 1993).

The inhibitory effect on synaptic transmission could be due to reduction of transmitter release, inhibition of the postsynaptic action of the transmitter, or reduction of the excitability of the postsynaptic cell. Though all three effects have been described, most studies suggest that reduced transmitter release and reduced postsynaptic response are the main factors. A reduction of acetylcholine release has been demonstrated directly in studies on peripheral synapses, and reduced sensitivity to excitatory transmitters (due to inhibition of ligand-gated ion channels) has been shown at both peripheral and central synapses.

The action of inhibitory synapses may be enhanced or reduced by anaesthetics. Enhancement of inhibitory synaptic action occurs particularly with barbiturates, though similar effects also occur with volatile anaesthetics (see Pocock & Richards 1993).

Much effort has gone into identifying a particular brain region on which anaesthetics act to produce their anaesthetic effect (see review by Richards 1980). Unconsciousness can be produced by damage to the brainstem reticular formation, the hypothalamus or the thalamus. Cortical damage produces profound sensory and motor disturbances, but not actual loss of consciousness. Activity of the reticular formation is responsible for cortical 'arousal' and also for facilitation of transmission through the thalamic sensory relay nuclei that lie en route from peripheral sensory receptors to the cortex. Inhibition of activity in this part of the reticular formation may thus be important in causing cortical inactivity together with a lack of awareness of sensory input.

Anaesthetics, even in low concentrations, cause short-term *amnesia*, i.e. experiences occurring during the influence of the drug are not recalled later even though the subject was responsive at the time. It is likely that interference with hippocampal function produces this effect, for it is known that the hippocampus is involved in short-term memory and that certain hippocampal synapses are highly susceptible to inhibition by anaesthetics.

Thus the reticular formation and the hippocampus may be the most important sites at which anaesthetics work in the brain. As the concentration is increased, however, many other functions are affected, including motor control and reflex activity, respiration and autonomic regulation. It is clear that the cellular effects produced by anaesthetics can influence the function of the nervous system in many different ways, and it is therefore unrealistic to seek a critical 'target site' in the brain responsible for all the phenomena of anaesthesia.

STAGES OF ANAESTHESIA

When a slowly acting anaesthetic, such as **ether**, is given on its own, certain well-defined stages are passed through as its concentration in the blood increases.

- *Stage I—Analgesia*. The subject is conscious but drowsy. Responses to painful stimuli are reduced. The degree of analgesia actually varies greatly with different agents; it is pronounced with ether and nitrous oxide, but not with halothane.
- *Stage II—Excitement*. The subject loses consciousness, and no longer responds to non-painful stimuli, but responds in a reflex fashion to painful stimuli. Other reflexes, for example the cough reflex, and gagging in response to pharyngeal stimulation, are present and often exaggerated. The subject may move, talk incoherently, hold his breath, choke or vomit. Irregular ventilation may affect the absorption of the anaesthetic agent. It is a dangerous state, and modern anaesthetic procedures are designed to eliminate it.
- *Stage III—Surgical anaesthesia*. Spontaneous movement ceases and respiration becomes regular. If anaesthesia is light, some reflexes (e.g. responses to pharyngeal and peritoneal stimulation) are still present, and muscles show appreciable tone. With deepening anaesthesia, these reflexes disappear, and the muscles relax fully. Respiration becomes progressively shallower, with the intercostal muscles failing before the diaphragm.
- *Stage IV—Medullary paralysis*. Respiration and vasomotor control cease, and death occurs within a few minutes.

The use of a single anaesthetic agent on its own is now uncommon, and the orderly progression through the above-listed stages of anaesthesia is seldom observed in practice. The anaesthetic state, for clinical purposes, consists of three main components, namely *loss of consciousness*, *analgesia*, and *muscle relaxation*, and in practice these effects are produced with a combination of drugs rather than with a single anaesthetic agent. Thus, a common procedure would be to produce unconsciousness rapidly with an intravenous induction agent (e.g. **thiopentone**), to maintain unconsciousness and produce analgesia with one or more inhalation agents (e.g. **nitrous oxide** and **halothane**), which might be supplemented with an intravenous analgesic agent (e.g. an opiate; see Ch. 31), and to produce muscle paralysis with a neuromuscular blocking drug (e.g. **tubocurarine**; see Ch. 6). Such a procedure results in much faster induction and recovery, avoiding long (and hazardous) periods of semiconsciousness, and it enables surgery to be carried out with relatively little impairment of homeostatic reflexes.

EFFECTS ON THE CARDIOVASCULAR AND RESPIRATORY SYSTEMS

Though all anaesthetics decrease the contractility of isolated heart preparations, their effects on cardiac output and blood pressure in man vary, mainly because of concomitant actions on the sympathetic nervous system. Some agents (e.g. nitrous oxide) cause an increased sympathetic discharge and increased plasma noradrenaline concentration and tend to increase blood pressure, whereas others (e.g. **halothane** and other halogenated anaesthetics) have the opposite effect.

Many anaesthetics, particularly halogenated agents, cause cardiac dysrhythmias, particularly ventricular extrasystoles. The mechanism is not well understood, but involves an interaction with catecholamines. Thus an injection of noradrenaline which would not normally produce dysrhythmia will do so if given in the presence of halothane. The usual manifestation is the appearance of ventricular ectopic beats, and careful ECG monitoring shows that these occur very commonly in patients under halothane anaesthesia, without producing any harmful effect. If catecholamine secretion is excessive, however, there is a risk of precipitating ventricular fibrillation, which is a particular hazard if stage II of the induction process is unduly prolonged.

With the exception of nitrous oxide and ketamine, all anaesthetics depress respiration markedly, and increase arterial P_{CO_2}. Nitrous oxide has much less effect, mainly because its low potency prevents very deep anaesthesia from being produced with this drug (see below).

Pharmacological effects of anaesthetic agents

- Anaesthesia involves three main neurophysiological changes: unconsciousness, loss of response to painful stimulation and loss of motor reflexes.
- At supra-anaesthetic doses, all anaesthetic agents can cause death by loss of cardiovascular reflexes and respiratory paralysis.
- At the cellular level, anaesthetic agents affect synaptic transmission rather than axonal conduction. Transmitter release and the response of the postsynaptic receptors are both inhibited. GABA-mediated transmission is enhanced by some anaesthetics.
- Though all parts of the nervous system are affected by anaesthetic agents, the state of unconsciousness is probably associated with inhibition of activity in the reticular formation and hippocampus.
- Most anaesthetic agents (with exceptions, such as ketamine and benzodiazepines) produce similar neurophysiological effects, and differ mainly in respect of their pharmacokinetic properties and toxicity.
- Most anaesthetic agents cause cardiovascular depression, by effects on the myocardium and blood vessels, as well as on the nervous system. Halogenated anaesthetic agents are likely to cause cardiac dysrhythmias, accentuated by circulating catecholamines.

INHALATION ANAESTHETICS

PHARMACOKINETIC ASPECTS

An important characteristic of an inhalation anaesthetic is the speed at which the arterial blood concentration, on which the pharmacological effect closely depends, follows changes in the concentration of the drug in the inspired air. Ideally, the blood concentration should follow as quickly as possible, so that the depth of anaesthesia can be controlled rapidly. In particular, it is important that the blood concentration should fall to a subanaesthetic level rapidly when administration is stopped, so that the patient recovers consciousness without delay. A prolonged semicomatose state, in which respiratory reflexes are weak or absent, represents a distinct hazard to life.

The only quantitatively important route by which inhalation anaesthetics enter and leave the body is via the lungs. Metabolic degradation of anaesthetics (see below), though important in relation to their toxicity, is generally insignificant in determining their duration of action. Anaesthetics are all small, lipid-soluble molecules, which cross the alveolar membrane with great ease. It is therefore the rate of delivery of drug to and from the lungs, via the inspired air and the bloodstream, that determines the overall kinetic behaviour of an anaesthetic. The reason that anaesthetics vary in their kinetic behaviour is that their relative solubilities in blood, and in body fat, vary between one drug and another.

The main factors that determine the speed of induction and recovery (and also the speed with which the level of anaesthesia responds to changes in the concentration added by the anaesthetist to the inspired air) can be summarised as follows:

- Properties of the anaesthetic
  —blood : gas partition coefficient
  —oil : gas partition coefficient
- Physiological factors
  —alveolar ventilation rate
  —cardiac output.

Table 26.1 Characteristics of inhalation anaesthetics

Drug	Partition coefficient		MAC (% v/v)	Induction	Metabolism	Flammability
	blood : gas	oil : gas				
Ether	12.0	65	1.9	Slow	Some oxidation → ethanol, acetaldehyde, acetic acid	++
Halothane	2.4	220	0.8	Medium	About 30% → trifluoroacetic acid, bromide	–
Nitrous oxide	0.47	1.4	100*	Fast	Not metabolised	–
Enflurane	1.9	98	0.7	Medium	About 5% → fluoride	–
Isoflurane	1.4	91	1.15	Medium	< 2% → fluoride	–
Methoxyflurane	13.0	950	0.16	Slow	About 50% → fluoride, oxalate	–
Cyclopropane	0.55	11.5	9.2	Fast	Not known	++

*Theoretical value based on measurements under hyperbaric conditions.

THE SOLUBILITY OF ANAESTHETICS

For practical purposes anaesthetics can be regarded physicochemically as ideal gases: their solubility in different media can thus be expressed as *partition coefficients*, defined as the ratio of the concentration of the agent in two phases at equilibrium.

The blood : gas partition coefficient is the main factor that determines the *rate of induction and recovery* of an inhalation anaesthetic, and the lower the blood : gas partition coefficient the faster the induction and recovery.

The oil : gas partition coefficient, or lipid solubility, is the main determinant of the *potency* of an anaesthetic (as already discussed) and also influences the kinetics of its distribution in the body, the main effect being that high lipid solubility tends to delay recovery from the effects of anaesthesia. Values of blood : gas and oil : gas partition coefficients for some anaesthetics are given in Table 26.1.

INDUCTION AND RECOVERY

The brain has a large blood flow, and the blood–brain barrier is freely permeable to anaesthetics. Thus, the concentration of anaesthetic in the brain remains virtually in equilibrium with the concentration in the arterial blood (i.e. with the concentration in the blood leaving the lungs). The kinetics of transfer of anaesthetic between the inspired air and the arterial blood therefore determine the kinetics of the pharmacological effect.

If an anaesthetic is added to the inspired air at a concentration which, at *equilibrium*, will produce surgical anaesthesia, the rate at which this equilibrium is approached depends mainly on the blood : gas partition coefficient. Contrary to what one might intuitively suppose, the *lower* the solubility in blood, the *faster* the process of equilibration. This is because, with a low-solubility agent, less has to be transferred via the lungs to the blood in order to achieve a given partial pressure. Thus a single lungful of air containing a low-solubility agent will bring the partial pressure in the blood closer to that of the inspired air than is the case for a high-solubility agent, and a smaller number of breaths (i.e. a shorter time) will be needed to reach equilibrium. The same principle applies in reverse for washout of the drug—with a low-solubility agent, the arterial partial pressure will fall more quickly, and recovery will be faster, than with a high-solubility agent. Figure 26.3 shows the much faster equilibration for nitrous oxide—a low-solubility agent—than for ether—a high-solubility agent (now clinically obsolete).

In addition to the exchanges between air and blood, the transfer of anaesthetic between blood and tissues also affects the kinetics of equilibration. Figure 26.2 shows a very simple model of the circulation in which two tissue compartments are included. Body fat is particularly important, since it has a low blood flow and often a high anaesthetic solubility (see Table 26.1). Body fat constitutes about 20% of the volume of a normal male. Thus for a drug such as halothane, the solubility of which in fat is about 100 times as great as its solubility in water, the amount present in the fat after complete equilibration would be roughly 95% of the total

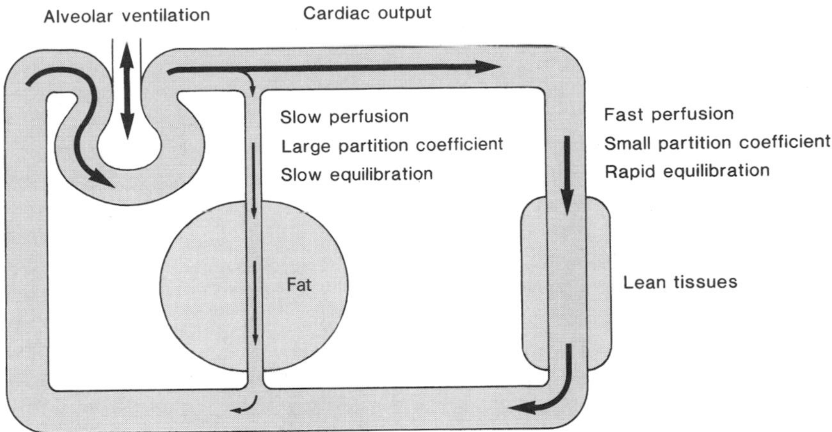

Fig. 26.2 Factors affecting the rate of equilibration of inhalation anaesthetics in the body. The body is represented as two compartments. Lean tissues have a large blood flow and low partition coefficient for anaesthetics, and therefore equilibrate rapidly with the blood. Fat tissues have a small blood flow and large partition coefficient, and therefore equilibrate slowly, acting as a reservoir of drug during the recovery phase.

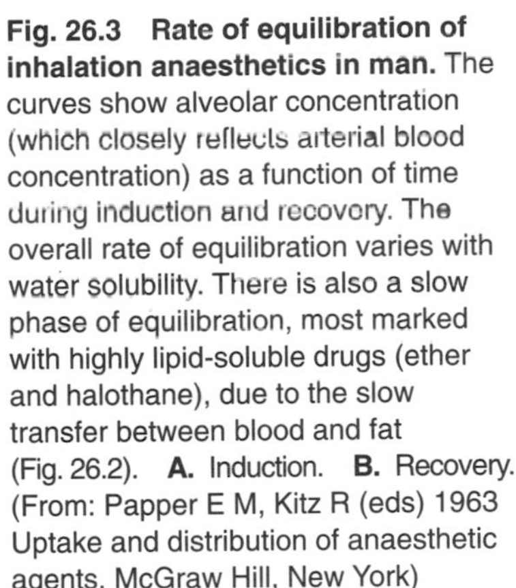

Fig. 26.3 Rate of equilibration of inhalation anaesthetics in man. The curves show alveolar concentration (which closely reflects arterial blood concentration) as a function of time during induction and recovery. The overall rate of equilibration varies with water solubility. There is also a slow phase of equilibration, most marked with highly lipid-soluble drugs (ether and halothane), due to the slow transfer between blood and fat (Fig. 26.2). **A.** Induction. **B.** Recovery. (From: Papper E M, Kitz R (eds) 1963 Uptake and distribution of anaesthetic agents. McGraw Hill, New York)

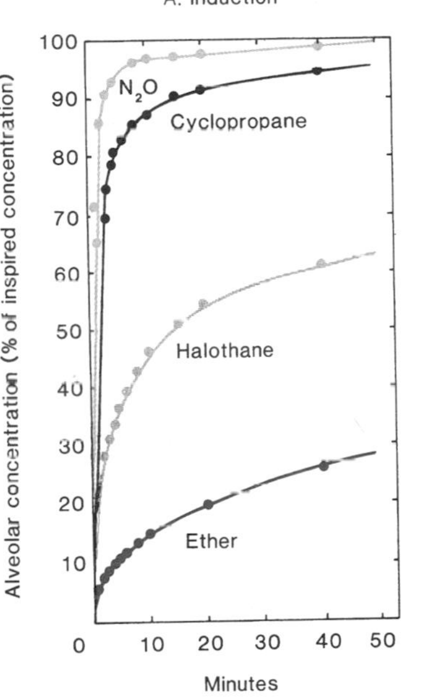

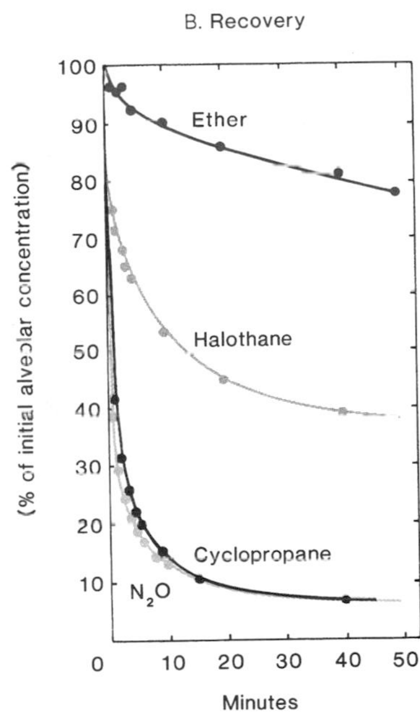

amount in the body. Because of the low blood flow it takes many hours for the drug to enter and leave the fat, which results in a pronounced slow phase of equilibration following the rapid phase associated with the blood–gas exchanges (Fig. 26.3). The more fat soluble the anaesthetic and the fatter the patient, the more pronounced this slow phase becomes.

Of the physiological factors affecting the rate of equilibrium of inhalation anaesthetics, alveolar ventilation is the most important. The greater the ventilation rate, the faster is the process of equilibration, particularly for drugs that have high blood : gas partition coefficients. The use of analgesic drugs, such as **morphine** (see Ch. 31), which reduce alveolar ventilation, can thus retard recovery from anaesthesia. Changes in cardiac output produce complex effects. Increasing the cardiac output increases the rate of extraction of anaesthetic from the alveoli and thus *retards* the rise in arterial anaesthetic content, slowing down the early phase of induction. It also increases the rate of delivery of anaesthetic to the tissues, so tends to speed up the later phase of equilibration.

Recovery from anaesthesia involves the same processes as induction but in reverse (Fig. 26.3). There is a rapid decrease in arterial anaesthetic concentration, which is mirrored in the brain, followed by a slower decline as the anaesthetic is transferred from the tissues into the bloodstream. If anaesthesia with a highly fat-soluble drug has been maintained for a long time, so that the fat has had time to accumulate a substantial amount, this slow phase of recovery can become very pronounced and the patient may remain drowsy for some hours. Because of these kinetic factors, the search for improved inhalation anaesthetics has focused on agents with low blood and tissue solubility. Recent introductions, which show kinetic properties similar to those of nitrous oxide, but have higher potency, include **sevoflurane** and **desflurane** (see below).

METABOLISM OF INHALATION ANAESTHETICS

It was originally thought that anaesthetics were too unreactive to be metabolised in the body, but in fact the metabolism of halogenated anaesthetics can be considerable, and the resulting metabolites contribute appreciably to certain toxic effects. Only with **methoxyflurane** (approximately 50% metabolised) and **halothane** (approximately 30% metabolised) does metabolism contribute appreciably to the inactivation of the drug. In other cases, the fraction of the absorbed drug that undergoes biotransformation is too small (20% or less) appreciably to affect its pharmacokinetic properties.

Metabolism in relation to toxicity

Certain types of anaesthetic-related toxicity, particularly *renal* and *hepatic* damage, are clearly associated with the formation of metabolites (see Ch. 43). These may be free radicals (e.g. $CCl_3^{\cdot}$ and $CCl_2^{\cdot}$ formed from chloroform in liver cells) or other products (e.g. fluoride ion and oxalate formed from methoxyflurane). Halothane is metabolised to bromide ion and also to trifluoroacetic acid. Following anaesthesia with methoxyflurane, the plasma fluoride concentration increases from the normal value of about 2 μmol/l to 40–80 μmol/l, and remains raised for 5–10 days (Fig. 26.4). At these levels fluoride causes detectable renal impairment, and this is the main reason why methoxyflurane has been

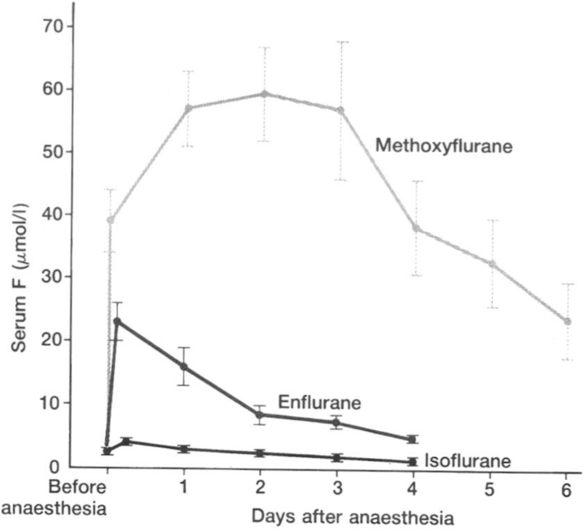

Fig. 26.4 Fluoride production following anaesthesia with methoxyflurane, isoflurane and enflurane. (From: Mazze R I 1983 Clin Anesthesiol 1(2): 469–483)

Pharmacokinetic properties of inhalation anaesthetics

- Rapid induction and recovery are important properties of an anaesthetic agent, allowing flexible control over the depth of anaesthesia.
- Speed of induction and recovery are determined by two properties of the anaesthetic: solubility in blood (blood : gas partition coefficient) and solubility in fat (lipid solubility).
- Agents with low blood : gas partition coefficients produce rapid induction and recovery (e.g. nitrous oxide, enflurane); agents with high blood : gas partition coefficients show slow induction and recovery (e.g. halothane).
- Agents with high lipid solubility (e.g. halothane and methoxyflurane) accumulate gradually in body fat, and may produce a prolonged hangover if used for a long operation.
- Some halogenated anaesthetics (especially halothane and methoxyflurane) are metabolised. This is not very important in determining their duration of action, but contributes to toxicity.

largely superseded by **enflurane** and **isoflurane**, which cause less fluoride production (Fig. 26.4), as do the newer fast-acting agents **sevoflurane** and **desflurane**.

The relationship of halothane metabolites to the occurrence of liver toxicity (see below) is not clearly established.

The problem of toxicity of low concentrations of anaesthetics inhaled over long periods by operating theatre staff causes much concern, following the demonstration that such chronic low-level exposure leads to liver toxicity (associated with metabolite formation) in experimental animals. Epidemiological studies of operating theatre staff have shown increased incidence of liver disease and of certain types of leukaemia, and of spontaneous abortion and congenital malformations, compared with similar groups of subjects not exposed to anaesthetic agents.

Causation has not been clearly established, but much effort has gone into reducing the escape of anaesthetics into the air of operating theatres.

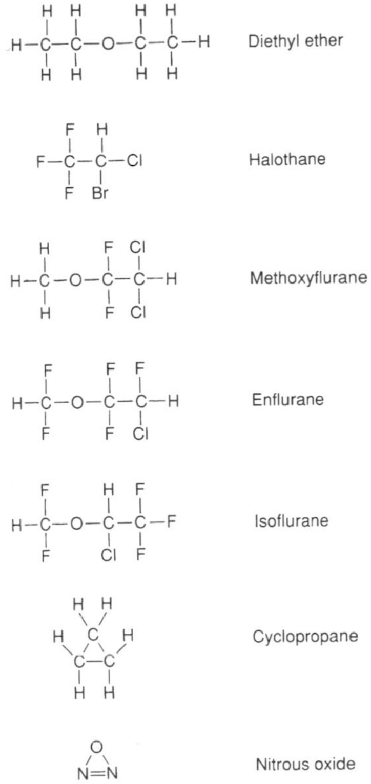

INDIVIDUAL INHALATION ANAESTHETICS

The structures of the most important inhalation anaesthetics are shown in Figure 26.5. The agents currently used in developed western countries are **halothane**, **nitrous oxide**, **enflurane** and **isoflurane**. **Ether** and **cyclopropane** are still used in some parts of the world; **methoxyflurane** (see above) has been largely superseded by enflurane and isoflurane because of its renal toxicity.

Diethyl ether

Halothane

Methoxyflurane

Enflurane

Isoflurane

Cyclopropane

Nitrous oxide

Fig. 26.5 Structures of inhalation anaesthetics.

HALOTHANE

Halothane is probably the most widely used inhalation anaesthetic. It is non-explosive and nonirritant; induction and recovery are relatively fast; it is highly potent, and can easily produce respiratory and cardiovascular failure. To control its concentration accurately, therefore, a special vaporisation chamber is used. Even in normal anaesthetic concentrations, halothane causes a fall in blood pressure, partly due to myocardial depression and partly to vasodilatation. Halothane has a relaxant effect on the uterus, which limits its usefulness for obstetric purposes. In common with other halogenated anaesthetics, halothane tends to cause cardiac dysrhythmias, particularly ventricular extrasystoles, though this does not appear to matter much in routine practice.*

The main adverse effect that has been attributed to halothane is liver damage. In a major study in 1986 of 850 000 cases involving anaesthesia with different agents, nine patients died from liver failure not attributable to any other recognisable cause, seven of whom had received halothane. Subsequent reports have suggested that the risk of liver damage is associated with repeated administration of halothane. Thus a study by the UK Committee on the Safety of Medicines of 62 cases of unexplained serious liver disease, in which drug histories were available, showed that 66% were associated with *repeated* halothane administration. About 30% of the absorbed dose of halothane undergoes metabolism, mainly by oxidation to trifluoroacetic acid, Br^- and

*It can be important in special circumstances, for example in operations for phaeochromocytoma (see Ch. 7), where there is a risk of precipitating ventricular fibrillation, and halothane must be avoided.

Cl^- ion. Trifluoroacetic acid reacts with many proteins to produce fluoroacetyl derivatives. This happens particularly in liver cells, where halothane metabolism takes place, and the mechanism of hepatotoxicity is thought to involve an immune response to certain fluoroacetylated liver enzymes (Kenna et al. 1993).

NITROUS OXIDE

Nitrous oxide is an odourless and non-explosive gas with many advantageous features for anaesthesia, and is in widespread use. It is particularly rapid in action, because of its low blood : gas partition coefficient (Table 26.1), and is also an effective analgesic agent in concentrations too low to cause unconsciousness. It is used in this way to reduce pain during childbirth. One serious drawback of nitrous oxide is its low potency. Even at a concentration of 80% in the inspired gas mixture (the maximum possible without reducing the oxygen content) nitrous oxide does not produce surgical anaesthesia. It cannot therefore be used on its own, but is very often used in conjunction with a more powerful agent such as halothane. During recovery from nitrous oxide anaesthesia, the transfer of the gas from the blood into the alveoli can be sufficient to reduce, by dilution, the alveolar partial pressure of oxygen, producing a transient hypoxia, but this is only important in patients with respiratory disease.

Nitrous oxide was for long thought to be devoid of any serious toxic effects, but has now been shown to produce significant metabolic abnormalities, resulting from the oxidation of cobalt in vitamin B_{12} (see Nunn 1984). Vitamin B_{12} (cobalamin; see Ch. 23) is required for reactions in which methionine serves as a methyl donor in the synthesis of DNA and many proteins, and exposure to nitrous oxide causes a marked inhibition of these reactions, which takes several days to recover, and has many consequences, including inhibition of cell division, which results in anaemia and leucopenia. With a single administration of nitrous oxide, these effects are not usually detectable in man, because the bone marrow has a sufficient reserve to cope with a temporary suppression of cell division, but repeated or excessively prolonged administration is known to cause leucopenia and megaloblastic anaemia. Prolonged exposure to very low concentrations of nitrous oxide, far below the level causing anaesthesia, affects protein and DNA synthesis very markedly, and nitrous oxide has been suspected to be a cause of the increased frequency of abortion and foetal abnormality among operating theatre staff.

On the basis of epidemiological evidence, nitrous oxide appears to be safe for routine purposes, but its use for prolonged anaesthesia, or in patients with B_{12}-related anaemia, is agreed to be undesirable.

METHOXYFLURANE

Methoxyflurane is a fluorinated ether (Fig. 26.5) introduced in 1960 with the aim of producing a non-explosive agent without some of the drawbacks of halothane. It is exceptionally potent (MAC 0.16%), due to its very high lipid solubility. Its blood : gas partition coefficient is considerably higher than that of halothane (Table 26.1), so induction and recovery are slower. Very high fat solubility leads to a gradual accumulation in body fat, which results in slow recovery from anaesthesia if methoxyflurane is administered for a long time. In most respects, methoxyflurane is similar to halothane, producing a similar degree of cardiovascular and respiratory depression, and a similar likelihood of cardiac dysrhythmias. It is, however, a more effective analgesic, and produces less uterine relaxation, which may be an advantage. 50% or more of the drug is metabolised to fluoride (Fig. 26.4), and this is responsible for a high incidence of renal damage, which can progress to renal failure. Oxalate, another metabolic product of methoxyflurane, also appears in the urine, but is not responsible for the toxic effect. Renal toxicity severely limits the usefulness of methoxyflurane for anything but brief administration, and it has been largely replaced by enflurane and isoflurane.

ENFLURANE

Enflurane is another halogenated ether introduced in 1973, which is much faster in its actions than methoxyflurane, is less liable to accumulate in body fat, and is metabolised to only a very minor extent, and is much less prone than methoxyflurane to cause renal damage. The main drawback to enflurane, which otherwise has many favourable characteristics, is that it can cause seizures, either during induction or following recovery from anaesthesia. In this connection it is interesting that a related substance, the fluorine-substituted diethyl-ether, hexafluoroether, is a powerful convulsant agent, though the mechanism is not understood.

ISOFLURANE

Isoflurane is similar to enflurane in many respects. It is not appreciably metabolised, and shows little sign of toxicity; it also lacks the proconvulsive property of enflurane. Its main drawbacks are high cost, associated with difficulty in separating isomers formed during synthesis, and a reported tendency to increased incidence of coronary ischaemic attacks, which means that its use should be avoided in patients with coronary disease.

Desflurane, introduced recently, is chemically similar to isoflurane, but its lower solubility in blood and fat means that induction and recovery are faster. **Sevoflurane** is intermediate in its properties. Neither of these agents produces appreciable quantities of fluoride ion.

Individual inhalation anaesthetics

- The main agents in current use in developed western countries are halothane, nitrous oxide, enflurane and isoflurane. Ether and cyclopropane are in use elsewhere in the world.
- **Halothane:**
  - —the most widely used agent
  - —potent, non-explosive and non-irritant hypotensive; may cause dysrhythmias; about 30% metabolised hangover likely, due to high lipid solubility
  - —risk of liver damage if used repeatedly.
- **Nitrous oxide:**
  - —low potency, therefore must be combined with other agents
  - —rapid induction and recovery analgesic
  - —until recently, thought to be free of serious unwanted effects; however, inhibition of methionine synthase (risk of bone marrow depression) occurs with prolonged administration.
- **Enflurane:**
  - —halogenated anaesthetic similar to halothane
  - —less metabolism than halothane or methoxyflurane, therefore less risk of toxicity
  - —faster induction and recovery than halothane
  - —some risk of epilepsy-like seizures
  - —isoflurane is similar, lacks epileptogenic property, but may precipitate myocardial ischaemia. Desflurane and sevoflurane (recently introduced) are similar, and may have advantages.
- **Ether:**
  - —easy to administer and control
  - —analgesic and muscle relaxant properties
  - —highly explosive
  - —liable to cause respiratory tract irritation
  - —long and hazardous stage II if used on its own
  - —postoperative nausea and vomiting.

Many inhalation anaesthetics have been introduced and gradually superseded, mainly because of their inflammable nature or because of toxicity. They include **chloroform** (abandoned because of hepatotoxicity and cardiac dysrhythmias), **diethyl ether** (explosive and highly irritant to the respiratory tract, leading to postoperative complications), **vinyl ether** (explosive), **cyclopropane** (explosive, strongly depressant to respiration, and hypotensive) and **trichloroethylene** (chemically unstable, no special advantages).

Further information is available in many excellent textbooks of anaesthesia (e.g. Nimmo & Smith 1989, Nunn et al. 1989, Miller 1990).

INTRAVENOUS ANAESTHETIC AGENTS

Even the fastest-acting inhalation anaesthetics, such as nitrous oxide, take a few minutes to act, and cause a period of excitement before anaesthesia is produced. Intravenous anaesthetics act much more rapidly, producing unconsciousness in about 20 seconds, as soon as the drug reaches the brain from its site of injection. These drugs are normally used for *induction of anaesthesia*. They are preferred by patients, since injection generally lacks the menacing quality associated with a face-mask in an apprehensive individual.

Other agents (e.g. **diazepam**; see Ch. 25), which are known as *basal anaesthetics*,* act rather less rapidly, but can be used to produce sedation prior to anaesthesia, thus reducing the amount of the inhalation anaesthetic that is required. In general, intravenous anaesthetics on their own are unsatisfactory for producing maintained anaesthesia

*Basal anaesthesia does not, as some students have averred, imply a rectal route of administration.

Table 26.2 Properties of intravenous anaesthetic agents

Drug	Speed of induction and recovery	Main unwanted effects	Notes
Thiopentone	Fast (cumulation occurs, giving slow recovery)	Cardiovascular and respiratory depression Hangover	Widely used as induction agent for routine purposes
Etomidate	Fast onset. Fairly fast recovery	Excitatory effects during induction and recovery Adrenocortical suppression	Less cardiovascular and respiratory depression than with thiopentone
Propofol	Fast onset. Very fast recovery	Cardiovascular and respiratory depression	Rapidly metabolised. Possible to use as continuous infusion
Ketamine	Slow onset. After-effects common during recovery	Psychotomimetic effects following recovery	Produces good analgesia and amnesia
Midazolam	Slower than other agents		Little respiratory or cardiovascular depression

because their elimination from the body is usually much slower than that of an inhalation agent, so that they do not provide the rapid control of the depth of anaesthesia that is required for surgery. However, some drugs (e.g. **ketamine**; see below) act for sufficiently long (10–20 minutes) that they can be used for short operations without the need for an inhalation agent.

The main induction agents in current use are **thiopentone, etomidate** and **propofol. Ketamine** and the short-acting benzodiazepine **midazolam** (see Ch. 27) are also used. Their main properties are summarised in Table 26.2. Agents now withdrawn because of a high incidence of acute allergic reactions, producing hypotension and bronchoconstriction, include **propanidid** and **althesin.**

The main intravenous basal anaesthetics are **ketamine** and **diazepam.**

Various other combined formulations of neuroleptic drugs (Ch. 28) and analgesics (Ch. 31) may also be used to produce a state of deep sedation and analgesia (known as neuroleptanalgesia) in which the patient remains responsive to simple commands and questions, but does not respond to painful stimuli or retain any memory of the procedure.

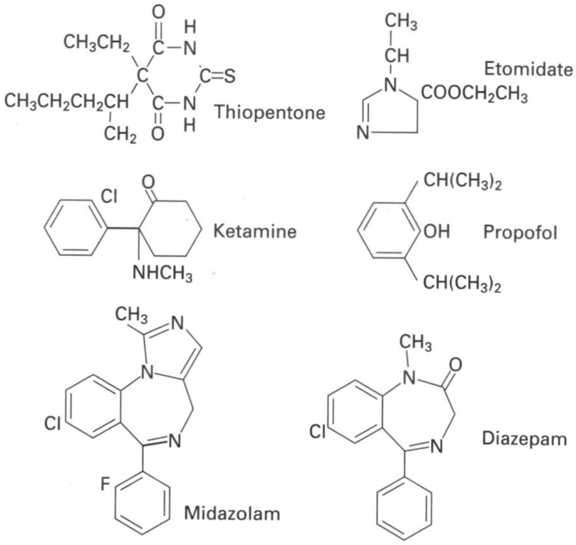

Fig. 26.6 Structures of intravenous anaesthetics.

THIOPENTONE

Thiopentone (Fig. 26.6) is a member of the barbiturate group of central nervous system depressants. Many of these have been produced and tested, but thiopentone is the only one of major importance in anaesthesia. It has very high lipid solubility, which is the main factor responsible for the speed and transience of its effect when it is injected intravenously (see below). The free acid is insoluble in water, so thiopentone is given as the sodium salt. This solution is strongly alkaline, and is unstable, so the drug must be dissolved immediately before it is used.

Pharmacokinetic aspects

On intravenous injection, thiopentone causes unconsciousness within about 20 seconds, which lasts for 5–10 minutes. The anaesthetic effect closely parallels the concentration of thiopentone in the blood reaching the brain, because its high lipid solubility allows it to cross the blood–brain barrier without appreciable hindrance.

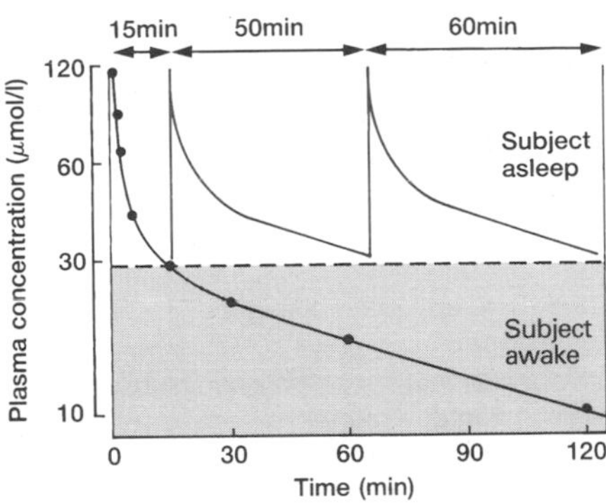

Fig. 26.7 Pharmacokinetics of intravenous thiopentone in man. Plasma concentration (logarithmic scale) following a single intravenous injection is shown as the experimental points. The concentration falls from a peak of 120 μmol/l to 30 μmol/l in about 15 minutes, due to redistribution of the drug into well-perfused tissues, and then falls much more slowly as it is distributed into fatty tissues. The red curves show the predicted time-course of the plasma concentration if subsequent injections are given each time the patient recovers consciousness. The duration of action becomes much longer as the slow phase of equilibration becomes more pronounced.

The rapid decline in the blood concentration of thiopentone following the initial peak (Fig. 26.7) occurs because of redistribution of the drug, first of all to tissues with a large blood flow (liver, kidneys, brain, etc.) and more slowly to muscle. Uptake into body fat, though favoured by the high lipid solubility of thiopentone, occurs only slowly, because of the low blood flow to this tissue. After several hours, however, most of the thiopentone present in the body will have accumulated in body fat, the rest having been metabolised. Recovery from the anaesthetic effect depends entirely on redistribution of the drug, since very little is metabolised in the first 10 minutes after injection. The blood concentration drops rapidly from its peak, but then declines only slowly as the drug is taken up by body fat and metabolised (Fig. 26.7). This means that thiopentone produces a long-lasting 'hangover', and also that repeated intravenous doses cause progressively longer periods of anaesthesia, since this plateau in blood concentration becomes progressively more elevated as more drug accumulates in the body. For this reason, thiopentone cannot be used to maintain surgical anaesthesia, but only as an induction agent.

Thiopentone binds to plasma albumin (roughly 70% of the blood content normally being bound). The fraction bound is less in states of malnutrition, liver disease or renal disease, which affect the concentration and drug-binding properties of plasma albumin, and this can appreciably reduce the dose needed for induction of anaesthesia.

Actions and side effects

The actions of thiopentone on the nervous system are very similar to those of inhalation anaesthetics, though it has no analgesic effect, and can cause profound respiratory depression even in amounts that fail to abolish reflex responses to painful stimuli. It is thus unsatisfactory as an agent for producing surgical anaesthesia and is used only for induction, before administration of an inhalation anaesthetic.

Its long after-effect, associated with a slowly declining plasma concentration, means that drowsiness and some degree of respiratory depression persist for some hours.

A danger with thiopentone is that it may accidentally be injected around, rather than into, the vein, or into an artery. This can cause local tissue necrosis and ulceration or severe arterial spasm which can result in gangrene. Immediate injection of procaine, through the same needle, is the recommended procedure if this accident occurs. The risk is nowadays small, since lower concentrations of thiopentone are now preferred for intravenous injection. Thiopentone, like other barbiturates, can precipitate an attack of porphyria in susceptible individuals (see Ch. 43).

ETOMIDATE

The intravenous induction agent etomidate was introduced in the mid-1970s, and gained favour over thiopentone on account of the larger margin between the anaesthetic dose and the dose needed to produce respiratory and cardiovascular depression. It is also more rapidly metabolised than thiopentone, and thus less likely to cause a prolonged hangover. In other respects, etomidate is very similar to thiopentone, though it appears more likely to cause involuntary movements during induction, and to cause postoperative nausea and vomiting. With prolonged use, etomidate appears to suppress the adrenal cortex, which has been associated with an increase in mortality in severely ill patients. It is therefore only used as an induction agent, and is preferable to thiopentone in patients at risk of circulatory failure.

PROPOFOL

Propofol, introduced in 1983, is also similar in its properties to thiopentone, but has the advantage of being very rapidly metabolised, and therefore giving rapid recovery without any hangover effect. The use of propofol as a continuous infusion to maintain surgical anaesthesia without the need for any inhalation agent is a possibility that is being investigated. Propofol lacks the tendency to cause involuntary movement and adrenocortical suppression seen with etomidate.

OTHER INDUCTION AGENTS

Ketamine

Ketamine (Fig. 26.6) closely resembles, both chemically and pharmacologically, **phencyclidine**, which is a 'street-drug' with a pronounced effect on sensory perception (see Ch. 32). Both drugs produce a similar anaesthesia-like state, but ketamine produces considerably less euphoria and sensory distortion than phencyclidine and is thus more useful in anaesthesia. Both drugs are believed to act by blocking activation of one type of excitatory amino acid receptor (the NMDA receptor; see Ch. 24).

Given intravenously, ketamine takes effect more slowly (2–5 minutes) than thiopentone, and produces a different effect, known as 'dissociative anaesthesia' in which there is a marked sensory loss and analgesia, as well as amnesia and paralysis of movement, without actual loss of consciousness. During induction and recovery, involuntary movements and peculiar sensory experiences often occur. Ketamine does not act simply as a depressant, and it produces cardiovascular and respiratory effects quite different from those of most anaesthetics. Blood pressure and heart rate are usually increased, and respiration is unaffected by effective anaesthetic doses. The main drawback of ketamine, in spite of the safety associated with a lack of overall depressant activity, is that hallucinations, and sometimes delirium and irrational behaviour, are common during recovery. These after-effects limit the usefulness of ketamine, but are said to be less marked in children; thus, ketamine, often in conjunction with a benzodiazepine, is frequently used for minor procedures in paediatrics.

Intravenous anaesthetic agents

- Most commonly used for induction of anaesthesia, followed by inhalation agent.
- Thiopentone is most commonly used; etomidate and propofol are alternatives; all act within 20–30 seconds if given intravenously.
- **Thiopentone:**
  —barbiturate with very high lipid solubility
  —rapid action due to rapid transfer across blood–brain barrier
  —short duration (about 5 min) due to redistribution, mainly to muscle
  —slowly metabolised, and liable to accumulate in body fat; therefore may cause prolonged effect if given repeatedly
  —no analgesic effect
  —narrow margin between anaesthetic dose and dose causing cardiovascular depression
  —risk of severe vasospasm if accidentally injected into artery.
- **Etomidate:**
  —similar to thiopentone, but more quickly metabolised
  —less risk of cardiovascular depression
  —may cause involuntary movements during induction
  —possible risk of adrenocortical suppression.
- **Propofol:**
  —recently introduced
  —rapidly metabolised
  —very rapid recovery; no cumulative effect.
- **Ketamine:**
  —analogue of phencyclidine, with similar properties
  —action differs from other agents; probably related to effect on NMDA-type glutamate receptors
  —onset of effect is relatively slow (2–5 min)
  —produces 'dissociative' anaesthesia, in which patient may remain conscious, though amnesic and insensitive to pain
  —high incidence (less in children) of dysphoria, hallucinations, etc. during recovery; therefore used mainly for minor procedures in children.

Midazolam

Midazolam is appreciably slower in its action, both induction and recovery, than the drugs discussed above, but lacks the tendency to cause respiratory and cardiovascular depression, which can be an advantage in some patients.

REFERENCES AND FURTHER READING

Franks N P, Lieb W R 1987 What is the molecular nature of general anaesthetic target sites? Trends Pharmacol Sci 8: 169–174

Franks N P, Lieb W R 1994 Molecular and cellular mechanisms of general anaesthesia. Nature 367: 607–614

Halsey M J 1989 Physicochemical properties of inhalation anaesthetics. In: Nunn J F, Utting J E, Brown B R (eds) General anaesthesia. Butterworth, London

Kenna J G, Knight T L, van Pelt F N A M 1993 Immunity to halothane metabolite-modified proteins in halothane hepatitis. Ann NY Acad Sci 685: 646–661

Miller K W, Paton W D M, Smith R A, Smith E B 1973 The pressure reversal of general anaesthesia and the critical volume hypothesis. Mol Pharmacol 9: 131–143

Miller R D (ed) 1990 Anaesthesia. Churchill Livingstone, New York

Nimmo W S, Smith G (eds) 1989 Anaesthesia. Blackwell, Oxford

Nunn J F 1984 Interaction of nitrous oxide and vitamin B_{12}. Trends Pharmacol Sci 5: 225–227

Nunn J F, Utting J E, Brown B R (eds) 1989 General anaesthesia. Butterworth, London

Pocock G, Richards C D 1993 Excitatory and inhibitory synaptic mechanisms in anaesthesia. Br J Anaesth 71: 134–147

Richards C D 1980 The mechanism of general anaesthesia. In: Norman J, Whitwam J (eds) Topical reviews in anaesthesia. Wright, Bristol, vol 1

Wann K T, Macdonald A G 1988 Actions and interactions of high pressure and general anaesthetics. Prog Neurobiol 30: 271–307

27
ANXIOLYTIC AND HYPNOTIC DRUGS

In this chapter we discuss **anxiolytic drugs** (used to treat the symptoms of anxiety) and **hypnotic drugs** (used to treat insomnia). Though the clinical objectives are different, the same drugs are often used for both purposes. This is a reflection of the fact that drugs that relieve anxiety generally cause a degree of sedation and drowsiness, which is one of the main drawbacks in the clinical use of anxiolytic drugs. Until about 30 years ago, the sedatives that were in clinical use (mainly barbiturates and related compounds) were pharmacologically indistinguishable from general anaesthetics (see Ch. 26). In high doses, all of these drugs cause unconsciousness, and eventually death from respiratory and cardiovascular depression. In 1961 the benzodiazepines were discovered, and these drugs quickly replaced most of the earlier anxiolytic and hypnotic agents. In recent years, a number of drugs that act on 5-HT receptors in the brain, and do not have strong sedative activity, have been introduced as anxiolytic agents

THE NATURE OF ANXIETY AND MEASUREMENT OF ANXIOLYTIC ACTIVITY

The distinction between a 'pathological' and a 'normal' state of anxiety is hard to draw, but in spite of (or perhaps because of) this diagnostic vagueness, anxiolytic drugs are among the most frequently prescribed substances. A study in Western European countries in the mid-1980s showed that the proportion of the total population using anxiolytic drugs regularly was 17% in Belgium and France, 14% in the UK and 10% in Spain. The chief manifestations of anxiety (see Dews 1981) are:

- *Verbal complaint.* The patients says that he or she is excessively anxious.
- *Somatic and autonomic effects.* The patient is restless and agitated, has tachycardia, increased sweating, weeping and often gastrointestinal disorders.
- *Interference with normal productive activities.*

Clinical conditions related to anxiety include *phobic anxiety* and *panic disorder.* In phobic states, anxiety is triggered by specific circumstances, such as open spaces, social interactions or spiders. In panic disorder, attacks of unbearable fear occur in association with marked somatic symptoms, such as sweating, tachycardia, chest pains, trembling, choking, etc. Such attacks can be induced even in normal individuals by infusion of sodium lactate, and the condition appears to have a genetic component, so an underlying biochemical abnormality is suspected. The distinction between these conditions and generalised anxiety disorders is not a sharp one, and anxiolytic drugs are used to treat all of them.

Anxiety is a subjective human phenomenon and, except for some of the associated somatic and autonomic changes, it has no obvious counterpart in experimental animals. In biological terms, anxiety may be regarded as a particular form of behavioural inhibition that occurs in response to environmental events that are *novel, non-rewarding* (under conditions where reward is expected) or *punishing.* In animals this behavioural inhibition may take the form of immobility, or suppression of a behavioural response such as bar-pressing to obtain food (see below). To develop new anxiolytic drugs it is essential to have animal tests that give a good guide to activity in man, and considerable effort has gone into developing and validating such tests.

ANIMAL MODELS OF ANXIETY

Various types of behavioural test may be used to measure anxiolytic activity. For example, a rat placed in an unfamiliar environment normally responds by remaining immobile, though alert, ('behavioural suppression') for a time, which may represent 'anxiety' produced by the strange environment. This immobility is reduced if anxiolytic drugs are administered. The 'elevated cross' is a widely-used test model. Two arms of the cross are closed in, and the others are open. Normally rats spend most of their time in the closed arms and avoid the open arms (afraid, possibly, of falling off). Administration of anxiolytic drugs increases the time spent in the open arms, and also increases the mobility of the rats as judged by the frequency of crossing the transection.

Conflict tests can also be used. For example, a rat trained to press a bar repeatedly to obtain a food pellet normally achieves a high and consistent response rate. A conflict element is then introduced: at intervals, indicated by an auditory signal, bar-pressing results in an occasional 'punishment' in the form of an electric shock in addition to the reward of a food pellet. Normally, the rat ceases pressing the bar (behavioural inhibition), and thus avoids the shock, during the period when the signal is sounding. The effect of an anxiolytic drug is to relieve this suppressive effect, so that the rats continue bar-pressing for reward in spite of the 'punishment'. Surprisingly, analgesic drugs, which presumably make the punishment less painful, are ineffective in this test in animals, as are other types of psychotropic drug. Other evidence confirms that it is the behavioural inhibition produced by the conflict situation, rather than an elevation of the pain threshold, that is changed by anxiolytic drugs.

In other tests, aggressive behaviour is produced experimentally by lesions of the midbrain septum, or by housing mice in individual cages and then introducing a stranger. Anxiolytic drugs reduce the amount of aggressive behaviour displayed, in a quantifiable way. They also increase the amount of social interaction occurring between pairs of rats placed in an unfamiliar environment, this being a situation in which social interaction is greatly decreased in control animals. In most of these tests, the response is an increase in behavioural activity, so it is clear that the anxiolytic drugs are producing something more than a non-specific sedation.

TESTS ON HUMANS

Various 'anxiety scale' tests have been devised in which a patient's responses to a standard battery of questions are scored, and these are widely used to assay the clinical effectiveness of anxiolytic drugs. Effects have been clearly demonstrated in tests of this kind, but placebo treatment often also produces highly significant responses.

Other tests rely on measurement of the somatic and autonomic effects associated with anxiety. An example is the *galvanic skin response* (GSR) in which the electrical conductivity of the skin is used as a measure of sweat production. Any novel stimulus, whether pleasant or unpleasant, causes a brief reduction of resistance. This forms the basis of the lie-detector test. If an innocuous stimulus is repeated at intervals, the magnitude of the response decreases (habituation). The rate of habituation is less in anxious patients than in normal subjects, and is increased by anxiolytic drugs. GSR habituation seems to be a particularly sensitive measure, for many tests of autonomic function in anxious subjects (e.g. heart rate changes) show no clear-cut change in response to anxiolytic drugs.

A human version of the conflict test described above involves the substitution of money for food

Measurement of anxiolytic activity

- Behavioural tests in animals are based on measurements of the behavioural inhibition (considered to reflect 'anxiety') in response to conflict or novelty.
- Human tests for anxiolytic drugs employ psychiatric rating scales or measures of autonomic responses, such as the galvanic skin response.
- Tests such as these can distinguish between anxiolytic drugs (benzodiazepines, 5-HT agonists, etc.) and other types of psychotropic drug.

pellets, and the use of graded electric shocks as punishment. As with rats, administration of diazepam increases the rate of button-pressing for money during the periods when the punishment was in operation, though the subjects reported no change in the painfulness of the electric shock. Subtler forms of torment and reward could easily be envisaged.

CLASSIFICATION OF ANXIOLYTIC AND HYPNOTIC DRUGS

The main groups of drugs are:

- *Benzodiazepines*. This is the most important group, used as anxiolytic and hypnotic agents.
- *5-HT_{1A}-receptor agonists* (e.g. **buspirone**). These agents, recently introduced, are anxiolytic but not appreciably sedative.
- *Barbiturates*. These are now largely obsolete, superseded by benzodiazepines. Their use is now more-or-less confined to anaesthesia (Ch. 26) and the treatment of epilepsy (Ch. 30).
- *β-adrenoceptor antagonists* (e.g. **propranolol**; Ch. 7). These are used to treat some forms of anxiety, particularly where physical symptoms, such as sweating, tremor and tachycardia, are troublesome. Their effectiveness depends on block of peripheral sympathetic responses rather than on any central effects, though they may cause drowsiness. They are often used by actors and musicians to reduce the symptoms of stage fright, but their use by professional snooker players to minimise tremor is banned as unsportsmanlike.
- *Miscellaneous other drugs* (e.g. **chloral hydrate**, **meprobamate** and **paraldehyde**). They are no longer recommended, but therapeutic habits die hard, and chloral hydrate and paraldehyde are still used, mainly in hospitals. Sedative antihistamines (see Ch. 12), such as **diphenhydramine**, are sometimes used as sleeping pills, particularly for wakeful children.

Classes of anxiolytic and hypnotic drugs

- Benzodiazepines: the most important class, used for treating both anxiety states and insomnia.
- 5-HT_{1A}-receptor agonists: recently introduced, showing anxiolytic activity with little sedation.
- Barbiturates: now largely obsolete as anxiolytic/sedative agents, though still occasionally prescribed.
- β-adrenoceptor antagonists: used mainly to reduce physical symptoms of anxiety (tremor, palpitations, etc.); no effect on affective component.
- Miscellaneous other agents are still used occasionally to treat insomnia (benzodiazepines are preferable in most cases).

BENZODIAZEPINES

The first compound of the benzodiazepine group, **chlordiazepoxide**, was synthesised by accident in 1961, the unusual 7-membered ring having been produced as a result of an unplanned reaction in the laboratories of Hoffman la Roche. Its unexpected pharmacological activity was recognised as a result of a routine screening procedure. This series of compounds quite soon became the most widely prescribed drugs in the pharmacopoeia—a potent reminder to advocates of rational drug design that historical examples do not always support their view.

Chemistry and structure–activity relationships

The basic chemical structure of all benzodiazepines consists of an unusual 7-membered ring fused to an aromatic ring, with four main substitutent groups which can be modified without loss of activity. Thousands of compounds have been made and tested, and about 20 are available for clinical use, the most important ones being listed in Table 27.1. They are basically similar in their pharmacological actions, though some degree of selectivity has been reported. For example, it is claimed that some compounds show a greater anticonvulsant activity than others in relation to their sedative and anxiolytic effects. Results from different laboratories, however, show wide variations, probably because of variations in experimental methodology.* It is therefore risky

*For example, the ED_{50} for diazepam in mice, measured by a standard laboratory test for motor coordination (the rotarod test) varied between 2.1 and 30 mg/kg in seven different laboratories (see Haefely et al. 1981).

to assume that the differences in pharmacological specificity that have been reported will be reflected in clinical use. From a clinical point of view, differences in pharmacokinetic behaviour among different benzodiazepines (see below) are more important than differences in profile of activity. Recently, drugs with a similar structure have been discovered which specifically antagonise the effects of the benzodiazepines, for example **flumazenil** (see below).

Pharmacological effects

The most important effects of the benzodiazepines are on the central nervous system and consist of:

- reduction of anxiety and aggression
- sedation and induction of sleep
- reduction of muscle tone and coordination
- anticonvulsant effect.

Reduction of anxiety and aggression

The measurement of anxiolytic effects in animals and man has been discussed above. Benzodiazepines show activity in this type of assay, and also exert a marked 'taming' effect, allowing animals to be handled much more easily. If given to the dominant member of a pair of animals (e.g. mice or monkeys) housed in the same cage, benzodiazepines reduce the number of attacks by the dominant individual and increase the number of attacks made upon him. With the possible exception of **alprazolam** (Table 27.1), benzodiazepines do not have specific antidepressant effects, though the relief of anxiety may be beneficial in depressed patients. Benzodiazepines may paradoxically produce an increase in irritability and aggression in some individuals. This appears to be particularly pronounced with the ultra-short-acting drug **triazolam** (and led to its withdrawal in the UK and some other countries), and is generally more common with short-acting compounds. It is probably a manifestation of the benzodiazepine withdrawal syndrome, which occurs with all of these drugs (see below), but is more acute with drugs whose action wears off rapidly.

The use of benzodiazepines as anxiolytic agents is reviewed by Shader & Greenblatt (1993).

Sedation and induction of sleep

Benzodiazepines decrease the time taken to get to sleep, and increase the total duration of sleep, though the latter effect occurs only in subjects who normally sleep for less than about 6 hours each night. Both effects tend to decline when benzodiazepines are taken regularly for 1–2 weeks.

On the basis of EEG measurements, several levels of sleep can be recognised. Of particular psychological importance are 'rapid eye movement' (REM) sleep, which is associated with dreaming, and 'slow wave' (SW) sleep, which corresponds to the deepest level of sleep when the metabolic rate and adrenal steroid secretion are at their lowest and the secretion of growth hormone is at its highest (see Ch. 21). All hypnotic drugs reduce the proportion of REM sleep, though benzodiazepines affect it less than other hypnotics. Artificial interruption of REM sleep causes irritability and anxiety, even if the total amount of sleep is not reduced, and the lost REM sleep is made up for at the end of such an experiment by a rebound increase. The same pattern of rebound in REM sleep is seen at the end of a period of administration of benzodiazepines or other hypnotics. It is therefore assumed that REM sleep has a function, and that the lesser reduction of REM sleep by benzodiazepines is a point in their favour.

The proportion of SW sleep is significantly reduced by benzodiazepines, though a recent study showed no change in growth hormone secretion.

Insomnia (see Gillin & Byerley 1990) is subjectively unpleasant rather than objectively harmful, so the best guide to the usefulness of hypnotic drugs in improving the quality of sleep may be the patient's own judgement. Figure 27.1 shows the improve-

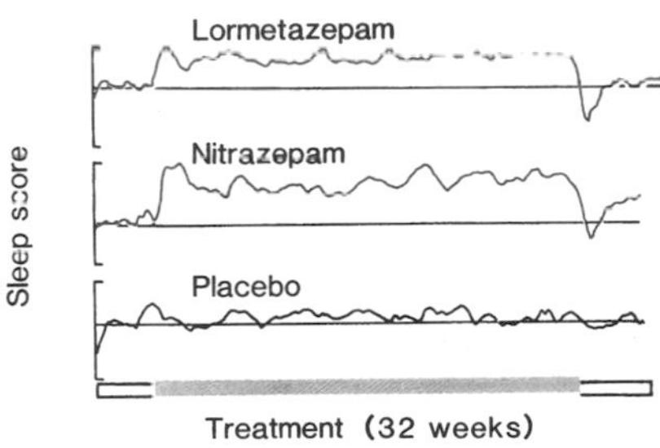

Fig. 27.1 Effects of long-term benzodiazepine treatment on sleep quality. 100 poor sleepers were given, under double-blind conditions, lormetazepam 5 mg, nitrazepam 2 mg, or placebo nightly for 24 weeks, the test period being preceded and followed by 4 weeks of placebo treatment. They were asked to assess, on a subjective rating scale, the quality of sleep during each night, and the results are expressed as a 5-day rolling average of these scores. The improvement in sleep quality was maintained during the 24-week test period, and was followed by a 'rebound' worsening of sleep when the test period ended. (From: Oswald I et al. 1982 Br Med J 284: 860–864)

ment of subjective ratings of sleep quality produced by a benzodiazepine, and the rebound decrease at the end of a 32-week period of drug treatment. It is notable that, though tolerance to objective effects such as reduced sleep latency occurs within a few days, this is not obvious in the subjective ratings.

In general, the sedative effects of benzodiazepines appear to go hand in hand with their anxiolytic effects, so it has not yet been possible to develop a non-sedative anxiolytic agent of this class.

Reduction of muscle tone and coordination

Benzodiazepines appear to reduce muscle tone by a central action that is independent of their sedative effect. Cats are particularly sensitive to this action, and some benzodiazepines (e.g. **clonazepam**, **flunitrazepam**) reduce decerebrate rigidity in doses that are much smaller than those needed to produce behavioural effects. In other species, the effect is less clear. Coordination can be tested by measuring the length of time for which mice can stay on a slowly rotating horizontal plastic rod, or the time taken for them to escape from confinement by climbing up the inside of a tubular chimney. Performance in these acrobatic tricks is impaired by benzodiazepines and other sedatives, but it is not clear that particular drugs show selectivity in this respect in species other than the cat. Studies in man have failed to show differences between benzodiazepines.

Increased muscle tone is a common feature of anxiety states in man, and may contribute to the aches and pains, including headache, which often trouble anxious patients. The relaxant effect of benzodiazepines may therefore be clinically useful. A reduction of muscle tone appears to be possible without producing appreciable incoordination.

Anticonvulsant effects

All of the benzodiazepines have anticonvulsant activity in experimental animal tests. They are generally more effective against chemically induced convulsions caused by leptazol, bicuculline and like drugs (see Chs 30 and 32) than against electrically induced convulsions, and are among the most potent agents known in preventing leptazol-induced convulsions. Benzodiazepines do not affect strychnine-induced convulsions in experimental animals. Both bicuculline and strychnine are believed to act by blocking the action of inhibitory transmitters in the central nervous system; strychnine exerts its effect on glycine receptors (see Ch. 32), whereas bicuculline and several other chemical convulsant agents act on $GABA_A$ receptors. Since benzodiazepines enhance the action of GABA but not glycine, the selectivity of their anticonvulsant action is explicable. There is some evidence that **clonazepam** is relatively more effective as an anticonvulsant in relation to its behavioural effects than other benzodiazepines, and this drug is sometimes used clinically, particularly for the treatment of absence seizures and myoclonic seizures in children (see Ch. 30). **Diazepam**, given intravenously, is an effective way of terminating the repeated seizures that constitute *status epilepticus*.

Mechanism of action

Benzodiazepines were originally assumed, in the absence of evidence to the contrary, to be acting as 'non-specific depressants'. In 1977, however, it was found that benzodiazepines interact with specific binding sites in the brain. Binding to tissues other than the brain is weak or absent* and, within the brain, diazepam binding shows a distinct regional distribution. Binding is highest in the cerebral cortex, less in the limbic system and midbrain, and still less in the brainstem and spinal cord. It roughly, but not exactly, agrees with counts of $GABA_A$ receptors, though the number of benzodiazepine sites is consistently less. The correlation between affinity for binding sites and pharmacological potency among a range of benzodiazepines is reasonable but not perfect (Fig. 27.2; data summarised in Braestrup & Nielsen 1986). The discrepancies are up to 10-fold for some compounds. This may be partly due to the fact that the pharmacological measurements were made in vivo, so that the drugs were subject to metabolic alteration. It is known that benzodiazepines are metabolised at very variable rates, and that in some cases the metabolites are pharmacologically active. Alternatively, the heterogeneity among binding sites (see below) may well obscure a simple correlation of overall binding with activity.

About the same time that the existence of specific benzodiazepine binding was discovered, evidence was accumulating that these drugs specifically augment the actions of GABA (Fig. 27.3). This aug-

*Peripheral benzodiazepine-binding sites, not associated with GABA receptors, are known to exist in many tissues, but their function and pharmacological significance are unknown.

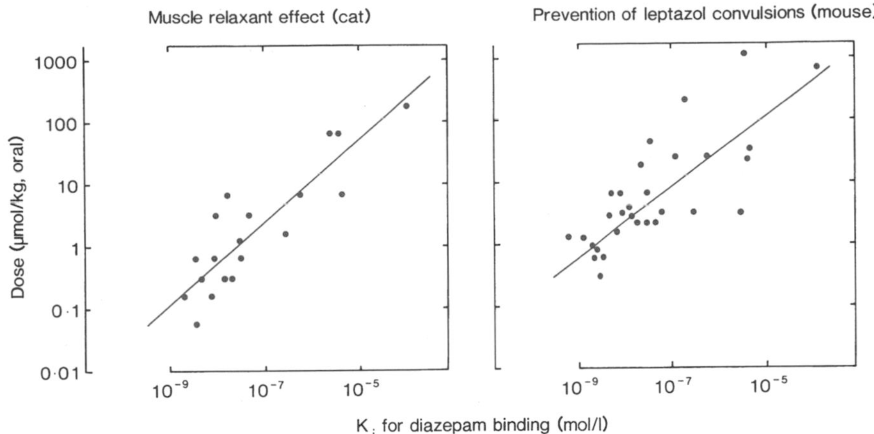

Fig. 27.2 Correlation of binding affinity and pharmacological potency among benzodiazepines. Binding affinity is expressed as an equilibrium constant, and was calculated by measuring the concentration of drug needed to inhibit the binding of ^{3}H-diazepam to brain membranes. The ordinates show equipotent doses in two biological test systems. (Data from: Braestrup C, Squires R F 1978 Eur J Pharmacol 78: 263)

mentation of the pharmacological effects of GABA is confined to $GABA_A$ receptors in the central nervous system, which produce an increased chloride conductance (see Ch. 24); actions produced by $GABA_B$ receptors (reduction of calcium currents and increased potassium permeability) are not affected, nor are most $GABA_A$ responses in peripheral neurons.

Binding studies have revealed something of the mechanism of this interesting interaction. There is a mutual augmentation of binding between GABA and benzodiazepines. The two agents bind to independent sites on the same receptor–ion-channel complex, and each increases the affinity of the sites for the other, without affecting the total number of sites. Benzodiazepines do not open chloride channels by themselves, but they act allosterically to increase the affinity of the receptors for GABA. Enhancement of the GABA effect has been shown by a noise analysis (see Ch. 2) to be associated with an increase in the number of channels that are opened by a given concentration of GABA, rather than with an increase in channel conductance or average open time (Fig. 27.3).

Cloning of the $GABA_A$ receptor (see Lüddens & Wisden 1991, Doble & Martin 1992) has given some insights into the molecular interaction between benzodiazepine binding and GABA action, though the details are dauntingly complex and still far from clear. The receptor is of the ligand-gated ion channel type, similar to the nicotinic ACh receptor (Ch. 2). It consists of several subunits (probably five in the native receptor), surrounding a central channel. The main subunits (α, β, γ, δ) each exist in various subtypes; for example, six different α-subtypes have been defined, and four different β-subtypes. Controlled expression of different combinations of receptor subunits in toad oocytes (see Ch. 2) has allowed the functions of each to be understood more clearly. 'Receptors' consisting of only one type of subunit (α or β or γ) are able to respond to GABA, so it appears that all of these subunits possess GABA-binding sites. Optimal function, however, requires the presence of all three subtypes. The α-subunit is essential for modulation by benzodiazepines, and is believed to contain the benzodiazepine-binding site. One variant of the α-subunit (α_6) lacks this site, and receptors containing this subunit, which are present in various brain regions, are insensitive to benzodiazepines. Other variants of this subunit may give rise to two distinct types of benzodiazepine receptor (BZ_1 and BZ_2) which differ in their pharmacological properties and distribution within the brain (see Doble & Martin 1992). The γ-subunit must also be present for benzodiazepines to act, and variants of it affect the selectivity for different benzodiazepine ligands. The emergence of multiple molecular subtypes of the GABA and benzodiazepine receptors is an example of an increasingly familiar pharmacological scenario. In time,

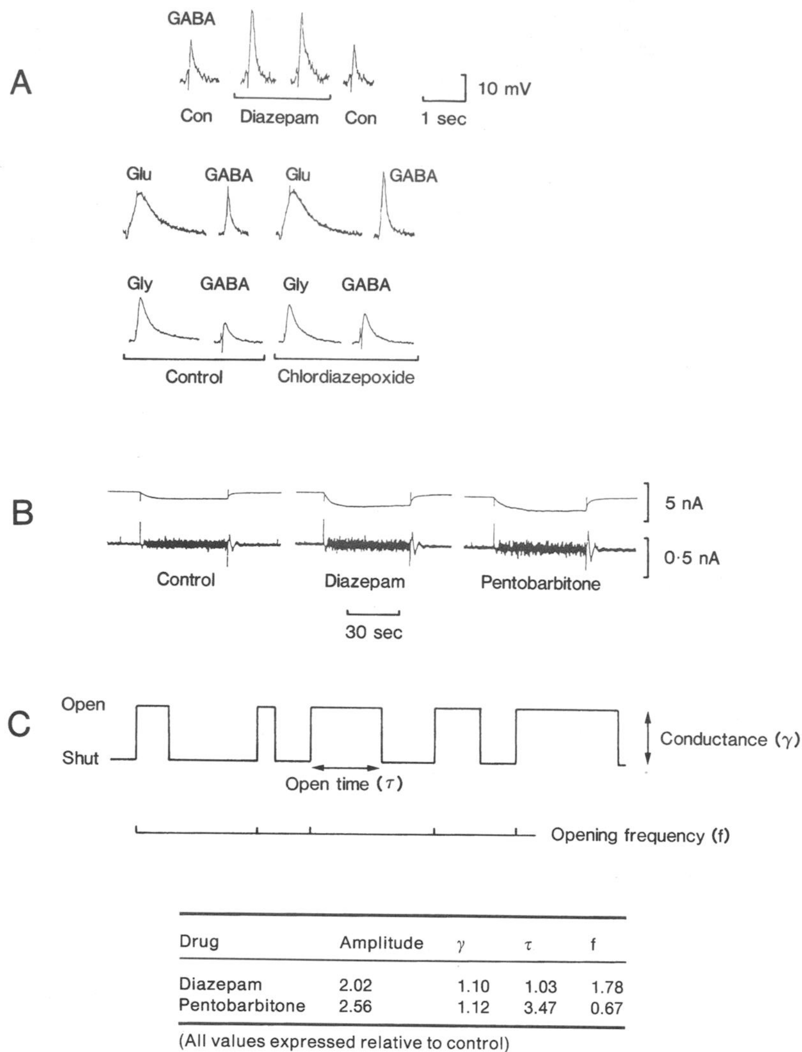

Drug	Amplitude	γ	τ	f
Diazepam	2.02	1.10	1.03	1.78
Pentobarbitone	2.56	1.12	3.47	0.67

(All values expressed relative to control)

Fig. 27.3 Potentiating effect of benzodiazepines and pentobarbitone on the action of GABA in mouse spinal cord neurons grown in tissue culture. Drugs were applied by ionophoresis to mouse spinal cord neurons grown in tissue culture, from micropipettes placed close to the cells. The membrane was hyperpolarised to –90 mv, and the cells were loaded with chloride ions from the recording microelectrode, so inhibitory amino acids (GABA and glycine), as well as excitatory ones (glutamate), caused depolarising responses. **A.** The potentiating effect is restricted to GABA responses, glutamate and glycine responses being unaffected. **B.** Enhancement of GABA responses by diazepam and pentobarbitone, recorded with a voltage-clamp technique. Inward current (i.e. outward flux of chloride ions) is shown as a downward deflection in the upper records. The lower records are at higher gain, and are filtered to remove the DC component, leaving the high-frequency noise signal (see Ch. 2) which was analysed to provide estimates of channel conductance, mean channel lifetime and opening frequency. **C.** Schematic diagram of channel-opening parameters. The table below shows the effects of diazepam and pentobarbitone. (From: MacDonald R, Barker J L 1978 Nature 271: 563; Study R E, Barker J L 1981 Proc Natl Acad Sci 78: 7180)

some of the pharmacological complexities will probably be explained in terms of this molecular diversity, but at this stage the insights remain elusive. However, being lost in an elaborate citadel is surely an advance on being lost in a featureless fog.

The $GABA_A$ receptor is responsive to an extraordinarily wide range of chemical modulators (see Sieghart 1992), including various CNS depressants, such as barbiturates (see below), ethanol (Ch. 33) and anaesthetic steroids (Ch. 26), and these interactions may account for the effects of many of these drugs on brain function.

Is there an endogenous benzodiazepine-like mediator?

The existence of specific benzodiazepine receptors suggested that there might be an endogenous ligand (analogous to endorphins in relation to the morphine receptor) whose function was to regulate the inhibitory effect of GABA. So far no such substance has been definitely identified, though there has been much speculation (see Barbaccia et al. 1988). One candidate, now known to be an artefact, was ethyl β-carboline 3-carboxylate (β-CCE), which was discovered by assaying urine samples for activity in inhibiting benzodiazepine binding. Another candidate is a 10 kDa peptide, *diazepam-binding inhibitor* (DBI) isolated from rat brain. This peptide binds strongly to the benzodiazepine-binding site of the $GABA_A$ receptor, but, like β-CCE, has the opposite effect to benzodiazepines; i.e. these compounds inhibit chloride channel opening by GABA, and have an anxiogenic and pro-convulsant effect. Other evidence suggests that benzodiazepines themselves may occur naturally in the brain. At present there is no general agreement on the nature of the putative endogenous ligand.

Benzodiazepine inverse agonists and antagonists

The term 'inverse agonist' is applied to drugs which bind to benzodiazepine receptors and exert the opposite effect to that of conventional benzodiazepines, producing signs of increased anxiety and convulsions. β-CCE is an example, and other benzodiazepine-like molecules have also been discovered. It may be possible (see Fig. 27.4) to explain these complexities in terms of the two-state model discussed in Chapter 1, by postulating that the benzodiazepine receptor exists in two distinct conformations, only one of which (A) can bind a GABA molecule and open the chloride channel. The other conformation (B) cannot bind GABA. Normally, with no benzodiazepine receptor ligand present, there is an equilibrium between these two conformations; sensitivity to GABA is present, but submaximal. Benzodiazepine agonists (e.g. diazepam) are postulated to bind only to conformation A, thus shifting the equilibrium in favour of A and enhancing GABA sensitivity. Inverse agonists bind selectively to B, and have the opposite effect. Competitive antagonists, such as flumazenil, bind equally to A and B, and consequently do not disturb the conformational equilibrium but prevent the binding of other substances to the benzodiazepine receptor, thus antagonising the effect of both agonists and inverse

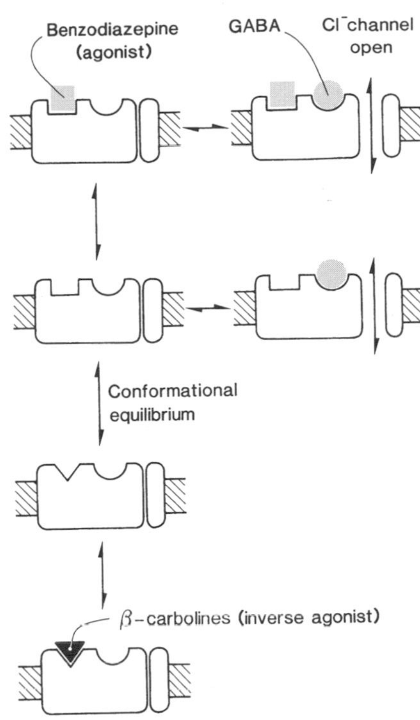

Fig. 27.4 Model of benzodiazepine/GABA-receptor interaction. Benzodiazepine agonists (e.g. diazepam) and antagonists (e.g. flumazenil) are believed to bind to a site on the GABA receptor distinct from the GABA-binding site. A conformational equilibrium exists between states in which the benzodiazepine receptor exists in its agonist-binding conformation (above) and in its antagonist-binding conformation (below). In the latter state, the GABA receptor has a much reduced affinity for GABA, so that the chloride channel remains closed.

Table 27.1 Characteristics of benzodiazepines in man

Drug	Half-life of parent compound (h)	Active metabolite	Half-life of metabolite (h)	Overall duration of action	Main uses
Triazolam	2–4	Hydroxylated derivative	2	Ultra-short (< 6h)	Hypnotic*
Lorazepam **Oxazepam** **Temazepam** **Lormetazepam**	8–12	No		Short (12–18 h)	Anxiolytic, hypnotic
Alprazolam	6–12	Hydroxylated derivative	6	Medium (24 h)	Anxiolytic, antidepressant
Nitrazepam	16–40	No		Medium	Hypnotic, anxiolytic
Diazepam **Chlordiazepoxide**	20–40	Nordiazepam	60	Long (24–48 h)	Anxiolytic, anticonvulsant
Flurazepam	1	Desmethyl-flurazepam	60	Long	Anxiolytic
Clonazepam	50	No		Long	Anticonvulsant, anxiolytic

* Triazolam has been withdrawn from use in the UK on account of side effects.

agonists. Some of the molecular variants of the $GABA_A$ receptor (see above) seem to show different relative affinities for agonists, antagonists and inverse agonists, and it is possible that this reflects differences in the equilibrium between the A and B states among these variants.

Pharmacokinetic aspects

Benzodiazepines are well absorbed when given orally, usually giving a peak plasma concentration in about 1 hour. Some (e.g. oxazepam, lorazepam) are absorbed more slowly. They bind strongly to plasma protein, but their high lipid solubility causes many of them to accumulate gradually in body fat.

These two factors result in distribution volumes not far from 1 l/kg body weight for most benzodiazepines. They are normally given by mouth, but can be given intravenously (e.g. diazepam in status epilepticus). Intramuscular injection often results in slow absorption.

Benzodiazepines are all inactivated by metabolic processes, and are eventually excreted as glucuronide conjugates in the urine. They vary greatly in duration of action, and can be roughly divided into short-, medium- and long-acting compounds (Table 27.1). The distinction between these categories depends partly on whether or not the drug forms a long-lasting pharmacologically active metabolite, such as N-desmethyldiazepam (**nordiazepam**). The half-life of this compound, which lies on the metabolic pathway of several of the benzodiazepines, is about 60 hours, and this accounts for the tendency of many benzodiazepines to produce cumulative effects and long hangovers when they are given at regular intervals. The short-acting compounds are those that are metabolised directly by conjugation with glucuronide. The main pathways are shown in Figure 27.5. Figure 27.6 shows the gradual build-up and slow disappearance of nordiazepam from the plasma of a human subject given diazepam daily for 15 days.

Advancing age affects the rate of oxidative reactions more than that of conjugation reactions. Thus the effect of the long-acting benzodiazepines, which are sometimes (though inadvisably) used regularly as hypnotics or anxio-lytic agents for many years, tends to increase with age, and it is common for drowsiness and confusion to develop insidiously for this reason.*

Clinical uses

There are summarised on page 558.

*At the age of 91, the grandmother of one of the authors was growing increasingly forgetful and mildly dotty, having been taking nitrazepam for insomnia regularly for years. To the author's lasting shame, it took a canny general practitioner to diagnose the problem. Cancellation of the nitrazepam prescription produced a dramatic improvement.

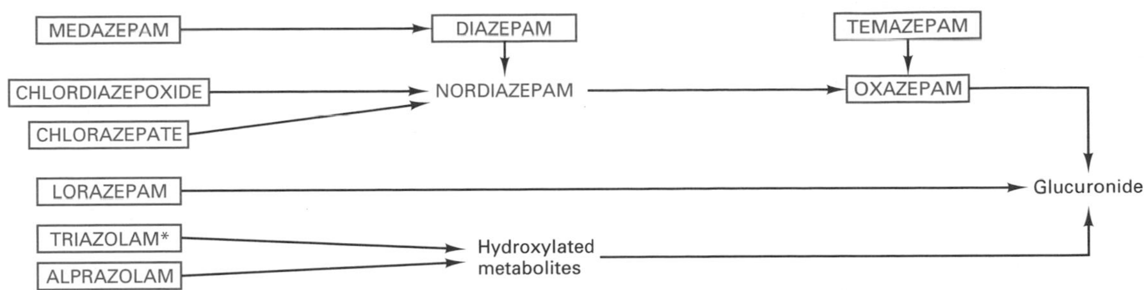

Fig. 27.5 The metabolism of benzodiazepines. The N-demethylated metabolite, nordiazepam, is formed from many benzodiazepines, and is important because it is biologically active and has a very long half-life. Compounds in red have pharmacological activity. Boxed compounds are administered as drugs.

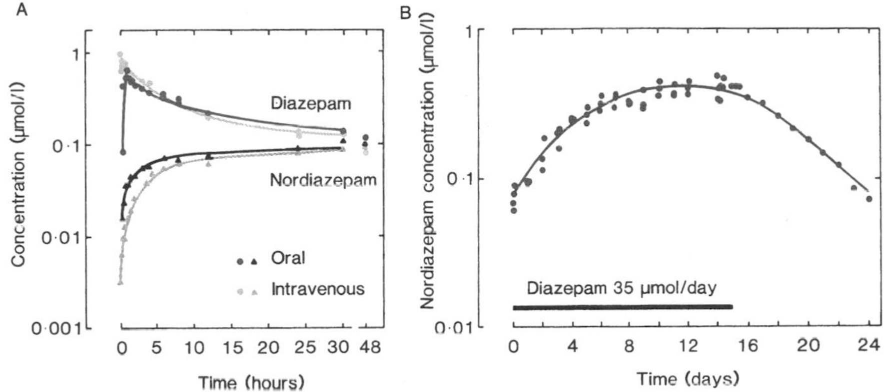

Fig. 27.6 Pharmacokinetics of diazepam in man. A. Concentrations of diazepam and nordiazepam following a single oral or intravenous dose. Note the very slow disappearance of both substances after the first 20 hours. **B.** Accumulation of nordiazepam during 2 weeks of daily administration of diazepam, and slow decline (half-life about 3 days) after cessation of diazepam administration. (Data from: Kaplan S A et al. 1973 J Pharmacol Sci 62: 1789)

Unwanted effects

These may be divided into:

- toxic effects resulting from acute overdosage
- unwanted effects occurring during normal therapeutic use
- tolerance and dependence.

Acute toxicity

Benzodiazepines in acute overdose are considerably less dangerous than other anxiolytic/hypnotic drugs. Since such agents are often used in attempted suicide, this is an important advantage. The effect of an overdose is to cause prolonged sleep, with the patient normally remaining rousable, without serious depression of respiration or cardiovascular function. However, in the presence of other CNS depressants, particularly alcohol, benzodiazepines can cause severe, even life-threatening, respiratory depression. The availability of an effective antagonist, **flumazenil**, means that the effects of an acute overdose can be counteracted, which is not possible for most CNS depressants.

Side effects during therapeutic use

The main side effects of benzodiazepines are drow-

Clinical uses of benzodiazepines

- As hypnotics (for insomnia): short term use, e.g. temazepam, flurazepam.
- As anxiolytics (for severe anxiety: short term use, e.g. diazepam, chlordiazepoxide). Shorter acting compounds (e.g. oxazepam) may be preferred in the presence of liver disease, but have greater risk of withdrawal symptoms and dependency.
- For preoperative sedation.
- For acute alcohol withdrawal.
- As anticonvulsants (Ch. 28)
- As muscle relaxants in chronic muscle spasm and spasticity (Ch. 30).

siness, confusion, amnesia and impaired motor coordination, which considerably impairs manual skills such as driving performance. An interaction with alcohol is often claimed, whereby a low plasma concentration of a benzodiazepine can enhance the depressant effect of alcohol in a more additive way. The long and unpredictable duration of action of many benzodiazepines is important in relation to side effects. Drugs such as nitrazepam that are used as hypnotics have been shown to produce a substantial day-after impairment of job performance and driving skill.

Tolerance and dependence

Benzodiazepines seem to have much the same tendency to produce dependence as do other hypnotics such as barbiturates, though they are less liable to produce tolerance.

Tolerance has two components. *Pharmacokinetic tolerance* (i.e. the production of a lower blood concentration with prolonged usage) is not important for benzodiazepines, since they have little inducing effect on hepatic microsomal enzymes. They do, however, produce some degree of *tissue tolerance*; this seems to be similar in degree to that occurring with the barbiturates, though objective measurements are few. The sleep-inducing effect shows relatively little tolerance (Fig. 27.1). Lader (1983) found that in normal subjects, the euphoria associated with an intravenous injection of diazepam disappeared in those taking oral diazepam daily, as did the surge in growth hormone release. It is not clear whether tolerance to the anxiolytic effect is significant.

Early claims that benzodiazepines cannot produce *dependence* have now been recognised as false (see reviews by Lader 1983, Woods et al. 1987). In human subjects and patients, stopping benzodiazepine treatment after weeks or months causes an increase in symptoms of anxiety, together with tremor and dizziness (Marks 1978). In experimental animals, withdrawal causes clear signs of physical dependence, namely nervousness, tremor, loss of appetite and sometimes convulsions, though animals show only a weak tendency to self-administration of benzodiazepines. The withdrawal syndrome, in both animals and man, is generally slower in onset and less intense than with barbiturates, probably because of the long plasma half-life of most benzodiazepines. Short-acting benzodiazepines cause more abrupt withdrawal effects. With triazolam, a very short-acting drug, the withdrawal effect becomes apparent within a few hours, even after a single dose, resulting in early-morning insomnia and reports of daytime anxiety when the drug is used as a hypnotic.

It is recognised clinically that patients who are anxious to give up the regular taking of benzodiazepines may have difficulty in doing so, principally because of the physical withdrawal effects (see Nutt 1986), but severe psychological dependence, such as readily occurs with many drugs of abuse (Ch. 33), is not a major problem, as evidenced by the fact that there is little illicit traffic in benzodiazepines.

BENZODIAZEPINE ANTAGONISTS

Competitive antagonists of benzodiazepines were first discovered in 1981. The best-known compound is **flumazenil**. This compound was originally reported to lack effects on behaviour or on drug-induced convulsions when given on its own, though it was later found to possess some 'anxiogenic' and pro-convulsant activity. Flumazenil has been introduced for clinical use (see Broaden & Goa 1988), mainly to reverse the sedative action of benzodiazepines used during anaesthesia, and also in the treatment of acute benzodiazepine overdose. Flumazenil acts quickly and effectively when given by injection, but its action lasts for only about 2 hours, so drowsiness tends to return. It is often used in treating comatose patients suspected of having overdosed with benzodiazepines even before the diagnosis is confirmed on the basis of a blood sample. Convulsions may rarely occur in patients treated with flumazenil, and this is apparently more

Benzodiazepines

- Act by binding to a specific regulatory site on the $GABA_A$ receptor, thus enhancing the inhibitory effect of GABA. Subtypes of the $GABA_A$ receptor exist in different regions of the brain, and differ in their sensitivity to benzodiazepines.
- Anxiolytic benzodiazepines are *agonists* at this regulatory site. Other benzodiazepines (e.g. flumazenil) are *antagonists*, and prevent the actions of the anxiolytic benzodiazepines. A further class of *inverse agonists* is recognised, which reduce the effectiveness of GABA and are anxiogenic; they are not used clinically.
- An endogenous ligand for the benzodiazepine-binding site is believed to exist, and certain peptides have been tentatively identified. The physiological function of this regulatory system is not yet understood.
- Benzodiazepines cause:
  - —reduction of anxiety and aggression
  - —sedation, leading to improvement of insomnia
  - —muscle relaxation and loss of motor coordination
  - —suppression of convulsions (antiepileptic effect).
- Differences in the pharmacological profile of different benzodiazepines are minor; clonazepam appears to have more anticonvulsant action in relation to its other effects.
- Benzodiazepines are active orally, and differ mainly in respect of their duration of action. Short-acting agents (e.g. lorazepam and temazepam, $t_{½}$ 8–12 h) are metabolised to inactive compounds, and are used mainly as sleeping pills. Many long-acting agents (e.g. diazepam and chlordiazepoxide) are converted to a long-lasting active metabolite (nordiazepam); with others (e.g. nitrazepam), the parent drug is slowly metabolised.
- Benzodiazepines are relatively safe in overdose (in contrast to many sedatives, e.g. barbiturates). Their main disadvantages are long-lasting hangover effects and the development of dependence.

common in patients receiving tricyclic antidepressants (Ch. 29). Flumazenil has recently been reported to be effective in two unexpected situations, namely in counteracting the drowsiness and coma associated with severe liver disease (hepatic encephalopathy) and alcohol intoxication. These findings suggest that there may be involvement of an endogenous benzodiazepine-like substance in causing CNS depression in these conditions, but this remains speculative.

5-HT AGONISTS AS ANXIOLYTIC DRUGS

Work on the neurochemical effects of benzodiazepines has drawn attention to the role of other 'downstream' neurotransmitter systems that may be controlled by GABA pathways, through which manipulation of the GABA transmission may result in behavioural effects. In relation to the control of anxiety and aggression, there is considerable evidence of a role for 5-HT (see Kahn et al. 1988, Blackburn 1992). Thus, benzodiazepines inhibit the firing of 5-HT neurons in the raphe nuclei (see Ch. 24), and chemical destruction of 5-HT neurons in specific parts of the raphe nuclei causes a release from the type of behavioural suppression that is used as a model for anxiety. However, behavioural studies—based on anxiety models in animals and clinical observations in man—with drugs that affect 5-HT function, including various agonists, synthesis inhibitors, antagonists and uptake blockers, have given equivocal results, so there did not seem to be a strong basis for attempting to develop anxiolytic drugs on this principle.

The potent anxiolytic activity of **buspirone**, now in clinical use (Ch. 8) has rekindled interest in the role of 5-HT. Buspirone has high affinity for $5\text{-}HT_{1A}$ receptors which are abundant in parts of the brain (e.g. the septohippocampal region) which receive a projection from the 5-HT neurons of the midbrain raphe. It also binds to dopamine receptors, but it is likely that its 5-HT-related actions are important in relation to anxiety suppression, since related anxiolytic compounds (e.g. **ipsapirone** and **gepirone**; see Traber & Glaser 1987) show high specificity for $5\text{-}HT_{1A}$ receptors. Exactly how these 5-HT anxiolytic drugs work is still unclear (see Lucki 1992). They are agonists at $5\text{-}HT_{1A}$ receptors, and thus might be thought to mimic hyperactivity of 5-HT neurons, whereas benzodiazepine action leads to inhibition of these neurons. It is possible that they act on inhibitory presynaptic receptors, thus reducing 5-HT release. However, they take days or weeks to produce their effects in man, suggesting a more complex indirect mechanism of action.

Buspirone, ipsapirone and gepirone have side effects quite different from those of benzodiazepines. They do not cause sedation or motor incoordination, nor have withdrawal effects been reported. Their main side effects are nausea, dizziness, head-

5-HT$_{1A}$ agonists as anxiolytic drugs

- **Buspirone** is a potent (though non-selective) agonist at 5-HT$_{1A}$ receptors. **Ipsapirone** and **gepirone** are similar.
- Anxiolytic effects take days or weeks to develop.
- Side effects appear less troublesome than with benzodiazepines; they include dizziness, nausea, headache, but not sedation or loss of coordination.

ache and restlessness, which generally seem to be less troublesome than the side effects of benzodiazepines.

BARBITURATES

The sleep-inducing properties of barbiturates were discovered early in this century, and hundreds of compounds were made and tested. Until the 1960s, they formed the largest group of hypnotics and sedatives in clinical use. Barbiturates all have depressant activity on the central nervous system, producing effects similar to those of inhalation anaesthetics. They cause death from respiratory and cardiovascular depression if given in large doses, which is one of the main reasons that they are now little used as anxiolytic and hypnotic agents. **Pentobarbitone**, and similar typical barbiturates with a duration of action of 6–12 hours are still very occasionally used as sleeping pills and anxiolytic drugs, but they are less safe than benzodiazepines.

Barbiturates that remain in widespread use are those which have specific properties, such as **phenobarbitone**, used for its anticonvulsant activity (see Ch. 30), and **thiopentone**, which is widely used as an intravenous anaesthetic agent (see Ch. 26). The very high lipid solubility of thiopentone allows it to cross the blood–brain barrier very quickly, and accounts for the rapid and brief action which makes it useful in anaesthesia.

Barbiturates share with benzodiazepines the ability to enhance the action of GABA, but they bind to a different site on the GABA-receptor/chloride channel, and their action seems to be much less specific.

Apart from the risk of dangerous overdose, the main disadvantages of barbiturates are that they induce a high degree of tolerance and dependence, and that they strongly induce the synthesis of hepatic cytochrome P-450 and conjugating enzymes (Ch. 42) and thus increase the rate of metabolic degradation of many other drugs, giving rise to a number of potentially troublesome drug interactions.

Barbiturates

- Non-selective CNS depressants which produce effects ranging from sedation and reduction of anxiety, to unconsciousness and death from respiratory and cardiovascular failure. Therefore dangerous in overdose.
- Act partly by enhancing action of GABA, but less specific than benzodiazepines.
- Mainly used in anaesthesia and treatment of epilepsy; use as sedative/hypnotic agents is no longer recommended.
- Potent inducers of hepatic drug metabolising enzymes, especially cytochrome P-450 system, so liable to cause drug interactions. Also precipitate attacks of acute porphyria in susceptible individuals.
- Tolerance and dependence occur, similar to benzodiazepines.

OTHER POTENTIAL ANXIOLYTIC DRUGS

In addition to the 5-HT$_{1A}$ agonists described above, drugs acting on other 5-HT receptors may also be useful as anxiolytic agents (see Blackburn 1992). In particular, 5-HT$_3$-receptor antagonists, such as **ondansetron** (Ch. 9) show activity in animal models and are currently being tested clinically.

Another interesting approach is the possible use of antagonists to the neuropeptide, cholecystokinin (CCK; see Ch. 9). CCK has been implicated particularly as a possible mediator of panic attacks (see Harro et al. 1993), since intravenous injection of a CCK-related tetrapeptide (small enough to cross the blood–brain barrier) induces panic attacks in patients with this condition. Non-peptide CCK antagonists are currently being developed as potential anxiolytic drugs, but have not yet been tested clinically.

REFERENCES AND FURTHER READING

Barbaccia M L, Costa E, Guidotti A 1988 Endogenous ligands for high-affinity recognition sites of psychotropic drugs. Annu Rev Pharmacol 28: 451–476

Blackburn T P 1992 5-HT receptors and anxiolytic drugs. In: Marsden C A, Heal D J (eds) Central serotonin receptors and psychotropic drugs. Blackwell Scientific Publications, Oxford, p 175–197

Braestrup C, Nielsen M 1986 Benzodiazepine receptor binding in vivo and efficacy. In: Olse R W, Venter J C (eds) Benzodiazepine/GABA receptors and chloride channels. Receptor biochemistry and methodology. Liss, New York, vol 5

Broaden R N, Goa K L 1988 Flumazenil. A preliminary review of its benzodiazepine antagonist properties, intrinsic activity and clinical use. Drugs 35: 448–467

Dews P B 1981 Behavioural pharmacology of anxiolytics. Handbook of experimental pharmacology. Springer-Verlag, Berlin, vol 55(II): 285–293

Doble A, Martin I L 1992 Multiple benzodiazepine receptors: no reason for anxiety. Trends Pharmacol Sci 13: 76–81

File S E 1983 Behavioural actions of benzodiazepine antagonists. In: Trimble M R (ed) Benzodiazepines divided. John Wiley & Sons, Chichester

Gillin J C, Byerley W F 1990 The diagnosis and management of insomnia. N Engl J Med 322: 239–248

Haefely W, Schaffner R, Polc P, Pieri L 1981 General pharmacology and neuropharmacology of propanediol carbamates. Handbook of experimental pharmacology. Springer-Verlag, Berlin, vol 55(II): 263–283

Harro J, Vasar E, Bradwejn J 1993 CCK in animal and human research on anxiety. Trends Pharmacol Sci 14: 244–249

Kahn R S, van Praag H M, Wetzler S, Asnis G M, Barr G 1988 Serotonin and anxiety revisited. Biol Psychiatry 23: 189–208

Lader M H 1983 Benzodiazepine withdrawal states. In: Trimble (ed) Benzodiazepines divided. John Wiley & Sons, Chichester

Lader M H, Wing L 1966 Physiological measurements, sedative drugs and morbid anxiety. Oxford University Press, Oxford

Lucki I 1992 5-HT_1 receptors and behaviour. Neurosci Behav Rev 16: 83–93

Lüddens H, Wisden W 1991 Function and pharmacology of multiple $GABA_A$ receptor subunits. Trends Pharmacol Sci 12: 49–51

Marks J 1978 The benzodiazepines. Use, overuse, misuse, abuse. MTP Press, Lancaster

Nutt D 1986 Benzodiazepine dependence in the clinic: reason for anxiety? Trends Pharmacol Sci 7: 457–460

Shader R I, Greenblatt D J 1993 Use of benzodiazepines in anxiety disorders. New Engl J Med 328: 1398–1405

Sieghart W 1992 $GABA_A$ receptors: ligand-gated Cl^- channels modulated by multiple drug-binding sites. Trends Pharmacol Sci 13: 446–450

Traber J, Glaser T 1987 5-HT_{1A} receptor-related anxiolytics. Trends Pharmacol Sci 8: 432–437

Woods J H, Katz J L, Winger G 1987 Abuse liability of benzodiazepines. Pharm Rev 39: 251–413

28 NEUROLEPTIC DRUGS

Neuroleptic drugs are also known as *antischizophrenic drugs, antipsychotic drugs* or *major tranquillisers* (see Ch. 24). Although originally defined in terms of their clinical usefulness in the treatment of psychotic illness and their behavioural effects in animals, these drugs have in common the pharmacological property of antagonising the actions of dopamine, and this is responsible for most of their effects on the nervous system.

The most important types of psychosis are:

- schizophrenia
- affective disorders (e.g. depression, mania)
- organic psychoses (mental disturbances caused by head injury, alcoholism, or other kinds of organic disease).

Neuroleptic drugs are used mainly in the treatment of schizophrenia and other behavioural emergencies, but they are also used for other psychotic illnesses. The principal drugs used to treat affective disorders are discussed in Chapter 29.

THE NATURE OF SCHIZOPHRENIA

Schizophrenia (see Crow 1982, Ashton 1992) is estimated to affect about 1% of the population. It is one of the most important forms of psychiatric illness because it often affects people from an early age, and may be chronic and highly disabling. There is a strong hereditary factor in its aetiology, which points to the possibility of a fundamental biochemical abnormality. The main clinical features of the disease are as follows:

- Positive symptoms:
  - *delusions* (often paranoid in nature)
  - *hallucinations*, usually in the form of voices, and often exhortatory in their message
  - *thought disorder*, which causes the individual to draw irrational conclusions, and may be associated with the feeling that thoughts are inserted or withdrawn by an outside agency.
- Negative symptoms:
  - withdrawal from social contacts and flattening of emotional responses.

Most cases of schizophrenia begin in adolescence or young adult life, and tend either to follow a relapsing and remitting course, or to be chronic and progressive. Chronic schizophrenia accounts for most of the patients in long-stay psychiatric hospitals.

It has been suggested (see Crow 1982) that the positive symptoms result from some specific neurochemical abnormality (see below) whereas the negative symptoms may reflect a structural brain abnormality. Brain imaging studies have shown a degree of atrophy of specific brain regions, mainly temporal lobe structures, in chronic schizophrenia, and it was thought that progressive neurodegeneration might be occurring as the disease progressed. However, this now seems unlikely, since pre-schizophrenic subjects show the same phenomenon, and it does not appear to be progressive. In general, the positive symptoms respond to drug treatment, whereas negative symptoms are more refractory.

THEORIES OF SCHIZOPHRENIA

This topic has been briefly discussed in Chapter

24. The cause of schizophrenia remains mysterious (see Crow 1982). The disease shows a strong, but by no means invariable, hereditary tendency. In first-degree relatives, the risk is about 10%; even in monozygotic twins, one of whom has schizophrenia, the probability of the other being affected is only about 50%. No defined biochemical disorder has been identified. Hypotheses include the suggestions that schizophrenia may be due to a slow virus infection, possibly associated with an autoimmune process, or to a developmental abnormality involving the temporal lobes. The main anatomical changes that have been described are in the region of the temporal lobes (entorhinal cortex, hippocampus) and the amygdala, which collectively comprise the limbic system.

The search for an underlying neurochemical disorder has gone on unsuccessfully for many years (for a catalogue of the many unsuccessful attempts to discover specific biochemical abnormalities in schizophrenic patients, see Lieberman & Koreen 1993), the hope being that a biochemical understanding of the mechanism would provide the basis for rational drug treatment. In fact, the biochemical theories have come mainly from analysis of the actions of drugs found by chance to be effective, rather than vice versa.

There is general (though certainly not universal) agreement that dopamine hyperactivity underlies at least the positive symptoms of schizophrenia. However, several other transmitters, particularly 5-HT and noradrenaline, interact strongly with dopamine pathways, and may be important in relation to the actions of neuroleptic drugs, and possibly also in the aetiology of schizophrenia. The complexity of neurotransmitter interactions, and the ingenuity of theorists, are such that the possibilities tend to outnumber the facts in a somewhat dispiriting way.

The fragmentary understanding of how CNS function is altered in schizophrenia means that animal models of the disease, which can be used to test prospective therapies, are generally unsatisfactory. From a psychological point of view, one characteristic feature of schizophrenia is a defect in 'selective attention'. Whereas a normal individual quickly accommodates to stimuli of a familiar or inconsequential nature, and responds only to stimuli that are unexpected or significant, the ability of schizophrenic patients to discriminate between significant and insignificant stimuli seems to be impaired. Thus, the ticking of a clock may command as much attention as the words of a companion; a chance thought, which a normal person would dismiss as inconsequential, may become an irresistible imperative. 'Latent inhibition' is a form of behavioural testing in animals which can be used as a model for this type of sensory habituation. Latent inhibition is reduced by drugs such as **amphetamine** (see below), and this effect is inhibited by many antischizophrenic drugs (see Ellenbroek & Cools 1990).

Dopamine theory

The dopamine theory was proposed in 1965 (see Meltzer & Stahl 1976), and is supported by a good deal of indirect evidence. The best evidence comes from pharmacological observations in man and experimental animals. **Amphetamine**, which releases dopamine in the brain (see Ch. 32), can produce in man a syndrome indistinguishable from the 'positive' symptoms of schizophrenia. In animals it causes behavioural disturbances (especially stereotyped behaviour) which have clearly been shown to result from dopamine release. Potent D_2-receptor agonists (e.g. **apomorphine** and **bromocriptine**) produce similar effects in animals, and these drugs, like amphetamine, exacerbate the symptoms of schizophrenic patients. Furthermore, dopamine antagonists and drugs that cause dopamine depletion (e.g. **reserpine**) are effective in controlling the positive symptoms of schizophrenia, and in preventing amphetamine-induced behavioural changes. There is a striking correlation between clinical neuroleptic potency and activity in blocking D_2-receptors, measured by inhibition of specific binding of ^{3}H-haloperidol to brain tissue (Fig. 28.1).

This pharmacological evidence provides no more than indirect support for the theory that hyperactivity of dopamine, specifically at D_2-receptors, occurs in schizophrenia, and many efforts have been made to find more direct biochemical evidence, mostly with negative or inconsistent results. The amount of homovanillic acid (HVA, the main dopamine metabolite; see Ch. 24) in the CSF of schizophrenic patients is normal or low, rather than high. In post-mortem brains, many studies have failed to demonstrate that either dopamine or its metabolites are present in abnormally high concentrations, nor is the activity of dopamine-metabolising enzymes abnormal. Furthermore, the production of prolactin, which might be expected to be abnormally low if dopaminergic transmission

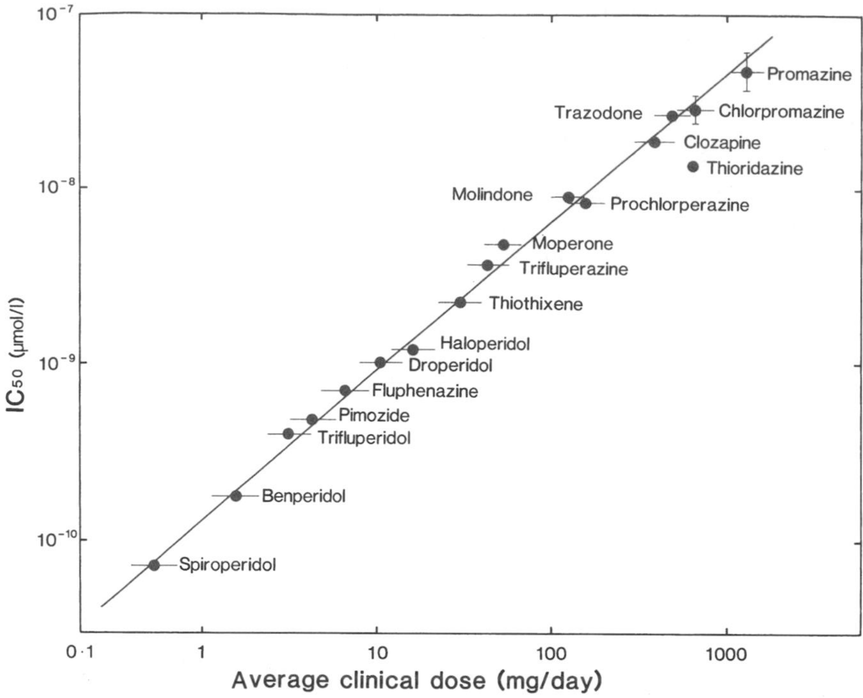

Fig. 28.1 Correlation between the clinical potency and affinity for dopamine receptors among neuroleptic drugs. Clinical potency is expressed as the daily dose used in treating schizophrenia, and binding activity is expressed as the concentration needed to produce 50% inhibition of haloperidol binding. (From: Seeman P et al. 1976 Nature 261: 717)

was facilitated, is normal in schizophrenic patients. One difficulty in interpreting such studies is that nearly all schizophrenic patients are treated with drugs (e.g. **chlorpromazine**) that are known to affect dopamine metabolism, whereas the non-schizophrenic control group are not. In some studies it has been possible to allow for this factor, but the results are still generally negative. A well-controlled study by Reynolds (1983), however, showed an abnormally high dopamine content post-mortem in a restricted area of the temporal lobe of schizophrenic subjects. The amygdala, which receives a dopaminergic innervation from the midbrain via part of the mesolimbic dopaminergic pathway, was consistently richer in dopamine in schizophrenic than in control brains. The noradrenaline content was not affected. Most surprisingly the abnormally high dopamine content was confined to the left side of the brain, which makes it most unlikely that it could have been the result of neuroleptic drug treatment. This finding accords with other evidence suggesting asymmetry in the neurological abnormality in schizophrenia (e.g. the greater than expected frequency of left-sided temporal lobe epilepsy in schizophrenic patients). There also appears to be an increase (roughly twofold) in the number of spiroperidol binding sites, initially believed to represent D_2-receptors (see Seeman 1987); D_1-receptors are unchanged. These findings have been confirmed in some, though not all, studies with positron emission tomography (PET scanning) in living subjects (see Seeman 1987). The reported increase in D_2-receptor binding was seen to be consistent with the fact that the antischizophrenic effect of most neuroleptic drugs relates more closely to their activity on D_2- than D_1-receptors.

It was subsequently discovered that spiroperidol binds, not only to the D_2-receptor, but also to the newly discovered D_4-receptor (see Ch. 24) and, when the two were measured independently, it was found that D_4-receptors were increased about sixfold in the striatum of schizophrenic, compared with control, subjects, whereas D_2-receptors were unchanged (Seeman et al. 1993). The D_4-receptor has also attracted attention on account of the remarkable genetic polymorphism that it shows in human subjects, and because some of the newer antipsychotic drugs (e.g. clozapine; see below) turn out to have a high affinity for this receptor subtype. The possibility that schizophrenia might be associated with a particular genetic variant of the D_4-receptor remains to be investigated.

5-HT theories

A suggestion that 5-HT deficiency might be the underlying cause of schizophrenia was based on the observation that lysergic acid diethylamide (LSD; see Ch. 32) produces hallucinations and sensory disturbances. Though there is no clear biochemical evidence suggesting any alteration in 5-HT metabolism or 5-HT receptor function in schizophrenia, many effective neuroleptic drugs, in addition to blocking dopamine receptors (see below) also act as 5-HT_2-receptor antagonists (see Siever et al. 1991). 5-HT has a modulatory effect on dopamine pathways, so the two theories are not incompatible. Excessive production of a normal 5-HT metabolite, dimethyltryptamine (DMT), which has an LSD-like hallucinogenic effect in man, has been proposed as a mechanism in schizophrenia, but the biochemical evidence for this, or other theories based on endogenously produced hallucinogens, is very weak.

The nature of schizophrenia

- Psychotic illness characterised by delusions, hallucinations and thought disorder (positive symptoms), together with social withdrawal, flattening of emotional responses, and often dementia (negative symptoms).
- Acute episodes (mainly positive symptoms) frequently recur and develop into chronic schizophrenia, with predominantly negative symptoms.
- Incidence is about 1% of population, with a strong, but not invariable, hereditary component.
- Pharmacological evidence is generally consistent with dopamine overactivity hypothesis, but most neurochemical evidence is negative or equivocal. Increase in dopamine receptors in limbic system (especially in left hemisphere) is consistently found. D_4-receptor subtype may be specifically increased.
- Some evidence for involvement of 5-HT.

NEUROLEPTIC DRUGS

CLASSIFICATION OF NEUROLEPTIC DRUGS

More than 20 different neuroleptic drugs are available for clinical use. They fall into several chemical groups (Table 28.1; see Reynolds 1992), but with certain exceptions the differences between them are minor. Some representative chemical structures are shown in Figure 28.2.

Phenothiazines and related **thioxanthines**, together with the **butyrophenones**, form the most important group, often referred to as *classical* or *typical neuroleptics*, as distinct from the more recently developed agents (e.g. dibenzodiazepines, diphenylbutylpiperazines and benzamides) which are referred to as *atypical neuroleptics*. These terms are widely used, but not clearly defined. The distinction rests partly on the claimed freedom of the newer compounds from certain unwanted effects (especially motor disturbances; see below), and partly on the pharmacological profile. Thus, it is suggested that atypical neuroleptics may, in addition to blocking D_2-receptors, also block presynaptic D_1-receptors and/or D_4-receptors.

The phenothiazines are further subdivided according to the nature of the side-chain into the following:

- aliphatic derivatives (e.g. **chlorpromazine**)
- piperazine derivatives (e.g. **fluphenazine**)
- piperidine derivatives (e.g. **thioridazine**).

Phenothiazines block many different types of neurotransmitter receptor, and the nature of the side-chain determines both the potency and the pharmacological specificity. Thus, the piperazine compounds are much more potent than aliphatic compounds at D_2-receptors, and have relatively less α-adrenoceptor-blocking activity, while the piperidine group is intermediate in potency and possesses more antimuscarinic activity than chlorpromazine (see below).

The thioxanthenes (e.g. flupenthixol) closely resemble the aliphatic phenothiazines, both chemically and pharmacologically. The butyrophenones (e.g. haloperidol) are unrelated chemically, having been discovered accidentally as a result of screening pethidine analogues for analgesic activity, but resemble the piperazine-type phenothiazines in their biological activity.

Table 28.1 Properties of neuroleptic drugs

Chemical type	Examples	Receptors blocked*						Actions/unwanted effects†					Notes
		D_1	D_2	α-Ad	H_1	Musc	5-HT_2	Anti-emetic	Sed	EP	Hypo	Other	
Typical neuroleptics													
Phenothiazine													
aliphatic	Chlorpromazine	++	+++	+++	++	++	+	+	++	++	++	Hypothermia, obst. jaundice (esp. chlorpromazine), dry mouth, blurred vision, urinary retention, hypersensitivity, incr. prolactin, causing gynaecomastia etc.	Fluphenazine used as depot preparation; trifluoperazine blocks calmodulin
piperazine	Fluphenazine	+	+++	++	++	++	+	+	+	+++	+		
	Trifluoperazine	+	+++	++	++	++	+	+	+	+++	+		
piperidine	Thioridazine	+	++	+++	–	++	++	–	++	+	++		
Butyrophenone	Haloperidol	+	+++	±	+	±	+	+	–	+++	+	Incr. prolactin	
Thioxanthines	Flupenthixol	++	+++	++	–	–	+++	–	+	++	+	Restlessness	Available as depot preparations
	Clopenthixol	+	+++	++	–	–	+++	–	+	++	+	Incr. prolactin	
Atypical neuroleptics													
Benzamide	Sulpiride, Remoxipride	–	+++	–	–	–	–	+	+	+	–	Incr. prolactin	Sulpiride is poorly absorbed
Diphenylbutyl-piperazine	Pimozide	–	+++	–	–	–	–	+	+	+	–	Incr. prolactin	Long-acting
Dibenzodiazepine	Clozapine	+	++	+++	++	+++	+++	–	++	±	+	Agranulocytosis, salivation, hypertension, convulsions	Effective in some 'neuroleptic-resistant' patients Regular blood-counts needed No effect on prolactin Risperidone is similar, but does not cause agranulocytosis

* D = dopamine receptors; α-Ad = α-adrenoceptors; H_1 = histamine receptors; Musc = mACh receptors

† Sed = sedation; EP = extrapyramidal motor disturbances; Hypo = hypotension

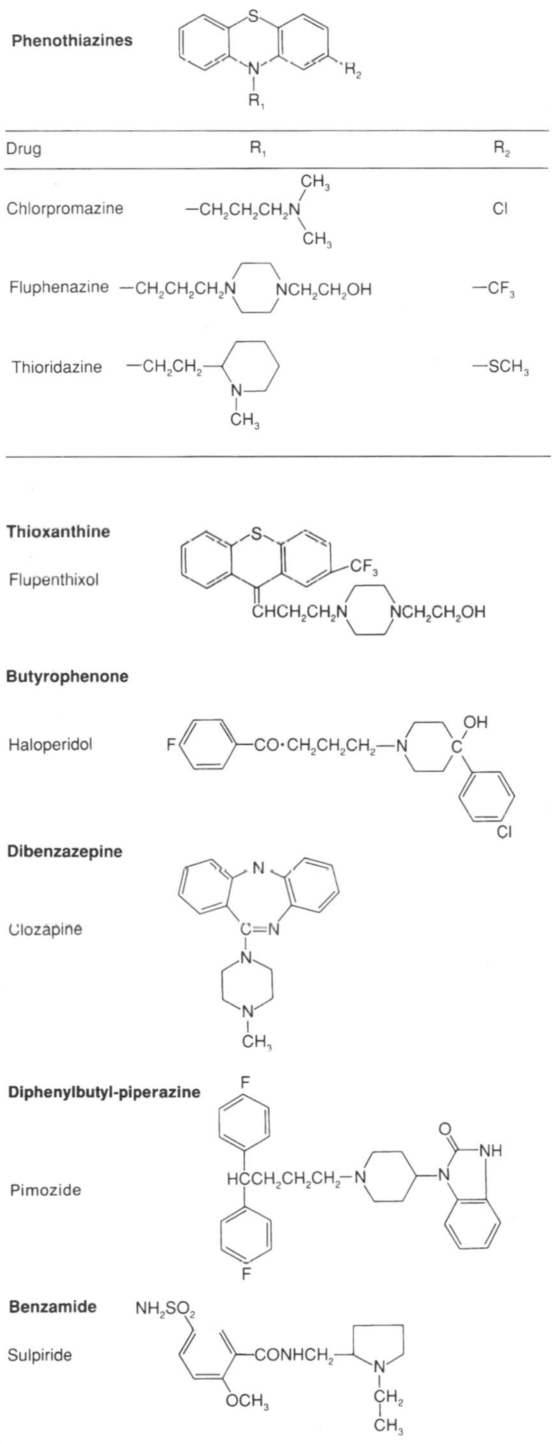

Phenothiazines

S, N, R_1, R_2

Drug	R_1	R_2
Chlorpromazine	$-CH_2CH_2CH_2N(CH_3)_2$	Cl
Fluphenazine	$-CH_2CH_2CH_2N$ NCH_2CH_2OH	$-CF_3$
Thioridazine	$-CH_2CH_2-$ N–CH_3	$-SCH_3$

Thioxanthine

Flupenthixol

S, CF_3, $CHCH_2CH_2N$ NCH_2CH_2OH

Butyrophenone

Haloperidol

F, $CO\cdot CH_2CH_2CH_2-N$, C, OH, Cl

Dibenzazepine

Clozapine

N, C=N, N, N, CH_3

Diphenylbutyl-piperazine

Pimozide

F, $HCCH_2CH_2CH_2-N$, N, O, NH, F

Benzamide

Sulpiride

NH_2SO_2, $CONHCH_2$, N, OCH_3, CH_2, CH_3

Fig. 28.2 Structures of neuroleptic drugs.

Classification of neuroleptic drugs

Main chemical categories are:

- **Typical neuroleptics:**
  - —Phenothiazines (e.g. chlorpromazine, fluphenazine, thioridazine)
  - —Butyrophenones (e.g. haloperidol, droperidol)
  - —Thioxanthines (e.g. flupenthixol, clopenthixol)
- **Atypical neuroleptics:**
  - —Benzamides (e.g. sulpiride, remoxipride)
  - —Diphenybutylpiperazines (e.g. pimozide)
  - —Dibenzodiazepines (e.g. clozapine).

Distinction between 'typical' and 'atypical' groups is not clearly defined, but rests partly on incidence of extrapyramidal side effects (less in 'atypical' group) and partly on receptor specificity.

In this chapter, the common pharmacological properties of neuroleptic drugs are discussed first, followed by notes on the special features of some individual compounds.

GENERAL PROPERTIES OF NEUROLEPTIC DRUGS

The therapeutic activity of chlorpromazine in schizophrenic patients was discovered through the acute observations of a French surgeon, Laborit, in 1947. He tested various substances, including promethazine, for their ability to alleviate signs of stress in patients undergoing surgery, and concluded that promethazine had a calming effect that was different from mere sedation. Elaboration of the phenothiazine structure produced **chlorpromazine,** the antipsychotic effect of which was demonstrated, at Laborit's instigation, by Delay & Deniker in 1953. This drug was quickly found to be much more effective than any hitherto available in controlling the symptoms of psychotic patients without excessively sedating them. Thus the clinical efficacy of phenothiazines was demonstrated long before their mechanism of action was understood.

Pharmacological investigation showed that phenothiazines blocked the actions of many different mediators, including histamine, catecholamines, acetylcholine and 5-HT, and this multiplicity of actions led to the trade name Largactil for chlorpromazine. It is now clear (see Fig. 28.1) that antagonism at dopamine receptors is the main determinant of antipsychotic action.

MECHANISM OF ACTION

DOPAMINE RECEPTORS AND DOPAMINERGIC NEURONS

The classification of dopamine receptors in the CNS is discussed in Chapter 24 (see Table 24.1) There appear to be two distinct receptor types: D_1, which increases adenylate cyclase activity, and D_2, which mediates the main presynaptic and postsynaptic actions of dopamine. The recently discovered D_4-receptor (see above) resembles the D_2 type, and may be specially implicated in schizophrenia. The neuroleptic drugs probably owe their antipsychotic effects mainly to blockade of D_2 (and possibly D_4) receptors. Receptor block can be assessed directly in patients by scanning techniques with labelled dopamine antagonists (see Fig. 1.8). Effective neuroleptic therapy consistently results in approximately 80% block of dopamine receptors measured by this technique. Antagonism at D_2-receptors can be measured in experimental animals by various tests, such as inhibition of amphetamine-induced stereotypic behaviour, or of apomorphine-induced turning behaviour in animals with unilateral striatal lesions (see Ch. 24), and in vitro by ability to inhibit the binding of a radioactive D_2-antagonist (e.g. spiroperidol) to brain membrane fragments. The main groups, phenothiazines, thioxanthines and butyrophenones, show preference for D_2-receptors over D_1-receptors; some of the newer agents (e.g. **sulpiride, remoxipride**) are highly selective for D_2-receptors, whereas **clozapine** is relatively non-selective between D_1 and D_2, but has high affinity for D_4.

All neuroleptic drugs have been found initially to increase the rate of production of dopamine in areas of the brain containing dopaminergic nerve terminals, such as the striatum and components of the limbic system (see Seeman 1987). This is detectable by an increase in tyrosine hydroxylase activity, and an increase in the concentration of the dopamine metabolites, homovanillic acid and DOPAC. At the same time, electrical recording has shown that the activity of dopaminergic neurons (e.g. in the A9 and A10 areas; see Ch. 24) is initially increased by these drugs (Bunney et al 1973, Coward et al 1989). Effects on the A10 cell group (the mesolimbic system) are believed to correlate with antipsychotic effects, whereas the A9 cell group (the nigrostriatal system) is involved mainly in the motor effects produced by neuroleptic drugs (see below). The increase in activity of dopaminergic neurons is not maintained when neuroleptic drugs are administered chronically. Both the biochemical and electrophysiological hyperactivity decline in rats after about three weeks' treatment (Fig. 28.3).

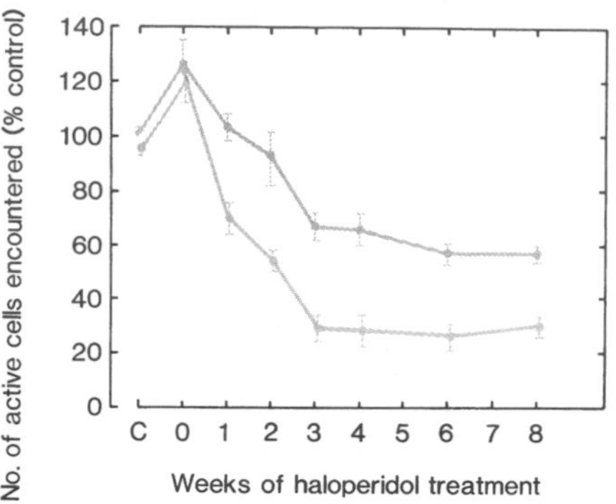

Fig. 28.3 Effect of chronic haloperidol treatment on the activity of dopaminergic neurons in the rat brain. In both A9 (grey line) and A10 (light pink line) regions the activity of dopaminergic neurons, recorded with microelectrodes from anaesthetised animals, declines for 3 weeks before reaching a steady level. (From: White F J, Wang R Y 1983 Life Sci 32: 983)

Another late effect seen only when neuroleptic drugs are given chronically is a significant proliferation of dopamine receptors, detectable as an increase in haloperidol binding (see Seeman 1987), and also

Mechanism of action of neuroleptic drugs

- All neuroleptic drugs are antagonists at dopamine D_2-receptors, but most also block other monoamine receptors, especially 5-HT_2. Clozapine also blocks D_4-receptors.
- Neuroleptic potency generally runs parallel to activity on D_2-receptors, but other activities may determine side-effect profile.
- Neuroleptics take days or weeks to work, suggesting that secondary effects (e.g. increase in number of D_2-receptors in limbic structures) may be more important than direct effect of D_2-receptor block.

a pharmacological supersensitivity to dopamine, somewhat akin to the phenomenon of denervation supersensitivity. These late effects of chronic neuroleptic treatment have received considerable attention, for it is well-established that some of the major beneficial and adverse clinical effects are delayed in their onset, even though the primary action of the drugs in blocking dopamine receptors occurs immediately. At present neither the mechanism of the delayed effects, nor their relationship to the clinical response is at all well understood.

Many neuroleptic drugs block 5-HT_2 receptors at concentrations similar to those effective on dopamine receptors (Table 28.1).

PHARMACOLOGICAL EFFECTS OF NEUROLEPTIC DRUGS

BEHAVIOURAL EFFECTS

Neuroleptic drugs produce many different behavioural effects in experimental animals (see Ashton 1992), but no single test is known that distinguishes them clearly from other types of psychotropic drug. Most kinds of motor behaviour are inhibited. Thus chlorpromazine reduces spontaneous activity and in larger doses causes catalepsy, a state in which the animal remains immobile though it will still respond to stimulation. Neuroleptics were shown to be particularly active in suppressing conditioned avoidance responses. Thus if a rat is trained to respond to an innocuous stimulus by behaviour (e.g. climbing a pole) that enables it to escape from an electric shock delivered a few seconds after this stimulus, chlorpromazine will inhibit the response to the innocuous stimulus, though the animal will continue to respond when the painful shock is applied. Behaviour maintained by either reward or punishment is inhibited. Many of these effects are probably the result of suppression of motor activity by dopamine antagonism in the basal ganglia, but there is also evidence for behavioural effects that are not the result of overall motor inhibition. For example, in a variant of the conditioned avoidance response, a rat may be trained to respond to a stimulus by remaining immobile, thereby avoiding a painful shock, and chlorpromazine impairs this response as well as responses that demand active motor participation. Furthermore, in doses too small to reduce spontaneous motor activity, chlorpromazine reduces social interactions (grooming, mating, fighting, etc.) in mice. It is also found that chlorpromazine reduces the ability of rats to discriminate between two conditioned stimuli (e.g. a red and a green light).

The antidopamine activity of neuroleptics can be revealed in tests in which they are used to antagonise the behavioural effects of amphetamine, which are due mainly to dopamine release (see Chs 24 and 32) or of apomorphine, which is a dopamine agonist. Various forms of stereotyped behaviour in rats and mice induced by amphetamine are strongly inhibited by neuroleptic drugs in doses too small to produce overt behavioural effects. Interestingly, some neuroleptics, such as **clozapine** and **thioridazine**, do not antagonise amphetamine in these tests. These particular drugs are notable in having less tendency than other neuroleptics to cause extrapyramidal side effects in man (see below), and it appears that the amphetamine tests reflect the activity of the neuroleptics mainly on the nigrostriatal (A9) neurons, whereas other behavioural tests may relate to activity on the mesolimbic (A10) system.

In man, the effect of neuroleptic drugs is to produce a state of apathy and reduced initiative. The subject displays few emotions, is slow to respond to external stimuli and tends to drowse off. He is, however, easily aroused and can respond to questions accurately, showing no obvious confusion or loss of intellectual function. Aggressive tendencies are strongly inhibited. The effects in man are quite distinct from those of hypnotic and anxiolytic drugs, which cause drowsiness and confusion, with euphoria rather than apathy.

Because of the lack of any single animal test that reliably predicts antipsychotic activity in man, the screening of potential new antipsychotic drugs generally requires a battery of animal tests and the construction of an 'activity profile' for each compound. The most useful tests for predicting antipsychotic activity in man are those that measure dopamine antagonism (e.g. inhibition of abnormal behaviour induced by apomorphine, enhancement of dopamine turnover).

OTHER EFFECTS RELATED TO DOPAMINE ANTAGONISM

Anti-emetic activity

Anti-emetic activity is a property of many neuroleptic drugs (see Ch. 19), and seems to be partly a function of their ability to antagonise dopamine, since dopamine agonists (e.g. apomorphine) act on the chemoreceptor trigger zone in the medulla to cause nausea and vomiting, and this action is blocked by neuroleptic drugs. The presence of antihistamine activity in many phenothiazines is probably also important, though the reason for the pharmacological correlation between H_1-receptor antagonism and anti-emetic action is not understood. The neuroleptic phenothiazines are effective in controlling nausea and vomiting produced by drugs (e.g. cancer chemotherapeutic agents) and also in conditions such as pregnancy and renal failure, but not against motion sickness, whereas antihistamines (and muscarinic antagonists) are effective in motion sickness (see Ch. 19).

Tardive dyskinesia and extrapyramidal motor disturbances

Neuroleptic drugs produce two main kinds of motor disturbance in man which are clearly related to their action as dopamine antagonists and closely resemble the syndromes that occur when patients with parkinsonism are treated with levodopa (Ch. 25). The two syndromes are *parkinsonism-like symptoms* and *tardive dyskinesia* (see Crane 1978, Klawans et al. 1988, Jenner & Marsden 1988). Since parkinsonism (see Ch. 25) is the result of a deficiency of dopaminergic neurons in the nigrostriatal pathway, it is not surprising that neuroleptic drugs produce a similar syndrome with muscle rigidity, loss of mobility and tremor. Acute symptoms of this kind occur in a large proportion of patients treated with neuroleptics. The symptoms are closely related to the dose used, develop quite rapidly and are reversible, often declining as treatment progresses.

Tardive dyskinesia is a much more puzzling and serious form of movement disorder. The syndrome consists of involuntary movements, often of the face and tongue, but also of the trunk and limbs, which can be severely disabling. The syndrome, which closely resembles the dyskinesia resulting from prolonged treatment with levodopa of patients with parkinsonism, appears after an interval of a few months to several years after neuroleptic treatment has been started (hence the description 'tardive') and is not usually reversible. The incidence has been estimated at 20–40% of neuroleptic-treated patients, but this depends greatly on the drug dosage, the age of the patient (commonest in patients over 50 years) and partly on the particular drug used. Tardive dyskinesia is often disabling, and treatment is ineffective; it is one of the main problems of neuroleptic therapy. Some neuroleptics (e.g. **sulpiride**, **clozapine**) have much less tendency to produce this effect. The reason for this is not clear. Sulpiride is claimed to exert a selective effect on the mesolimbic dopaminergic pathway with sparing of the nigrostriatal pathway. Clozapine has relatively high affinity for D_1- and D_4-receptors, thus producing relatively less block of the striatal D_2-receptors; it also has marked antimuscarinic activity, as do other neuroleptics, such as thioridazine, and this may counteract its effects on the motor system.

There is evidence that the occurrence of tardive dyskinesia may correlate with a gradual increase in the number of D_2-receptor sites in the striatum (see Jenner & Marsden 1988). This receptor proliferation may be similar to that which occurs following physical denervation (see Ch. 5), representing the postsynaptic response to inhibition of transmission. The drugs that are less likely to cause tardive dyskinesia also cause less receptor proliferation and dopamine supersensitivity, but the reason for this is still unclear. It seems unlikely that D_1/D_2-receptor selectivity provides an explanation, since sulpiride and clozapine differ markedly in this respect (see Table 28.1). More likely, these drugs show a greater

Neuroleptic-induced motor disturbances

- Two main types of disturbance occur: acute, reversible Parkinson-like symptoms, and slowly developing tardive dyskinesia, often irreversible.
- Tardive dyskinesia is one of the most serious problems with neuroleptic drug treatment.
- Acute Parkinson-like syndrome consists of tremor and rigidity, and is probably the direct consequence of block of nigrostriatal dopamine receptors.
- Tardive dyskinesia comprises mainly involuntary movements of face and limbs, appearing after months or years of neuroleptic treatment. It may be associated with proliferation of dopamine receptors (possibly presynaptic) in corpus striatum. Treatment is generally unsuccessful.
- Incidence of tardive dyskinesia is less with atypical neuroleptics, and particularly low with clozapine. This may reflect relatively strong muscarinic receptor block with these drugs, or a degree of selectivity for the mesolimbic, as opposed to the nigrostriatal, dopamine pathways.

degree of selectivity with respect to mesolimbic, as opposed to nigrostriatal, neurons, but the reason for this is uncertain.

Endocrine effects

Dopamine, released in the median eminence by neurons of the tubero-infundibular pathway (see Chs 21 and 24) acts physiologically via D_2-receptors as an inhibitor of prolactin secretion, being transported from its site of release in the median eminence to the anterior pituitary gland via the hypophyseal portal system. The result of blocking D_2-receptors by neuroleptic drugs is thus to increase the serum prolactin concentration (Fig. 28.4), the main effect of which is to cause breast enlargement and sometimes lactation, in men as well as women (see Ch. 21). As can be seen from Figure 28.4, the effect is maintained during chronic neuroleptic administration, without any habituation. Other less-pronounced endocrine changes have also been reported, including a decrease of growth hormone secretion, but these, unlike the prolactin response, are unimportant clinically.

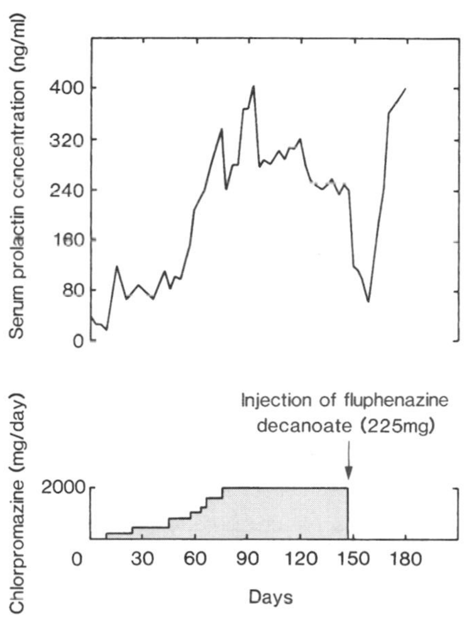

Fig. 28.4 Effect of neuroleptics on prolactin secretion in a schizophrenic patient. When daily dosage with chlorpromazine was replaced with a depot injection of fluphenazine the plasma prolactin initially dropped, because of the delay in absorption, and then returned to a high level. (From: Meltzer H Y et al. 1978 In: Lipton et al. (eds) Psychopharmacology. A generation of progress. Raven Press, New York)

ACTIONS UNRELATED TO DOPAMINE ANTAGONISM

Phenothiazines and, to a variable extent, other neuroleptic drugs, block a variety of receptors, particularly acetylcholine (muscarinic), histamine (H_1), noradrenaline (α) and 5-HT (Table 28.1).

Blocking muscarinic receptors produces a variety of peripheral effects, including blurring of vision and increased intraocular pressure, dry mouth and eyes, constipation and urinary retention (see Ch. 6). It may, however, also be beneficial in relation to extrapyramidal side effects. Acetylcholine acts in opposition to dopamine in the basal ganglia (see Ch. 25) and it is possible that the relative lack of extrapyramidal side effects with **clozapine** and **thioridazine** is due to their high antimuscarinic potency.

Blocking α-adrenoceptors results in the important side effect in man of orthostatic hypotension (see Ch. 14). It does not seem to be important for their antipsychotic action. Different neuroleptics vary greatly in their relative α-receptor- and dopamine-receptor-blocking activity. Thus **haloperidol, flupenthixol** and **fluphenazine** cause less postural hypotension than other drugs, such as **chlorpromazine, clozapine** and **thioridazine.**

Antihistamine (H_1) activity is a property of many phenothiazines, including a number that have no antipsychotic effect, and some other neuroleptic drugs (e.g. **thioridazine**). All H_1-receptor antagonists have sedative and anti-emetic properties (see above), though the mechanism of these actions is not understood.

Some neuroleptic drugs, particularly chlorpromazine and thioridazine, have direct effects on the myocardium, and can reduce contractility and cause dysrhythmias. These effects are rarely important from the clinical point of view.

UNWANTED EFFECTS

The major unwanted effects of neuroleptics can be inferred from their pharmacological actions, as discussed above, though individual drugs differ somewhat (see Table 28.1). Acute toxicity is not a problem in clinical practice, doses up to 100 times the therapeutic dose usually being non-fatal.

The important side effects are as follows:

- *Cardiovascular effects.* Postural hypotension results partly from α-adrenoceptor block and partly from a direct vasodilator action. Apart from clozapine, most non-phenothiazine neuroleptics do not cause hypotension.

- *Sedation*, which tends to decrease with continued use.
- *Weight gain* is a common and troublesome side effect, the mechanism for which is unknown.
- *Autonomic effects*. In addition to α-receptor block, many neuroleptics have atropine-like actions, causing visual disturbance, dry mouth, constipation, etc.
- *Extrapyramidal effects* (see above). These consist of:
  - Acute, reversible effects, namely, *parkinsonian syndrome* consisting of rigidity, tremor and akinesia (tending to occur in elderly patients); and *motor restlessness and anxiety* (akathisia), the mechanism of which is not well understood.
  - Chronic effects, the most important of which is *tardive dyskinesia* (see above). This usually develops after months or years of treatment, tends to get worse if the neuroleptic is stopped, and is unresponsive to most forms of drug treatment. It is the most serious side effect of neuroleptic drugs, and can occur at any age.
- *Endocrine disturbances* resulting from increased prolactin secretion (gynaecomastia, lactation and painful breasts).
- *Idiosyncratic and hypersensitivity reactions:*
  - *Jaundice*. This occurs with older phenothiazines, such as chlorpromazine. The jaundice is usually mild, and of obstructive origin. The exact mechanism is uncertain, but it is believed to be a type of hypersensitivity reaction. The effect disappears quickly when the drug is stopped or substituted by a neuroleptic of a different class.
  - *Leucopenia and agranulocytosis*. This is a rare, but potentially fatal reaction, which can occur in the first few weeks of treatment. It probably represents a type of hypersensitivity reaction (see Ch. 43). The incidence of leucopenia (usually reversible) is less than 1 in 10 000 for most neuroleptics, but much higher (1–2%) with clozapine, whose use requires regular monitoring of blood cell counts. Provided the drug is stopped at the first sign of leucopenia or anaemia, the effect is reversible.
  - *Skin reactions*. Urticarial reactions are common in the first few weeks of treatment, but are not serious. Recovery may occur even if the drug is continued. Excessive sensitivity to ultraviolet light may also occur.
  - *Neuroleptic malignant syndrome* is a rare but serious complication, similar to the malignant hyperthermia syndrome seen with certain anaesthetics (see Ch. 26). Muscle rigidity is accompanied by a rapid rise in body temperature and mental confusion. It is usually reversible, but death from renal or cardiovascular failure occurs in 10–20% of cases.

Unwanted effects of neuroleptic drugs

- Important side effects common to most drugs are extrapyramidal motor disturbances and endocrine disturbances (increased prolactin release); these are secondary to dopamine-receptor block. Sedation and weight gain are also common.
- Obstructive jaundice sometimes occurs with phenothiazines.
- Other side effects (dry mouth, blurred vision, hypotension, etc.) are due to block of muscarinic and α-adrenoceptors.
- Some neuroleptics cause agranulocytosis as a rare and serious idiosyncratic reaction. With clozapine, leucopenia is common, and requires routine monitoring.
- Neuroleptic malignant syndrome is a rare but potentially dangerous idiosyncratic reaction.

PHARMACOKINETIC ASPECTS

Chlorpromazine, which is typical of many phenothiazines, is erratically absorbed into the bloodstream after oral administration. Figure 28.5 shows the wide range of variation of the peak plasma concentration as a function of dosage in 14 patients. Among four patients treated at the high dosage level of 6–8 mg/kg, the variation in peak plasma concentration was nearly 90-fold; two showed marked side effects, one was correctly controlled and one showed no clinical response. The main factor in this variability is not poor absorption from the gut or rapid first-pass metabolism in the liver. It seems instead to be due to a large and variable amount of tissue binding. In accordance with this, the volume of distribution of many neuroleptics greatly exceeds

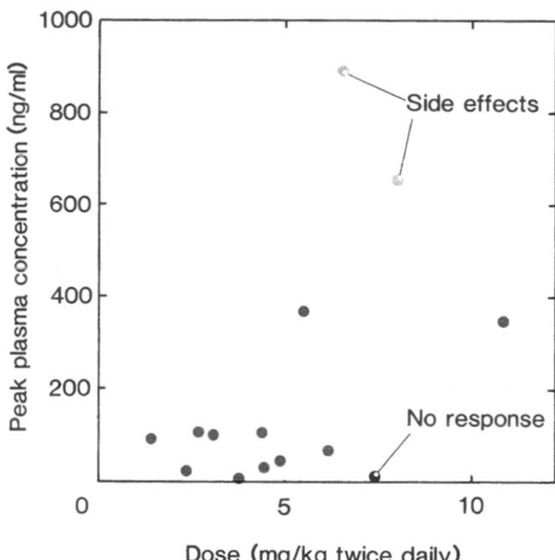

Fig. 28.5 Individual variation in the relation between dose and plasma concentration of chlorpromazine in a group of schizophrenic patients. (Data from: Curry S H et al. 1970 Arch Gen Psychiat 22: 289)

the total body volume (see Table 4.2), indicative of considerable extravascular sequestration of the drug. They are also bound (usually about 90%) to plasma protein.

The relationship between the plasma concentration and the clinical effect of neuroleptic drugs is also highly variable; the therapeutic range of plasma concentration of chlorpromazine (30–300 ng/ml) is unusually wide. Thus, dosage of neuroleptics has to be adjusted on a trial-and-error basis, without useful guidance from pharmacokinetic data. Adjustment of the dose is made even more difficult by the fact that at least 40% of schizophrenic patients fail to take drugs as prescribed. It is remarkably fortunate that the acute toxicity of neuroleptic drugs is slight, given the unpredictability of the clinical response.

The half-time for removal of most neuroleptics from the plasma is 15–30 hours, clearance depending entirely on hepatic transformation by a combination of oxidative and conjugative reactions. The metabolism of phenothiazines is complex, but metabolites do not appear to contribute much to the pharmacological response.

Most neuroleptic drugs can be given orally or by intramuscular injection, once or twice a day. Slow-release (depot) preparations of many neuroleptics are available, in which the active drug is esterified with heptanoic or decanoic acid and dissolved in oil. Given as an intramuscular injection, the drug acts for 2–4 weeks, but initially may produce acute side effects. These preparations are widely used as a means of overcoming compliance problems.

CLINICAL USE AND CLINICAL EFFICACY

The clinical uses of neuroleptic drugs are summarised on page 574.

The clinical efficacy of neuroleptic drugs in enabling schizophrenic patients to lead more normal lives is evident from the sharp decline in the in-patient population (mainly comprised of chronic schizophrenics) of mental hospitals since the later 1950s (Fig. 28.6). Undoubtedly the major decline between 1960 and 1970 reflects changing public and professional attitudes towards hospitalisation of the mentally ill, but it is generally acknowledged that the efficacy of neuroleptics was an essential enabling factor. Many double-blind trials have been carried out which show objectively that neuroleptics reduce schizophrenic symptoms more effectively than does placebo treatment (see Davis & Garver 1978). In one large multicentre trial organised by the National Institutes of Health in 1964, three phenothiazines were tested against a placebo over a 6-week period in 344 newly diagnosed schizophrenic patients, clinical improvement being assessed by ratings of several schizophrenic symptoms. Figure 28.7 summarises the results. Although 60% of the group taking placebo showed improvement, the group taking phenothiazine fared significantly better, 94% showing improvement. At the end of the trial period the median rating for the placebo group was 4.5 (moderately to markedly ill) compared with 3.0 (mildly ill) for the treated group. This trial showed no differences between the three phenothiazines

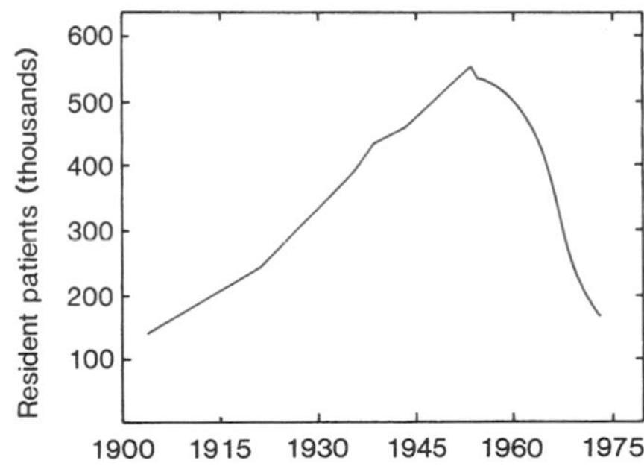

Fig. 28.6 Patient population in public mental hospitals in the USA. (From: Bassuk E L, Gerson S 1978 Scientific American 238: 46)

Clinical efficacy of neuroleptic drugs

- Neuroleptic drugs are effective in controlling symptoms of acute schizophrenia, when large doses may be needed.
- Long-term neuroleptic treatment is often effective in preventing recurrence of schizophrenic attacks, and is a major factor in allowing schizophrenic patients to lead normal lives.
- Depot preparations are often used for maintenance therapy.
- Neuroleptic drugs are not generally effective in improving negative schizophrenic symptoms.
- Approximately 40% of chronic schizophrenic patients are poorly controlled by neuroleptic drugs; clozapine may be effective in some of these 'neuroleptic-resistant' cases.

tested, either in the assessment of their overall efficacy or in a more detailed analysis of their ability to control specific symptoms. Crow (1982) has, however, concluded that all neuroleptics control the 'positive' symptoms (e.g. delusions, paranoia and aggression) more effectively than the 'negative' symptoms (e.g. apathy and reduction in speech).

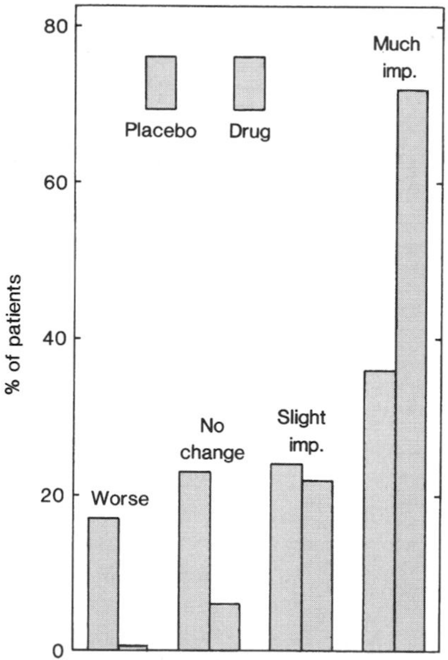

Fig. 28.7 Clinical trial of phenothiazines in acute schizophrenia. (Results of NIMH Collaborative Study 1964 Arch Gen Psychiat 10: 246)

Clinical uses of neuroleptic drugs

- Schizophrenia (e.g. chlorpromazine, haloperidol, flupenthixol). Clozapine is used in patients unresponsive to other drugs.
- Mania.
- Behavioural emergencies (e.g. violent impulsive behaviour).
- For treatment of emesis (e.g. prochlorperazine; see Ch. 19).
- Huntington's disease, to suppress involuntary movements (Ch. 25).
- Occasionally used in depression (especially sulpiride).

In general, clinical trials have shown no significant differences in the therapeutic efficacy of different neuroleptics, the main difference being in the incidence and type of the major side effects.

SOME NEWER 'ATYPICAL' NEUROLEPTIC DRUGS

The term 'atypical' is used loosely; usually it implies that the drugs are less prone to produce motor disorders than the conventional drugs, but sometimes it merely means that the pharmacological profile differs in an unspecified way. In fields where me-too drugs abound, there is a tendency to invent labels such as 'atypical' and 'second-generation' compounds to give the impression that the new represents a qualitative advance on the old. Be suspicious of such terms unless they are clearly defined.

Sulpiride, and the newer agents **pimozide** and **remoxipride**, show high selectivity for D_2-receptors compared with D_1- or other neurotransmitter receptors. Sulpiride and remoxipride have less tendency to cause extrapyramidal motor disorders than do conventional neuroleptic drugs. It has been suggested that sulpiride acts specifically on presynaptic, rather than postsynaptic, D_2-receptors, and that it does not cause the secondary increase in overall D_2-receptor numbers that occurs with other agents (see above), but actually causes D_1-receptors to increase. How this relates to its pharmacological profile is not clear.

Pimozide appears similar to conventional neuroleptic drugs, but has a longer duration of action, allowing once-daily dosage.

Clozapine is a recently introduced neuroleptic drug that has a different pharmacological spectrum from other neuroleptics (see Coward et al. 1989, Gudelsky et al. 1989), being a relatively weak D_2-receptor antagonist, but blocking D_1- and D_4-receptors, as well as α-adrenoceptors, 5-HT_2 receptors and muscarinic acetylcholine receptors. It is an effective antischizophrenic drug, with little tendency to cause extrapyramidal motor disorders or to increase prolactin release. Its main advantages are: (a) that it is often effective in the substantial proportion of chronic schizophrenic patients who fail to respond to conventional neuroleptic drugs (Kane et al. 1989); (b) that it appears to improve negative as well as positive symptoms. The main problem with clozapine is its tendency to cause agranulocytosis (see above), which currently limits its use to cases in which other treatment has failed, and in which regular blood-count monitoring is feasible. Other side effects include postural hypotension (though, paradoxically, hypertension in some patients), salivation and occasionally convulsions.

Other potential new approaches to treating schizophrenia, not yet tested in practice, are discussed by Tricklebank et al. (1992) and by Reynolds (1992).

REFERENCES AND FURTHER READING

Ashton H 1992 Brain systems disorders and psychotropic drugs. Blackwell, Oxford

Bunney B S, Walters J R, Roth R H, Aghajanian G K 1973 Dopaminergic neurons: effect of antipsychotic drugs and amphetamine on single cell activity. J Pharmacol Exp Ther 185: 560–571

Coward D M, Imperato A, Urwyler S, White T G 1989 Biochemical and behavioural properties of clozapine. Psychopharmacology 99 (Suppl): 6–12

Crane G F 1978 Tardive dyskinesia and related neurologic disorders. Handbook of psychopharmacology. Plenum Press, New York, vol 10: 165–196

Crow T J 1982 Schizophrenia. In: Crow T J (ed) Disorders of neurohumoral transmission. Academic Press, London

Davis J M, Garver D L 1978 Neuroleptics: clinical use in psychiatry. Handbook of psychopharmacology. Plenum Press, New York, vol 10: 29–164

Ellenbroek B A, Cools A R 1990 Animal models with construct validity for schizophrenia. Behav Pharmacol 1: 469–490

Gudelsky G A, Nash J F, Berry S A, Meltzer H Y 1989 Basic biology of clozapine: electrophysiological and neuroendocrinological studies. Psychopharmacology 99 (Suppl): 13–17

Jenner P, Marsden C D 1988 Adaptive changes in brain dopamine function as a result of neuroleptic treatment. Adv Neurol 49: 417–431

Kane J M, Honigfeld G, Singer J, Meltzer H, Clozaril Collaborative Study Group 1989 Clozapine for the treatment-resistant schizophrenic: results of a US multicenter trial. Psychopharmacology 99 (Suppl): 60–63

Klawans H L, Tanner C M, Goetz C G 1988 Epidemiology and pathophysiology of tardive dyskinesias. Adv Neurol 49: 185–197

Lieberman J A, Koreen A R 1993 Neurochemistry and neuroendocrinology of schizophrenia: a selective review. Schizophr Bull 19: 371–429

Mason S T 1983 Designing a non-neuroleptic antischizophrenic drug: the noradrenergic strategy. Trends Pharmacol Sci 4: 353–355

Meltzer H, Stahl S M 1976 The dopamine hypothesis of schizophrenia: a review. Schizophr Bull 2: 19–76

Reynolds G P 1983 Increased concentrations and lateral asymmetry of amygdala dopamine in schizophrenia. Nature 305: 527–529

Reynolds G P 1992 Developments in the drug treatment of schizophrenia. Trends Pharmacol Sci 13: 116–121

Seeman P 1987 Dopamine receptors and the dopamine hypothesis of schizophrenia. Synapse 1: 133–152

Seeman P, Guan H-C, Van Tol H H M 1993 Dopamine D_4 receptors elevated in schizophrenia. Nature 365: 441–445

Siever L J, Kahn R S, Lawlor B A, Trestman R L, Lawrence T L, Coccaro E F 1991 Critical issues in defining the role of serotonin in psychiatric disorders. Pharm Rev 43: 509–525

Tricklebank M D, Bristow L J, Hutson P H 1992 Alternative approaches to the discovery of novel antipsychotic agents. Prog Drug Res 38: 299–337

29

DRUGS USED IN AFFECTIVE DISORDERS

THE NATURE OF AFFECTIVE DISORDERS

Affective disorders are characterised primarily by changes of mood (depression or mania) rather than by thought disturbances. Depression is the most common manifestation, and it may range from a very mild condition, bordering on normality, to severe depression—sometimes called psychotic depression—accompanied by hallucinations and delusions.

The symptoms of depression include:

- a general feeling of misery, apathy and pessimism
- low self-esteem—feelings of guilt, inadequacy and ugliness
- indecisiveness, loss of motivation
- retardation of thought and action
- sleep disturbance and loss of appetite.

Mania is in most respects exactly the opposite, with excessive exuberance, enthusiasm and self-confidence, and excessive physical activity, these signs often being combined with irritability, impatience and anger. As with depression, the mood is generally inappropriate to the circumstances. There may be grandiose delusions of the Napoleonic kind.

There are two distinct types of depressive syndrome, namely *bipolar* and *unipolar* depression. In bipolar depression, the patient oscillates between depression and mania. There is strong evidence for an hereditary link in the condition, suggesting that a biochemical abnormality underlies the disorder. Patients with unipolar depression do not swing into bouts of mania. They tend to be older than bipolar depressives when the illness first occurs, and their depression is more often mixed with symptoms of anxiety and agitation than is the case with patients with bipolar depression, who tend to be inert and apathetic during their depressive phase. There is some evidence (see below) that these two types of depressive illness respond differently to antidepressant drugs. Either type may be associated with symptoms of anxiety and agitation, or with retardation and stupor. If severe, either type may be accompanied by psychotic symptoms.

THE MONOAMINE THEORY OF DEPRESSION

The main biochemical theory that has been put forward is the monoamine hypothesis (Schildkraut 1965; for reviews, see Ashton 1992, Siever 1987, Meltzer & Lowy 1987), which states that depression is caused by a functional deficit of monoamine transmitters at certain sites in the brain, while mania results from a functional excess.

The monoamine hypothesis grew originally out of associations between the clinical effects of various drugs which cause or alleviate symptoms of depression and their known neurochemical effects on monoaminergic transmission in the brain. Depressive illness, particularly bipolar illness, has a strong genetic component, and tends to run in families, strengthening the idea of an underlying biochemical abnormality. Initially the monoamine hypothesis was formulated in terms of noradrenaline, but subsequent work showed that most of the observations were equally consistent with 5-HT being the key substance. This pharmacological evidence, which is summarised below, gives general support to the monoamine hypothesis, though there are several anomalies. Attempts to obtain more direct evidence, by studying monoamine metabolism in depressed patients, or by measuring changes in the number of monoamine receptors in postmortem brain tissue, have in general provided only very equivocal support for the theory, and the interpretation of these studies is often problematic. Similarly, investigation by functional tests of the activity of known monoaminergic pathways (e.g. those controlling pituitary hormone release) in depressed patients have also given equivocal results. The evidence relating to the monoamine theory is well reviewed by Johnstone (1982), Baker & Dewhurst (1985).

Pharmacological evidence

Table 29.1 summarises the main drugs that are known to affect monoamine metabolism, and compares their predicted effect on mood with the observed effect. In general, there is reasonable support for the theory, though there are several examples of drugs that might have been predicted to improve or worsen depressive symptoms, but fail to do so convincingly. It has to be recognised that the basis for predicting the effects of drugs on mood is, at best, very simple-minded. Thus, supplying a transmitter precursor will not actually increase the release of transmitter unless availability of the precursor is rate-limiting. Similarly, a drug that releases monoamines from normal nerve terminals may fail to do so if the nerve terminals are functionally defective. The absence of a useful antidepressant action of amphetamine is therefore not strong evidence against the monoamine theory.

More difficult to reconcile with the monoamine theory in any simple way is the fact that the biochemical actions of antidepressant drugs appear very rapidly, whereas their antidepressant effects usually take days or weeks to develop. A similar situation exists in relation to antischizophrenic drugs (Ch. 28) and some anxiolytic drugs (Ch. 27), and it strongly suggests that it may be the secondary, adaptive changes in the brain, rather than the primary drug effect, that are important in producing the clinical improvement. Evidence for such adaptive changes in adrenoceptor function is discussed below (p. 583). This change in the interpretation of the mechanism of action of antidepressant drugs clearly undermines one of the original key arguments on which the monoamine theory was based. The general conclusion that monoamines are in some way important remains plausible, but recent studies have tended more to confuse than to clarify the original theory.

Table 29.1 Pharmacological evidence relating to the monoamine hypothesis of depression

Drug	Principal action	Effect in depressed patients
Effects consistent with the hypothesis		
Tricyclic antidepressants	Block NA and 5-HT re-uptake	Mood ↑
MAO inhibitors	Increase stores of NA and 5-HT	Mood ↑
α-methyltyrosine	Inhibits NA synthesis	Mood ↓ Calming of manic patients
Methyldopa	Inhibits NA synthesis	Mood ↓
Reserpine	Inhibits NA and 5-HT storage	Mood ↓
Electroconvulsive therapy	?Increases CNS responses to NA and 5-HT	Mood ↑
Effects that do not support hypothesis		
Amphetamine	Releases NA and blocks re-uptake	None. Euphoria in normal subjects
Cocaine	Inhibits NA re-uptake	None. Euphoria in normal subjects
Tryptophan (5-hydroxytryptophan)	Increases 5-HT synthesis	Mood? ↑ in some studies
α- and β-adrenoceptor antagonists	Block actions of NA	Mood slightly ↓ with β-antagonists No effect on manic patients
Methysergide	5-HT antagonist	None
L-dopa	Increases NA synthesis	None
Iprindole	No effect on amine metabolism	Mood ↑

Biochemical studies

The most direct way of testing the amine hypothesis is to look for biochemical abnormalities in CSF, blood or urine, or in post-mortem brain tissue, from depressed or manic patients. The major metabolites of noradrenaline, 5-HT and dopamine that appear in the CSF, blood and urine (see Chs 7, 8 and 24) are, respectively, 3-methoxy-4-hydroxyphenylglycol (MOPEG), 5-hydroxyindoleacetic acid (5-HIAA) and homovanillic acid (HVA). There are two fundamental problems in relating changes in the concentration of these metabolites in body fluids to changes in transmitter function in the brain. One is that many secondary factors can affect their concentration, such as diet, transport between CSF, blood and urine, or release of monoamines from non-cerebral sites. The second is that many patients receive drug treatment, which affects the metabolite concentrations markedly.

Among a variety of clinical studies, there is now a general consensus that MOPEG in urine and CSF is reduced (by roughly 25% compared with normal subjects) in depression, and that it shows a cyclic change in patients who are switching between depressive and manic states (see reviews by Johnstone 1982, Siever 1987). These changes do not seem to be due to variations in peripheral sympathetic activity associated with greater excitability and activity in the manic state, since exercise has little effect on the results. Plasma noradrenaline actually tends to be higher in depressed than in normal subjects, though it too shows a cyclic variation in bipolar depressive patients.

Results obtained with 5-HIAA are more variable (see Meltzer & Lowy 1987). Urinary excretion of 5-HIAA does not change in depression, but several studies have shown lower CSF 5-HIAA concentrations in depressed patients (see Åsberg & Wågner 1986). The results of one thorough study, shown in Figure 29.1, showed an equal (50%) reduction of 5-HIAA in lumbar CSF in depressed, manic and recovered depressed patients. It is believed that CSF 5-HIAA concentrations in depressed patients actually show a bimodal distribution, being normal in about 50% of cases and reduced in the rest. There is evidence that patients with low values have a greater suicide risk and poorer response to treatment than those with normal values. There is no consistent evidence that the 5-HIAA or 5-HT content of post-mortem brain tissue is reduced in depression, though lower levels have been reported in the brains of suicide victims (assumed to be suffering from severe depression) than in the brains of victims of other forms of sudden death.

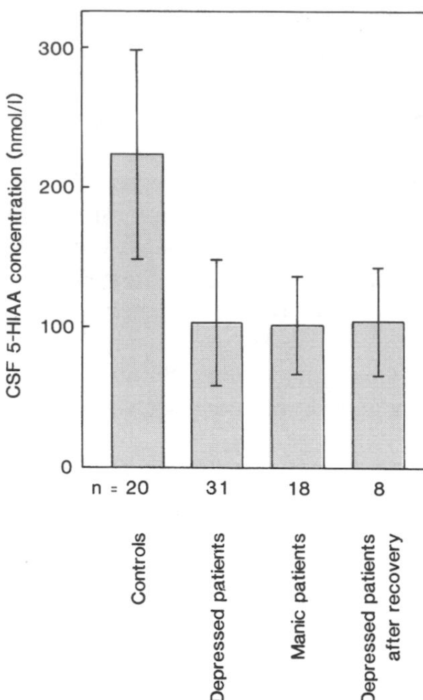

Fig. 29.1 Reduced concentration of a 5-HT metabolite in CSF of patients with affective disorders. 5-hydroxyindoleacetic acid (5-HIAA) is the main metabolite of 5-HT found in CSF. The error bars show standard deviations, and the reduction compared with control is significant ($p < 0.001$) in all three groups.

Studies on blood platelets have been widely used to investigate possible biochemical abnormalities underlying mental disease. This is because the platelets (which, unlike the brain, are easily studied in man) possess mechanisms for the uptake and metabolism of 5-HT very similar to those found in the brain. The main results so far reported in depressed patients are that 5-HT uptake by platelets is reduced in comparison to control patients (an effect not attributable to drug treatment). Platelet MAO activity, however, is not consistently altered, though there are suggestions that it is reduced in some bipolar depressive patients. The finding of an abnormality in 5-HT uptake by platelets is generally consistent with the monoamine theory, though it requires some special pleading (readily forthcoming) to explain how this could lead to a deficit, rather than an enhancement, of 5-HT-mediated transmission in the brain.

Functional studies

Various attempts have been made to test for a functional deficit of monoamine pathways in depression. Hypothalamic neurons controlling pituitary function receive noradrenergic and 5-HT inputs, which control the discharge of these cells and thus regulate the secretion of pituitary hormones such as ACTH and growth hormone. The plasma cortisol concentration is usually high in depressed patients and it fails to respond with the normal fall when a synthetic steroid, such as dexamethasone, is given. This formed the basis of a clinical test, the *dexamethasone suppression test* (also used in the diagnosis of Cushing's syndrome; see p. 441), which was proposed to be indicative of severe depression, but is now largely discredited. Other hormones in plasma are also affected; for example, growth hormone concentration is reduced and prolactin is increased. In general, these changes are consistent with deficient monoamine transmission, but they are not specific to depressive syndromes.

Monoamine theory of depression

- The monoamine theory, proposed in 1965, suggests that depression results from functionally deficient monoaminergic (noradrenaline and/or 5-HT) transmission in the CNS.
- The theory was based on the ability of known antidepressant drugs (TCA and MAOI) to facilitate monoaminergic transmission, and of drugs such as reserpine to cause depression.
- Other pharmacological evidence fails to support the monoamine hypothesis.
- Biochemical studies on depressed patients do not, in general, support the monoamine hypothesis, except that consistently low concentrations of 5-HIAA in the CSF are found.
- An abnormally weak response of plasma cortisol to exogenous steroid (dexamethasone suppression test) is common in depression, and may reflect defective monoamine transmission in the hypothalamus.
- Though the monoamine hypothesis in its simple form is no longer tenable as an explanation of depression, pharmacological manipulation of monoamine transmission remains the most successful therapeutic approach.

Current status of monoamine theory

In summary, there is a good deal of circumstantial evidence to suggest that Schildkraut's monoamine theory is basically correct. (Johnstone (1982) puts it more circumspectly: 'Thus the body of circumstantial evidence . . . is such that it is unlikely that the hypothesis is incorrect.') There are, however, some glaring inconsistencies, of which the most obvious are the following:

- Neither amphetamine, cocaine or L-dopa have antidepressant actions.
- Antidepressant drugs have a delayed therapeutic effect, which coincides in time with an apparent inhibition rather than facilitation of monoaminergic transmission.
- Some clinically effective antidepressants seem to lack any actions that could enhance monoamine transmission.
- The biochemical changes associated with depression have, in several studies, been identical with changes observed in manic patients.

Recognising these inconsistencies, many authors (see reviews by Maj et al. 1984, Ashton 1992) have suggested more complicated mechanisms than a simple transmitter deficit, and have invoked dopamine, acetylcholine and peptides in delicately balanced arrays in attempts to account for all the facts. Receptor down-regulation and its counterpart, denervation supersensitivity, as long-term effects of agents that enhance or inhibit transmitter function are also often invoked.

It seems clear that Schildkraut's basic idea will need to be modified and elaborated, but the last few years have seen little progress in this direction.

ANIMAL MODELS OF DEPRESSION

Progress in unravelling the neurochemical mechanisms is, as in so many areas of psychopharmacology, considerably limited by the lack of good animal models of the clinical condition. There is no known animal condition corresponding to the inherited condition of depression in man, but various procedures have been described which produce in animals behavioural states (withdrawal from social interaction, loss of appetite, reduced motor activity, etc.) typical of human depression (see review by

Porsolt 1985). For example, the delivery of repeated inescapable painful stimuli leads to a state of 'learned helplessness', in which even when the animal is free to escape it fails to do so. Mother–infant separation in monkeys, and administration of amine-depleting drugs, such as reserpine, also produce states that superficially resemble human depression. As well as being inherently distasteful, these experiments often require elaborate and expensive experimental protocols, and there is only a limited amount of information about the similarity of these states to human depression. However, it has been reported that the learned helplessness state and the effect of mother–infant separation can be reversed by tricyclic antidepressants, and increased by small doses of α-methyl p-tyrosine (which inhibits noradrenaline synthesis), suggesting a basic similarity to the human state.

ANTIDEPRESSANT DRUGS

TYPES OF ANTIDEPRESSANT DRUG

The major classes of drug that are used to treat depressive illness are:

- *Tricyclic antidepressants* (TCA) (e.g. **imipramine**, **amitriptyline**).
- *Monoamine oxidase inhibitors* (MAOI) (e.g. **phenelzine**, **tranylcypromine**, together with newer compounds such as **moclobemide**).
- *Selective 5-HT uptake inhibitors* (e.g. **fluoxetine**, **fluvoxamine**).
- *'Atypical' antidepressants.* This group includes compounds that act similarly to TCA but have a different chemical structure (e.g. **nomifensine** and **maprotiline**), and also compounds with different pharmacological actions (e.g. **mianserin, iprindole** and **trazodone**).
- **Lithium.** This is used mainly for bipolar depression, as prophylaxis or to control the manic phase; it may also be used in unipolar depression.

Table 29.2 summarises the main features of these types of drug. A recent update is provided by Hollister & Claghorn (1993).

Mention should also be made of electroconvulsive therapy (ECT) which is very effective, and usually acts more rapidly than antidepressant drugs (see later section).

MEASUREMENT OF ANTIDEPRESSANT ACTIVITY

The clinical effectiveness of the first MAOI and TCA drugs was discovered by chance when these drugs were given to patients for other reasons. **Iproniazid**, the first MAOI, was originally used to treat tuberculosis, being chemically related to isoniazid (see Ch. 37); **imipramine**, the first TCA, resembles chlorpromazine (see Ch. 28) and was first tried as an antischizophrenic drug. Later, the monoamine hypothesis of depression produced a kind of biochemical rationale for their antidepressant actions and, hence, ways of testing new compounds as a preliminary to clinical trials. The results of such biochemical tests are successful in predicting clinical efficacy for conventional TCA and MAOI, but fail to predict efficacy with the newer group of atypical antidepressant drugs. Various behavioural tests have also been used (see above), though there is no animal model that satisfactorily resembles depressive illness in man. Some of the most useful tests are the following:

- *Potentiation of noradrenaline effects in the periphery.* Stimulation of sympathetic nerves or administration of noradrenaline causes contraction of smooth muscle, which is enhanced if the noradrenaline re-uptake mechanism of the nerve terminal is blocked (see Ch. 7). This test gives positive results with TCA, but does not reveal MAOI or atypical antidepressant activity.
- *Potentiation of the central effects of amphetamine.* Amphetamine works partly by releasing noradrenaline in the brain, and its actions are enhanced both by MAOI (which increase noradrenaline stores) and by TCA (which block re-uptake). Atypical antidepressants also give a positive response, for uncertain reasons, making it a useful test for predicting activity in man.
- *Antagonism of reserpine-induced depression.* Reserpine depletes the brain of both noradrenaline and 5-HT, causing various measurable effects (hypothermia, bradycardia, reduced motor activity, etc.) which are reduced by antidepressant drugs. This test also reveals activity among the atypical drugs which do not affect MAO or transmitter re-uptake in biochemical assays.
- *Block of amine uptake in vitro.* Radioactive noradrenaline or 5-HT can be used to measure neuronal uptake in the brain or peripheral tissues.

Table 29.2 Characteristics of the main classes of antidepressant drugs

	TCA	MAOI	5-HT uptake inhibitors	Atypical (see Table 29.5)	Lithium
Examples	Imipramine Desipramine Amitriptyline Protriptyline Clomipramine	Phenelzine Tranylcypromine Isocarboxazid Moclobemide	Fluoxetine Fluvoxamine Paroxetine Sertraline	Maprotiline Nomifensine Mianserin Trazodone Iprindole	Lithium carbonate
Duration of action	1–3 days	2–4 weeks (except meclobemide ~ 12 hours)	1–3 days	12–24 hours	1 day
Delay in therapeutic effect	2–4 weeks	2–4 weeks	2–4 weeks	2–4 weeks (some claimed faster)	1–2 weeks
Immediate effect on mood	Sedation, dysphoria	Euphoria	None	Variable, usually slight	None
Main unwanted effects	Sedation Anticholinergic effects (dry mouth, constipation, blurred vision) Postural hypotension Seizures Mania Impotence	Sedation Postural hypotension Insomnia Weight gain Liver damage (rare)	Nausea Diarrhoea Anxiety and restlessness Insomnia	Variable Generally no anticholinergic effects. Hypotension (trazodone) Sedation (mianserin, trazodone) Seizures (maprotiline)	Tremor Thirst and polyuria Weakness Hypothyroidism Weight gain Teratogenic risk (Monitoring required)
Risk with acute overdose	High (cardiac dysrhythmias, seizures, mania)	Moderate (seizures, mania)	Low	Variable. Some cause seizures or dysrhythmias	Dysrhythmias, seizures, confusion.
Risk of drug interactions	Many (e.g. alcohol)	Many (e.g. ephedrine, pethidine)	Must not be used with MAOI	Few	Diuretics

Testing of antidepressant drugs

- Animal models of depression include:
  - —learned helplessness model
  - —reversal of reserpine-induced behavioural syndrome
  - —mother–infant separation in primates.

  None is a good model for human depressive illness, but they are the best available for testing new drugs.
- Biochemical and pharmacological measures include inhibition of monoamine uptake, receptor-blocking activity, enhancement of peripheral noradrenergic transmission.
- Clinical testing of antidepressant drugs necessitates allowance for large placebo effects.

If brain tissue is homogenised, the nerve terminals are broken off, but reseal spontaneously to form vesicular structures (synaptosomes) which can be separated from the rest of the cellular components by differential centrifugation. Synaptosomes can accumulate and release transmitters much like intact nerve terminals, and form a convenient preparation for measuring the effect of amine-uptake inhibitors. Among TCA there is a fairly good correlation between antidepressant activity and potency in inhibiting noradrenaline or 5-HT uptake, but MAOI and many atypical antidepressants have no effect.

A general point that has to be borne in mind when using in vitro tests to assess potential antidepressants is that many drugs (particularly TCA) are metabolised to pharmacologically active substances in vivo. In several cases (see below), the metabolite has a different ratio of selectivity with respect to noradrenaline and 5-HT uptake, and it is often unclear whether the parent drug or the metabolite is actually responsible for the clinical effect.

MECHANISM OF ACTION OF ANTIDEPRESSANT DRUGS

The view that antidepressant drugs work simply by enhancing monoamine neurotransmission at some key site in the brain (which formed the basis of the original monoamine theory of depression) is no longer tenable, having been effectively demolished by two facts already discussed, namely:

- the temporal discrepancy between the pharmacodynamic and the therapeutic actions of antidepressant drugs
- the discovery of many 'atypical' antidepressant drugs which do not facilitate monoaminergic transmission.

Unfortunately, despite much experimental work and an overwhelming volume of prose directed at the problem, there is still no convincing mechanistic theory with which to replace the monoamine hypothesis.

In the absence of a simple mechanistic theory to account for antidepressant action, it is useful to look for pharmacological effects that the various drugs have in common, concentrating more on the slow adaptive changes that follow a similar time-course to the therapeutic effect, rather than on the immediate biochemical effects. This approach (see Enna et al. 1981, Stahl & Palazidou 1986) has led to the discovery that certain monoamine receptors, in particular β- and α_2-adrenoceptors, are consistently down-regulated following chronic antidepressant treatment. This can be demonstrated as a reduction in the number of binding sites in experimental animals, as well as by a reduction in the functional response to agonists (e.g. stimulation of cAMP formation by β-adrenoceptor agonists). Receptor down-regulation probably also occurs in man, since responses to **clonidine**, an α_2-adrenoceptor agonist, are reduced by long-term antidepressant treatment. Other receptors have also been studied; α_1-adrenoceptors are not consistently affected, but 5-HT_2 receptors are also down-regulated.

How these findings relate to the monoamine theory is far from clear at present. Loss of β-adrenoceptors as a factor in alleviating depression does not fit comfortably with theory, since β-adrenoceptor antagonists are not antidepressant, though it is the most consistent change reported. Impaired presynaptic inhibition, secondary to down-regulation of α_2-adrenoceptors might, it is argued, facilitate monoamine release and thus facilitate transmission.

The antidepressant effects of many drugs correlate closely with their ability to compete with ^{3}H imipramine for binding sites in the brain and on blood platelets. These binding sites do not correspond to any known neurotransmitter receptors, and are probably associated with the 5-HT uptake mech-

Types of antidepressant drugs

- Main types are:
  —tricyclic antidepressants (TCA)
  —monoamine oxidase inhibitors (MAOI)
  —5-HT uptake inhibitors
  —'atypical' antidepressants
  —lithium.
- TCA act by inhibiting uptake of noradrenaline and/or 5-HT by monoaminergic nerve terminals, thus acutely facilitating transmission.
- MAOI inhibit one or both forms of brain MAO, thus increasing the cytosolic stores of noradrenaline, dopamine and 5-HT in nerve terminals. Inhibition of type A MAO correlates with antidepressant activity. Selective type A MAOI have recently been introduced.
- Atypical antidepressants act by various mechanisms, often poorly understood.
- All types of antidepressant drug take about 2 weeks to produce any beneficial effects, even though their pharmacological effects are produced immediately, suggesting that secondary adaptive changes are important.
- The most consistent adaptive change seen with different types of antidepressant drugs is down-regulation of β- and α_2-adrenoceptors, as well as 5-HT_2 receptors. How this is related to therapeutic effect is not clear.
- Lithium is mainly used prophylactically; it prevents the manic phase of bipolar depression, as well as having antidepressant activity.

anism which is common to platelets and 5-HT-releasing nerve terminals. It is interesting that electroconvulsive therapy, as well as antidepressant drug treatment, reduces the number of these binding sites in the brain. Some of the 'atypical' antidepressants (see later section), such as mianserin, do not, however, affect these binding sites, arguing against a simple unitary hypothesis of how antidepressant drugs work.

TRICYCLIC ANTIDEPRESSANT DRUGS

Tricyclic antidepressants form the most important group of antidepressants in current clinical use. They are, however, far from ideal in practice, and it is the need for drugs which act more quickly and reliably and produce fewer side effects that has led to the introduction of newer 'atypical' antidepressants.

Chemical aspects

TCA are closely related in structure to the phenothiazines (Ch. 28) and were initially produced (in 1949) as potential neuroleptic drugs. **Imipramine** was found to be of no use in schizophrenia, but effective in relieving depression, so other compounds were synthesised, following much the same pattern as the development of the neuroleptic drugs. They differ from phenothiazines principally in the incorporation of an extra atom into the central ring (Fig. 29.2). The ring structure is considerably distorted by this change, and the two outer rings become twisted out of alignment so that the molecule is no longer planar as in phenothiazines.

Similar changes to the structure of thioxanthine-

Dibenzazepines

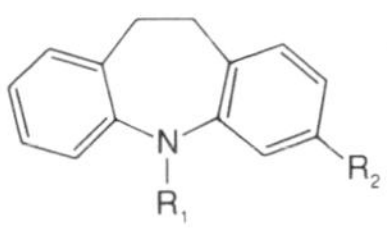

Drug	R_1	R_2
Imipramine	$-CH_2CH_2CH_2N(CH_3)_2$	H
Desipramine	$-CH_2CH_2CH_2NHCH_3$	H
Clomipramine	$-CH_2CH_2CH_2N(CH_3)_2$	Cl

Dibenzcycloheptenes

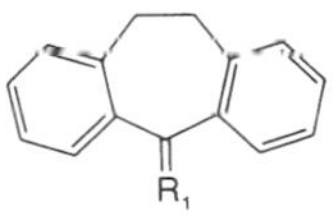

Drug	R_1
Amitriptyline	$=CHCH_2CH_2N(CH_3)_2$
Nortriptyline	$=CHCH_2CH_2NHCH_3$
Protriptyline	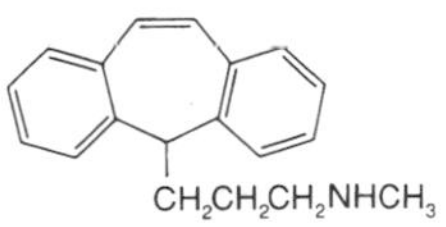 $CH_2CH_2CH_2NHCH_3$

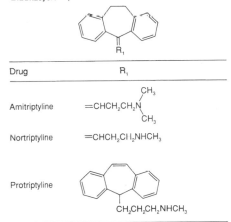

Fig. 29.2 Chemical structures of tricyclic antidepressants.

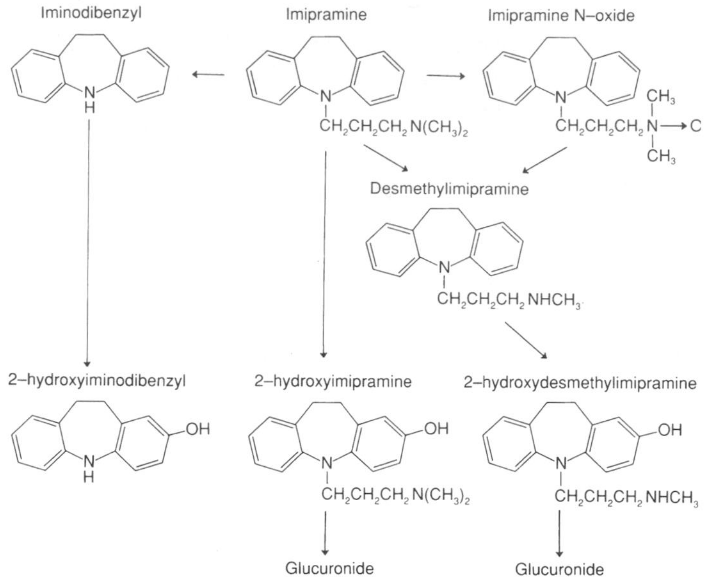

Fig. 29.3 Metabolism of imipramine, which is typical of that of other tricyclic antidepressants.

type neuroleptics resulted in drugs such as **amitriptyline,** while addition of a chlorine atom to imipramine, as in chlorpromazine, led to another useful drug, **clomipramine**. All of these compounds are tertiary amines, with two methyl groups attached to the basic nitrogen atom. They are quite rapidly demethylated in vivo (Fig. 29.3) to the corresponding secondary amines (**desipramine, nortriptyline,** etc.; Fig. 29.2), which are themselves active and may be administered as drugs in their own right. Other tricyclic derivatives with slightly modified bridge structures include **protriptyline** and **doxepin.** The pharmacological differences between these drugs are not very great, and relate mainly to their side effects, which are discussed below.

Mechanism of action

As discussed above, the main effect of TCA is to block the uptake of amines by nerve terminals, probably by competition for the carrier which forms part of this membrane transport system (Ch. 7). Synthesis of amines, storage in synaptic vesicles, and release are not directly affected, though some TCA appear to increase transmitter release indirectly by blocking presynaptic α_2-adrenoceptors. Most TCA inhibit noradrenaline and 5-HT uptake by brain synaptosomes, but have much less effect on dopamine uptake. Among the conventional TCA, there is relatively little selectivity between noradrenaline and 5-HT uptake (Fig. 29.4), and it is not at all clear which type of activity is most important in relation to their antidepressant effects. It has been suggested that improvement of mood reflects mainly an enhancement of 5-HT-mediated transmission, whereas increased motor activity ('psychomotor stimulation') results from facilitation of noradrenergic transmission (see reviews by Iversen & Mackay 1979, Carlsson 1984). Interpretation is made difficult by the fact that the major metabolites of TCA have considerable pharmacological activity (in some cases greater than that of the parent drug) and often differ from the parent drug in respect of their noradrenaline/5-HT selectivity (Table 29.3). Evidence that effects on 5-HT-mediated transmission may be the major factor comes from clinical studies in which either administration of the 5-HT-synthesis inhibitor, PCPA (see Ch. 8), or rigorous exclusion of the precursor, 5-HTP, from the diet have been shown to cause relapse in depressed patients (Delgado et al. 1990).

In addition to their effects on amine uptake, most TCA affect one or more types of neurotransmitter receptor, including muscarinic ACh receptors, histamine receptors and 5-HT receptors. The anti-

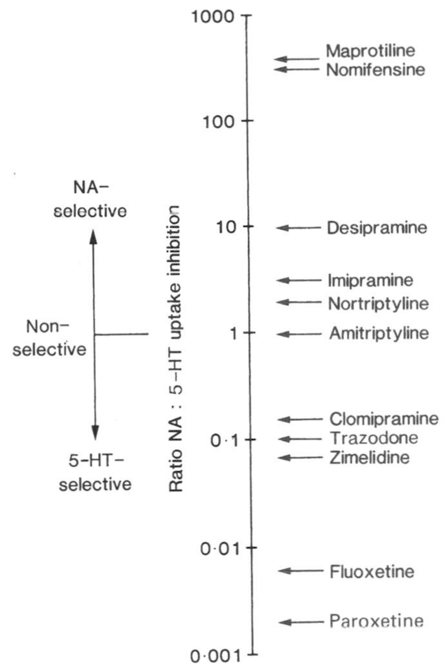

Fig. 29.4 Selectivity of inhibition of noradrenaline and 5-HT uptake by various antidepressants.

muscarinic effects of TCA do not contribute to their antidepressant effects, but are responsible for various troublesome side effects (see below). The antihistamine actions were revealed in a study of histamine activated adenylate cyclase activity in guinea-pig brain (Kanof & Greengard 1978) which showed a close correlation between the blocking of this response (mediated by H_2-receptors; see Ch. 11) and antidepressant activity. This correlation

Table 29.3 Inhibition of neuronal noradrenaline and 5-HT uptake by tricyclic antidepressants and their metabolites

Drug/metabolite	NA uptake	5-HT uptake
Imipramine	+++	++
Desmethylimipramine (DMI)	++++	+
Hydroxy-DMI	+++	–
Clomipramine (CMI)	++	+++
Desmethyl-CMI	+++	+
Amitriptyline (AMI)	++	++
Nortriptyline (desmethyl-AMI)	+++	++
Hydroxy-nortriptyline	++	++

was not confined to TCA but extended also to other groups of antidepressants. Its significance is still very uncertain.

Other studies (see Sulser 1983) have suggested that the down-regulation of β-adrenoceptors and 5-HT_2 receptors that is consistently produced by antidepressant drugs may be essential for their clinical effects, but the mechanism has not been elucidated.

Actions and unwanted effects

In non-depressed human subjects, TCA cause sedation, confusion and motor incoordination. These effects occur also in depressed patients in the first few days of treatment, but tend to wear off in 1–2 weeks as the antidepressant effect develops. In experimental animals, TCA produce sedation, but they are able to reverse the depressant effect of reserpine treatment.

Unwanted effects with normal clinical dosage

TCA produce a number of troublesome side effects, mainly due to interference with autonomic control.

Atropine-like effects include dry mouth, blurred vision, constipation and urinary retention. These effects are strong with **amitriptyline**, and much weaker with **desipramine**. *Postural hypotension* occurs with TCA. This may seem anomalous for drugs which enhance noradrenergic transmission. The effect possibly results from an effect on noradrenergic transmission in the medullary vasomotor centre. The other common side effect is sedation (see above). Since many depressed patients have difficulty in sleeping, this effect may actually be helpful, but the long duration of action means that daytime performance is often affected by drowsiness and difficulty in concentrating.

Interactions with other drugs

TCA are particularly likely to cause adverse effects when given in conjunction with other drugs (see Ch. 42). They rely on hepatic microsomal metabolism for elimination from the body, and this may be inhibited by competing drugs (e.g. neuroleptics and some steroids).

TCA cause a strong potentiation of the effects of alcohol, for reasons that are not well understood, and respiratory depression may follow a bout of drinking. TCA also interact with various antihypertensive drugs (see Ch. 14). Dangerous consequences can result from an excessive rise or a fall in blood pressure, so the use of TCA in patients being treated for hypertension requires close monitoring.

Acute toxicity

Antidepressant drugs (most commonly TCA) are now one of the most frequently used methods for attempted suicide, so their acute toxic effects are a matter of some practical importance. In the United Kingdom, an estimated 1 000 000 cases of TCA overdose occur annually, with about 400 deaths. The main effects are on the central nervous system and the heart. The initial effect of TCA overdosage is to cause excitement and delirium, which may be accompanied by convulsions. This is followed by coma and respiratory depression lasting for some days before a gradual recovery. Pronounced atropine-like effects are produced, with flushing, dry mouth and skin, and inhibition of gut and bladder.

Cardiac dysrhythmias are common, usually atrial or ventricular extrasystoles, and sudden death may occur from ventricular fibrillation. The mechanism is not understood, but the dysrhythmias often fail to respond to β-adrenoceptor-blocking drugs, so it is not very likely that enhanced noradrenaline effects on the heart are responsible.

One form of treatment that has been reported to control the main CNS effects is the use of the anticholinesterase, **physostigmine** (see Ch. 6), though this is not recommended routinely. This suggests that the antimuscarinic effects of TCA may be partly responsible, and indeed the symptoms produced closely resemble those of atropine poisoning.

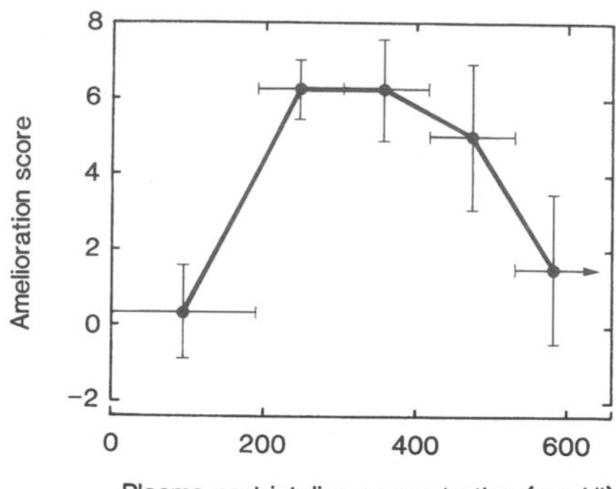

Fig. 29.5 'Therapeutic window' for nortriptyline. The antidepressant effect, determined from subjective rating scales, is optimal at plasma concentrations between 200 nmol/l and 400 nmol/l, and declines at higher levels.

> **Tricyclic antidepressants**
>
> - TCA are chemically related to phenothiazines, and some have similar receptor-blocking actions.
> - Important examples are: imipramine, amitriptyline and clomipramine.
> - The most widely used type of antidepressant, though ineffective in 30–40% of cases.
> - Most are eliminated slowly, and they are often converted to active metabolites.
> - Important side effects: sedation (H_1-block); postural hypotension (α-block); dry mouth, blurred vision, constipation (muscarinic block); occasionally mania and convulsions.
> - Dangerous in acute overdose: confusion and mania; cardiac dysrhythmias.
> - Liable to interact with other drugs: e.g. alcohol, anaesthetics, and hypotensive drugs should not be given with MAOI.

Pharmacokinetic aspects

TCA are all rapidly absorbed when given orally and bind strongly to plasma albumin, most being 90–95% bound at therapeutic plasma concentrations. They bind to extravascular tissues, which accounts for their generally large distribution volumes (usually 10–50 l/kg; see Ch. 4) and low rates of elimination. This extravascular sequestration and high plasma protein binding mean that extra-corporeal dialysis is ineffective in acute overdosage.

TCA are metabolised in the liver by two main routes (Fig. 29.3), namely *N-demethylation*, whereby tertiary amines are converted to secondary amines (e.g. **imipramine** to **desmethylimipramine**, **amitriptyline** to **nortriptyline**) and *ring hydroxylation*. Both the desmethyl and the hydroxylated metabolites commonly retain biological activity (see Table 29.3). During prolonged treatment with TCA, the plasma concentration of these metabolites is usually comparable to that of the parent drug, though there is wide variation between individuals. Inactivation of the drugs occurs by glucuronide conjugation of the hydroxylated metabolites, the glucuronides being excreted in the urine.

The overall half-times for elimination of TCA are generally long, ranging from 10–20 hours for **imipramine** and **desipramine** to about 80 hours for **protriptyline**. They are even longer in elderly

Clinical uses of tricyclic antidepressants (TCA)

- Endogenous depression; agitated and anxious patients with disturbed sleep benefit from TCA with sedative properties (e.g. amitriptyline); withdrawn and apathetic patients require less sedative drugs (e.g. imipramine).
- Panic attacks (Ch. 27).
- Phobic and obsessional states (e.g. clomipramine).
- Neuropathic pain states (Ch. 31).
- Bed-wetting in children (e.g. amitriptyline).

patients. Thus, gradual accumulation is possible, leading to slowly developing side effects. The relationship between plasma concentrations and the therapeutic effect may not be simple, according to a study on **nortriptyline** (Fig. 29.5) which shows that too high a plasma concentration actually reduces the antidepressant effect, and there is quite a narrow 'therapeutic window'. Whether this is true for other antidepressant drugs is not known.

Clinical uses

The clinical uses of tricyclic antidepressants are summarised above.

MONOAMINE OXIDASE INHIBITORS (MAOI)

Drugs of the MAOI type were among the first to be introduced clinically as antidepressants, but were largely superseded by tricyclic and other types of antidepressants whose clinical efficacies were considered better and whose side effects are generally less than those of MAOI. The main examples are **phenelzine**, **tranylcypromine** and **iproniazid**. These drugs cause irreversible inhibition of the enzyme, and do not distinguish between the two main isozymes (see below). Recently, the discovery of reversible inhibitors that show isozyme selectivity has rekindled interest in this class of drug. Though several studies have shown a reduction in platelet MAO activity in certain groups of depressed patients, there is no clear evidence that abnormal MAO activity is involved in the pathogenesis of depression.

MAO (see Benedetti & Dostert 1992; also Ch. 7) is found in nearly all tissues, and exists in two similar but distinct molecular forms (see Table 29.4). MAO-A has a substrate preference for 5-HT, and is the main target for the antidepressant MAOI. MAO-B has a substrate preference for phenylethylamine, and both enzymes act on noradrenaline and dopamine. Type B is selectively inhibited by **selegiline** (alternative name: **deprenyl**), which has been used clinically in the treatment of parkinsonism (see Ch. 25). Most of the current antidepressant MAOI act on both forms of MAO, but clinical studies with subtype-specific inhibitors have shown clearly that antidepressant activity, as well as the main side effects of MAOI, is associated with MAO-A inhibition. MAO is located intracellularly, mostly associated with mitochondria, and has two main functions:

- Within noradrenergic and 5-HT-containing nerve terminals, MAO has the effect of regulating the free intraneuronal concentration of noradrenaline

Table 29.4 Substrates and inhibitors for type A and type B monoamine oxidase

	Type A-selective	Non-selective	Type B-selective
Substrates	Noradrenaline 5-HT	Dopamine Tyramine	Phenylethylamine Benzylamine
Inhibitors	Clorgyline Moclobemide	Pargyline Tranylcypromine Iproniazid	Selegiline

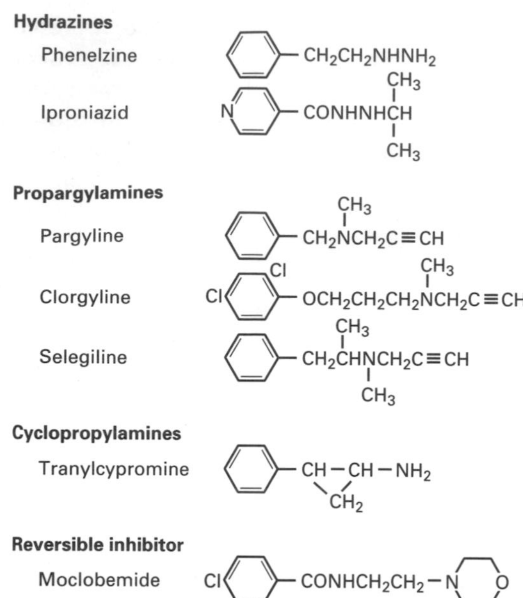

Fig. 29.6 Chemical structures of monoamine oxidase inhibitors. Most of the clinically used MAOI are non-selective between MAO-A and MAO-B. Exceptions are **selegiline** (MAO-B-specific, and not used as an antidepressant) and **clorgyline** (MAO-A-specific and effective in depression).

or 5-HT and hence the releasable stores of these transmitters. It is not involved in the inactivation of released transmitter. The biochemical role of MAO in noradrenergic nerves, and the effect of MAOI on transmitter metabolism are discussed in Chapter 7.

- MAO is important in the inactivation of endogenous and ingested amines which would otherwise produce unwanted effects. An example is tyramine, an ingested amine which is a substrate for both MAO-A and MAO-B, and is important in producing some of the side effects of MAOI (see below).

Chemical aspects

Many substances similar to phenylethylamines act as weak competitive inhibitors of MAO. **Amphetamine** is an example, though its actions on noradrenergic transmission (Ch. 7) are not primarily the result of this mechanism. MAOI possess a phenylethylamine-like structure, similar to MAO substrates (Fig. 29.6); most contain a reactive group which enables the inhibitor to bind covalently to the enzyme, resulting in a non-competitive and long-lasting inhibition. In many MAOI (e.g. **iproniazid** and **phenelzine**), this reactive moiety is a hydrazine group. It can also be a propargylamine (as in **pargyline** or **selegiline**) or a cyclopropylamine (as in **tranylcypromine**). Recovery of MAO activity after inhibition takes several weeks with most drugs, but is quicker after tranylcypromine which forms a less stable bond with the enzyme. **Moclobemide** acts as a reversible competitive inhibitor and is relatively selective for MAO-A.

MAOI are not particularly specific in their actions and inhibit a variety of other enzymes as well as MAO, including many enzymes involved in the metabolism of other drugs. This is responsible for some of the many clinically important drug interactions associated with MAOI.

Pharmacological effects

MAOI cause a rapid and sustained increase in the 5-HT, noradrenaline and dopamine content of the brain, 5-HT being affected most and dopamine least. Similar changes occur in peripheral tissues such as heart, liver and intestine, and increases in the plasma concentrations of these amines are also detectable. Although these increases in tissue amine content are largely due to accumulation within neurons, transmitter release in response to nerve activity is not increased. In contrast to the effect of TCA, MAOI do not increase the response of peripheral organs, such as the heart and blood vessels, to sympathetic nerve stimulation. The main effect of MAOI is to increase the cytoplasmic concentration of monoamines in nerve terminals, without greatly affecting the vesicular stores which form the pool that is releasable by nerve stimulation. The increased cytoplasmic pool results in an increased rate of spontaneous leakage of monoamines, and also an increased release by indirectly acting sympathomimetic amines such as amphetamine and tyramine (see Ch. 7). This occurs because these amines work by displacing noradrenaline from the vesicles into the nerve terminal cytoplasm, from which it may either leak out and produce a response, or be degraded by MAO (see Fig. 7.11). Inhibition of MAO increases the proportion that escapes, and thus enhances the response. Tyramine thus causes a much greater rise in blood pressure in MAOI-treated animals than in controls. This mechanism is important in relation to the 'cheese reaction' produced by MAOI in man (see later section).

In normal human subjects, MAOI causes an immediate increase in motor activity, and euphoria and excitement develop over the course of a few days. This is in contrast to TCA which cause only sedation and confusion when given to non-depressed subjects. Experimental animals show a similar pattern of increased motor activity, and MAOI (like TCA) are effective in reversing the behavioural effects of reserpine treatment. The effects of MAOI on amine metabolism develop rapidly, and the effect of a single dose lasts for several days. There is a clear discrepancy, as with TCA, between the rapid biochemical response and the delayed antidepressant effect.

The mechanisms underlying the antidepressant effects of MAOI are not well understood; as discussed above, the superficially similar actions of MAOI and TCA in protecting monoamines from removal or destruction may be misleading, since their effects on neurotransmission appear to be very different. Some evidence for a common, if poorly understood, mechanism of action comes from studies demonstrating that MAOI and TCA produce a similar delayed down-regulation of β-adrenoceptors and 5-HT_2 receptors (see Heninger & Charney 1987).

Unwanted effects and toxicity

Many of the unwanted effects of MAOI result directly from MAO inhibition, but some are produced by other mechanisms.

Hypotension is a common side effect; indeed **pargyline** was at one time used as an antihypertensive drug. At first sight, it seems surprising in view of the increase in noradrenaline storage and release that occurs. One possible explanation is that amines such as dopamine or octopamine are able to accumulate within peripheral sympathetic nerve terminals and displace noradrenaline from the storage vesicles, thus reducing noradrenaline release associated with sympathetic activity.

Excessive central stimulation may cause tremors, excitement, insomnia, and, in overdose, convulsions.

Weight gain, associated with increased appetite, occurs in a proportion of patients, and can be so extreme as to require the drug to be discontinued.

Atropine-like side effects (dry mouth, blurred vision, urinary retention, etc.) are common with MAOI, though they are less of a problem than with TCA.

MAOI of the hydrazine type (e.g. **phenelzine** and **iproniazid**) produce, very rarely (less than 1 in 10 000), *severe hepatotoxicity* which seems to be due to the hydrazine moiety of the molecule. Their use in patients with liver disease is therefore unwise.

Interaction with other drugs and foods

Interaction with other drugs and foods is the most serious problem with MAOI, and is the main factor that caused their clinical use to decline. The main advantage claimed for the new reversible MAOI, such as moclobemide, is that these interactions are reduced (though the reason for this is not clear).

The *'cheese reaction'* is a direct consequence of MAO inhibition, and occurs when normally innocuous amines (mainly **tyramine**) are ingested. Tyramine is normally metabolised by MAO in the gut wall and liver and, so, little dietary tyramine reaches the systemic circulation. When this is prevented, tyramine is absorbed, and moreover its sympathomimetic effect is enhanced (see above). The result is acute hypertension, giving rise to a severe throbbing headache, and occasionally even

Monoamine oxidase inhibitors

- Main examples are phenelzine, tranylcypromine, iproniazid and moclobemide.
- Have tended to be superseded by TCA, mainly because of interactions and doubts about efficacy; currently undergoing a revival.
- Action is long-lasting (weeks) because of irreversible inhibition of MAO. Moclobemide has a short duration of action.
- Main side effects: postural hypotension (sympathetic block); atropine-like effects (as with TCA); weight gain; CNS stimulation, causing restlessness, insomnia, liver damage (rare).
- Acute overdose causes CNS stimulation, sometimes convulsions.
- May cause severe hypertensive response to tyramine-containing foods ('cheese reaction'); should not be given simultaneously with TCA. This does not occur with moclobemide.
- Interact with pethidine, causing hyperpyrexia and hypotension.

Clinical uses of monoamine oxidase inhibitors (MAOI)

- Severe depression refractory to other treatment. Also depression with atypical/hysterical features.
  — Caution needed to avoid hypertensive 'cheese reaction'. Less risk with moclobemide than with older MAOI (e.g. phenelzine).
- Treatment of phobias.
- Selegiline (selective MAO-B inhibitor) used in Parkinson's disease (Ch. 25).

to intracranial haemorrhage. Though many foods contain some tyramine, it appears that at least 10 mg of tyramine needs to be ingested to produce such a response and the main danger is from mature cheeses and from concentrated yeast products such as Marmite. Administration of indirectly acting sympathomimetic amines (e.g. **ephedrine, amphetamine**) is also likely to cause severe hypertension in patients receiving MAOI; directly acting agents, such as **noradrenaline** used in conjunction with local anaesthetic injection (see Ch. 34), are not hazardous.

Hypertensive episodes have also been reported in patients given TCA and MAOI simultaneously. The probable explanation is that inhibition of noradrenaline re-uptake further enhances the cardiovascular response to dietary tyramine, thus accentuating the cheese reaction. This combination of drugs can also produce excitement and hyperactivity.

MAOIs interact with some drugs to cause not merely an enhancement of their action, but an abnormal syndrome. An important example is the opioid analgesic **pethidine** (see Ch. 31) which may cause severe hyperpyrexia, with restlessness, coma and hypotension when given in combination with MAOI. The mechanism is not known for certain, but it is likely that an abnormal pethidine metabolite is produced because of inhibition of the normal demethylation pathway.

A comparison of the main characteristics of MAOI and other antidepressant drugs is given in Table 29.2.

Clinical uses

The clinical uses of MAOI are summarised above.

SELECTIVE 5-HT UPTAKE INHIBITORS

Several drugs of this type have been introduced recently, the main ones being **fluoxetine, fluvoxamine, paroxetine** and **sertraline** (see Table 29.2). Fluoxetine is currently the most prescribed antidepressant. As well as showing selectivity with respect to 5-HT over noradrenaline uptake, their side effect profile differs from that of TCA, and this may be a significant advantage. Clinical trials have shown these drugs to be as effective as TCA in treating depression, though no more so. The delay of 2–4 weeks before the therapeutic effect develops is similar to that seen with other antidepressants.

The main advantages of 5-HT uptake inhibitors compared with TCA and MAOI are:

- Lack of anticholinergic and cardiovascular side effects. No problem with weight gain.
- Low acute toxicity (low risk of overdose).
- No food reactions.

The main drawbacks of 5-HT uptake inhibitors, apart from their high cost, are:

- Common side effects are nausea, anorexia and insomnia.
- In combination with MAOI, they can result in 'serotonin syndrome' associated with tremor, hyperthermia and cardiovascular collapse, from which deaths have occurred.
- There have been reports of increased aggression, and occasionally violence, in patients treated with

5-HT uptake inhibitors

- Examples include fluoxetine, fluvoxamine, paroxetine, sertraline.
- Antidepressant actions are similar in efficacy and time-course to those of TCA.
- Acute toxicity is less than that of MAOI or TCA, so overdose risk is reduced.
- Side effects include nausea and insomnia.
- No food reactions, but dangerous 'serotonin reaction' (hyperthermia, muscle rigidity, cardiovascular collapse) can occur if given with MAOI.
- Increased aggression has been reported.
- Currently the most commonly prescribed antidepressants; also used for some other psychiatric indications.

Table 29.5 Properties of 'atypical' antidepressant drugs

Drug	Mechanism	Unwanted effects	Advantages	Pharmacokinetics	Notes
Nomifensine	NA, DA* uptake blocker	Behavioural stimulation Insomnia Dyskinesias Allergic reactions	No sedation No atropine-like effects No cardiovascular effects Safe in overdose	Short-acting $t_{½} \sim 4$ h Needs twice-daily dosage	'Stimulant' profile
Maprotiline	Selective NA uptake blocker	Atropine-like effects Sedation Seizures Allergic rashes Acute toxicity similar to TCA†	No major advantages	Long-acting $t_{½} \sim 40$ h	Similar to imipramine, with long duration of action
Trazodone	Weak 5-HT uptake blocker Also blocks 5-HT_2 and α_2-receptors	Sedation Confusion Hypotension Cardiac dysrhythmias	No atropine-like effects Safe in overdose	Fairly short-acting $t_{½}$ 6–12 h	Doubtful clinical efficacy Anxiolytic activity
Mianserin	Blocks α_2, 5-HT_2, and H_1-receptors No effect on monoamine uptake	Sedation Seizures Hypersensitivity reactions including agranulocytosis	No atropine-like effects No cardiovascular effects Safe in overdose	Medium duration of action $t_{½} \sim 12$ h	
Iprindole	Not known No effect on monoamine uptake	No major unwanted effects	No sedation No atropine-like effects	Short-acting Needs thrice-daily dosage	Doubtful clinical efficacy

* NA = noradrenaline; DA = dopamine
† TCA = tricyclic antidepressant drugs

fluoxetine. It was claimed to be responsible for an increased suicide rate, but this has not been confirmed by controlled studies.

In spite of the apparent advantages of 5-HT uptake inhibitors over TCA in terms of side effects, the combined results of many trials show no overall difference in terms of patient acceptability (Song et al. 1993).

5-HT uptake inhibitors are used in a variety of psychiatric disorders, as well as in depression; these include anxiety and panic disorder (see Ch. 27), as well as eating disorders, such as bulimia.

Nefopan is a 5-HT uptake inhibitor used mainly as an analgesic (see Ch. 31).

Atypical antidepressant drugs

- Heterogeneous group, including maprotiline, nomifensine, trazodone, mianserin and iprindole.
- No common mechanism of action. Some are monoamine uptake blockers, but others (e.g. mianserin and iprindole) act by unknown mechanisms.
- Delay in therapeutic response is similar to TCA and MAOI.
- Most are fairly short-acting.
- Unwanted effects and acute toxicity vary, but are generally less than with TCA.

'ATYPICAL' ANTIDEPRESSANT DRUGS

Uncertainty about the exact biochemical mode of action of antidepressants has meant that the development of new drugs has often been empirical. This has resulted in the introduction of a heterogeneous group of compounds, only distantly related to conventional TCA though sharing some of their biochemical actions. The main claims made for these newer agents are:

- fewer side effects (e.g. sedation and anticholinergic effects)
- lower acute toxicity in overdose
- action with less delay
- efficacy in patients non-responsive to TCA or MAOI.

In practice, the newer drugs may definitely be better than TCA in respect of side effects and acute toxicity, but have not proved to be more rapid in action, nor more efficacious.

The properties of some of the more important drugs in this class are summarised in Table 29.5.

They can be divided into two broad categories:

- Non-tricyclic structures with similar noradrenaline-uptake-blocking effects to TCA (e.g. **nomifensine** and **maprotiline**). These drugs are all relatively inactive against 5-HT uptake (see Fig. 29.4), but nomifensine is unusual in being highly active as a dopamine uptake inhibitor.
- Drugs that do not affect amine re-uptake (e.g. **mianserin** and **iprindole**). The mechanism of action of these drugs is uncertain. One possibility is that mianserin increases noradrenaline release by blocking α_2-adrenoceptors on noradrenergic nerve terminals, thus reducing the inhibitory feedback control of noradrenaline release. Iprindole does not, however, work in this way, and tantalisingly seems to lack every expected property of an antidepressant drug except for clinical efficacy.

ELECTROCONVULSIVE THERAPY (ECT)

A tortuous line of reasoning, namely that schizophrenia and epilepsy were considered to be mutually exclusive, led to the use of induced convulsions as therapy for psychological disorders in the 1930s, and its efficacy in treating severe depression has been repeatedly confirmed. ECT in man involves stimulation through electrodes placed on either side of the head, with the patient lightly anaesthetised, paralysed with a neuromuscular-blocking drug so as to avoid physical injury, and artificially ventilated. Controlled trials have shown ECT to be at least as effective as antidepressant drugs, with response rates ranging between 60% and 80% in most studies (see Kiloh 1982); it appears to be the most effective treatment for severe suicidal depression. The main disadvantage of ECT is that it often causes confusion and memory loss lasting for days or weeks.

The effect of ECT on experimental animals has been carefully analysed to see if it provides clues as to the mode of action of antidepressant drugs (see Grahame-Smith 1984), but the clues it gives are distinctly enigmatic. 5-HT synthesis and uptake are unaltered, and noradrenaline uptake is somewhat increased (in contrast to the effect of TCA). Decreased β-adrenoceptor responsiveness, both biochemical and behavioural, occurs with both ECT and long-term administration of antidepressant drugs, but changes in 5-HT-mediated responses tend to go in opposite directions (see Lerer 1987).

CLINICAL EFFECTIVENESS OF ANTIDEPRESSANT TREATMENTS

The overall clinical efficacy of antidepressants has been established in many well-controlled clinical trials. However, it is clear that a substantial proportion of patients recover spontaneously, and that 30–40% of patients fail to improve with drug treatments. The effects of the drugs are significant, but not miraculous.

The results of a Medical Research Council trial in 1965 showed ECT to be the most effective treatment. **Imipramine** also produced significant improvement, but the MAOI **phenelzine** appeared to be no better than the placebo. The reported ineffectiveness of phenelzine in this trial (together with the incidence of severe hypertensive episodes) caused MAOI to lose favour clinically. Subsequent trials (see Nies & Robinson 1982, Murphy et al. 1987) showed that with larger dosage, MAOI may be significantly better than TCA for patients with mild depression, particularly those with neurotic symptoms (anxiety, etc.) as opposed to psychotic symptoms (withdrawal, delusions, etc.) where TCA appear to be more successful. The overall conclusion of many individual trials is that there is little to choose in efficacy between any of the drugs currently in use.

Even the most favourable trials, however, show that about 30% of depressed patients fail to improve. Attempts to identify which patients will respond on the basis of behavioural or biochemical measurements (e.g. platelet MAO activity, MHPG excretion) have not been successful.

LITHIUM

Lithium is different in its effects from the antidepressant drugs discussed so far, in that it controls the manic phase of manic-depressive (bipolar) illness and is also effective in unipolar depression. Used prophylactically in bipolar depression, lithium is able to prevent the swings of mood and thus to reduce both the depressive and the manic phases of the illness. Given in an acute attack, lithium is effective only in reducing mania and has no effect during the depressive phase. Other drugs (e.g. neuroleptics) are equally effective in treating acute mania; they act more quickly and are considerably safer, so the clinical use of lithium is mainly confined to prophylactic control of manic-depressive illness. The anticonvulsant **carbamazepine** (Ch. 30) has a similar prophylactic effect against mood swings in patients with manic-depressive illness, and is used clinically in patients who are unresponsive to lithium.

The psychotropic effect of lithium was discovered in 1949 by Cade, who had predicted that urate salts should prevent the induction by uraemia of a hyperexcitability state in guinea pigs. He found lithium urate to produce an effect, quickly discovered that it was due to lithium rather than urate, and went on to show that lithium produced a rapid improvement in a group of manic patients.

Pharmacological effects and mechanism of action

The main features of lithium are summarised in Table 29.2. Lithium is clinically effective at a plasma concentration of 0.5–1 mmol/l, and above 1.5 mmol/l it produces a variety of toxic effects, so the therapeutic window is narrow. In normal subjects, 1 mmol/l lithium in plasma has no appreciable psychotropic effects. It does, however, produce many detectable biochemical changes, and it is still extremely unclear how these may be related to its therapeutic effect.

Lithium is a monovalent cation, which partially mimics the effects of a variety of other cations in cellular processes. Thus, it resembles sodium in excitable tissues, being able to permeate the fast voltage-sensitive channels that are responsible for action potential generation (see Ch. 34). It is not, however, pumped out nearly so quickly as sodium by the Na^+/K^+-ATPase and tends to accumulate inside excitable cells to a greater extent than sodium. This leads to a partial loss of intracellular potassium, and partial depolarisation of the cell. Its effects on monoamine metabolism are complex. Given acutely, lithium increases noradrenaline and 5-HT turnover in the brain, but seems to inhibit depolarisation-evoked release. These changes apparently subside during long-term administration, though, clinically, the drug remains effective, so their significance is unclear.

The biochemical effects of lithium are complex, but its therapeutic actions are generally ascribed to two mechanisms (see Bunney & Garland-Bunney 1987, Nahorski et al. 1991):

- Hormone-induced cAMP production is usually reduced (e.g. the response of renal tubular cells to ADH, see Ch. 18; the response of thyroid follicle cells to thyrotrophin, see Ch. 21). This is not, however, a pronounced effect in the brain.
- The phosphatidylinositol (PI) pathway (see Ch. 2) is blocked at the point where inositol phosphate is hydrolysed to free inositol (see Nahorski et al. 1991). This step is required for the regeneration of PI in the membrane after it has been hydrolysed by agonist action, as described in Chapter 2. Lithium thus causes a depletion of membrane PI and accumulation of intracellular inositol phosphate. The result is inhibition of agonist-stimulated $InsP_3$ formation through various PI-linked receptors, and therefore block of many receptor-mediated effects.

It seems quite possible that the effects of lithium on these two important second messenger systems somehow underlie its therapeutic effect, and that its cellular selectivity depends on the uptake of lithium in varying amounts reflecting the activity of sodium channels in different cells. This could account for its relatively selective action in the brain and kidney, even though many other tissues use the same second messengers.

Pharmacokinetic aspects and toxicity

Lithium excretion by the kidney occurs in two phases. About half of an oral dose is excreted within about 12 hours—the remainder, which presumably represents lithium taken up by cells, is excreted over the next 1–2 weeks. This very slow phase means that, with regular dosage, lithium accumulates slowly over approximately 2 weeks before a steady state is reached. The narrow therapeutic limit for the plasma concentration (approximately 0.5–1.5 mmol/l) means that monitoring is essential. Factors such as renal disease or sodium depletion reduce the rate of excretion and thus increase the likelihood of toxicity. Diuretics also have this effect.

The main toxic effects that may occur during treatment are:

- Nausea, vomiting and diarrhoea.
- Tremor.
- Renal effects: polyuria (with resulting thirst) resulting from inhibition of the action of antidiuretic hormone. At the same time there is some sodium retention, associated with increased aldosterone secretion. With prolonged treatment, serious renal tubular damage may occur, making it essential to monitor renal function regularly in lithium-treated patients.
- Thyroid enlargement, sometimes associated with hypothyroidism, resulting from inhibition of the action of thyrotrophin.
- Weight gain.

Acute lithium toxicity results in various neurological effects, progressing from confusion and motor impairment, to coma, convulsions and death if the plasma concentration reaches 3–5 mmol/l.

Lithium

- Inorganic ion taken orally as lithium carbonate.
- Mechanism of action is not understood. The main biochemical possibilities are:
  —interference with cAMP formation
  —interference with $InsP_3$ formation.
- Effects on neurotransmitter systems are numerous and complex.
- Acts to control mania as well as depression; mainly used prophylactically in bipolar depression.
- Long plasma half-life and narrow therapeutic window. Hence, side effects are common, and monitoring of plasma concentration essential.
- Main unwanted effects: nausea, thirst and polyuria, hypothyroidism, tremor, weakness, mental confusion, teratogenesis. Acute overdose causes confusion, convulsions and cardiac dysrhythmias.
- Action enhanced by diuretic drugs.

REFERENCES AND FURTHER READING

Åsberg M, Wågner A 1986 Biochemical effects of antidepressant treatment—studies of monoamine metabolites in cerebrospinal fluid and platelet [^{3}H] imipramine binding. In: Antidepressants and receptor function. Ciba Foundation Symposium 123: 57–83

Ashton H 1992 Brain systems, disorders and psychotropic drugs. Blackwell Scientific Publications, Oxford

Baker G B, Dewhurst W G 1985 Biochemical theories of affective disorders. In: Dewhurst W G, Baker G B (eds) Pharmacotherapy of affective disorders. Croom Helm, Beckenham

Benedetti M S, Dostert P 1992 Monoamine oxidase: from physiology and pathophysiology to the design and clinical application of reversible inhibitors. Adv Drug Res 23: 66–125

Bunney W E, Garland-Bunney B L 1987 Mechanisms of action of lithium in affective illness: basic and clinical implications. In: Meltzer H Y (ed) Psychopharmacology. Raven Press, New York, p 553–565

Carlsson A 1984 Current theories on the mode of action of antidepressant drugs. Adv Biochem Psychopharmacol 39: 213–221

Delgado P L, Charney D S, Price L H, Aghajanian G K, Landis H, Heninger G R 1990 Serotonin function and the mechanism of antidepressant action: reversal of antidepressant-induced remission by rapid depletion of plasma tryptophan. Arch Gen Psychiatry 47: 411–418

Enna S J, Malick J B, Richelson E 1981 Antidepressants: neurochemical, behavioural and clinical perspectives. Raven Press, New York

Grahame-Smith D G 1984 The neuropharmacological effects of electroconvulsive shock and their relationship to the therapeutic effect of electroconvulsive therapy in depression. In: Usdin E et al. (eds) Frontiers in biochemical and pharmacological research in depression. Raven Press, New York

Heninger G R, Charney D S 1987 Mechanism of action of antidepressant treatments: implications for the etiology and treatment of depressive disorders. In: Meltzer H Y (ed) Psychopharmacology. Raven Press, New York, p 513–526

Hollister L E, Claghorn J L 1993 New antidepressants. Ann Rev Pharmacol Toxicol 32: 165 177

Iversen L L, Mackay A V P 1979 Pharmacodynamics of antidepressants and antimanic drugs. In: Paykel E S, Coppen A (eds) Psychopharmacology of affective disorders. Oxford University Press, Oxford

Johnstone E C 1982 Affective disorders In: Crow T J (ed) Disorders of neurohumoral transmission. Academic Press, London, p 255–286

Kanof P D, Greengard P 1978 Brain histamine receptors as targets for antidepressant drugs. Nature 272: 329–333

Kiloh L G 1982 Electroconvulsive therapy. In: Paykel F S (ed) Handbook of affective disorders. Churchill Livingstone, Edinburgh, p 262–275

Lerer B 1987 Neurochemical and other neurobiological consequences of ECT: implications for the pathogenesis and treatment of affective disorders. In: Meltzer H Y (ed) Psychopharmacology. Raven Press, New York, p 577–588

Maj J, Przegalinski E, Mogilnicka E 1984 Hypotheses concerning the mechanism of action of antidepressant drugs. Rev Physiol Biochem Pharmacol 100: 1–74

Meltzer H Y, Lowy M T 1987 The serotonin hypothesis of depression. In: Meltzer H Y (ed) Psychopharmacology. Raven Press, New York, p 513–526

Murphy D L, Aulakh C S, Garrick N A, Sunderland T 1987 Monoamine oxidase inhibitors as antidepressants: implications for the mechanism of action of antidepressants and the psychobiology of the affective disorders and some related disorders. In: Meltzer H Y (ed) Psychopharmacology. Raven Press, New York, p 545–552

Nahorski S R, Ragan C I, Challiss R A J 1991 Lithium and the phosphoinositide cycle: an example of uncompetitive inhibition and its pharmacological consequences. Trends Pharmacol Sci 12: 297–303

Nies A, Robinson D S 1982 Monoamine oxidase inhibitors. In: Paykel E S (ed) Handbook of affective disorders. Churchill Livingstone, Edinburgh, p 246–261

Porsolt R D 1985 Animal models of affective disorders. In: Dewhurst W G, Baker G B (eds) Pharmacotherapy of affective disorders. Croom-Helm, Beckenham

Schildkraut J J 1965 The catecholamine hypothesis—a review of the supporting evidence. Am J Psychiatry 122: 509–522

Siever L J 1987 Role of noradrenergic mechanisms in the etiology of the affective disorders. In: Meltzer H Y (ed) Psychopharmacology. Raven Press, New York, p 393–504

Song F, Freemantle N, Sheldon T A, House A, Watson P, Long A, Mason J 1993 Selective serotonin reuptake inhibitors: meta-analysis of efficacy and acceptability. Br Med J 306: 683–687

Stahl S M, Palazidou L 1986 The pharmacology of depression: studies of neurotransmitter receptors lead the search for biochemical lesions and new drug therapies. Trends Pharmacol Sci 7: 349–354

Sulser F 1983 Mode of action of antidepressant drugs. J Clin Psychiatry 44: 14–20

30

ANTIEPILEPTIC DRUGS AND CENTRALLY ACTING MUSCLE RELAXANTS

EPILEPSY

Epilepsy is a very common disorder, affecting approximately 0.5% of the population. Usually there is no recognisable cause, although it may develop as a consequence of various kinds of brain damage, such as trauma, infection or tumour growth. Detailed coverage is given in the textbook by Laidlaw et al. (1988).

The characteristic event in epilepsy is the *seizure*, which is associated with the episodic high frequency discharge of impulses by a group of neurons in the brain. What starts as a local abnormal discharge may then spread to other areas of the brain. The site of the primary discharge and the extent of its spread determines the symptoms that are produced, which range from a brief lapse of attention to a full-blown convulsive fit lasting for several minutes. The particular symptoms produced depend on the function of the region of the brain that is affected. Thus involvement of the motor cortex causes convulsions; involvement of the hypothalamus causes peripheral autonomic discharge, and involvement of the reticular formation in the upper brainstem leads to loss of consciousness.

Abnormal electrical activity during a seizure can be detected by electroencephalograph (EEG) recording from electrodes distributed over the surface of the scalp. Various types of seizure can be recognised on the basis of the nature and distribution of the abnormal discharge (Fig. 30.1).

TYPES OF EPILEPSY

The agreed clinical classification of epilepsy recognises two major categories, namely *partial* and *generalised* seizures, though there is some overlap and many varieties of each.

Partial seizures

Partial seizures are those in which the discharge begins locally, and often remains localised. These may produce relatively simple symptoms without loss of consciousness, such as involuntary muscle contractions, abnormal sensory experiences or autonomic discharge, or they may cause more complex effects on consciousness, mood and behaviour, often termed psychomotor epilepsy. The localised EEG discharge in this type of epilepsy is shown in Figure 30.1D. Partial seizures can often be attributed to local cerebral lesions, and their incidence increases with age.

An epileptic focus in the motor cortex results in attacks, sometimes called *Jacksonian epilepsy*, consisting of repetitive jerking of a particular muscle group, which spreads and may involve much of the body within about 2 minutes before dying out. Though the patient loses voluntary control of the affected parts of the body, he does not lose consciousness. In *psychomotor epilepsy*, which is often associated with a focus in the temporal lobe, the attack may consist of stereotyped purposive movements such as rubbing or patting movements, or much more complex behaviour such as dressing or walking or hair-combing. The seizure usually lasts

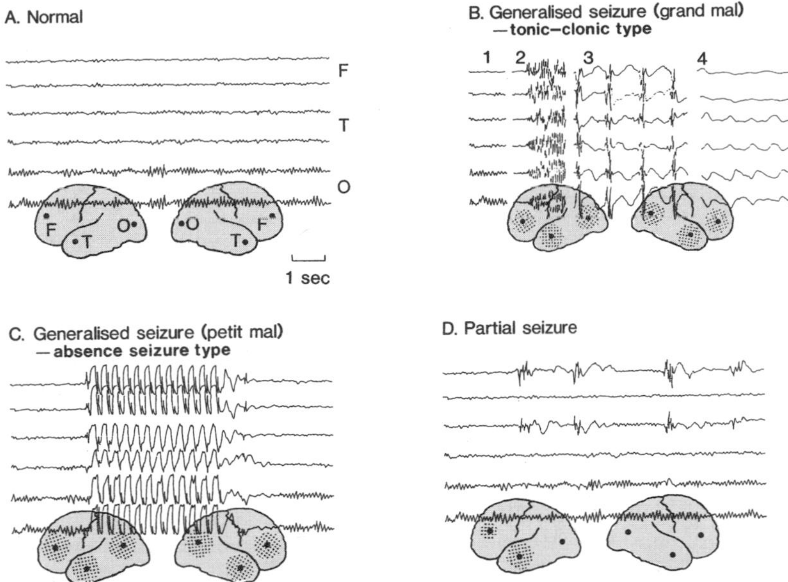

Fig. 30.1 EEG records in epilepsy. A. Normal EEG recorded from frontal (F), temporal (T) and occipital (O) sites on both sides, as shown in the inset diagram. The α-rhythm (10/second) can be seen in the occipital region. **B.** Sections of EEG recorded during a generalised tonic–clonic (grand mal) seizure. 1. Normal record. 2. Onset of tonic phase. 3. Clonic phase. 4. Post-convulsive coma. **C.** Generalised absence seizure (petit mal) showing sudden brief episode of 3/second 'spike and wave' discharge. **D.** Partial seizure with synchronous abnormal discharges in left frontal and temporal regions. (From: Eliasson S G et al. 1978 Neurological pathophysiology, 2nd edn. Oxford University Press, New York)

for a few minutes, after which the patient recovers with no recollection of the event. The behaviour during the seizure can be bizarre and accompanied by a strong emotional response.

Generalised seizures

Generalised seizures involve the whole brain, including the reticular system, thus producing abnormal electrical activity throughout both hemispheres. Immediate loss of consciousness is characteristic of generalised seizures. The main categories are *tonic–clonic seizures* (*grand mal*) and *absences* (*petit mal*). A tonic–clonic seizure consists of an initial strong contraction of the whole musculature, causing a rigid extensor spasm. Respiration stops and defaecation, micturition and salivation often occur. This tonic phase lasts for about 1 minute and is followed by a series of violent, synchronous jerks which gradually dies out in 2–4 minutes. The patient stays unconscious for a few more minutes and then gradually recovers, feeling ill and confused. Injury may occur during the convulsive episode. The EEG shows generalised continuous high frequency activity in the tonic phase, and an intermittent discharge in the clonic phase (Fig. 30.1B).

Absence seizures occur in children; they are much less dramatic, but may occur more frequently (many seizures each day), than tonic–clonic seizures. The patient abruptly ceases whatever he was doing, sometimes stopping speaking in mid-sentence, and stares vacantly for a few seconds, with little or no motor disturbance. The patient is unaware of his surroundings, and recovers abruptly with no after-effects. The EEG pattern shows a characteristic synchronous discharge during the period of the seizure (Fig. 30.1C). A particularly severe kind of epilepsy (Lennox–Gastaut syndrome) that occurs in children is associated with progressive mental retardation, possibly a reflection of excitotoxic neurodegeneration (see Ch. 25).

Pharmacologically there is a clear distinction between drugs that are effective in absence seizures and those that are effective in other types of epilepsy, though most drugs show little selectivity with respect to the other clinical subdivisions.

With optimal drug therapy, epilepsy is controlled completely in about 75% of patients, and about 10% (50 000 in Britain) continue to have seizures at intervals of 1 month or less, which severely disrupts their life and work. There is therefore a need to improve the efficacy of therapy.

CELLULAR MECHANISMS UNDERLYING EPILEPSY

The underlying neuronal abnormality in epilepsy is poorly understood. Because detailed studies are difficult or impossible to carry out on epileptic patients, many different animal models of epilepsy have been investigated. These include a variety of genetic strains that show epilepsy-like characteristics (e.g. mice that convulse briefly in response to certain sounds, baboons that show photically induced seizures, and beagles with an inherited abnormality that closely resembles human epilepsy). Local cortical damage (e.g. by applying aluminium oxide paste or crystals of a cobalt salt) results in a type of focal epilepsy. Local application of penicillin crystals has a similar effect, probably by interfering with inhibitory synaptic transmission. Convulsant drugs, such as **leptazol** (see Ch. 32), are often used, particularly in the testing of anticonvulsant agents, and seizures caused by electrical stimulation of the whole brain are used for the same purpose. It has been found empirically that activity in inhibiting leptazol-induced convulsions and in raising the *threshold* for production of electrically induced seizures is a fairly good index of effectiveness against absence seizures, whereas activity in reducing the *duration* and *spread* of convulsions induced by maximal electrical stimuli correlates with effectiveness in controlling other types of epilepsy, such as tonic–clonic seizures.

An interesting form of experimental epilepsy is the so-called *kindling response* (see review by Mosh & Ludvig 1988). Low-intensity electrical stimulation of certain regions of the limbic system, such as the amygdala, with implanted electrodes normally produces no seizure response. If a brief period of stimulation is repeated daily for several days, however, the response gradually increases until very low levels of stimulation will evoke a full seizure. The mechanism by which this change occurs is not clear, but it is prevented by NMDA-receptor antagonists, and may involve processes similar to those that cause long-term potentiation of synaptic transmission in the hippocampus (see Ch. 24). Kindling may be relevant to human epilepsy (see Mosh & Ludvig 1988). Thus it is often found that surgical removal of a damaged region of cortex fails to cure the epilepsy, as though the abnormal discharge from the region of primary damage had somehow produced a secondary hyperexcitability elsewhere in the brain. Prophylactic treatment with anticonvulsant drugs for 2 years following severe head injury reduces the subsequent incidence of post-traumatic epilepsy (Servit & Musil 1981), which suggests that a phenomenon similar to kindling may underlie this form of epilepsy.

By intracellular recording techniques it was shown in 1963 that the group of neurons from which the epileptic discharge originates display an unusual type of electrical behaviour, termed the '*paroxysmal depolarising shift*' (PDS), during which the membrane potential suddenly decreases by about 30 mV and remains depolarised for up to a few seconds before returning to normal. A burst of action potentials often accompanies this depolarisation (Fig. 30.2). This event probably results from the abnormally exaggerated and prolonged action of an excitatory transmitter, and it is interesting that activation of glutamate receptors of the NMDA type (see Ch. 24) produces 'plateau-shaped' depolarising responses very similar to the PDS (Fig. 30.2). This type of response probably occurs because of the voltage-dependent blocking action of Mg^{2+} on channels operated by NMDA receptors (see Ch. 24), and it is interesting that local injection of NMDA-receptor agonists can initiate seizure activity. It is possible that hyperactivity of glutamate or another excitatory amino acid is responsible for the discharge of epileptic neurons, and efforts to develop glutamate antagonists as anticonvulsant drugs appear to be promising (see below). It is known that repeated seizure activity can lead to neuronal degeneration, possibly due to 'excitotoxicity' (Ch. 25). Attention is currently focused mainly on an abnormal balance of excitatory and inhibitory synaptic influences as the mechanism underlying epilepsy, though a primary defect leading to membrane instability, such as altered potassium or sodium channel function, cannot be ruled out.

Attempts to find a common neurochemical basis

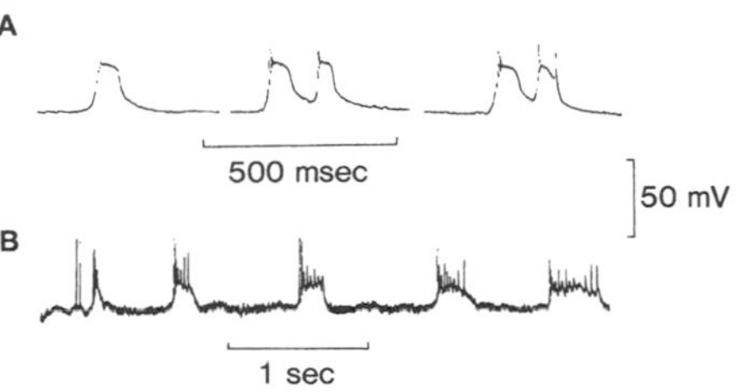

Fig. 30.2 'Paroxysmal depolarising shift' compared to experimental activation of glutamate receptors of the N-methyl D-aspartate type. A. PDS recorded with an intracellular microelectrode from cortical neurons of anaesthetised cats. Seizure activity was induced by topical application of penicillin. **B.** Intracellular recording from caudate nucleus of anaesthetised cat. The glutamate analogue, N-methyl D-aspartate was applied by ionophoresis from a nearby micropipette. Note the periodic waves of depolarisation, associated with a burst of action potentials, which closely resemble the paroxysmal depolarising shift. (From: (A) Matsumoto H, Marsan C A 1964 Exp Neurol 9: 286, (B) Herrling P L et al. 1983 J Physiol 339: 207)

for human or experimental epilepsy have been disappointing, though there are some clues. The quest has focused mainly on a possible deficit in GABA-mediated inhibitory transmission, or on an excess of excitatory amino acids (see reviews by Chapman 1988, Porter et al. 1992). The epileptic focus has been reported to contain more glutamate than normal, though the GABA content is not affected. Potassium-stimulated glutamate release from slices of cortex removed surgically from epileptic patients is increased in the epileptic focus compared with normal tissue. There are, however, no major abnormalities in the activity of enzymes involved in amino acid synthesis or degradation, or in the number of glutamate or GABA receptors, either in the brains of epileptic patients or in the various animal models of epilepsy. Direct evidence favouring an abnormality of amino acid transmission as the underlying cause of seizures is therefore limited.

Nature of epilepsy

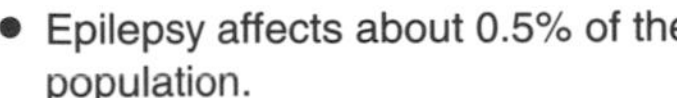
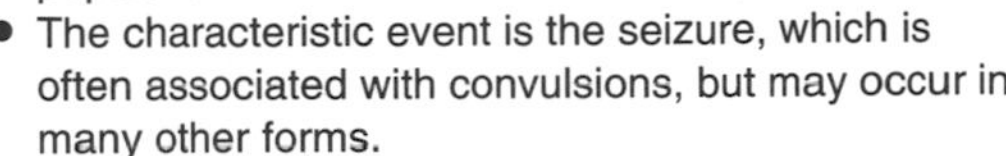

- Epilepsy affects about 0.5% of the population.
- The characteristic event is the seizure, which is often associated with convulsions, but may occur in many other forms.
- The seizure is caused by an abnormal high frequency discharge of a group of neurons, starting locally and spreading to a varying extent to affect other parts of the brain.
- Seizures may be partial or generalised depending on the location and spread of the abnormal neuronal discharge. The attack may involve mainly motor, sensory or behavioural phenomena. Unconsciousness occurs when the reticular formation is involved.
- Partial seizures are often associated with damage to the brain, whereas generalised seizures occur without obvious cause.
- Two common forms of generalised epilepsy are the tonic–clonic fit (grand mal) and the absence seizure (petit mal).
- Many animal models have been devised, including electrically and chemically induced generalised seizures, production of local chemical damage, and kindling. These provide good prediction of anticonvulsant drug effects in man.
- The neurochemical basis of the abnormal discharge is not well understood. It may be associated with enhanced excitatory amino acid transmission, impaired inhibitory transmission, or abnormal electrical properties of the affected cells. The glutamate content in areas surrounding an epileptic focus is often raised.
- Prolonged epileptic discharge (status epilepticus) can cause neuronal death (excitotoxicity).
- Current drug therapy is effective in 70–80% of patients.

MECHANISM OF ACTION OF ANTICONVULSANT DRUGS

The current anticonvulsant drugs were developed empirically, on the basis of activity in animal models, such as the electroshock seizure test, and their mechanism of action at the cellular level is not generally well understood. Two main mechanisms appear to be important, however:

- enhancement of GABA action
- inhibition of sodium channel function.

A third mechanism that may be relevant is inhibition of calcium channel function (see Macdonald & Kelly 1993).

Enhancement of GABA action

Many of the clinically effective anticonvulsants (e.g. **phenobarbitone** and **benzodiazepines**) enhance the inhibitory effect of GABA by facilitating the

GABA-mediated opening of chloride channels (see Ch. 27). A recently introduced drug, **vigabatrin** (see below), acts by inhibiting the enzyme GABA-transaminase which is responsible for inactivating GABA, thereby increasing the GABA content of the brain, and enhancing its action as an inhibitory transmitter. **Valproate** (see below) appears to act partly by this mechanism. Another recently introduced drug is **progabide**, a directly acting $GABA_A$ agonist, which has yet to be assessed clinically. **Gabapentin** (see below) was designed as an agonist at $GABA_A$ receptors, but ironically was found to be an effective antiepileptic drug in spite of having little or no effect on GABA receptors; its mechanism of action remains uncertain (see Macdonald & Kelly 1993).

Inhibition of sodium channel function

Two of the most important antiepileptic drugs, **phenytoin** and **carbamazepine**, affect membrane excitability by an action on voltage-dependent sodium channels (see Ch. 34) which carry the inward membrane current necessary for the generation of an action potential. Their blocking action shows the property of *use-dependence* (see Chs 13 and 34); in other words they block preferentially the excitation of cells that are firing repetitively, and the higher the frequency of firing, the greater the block produced. This characteristic, which is relevant to the ability of drugs to block the high frequency discharge that occurs in an epileptic fit without unduly interfering with the low frequency firing of neurons in the normal state, arises from the ability of blocking drugs to discriminate between sodium channels in their *resting*, *open* and *inactivated* states. Depolarisation of a neuron (such as occurs in the PDS described above) increases the proportion of the sodium channels in the inactivated state. Phenytoin and carbamazepine bind preferentially to channels in this state, preventing them from returning to the resting state, and thus reducing the number of functional channels available to generate action potentials. The same mechanism accounts for the actions of some antidysrhythmic drugs (see Ch. 13), and indeed, phenytoin is used for its cardiac effects as well as for its antiepileptic effect.

Other mechanisms

In many cases the mechanism of action of anticonvulsant drugs remains poorly understood (see Woodbury et al. 1982, Macdonald & McLean 1986, Macdonald & Kelly 1993 for further information). **Phenobarbitone** is a barbiturate (see Ch. 27) which has a considerably greater anticonvulsant effect in relation to its sedative action than most other barbiturates, though it is no more effective than other barbiturates in potentiating the action of GABA. Furthermore, phenobarbitone is as effective against electrically induced convulsions as it is against leptazol-induced convulsions in rats or mice, whereas benzodiazepines, which are known to work by increasing the action of GABA (see Ch. 27), are without effect on electrically induced convulsions. Phenobarbitone reduces the electrical activity of neurons within an artificially induced epileptic focus within the cortex, whereas diazepam (a benzodiazepine) does not much alter the focal activity but appears to prevent it from spreading. The action of phenobarbitone cannot therefore be due solely to its interaction with GABA, and there is good evidence that it can also act by inhibiting excitatory synaptic responses, though little is known about the mechanism.

Phenytoin has been studied in great detail, but its mechanism of action remains rather mysterious. It causes use-dependent block of sodium channels (see above), but also affects other aspects of membrane function, including inhibition of calcium entry, and post-tetanic potentiation, as well as intracellular

Mechanism of action of anticonvulsant drugs

- Current anticonvulsant drugs are thought to act by two main mechanisms:
  - —reducing electrical excitability of cell membranes, possibly through use-dependent block of sodium channels
  - —enhancing GABA-mediated synaptic inhibition. This may be achieved by an enhanced postsynaptic action of GABA, by inhibiting GABA-transaminase, or by drugs with direct GABA-agonist properties.
- Newer drugs act by other mechanisms, yet to be elucidated.
- Drugs that block excitatory amino acid receptors are effective in animal models, but not yet developed for clinical use.

The rather scant information available on the mechanism of action of anticonvulsant drugs is summarised in Table 30.1.

protein phosphorylation by calmodulin-activated kinases, which could also interfere with membrane excitability as well as synaptic mechanisms.*

Obvious targets for potential antiepileptic drugs are the receptors for excitatory amino acids (see Ch. 24), and experimental studies have shown that antagonists acting on NMDA, AMPA or metabotropic glutamate receptors all show anticonvulsant activity in various animal models (see Chapman & Meldrum 1993). Few of these drugs have yet been tested in man, and there is a risk that they will show unacceptable side effects.

ANTIEPILEPTIC DRUGS

It is estimated that antiepileptic drugs are fully effective in controlling seizures in 50–80% of patients, though unwanted effects are common (see below). There is clearly a need for more specific and effective drugs, and a number of new drugs are in development, or have been recently introduced for clinical use. The main well-established antiepileptic drugs (see Table 30.1) are **phenytoin**, **carbamazepine**, **valproate**, **ethosuximide** and **phenobarbitone**, together with various benzodiazepines, such as **diazepam**, **clonazepam** and **clobazam**. The newer drugs, whose place in therapy is still being evaluated, include **vigabatrin**, **gabapentin**, **lamotrigine** and **felbamate**.

PHENYTOIN

Phenytoin is the most important member of the hydantoin group of compounds, which are structurally related to the barbiturates. It was found to be highly effective in reducing the intensity and duration of electrically induced convulsions in mice, though ineffective against leptazol-induced convulsions. Clinically, in spite of its many side effects and unpredictable pharmacokinetic behaviour, phenytoin remains a useful antiepileptic drug, being effective against various forms of partial and generalised seizures, but not against absence seizures, which may even get worse.

Pharmacokinetic aspects

Phenytoin has certain pharmacokinetic peculiarities that need to be taken into account when it is used clinically (see Perucca & Richens 1982). It is well absorbed when given orally, and about 80–90% of the plasma content is bound to albumin. Other drugs, such as **salicylates**, **phenylbutazone** and **valproate**, inhibit this binding competitively (see Ch. 42). This increases the free phenytoin concentration, but also increases hepatic clearance of phenytoin, so may enhance or reduce the effect of the phenytoin in an unpredictable way. Phenytoin is metabolised by the hepatic mixed function oxidase system and excreted mainly as glucuronide. It causes enzyme induction, and thus increases the rate of metabolism of other drugs (e.g. oral anticoagulants). The metabolism of phenytoin itself can be either enhanced or competitively inhibited by various other drugs that share the same hepatic enzymes. **Phenobarbitone** produces both effects, and since competitive inhibition is immediate whereas induction takes time, it initially enhances and later reduces the pharmacological activity of phenytoin. **Ethanol** has a similar dual effect.

The metabolism of phenytoin shows the characteristic of *saturation* (see Ch. 4), which means that over the therapeutic plasma concentration range the rate of inactivation does not increase in proportion to the plasma concentration. The consequences of this are:

- the plasma half life (approximately 20 hours) increases as the dose is increased
- the steady-state mean plasma concentration, achieved when a patient is given a constant daily dose, varies disproportionately with the dose.

This can be a striking phenomenon. Figure 30.3 shows that in one patient increasing the dose by 50% caused the steady-state plasma concentration to increase more than fourfold.

The range of plasma concentration over which phenytoin is effective without causing excessive unwanted effects is approximately 40–100 μmol/l. The very steep relationship between dose and plasma concentration, and the many interacting factors, mean that there is considerable individual variation in the plasma concentration achieved with a given dose. A radioimmunoassay for phenytoin

*The highly complex actions of established antiepileptic drugs are apt to make discouraging reading for those engaged in trying to develop new drugs on simple rational principles. Serendipity, not science, appears to have been the path to therapeutic success.

Table 30.1 Properties of the main antiepileptic drugs

Drug	Cellular mechanisms	Effect on discharge	Main uses	Main unwanted effects	Pharmacokinetics
Phenytoin	Use-dependent block of Na^+ channels	Inhibits spread	All types **except** absence seizures	Ataxia, vertigo Gum hypertrophy Hirsutism Megaloblastic anaemia Foetal malformation Hypersensitivity reactions	Half-life approx. 24 h Saturation kinetics; therefore unpredictable plasma levels Plasma monitoring often required
Carbamazepine	Use-dependent block of Na^+ channels	Inhibits spread	All types **except** absence seizures Especially temporal lobe epilepsy (Also used in trigeminal neuralgia) Most widely used antiepileptic drug	Sedation, ataxia Blurred vision Water retention Hypersensitivity reactions Leucopenia, liver failure (rare)	Half-life 12–18 h (longer initially) Strong induction of microsomal enzymes; therefore risk of drug interactions
Valproate	Uncertain. Weak effect on GABA transaminase and on Na^+ channels	Unknown	Most types, especially absence seizures	Generally less than with other drugs Nausea Hair loss Weight gain Foetal malformations	Half-life 12–15 h
Ethosuximide*	Unknown ? Inhibition of Ca^{2+} channel function	Unknown	Absence seizures May exacerbate tonic–clonic seizures	Nausea, anorexia Mood changes Headache	Long plasma half-life (approx. 60 h)
Phenobarbitone†	Enhanced GABA action ? Inhibition of synaptic excitation	Inhibits initiation of discharge	All types **except** absence seizures	Sedation, depression	Long plasma half-life (> 60 h) Strong induction of microsomal enzymes; therefore risk of drug interactions (e.g. with phenytoin)
Benzodiazepines: e.g. **clonazepam** **clobazam** **diazepam**	Enhanced GABA action	Inhibits spread	All types Diazepam used i.v. to control *status epilepticus*	Sedation Withdrawal syndrome (see Ch. 27)	See Ch. 27
Vigabatrin	Inhibits GABA transaminase	Inhibits spread	All types Appears to be effective in patients resistant to other drugs	Sedation Behavioural and mood changes (occasionally psychosis)	Short plasma half-life, but enzyme inhibition is long-lasting

* **Trimethadione** is similar to ethosuximide in that it acts selectively against absence seizures. Its greater toxicity (especially the risk of severe hypersensitivity reactions) means that ethosuximide has largely replaced it in clinical use.

† **Primidone** is pharmacologically similar to phenobarbitone, and is converted to phenobarbitone in the body. It has no clear advantages, and is more liable to produce hypersensitivity reactions, so is now rarely used.

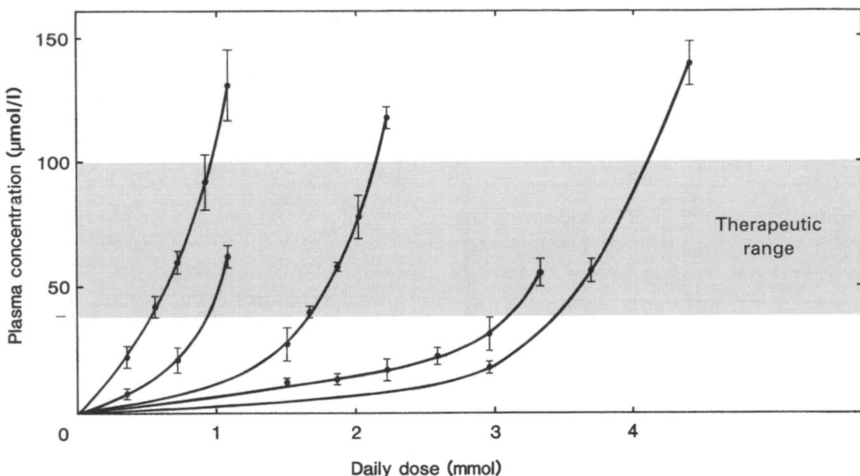

Fig. 30.3 Non-linear relationship between daily dose of phenytoin and steady-state plasma concentration in five individual human subjects. Although the therapeutic range is quite broad (40–100 µmol/l) the daily dose required varies greatly between individuals, and for any one individual the dose has to be adjusted rather precisely to keep within the acceptable plasma concentration range. (Redrawn from: Richens A, Dunlop A 1975 Lancet 2: 247)

in plasma is available, and its use has helped considerably in achieving an optimal therapeutic effect. The past tendency was to use complex multiple prescriptions in cases where a single drug failed to give adequate control. Now that phenytoin dosage can be monitored quite precisely, the use of polypharmacy in treating epilepsy is declining.

Unwanted effects

Side effects of phenytoin begin to appear at plasma concentrations exceeding 100 µmol/l and may be severe above about 150 µmol/l. The milder side effects include vertigo, ataxia, headache and nystagmus, but not sedation. At higher plasma concentrations, marked confusion with intellectual deterioration occur; these effects occur acutely and are quickly reversible. Hyperplasia of the gums, which is disfiguring rather than harmful, often develops gradually, as does hirsutism, which probably results from increased androgen secretion. Megaloblastic anaemia, associated with a disorder of folate metabolism, sometimes occurs, and can be corrected by giving folic acid (Ch. 23). Hypersensitivity reactions, mainly skin rashes, are quite common; hepatitis (which can be severe) and lymph node enlargement are less common. Phenytoin has also been implicated as a cause of the increased incidence of foetal malformations in children born to epileptic mothers, particularly the occurrence of cleft palate; this appears to be due to the formation of an epoxide metabolite (see Yerby 1988).

CARBAMAZEPINE

Carbamazepine is chemically derived from the tricyclic antidepressant drugs (see Ch. 29), and was found in a routine screening test to inhibit electrically evoked seizures in mice. Pharmacologically and clinically its actions resemble those of phenytoin (see Suria & Killam 1980), though it appears to be particularly effective in treating complex partial seizures (e.g. psychomotor epilepsy). It is also used to treat trigeminal neuralgia, an exceedingly painful condition believed to result from a paroxysmal discharge of neurons associated with the trigeminal sensory pathway, which is triggered by slight sensory stimulation. Though not obviously associated with epilepsy, this condition probably involves similar neuronal mechanisms. Carbamazepine is now one of the most widely used antiepileptic drugs; it also has a special place in the treatment of trigeminal neuralgia, and is occasionally used in treating manic-depressive illness (see Ch. 29).

Pharmacokinetic aspects

Carbamazepine is well absorbed. Its plasma half-life

is about 30 hours when it is given as a single dose, but it is a strong inducing agent, and the plasma half-life shortens to about 15 hours when it is given repeatedly.

Unwanted effects

Carbamazepine produces a variety of unwanted effects, ranging from drowsiness, dizziness and ataxia to more severe mental and motor disturbances. These effects are less with a slow-release formulation, which avoids the occurrence of a high peak plasma concentration after each dose. It can also cause water retention, and a variety of gastrointestinal and cardiovascular side effects. The incidence and severity of these effects is relatively low, however, compared with other drugs. Dangerous or fatal bone marrow depression and other severe forms of hypersensitivity reaction have occurred but are very rare.

Carbamazepine is a powerful inducer of hepatic microsomal enzymes, and thus accelerates the metabolism of many other drugs, such as phenytoin, oral contraceptives, warfarin, corticosteroids, etc. In general it is inadvisable to combine it with other antiepileptic drugs.

VALPROATE

Valproate is a simple monocarboxylic acid, chemically unrelated to any other class of anticonvulsant drug, and in 1963 it was discovered quite accidentally to have anticonvulsant properties in mice. It inhibits most kinds of experimentally induced convulsions, and is effective in many kinds of epilepsy, being particularly useful in certain types of infantile epilepsy, where its low toxicity and lack of sedative action are important.

Mechanism of action

Valproate has many effects, and probably works by several mechanisms (a familiar refrain in many areas of neuropharmacology).

Valproate causes a significant increase in the GABA content of the brain, and also decreases aspartate (see Chapman et al. 1982), but the turnover of GABA is reduced. It is a weak inhibitor of two enzyme systems that inactivate GABA, namely GABA-transaminase and succinic semialdehyde dehydrogenase, but in vitro studies suggest that these effects would be very slight at clinical dosage. Other more potent inhibitors of these enzymes (e.g. **vigabatrin**; see below) also increase GABA content and have an anticonvulsant effect in experimental animals, but the precise mode of action of valproate remains uncertain (see Chapman et al. 1982, Johnston & Slater 1982). There is some evidence that it enhances the action of GABA by a postsynaptic action, but no clear evidence that it affects inhibitory synaptic responses. It has also been shown to have direct effects on membrane excitability similar to those of phenytoin.

Valproate is well absorbed orally and excreted, mainly as the glucuronide, in the urine, the plasma half-life being about 15 hours.

Unwanted effects

Compared with most antiepileptic drugs, valproate is relatively free of unwanted effects. It causes thinning and curling of the hair in about 10% of patients. Potentially the most serious side effect is hepatotoxicity. An increase in serum glutamic oxaloacetic transaminase (SGOT), which signals liver damage of some degree, commonly occurs, but proven cases of valproate-induced hepatitis are rare. The few cases of fatal hepatitis in valproate-treated patients may well have been caused by other factors. There is also evidence of teratogenicity, with increased incidence of spina bifida.

ETHOSUXIMIDE

Ethosuximide, which belongs to the succinimide class, is yet another drug developed empirically by modifying the barbituric acid ring structure. Pharmacologically and clinically, however, it is different from the drugs so far discussed, in that it is active against leptazol-induced convulsions in animals and against absence seizures in man, with little or no effect on other types of epilepsy. **Trimethadione,** the first drug found to be effective in absence seizures, has now been supplanted by **ethosuximide**, which has fewer unwanted effects, especially sedation and hypersensitivity reactions, which were a major problem with trimethadione. Ethosuximide is used clinically for its selective effect on absence seizures, but is said to precipitate tonic–clonic seizures in susceptible patients.

The mechanism of action of ethosuximide is not understood. It is well absorbed, and metabolised and excreted much like phenobarbitone, with a plasma half-life of about 50 hours. Its main side effects are nausea and anorexia, sometimes lethargy and dizziness. Very rarely it can cause severe hypersensitivity reactions.

PHENOBARBITONE

Phenobarbitone was one of the first barbiturates to be developed and its anticonvulsant properties were recognised in 1912. In its action against experimentally induced convulsions and clinical forms of epilepsy it closely resembles phenytoin; it affects the duration and intensity of artificially induced seizures, rather than the seizure threshold, and is correspondingly (like phenytoin) ineffective in treating absence seizures. **Primidone**, now rarely used, acts by being metabolised to phenobarbitone. It often causes hypersensitivity reactions. The clinical uses of phenobarbitone are virtually the same as those of phenytoin, though phenytoin is preferred because of the absence of sedation.

Pharmacokinetic aspects

The pharmacokinetic behaviour of phenobarbitone is straightforward. It is well absorbed and about 50% of the drug in the blood is bound to plasma albumin. It is eliminated slowly from the plasma (half-life, 50–140 hours). About 25% is excreted unchanged in the urine, its lipid solubility being sufficiently low for it to be incompletely reabsorbed from the renal tubules. Since phenobarbitone is a weak acid, its ionisation and hence renal elimination are increased if the urine is made alkaline (see Ch. 4). The remaining 75% is metabolised, mainly by oxidation and conjugation, by the hepatic microsomal enzymes. Phenobarbitone is a particularly effective inducer, and by this mechanism it lowers the plasma concentration of several other drugs (e.g. steroids, oral contraceptives, warfarin, tricyclic antidepressants) to an extent that is clinically important.

Unwanted effects

The main unwanted effect of phenobarbitone is sedation, which often occurs at plasma concentrations within the therapeutic range for seizure control. This is a serious drawback, since the drug may have to be used for years on end. Some degree of tolerance to the sedative effect seems to occur, but objective tests of cognition and motor performance show impairment even after long-term treatment. Impaired school performance has been shown to result from treatment of children with phenobarbitone. Other unwanted effects that may occur with clinical dosage include megaloblastic anaemia (similar to that caused by phenytoin), mild hypersensitivity reactions and osteomalacia. Like other barbiturates (see Ch. 42) it must not be given to patients with porphyria. In overdose, phenobarbitone produces coma and respiratory and circulatory failure, as do all barbiturates.

BENZODIAZEPINES

Diazepam, given intravenously, is used to treat *status epilepticus*, a life-threatening condition in which epileptic seizures occur almost without a break. Its advantage in this situation is that it acts very rapidly compared with other antiepileptic drugs. With most benzodiazepines (see Ch. 27), the sedative effect is too pronounced for them to be used as maintenance anticonvulsant therapy. **Clonazepam**, and the related compound, **clobazam**, are claimed to be relatively selective as anticonvulsants. Sedation is the main side effect of these compounds, and an added problem may be the withdrawal syndrome, which results in an exacerbation of seizures if the drug is stopped.

NEW ANTIEPILEPTIC DRUGS

In recent years, many new agents have been proposed, the motivation being that existing antiepileptic drug therapy fails to achieve control of seizures in about 25% of cases, and is often associated with unwanted effects. Many of these drugs are currently undergoing clinical testing, but are not yet fully evaluated (reviewed by Vajda 1992, Ramsay 1993). A detailed account is given by Meldrum & Porter (1986).

Vigabatrin

Vigabatrin (see Reynolds 1990) is a γ-vinyl-substituted analogue of GABA, which was designed as an inhibitor of the GABA metabolising enzyme, GABA-transaminase. Vigabatrin is extremely specific for this enzyme, and works by forming an irreversible covalent bond. In animal studies, vigabatrin increases the GABA content of the brain, and also increases the stimulation-evoked release of GABA, implying that GABA-transaminase inhibition can increase the releasable pool of GABA and effectively enhance inhibitory transmission. In man, vigabatrin increases the content of GABA in the

The major anticonvulsant drugs

- The main drugs in current use are: phenytoin, carbamazepine, valproate and ethosuximide.
- **Phenytoin**
  - —Mode of action poorly understood, mainly by use-dependent block of sodium channels.
  - —Effective in many forms of epilepsy, but not absence seizures.
  - —Metabolism shows saturation kinetics, therefore plasma concentration can vary widely; monitoring is often needed.
  - —Drug interactions are common.
  - —Main unwanted effects are sedation, confusion, gum hyperplasia, skin rashes, anaemia, teratogenesis.
  - —Widely used in treatment of epilepsy; also used as antidysrhythmic agent.
- **Carbamazepine**
  - —Derivative of tricyclic antidepressants.
  - —Similar profile to that of phenytoin, but with fewer unwanted effects.
  - —Effective in most forms of epilepsy (except absence seizures); particularly effective in psychomotor epilepsy; also useful in trigeminal neuralgia.
  - —Strong inducing agent; therefore many drug interactions.
  - —Low incidence of unwanted effects; principally sedation, ataxia, mental disturbances, water retention.
- **Valproate**
  - —Chemically unrelated to other anticonvulsants.
  - —Mechanism of action not clear; weak inhibition of GABA-transaminase; some effect on sodium channels.
  - —Relatively few unwanted effects; baldness, teratogenicity, liver damage (rare, but serious).
- **Ethosuximide**
  - —The main drug used to treat absence seizures, may exacerbate other forms.
  - —Mechanism of action is unknown.
  - —Relatively few unwanted effects, mainly nausea and anorexia.
- Secondary drugs include:
  - —Phenobarbitone: highly sedative
  - —Various benzodiazepines (e.g. clonazepam); diazepam used in treating status epilepticus.

CSF. Its side effects, mainly sedation, dizziness and behavioural changes, are similar to those of other drugs, such as phenytoin. Evidence of neurotoxicity was found in animals, but has not been found in man, removing one of the main question marks hanging over this drug. Vigabatrin has been reported to be effective in a substantial proportion of patients resistant to the established drugs, and may represent an important therapeutic advance.

Lamotrigine

Lamotrigine (see Vajda 1992, Goa et al. 1993) resembles phenytoin in its pharmacological effects, acting on sodium channels. It appears to cause a selective inhibition of the release of excitatory amino acids, but it is not clear how this selectivity occurs. Lamotrigine has similar side effects to phenytoin (mainly sedation and skin rashes), a plasma half-life of about 24 hours, and no particular pharmacokinetic anomalies. It is effective in several kinds of epilepsy, but has not yet been fully evaluated.

Felbamate

Felbamate (see Palmer & McTavish 1993) is an analogue of an obsolete anxiolytic drug, meprobamate. It is active in many animal seizure models, but its mechanism of action at the cellular level is unknown. It does not affect sodium channels or GABA activity, and has only a very weak activity against NMDA receptors. It has side effects similar to those of phenytoin, with a tendency to cause nausea and vomiting, as well as sedation. Its plasma half-life is about 24 hours. Clinically, felbamate appears to be effective against both partial and generalised seizures; its main use currently is in the treatment of intractable seizures in children, associated with mental retardation (Lennox–Gastaut syndrome).

Gabapentin

Gabapentin (see Goa & Sorkin 1993) was designed as a simple analogue of GABA that would be sufficiently lipid-soluble to penetrate the blood–brain barrier. It turned out to be an effective anticonvulsant in several animal models, but, surprisingly, not a GABA-mimetic. It has no effect on any of the major neurotransmitter mechanisms, or on sodium channels, but binds with high affinity to a specific site in the brain, which appears to be the amino acid transporter system that occurs in many neurons and other cells. The mechanistic implications of this are unknown, and its mode of action remains an intriguing mystery. The side effects of gabapentin (mainly sedation and ataxia) appear to be less severe than with many antiepileptic drugs. The absorption of gabapentin from the intestine depends on the

New antiepileptic drugs

- **Vigabatrine**
  - —Acts by inhibiting GABA transaminase.
  - —Effective in patients unresponsive to conventional drugs.
  - —Main side effects: drowsiness, behavioural and mood changes.
- **Lamotrigine, felbamate, gabapentin**
  - —Mechanisms of action unknown. Not yet fully evaluated clinically.
  - —Lamotrigine is similar to phenytoin, but appears to have fewer side effects.
  - —Felbamate is used to treat intractable epilepsy in children; side effects similar to phenytoin.
  - —Gabapentin shows saturable absorption; relatively free of side effects.

amino acid carrier system (see Ch. 4), and shows the property of saturability, which means that increasing the dose does not proportionately increase the amount absorbed. This makes gabapentin relatively safe, and free of side effects associated with overdosing. It is also free of problems associated with drug interactions. Efficacy in patients resistant to conventional drugs has been claimed, but the clinical role of gabapentin remains to be established.

Drugs currently used to treat the major forms of epilepsy are summarised in the box below.

Uses of antiepileptic drugs

- *Tonic–clonic (grand mal) seizures:* **carbamazepine** (preferred because of low incidence of side effects), **phenytoin**, **valproate**. Use of single drug is preferred when possible, because of risk of pharmacokinetic interactions. Newer agents (not yet fully assessed) include **vigabatrin, lamotrigine, felbamate, gabapentin.**
- *Partial (focal) seizures:* **carbamazepine, valproate. Clonazepam** or **phenytoin** are alternatives.
- *Absence seizures (petit mal):* **ethosuximide** or **valproate.** Valproate is used when absence seizures coexist with tonic–clonic seizures, since most drugs used for tonic–clonic seizures may worsen absence seizures.
- *Myoclonic seizures:* **valproate** or **clonazepam**.
- *Status epilepticus:* must be treated as an emergency, with **diazepam** intravenously or (in infants with no accessible veins) rectally.

MUSCLE SPASM AND CENTRALLY ACTING MUSCLE RELAXANTS

Many diseases of the brain and spinal cord produce an increase in muscle tone which can be painful and disabling. Spasticity, resulting from birth injury or cerebral vascular disease, and the paralysis produced by spinal cord lesions are examples. Local injury or inflammation, as in arthritis, can have the same effect, and chronic back pain is also often associated with local muscle spasm.

Though skeletal muscle can be relaxed by neuromuscular-blocking drugs (Ch. 6) these are too non-selective to be useful in treating muscle spasm. Instead, certain centrally acting drugs are available which have the effect of reducing the background tone of the muscle without seriously affecting its ability to contract transiently under voluntary control. The distinction between voluntary movements and 'background tone' is not clear-cut, and the selectivity of those drugs is not complete. Postural control, for example, is usually jeopardised by centrally acting muscle relaxants. Furthermore, drugs that affect motor control generally produce rather widespread effects on the central nervous system, and drowsiness and confusion turn out to be very common side effects of these agents. The main group of drugs that have been used to control muscle tone are:

- **mephenesin** and related drugs
- **baclofen**
- **benzodiazepines** (see Ch. 27).

Mephenesin

Mephenesin is an aromatic ether, selected as the most active member of a series of such compounds. All of these drugs cause, in large doses, muscular paralysis, without loss of consciousness, by an action on the central nervous system. Mephenesin acts mainly on the spinal cord, causing a selective inhibition of polysynaptic excitation of motor neurons. Thus it strongly inhibits the flexor reflex without affecting the tendon jerk reflex, which is monosynaptic, and it abolishes decerebrate rigidity. Its mechanism of action at the cellular level is unknown. Mephenesin is little used clinically, though it is sometimes given as an intravenous injection to reduce acute muscle spasm resulting from injury.

Baclofen

Baclofen (see Ch. 23) is a chlorophenyl derivative

of GABA, originally prepared as a lipophilic GABA-like agent in order to assist penetration of the blood–brain barrier, which GABA itself does not do. Baclofen is a selective agonist at presynaptic $GABA_B$ receptors (see Bowery 1982; Ch. 24). The antispastic action of baclofen is exerted mainly on the spinal cord, where it inhibits both monosynaptic and polysynaptic activation of motor neurons (Davies 1981). It is effective when given by mouth, and is widely used in the treatment of spasticity associated with multiple sclerosis or spinal injury. However, it is ineffective in cerebral spasticity caused by birth injury.

Baclofen produces various unwanted effects, particularly drowsiness, motor incoordination and nausea, and it may also have behavioural effects. It is not useful in epilepsy.

REFERENCES AND FURTHER READING

Bowery N G 1982 The kindling model of epilepsy. Trends Pharmacol Sci 3: 400–403

Chapman A G 1988 Amino acid abnormalities in plasma, CSF and brain in epilepsy. In: Pedley T A, Meldrum B S (eds) Recent advances in epilepsy. Churchill Livingstone, Edinburgh, vol 4

Chapman A G, Keane P E, Meldrum B S, Simiand J, Vernieres J C 1982 Mechanism of action of valproate. Prog Neurobiol 19: 315–359

Chapman A G, Meldrum B S 1993 Excitatory amino acid antagonists and epilepsy. Biochem Soc Trans 21: 106–110

Davies J 1981 Selective depression of synaptic excitation in cat spinal neurones by baclofen: an ionophoretic study. Br J Pharmacol 72: 373–384

Goa K L, Sorkin E M 1993 Gabapentin: a review of its pharmacological properties and clinical potential in epilepsy. Drugs 46: 409–427

Goa K L, Ross S R, Chrisp P 1993 Lamotrigine: a review of its pharmacological properties and clinical efficacy in epilepsy. Drugs 46: 152–176

Janz D 1975 The teratogenic risk of anti-epileptic drugs. Epilepsia 16: 159–169

Johnston D, Slater G E 1982 Valproate mechanisms of action. In: Woodbury D M, Penry J K, Pippenger C E (eds) Antiepileptic drugs. Raven Press, New York, ch 50

Laidlaw J, Richens A, Oxley J 1988 Textbook of epilepsy. Churchill Livingstone, Edinburgh

Macdonald R L, Kelly K M 1993 Antiepileptic drug mechanisms of action. Epilepsia 34 (Suppl 5): S1–S8

Macdonald R L, McLean M J 1986 Anticonvulsant drugs: mechanisms of action. Adv Neurol 44: 713–736

Meldrum B S, Porter R J (eds) 1986 New anticonvulsant drugs. Current problems in epilepsy. John Libby, London, vol 4

Mosh S L, Ludvig N 1988 Kindling. In: Pedley T A, Meldrum B S (eds) Recent advances in epilepsy. Churchill Livingstone, Edinburgh, vol 4

Palmer K J, McTavish D 1993 Felbamate: a review of its pharmacodynamic and pharmacokinetic properties, and therapeutic efficacy in epilepsy. Drugs 45: 1041–1065

Perucca E, Richens A 1982 Biotransformation. In: Woodbury D M, Penry J K, Pippenger C E (eds) Antiepileptic drugs. Raven Press, New York, ch 3

Porter R J, Schmidt D, Treiman D M, Nadi N S 1992 Pharmacologic approaches to the treatment of focal seizures. Adv Neurol 57: 607–634

Ramsay R E 1993 Advances in the pharmacotherapy of epilepsy. Epilepsia 34 (Suppl 5): S9–S16

Reynolds E H 1990 Vigabatrin. Br Med J 300: 277–278

Servit Z, Musil F 1981 Prophylactic treatment of post-traumatic epilepsy: results of a long-term follow-up in Czechoslovakia. Epilepsia 22: 15–20

Suria A, Killam E K 1980 Carbemazepine. Adv Neurol 27: 563–575

Vajda F J E 1992 New anticonvulsants. Curr Opin Neurol Neurosurg 5: 519–525

Woodbury D M, Penry J K, Pippenger C E (eds) 1982 Antiepileptic drugs. Raven Press, New York

Yerby M S 1988 Teratogenicity of antiepileptic drugs. In: Pedley T A, Meldrum B S (eds) Recent advances in epilepsy. Churchill Livingstone, Edinburgh, vol 4

31
ANALGESIC DRUGS

The control of pain is one of the most important uses to which drugs are put. Analgesic drugs fall into the following main categories:

- morphine-like drugs (**opioids**)
- non-steroidal anti-inflammatory drugs (**aspirin** and related substances; see Ch. 12)
- **local anaesthetics** (see Ch. 34)
- various centrally acting non-opioid drugs, for example:
  - — Antidepressants (e.g. **amitriptyline**), which appear to have an analgesic action in patients who are not suffering from depression. This may be related to their effect of enhancing monoaminergic transmission (see Ch. 29), since inhibitory monoaminergic pathways are known to be important in modulating pain transmission (see below).
- Drugs used for specific painful conditions, for example, **carbamazepine** (used in trigeminal neuralgia; Ch. 30), **ergotamine** (used in migraine, Ch. 8).

Morphine-like drugs, as well as most of the drugs in the last group, produce analgesia by acting on the central nervous system; local anaesthetics act peripherally, while aspirin-like drugs appear to act by both central and peripheral effects. In this chapter we consider first some physiological aspects of pain perception, and then present the pharmacology of the opioid drugs in detail.

NEURAL MECHANISMS OF PAIN SENSATION

Excellent detailed accounts of the neural basis of pain can be found in Fields (1987), Besson & Chaouch (1987), and Wall & Melzack (1994).

NOCICEPTIVE AFFERENT NEURONS

Under normal conditions, pain is associated with electrical activity in small diameter primary afferent fibres of peripheral nerves. These nerves have sensory endings in peripheral tissues, and are activated by stimuli of various kinds (mechanical, thermal, chemical; see Rang et al. 1991). They are distinguished from other sorts of mechanical and thermal receptors by their higher threshold, since they are normally activated only by stimuli of noxious intensity—sufficient to cause some degree of tissue damage. Recordings of activity in single afferent fibres in human subjects have shown that stimuli sufficient to excite these small afferent fibres also evoke a painful sensation. Many of these fibres are non-myelinated C-fibres with low conduction velocities (< 1 m/s); this group is known as *C-polymodal*

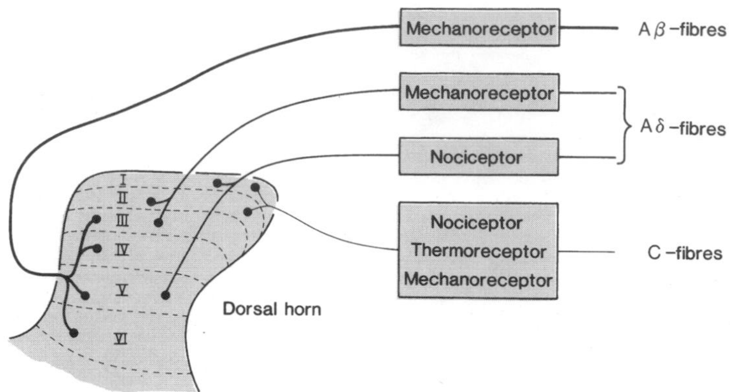

Fig. 31.1 The termination of afferent fibres in the six laminae of the dorsal horn of the spinal cord.

nociceptors (PMN). Others are fine myelinated (Aδ) fibres, which conduct more rapidly but respond to similar peripheral stimuli. Though there are some species differences, the majority of the C-fibres are associated with polymodal nociceptive endings. Afferents from muscle and viscera also convey nociceptive information. In the nerves from these tissues, the small myelinated fibres are connected to high threshold mechanoreceptors, while the unmyelinated fibres are connected to polymodal nociceptors as in the skin.

Experiments on human subjects, in which recording or stimulating electrodes are applied to cutaneous sensory nerves, have shown that activity in the Aδ-fibres causes a sensation of sharp, well-localised pain, whereas C-fibre activity causes a dull burning pain.

The mechanism by which a variety of different stimuli can evoke activity in nociceptive nerve terminals is only dimly understood. With many pathological conditions, tissue injury is the immediate cause of the pain, and this results in the local release of a variety of chemical agents which are assumed to act on the nerve terminals, either activating them directly or enhancing their sensitivity to other forms of stimulation. The pharmacological properties of nociceptive nerve terminals are discussed in more detail below.

The cell bodies of spinal nociceptive afferent fibres lie in dorsal root ganglia; fibres enter the spinal cord via the dorsal roots, ending in the grey matter of the dorsal horn (Fig. 31.1). Most of the nociceptive afferents terminate in the superficial region of the dorsal horn, the C-fibres and some Aδ-fibres innervating cell bodies in laminae I and II, while other A-fibres penetrate deeper into the dorsal horn (lamina V). Cells in laminae I and V give rise to the main projection pathways from the dorsal horn to the thalamus.

The non-myelinated afferent neurons contain several neuropeptides (see Ch. 9), particularly substance P and calcitonin gene-related peptide (CGRP). These are released as mediators at both the central and peripheral terminals, and play an important role in the pathology of pain.

MODULATION IN THE NOCICEPTIVE PATHWAY

Acute pain is generally well accounted for in terms of *nociception*—an excessive noxious stimulus giving rise to an intense and unpleasant sensation. In contrast, most chronic pain states* are associated with aberrations of the normal physiological pathway, giving rise to *hyperalgesia* (an increased amount

*Defined as pain which outlasts the precipitating tissue injury. Many clinical pain states fall into this category. The dissociation of pain from noxious input is most evident in 'phantom limb' pain which occurs after amputations and may be very severe. The pain is usually not relieved by local anaesthetic injections, implying that electrical activity in afferent fibres is not an essential component. At the other extreme, noxious input with no pain, there are many well-documented reports of mystics and showmen who subject themselves to horrifying ordeals with knives, burning embers, nails and hooks (undoubtedly causing massive afferent input) without apparently suffering pain.

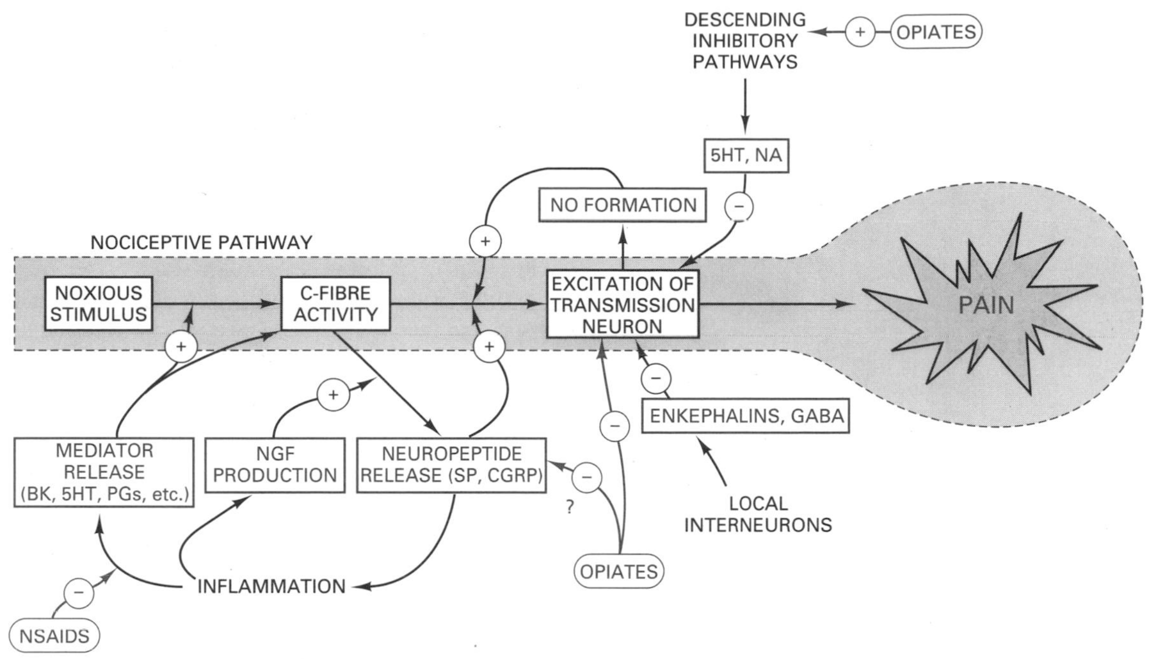

Fig. 31.2 Summary of modulatory mechanisms in the nociceptive pathway.

of pain associated with a mild noxious stimulus), *allodynia* (pain evoked by a non-noxious stimulus), or spontaneous spasms of pain with no precipitating stimulus. An analogy is with an old radio set that plays uncontrollably loudly (hyperalgesia), receives two stations at once (allodynia), or produces random shrieks and whistles (spontaneous pain spasms). These distortions in the transmission line are beginning to be understood in terms of various types of positive and negative modulation in the nociceptive pathway, discussed in more detail below. Some of the main mechanisms are summarised in Figure 31.2.

HYPERALGESIA AND ALLODYNIA

Anyone who has burned himself or sprained an ankle has experienced hyperalgesia and allodynia. Hyperalgesia involves both sensitisation of peripheral nociceptive nerve terminals and central facilitation of transmission at the level of the dorsal horn and thalamus—changes defined by the 90s buzz-word *neuroplasticity*. The peripheral component is due to the action of mediators such as bradykinin, prostaglandins, etc. acting on the nerve terminals (see below). The central component reflects facilitation of synaptic transmission. This has been well studied in the dorsal horn (see McMahon et al. 1993). The synaptic responses of dorsal horn neurons to nociceptive inputs display the phenomenon of 'wind-up'—i.e. the synaptic potentials steadily increase in amplitude with each stimulus—when repeated stimuli are delivered at physiological frequencies (see Fig. 31.6). This activity-dependent facilitation of transmission has many features in common with the phenomenon of long-term potentiation (LTP) in the hippocampus, described in Chapter 24, and the chemical mechanisms underlying it also appear to be similar (see McMahon et al. 1993; Fig. 24.13). In the dorsal horn, the facilitation is blocked by NMDA-receptor antagonists, also by antagonists of substance P, a slow excitatory transmitter released by nociceptive afferent neurons (see above), and by inhibitors of NO synthesis. Substance P produces a slow depolarising response in the postsynaptic cell, which builds up during repetitive stimulation, and (as with LTP; see Fig. 24.13) is believed to enhance NMDA-receptor-mediated transmission (see Ch. 24). This results in calcium influx and activation of NO synthase (see Ch. 10), the released NO acting to facilitate transmission by mechanisms that have yet to be elucidated. Substance P and CGRP released from primary afferent neurons also act in the periphery, promoting inflammation by their effects on blood vessels and cells

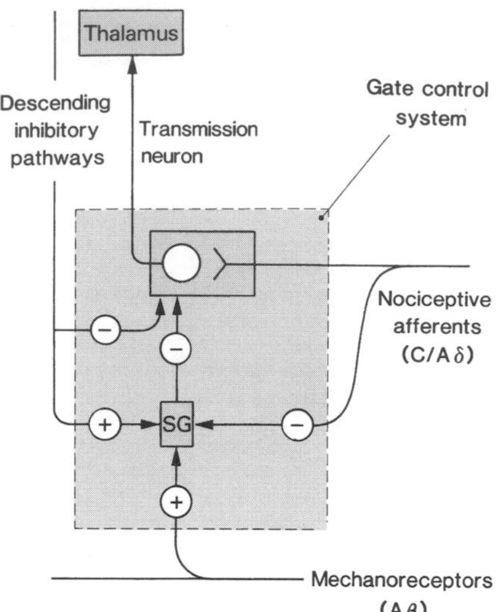

Fig. 31.3 Schematic diagram of the gate control system. This system regulates the passage of impulses from the peripheral afferent fibres to the thalamus via transmission neurons originating in the dorsal horn. Neurons in the *substantia gelatinosa* (SG) of the dorsal horn act to inhibit the transmission pathway. Inhibitory interneurons are activated by descending inhibitory neurons or by non-nociceptive afferent input. They are inhibited by nociceptive C-fibre input, so that persistent C-fibre activity facilitates excitation of the transmission cells by either nociceptive or non-nociceptive inputs. This autofacilitation causes successive bursts of activity in the nociceptive afferents to become increasingly effective in activating transmission neurons. Details of the interneuronal pathways are not shown. (From: Melzack R, Wall P D 1982 The challenge of pain. Penguin, Harmondsworth)

of the immune system (Ch. 11). This mechanism, known as *neurogenic inflammation*, acts to amplify and sustain the inflammatory reaction, and the accompanying activation of nociceptive afferent fibres. There is evidence that these processes (summarised in Fig. 31.2) are also involved in pathological hyperalgesia (e.g. that associated with inflammatory processes), in which central facilitation is known to occur (see Coderre et al. 1993). The importance of repetitive C-fibre activity in setting up a long-lasting state of hyperexcitability in the spinal cord has led to the concept of *pre-emptive analgesia*, whereby, in the anaesthetised patient, the field of a surgical operation is treated with local anaesthetic in order to block the intense C-fibre discharge associated with the incision and operation, thus preventing, it is argued, the spinal cord hyperexcitability from being established, and thereby reducing postoperative pain. Clinical reports on the efficacy of this procedure give conflicting views (see Dahl & Kehlet 1993). Other mechanisms can also contribute to central facilitation. Nerve growth factor (NGF), a cytokine-like mediator produced by peripheral tissues, particularly in inflammation, acts specifically on nociceptive afferent neurons, increasing their electrical excitability, chemosensitivity and peptide content, and also promoting the formation of synaptic contacts. Increased NGF production may be an important mechanism by which nociceptive transmission becomes facilitated by tissue damage, leading to hyperalgesia (see Lewin & Mendell 1993). Increased gene expression in dorsal horn neurons (particularly of the opioid peptide dynorphin) accompanies peripheral inflammation and activity in the nociceptive pathway; this peptide, which has both excitatory and inhibitory effects in the spinal cord, also plays a part in long-term modulation, though its exact role is unclear (see Dubner & Ruda 1992).

THE SUBSTANTIA GELATINOSA AND THE GATE CONTROL THEORY

Cells of lamina II of the dorsal horn (the substantia gelatinosa, SG) are mainly short inhibitory interneurons projecting to lamina I and lamina V, and they regulate transmission at the first synapse of the nociceptive pathway, between the primary afferent fibres and the spinothalamic tract transmission neurons. This gatekeeper function gave rise to the term 'gate control theory', proposed by Wall & Melzack in 1965. According to this view (summarised in Fig. 31.3) the SG cells respond both to the activity of afferent fibres entering the cord (thus allowing the arrival of impulses via one group of afferent fibres to regulate the transmission of impulses via another pathway) and to the activity of descending pathways (see below). The SG is rich in both opioid peptides and opioid receptors and may be an important site of action for morphine-like drugs (see later section). Further studies have added extra detail to the dorsal horn circuitry shown schematically in Figure 31.3 (see Fields & Basbaum 1989), and it is evident that similar 'gate' mechanisms also operate in the thalamus.

From the spinothalamic tracts, the projection fibres form synapses mainly in the ventral and medial parts of the thalamus with cells whose axons

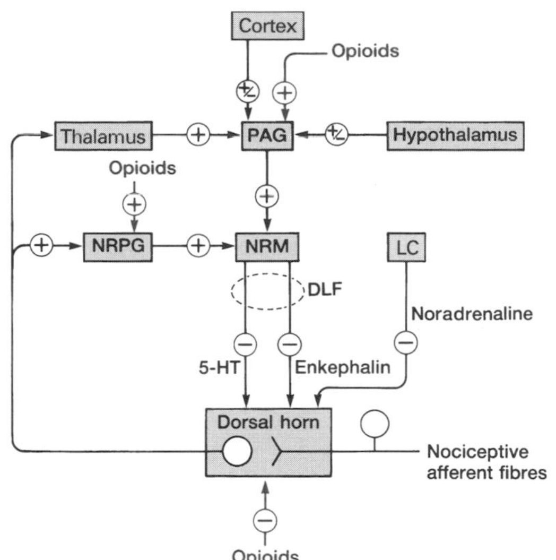

Fig. 31.4 The descending control system, showing postulated sites of action of opioids on pain transmission. Opioids excite neurons in the *periaqueductal grey matter* (PAG) and in the *nucleus reticularis paragigantocellularis* (NRPG), which in turn project to the rostroventral medulla, which includes the *nucleus raphe magnus* (NRM). From the NRM, 5-HT- and enkephalin-containing neurons run to the *substantia gelatinosa* of the dorsal horn, and exert an inhibitory influence on transmission. Opioids also act directly on the dorsal horn. The *locus ceruleus* (LC) sends noradrenergic neurons to the dorsal horn, which also inhibit transmission. The pathways shown in this diagram represent a considerable over-simplification, but depict the general organisation of the supraspinal control mechanisms. Light pink boxes represent areas rich in opioid peptides. (DLF = dorsolateral funiculus) (For more detailed information, see Fields & Basbaum 1989)

run to the somatosensory cortex. In the medial thalamus in particular, many cells respond specifically to noxious stimuli in the periphery and lesions in this area cause analgesia. Pain sensation does not require that impulses should reach the somatosensory cortex via the thalamic relay. There is no clear evidence of specifically nociceptive cells in the cortex, and lesions of the somatosensory areas do not prevent the sensation of pain, though they can alter its quality. It appears to be the affective, discriminatory and motivational aspects of pain, rather than the sensation itself, that depend on the cerebral cortex.

DESCENDING INHIBITORY CONTROLS

As mentioned above, descending pathways constitute one of the gating mechanisms that control impulse transmission in the dorsal horn (see Lewis & Liebeskind 1983, Fields & Basbaum 1989). A key part of this descending system is the *periaqueductal grey* (PAG) area of the midbrain, a small area of grey matter surrounding the central canal. In 1969, Reynolds found that electrical stimulation of this brain area in the rat caused analgesia sufficiently intense that abdominal surgery could be performed without anaesthesia and without eliciting any marked response. Non-painful sensations are unaffected. The PAG receives inputs from many other brain regions, including the hypothalamus, cortex and thalamus, and is thought to represent the mechanism whereby cortical and other inputs act to control the nociceptive 'gate' in the dorsal horn.

The main neuronal pathway activated by PAG stimulation runs first to an area of the medulla close to the midline, known as the *nucleus raphe magnus* (NRM), and thence via fibres running in the dorsolateral funiculus of the spinal cord, which form synaptic connections on dorsal horn interneurons. The major transmitter at these synapses is 5-HT, and the interneurons in turn act to inhibit the discharge of spinothalamic neurons (Fig. 31.4). The NRM itself receives an input from spinothalamic neurons, via the adjacent *nucleus reticularis paragigantocellularis* (NRPG), so this descending inhibitory system may form part of a regulatory feedback loop whereby transmission through the dorsal horn is controlled according to the amount of activity reaching the thalamus.

The descending inhibitory pathway is probably an important site of action for opioid analgesics (see below). Both PAG and SG are particularly rich in enkephalin-containing neurons, and opioid antagonists, such as naloxone (see p. 630), can prevent electrically induced analgesia, which would suggest that opioid peptides may function as transmitters in this system. The physiological role of opioid peptides in regulating pain transmission has been controversial, mainly because under normal conditions naloxone has relatively little effect on pain threshold. Under pathological conditions, however, when stress is present, naloxone causes hyperalgesia, implying that the opioid system is active.

There is also a noradrenergic pathway from the *locus ceruleus* (see Ch. 24), which has a similar inhibitory effect on transmission in the dorsal horn (Fig. 31.4).

NEUROPATHIC PAIN

Neurological disease affecting the sensory pathway can produce severe chronic pain—termed *neuropathic pain*—unrelated to any peripheral tissue injury. This occurs with CNS disorders, such as stroke and multiple sclerosis, or with conditions associated with peripheral nerve damage, such as diabetic neuropathy or herpes zoster infection (shingles). Chronic neuropathic pain is often a sequel of injury. The pathophysiological mechanisms underlying this kind of pain are poorly understood, though spontaneous activity in damaged sensory neurons is thought to be a factor. The sympathetic nervous system also plays a part, since damaged sensory neurons can apparently express α-adrenoceptors, and develop a sensitivity to noradrenaline that they do not possess under normal conditions. Thus physiological stimuli that evoke sympathetic responses can produce severe pain, a phenomenon described clinically as *sympathetically mediated pain*. Neuropathic pain, which appears to be a component of many types of clinical pain (including common conditions such as back pain, cancer pain, as well as amputation pain) is generally difficult to control with conventional analgesic drugs. A better understanding of its mechanism should provide more rational therapeutic approaches.

CHEMICAL MEDIATORS AND THE NOCICEPTIVE PATHWAY

CHEMOSENSITIVITY OF NOCICEPTIVE NERVE ENDINGS

In most cases, stimulation of nociceptive endings in the periphery is chemical in origin. Excessive mechanical or thermal stimuli can obviously cause acute pain, but the persistence of such pain after the stimulus has been removed, or the pain resulting from inflammatory or ischaemic changes in tissues, generally reflects a chemical stimulation of the pain afferents. Much of our current knowledge comes from the work of Keele & Armstrong (1964), who developed a simple method for measuring the pain-producing effect of various substances that act on cutaneous nerve endings. By applying cantharidin to the skin of the forearm of human subjects a small blister is produced, the base of which may be bathed in drug solutions which gain access to the nerve terminals in the dermis. Pain is recorded subjectively, and with practice the subjects are able to achieve quite reproducible responses.

The main groups of substances that stimulate pain endings in the skin (see Rang et al. 1991) are discussed below.

Various neurotransmitters including 5-HT, histamine and acetylcholine

5-HT is the most active; histamine is much less active and tends to cause itching rather than actual pain. Both of these substances are known to be released locally in inflammation (see Ch. 11).

Kinins

The most active substances are *bradykinin* and *kallidin* (see Ch. 11), two closely related peptides produced under conditions of tissue injury by the proteolytic cleavage of the active kinins from a precursor protein contained in the plasma (reviewed by Dray & Perkins 1993). Bradykinin is a potent pain-producing substance, acting partly by release of prostaglandins, which strongly enhance the direct action of bradykinin on the nerve terminals (Fig. 31.5). Bradykinin acts by combining with specific receptors of the G-protein-coupled type (Ch. 2), and produces its cellular effects through production of various intracellular messengers. Specific competitive antagonists, based on the peptide structure of bradykinin, such as **icatibant** (Ch. 11) have recently been developed, and these show analgesic and anti-inflammatory properties. Such peptides are not suitable for clinical use as analgesics, but may provide a new principle on which to base future analgesic drugs.

Various metabolites and substances released from active cells, such as lactic acid, ATP and ADP, K^+

Low pH excites nociceptive afferent neurons specifically by opening proton-activated cation channels similar or identical to those activated by capsaicin (see below). ATP acts similarly. These agents are mainly of interest as potential mediators of ischaemic pain.

Prostaglandins

Prostaglandins do not themselves cause pain, but they strongly enhance the pain-producing effect of other agents such as 5-HT or bradykinin (Fig. 31.5). Prostaglandins of the E and F series are known to be released in inflammation (Ch. 11) and also during

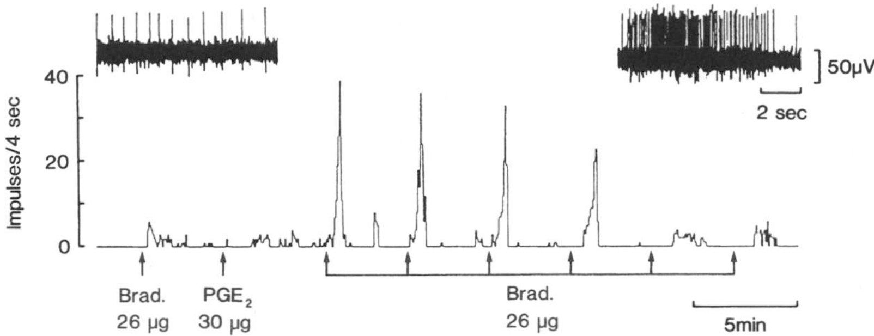

Fig. 31.5 Response of a nociceptive afferent neuron to bradykinin and prostaglandin. Recordings were made from a nociceptive afferent fibre supplying a muscle, and drugs were injected into the arterial supply. *Upper records:* single fibre recordings showing discharge caused by bradykinin alone (left), and by bradykinin following injection of prostaglandin (right). *Lower trace:* ratemeter recording of single fibre discharge showing long-lasting enhancement of response to bradykinin after an injection of prostaglandin E_2. Prostaglandin itself did not evoke a discharge. (From: Mense S 1981 Brain Res 225: 95)

tissue ischaemia. How they act to sensitise the nerve terminals to other agents is not known at present. It is of interest that bradykinin itself causes prostaglandin release, and thus has a powerful 'self-sensitising' effect on nociceptive afferents. Other eicosanoids, including prostacyclins, leukotrienes and the unstable HETE derivatives (Ch. 11), may also be important, but information is sparse.

Capsaicin and related irritant substances

Capsaicin is the active substance in chili peppers and is responsible for their burning taste. Other spicy plants (ginger, black pepper, etc.) also contain similar agents, but capsaicin is the most potent and most thoroughly studied. It is a highly potent pain-producing substance, which selectively stimulates nociceptive and temperature-sensitive nerve endings in tissues, apparently by acting on a specific membrane receptor (see James et al. 1993).

There are several very interesting features of the action of capsaicin (for reviews, see Wood 1993).

- Capsaicin acts on membrane receptors that are specifically expressed by nociceptive sensory neurons, and are directly coupled to cation channels (see Ch. 2), which have a high permeability to calcium. Calcium entry may account for many of the cellular effects produced.
- After a few applications the pain-producing effect disappears and nociceptive responses to other stimuli disappear as well; capsaicin applied topically to the skin is sometimes used to treat certain kinds of neuropathic pain.
- It causes release of substance P from afferent neurons (see above), both peripherally and within the spinal cord. In adult animals the afferent neurons are depleted of substance P and take days or weeks to recover.
- In newborn animals, capsaicin selectively destroys C-fibre neurons in the periphery, and the animals grow up with a greatly reduced response to painful and thermal stimuli. It has therefore been widely used as an experimental tool for investigating the function of C-fibre afferents.

TRANSMITTERS IN THE NOCICEPTIVE PATHWAY

Glutamate, released from primary afferent neurons and acting on AMPA receptors (see Ch. 24), is responsible for fast synaptic transmission at the first synapse in the dorsal horn. There is also a slower NMDA-receptor-mediated response, which is important in relation to the wind-up phenomenon (see Fig. 31.6). Substance P, acting on NK_1 receptors, and a related tachykinin, neurokinin A, acting on NK_2 receptors (see Ch. 9), elicit very slow excitatory synaptic potentials, which are insufficient on their own to excite the postsynaptic neuron, but may build up during repetitive activity to produce a burst of action potentials lasting for a few seconds in response to each stimulus. Inflammation appears to

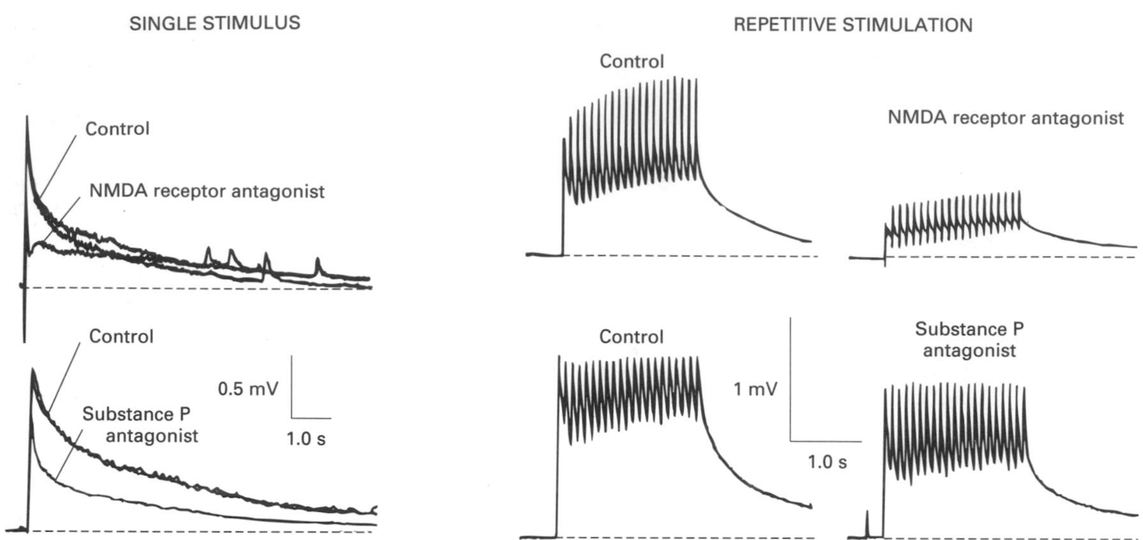

Fig. 31.6 Effect of antagonists of glutamate and substance P on nociceptive transmission in the rat spinal cord. The rat paw was inflamed by ultraviolet irradiation 2 days before the experiment, a procedure which induces hyperalgesia and spinal cord facilitation. The synaptic response was recorded from the ventral root, in response to stimulation of C-fibres in the dorsal root with single stimuli (left) or repetitive stimuli (right). The effect of the NMDA-receptor antagonist D-AP5 (see Ch. 24) and the substance P antagonist RP 67580 (NK_2-receptor selective; see Ch. 9) are shown. The slow component of the synaptic response is reduced by both antagonists (left-hand traces), as is the 'wind-up' in response to repetitive stimulation (right-hand traces). These effects are much less pronounced in the normal animal. Thus both glutamate, acting on NMDA receptors, and substance P, acting on NK_2 receptors, are involved in nociceptive transmission, and their contribution increases as a result of inflammatory hyperalgesia. (Records kindly provided by L Urban and S W Thompson)

enhance the contribution of substance P to synaptic responses in the spinal cord, an adaptive change which may be an important factor in hyperalgesia.

Transmitters that are known to play a part in the modulation of transmission in the nociceptive pathway (see Fig. 31.2) include the following:

- Opioid peptides (see Ch. 9), mainly met-enkephalin and β-endorphin. Both peptides are found in the periaqueductal grey matter, and met-enkephalin is also found in the *nucleus raphe magnus* (NRM) and in superficial layers of the dorsal horn.
- 5-HT, the transmitter of inhibitory neurons running from NRM to the dorsal horn.
- Noradrenaline, the transmitter of the inhibitory pathway from the locus ceruleus to the dorsal horn, and possibly also in other antinociceptive pathways.

Several species differences exist among these systems, so studies of analgesic action in animals may not relate directly to man.

PAIN AND NOCICEPTION

As emphasised above, the perception of noxious stimuli (termed 'nociception' by Sherrington) is not the same thing as pain, which is a subjective experience and includes a strong affective component. The amount of pain that a particular stimulus produces depends on many factors other than the stimulus itself. A stabbing sensation in the chest will cause much more pain if it occurs spontaneously in a middle-aged man than a similar sensation produced by a 2-year-old poking him with a sharp stick. The nociceptive component may be much the same, but the affective component is quite different. Animal tests of analgesic drugs commonly measure nociception, and involve testing the reaction of an animal to a mildly painful stimulus, often mechanical or thermal. Such measures include the tail-flick test (measuring the time taken for a rat to withdraw its tail when a standard radiant heat stimulus is applied) or the paw pressure test (mea-

> **Mechanisms of pain and nociception**
>
> - Nociception is the mechanism whereby noxious peripheral stimuli are transmitted to the central nervous system. Pain is a subjective experience, not always associated with nociception.
> - Polymodal nociceptors (PMN) are the main peripheral sense organs that respond to noxious stimuli. The majority are non-myelinated C-fibres whose endings respond to thermal, mechanical and chemical stimuli.
> - Chemical stimuli acting on PMN to cause pain include bradykinin, 5-HT, and capsaicin. PMN are sensitised by prostaglandins, which explains the analgesic effect of aspirin-like drugs, particularly in the presence of inflammation.
> - Nociceptive fibres terminate in the superficial layers of the dorsal horn, forming synaptic connections with transmission neurons running to the thalamus.
> - PMN neurons release glutamate (fast transmitter) and various peptides (especially substance P) which act as slow transmitters. Peptides are also released peripherally and contribute to neurogenic inflammation.
> - Neuropathic pain, associated with damage to neurons of the nociceptive pathway rather than an excessive peripheral stimulus, is frequently a component of chronic pain states, and may respond poorly to opioid analgesics.

> **Modulation of pain transmission**
>
> - Transmission in the dorsal horn is subject to various modulatory influences, constituting the 'gate control' mechanism.
> - Descending pathways from the midbrain and brainstem exert a strong inhibitory effect on dorsal horn transmission. Electrical stimulation of the midbrain PAG causes analgesia through this mechanism.
> - The descending inhibition is mediated by enkephalins, 5-HT and noradrenaline. Opioids cause analgesia partly by activating these descending pathways, and partly by inhibiting transmission in the dorsal horn.
> - Repetitive C-fibre activity facilitates transmission through the dorsal horn ('wind-up') by mechanisms involving activation of NMDA and substance P receptors.

suring the withdrawal threshold when the paw is pinched with increasing force). Similar tests can be used on human subjects, who simply indicate when a stimulus begins to feel painful, but the pain in these circumstances lacks the affective component. Clinically, spontaneous pain of neuropathic origin is coming to be recognised as particularly important, but this is difficult to model in animal studies for both technical and ethical reasons.

It is recognised clinically that many analgesics, particularly those of the morphine-type, can greatly reduce the distress associated with pain even though the patient reports no great change in the intensity of the actual sensation. It is much more difficult to devise tests that measure this affective component, and important to realise that this may be at least as significant as the antinociceptive component in the action of these drugs. There is often a poor correlation between the activity of analgesic drugs in animal tests (which mainly assess antinociceptive activity) and their clinical effectiveness.

ANALGESIC DRUGS

MORPHINE-LIKE DRUGS

The term **opioid** applies to any substance that produces morphine-like effects that are blocked by antagonists such as naloxone; it includes various neuropeptides and synthetic analogues, the structure of which may be quite different from morphine. The older term, **opiate**, is more restrictive, meaning morphine-like drugs with a close structural similarity to morphine, thus excluding peptides and many synthetic analogues. The field is reviewed exhaustively by Herz (1993).

Opium is an extract of the juice of the poppy *Papaver somniferum*, which has been used for social and medicinal purposes for thousands of years, as an agent to produce euphoria, analgesia and sleep, and to prevent diarrhoea. It was introduced in Britain at the end of the seventeenth century, usually taken orally as 'tincture of laudanum', addiction to which acquired a certain social cachet during the next 200 years. The situation changed when the hypodermic syringe and needle was invented in the mid-nineteenth century and opiate dependence began to take on a more sinister significance.

CHEMICAL ASPECTS

Opium contains many alkaloids related to morphine. The structure of morphine (Fig. 31.7) was determined in 1902 and since then many semisynthetic compounds (produced by chemical modification of morphine) and fully synthetic analgesics have been studied. In addition to morphine-like compounds, opium also contains **papaverine**, a smooth muscle relaxant (see Ch. 14).

The main groups of drugs that are discussed in this section are:

- *Morphine analogues.* These are compounds closely related in structure to morphine, and often synthesised from it. They may be agonists (e.g. **morphine, heroin** and **codeine**), partial agonists (e.g. **nalorphine** and **levallorphan**), or antagonists (e.g. **naloxone**).
- *Synthetic derivatives with structures unrelated to morphine.*
  - — phenylpiperidine series (e.g. **pethidine** and **fentanyl**)
  - — methadone series (e.g. **methadone** and **dextropropoxyphene**)
  - — benzomorphan series (e.g. **pentazocine** and **cyclazocine**)
  - — semisynthetic thebaine derivatives (e.g. **etorphine** and **buprenorphine**).

Morphine analogues

Morphine is a **phenanthrene** derivative, with two planar rings (A and B) and two aliphatic ring structures (C and D), which occupy a plane roughly at right angles to A and B. Variants of the morphine molecule have been produced by substitution at one or both of the hydroxyl groups (the phenolic OH at position 3 and the alcoholic OH at position 6), and by substitution at the nitrogen atom at position 17. Some of the most important analogues are shown in Table 31.1.

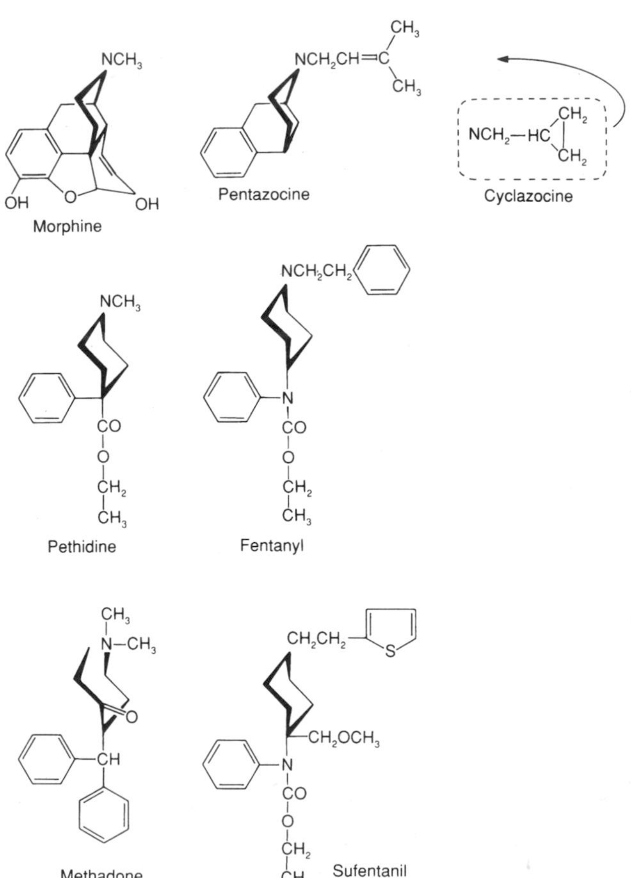

Fig. 31.7 Structures of some opiate analgesics.

Table 31.1 Morphine analogues

Morphine

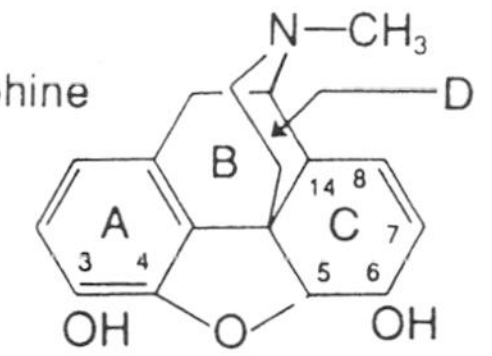

Drug	Substituents 3	6	N	14
Morphine	—OH	—OH	$—CH_3$	—H
Heroin	—OCO · CH_3	—OCO · CH_3	$—CH_3$	—H
Codeine	$—OCH_3$	—OH	$—CH_3$	—H
Levorphanol	—OH	—H	$—CH_3$	—H (lacks —O— at C_4–C_5)
Dihydrocodeine	$—OCH_3$	—OH	$—CH_3$	—H (lacks double bond C_7–C_8)
Nalorphine	—OH	—OH	$—CH_2CH{=}CH_2$	—H
Nalbuphine	—OH	—OH	$—CH_2$—cyclobutyl	—OH (lacks double bond C_7–C_8)
Butorphanol	—OH	—H	$—CH_2$—cyclobutyl	—H (lacks —O— at C_4–C_5 & double bond C_7–C_8)
Naloxone	—OH	=O	$—CH_2CH{=}CH_2$	—HO (lacks double bond C_7–C_8)

Buprenorphine

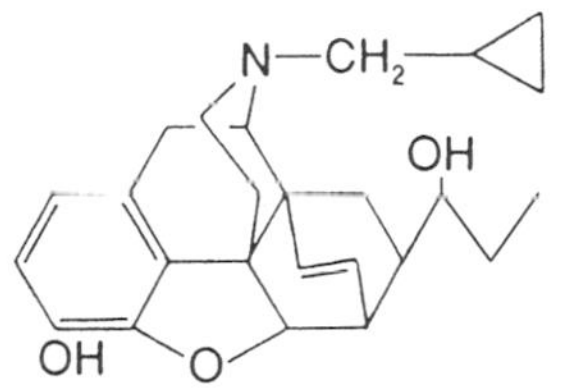

Synthetic derivatives

Phenylpiperidine series

Pethidine (known as meperidine in USA), the first fully synthetic morphine-like drug, was discovered accidentally when new atropine-like drugs were being sought. It is chemically simpler than morphine, though its pharmacological actions are very similar.

Fentanyl and **sufentanil** are more potent and shorter-acting derivatives which are used intravenously to treat severe pain or as an adjunct to anaesthesia.

Methadone series

Methadone, though its structural formula bears no obvious chemical relationship to that of morphine, assumes a similar configuration in solution, and was designed by reference to the common three-dimensional structural features of morphine and pethidine (Fig. 31.7). It is longer-acting than morphine, but otherwise very similar to it. **Dextropropoxyphene** is very similar and used clinically for treating mild or moderate pain.

Benzomorphan series

The most important members of this class are **pentazocine** and **cyclazocine** (Fig. 31.7). These drugs differ from morphine in the way in which they interact with their receptors (see below), and so have somewhat different actions and side effects.

Thebaine derivatives

Etorphine is a highly potent morphine-like drug, used mainly in veterinary practice. **Buprenorphine** resembles morphine, but appears to act as a partial agonist (see below); thus, although very potent, its maximal effect is less than that of morphine, and it can act as an antagonist of other opioids.

Opioid analgesics

- There are three main families of endogenous opioid peptides; these have analgesic activity and have many physiological functions, but they are not used as drugs.
- Opioid drugs include:
  - —phenanthrene derivatives, structurally related to morphine
  - —synthetic compounds with dissimilar structures but similar pharmacological effects.
- Important morphine-like agonists include heroin, codeine; other structurally related compounds are partial agonists (e.g. nalorphine and levallorphan) or antagonists (e.g. naloxone).
- The main groups of synthetic analogues are the piperidines (e.g. pethidine and fentanyl), the methadone-like drugs, the benzomorphans (e.g. pentazocine) and the thebaine derivatives (e.g. buprenorphine).
- Many opiate analgesics may be given intrathecally to produce analgesia with limited side effects.

OPIOID RECEPTORS

Direct evidence that opioids are recognised by specific receptors came from binding studies (see Snyder et al. 1973, Brownstein 1993), though the existence of specific antagonists had earlier suggested that such receptors must exist. Various pharmacological observations implied that more than one type of receptor was involved, the original suggestion of multiple receptor types arising from in vivo studies of the spectrum of actions (analgesia, sedation, pupillary constriction, bradycardia, etc.) produced by different drugs. It was also found that some opioids, but not all, were able to relieve withdrawal symptoms in morphine-dependent animals, and this was interpreted in terms of distinct receptor subtypes. The conclusion from these and many subsequent pharmacological studies (see Wood & Iyengar 1988) is that three receptors, termed μ, δ and κ, mediate the main pharmacological effects of opiates, as shown in Table 31.2. A fourth subtype, σ, was also postulated in order to account for the 'dysphoric' effects (anxiety, hallucinations, bad dreams, etc.) produced by some opiates. These are now considered not to be true opioid receptors, since many other types of psychotropic drug also interact with them, and their biological role remains unclear (see Walker et al. 1990). Of the opioid drugs, only benzomorphans, such as **pentazocine** and **cyclazocine**, bind appreciably to σ-receptors, which is consistent with their known psychotomimetic properties. The three main subtypes have been shown by receptor cloning to belong to the G-protein-coupled family of receptors (see Ch. 2). There is evidence for further subdivisions of each of these subtypes, but the pharmacological significance of this is uncertain.

The interaction of various opioid drugs and peptides (see Ch. 9) with the various receptor types is summarised in Table 31.3.

AGONISTS AND ANTAGONISTS

Opioids vary not only in their receptor specificity, but also in their efficacy at the different types of receptor. Thus some agents act as agonists on one type of receptor and antagonists or partial agonists at another, producing a very complicated pharmacological picture.

Table 31.2 Pharmacological effects associated with opioid receptor subtypes

Receptor type	μ/δ	κ	σ
Analgesia	Supraspinal/ spinal	Spinal	–
Respiratory depression	++	+	–
Pupil	Constriction	–	Dilatation
GI motility	Reduced	–	–
Smooth muscle spasm	++	–	–
Behaviour/affect	Euphoria ++ Sedation ++	Dysphoria + Sedation +	Dysphoria ++ Psychotomimetic
Physical dependence	++	+	–

Note that μ- and δ-receptors are known to be distinct molecular entities, though they appear to be functionally very similar. Selective agonists and antagonists have only recently been developed.

Table 31.3 Selectivity of opioid drugs and peptides for different receptors

Compound	Receptor type μ	δ	κ	σ
Opioid peptides				
β-endorphin	+++	+++	+++	–
Leu-enkephalin	+	+++	–	–
Met-enkephalin	++	+++	–	–
Dynorphin	++	+	+++	–
Opioid drugs				
Pure agonists				
Morphine	+++	+	++	–
Codeine	+	+	+	–
Pethidine	++	+	+	–
Etorphine	+++	+++	+++	–
Fentanyl	+++	+	–	–
Sufentanil	+++	+	–	–
Partial/mixed agonists				
Pentazocine	+	+	(++)	+
Nalbuphine	+	+	(++)	+
Nalorphine	++	(++)	(++)	+
Buprenorphine	(+++)	–	–	–
Meptazinol	(++)	–	–	–
Antagonists				
Naloxone	+++	++	++	–
Naltrexone	+++	++	++	–

+ agonist; + antagonist; (+) signifies partial agonist.

Three main categories may be distinguished (Table 31.3):

- *Pure agonists.* This group includes most of the typical morphine-like drugs. They all have high affinity for μ-receptors and varying affinity for δ- and κ-sites, and they lack appreciable activity at the σ-receptor. Some drugs of this type, notably **codeine**, **methadone** and **dextropropoxyphene**, are sometimes referred to as *weak agonists*, since their maximal effects, both analgesic and unwanted, are much less than those of morphine, and they do not cause dependence. Whether they are truly partial agonists is not established.
- *Partial agonists and mixed agonist–antagonists.* These drugs typified by **nalorphine** and **pentazocine** combine a degree of agonist and antagonist activity on different receptors. **Nalorphine**, for example, is an agonist when tested on guinea-pig ileum, but it also inhibits competitively the effect of morphine on this tissue (consistent with a partial agonist profile; see Ch. 1). In vivo it shows a similar mixture of agonist and antagonist actions. **Pentazocine** and **cyclazocine**, on the other hand, are antagonists at μ-receptors, but partial agonists on δ- and κ-receptors. Most of the drugs in this group tend to cause dysphoria, rather than euphoria, an effect which may be due to an interaction with the σ-receptor.
- *Antagonists.* These drugs produce very little effect when given on their own, but block the effects of opioids. The most important examples are **naloxone** and **naltrexone**.

MECHANISM OF ACTION OF OPIOIDS

The opioids have probably been studied more intensively than any other group of drugs in the effort to understand their powerful effects in molecular and biochemical and physiological terms, and to use this understanding to develop opioid drugs as analgesics with significant advantages over morphine. Despite the intense effort, and the huge volume of literature that has resulted, we remain surprisingly unsure of exactly how opioids produce their analgesic effects. Morphine, the prototype analgesic, remains the standard against which new analgesics are assessed. It is as though Ehrlich's salvarsan were still the standard for comparison of new anti-syphilitics. Useful reviews on the neuropharmacology of opiates include Duggan & North (1984), Duggan (1992) and Pasternak (1993).

Cellular actions

Opioid receptors, which have recently been cloned, belong to the family of G-protein-coupled receptors, and act to inhibit adenylate cyclase, so reducing the intracellular cAMP content (see West & Miller 1983, Childers 1993). All three receptor subtypes exert this effect, but its significance in relation to the functional effects of opioids is not clear, since opioids are known to exert effects on ion channels through a direct G-protein coupling to the channel, not involving any intracellular second messenger. By this means, opioids promote the opening of potassium channels and inhibit the opening of voltage-gated calcium channels (see review by North 1993), which are the main effects seen at the membrane level. These membrane effects act to reduce both neuronal excitability (since the increased potassium conductance causes hyperpolarisation of the membrane) and transmitter release (due to inhibition of calcium entry). The overall effect is therefore inhibitory at the cellular level. Nonetheless, opioids increase activity in some neuronal pathways (see below), presumably by suppressing the firing of inhibitory interneurons. At the cellular level, all three receptor subtypes mediate very similar effects, though the heterogeneous distribution of the receptors means that particular neurons and pathways are affected selectively by different agonists.

Effects on the nociceptive pathway

Opioid receptors are widely distributed in the brain, and their relationship to the nociceptive pathway is summarised in Figure 31.4. Opioids are effective as analgesics when given intrathecally, as well as by the systemic route, implying that an action on the spinal cord can account for their analgesic effect. However, injection of morphine into the PAG region also causes marked analgesia, which can be prevented by surgical interruption of the descending pathway to NRM or by blocking 5-HT synthesis pharmacologically with p-chlorophenylalanine. This latter procedure interrupts the 5-HT pathway running from NRM to the dorsal horn. Moreover, systemic morphine is rendered less effective in suppressing nociceptive spinal reflexes by transection of the spinal cord in the neck, and the firing of neurons associated with the descending inhibitory pathways is increased by morphine, findings that imply that there is a significant supraspinal component of the overall effect. Recent studies on the distribution of morphine and its active metabolites in the brain and spinal cord, however, suggests that the spinal cord is the principal site of action (see Duggan 1992), though the issue remains contentious.

Acting at the spinal level, morphine causes inhibition of transmission of nociceptive impulses through the dorsal horn, and suppresses nociceptive spinal reflexes in patients with spinal cord transection. It has been shown to inhibit release of substance P from dorsal horn neurons in vitro and in vivo (Fig. 31.8), by exerting a presynaptic inhibitory effect on the central terminals of nociceptive afferent neurons. Microinjection of morphine into the dorsal horn also produces this effect. However, measurement of substance P release by an antibody-covered microprobe inserted directly into the dorsal horn (see Ch. 3) failed to show any inhibition of release when morphine was given systemically in analgesic doses, implying that an action on primary afferent terminals may not be important.

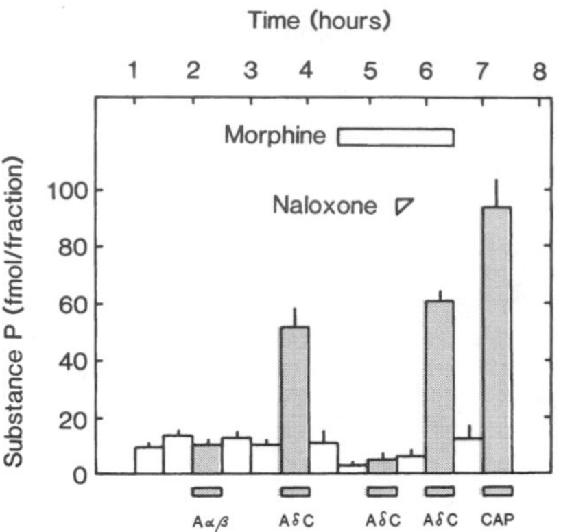

Fig. 31.8 Morphine inhibits the release of substance P from cat spinal cord. Substance P was measured by radioimmunoassay in the fluid superfusing the spinal cord. Stimulation of the sciatic nerve at low intensity stimulates large myelinated fibres (Aα and Aβ) only and evokes no release. Increasing the stimulus strength to recruit Aδ and C fibres causes substance P release. The release is blocked by morphine, this effect being antagonised by naloxone. Capsaicin (CAP) added to the fluid superfusing the spinal cord also releases substance P. (From: Yaksh et al. 1980)

Opioid receptors

- μ-receptors are thought to be responsible for most of the analgesic effects of opioids, and for some major unwanted effects (e.g. respiratory depression, euphoria, sedation and dependence). Most of the analgesic opioids are μ-receptor agonists.
- δ-receptors are probably more important in the periphery, but may also contribute to analgesia.
- κ-receptors contribute to analgesia at the spinal level, and may elicit sedation and dysphoria, but produce relatively few unwanted effects, and do not contribute to dependence. Some analgesics are relatively κ-selective.
- σ-receptors are not selective opioid receptors, but are also the site of action of psychotomimetic drugs, such as phencyclidine (Ch. 32). They are believed to be associated with glutamate-activated ion channels, and may account for the dysphoria produced by some opioids.
- All opioid receptors are linked through G-proteins to inhibition of adenylate cyclase. They also facilitate opening of K^+ channels (causing hyperpolarisation), and inhibit opening of Ca^{2+} channels (inhibiting transmitter release). These membrane effects are not linked to the decrease in cAMP formation.

PHARMACOLOGICAL ACTIONS

Morphine is typical of many opioid analgesics, and will be taken as the reference compound.

The most important effects of morphine are on the central nervous system and the gastrointestinal tract, though numerous effects of lesser significance on many other systems have been described.

Effects on the central nervous system

Analgesia

Morphine is effective in most kinds of acute and chronic pain, though opioids in general are less useful in various pain syndromes that are neuropathic in origin, such as phantom limb and other types of deafferentation pain, trigeminal neuralgia, etc. (see above).

As well as being antinociceptive, morphine also reduces the affective component of pain, an effect which must certainly involve supraspinal sites, possibly including the limbic system, which is probably involved in the euphoria-producing effect (see Koob & Bloom 1983). Drugs such as nalorphine and pentazocine share the antinociceptive actions of morphine but have much less effect on the psychological response to pain.

Euphoria

Morphine causes a powerful sense of contentment and well-being. This is an important component of its analgesic effect, since the agitation and anxiety associated with a painful illness or injury are thereby reduced. If morphine or heroin is given intravenously, the result is a sudden 'rush' likened to an 'abdominal orgasm'. The euphoria produced by morphine depends considerably on the circumstances. In patients who are distressed, it is a marked effect, but in patients who become accustomed to chronic pain, morphine usually causes no euphoria, though the pain is none the less relieved. Some patients report restlessness rather then euphoria under these circumstances.

Euphoria appears to be mediated through μ-receptors, and to be balanced by the dysphoria associated with κ-receptor activation. Thus, different opioid drugs vary greatly in the amount of euphoria that they produce. It does not occur with codeine or with pentazocine to any marked extent, and nalorphine, in doses sufficient to cause analgesia, produces dysphoria.

Respiratory depression

A measurable degree of respiratory depression, resulting in increased arterial $P\text{CO}_2$, occurs with a normal analgesic dose of morphine or related compounds. The two effects are both mediated by μ-receptors, and the balance between them is thus the same for most opioids.

The depressant effect is associated with a decrease in the sensitivity of the respiratory centre to $P\text{CO}_2$, the hypoxic drive mediated through peripheral chemoreceptors being unaffected. The site and mechanism of action of opioids on respiration is not certain (see McQueen 1983). Neurons in the medullary respiratory centre itself do not appear to be directly depressed, but opioids applied to the ventral surface of the medulla in the region where CO_2 chemosensitivity is maximal, have a powerful depressant effect on respiration.

Respiratory depression by opioids is not accompanied by depression of the medullary centres controlling cardiovascular function (in contrast to the action of anaesthetics and other general depressants). This means that respiratory depression produced by opioids is much better tolerated than a similar degree of depression caused by, say, a barbiturate; none the less respiratory depression is the most troublesome unwanted effect of these drugs, and, unlike that due to general CNS depressant drugs, it occurs at therapeutic doses. It is the commonest cause of death in acute opioid poisoning.

Depression of cough reflex

Cough suppression, surprisingly, does not correlate closely with the analgesic and respiratory depressant actions of opioids, and may represent an action on a different type of receptor. In general, increasing substitution on the phenolic –OH group of morphine (position 3; see Table 31.1) increases antitussive relative to analgesic activity. Thus **codeine** suppresses cough in subanalgesic doses, and is often used in cough medicines (see Ch. 17). **Pholcodine**, with a much larger substituent group at position 3, is even more selective, though these agents tend to cause constipation as an unwanted effect.

Nausea and vomiting

Nausea and vomiting occur in up to 40% of patients to whom morphine is given, and do not seem to be separable from the analgesic effect among a range of opioid analgesics. The site of action is the *area postrema* (*chemoreceptor trigger zone*), a region of the medulla where chemical stimuli of many kinds may initiate vomiting (see Ch. 19). A chemically related compound, **apomorphine** (a dopamine-receptor agonist; see Ch. 24), is more effective than morphine in causing vomiting, and lacks analgesic actions. The emetic effect of morphine, however, is prevented by the administration of an opioid antagonist, such as naloxone (see below), whereas that of apomorphine is not affected. On the other hand, dopamine antagonists (Chs 19 and 28) oppose the action of apomorphine much more effectively than that of morphine. Nausea and vomiting following morphine injection are usually transient, and disappear with repeated administration.

Pupillary constriction

Pupillary constriction is a centrally mediated effect, caused by μ- and κ-receptor-mediated stimulation of the oculomotor nucleus. Pinpoint pupils are an important diagnostic feature in overdosage with morphine and related drugs, because most other causes of coma and respiratory depression produce pupillary dilatation.

Effects on the gastrointestinal tract

Morphine causes a marked *increase in tone* and *reduced motility* in many parts of the gastrointestinal system, resulting in constipation which may be severe, and very troublesome to the patient. There is a delay in gastric emptying that can considerably retard the absorption of other drugs. Pressure in the biliary tract increases considerably because of contraction of the gall bladder and constriction of the biliary sphincter. This effect is harmful in patients suffering from biliary colic due to gallstones, in whom pain may be increased rather than relieved. The rise in intrabiliary pressure can cause a transient increase in the concentration of amylase and lipase in the plasma.

The action of morphine on visceral smooth muscle is probably mediated mainly through the intramural nerve plexuses, since the increase in tone is reduced or abolished by atropine. It is partly mediated by a central action of morphine, since intraventricular injection of morphine inhibits propulsive gastrointestinal movements. The local effect of morphine and other opioids on neurons of the myenteric plexus is inhibitory, there being hyperpolarisation resulting from an increased potassium conductance. The receptors involved in these effects are of the μ, κ and δ type, with much variation between different preparations and different species.

Other actions of opioids

Morphine releases histamine from mast cells, by an action unrelated to opioid receptors. This release of histamine can cause local effects, such as *urticaria* and *itching* at the site of the injection, or systemic effects, namely *bronchoconstriction* and *hypotension*. The bronchoconstrictor effect can have serious consequences for asthmatic patients, to whom morphine should not be given. Other opioids, except those closely related to morphine, do not release histamine.

Hypotension and bradycardia occur with large doses of most opioids, due to an action on the medulla. With morphine and similar drugs, histamine release may contribute to the hypotension.

Effects on smooth muscle other than that of the gastrointestinal tract and bronchi are slight, though spasm of the ureters, bladder and uterus sometimes occur. The Straub tail reaction, one of the more improbable phenomena in pharmacology, consists of a raising and stiffening of the tail of rats or mice given opioid drugs, and is due to spasm of a muscle at the base of the tail. It was through this effect that the analgesic action of pethidine was discovered.

Opioids also exert complex *immunosuppressant* effects, which may be important as a link between

Actions of morphine

- The main pharmacological effects are:
  - —analgesia
  - —euphoria and sedation
  - —respiratory depression and suppression of cough
  - —nausea and vomiting
  - —pupillary constriction
  - —reduced gastrointestinal motility, causing constipation
  - —histamine release, causing bronchoconstriction and hypotension.
- The most troublesome unwanted effects are constipation and respiratory depression.
- Morphine may be given by injection (intravenous or intramuscular), or by mouth, often as slow-release tablets.
- Acute overdosage with morphine produces coma and respiratory depression.
- Morphine is metabolised to morphine-6-glucuronide, which is more potent as an analgesic.

the nervous system and immune function (see Sibinga & Goldstein 1988). The pharmacological significance of this is not yet clear, but there is evidence in man that the immune system is depressed by long-term opioid abuse, leading to increased susceptibility to infections.

TOLERANCE AND DEPENDENCE

Tolerance to opioids (i.e. an increase in the dose needed to produce a given pharmacological effect) develops rapidly, and is readily demonstrated. *Dependence* is a different phenomenon, much more difficult to define and measure which involves two separate components, namely *physical* and *psychological dependence* (see Koob & Bloom 1988; Ch. 33). Physical dependence is associated with a clear-cut *physical withdrawal syndrome* (or *abstinence syndrome*), which can be reproduced in experimental animals, and appears to be closely related to tolerance. Morphine also produces *strong psychological dependence*, expressed as craving for the drug, which is probably more important than the physical withdrawal syndrome as a factor causing dependence in man, but is far harder to study.

Tolerance

Tolerance can be detected within 12–24 hours of morphine administration. Figure 31.9 shows the increase in the equianalgesic dose of morphine (measured by the hot-plate test) that occurred when a slow-release pellet of morphine was implanted subcutaneously in mice. The pellet was removed 8 hours before the test, to allow the drug to be eliminated before the test was carried out. Within 3 days the equianalgesic dose increased about five-fold. Sensitivity returned to normal within about 3 days of removing the pellet. More detailed studies have subsequently shown that a detectable level of tolerance may persist in rats for several months (see Martin & Sloan 1977). Tolerance extends to most of the pharmacological effects of morphine, including analgesia, euphoria, and respiratory depression, but affects the constipating and pupil-constricting actions much less. Thus, addicts who take up to 50 times the normal analgesic dose of morphine show relatively little respiratory depression, but marked constipation and pupillary constriction.

The mechanisms by which tolerance develops have been intensively studied (see Nestler 1993). Certain possibilities can be excluded, such as in-

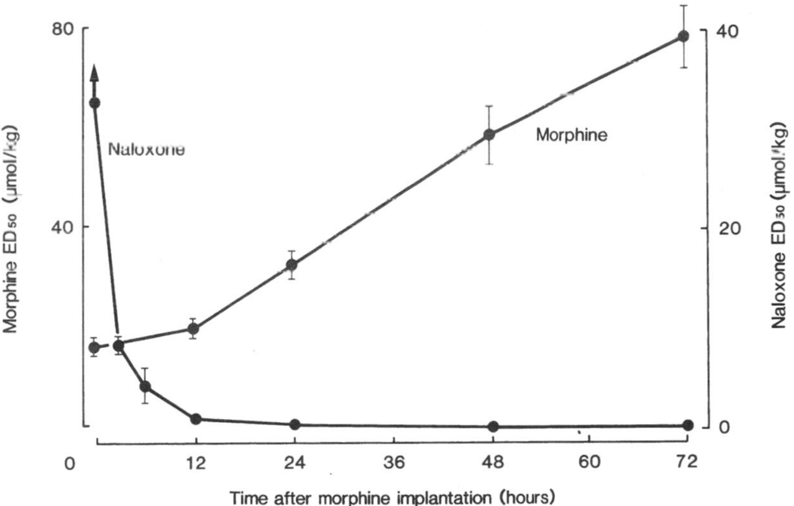

Fig. 31.9 Development of morphine tolerance in mice. The ED_{50} for analgesia (hot-plate test) produced by subcutaneous injection of a test dose of morphine (red circles) was measured at intervals after implantation of a slow-release pellet of morphine, the pellet being removed 8 hours before the assay in order to allow the circulating morphine concentration to fall to zero before the test dose was given. The ED_{50} increases about fivefold after 72 hours. Simultaneously, the dose of naloxone needed to precipitate withdrawal symptoms (black circles) decreases very markedly. (From: Way et al. 1969)

creased metabolic degradation, reduced affinity of opioids for their receptors, down-regulation of opioid receptors and inhibition of the release of endogenous opioids. Tolerance is a general phenomenon of opioid receptor ligands, irrespective of which type of receptor they act upon. Cross-tolerance occurs between drugs acting at the same receptor, but not between opioids that act on different receptors. Studies of opioid receptor distribution in the brains of opioid-tolerant animals show no consistent changes compared with normal controls. The expression of G-proteins and adenylate cyclase are, however, increased in certain brain areas, changes which show the same time-course as the development of tolerance. Both these biochemical changes and the development of tolerance are prevented by agents which block protein synthesis, suggesting that changes in gene expression are responsible. It is believed that the reduction of intracellular cAMP, acting through cAMP-dependent protein kinases (see Ch. 2), reduces the degree of phosphorylation of particular transcription factors, and thus enhances transcription of specific genes, including those coding for adenylate cyclase and certain G-proteins, as well as for other regulatory proteins. Similar changes occur in cells in culture exposed to opioids (Fig. 31.10). Addition of morphine to a culture of neuroblastoma-derived cells that express δ-opioid receptors causes a reduction in cAMP production for 2–3 days, after which it returns to normal, even though the morphine is still present. Removal of the morphine then causes the basal cAMP production to increase above the normal level, and the response of the cells to substances that activate adenylate cyclase (e.g. prostaglandin E_1) is similarly increased. Tolerance and dependence have been analysed in detail in opioid-sensitive brain regions such as the *locus ceruleus* (see Di Chiara & North 1992). The firing rate of *locus ceruleus* cells is inhibited by morphine, but recovers as tolerance develops. Removal of the morphine then increases the firing rate above the normal level, and addition of an antagonist, such as **naloxone**, causes a further increase, properties which exactly mirror those of the physical withdrawal syndrome. Thus, opiate tolerance and dependence are now fairly well understood at the cellular and molecular level. The relationship between these events and psychological dependence is much less clear, and is discussed further in Chapter 33.

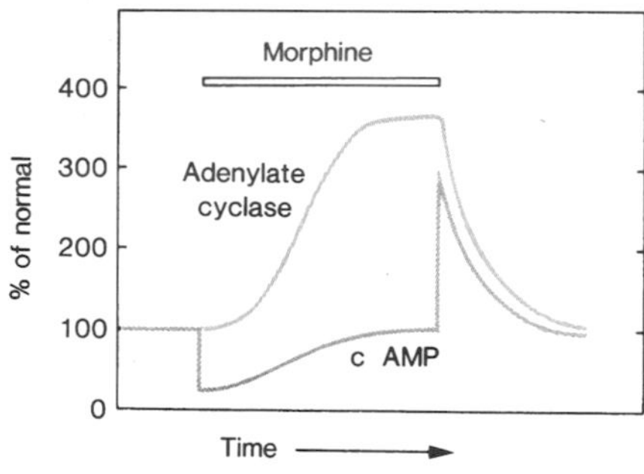

Fig. 31.10 Biochemical mechanism postulated to explain morphine tolerance and dependence. Morphine inhibits adenylate cyclase (grey line). A secondary rise in adenylate cyclase production occurs (pink line), so that cAMP production recovers in the presence of morphine (i.e. tolerance develops). On cessation of morphine treatment excessive cAMP production occurs, causing withdrawal symptoms, until the high level of adenylate cyclase returns to normal. (From: Sharma S K et al. 1975 Proc Natl Acad Sci USA 72: 3092)

Physical dependence

Physical dependence is characterised by a clear-cut *abstinence syndrome*. In experimental animals (for example, rats) abrupt withdrawal of morphine after chronic administration for a few days causes increased irritability, loss of weight and a variety of abnormal behaviour patterns, such as body shakes, writhing, jumping and signs of aggression. These reactions decrease after a few days, but abnormal irritability and aggression persist for many weeks. Human addicts show a similar abstinence syndrome, somewhat resembling severe influenza, with yawning, pupillary dilatation, fever, sweating, piloerection,* nausea, diarrhoea and insomnia.

Addicts are extremely restless and distressed during withdrawal and have a strong craving for the drug. The symptoms are maximal in about 2 days and largely disappear in 8–10 days, though some residual symptoms and physiological abnormalities persist for several weeks (Martin & Sloan 1977). Re-administration of morphine rapidly abolishes the abstinence syndrome.

Many physiological changes have been described in relation to the abstinence syndrome. For example, reflex hyperexcitability is demonstrable in the spinal

*Causing goose pimples. This is the origin of the phrase 'cold turkey' used to describe the effect of morphine withdrawal.

cord of morphine-dependent animals, and can be produced by chronic intrathecal as well as systemic administration of morphine. The noradrenergic pathways emanating from the *locus ceruleus* (see above) may also play an important role in causing the abstinence syndrome. The rate of firing of *locus ceruleus* neurons is inhibited by opioids, and increased during the abstinence syndrome. In this connection, it is interesting that **clonidine**, an α_2-adrenoceptor agonist (see Ch. 7) which inhibits cAMP formation, also inhibits firing of *locus ceruleus* neurons, and is effective in suppressing the morphine abstinence syndrome. Moreover, clonidine itself has analgesic activity (see later section) and cross-tolerance occurs between it and opioid analgesics. Similar changes occur in the *ventral tegmental area* where reside the cell bodies of the A10 group of dopaminergic neurons projecting to the *nucleus accumbens* (see Chs 24 and 33; Koob 1992). These cells receive input from opioid-containing neurons, and this dopaminergic pathway is believed to constitute the 'reward pathway' responsible for the strong reinforcing effect of opioids (see Ch. 33), and possibly for the euphoria experienced by human subjects.

PHARMACOKINETIC ASPECTS

Table 31.4 summarises the pharmacokinetic properties of the main opioid analgesics. The absorption of morphine congeners by mouth is variable. **Morphine** itself is slowly and erratically absorbed, and is commonly given by intravenous or intramuscular injection; oral morphine is, however, often used in treating chronic pain, and slow-release preparations are available to increase its duration of action. **Codeine** is well absorbed, and normally given by mouth. Most morphine-like drugs undergo considerable first-pass metabolism, and are therefore considerably less potent when taken orally than when injected.

The plasma half-life of most morphine analogues is 3–6 hours. Conjugation with glucuronide at the 3- and 6-OH groups occurs in the liver, and these glucuronides constitute a considerable fraction of the drug in the bloodstream. Morphine-6 glucuronide is, surprisingly, more active as an analgesic than morphine itself, and contributes substantially to the pharmacological effect. Morphine-3-glucuronide has been claimed to antagonise the analgesic effect of morphine, but the significance of this experimental finding is uncertain. Morphine glucuronides are excreted in the urine, so the dose needs to be reduced in cases of renal failure. Glucuronides also reach the gut via biliary excretion, where they are hydrolysed, most of the morphine being reabsorbed (enterohepatic circulation). Because of low conjugating capacity in neonates, morphine-like drugs have a much longer duration of action; because even a small degree of respiratory depression can be hazardous, morphine congeners should not be used in the neonatal period, nor used as analgesics during childbirth. **Pethidine** (see below) is a safer alternative for this purpose.

Analogues that have no free –OH in the 3-position (i.e. **heroin**, **codeine**) are metabolised to morphine, which accounts for at least part of their pharmacological activity.

Morphine produces very effective analgesia when administered intrathecally, and is often used in this way by anaesthetists, the advantage being that the sedative and respiratory depressant effects are reduced, though not completely avoided.

For the treatment of chronic or postoperative pain, opioids are being increasingly used 'on demand' (patient-controlled analgesia). The patients are provided with an infusion pump which they control, the maximum possible rate of administration being limited to avoid acute toxicity. Contrary to fears,

Tolerance and dependence

- Tolerance develops rapidly, accompanied by physical withdrawal syndrome.
- The mechanism of tolerance is poorly understood, but may involve adaptive up-regulation of adenylate cyclase. It is not pharmacokinetic in origin and receptor down-regulation is not a major factor.
- Dependence is satisfied by μ-receptor agonists, and the withdrawal syndrome is precipitated by μ-receptor antagonists.
- Dependence involves psychological as well as physical factors, and rarely occurs in patients being given opioids as analgesics.
- Weak, long-acting μ-receptor agonists, such as methadone, may be used to relieve withdrawal symptoms.
- Certain opioid analgesics, such as codeine, pentazocine and buprenorphine, are much less likely to cause physical or psychological dependence.

Table 31.4 Characteristics of the main opioid analgesic drugs

Drug	Uses	Route of admin.	Pharmacokinetic aspects	Main adverse effects	Notes
Morphine	Widely used for acute and chronic pain	Oral Injection* Intrathecal	Half-life 3–4 hours Converted to active metabolite (morphine-6-glucuronide)	Sedation, respiratory depression Constipation Nausea and vomiting Itching (histamine release) Tolerance and dependence Euphoria	Tolerance and withdrawal effects not common when used for analgesia
Heroin	Acute and chronic pain	Oral Injection	Acts more rapidly and more briefly than morphine Metabolised partly to morphine	As morphine	Not available in all countries Considered (irrationally) to be analgesic of last resort
Hydromorphone	Acute and chronic pain	Oral Injection	Half-life 2–4 hours No active metabolites	As morphine, but allegedly less sedative	**Levorphanol** is similar, with longer duration of action
Methadone	Chronic pain Maintenance of addicts	Oral	Long half-life (>24 hours) Slow onset	As morphine, but little euphoric effect Cumulation may occur due to long half-life	Slow recovery results in attenuated withdrawal syndrome
Pethidine	Acute pain	Oral Intramuscular injection	Half-life 2–4 hours Active metabolite (norpethidine) may account for stimulant effects	As morphine Anticholinergic effects Risk of excitement and convulsions	Known as **meperidine** in US
Buprenorphine	Acute and chronic pain	Sublingual Injection Intrathecal	Half-life about 12 hours Slow onset Inactive orally due to first-pass metabolism	As morphine but less pronounced Respiratory depression poorly reversed by naloxone (therefore not suitable for obstetric use)	Useful in chronic pain with patient-controlled injection systems
Pentazocine	Mainly acute pain	Oral Injection	Half-life 2–4 hours	Psychotomimetic effects (dysphoria) Irritation at injection site May precipitate morphine withdrawal syndrome (μ-antagonist effect)	**Butorphanol** (not available in UK) and **nalbuphine** are similar Butorphanol is not active orally
Fentanyl	Acute pain Anaesthesia	Intravenous Epidural Transdermal patch	Half-life 4–8 hours	As morphine	High potency allows transdermal administration **Sufentanil** is similar
Codeine	Mild pain	Oral	Acts as pro-drug. Metabolised to morphine and other active opioids	Mainly constipation No dependence liability	Effective only in mild pain Also used to suppress cough **Dihydrocodeine** is similar
Dextro-propoxyphene	Mild pain	Mainly oral	Half-life ~4 hours. Active metabolite (norpropoxyphene) with half-life ~24 hours	Respiratory depression May cause convulsions (possibly due to norpropoxyphene)	

* Injections may be given intravenously, intramuscularly or subcutaneously for most drugs.

patients show little tendency to use excessively large doses and become dependent; instead the dose is adjusted to achieve analgesia without excessive sedation, and is reduced as the pain subsides.

UNWANTED EFFECTS

The main unwanted effects of morphine and related drugs are listed in Table 31.4.

Acute overdosage with morphine results in coma and respiratory depression, with characteristically constricted pupils. It is treated by giving **naloxone** intravenously. This also serves as a diagnostic test, for failure to respond to naloxone indicates a cause other than opioid poisoning for the comatose state. There is a danger of precipitating a severe withdrawal syndrome with naloxone, since opioid poisoning occurs mainly in addicts.

OTHER OPIOID ANALGESICS

Diamorphine (heroin, diacetylmorphine) is produced from morphine by acetylation of both hydroxyl groups. A strong smell of vinegar commonly provides the lead to illicit heroin producers, at least in fiction. It is pharmacologically very similar to morphine, and is converted to morphine in the body, though heroin is itself more active than morphine. Because of its greater lipid solubility it crosses the blood–brain barrier more rapidly than morphine, and gives a greater 'rush' when injected intravenously. It is said to be less emetic than morphine, but the evidence for this is slight. It is still available in Britain for clinical use as an analgesic though its manufacture is banned in many countries. There is no evidence that heroin differs from morphine in either its respiratory depressant effect or in its liability to cause dependence. Its duration of action (about 2 hours) is shorter than that of morphine.

Codeine (3-methylmorphine) is also made commercially from morphine. It is more reliably absorbed by mouth than morphine, but has only about 20% of the analgesic potency. Furthermore, its analgesic effect does not increase appreciably at higher dose levels. It is therefore used mainly as an oral analgesic for mild types of pain (headache, backache, etc.). An important difference from morphine is that it causes little or no euphoria, and is rarely addictive, so is available without prescription. It is very frequently combined with aspirin-like drugs in proprietary analgesic preparations, but there is no evidence of any advantageous synergistic interaction between the two components. In relation to its analgesic effect, codeine produces the same degree of respiratory depression as morphine, but the limited response even at high doses means that it is seldom a problem in practice. It does, however, cause constipation. Codeine has some antitussive activity and is often used in cough mixtures (see Ch. 17). **Dihydrocodeine** is pharmacologically very similar, having no substantial advantages or disadvantages (apart from cost) over codeine.

Dextropropoxyphene is similar to codeine, but has a longer duration of action. It is commonly used in analgesic preparations, and was thought to be safe in overdose. Experience has shown, however, that it is not completely safe, nor free of dependence liability.

Pethidine is virtually identical to morphine in its pharmacological effects, except that it tends to cause restlessness rather than sedation, and it has an additional antimuscarinic action which may cause dry mouth and blurring of vision as side effects. It also has relatively less antitussive effect. It produces a very similar euphoric effect, and is equally liable to cause dependence. Its duration of action is appreciably shorter than that of morphine, and the route of metabolic degradation is different. Pethidine is partly N-demethylated in the liver to norpethidine, which has a hallucinogenic and convulsant effect. This becomes significant with large oral doses of pethidine, producing an overdose syndrome rather different from that of morphine. Pethidine is preferred to morphine for analgesia during labour, because it is shorter-acting. The difference in the duration of action of morphine and pethidine is particularly marked in the neonate. This is because the conjugation reactions, on which morphine excretion depends, are deficient in the newborn: pethidine does not rely on conjugation to be excreted, and any drug transferred from the maternal circulation is, in contrast to morphine, fairly quickly inactivated. Severe reactions, consisting of excitement, hyperthermia and convulsions, have been reported when pethidine is given to patients receiving monoamine oxidase inhibitors. This seems to be due to inhibition of an alternative metabolic pathway, leading to increased norpethidine formation, but the details are not known.

Fentanyl and **sufentanil** are highly potent

phenylpiperidine derivatives, with actions similar to morphine, but short-lasting, particularly sufentanil. Their main use is in anaesthesia, and they may be given intrathecally. They are also used in patient-controlled infusion systems, where a short duration of action is advantageous.

Etorphine is a morphine analogue of remarkable potency, more than 1000 times that of morphine, but otherwise very similar in its actions. Its high potency confers no particular clinical advantage, but it is used successfully to immobilise wild animals for trapping and research purposes, since the required dose, even for an elephant, is small enough to be incorporated into a dart or pellet.

Methadone is also pharmacologically similar to morphine, the main difference being that its duration of action is considerably longer (plasma half-life >24 hours) and it is claimed to have less sedative action. The increased duration seems to occur because the drug is bound in the extravascular compartment, and slowly released. One consequence is that the physical abstinence syndrome is less acute than with morphine or other short-acting drugs, though the psychological dependence is no less pronounced. For this reason, methadone is widely used as a means of treating morphine and heroin addiction. In the presence of methadone, an injection of morphine does not cause the normal euphoria, nor is there a physical abstinence syndrome, so it is often possible to wean addicts from morphine or heroin by giving regular oral doses of methadone—an improvement if not a cure.

Pentazocine is a mixed agonist–antagonist (see earlier section). In low doses its potency and effects are very similar to those of morphine, but increasing the dose does not cause a corresponding increase in the effects produced. Thus, at high doses, pentazocine causes only slight respiratory depression, and it causes marked dysphoria, with nightmares and hallucinations, rather than euphoria. It also tends to raise, rather than lower, arterial blood pressure. These differences mean that pentazocine has less tendency to cause dependence, and its acute toxicity is much less than that of morphine. Its antagonist activity is apparent in the fact that, given concurrently with morphine, pentazocine actually reduces the analgesic and other actions of morphine, and can even precipitate an abstinence syndrome in morphine addicts. Binding studies show that it has a higher affinity for κ- than for μ-receptors, and on behavioural criteria it is postulated to act on σ-receptors, this spectrum being somewhat different from that of conventional opioid drugs. Though clearly much less addictive than the conventional opioids, pentazocine still has an appreciable tendency to cause dependence, and is not quite the ideal morphine substitute that it was originally purported to be.

Buprenorphine acts as a partial agonist on μ-receptors. It appears less liable to cause dysphoria than pentazocine, but more liable to cause respiratory depression. It has a long duration of action. Its abuse liability is probably less than that of morphine.

Meptazinol and **dezocine** are recently introduced opiates of unusual chemical structure. Meptazinol can be given orally or by injection, and has a short plasma half-life. It seems to be relatively free of morphine-like side effects, causing neither euphoria nor dysphoria, nor causing severe respiratory depression. It does, however, produce nausea, sedation and dizziness, and has atropine-like side effects. Because of its short duration of action and lack of respiratory depression, it may have advantages for obstetric analgesia. Dezocine is a partial agonist at μ-receptors, with analgesic activity similar to that of morphine, but with respiratory depressant activity that reaches a 'ceiling' at high doses. It has not yet been fully evaluated.

For further information on the properties of clinically used opioids, see Hoskin & Hanks (1991).

OPIOID ANTAGONISTS

Nalorphine (Table 31.1) is closely related in structure to morphine, and was the first specific antagonist to be discovered. This was an important development, for it was the first clear evidence in favour of a specific receptor for morphine, recognition of which led to the successful search for endogenous mediators. Nalorphine has, in fact, a more complicated action than that of a simple competitive antagonist (Table 31.3). It antagonises most actions of morphine in whole animals or isolated tissues (e.g. analgesia, respiratory depression, and inhibition of electrically evoked contractions of guinea-pig ileum), and at low concentrations of nalorphine this interaction appears to be competitive. Higher concentrations of nalorphine, when tested alone, however, are analgesic, and mimic the effects of morphine. These effects probably reflect an antagonist action on μ-receptors, coupled with a partial agonist action on δ- and κ-receptors, the latter causing dysphoria, which makes it unsuitable for use as an analgesic. Nalorphine can itself produce physical dependence, but can also, in small doses, precipitate a withdrawal syndrome in morphine or heroin addicts. Nalorphine now has few clinical uses. At one time it was the most effective antidote available in cases of acute morphine or heroin overdosage, but had the disadvantage that, if large doses were needed, nalorphine itself caused respiratory depression. It has therefore been superseded by naloxone, which has no such effect.

Naloxone was the first pure opioid antagonist. On the basis of binding studies it appears to have a high affinity for μ-, δ- and κ-receptors. Naloxone blocks the actions of endogenous opioid peptides as well as those of morphine-like drugs, and has been extensively used as an experimental tool to determine the physiological role of these peptides, particularly in pain transmission.

Given on its own, naloxone produces very little effect, but in sufficiently high dose it rapidly reverses the effects of morphine and other opioids, including partial agonists such as pentazocine and nalorphine. It has little effect on pain threshold under normal conditions, but causes hyperalgesia under conditions of stress, when endogenous opioids are produced. This occurs, for example, in patients undergoing dental surgery, or in animals subjected to physical stress. Naloxone also inhibits acupuncture analgesia, which is known to be associated with the release of opioid peptides. Analgesia produced by PAG stimulation is also prevented.

The main clinical use of naloxone is to treat respiratory depression caused by opioid overdosage, and occasionally to reverse the effect of opioid analgesics, used during labour, on the respiration of the newborn baby. It is usually given intravenously and its effects are produced immediately. It is rapidly metabolised by the liver, and its effect lasts only 1–2 hours, which is considerably shorter than that of most morphine-like drugs. Thus it may have to be given repeatedly.

Naloxone has no important unwanted effects of its own, but precipitates withdrawal symptoms in addicts. It can be used to detect opioid addiction.

Naltrexone is very similar to naloxone but with the advantage of a much longer duration of action (half-life about 10 hours). It is used as an adjunct to prevent relapse of addicts following detoxification.

Specific antagonists at μ-, δ- and κ-receptors are available for experimental use, but not yet for clinical purposes.

Opioid antagonists

- Pure antagonists include naloxone (short-acting) and naltrexone (long-acting). They block μ-, δ- and κ-receptors more or less equally.
- Other drugs, such as nalorphine and pentazocine, produce a mixture of agonist and antagonist effects.
- Naloxone does not affect pain threshold normally, but blocks stimulation-induced analgesia, and can exacerbate clinical pain.
- Naloxone rapidly reverses opioid-induced analgesia and respiratory depression, and is used mainly to treat opioid overdose or to improve breathing in newborn babies affected by opioids given to the mother.
- Naloxone precipitates withdrawal symptoms in morphine-dependent patients or animals. Pentazocine may also do this.

Use of analgesic drugs

- The choice and route of administration of analgesic drugs depends on the nature and duration of the pain.
- A progressive approach is often used, starting with non-steroidal anti-inflammatory drugs, supplemented first by weak opioid analgesics, and then by strong opioids.
- In general, severe acute pain (e.g. trauma, burns, postoperative pain) is treated with strong opioid drugs (e.g. morphine, fentanyl) given by injection. Mild inflammatory pain (e.g. arthritis) is treated with non-steroidal anti-inflammatory drugs (e.g. aspirin) supplemented by weak opioid drugs (codeine, dextropropoxyphene, pentazocine) given orally if required. Severe pain (e.g. cancer pain, severe arthritis or back pain) is treated with strong opioids given orally, intrathecally, epidurally or by subcutaneous injection. Patient-controlled infusion systems are commonly used postoperatively.
- Chronic neuropathic pain is often unresponsive to opioids, and treated with tricyclic antidepressants (e.g. amitriptyline).

NEW APPROACHES

It can be seen from the earlier discussion of the neural mechanisms involved in pain and nociception that there are many potential sites at which drugs might act to inhibit transmission of information from the periphery to the thalamus and cortex. Attempts to develop new types of drug have tended to be dominated by opioid agonists on the one hand and NSAIDs on the other, but other possibilities are now being considered, and may find their way into clinical use.

Enkephalinase inhibitors, such as **thiorphan** (see Schwartz et al. 1985), act by inhibiting the metabolic degradation of endogenous opioid peptides, and have been shown to produce analgesia, together with other morphine-like effects, without causing dependence.

Various neuropeptides, such as **somatostatin** and **calcitonin** (see Ch. 21), produce powerful analgesia when applied intrathecally, and there are clinical reports suggesting that they may have similar effects when used systemically to treat endocrine disorders.

Non-peptide antagonists of substance P (see Ch. 9), which modulates transmission through the dorsal horn (see above), have recently been developed, and may prove to be useful analgesic drugs.

The clinical use of analgesic drugs is given on page 631.

REFERENCES AND FURTHER READING

Besson J-M, Chaouch A 1987 Peripheral and spinal mechanisms of nociception. Physiol Rev 67: 67–186

Brownstein M J 1993 A brief history of opiates, opioid peptides and opioid receptors. Proc Natl Acad Sci USA 90: 5391–5393

Chavkin C 1988 Electrophysiology of opiates and opioid peptides. In: Pasternak G W (ed) The opiate receptors. Humana Press, Clifton, NJ

Childers S R 1993 Opioid receptor-coupled second messenger systems. In: Herz A (ed) Opioids. Handbook of experimental pharmacology, Springer-Verlag, Berlin, vol 104

Coderre T J, Katz J, Vaccarino A L, Melzack R 1993 Contribution of central neuroplasticity to pathological pain: review of clinical and experimental evidence. Pain 52: 259–285

Dahl J B, Kehlet H 1993 The value of pre-emptive analgesia in the treatment of post-operative pain. Br J Anaesth 70: 434–439

Di Chiara G, North R A 1992 Neurobiology of opiate abuse. Trends Pharmacol Sci 13: 185–193

Dray A, Perkins M 1993 Bradykinin and inflammatory pain. Trends Neurosci 16: 99–104

Dubner R, Ruda M A 1992 Activity-dependent neuronal plasticity following tissue injury and inflammation. Trends Neurosci 15: 96–102

Duggan A W 1992 Neuropharmacology of pain. Curr Opin Neurol Neurosurg 5: 503–507

Duggan A W, North R A 1984 Electrophysiology of opioids. Pharmacol Rev 35: 219–281

Fields H L 1981 Pain: new approaches to therapy. Ann Neurol 9: 101–106

Fields H L 1987 Pain. McGraw Hill, New York

Fields H L, Basbaum A I 1989 Endogenous pain control mechanisms. In: Wall P D, Melzack R (eds) Textbook of pain. Churchill Livingstone, Edinburgh

Herz A (ed) 1993 Opioids. (2 vols) Handbook of experimental pharmacology. Springer-Verlag, Berlin, vol 104

Hoskin P J, Hanks G W 1991 Opioid agonist–antagonist drugs in acute and chronic pain states. Drugs 41: 326–344

James I F, Ninkina N, Wood J N 1993 The capsaicin receptor. In: Wood J N (ed) Capsaicin in the study of pain. Academic Press, London

Keele C A, Armstrong D M 1964 Substances causing pain and itch. Edward Arnold, London

Koob G F 1992 Drugs of abuse: anatomy, pharmacology and function of reward pathways. Trends Pharmacol Sci 13: 177–184

Koob G F, Bloom F E 1988 Cellular and molecular mechanisms of drug dependence. Science 242: 715–723

Lewin G R, Mendell L M 1993 Nerve growth factor and nociception. Trends Neurosci 16: 353–359

Lewis J W, Liebeskind J C 1983 Pain suppressive systems of the brain. Trends Pharmacol Sci 4: 73–75

McMahon S B, Lewin G R, Wall P D 1993 Central hyperexcitability triggered by noxious inputs. Curr Opin Neurobiol 3: 602–610

McQueen D S 1983 Opioid peptide interactions with respiratory and circulatory systems. Br Med Bull 39: 77–82

Martin W R, Sloan J W 1977 Neuropharmacology and neurochemistry of subjective effects, analgesia, tolerance and dependence produced by narcotic analgesics. Handbook of experimental pharmacology. Springer-Verlag, Berlin, vol 45: 43–158

Nestler E J 1993 Cellular responses to chronic treatment with drugs of abuse. Crit Rev Neurobiol 7: 23–39

North R A 1993 Opioid actions on membrane ion channels. In Herz A (ed) Opioids. Handbook of experimental pharmacology. Springer-Verlag, Berlin, vol 104

Pasternak G W (ed) 1988 The opiate receptors. Humana Press, Clifton, NJ

Pasternak G W 1993 Pharmacological mechanisms of opioid analgesics. Clin Neuropharm 16: 1–18

Rang H P, Bevan S, Dray A 1991 Chemical activation of nociceptive peripheral neurones. Br Med Bull 47: 534–548

Schwartz J-C, Costentin J, Lecomtet J-M 1985 Pharmacology

of enkephalinase inhibitors. Trends Pharmacol Sci 6: 472–476

Sibinga N E S, Goldstein A 1988 Opioid peptides and opioid receptors in cells of the immune system. Annu Rev Immunol 6: 219–249

Snyder S H, Pasternak G W, Pert C 1973 In: Iversen L L, Iversen S D, Snyder S H (eds) Handbook of psychopharmacology. Plenum, New York, vol 5: 329–360

Walker J M, Bowen W D, Walker F O, Matsumoto R R, De Costa B, Rice K C 1990 Sigma receptors: biology and function. Pharm Rev 42: 355–402

Wall P D, Melzack R (eds) 1994 Textbook of pain. Churchill Livingstone, Edinburgh

Way E L, Loh H H, Shen F H 1969 Simultaneous quantitative measurement of morphine tolerance and physical dependence. J Pharmacol Exp Ther 167: 1–8

West R E, Miller R J 1983 Opiates, second messengers and cell response. Br Med Bull 39: 53–58

Wood J N (ed) 1993 Capsaicin in the study of pain. Academic Press, London

Wood P L, Iyengar S 1988 Central actions of opiates and opioid peptides. In: Pasternak G W (ed) The opiate receptors. Humana Press, Clifton, NJ

Yaksh T L, Jessell T M, Gamse R, Mudge A W, Leeman S E 1980 Intrathecal morphine inhibits substance P release from mammalian spinal cord in vivo. Nature 286: 155–157

32 CENTRAL NERVOUS SYSTEM STIMULANTS AND PSYCHOTOMIMETIC DRUGS

Drugs that have a predominantly stimulant effect on the central nervous system fall into three broad categories:

- convulsants and respiratory stimulants
- psychomotor stimulants
- psychotomimetic drugs.

Drugs in the first category (e.g. **doxapram**, **nikethamide**, **leptazol** and **strychnine**) have relatively little effect on mental function, and appear to act mainly on the brainstem and spinal cord, producing exaggerated reflex excitability, an increase in activity of the respiratory and vasomotor centres, and with higher dosage, convulsions.

Drugs in the second category (e.g. **amphetamine**, **caffeine** and **cocaine**) have a marked effect on mental function and behaviour, producing excitement and euphoria, reduced sensation of fatigue and an increase in motor activity.

Drugs in the third category (e.g. **lysergic acid diethylamide** (LSD), **phencyclidine** and **cannabis**) mainly affect thought patterns and perception, distorting cognition in a complex way and producing effects that superficially resemble psychotic illness.

The distinctions between these three categories are not completely clear-cut. Amphetamine, for example, can produce thought disturbances very like schizophrenia as well as affecting motor behaviour. Table 32.1 summarises the classification of the drugs that are discussed in this chapter.

Cannabis (see Ch. 33) has predominantly depressant rather than stimulant actions; in addition, certain of its subjective effects resemble those of lysergic acid diethylamide and other psychotomimetics.

CONVULSANTS AND RESPIRATORY STIMULANTS

Convulsants and respiratory stimulants (sometimes called *analeptics*) are a chemically diverse group of substances whose mechanisms of action are, with some exceptions, not well understood. Such drugs were once used to treat patients in terminal coma or with severe respiratory failure. Although temporary restoration of function could often be achieved, mortality was not reduced, and the treatment carried a considerable risk of causing convulsions which left the patient more deeply comatose than before. They were used mainly to give the impression that something was being done for a patient *in extremis*. There remains a very limited clinical use for respiratory stimulants in treating acute ventilatory failure (see Ch. 17), **doxapram** (Table 32.1) being most commonly used since this drug carries less risk of causing convulsions than earlier compounds.

Also included in this group are various compounds, such as **strychnine**, **picrotoxin** and **leptazol**, which are of interest as experimental tools, but have no clinical uses.

Strychnine is an alkaloid found in the seeds of an Indian tree, which has been used for centuries as a poison (mainly vermin, but also human; it is much favoured in detective stories of a certain genre). It is a powerful convulsant, and acts throughout the central nervous system but particularly on the spinal cord, causing violent extensor spasms that are triggered by minor sensory stimuli, the head being

Table 32.1 Central nervous system stimulants and psychotomimetic drugs

Category	Examples	Mode of action	Clinical significance
Convulsants and respiratory stimulants (analeptics)			
Respiratory stimulants	Amiphenazole	Not known	Occasionally used as respiratory stimulant Risk of convulsions less than with nikethamide
	Doxapram	Not known	Short-acting respiratory stimulant sometimes given by intravenous infusion to treat acute respiratory failure
Miscellaneous convulsants	Strychnine	Antagonist of glycine Main action is to increase reflex excitability of spinal cord	No clinical uses
	Bicuculline	Competitive antagonist of GABA	No clinical uses
	Picrotoxin	Non-competitive antagonist of GABA	Clinical use as respiratory stimulant; now obsolete
	Nikethamide	Not known	Risk of convulsions
	Leptazol	Not known	No clinical use. Convulsant activity in experimental animals provides a useful model for testing anticonvulsant drugs (see Ch. 30)
Psychomotor stimulants			
	Amphetamine and related compounds e. g. dexamphetamine methylamphetamine methylphenidate fenfluramine	Release of catecholamines Inhibition of catecholamine uptake	Very limited clinical use owing to dependence liability and risk of peripheral sympathomimetic effects Some agents used as appetite suppressants Mainly important as drugs of abuse
	Cocaine	Inhibition of catecholamine uptake Local anaesthetic	Important as drug of abuse Occasionally used for nasopharyngeal and ophthalmic anaesthesia (see Ch. 34)
	Methylxanthines, e.g. caffeine theophylline	Inhibition of phosphodiesterase Antagonism of adenosine (relevance of these actions to central effects is not clear)	Clinical uses unrelated to stimulant activity, though caffeine is included in various 'tonics'. Theophylline used for action on cardiac and bronchial muscle. Constituents of beverages
Psychotomimetic drugs (hallucinogens)			
	Lysergic acid diethylamide (LSD)	Mixed agonist/antagonist at 5-HT receptors	No clinical use Important as drug of abuse
	Mescaline	Not known. Chemically similar to amphetamine	
	Psilocybin	Chemically related to 5-HT. Probably acts on 5-HT receptors	
	Cannabis	Acts as CNS depressant with mild psychotomimetic effects	No established clinical use* See Chapter 33
	Phencyclidine	Chemically similar to ketamine (see Ch. 26) Acts on σ-opiate receptors. Also blocks NMDA-receptor-operated ion channels (see Ch. 24)	Originally proposed as an anaesthetic, now important as drug of abuse and as a model for schizophrenia

* **Nabilone**, a synthetic cannabinoid, is sometimes used as an anti-emetic to reduce nausea during cancer chemotherapy.

thrown back and the face fixed, we are told, in a hideous grin. These effects result from blocking receptors for **glycine**, which is the main inhibitory transmitter acting on motoneurons. The action of strychnine superficially resembles that of **tetanus toxin**, a protein neurotoxin produced by the anaerobic bacterium *Clostridium tetani*. Tetanus toxin reaches the spinal cord from a site of infection by being transported along the axons of sensory neurons. Its action on the inhibitory interneurons is to block the release of glycine. This is very similar to the action of a closely related toxin, **botulinum toxin** (see Ch. 6), which is produced by another bacterium of the *Clostridium* genus, and causes paralysis by blocking acetylcholine release. In small doses, strychnine causes a measurable improvement in visual and auditory acuity; it was until quite recently included in various 'tonics', on the basis that CNS stimulation should restore both the weary brain and the enervated body.

Bicuculline is another plant alkaloid which somewhat resembles strychnine in its effects, but acts by blocking receptors for GABA rather than glycine. Its action is confined to $GABA_A$ receptors, which control chloride permeability, and it does not affect $GABA_B$ receptors (see Ch. 24). Its main effects are on the brain rather than the spinal cord, and it is a useful experimental tool for studying GABA-mediated transmission; it has no clinical uses.

Picrotoxin (literally 'fish poison') is also a plant toxin. The active substance, picrotoxinin, acts similarly to bicuculline in that it blocks the action of GABA on chloride channels, though not competitively. Its name reflects its use as a means of incapacitating fish by throwing berries into the water. Picrotoxin, like bicuculline, causes convulsions and has no clinical uses.

Nikethamide and **leptazol** are pharmacologically very similar, though their mode of action is unknown. They cause initial respiratory stimulation and also raise blood pressure by acting on the brainstem, at doses somewhat lower than those causing convulsions. Respiratory stimulation is short-lasting, and is followed by a period of depression. Inhibition of leptazol-induced convulsions by antiepileptic drugs (see Ch. 30) correlates quite well with their effectiveness against absence seizures, and leptazol has occasionally been used diagnostically in man, since it can precipitate the typical EEG pattern of absence seizures in susceptible patients.

Convulsants and respiratory stimulants

- This is a diverse group of drugs which have little clinical use.
- Certain short-acting respiratory stimulants (e.g. doxapram) can be used in respiratory failure.
- Strychnine is a convulsant poison that acts mainly on the spinal cord, by blocking receptors for the inhibitory transmitter, glycine.
- Picrotoxin and bicuculline act as $GABA_A$ antagonists; bicuculline blocks the $GABA_A$ receptor site, whereas picrotoxin appears to block the chloride channel coupled to it.
- Leptazol works by an unknown mechanism. Leptazol-induced convulsions provide an animal model for testing anticonvulsant drugs, giving good correlation with effectiveness in preventing absence seizures.

Doxapram is similar to the above drugs, but has a bigger margin of safety between respiratory stimulation and convulsions. Doxapram also causes nausea, coughing and restlessness, which limit its usefulness. Its action is very brief, and it is occasionally used as an intravenous infusion in patients with acute respiratory failure.

PSYCHOMOTOR STIMULANTS

AMPHETAMINES AND RELATED DRUGS

Amphetamine, and its active dextro-isomer **dextroamphetamine**, together with **methylamphetamine** and **methylphenidate**, comprise a group of drugs with very similar pharmacological properties (see Fig. 32.1). **Fenfluramine**, though chemically similar, has slightly different pharmacological effects. All of these drugs appear to act by releasing monoamines from nerve terminals in the brain. Noradrenaline and dopamine are the most important mediators in this connection, but 5-HT release also occurs, particularly with fenfluramine.

Pharmacological effects

The main central effects of amphetamine-like drugs are:

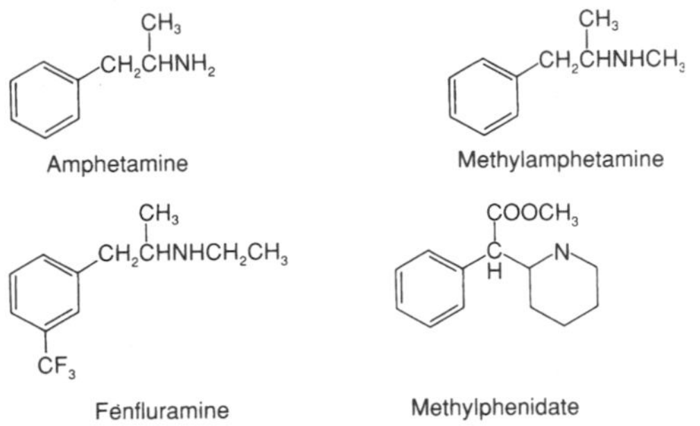

Amphetamine Methylamphetamine Fenfluramine Methylphenidate

Fig. 32.1 Structures of amphetamines.

- locomotor stimulation
- euphoria and excitement
- stereotyped behaviour
- anorexia.

In addition, amphetamines have peripheral sympathomimetic actions, producing a rise in blood pressure and inhibition of gastrointestinal motility.

In experimental animals, amphetamines cause increased alertness and locomotor activity, and increased grooming; they also increase aggressive activity. On the other hand, systematic exploration of novel objects by unrestrained rats is reduced by amphetamine. The animals run around more but appear less attentive to their surroundings. Studies of conditioned responses suggest that amphetamines increase the overall rate of responding without affecting the training process markedly. Thus, in a fixed-interval schedule where a reward for lever-pressing is forthcoming only after a fixed interval (say 10 minutes) following the last reward, trained animals normally press the lever very infrequently in the first few minutes after the reward, and increase the rate towards the end of the 10-minute interval when another reward is due. The effect of amphetamine is to increase the rate of unrewarded responses at the beginning of the 10-minute interval without affecting (or even reducing) the rate towards the end of the period. The effects of amphetamine on more sophisticated types of conditioned response, for example those involving discriminative tasks, are not clear-cut, and there is no clear evidence that either the rate of learning of such tasks or the final level of performance that can be achieved are affected by the drug. Crudely, it might be said that amphetamine tends to make animals busier rather than brighter.

With large doses of amphetamines, stereotyped behaviour occurs. This consists of repeated actions, such as licking, gnawing, rearing or repeated movements of the head and limbs. These activities are generally inappropriate to the environment, and with increasing doses of amphetamine they take over more and more of the behaviour of the animal. At the same time, the repertoire of stereotyped behaviour also becomes more limited. There is considerable evidence that these behavioural effects are produced by the release of catecholamines in the brain. Thus, treatment of newborn animals with **6-hydroxydopamine**, which greatly depletes the brain of both noradrenaline and dopamine, abolishes the effect of amphetamine, as does pretreatment with **α-methyltyrosine**, an inhibitor of catecholamine biosynthesis (see Ch. 7). **Tricyclic antidepressants** (see Ch. 29) potentiate the effects of amphetamine, presumably by blocking noradrenaline re-uptake. MAO inhibitors have a similar effect, resulting from an increase in the catecholamine content of the nerve terminals. Interestingly, **reserpine**, which inhibits vesicular storage of catecholamines and thus depletes nerve terminals of their catecholamine stores very markedly (see Ch. 7), does not block the behavioural effects of amphetamine. This is probably because amphetamine releases cytosolic rather than vesicular catecholamines (see Ch. 7). The behavioural effects of amphetamine are probably due mainly to release of dopamine rather than noradrenaline. The evidence for this is that destruction of the central noradrenergic bundle does not affect locomotor stimulation produced by amphetamine, whereas destruction of the dopamine-containing *nucleus accumbens* (see Ch. 24) or administration of neuroleptic drugs which antagonise dopamine (see Ch. 28) inhibit this response.

Amphetamine-like drugs cause marked anorexia, but with continued administration this effect wears off in a few days and food intake returns to normal. Amphetamine-like drugs differ in their relative activity in causing locomotor stimulation and anorexia (see Table 32.2). **Fenfluramine** and its D-isomer

Table 32.2 Behavioural effects of amphetamines

Drug	Locomotor stimulation	Stereotyped behaviour	Anorexia
Amphetamine	+++	+++	+++
Methylphenidate	+++	+++	+
Fenfluramine	–	–	+++

dexfenfluramine cause anorexia without stimulation (actually being somewhat sedative), and pharmacological studies suggest that this action may depend more on 5-HT release than on release of noradrenaline or dopamine. The same effect can be produced by local injection of amphetamine into the lateral hypothalamus.

In man, amphetamine causes euphoria; with intravenous injection, this can be so intense as to be described as 'orgasmic'. Subjects become confident, hyperactive and talkative, and sex drive is said to be enhanced. Fatigue, both physical and mental, is reduced by amphetamine, and many studies have shown improvement of both mental and physical performance in fatigued, though not in well-rested subjects. Mental performance is improved for simple tedious tasks much more than for difficult tasks, and amphetamines have been used to improve the performance of soldiers, military pilots and others who need to remain alert under extremely fatiguing conditions. It has also been in vogue as a means of helping students to concentrate before and during examinations, but it is likely that the improvement caused by reduction of fatigue is offset by the mistakes of over-confidence.* Amphetamine-like drugs bring about a small but significant improvement of athletic performance, particularly in endurance events, and their illicit use in competitive athletics poses a considerable problem. Fortunately, most amphetamines are excreted in the urine and are easily detected.

As appetite suppressants in man, for use in treating obesity, amphetamine derivatives have not generally been successful, mainly because their effectiveness is too short-lived and the risk of producing dependence is too great. However, a placebo-controlled trial on 822 obese Europeans showed that dexfenfluramine treatment significantly improved weight loss under a dietary and educational regime, measured over a 12-month period (Fig. 32.2), without serious side-effects.

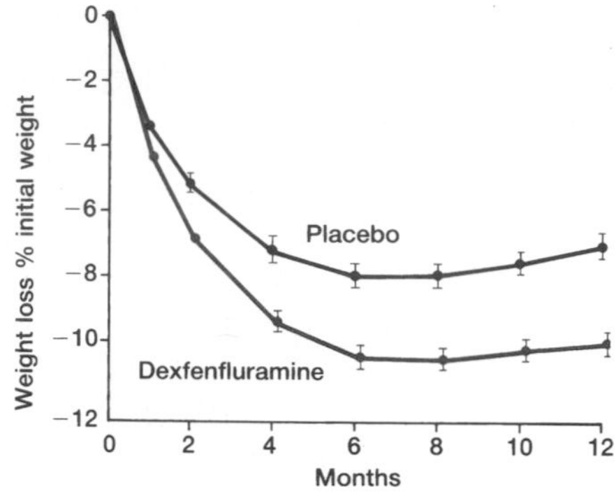

Fig. 32.2 Effect of an amphetamine analogue (dexfenfluramine) on weight loss by patients undergoing treatment for obesity. Dexfenfluramine (1–5 mg twice daily) or placebo were given under double-blind conditions. (From: Guy-Grand B et al. 1989 Lancet 1: 142–144)

Tolerance and dependence

If amphetamine is taken repeatedly over the course of a few days, which occurs when users seek to maintain the euphoric 'high' that a single dose produces, a state of 'amphetamine psychosis' often develops, which is almost indistinguishable from an acute schizophrenic attack (see Ch. 28). Visual and auditory hallucinations occur, accompanied by paranoid symptoms and aggressive behaviour. At the same time, repetitive stereotyped behaviour may develop (e.g. polishing shoes or stringing beads). The close similarity of this condition to acute paranoid schizophrenia, and the effectiveness of neuroleptic drugs in controlling it, is consistent with the dopamine theory of schizophrenia discussed in Chapter 28. When the drug is stopped after a few days, there is usually a period of deep sleep and, on awakening, the subject feels extremely lethargic, depressed and anxious (sometimes even suicidal), and is often very hungry. Even a single dose of amphetamine, which produces euphoria rather than acute psychotic symptoms, usually leaves the subject feeling tired and depressed. These after-effects may be the result of depletion of the normal stores of noradrenaline and dopamine, but the evidence for this is not clear-cut. A state of amphetamine dependence can be produced in experimental animals—thus, rats quickly learn to press a lever in order to obtain a dose of amphetamine, and also become inactive and irritable in the withdrawal phase. These effects do not occur with fenfluramine.

Tolerance to the peripheral sympathomimetic and anorexic effects of amphetamine develops rapidly, but it develops much more slowly to the other effects (locomotor stimulation and stereotyped behaviour). Dependence on amphetamine appears

*Pay heed to the awful warning of the medical student who, it is said, having taken copious dextroamphetamine, left the examination hall in confident mood, having spent 3 hours writing his name over and over again.

to be a consequence of the unpleasant after-effect that it produces, and the insistent recall of euphoria, which leads to a desire for a repeat dose. There is no clear-cut physical withdrawal syndrome such as occurs with opiates. It is estimated that only about 5% of users progress to full-blown dependence, the usual pattern being that the dose is increased as tolerance develops, and then uncontrolled 'binges' occur in which the user takes the drug repeatedly over a period of a day or more, remaining continuously intoxicated. Large doses may be consumed in such binges, with a high risk of acute toxicity, and the demand for the drug displaces all other considerations.

Experimental animals, given unlimited access to amphetamine, take it in such large amounts that they die from the cardiovascular effects within a few days. Given limited amounts, they too develop a 'binge' pattern of dependence.

Pharmacokinetic aspects

Amphetamine is readily absorbed from the gastrointestinal tract, and freely penetrates the blood–brain barrier. It does this more readily than other indirectly acting sympathomimetic amines, such as **ephedrine** or **tyramine** (Ch. 7), which probably explains why it produces more marked central effects than those drugs. It is also readily absorbed from the nasal mucosa, and is often taken by 'snorting'. Amphetamine is mainly excreted unchanged in the urine, and the rate of excretion is increased when the urine is made more acidic (see Ch. 4; Fig. 4.17). The plasma half-life of amphetamine varies from about 5 hours to 20–30 hours depending on urine flow and urinary pH.

Clinical use and unwanted effects

The uses of amphetamines are very few. Fenfluramine and dexfluramine may be useful in treating severe obesity, as discussed above. One paradoxical and controversial use is in the treatment of hyperkinetic children, who are calmed by amphetamine and by methylphenidate. The mechanism by which this happens is unknown, but the use of amphetamines for treating hyperactive children is widespread in some countries.

Narcolepsy is a disabling condition, probably a form of epilepsy, in which the patient suddenly and unpredictably falls asleep at frequent intervals during the day. Amphetamine is helpful but not completely effective.

The limited clinical usefulness of amphetamine is offset by its many unwanted effects, including hypertension, insomnia, tremors, risk of exacerbating schizophrenia and risk of dependence.

COCAINE

Cocaine (see reviews by Gawin & Ellinwood 1988, Johanson & Fischman 1989, Woolverton & Johnson 1992) is found in the leaves of a South American shrub, coca. These leaves are used for their stimulant properties by natives of South America, particularly those living at high altitude in the Andes. It appears that cocaine improves their ability to work at high altitude without excessive fatigue. Considerable mystical significance was attached to the powers of cocaine to boost the flagging human spirit, and Freud experimented with it on his patients. As a result of Freud's experiments with cocaine, his ophthalmologist colleague, Köller, obtained supplies of the drug and discovered its local anaesthetic action (Ch. 34), but the psychostimulant effects of cocaine have not proved to be clinically useful. They have, on the other hand, led to it becoming currently one of the most seriously abused substances in western countries, the incidence of its use having increased markedly during the last 10–15 years.*

Pharmacological effects

Cocaine is a potent inhibitor of catecholamine uptake by noradrenergic nerve terminals (uptake 1; see Ch. 7), and strongly enhances the effects of sympathetic nerve activity. This occurs also in the brain, and it is likely that its psychomotor stimulant effect depends on this mechanism. The effect of cocaine closely resembles that of amphetamine, causing euphoria, garrulousness, increased motor activity and a magnification of pleasure. Trained human subjects are unable to distinguish between the two drugs. With excessive dosage, tremors and convulsions, followed by respiratory and vasomotor depression, may occur, but cocaine has less tendency than amphetamines to produce stereotyped behaviour, delusions, hallucinations and paranoia. The peripheral sympathomimetic actions lead to

*In 1990, an official report estimated that 2 million Americans take cocaine regularly at least once a month. More than 10% of women attending urban prenatal clinics in US report using cocaine during pregnancy.

tachycardia, vasoconstriction and an increase in blood pressure. Body temperature may increase, owing to the increased motor activity coupled with reduced heat loss. Like amphetamine, cocaine produces no clear-cut physical dependence syndrome, but tends to cause depression and dysphoria following the initial stimulant effect. Withdrawal of cocaine after administration for a few days causes a marked deterioration of motor performance and learned behaviour, which are restored by resuming dosage with the drug. There is thus a considerable degree of psychological dependence. The pattern of dependence, evolving from occasional use through escalating dosage to compulsive binges, is identical to that seen with amphetamines.

The duration of action of cocaine (about 30 minutes when given intravenously) is much shorter than that of amphetamine.

Pharmacokinetic aspects

Cocaine is readily absorbed by many routes. For many years, illicit supplies consisted of the hydrochloride salt, which could be given by nasal inhalation or intravenously. The latter route produces an intense and immediate euphoria, but involves the danger and stigma of using a syringe. Nasal inhalation produces a less dramatic sensation, and also tends to cause atrophy and necrosis of the nasal mucosa and septum. Cocaine use increased dramatically when the free-base form ('crack') became available as a street drug. Unlike the salt, this can be smoked, giving a very rapid, intense effect with less risk and inconvenience than intravenous or nasal administration. The social, economic, and even political consequences of this small change in formulation have been far-reaching.

A cocaine metabolite is deposited in hair, and analysis of its content along the hair shaft allows the pattern of cocaine consumption to be monitored, a technique which has revealed a much higher incidence of cocaine use than was voluntarily reported. Cocaine exposure in utero can be estimated from analysis of the hair of neonates.

Cocaine is still occasionally used topically as a local anaesthetic, mainly in ophthalmology and minor nose and throat surgery, but has no other clinical uses. It is a valuable pharmacological tool for the study of catecholamine release and re-uptake, because of its relatively specific action in blocking uptake 1.

Adverse effects

Toxic effects occur commonly in cocaine abusers. The main acute dangers are cardiac dysrhythmias and coronary or cerebral thrombosis. Slowly developing damage to the myocardium can also occur, leading to heart failure, even in the absence of acute cardiac effects.

Recent evidence (see Volpe 1992) has shown that cocaine can severely impair brain development in utero. The brain size is significantly reduced in babies exposed to cocaine in pregnancy, and the incidence of neurological malformations is also increased. The incidence of ischaemic and haemorrhagic brain lesions, and of sudden infant death, is also higher in cocaine-exposed babies. Interpretation of the data is difficult because many cocaine abusers also take other illicit drugs which may affect foetal

Effects of amphetamines and cocaine

Amphetamines
- The main effects are:
  - —increased motor activity
  - —euphoria and excitement
  - —anorexia
  - —with prolonged administration, stereotyped and psychotic behaviour.
- Effects are due mainly to release of catecholamines, especially noradrenaline and dopamine.
- Stimulant effect lasts for a few hours, and is followed by depression and anxiety.
- Tolerance to the stimulant effects develops rapidly, though peripheral sympathomimetic effects may persist.
- Amphetamines may be useful in treating narcolepsy, and also (paradoxically) to control hyperkinetic children. **Dexfenfluramine** is used as an appetite-suppressant.

Cocaine
- Cocaine acts by inhibiting catecholamine uptake (especially dopamine) by nerve terminals.
- Behavioural effects of cocaine are very similar to those of amphetamines, though psychotomimetic effects are rarer. Duration of action is shorter.
- Cocaine used in pregnancy impairs foetal development, and may produce foetal malformations.

As drugs of abuse, amphetamines and cocaine produce strong psychological dependence, and carry a high risk of severe adverse reactions.

development, but the probability is that cocaine is highly detrimental.

METHYLXANTHINES

Various beverages, particularly tea, coffee and cocoa, contain methylxanthines to which they owe their mild central stimulant effects. The main compounds responsible are **caffeine** and **theophylline** (Fig. 17.4). The nuts of the cola plant also contain caffeine, which is present in cola-flavoured soft drinks. However, the most important sources, by far, are coffee and tea, which account for more than 90% of caffeine consumption. Among adults in tea and coffee drinking countries, the average daily caffeine consumption is about 200 mg. Further information on the pharmacology and toxicology of caffeine is presented by Arnaud (1987) and Nehlig et al. (1992).

Pharmacological effects

Methylxanthines have the following major pharmacological actions:

- CNS stimulation (including respiratory stimulation)
- diuresis (see Ch. 18)
- stimulation of cardiac muscle (see Ch. 13)
- relaxation of smooth muscle, especially bronchial muscle (see Ch. 17).

The latter two effects resemble those of β-adrenoceptor stimulation (see Ch. 7). This is thought to be because methylxanthines (especially theophylline) inhibit phosphodiesterase, which is responsible for the intracellular metabolism of cAMP (Ch. 2). They thus increase intracellular cAMP and produce effects that mimic those of mediators that stimulate adenylate cyclase. Methylxanthines also antagonise many of the effects of adenosine, acting on both A_1 and A_2 receptors (see Ch. 8), and it is possible, but unproven, that some of their effects result from this mechanism (see Nehlig et al. 1992). The concentration of caffeine reached in plasma and brain after 2–3 cups of strong coffee—about 100 μM—is sufficient to produce appreciable adenosine receptor block, and a small degree of phosphodiesterase inhibition. The diuretic effect probably results from vasodilatation of the afferent glomerular arteriole, causing an increased glomerular filtration rate.

Caffeine and theophylline have very similar stimulant effects on the central nervous system. Human subjects experience a reduction of fatigue, leading to insomnia, with improved concentration and a clearer flow of thought. This is confirmed by objective studies which have shown that caffeine reduces reaction time, and produces an increase in the speed at which simple calculations can be performed (though without much improvement in accuracy). Performance at motor tasks, such as typing and simulated driving, is also improved, particularly in fatigued subjects. Mental tasks, such as syllable-learning, association tests and so on, are also facilitated by moderate doses (up to about 200 mg caffeine, or about 3 cups of coffee) but inhibited by larger doses. By comparison with amphetamines, methylxanthines produce less locomotor stimulation and do not induce euphoria, stereotyped behaviour patterns or a psychotic state, but their effects on fatigue and mental function are similar.

Tolerance and habituation develop to a small extent, but much less than with amphetamines, and withdrawal effects are slight. Caffeine does not lead to self-administration in animals, and it cannot be classified as a dependence-producing drug.

Clinical use and unwanted effects

There are few clinical uses for **caffeine**. It is included with aspirin in some preparations for treating headaches and other aches and pains, and with

Methylxanthines

- Caffeine and theophylline produce psychomotor stimulant effects.
- Average caffeine consumption from beverages is about 200 mg/d.
- Main psychological effect is reduced fatigue and improved mental performance, without euphoria. Even large doses do not cause stereotyped behaviour or psychotomimetic effects.
- Methylxanthines may act partly by inhibiting phosphodiesterase, thus producing effects similar to those of β-adrenoceptor agonists, and partly by antagonism at purine receptors (A_1- and A_2-subtypes).
- Peripheral actions are exerted mainly on heart, bronchiolar smooth muscle and kidney.
- Theophylline is used clinically as a bronchodilator; caffeine is not used clinically.

ergotamine in some anti-migraine preparations, the object being to produce a mildly agreeable sense of alertness. **Theophylline** is used mainly as a bronchodilator in treating severe asthmatic attacks (see Ch. 17). Caffeine has few unwanted side effects, and is safe even in very large doses. In vitro tests show that it has a quite strong mutagenic effect, and there is evidence that large doses are teratogenic in animals. However, epidemiological studies have so far not revealed any carcinogenic or teratogenic effect of tea or coffee drinking in man.

PSYCHOTOMIMETIC DRUGS

Psychotomimetic drugs (also referred to as *psychedelic* or *hallucinogenic* drugs) are characterised by the fact that they affect thought, perception and mood, without causing marked psychomotor stimulation or depression. Thoughts and perceptions tend to become distorted and dream-like, rather than being merely sharpened or dulled, and the change in mood is likewise more complex than a simple shift in the direction of euphoria or depression. Not surprisingly, the categorisation of these drugs is very imprecise, and there is no sharp dividing line between the effects of, say, cocaine and those of LSD or cannabis. Psychotomimetic drugs fall broadly into two groups:

- Those with a chemical resemblance to known neurotransmitters (catecholamines or 5-HT). These include **LSD** and **psilocybin**, which are related to 5-HT, and **mescaline**, which is similar in structure to amphetamine.
- Drugs unrelated to monoamine neurotransmitters, for example **cannabis** and **phencyclidine**.

LSD, PSILOCYBIN AND MESCALINE

LSD is an exceptionally potent psychotomimetic drug, capable of producing very marked effects in man in doses less than 1 μg/kg. It is a chemical derivative of lysergic acid (see Fig. 9.4), which occurs in the cereal fungus, ergot (see Ch. 9), and was first synthesised by Hoffman in 1943. Hoffman deliberately swallowed about 250 μg of LSD, and wrote 30 years later of the experience: '. . . the faces of those around me appeared as grotesque coloured masks . . . marked motoric unrest, alternating with paralysis . . . heavy feeling in the head, limbs and entire body, as if they were filled with lead . . . clear recognition of my condition, in which state I sometimes observed, in the manner of an independent observer, that I shouted half insanely.' These effects lasted for a few hours, after which Hoffman fell asleep, 'and awoke next morning feeling perfectly well'. Despite these dramatic psychological effects, LSD has few physiological effects. **Mescaline**, which is derived from a Mexican cactus and has been known as a hallucinogenic agent for many centuries, was made famous by Aldous Huxley in *The Doors of Perception*. **Psilocybin** is obtained from a fungus, and has very similar properties. Both have basically similar effects to LSD but are much less potent.

Pharmacological effects

The main effects of these drugs are on mental function, most notably an alteration of perception in such a way that sights and sounds appear distorted and fantastic. Hallucinations—visual, auditory, tactile or olfactory—also occur, and sensory modalities may become confused, so that sounds are perceived as visions. Thought processes tend to become illogical and disconnected, but users generally retain insight into the fact that their disturbance is drug-induced. Occasionally, LSD produces a syndrome that is extremely disturbing to the subject (the 'bad trip') in which the hallucinatory experience takes on a menacing quality, and may be accompanied by paranoid delusions. This sometimes goes so far as to produce homicide or suicide attempts, and in many respects, the state has elements in common with acute schizophrenic illness. Furthermore, 'flashbacks' of the hallucinatory experience have been reported weeks or months later.

The main effects of psychotomimetic drugs are subjective, so it is not surprising that animal tests which reliably predict psychotomimetic activity in man have not been devised. Attempts to measure changes in perception by behavioural conditioning studies have given variable results, but some authors have claimed that effects consistent with increased sensory 'generalisation' (i.e. a tendency to respond similarly to any sensory stimulus) can be detected in this way. One of the more bizarre tests involves disorganisation of web-spinning patterns in spiders, whose normal elegantly symmetrical webs become jumbled and erratic if the animals are treated with LSD.

Dependence and adverse effects

Neither LSD nor other psychotomimetic agents (except for **phencyclidine**; see below) are self-administered by experimental animals. Indeed, they can be shown to have aversive rather than reinforcing properties in behavioural tests, which stands in marked contrast to most of the drugs that are widely abused by humans. Tolerance to the effects of LSD develops quite quickly, and there is cross-tolerance between it and most other psychotomimetics.

There is no physical withdrawal syndrome in animals or man. In peripheral tissues, LSD acts as an antagonist at 5-HT receptors, but in the central nervous system it is believed to work mainly as an agonist. Neurophysiological studies (see Cooper et al. 1991) show that LSD directly inhibits the firing of 5-HT-containing neurons in the raphe nuclei (see Ch. 24), apparently by acting as an agonist on the inhibitory autoreceptors of these cells (see Ch. 8). The action of mescaline is apparently different, however, and exerted mainly on noradrenergic neurons. It is still quite unclear how changes in cell firing rates might be related to the psychotomimetic action of these drugs.

There has been much concern over reports that LSD and other psychotomimetic drugs, as well as causing potentially dangerous 'bad trips', can lead to more persistent mental disorder. There are recorded instances in which altered perception and hallucinations have lasted for up to 3 weeks following a single dose of LSD. There are also reports of a persistent state resembling paranoid schizophrenia, which responds to antipsychotic drugs but may recur later (see Abraham & Aldridge 1993). It is now believed that LSD can occasionally give rise to long-lasting psychopathology. This, coupled with the fact that the occasional 'bad trip' can result in severe injury through violent behaviour, means that LSD and other psychotomimetics must be regarded as highly dangerous drugs, far removed from the image of peaceful 'experience enhancers' that the hippy subculture of the 1960s so enthusiastically espoused.

PHENCYCLIDINE

Phencyclidine was originally synthesised as a possible intravenous anaesthetic agent, but was found to produce in many patients a period of disorientation and hallucinations following recovery of consciousness. **Ketamine** (see Ch. 26), a close analogue of phencyclidine, is better as an anaesthetic, though it too can cause symptoms of disorientation. Phencyclidine is now of interest mainly as a drug of abuse (now declining in popularity), and because of some intriguing problems raised by its mode of action and possible relationship to schizophrenia (see Henderson 1982, Sonders et al. 1988, Johnson & Jones 1990).

Pharmacological effects

The effects of phencyclidine resemble those of other psychotomimetic drugs, but also include analgesia, which was one of the reasons for its introduction as an anaesthetic agent. It can also cause stereotyped motor behaviour, like amphetamine. It has the same reported tendency as LSD to cause occasional 'bad trips', and to lead to recurrent psychotic episodes. Its mode of action at a cellular level is not well

Psychotomimetic drugs

- The main types are:
  - —LSD, psilocybin and mescaline (actions related to 5-HT and catecholamines)
  - —phencyclidine.
- Their main effect is to cause sensory changes, hallucinations and delusions, partly resembling symptoms of acute schizophrenia.
- They are not used clinically, but are important as drugs of abuse.
- LSD is exceptionally potent, producing a long-lasting sense of dissociation and disordered thought, sometimes with frightening hallucinations and delusions which can lead to violence. Hallucinatory episodes can recur after a long interval.
- LSD and phencyclidine precipitate schizophrenic attacks in susceptible patients, and LSD may cause long-lasting psychopathological changes.
- LSD appears to act as an agonist at 5-HT receptors, and suppresses electrical activity in 5-HT raphe neurons, an action which appears to correlate with psychotomimetic activity.
- They do not cause physical dependence, and tend to be aversive, rather than reinforcing, in animal models.
- The mechanism of action of phencyclidine is complex; it binds to the σ-opioid receptor, and also blocks the glutamate-activated NMDA-receptor channel, as well as interacting with other neurotransmitter systems.

understood. Specific high-affinity binding sites occur on neuronal membranes, particularly in the frontal cortex and hippocampus, and it appears to have two distinct sites of action. One site is the σ-receptor described for various opioids of the benzomorphan type (Ch. 31), while the other is the glutamate-operated ion channel (the NMDA-receptor channel; see Ch. 24) which is blocked by phencyclidine, as well as by ketamine. The σ-opioid receptor is generally believed to mediate the effects of dysphoria and hallucinations produced by certain opiates, and may account for the psychotomimetic effects of phencyclidine. At present it is unclear whether the NMDA-channel action is important. However, studies with **dizocilpine**, a NMDA-channel-blocker (see Ch. 24) that lacks affinity for the σ-opioid receptor, suggest that it has much less psychotomimetic activity than phencyclidine, though other behavioural effects are similar. Which, if either, of the two phencyclidine-binding sites is the key to its behavioural effects remains undecided. One prominent question, however, is whether there may be an endogenous ligand for either of the phencyclidine-binding sites, and, if so, whether such substances might be involved in the causation of schizophrenia (see Debonnel 1993).

REFERENCES AND FURTHER READING

Abraham H D, Aldridge A M 1993 Adverse consequences of lysergic acid diethylamide. Addiction 88: 1327–1334

Arnaud M J 1987 The pharmacology of caffeine. Prog Drug Res 31: 273–313

Cooper J R, Bloom F E, Roth R H 1991 The biochemical basis of neuropharmacology. Oxford University Press, New York

Debonnel G 1993 Current hypotheses on sigma receptors and their physiological role: possible implications in psychiatry. J Psychiat Neurosci 18: 157–172

Gawin F H, Ellinwood E H 1988 Cocaine and other stimulants. N Engl J Med 318: 1173–1182

Lefebvre P, Turner P 1989 International trial of longterm dexfenfluramine in obesity. Lancet 1: 142–144

Henderson G 1982 Phenylcyclidine, a widely used but little understood psychotomimetic agent. Trends Pharmacol Sci 3: 248–250

Johanson C-E, Fischman M W 1989 The pharmacology of cocaine related to its abuse. Pharmacol Rev 41: 3–47

Johnson K M, Jones S M 1990 Neuropharmacology of phencyclidine: basic mechanisms and therapeutic potential. Annu Rev Pharmacol Toxicol 30: 707–750

Nehlig A, Daval J-L, Debry G 1992 Caffeine and the central nervous system: mechanisms of action, biochemical, metabolic and psychostimulant effects. Brain Res Rev 17: 139–170

Sonders M S, Keana J F W, Weber E 1988 Phencyclidine and psychotomimetic sigma opiates: recent insights into their biochemical and physiological sites of action. Trends Neurosci 11: 37–40

Volpe J J 1992 Effect of cocaine on the fetus. New Engl J Med 327: 399–407

Woolverton W L, Johnson K M 1992 Neurobiology of cocaine abuse. Trends Pharmacol Sci 13: 193–200

33

DRUG DEPENDENCE AND DRUG ABUSE

There are many drugs that human beings consume because they choose to, and not because they are advised to by doctors. Society in general disapproves, because in most cases there is a recognisable social cost; in some cases this cost is considered so far to outweigh the individual benefit that drug usage has been declared illegal. In western societies, the three most commonly-used non-therapeutic drugs are **caffeine**, **nicotine** and **ethanol**, all of which are legally and freely available. There is a much larger number of drugs which are widely used, though their manufacture, sale and consumption has been declared illegal in most western countries, except when it is under the control of the medical profession. A list of the more important ones is given in Table 33.1. This list does not include the increasing number of drugs that are used illicitly by body-builders and sportsmen to enhance their performance, an account of which is presented by Mottram (1988).

Table 33.1 The main drugs of abuse

Type	Examples	Dependence liability	Discussed in
Narcotic analgesics	Morphine	V. strong	Ch. 31
	Heroin	V. strong	Ch. 31
General CNS depressants	Ethanol	Strong	This chapter
	Barbiturates	Strong	Ch. 27
	Methaqualone	Moderate	Ch. 27
	Glutethimide	Moderate	Ch. 27
	Anaesthetics	Moderate	Ch. 26
	Solvents	Strong	–
Anxiolytic drugs	Benzodiazepines	Moderate	Ch. 27
Psychomotor stimulants	Amphetamines	Strong	Ch. 32
	Cocaine	V. strong	Ch. 32
	Caffeine	Weak	Ch. 32
	Nicotine	V. strong	This chapter
Psychotomimetic agents	LSD	Weak or absent	Ch. 32
	Mescaline	Weak or absent	Ch. 32
	Phencyclidine	Moderate	Ch. 32
	Cannabis	Weak or absent	This chapter

The reasons why a particular group of drugs should come to be used in a way that constitutes a problem to society are complex and largely outside the scope of this book. The drug and its pharmacological activity are only the starting point, for drug-taking is clearly seen by society in a quite different light from other forms of self-gratification, such as opera-going or sex. Furthermore, the 'drugs of abuse' form an extremely heterogeneous pharmacological group; we can find little in common between, say, morphine, cocaine and barbiturates. What links them together is that people enjoy the sensation that they produce and tend to want to repeat it. It becomes a problem when:

- the want becomes so insistent that it dominates the lifestyle of the individual and prevents him or her from living in a way that the rest of society can accept
- when the habit itself causes actual harm to the individual or the community.

Examples of the latter kind of problem are the mental incapacity and eventual liver damage caused by ethanol, the host of diseases associated with smoking, the serious danger of overdosage with most narcotics, and the criminal behaviour which often ensues when an addict needs to finance his habit.

In this chapter we discuss some general aspects of drug dependence and drug abuse, and describe the pharmacology of three important drugs which have no place in therapy but are consumed in large amounts, namely **nicotine**, **ethanol** and **cannabis**. Other drugs with abuse potential are described elsewhere in this book (see Table 33.1). For further information, including discussion of non-pharmacological aspects of drug abuse, see Hofmann (1983), Pratt (1991), Winger et al. (1992).

THE NATURE OF DRUG DEPENDENCE

Drug dependence is the term used to describe the state of affairs when administration of the drug is sought compulsively, leading to disturbed behaviour if necessary to secure its supply. Use continues despite the adverse psychological or physical effects produced by the drug.

The older term *drug addiction* generally refers to the state of physical dependence (see below), but is not clearly defined. *Drug abuse* and *substance abuse* are more general terms, meaning any use of illicit substances. *Tolerance*—the decrease in pharmacological effect on repeated administration of the drug—often accompanies the state of dependence, and it is possible that related mechanisms account for both phenomena (see below).

The common feature of the various types of psychoactive drugs that can engender dependence is that all produce a *rewarding* effect. In animal studies, where this cannot be inferred directly, it is manifest as a *reinforcing* property (i.e. an increase in the probability of occurrence of any behaviour that results in the drug being administered). Thus, with all dependence-producing drugs, the phenomenon of spontaneous self-administration can be demonstrated in animal studies. Coupled with the direct rewarding effect of the drug, there is usually also a process of *habituation*, or adaptation, when the drug is given repeatedly or continuously, such that cessation of the drug has an aversive effect, from which the subject will attempt to escape by self-administration of the drug. The physical withdrawal syndrome, associated with the state of physical dependence, is one manifestation of this type of habituation; the intensity and nature of physical withdrawal symptoms varies from one class of drug to another, being particularly marked with opioids, and is probably less important in sustaining drug-seeking behaviour than psychological habituation, which leads to a craving that is not related to physical symptoms. A degree of physical dependence is often produced when patients receive opioid analgesics in hospital for several days, but this almost never leads to addiction. On the other hand, addicts who recover fully from the physical abstinence syndrome are still extremely likely to revert to drug-taking later. Thus, physical dependence does not seem to be the major factor in long-term drug dependence.

In summary, three main factors are involved in drug dependence:

- the inherent *reward* property of the drug
- *habituation*, which leads to an aversive effect on termination of the drug (physical withdrawal syndrome)
- psychological *craving* associated with abstinence.

There is now some understanding of the neurobiological basis of reward and habituation, which is providing some hope of effective therapeutic intervention in the difficult problem of treating drug-

> **Drug dependence**
>
> - Dependence is defined as an excessive craving which develops as a result of repeated administration of the drug.
> - Dependence occurs with a wide range of psychotropic drugs, acting by many different mechanisms.
> - The common feature of dependence-producing drugs may be that they have a positive reinforcing action ('reward') associated with activation of the mesolimbic dopaminergic pathway.
> - Dependence is usually associated with (a) tolerance to the drug, which can arise by various biochemical mechanisms; (b) a physical abstinence syndrome, which varies in type and intensity for different classes of drug; (c) psychological dependence (craving), which may be associated with the tolerance-producing biochemical changes.
> - Psychological dependence, which usually outlasts the physical withdrawal syndrome, is the major factor leading to relapse among treated addicts.

dependence. In man, however, the drug habit is evidently sustained by processes that are more complex and long-lasting than any of the neurobiological changes that can be observed in experimental animals, for there is a very high rate of relapse among drug-takers long after the obvious withdrawal effects have subsided.

REWARD PATHWAYS

One reward pathway, which appears to be common to many types of dependence-producing drugs, involves the mesolimbic dopaminergic neurons (the A10 group; see Ch. 24) running, via the medial forebrain bundle, from the ventral midbrain to the *nucleus accumbens* and limbic region (see Fig. 24.3). Many dependence-producing drugs, such as opioids, nicotine, amphetamines, ethanol and cocaine, increase the release of dopamine in the nucleus accumbens, as shown by microdialysis and other techniques. Some of these increase the electrical activity of A10 cells, whereas others, such as amphetamine and cocaine, act to cause dopamine release or prevent its re-uptake (see Ch. 6). Chemical or surgical interruption of this dopaminergic pathway consistently impairs drug-seeking behaviours in many experimental situations (see Koob 1992). Administration of neuroleptic drugs with dopamine antagonist activity (see Ch. 28) reduces drug-seeking activity in some, though not all, animal models of dependence, though such drugs have not proved clinically useful in treating dependence. This dopaminergic pathway is certainly not the only reward pathway involved in drug dependence. There is evidence for a separate opioid-mediated reward pathway, as well as for involvement of other mediators, particularly 5-HT (see Sellers et al 1992) and GABA. Whether these act by modulation of the mesolimbic dopamine pathway, or by independent mechanisms, is not clear. In general, manipulations that increase 5-HT activity (e.g. 5-HT agonists or uptake blockers; see Chs 9 and 27), reduce drug-seeking behaviour. 5-HT uptake inhibitors (e.g. **zimeldine**) or 5-HT agonists (e.g. **buspirone**) reduce slightly the alcohol consumption in alcoholic patients, but long-term benefit has not been established (see Sellers et al. 1992). Thus the neurochemical manipulation of the reward pathway, though attractive in theory as an approach to treating drug dependence, has had relatively little success so far.

HABITUATION MECHANISMS

The cellular mechanisms involved in habituation to the effects of drugs such as opioids and cocaine have been studied in some detail (see Nestler 1993, Ch. 31). Both classes of drug produce, on chronic administration, an increase in the activity of adenylate cyclase in brain regions such as the *nucleus accumbens*, which compensates for their acute inhibitory effect on cAMP formation, and produces a rebound increase in cAMP when the drug is terminated (see Fig. 31.10). Chronic opioid treatment increases the amount, not only of adenylate cyclase itself, but also of other components of the signalling pathway, including the G-proteins and various protein kinases. This increase in cAMP affects many cellular functions through the increased activity of various cAMP-dependent protein kinases, which control the activity of ion channels (making the cells more excitable), as well as various enzymes and transcription factors. Similar effects also occur with cocaine, but much less is known about other dependence-producing drugs, so it is not known whether this type of cAMP up-regulation is a general property of such drugs.

GENETIC FACTORS

Epidemiological studies, particularly in alcoholism, show clear evidence of a genetic component in the pathogenesis of drug abuse. Twin studies suggest that genetic factors contribute up to 60% of an individual's susceptibility to alcohol abuse. There are also well-characterised genetic strains of rats and mice which differ in their tendency to self-administer alcohol, or in the incidence of withdrawal symptoms following chronic opioid administration. Genetic analysis of alcoholics and multiple drug abusers has shown a higher frequency of a particular mutation (termed A_1) of the dopamine D_2-receptor gene in these patients compared with controls (see Uhl et al. 1993). This is of interest in relation to the proposed role of dopaminergic pathways in drug-induced reward (see above), but its significance is not known at present.

NICOTINE AND TOBACCO

Tobacco growing, chewing and smoking was indigenous throughout the Americas and Australia at the time that European explorers first visited these places. Smoking spread through Europe during the sixteenth century, coming to England mainly as a result of its enthusiastic espousal by Raleigh at the court of Elizabeth I. James I strongly disapproved of both Raleigh and tobacco, and initiated the first anti-smoking campaign in the early seventeenth century with the support of the Royal College of Physicians. Parliament responded by imposing a substantial duty on tobacco, thereby setting up the dilemma (from which we show no sign of being able to escape) of giving the state an economic interest in the continuation of smoking at the same time that its official expert advisers were issuing emphatic warnings about its dangers.

Until the latter half of the nineteenth century, tobacco was smoked in pipes, and by men. Cigarette manufacture began at the end of the nineteenth century, and now cigarettes account for more than 90% of tobacco consumption. Cigarette smoking by women began after the First World War; the proportion of cigarette smokers is currently about 30% in both men and women. Cigarette sales have more or less levelled off (Fig. 33.1), possibly as a result of increasing adverse publicity, restrictions on advertising, and the compulsory publication of health warnings. Filter cigarettes (which give a somewhat lower delivery of tar and nicotine than standard cigarettes) and low-tar cigarettes (which

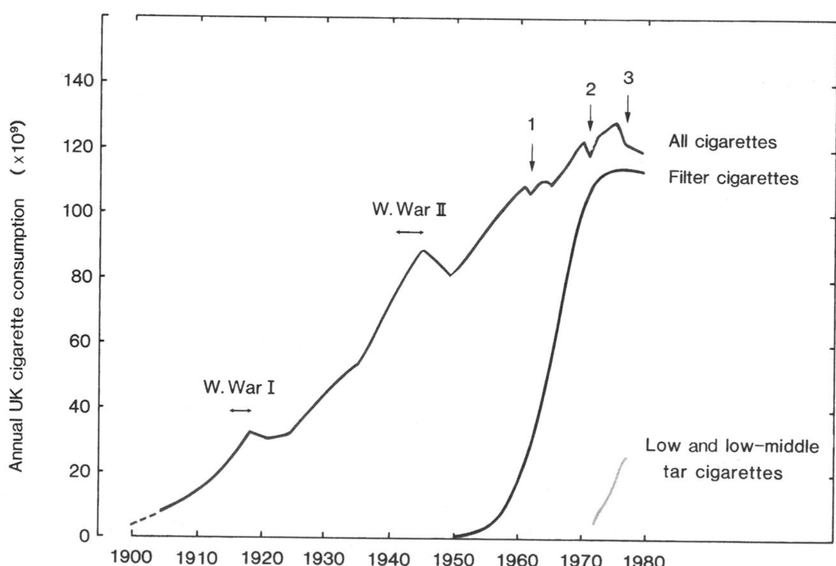

Fig. 33.1 Cigarette consumption in UK 1900–1980. Numbers 1, 2 and 3 refer to publication of Royal College of Physicians reports on smoking and health. (From: Ashton H, Stepney R 1982 Smoking psychology and pharmacology. Tavistock Publications, London)

are also low in nicotine) constitute an increasing proportion of the total. What is concealed by figures of total cigarette sales is a substantial change in individual smoking habits, with a trend towards fewer smokers each smoking more cigarettes. Furthermore, the decrease in the UK has happened mainly among middle-class adults; smoking by low-income adults and children of all income groups has not declined.

Useful reviews on nicotine and smoking include Benowitz (1988), Grenhoff & Svensson (1989), Stolerman & Shoaib (1991), Lee & D'Alonzo (1993).

PHARMACOLOGICAL EFFECTS OF SMOKING

Nicotine appears to be the only pharmacologically active substance in tobacco smoke, apart from carcinogenic tars and carbon monoxide (see below). The acute effects of smoking can be mimicked by injection of nicotine, and are blocked by **mecamylamine**, an antagonist at neuronal nicotinic acetylcholine receptors (see Ch. 6).

Effects on the central nervous system

The central effects of nicotine are complex and cannot be summed up overall simply in terms of stimulation or inhibition. At the cellular level, nicotine causes neuronal excitation by opening ion channels, exactly as it does in autonomic ganglia and the neuromuscular synapse (Ch. 6). The nicotinic receptors in the brain are slightly different from those at the neuromuscular junction, both in terms of their pharmacological specificity and their molecular structure, but they function in the same way as excitatory cholinergic receptors. It is possible that the overall effect of nicotine reflects a balance between activation of nicotinic acetylcholine receptors, causing neuronal excitation, and desensitisation, causing synaptic block. However, there is no direct evidence for the latter mechanism. Indeed, the ability of mecamylamine, a centrally acting nicotinic-receptor antagonist, to block rather than mimic the behavioural effects of nicotine suggests that desensitisation is not important.

At the spinal level, an inhibition of spinal reflexes occurs, and this produces skeletal muscle relaxation which can be measured by electromyography. It is probably due to stimulation of the Renshaw cells in the ventral horn of the spinal cord (see Ch. 25); these cells receive a cholinergic innervation from motoneuron collaterals and exert an inhibitory effect on the motoneurons. The higher level functioning of the brain, as reflected in the subjective sense of alertness or by the EEG pattern, can be affected in either direction by nicotine, according to dose and circumstances. Smokers report that smoking wakes them up when they are drowsy and calms them down when they are tense, and EEG recordings broadly bear this out. It also seems that small doses of nicotine tend to cause arousal, whereas large doses do the reverse. Tests of motor and sensory performance (e.g. reaction time measurements or vigilance tests) in humans have generally shown improvement after smoking, but the studies are difficult to interpret. This is because no satisfactory placebo, in the form of a nicotine-free smoking medium indistinguishable from tobacco, is available. Measures of learning in rats (e.g. in a maze-running test) generally show improvement in response to nicotine. Some extremely elaborate tests have been conducted to see, for example, whether the effect of nicotine on performance and aggression varies according to the amount of stress. In one, the subject first has to name the colours of a series of squares (low stress), and then has to name the colours in which the names of other colours are written (high stress). The difference between the scores, reflecting the extent by which performance is affected by stress, was diminished by smoking. Some tests border on nasty-mindedness, such as one in which subjects played a complicated logical game with a computer which initially played fair and then began to cheat randomly, causing stress and aggression in the subjects and a decline in their performance. Smoking, it was reported, did not reduce the anger, but did reduce the decline in performance.

Peripheral effects

The peripheral effects of small doses of nicotine result from stimulation of autonomic ganglia (see Ch. 6) and of peripheral sensory receptors, mainly in the heart and lungs. Stimulation of these receptors elicits various autonomic reflex responses, causing tachycardia, increased cardiac output and increased arterial pressure, reduction of gastrointestinal motility and sweating. When people smoke for the first time, they usually experience nausea and sometimes vomit, probably because of stimulation of sensory receptors in the stomach. All of these effects decline with repeated dosage, though the central effects remain. Secretion of adrenaline and noradrenaline from the adrenal medulla contribute to the cardiovascular effects, and release of antidiuretic hormone from the posterior pituitary causes a decrease in urine flow. The plasma concentration of free fatty acids is increased, probably due to sympathetic stimulation and adrenaline secretion.

Smokers weigh, on average, about 4 kg less than non-smokers, mainly because of reduced food intake; giving up smoking usually causes weight gain.

PHARMACOKINETIC ASPECTS

An average cigarette contains about 0.8 g of tobacco and 9–17 mg of nicotine, of which about 10% is normally absorbed by the smoker. This fraction varies greatly with the habits of the smoker and the type of cigarette. Nicotine is the only pharmacologically active constituent of tobacco smoke that is present in sufficient quantity to produce systemic effects. In heavy smokers, carbon monoxide may also be important.

Nicotine in cigarette smoke is rapidly absorbed from the lungs, but poorly from the mouth and nasopharynx. Thus, inhalation is required to give appreciable absorption of nicotine, each puff delivering a distinct bolus of drug to the central nervous system. Pipe or cigar smoke is less acidic than cigarette smoke, and the nicotine tends to be absorbed from the mouth and nasopharynx, rather than the lungs. Absorption is considerably slower than from inhaled cigarette smoke, and a later and longer-lasting peak in the plasma nicotine concentration occurs with pipe or cigar smoking than with cigarette smoking (Fig. 33.2). An average cigarette, smoked over 10 minutes, causes the plasma nicotine concentration to rise to 20–30 ng/ml (130–200 nmol/l), falling to about half within 10 minutes and then more slowly over the next 1–2 hours. The rapid decline results mainly from redistribution between the blood and other tissues; the slower decline is due to hepatic metabolism, mainly by oxidation to an inactive ketone metabolite, **cotinine**. This has a long plasma half-life, and measurement of plasma cotinine concentration provides a useful measure of smoking behaviour.

TOLERANCE AND DEPENDENCE

As with all drugs of abuse, three separate but related processes—tolerance, physical dependence and psychological dependence—contribute to the overall state of dependence, in which taking the drug becomes compulsive.

The effects of nicotine associated with peripheral

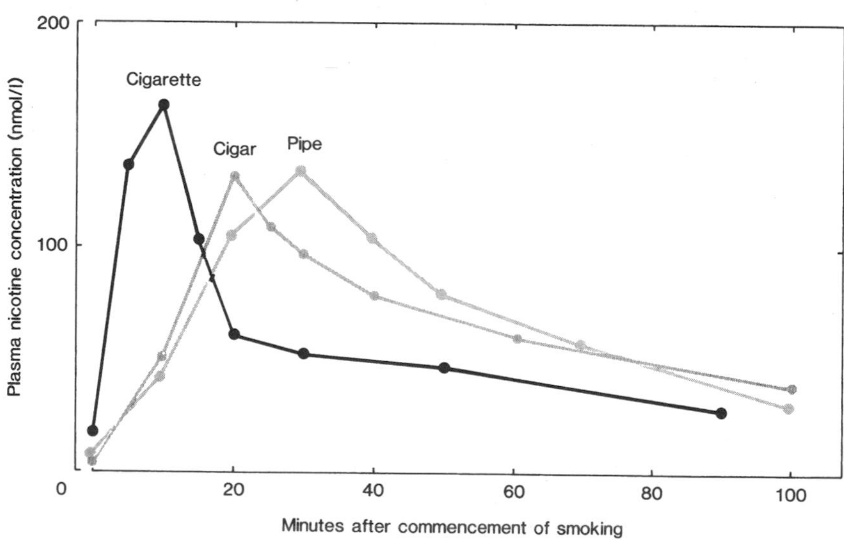

Fig. 33.2 Nicotine concentration in plasma during smoking. The subjects were habitual smokers who smoked a cigarette, cigar or pipe according to their usual habit. (From: Bowman W C, Rand M 1980 Textbook of pharmacology. Blackwell, Oxford, Ch. 4)

Tobacco smoking

- The total number of cigarettes smoked in Britain is now declining slowly, though the consumption per smoker is tending to increase.
- The prevalence of smoking is now 30–35% of the adult population, and equal in both sexes.
- Nicotine is the only pharmacologically active agent in tobacco, apart from carcinogenic tars and carbon monoxide.
- The amount of nicotine absorbed from an average cigarette is about 1.5 mg, which causes the plasma nicotine concentration to reach 130–200 nmol/l. These values depend greatly on the type of cigarette, and on the extent of inhalation of the smoke.

ganglionic stimulation show rapid tolerance, perhaps as a result of desensitisation of nicotinic acetylcholine receptors by nicotine. With large doses of nicotine this desensitisation produces a block of ganglionic transmission rather than stimulation (see Ch. 6). Tolerance to the central effects of nicotine (e.g. in the arousal response) is much less than in the periphery. Surprisingly, receptor-labelling studies have shown that chronic nicotine administration causes an *increase* in the number of nicotinic receptors in the brain. This also occurs in the brains of heavy smokers. It is in contrast to the usual effect of receptor agonists (for example β-adrenoceptor agonists), which is to down-regulate receptors. However, the cellular effects of nicotine are diminished, so it is possible that the additional binding sites represent desensitised, rather than functional, receptors.

The addictive nature of tobacco smoking is due to dependence on nicotine, and not to dependence on the act of smoking. Nicotine-free cigarettes have been found not to provide an acceptable alternative for habitual smokers. Various animal experiments confirm that nicotine is addictive. Thus, rats choose to drink dilute nicotine solution in preference to water if given a choice, and will perform various tasks to obtain nicotine as a reward. In a situation in which lever-pressing causes an injection of nicotine to be delivered, rats quickly learn to self-administer it. Similarly, monkeys who have been trained to smoke, by providing a reward in response to smoking behaviour, will continue to do so spontaneously (i.e. unrewarded) if the smoking medium contains nicotine, but not if nicotine-free tobacco is offered instead. The inherent 'reward' property of nicotine revealed in these tests is inhibited by mecamylamine, showing that it depends on receptor activation. Thus, if monkeys are habituated to tobacco smoking so that they choose to puff tobacco smoke in preference to warm air, administration of mecamylamine causes them to switch to puffing air instead of tobacco smoke. Like other dependence-producing drugs (see above) nicotine causes excitation of the mesolimbic pathway, and increased dopamine release in the *nucleus accumbens*.

A physical withdrawal syndrome occurs in both humans and experimental animals accustomed to regular nicotine administration. Its main features are increased irritability, impaired performance of psychomotor tasks, aggressiveness and sleep disturbance. The withdrawal syndrome is much less severe than that produced by opiates, and it can be alleviated not only by nicotine but also by amphetamine, a

Pharmacology of nicotine

- At a cellular level, nicotine acts on nicotinic acetylcholine receptors to cause neuronal excitation. Its central effects are blocked by receptor antagonists such as mecamylamine.
- The overall effects of nicotine consist of a mixture of inhibitory and excitatory effects.
- Nicotine shows reinforcing properties, associated with increased activity in the mesolimbic dopaminergic pathway, and self administration can be elicited in animal studies.
- EEG changes show an arousal response, and subjects report increased alertness. At the same time, subjects report a reduction of anxiety and tension.
- Learning, particularly under stress, is facilitated by nicotine.
- Peripheral effects of nicotine are due mainly to ganglionic stimulation: tachycardia, increased blood pressure and reduced gastrointestinal motility. Tolerance develops rapidly to these effects.
- Nicotine is metabolised, mainly in the liver, within 1–2 hours. The inactive product, cotinine, has a long plasma half-life, and can be used as a measure of smoking habits.
- Nicotine gives rise to tolerance, physical dependence and psychological dependence (craving), and is highly addictive.
- Nicotine replacement therapy (chewing gum or skin patch preparations) improves the chances of giving up smoking, but only when combined with active counselling.

finding consistent with the postulated role of dopamine in the reward pathway. The physical withdrawal syndrome is probably important in the short-term maintenance of the smoking habit, but it disappears in 2–3 weeks, though the craving for cigarettes persists for much longer than this; relapses during attempts to give up cigarette smoking occur most commonly at a time when the physical withdrawal syndrome has long since subsided.

HARMFUL EFFECTS OF SMOKING

It is well established that the life expectation of smokers is shorter than that of non-smokers. For example, in a study of British doctors (see Report of Royal College of Physicians 1971), the proportion of heavy smokers dying between the ages of 35 and 65 years was estimated to be 40% compared with 15% for non-smokers. Many studies have concluded that smoking constitutes a major risk to health (see Report of Royal College of Physicians 1977, US Public Health Service Reports 1981, 1982, 1983).

The main health risks are:

- *Cancer*, particularly of the lung, but also of the mouth, throat, oesophagus, pancreas and kidney. Smoking 20 cigarettes per day is estimated to increase the risk of lung cancer about 10-fold. Lung cancer accounts for about half of the total cancer deaths in men, and about 90% is estimated to be caused by smoking. Pipe and cigar smoking carry much less risk than cigarette smoking, though the risk is still appreciable. Leukaemia is also more common in smokers.
- *Coronary heart disease*, and other forms of peripheral vascular disease. The mortality among men aged 55–64 from coronary thrombosis is about 60% greater in men who smoke 20 cigarettes per day than in non-smokers. Even though the adverse effect of smoking is less striking than it is with lung cancer, the actual number of excess deaths associated with smoking is larger, because coronary heart disease is so common. Other kinds of peripheral vascular disease (e.g. stroke, intermittent claudication and diabetic gangrene) are also strongly smoking-related. Many studies have suggested that nicotine is mainly responsible for the adverse effect of smoking on the incidence of cardiovascular disease. Another factor may be carbon monoxide (see below). Surprisingly, there is no clear increase in ischaemic heart disease in pipe and cigar smokers, even though similar blood nicotine and carboxyhaemoglobin concentrations are reached, suggesting that nicotine and carbon monoxide may not be the only causative factors.
- *Chronic bronchitis*. Many studies have shown a much higher incidence of chronic bronchitis in smokers than non-smokers. None the less, in contrast to lung cancer, chronic bronchitis has declined in prevalence over the past 50 years. This is generally attributed to cleaner air and other social changes, and smoking now appears to be the most important remaining cause. Its effect is probably due to tar and other irritants, rather than nicotine.
- *Deleterious effects in pregnancy*. Smoking, particularly during the latter half of pregnancy, significantly reduces birth weight (by about 8% in women who smoke 25 or more cigarettes per day during pregnancy) and increases perinatal mortality (by an estimated 28% in babies born to mothers who smoke in the last half of pregnancy). There is evidence that children born to smoking mothers remain backward, in both physical and mental development, for at least 7 years. By 11 years of age, the difference has decreased. These effects of smoking, though measurable, are much smaller than the effects of other factors, such as social class and birth order. Various other complications of pregnancy are also more common in women who smoke, including spontaneous abortion (increased 30–70% by smoking), premature delivery (increased about 40%) and placenta praevia (increased 25–90%). Nicotine is excreted in breast milk in sufficient amounts to cause tachycardia in the infant.

The agents probably responsible for these effects are:

- *Tar and irritants*, such as NO_2, formaldehyde and so on. Cigarette smoke tar contains many known carcinogenic hydrocarbons (see p. 806), as well as tumour promoters, which account for the high cancer risk. It is likely that the various irritant substances are also responsible for the increase in bronchitis and emphysema.
- *Nicotine*. There is no evidence that nicotine contributes to the cancer risk. (Indeed, the lower cancer risk in pipe or cigar smokers suggests that it does not.) It is an obvious candidate for

causing peripheral vascular disease and retarding foetal development, because of its vasoconstrictor properties, but there is no clear evidence implicating it.

- *Carbon monoxide*. The average carbon monoxide content of cigarette smoke is about 3%. Carbon monoxide has a high affinity for haemoglobin and the average carboxyhaemoglobin content in the blood of cigarette smokers has been estimated at about 2.5% (compared with 0.4% for non-smoking urban dwellers). In very heavy smokers, up to 15% of haemoglobin may be complexed with carbon monoxide, a level which has been shown to cause retardation of foetal development in rats. It is possible that this factor also contributes to the increased incidence of heart and vascular disease. Foetal haemoglobin has a higher affinity for carbon monoxide than adult haemoglobin, and the proportion of carboxyhaemoglobin is higher in foetal than maternal blood. 'Low tar' cigarettes give a lower yield of both tar and nicotine than standard cigarettes. However, it has been shown that smokers puff harder, inhale more, and smoke more cigarettes when low tar brands are substituted for standard brands. The end result may be a reduced intake of tar and nicotine, but an increase in carbon monoxide intake.

Many studies have confirmed a reduced lung cancer risk with low tar cigarettes, but the risk of coronary heart disease is unchanged or even increased compared with that associated with standard cigarettes, suggesting that carbon monoxide may be important.

Pharmacological approaches to treatment of nicotine dependence

Most smokers would like to quit, but few succeed. The most successful smoking-cure clinics, using a combination of psychological and pharmacological treatments, achieve a success rate of about 25%, measured as the percentage of patients still abstinent after 1 year. The main pharmacological approach used is **nicotine replacement therapy** (see Benowitz 1993), though **clonidine** and the nicotinic receptor antagonist, **mecamylamine**, have also been used.

The aim of nicotine replacement therapy is to relieve the psychological and physical withdrawal syndrome associated with stopping smoking. Because nicotine is relatively short-acting, and not well absorbed from the gastrointestinal tract, it is given either in the form of chewing gum, or as a transdermal patch which is replaced daily. The latter gives a relatively steady plasma concentration for about 24 hours. These preparations cause various side effects, particularly nausea and gastrointestinal cramps, cough, insomnia and muscle pains. Because of the risk of coronary spasm, nicotine should not be used in patients with heart disease. Transdermal patches often cause local irritation and itching. The conclusion of many double-blind trials of nicotine against placebo is that these preparations, combined with professional counselling and supportive therapy, roughly double the chances of successfully breaking the smoking habit, from about 12 to 25%, measured 1 year after ceasing treatment. This may seem unimpressive, but in economic terms, nicotine replacement therapy, though expensive (approximately £150 for 3-months' supply), is a cheap form of preventive medicine, given the high morbidity and mortality of smoking-related disease. Nicotine on its own, without counselling and support, has been found to be no more effective than placebo, so its use as an over-the-counter smoking remedy has little justification.

Clonidine, an α_2-adrenoceptor agonist (see Ch. 7), has been shown in animal and human studies to reduce the withdrawal effects of several dependence-producing drugs, including opioids and cocaine, as well as nicotine. In patients, clonidine may be given orally or as a transdermal patch, and appears to be about as effective as nicotine substitution in assisting abstinence. The side effects of

Harmful effects of smoking

- Smoking reduces life expectancy, mainly through increased risk of:
  - —cancer, especially lung cancer, of which about 90% of cases are smoking related; carcinogenic tars are responsible
  - —ischaemic heart disease; both nicotine and CO may be responsible
  - —chronic bronchitis; tars are mainly responsible.
- Smoking in pregnancy reduces birth weight and retards childhood development. It also increases abortion rate and perinatal mortality. Nicotine, and possibly carbon monoxide, are responsible.

clonidine (hypotension, dry mouth, drowsiness) are troublesome, however, and it is not widely used.

The use of **mecamylamine**, which antagonises the effects of nicotine, is not promising. Small doses actually increase smoking, presumably because the nicotine effect can overcome the antagonism if the amount of nicotine is increased. Larger doses of mecamylamine, which abolish the effects of nicotine more effectively, have so many autonomic side effects (see Ch. 6) that subjects are unwilling to comply.

ETHANOL

Judged on a molar basis, the consumption of ethanol far exceeds that of any other drug. The ethanol content of various drinks ranges from about 2.5% (weak beer) to about 55% (strong spirits), and the size of the normal measure is such that a single drink usually contains about 8–12 g (0.17–0.26 moles) of ethanol. It is by no means unusual to consume 1–2 moles at a sitting, equivalent to about 0.5 kg of most other drugs. Its low pharmacological potency is reflected in the range of plasma concentrations needed to produce pharmacological effects: minimal effects occur at about 10 mmol/l (46 mg/100 ml), and 10 times this concentration may be lethal.

For calculation of ethanol consumption in the community, ethanol intake is often expressed in terms of units. One unit is equal to 8 g of ethanol, and is the amount contained in ½ pint of normal strength beer, 1 measure of spirits or 1 standard glass of wine.

The changing pattern of ethanol consumption in the UK up to 1986 is shown in Figure 33.3. The steady increase since the mid-1950s, particularly in wine and spirit consumption, correlates closely with a reduction in the real cost of alcoholic drinks over the same period. In Britain, more money (£11 billion in 1981) is spent on alcoholic drinks than on hospitals.

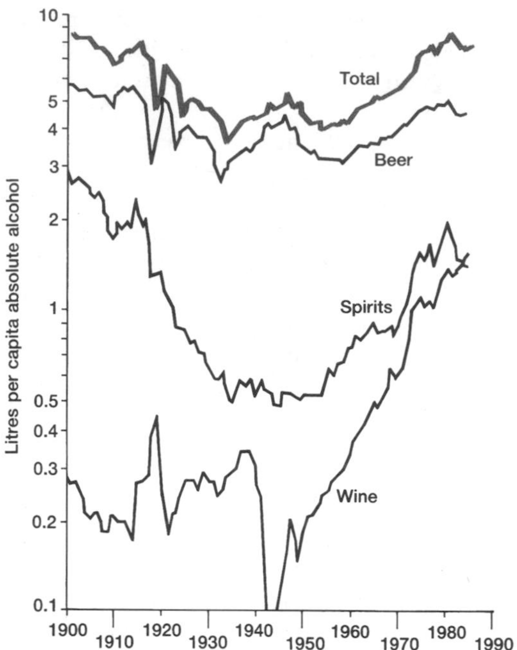

Fig. 33.3 Changes in ethanol consumption per person from 1900 to 1986. (From: Royal College of Physicians 1987 A great and growing evil: the medical consequences of alcohol abuse. Tavistock Publications, London)

PHARMACOLOGICAL EFFECTS OF ETHANOL

Effects on the central nervous system

The main effects of ethanol are on the central nervous system (see review by Charness et al. 1989), where its depressant actions resemble those of volatile anaesthetics (Ch. 26). Though ethanol, at pharmacologically effective concentrations, produces a measurable increase in the structural disorder (i.e. increased fluidity) of lipid membranes, similar to the effect of volatile anaesthetics, it is likely that its actions depend mainly on its effects on specific membrane ion channels and receptors. At a cellular level, the effect of ethanol is purely depressant, though it increases impulse activity—presumably by disinhibition—in some parts of the CNS, notably in the mesolimbic dopaminergic neurons that are involved in the reward pathway described above. The main theories of ethanol action (see reviews by Little 1991, Samson & Harris 1992) are:

- enhancement of GABA-mediated inhibition, similar to the action of benzodiazepines (see Ch. 25)
- inhibition of calcium entry through voltage-gated calcium channels
- inhibition of glutamate receptor function.

Ethanol enhances the action of GABA acting on $GABA_A$ receptors in a similar way to benzodiazepines (see Ch. 25). Its effect is, however, smaller and less consistent than that of benzodiazepines, and no clear effect on inhibitory synaptic transmission in the CNS has been demonstrated for ethanol. The benzodiazepine antagonist, **flumazenil**, has been found to reverse the central depressant actions of ethanol (see Lister & Nutt 1987), but this appears to result from physiological antagonism due to the contrary effects of flumazenil and ethanol on CNS function, rather than to a direct pharmacological interaction. The use of flumazenil to reverse ethanol intoxication and treat dependence has not found favour for several reasons, the main one being the danger that it could cause an increase in ethanol consumption and thus increase long-term toxic manifestations.

Ethanol inhibits transmitter release in response to nerve terminal depolarisation, without affecting release evoked by calcium ionophores (see Littleton 1984). Consistent with this action, it has been shown to inhibit the opening of voltage-sensitive Ca^{2+} channels in neurons.

The excitatory effects of glutamate are inhibited by ethanol at concentrations similar to those that produce CNS effects. NMDA-receptor activation is inhibited at lower ethanol concentrations than are required to affect AMPA receptors (see Ch. 24); these effects may contribute to its depressant actions, including, perhaps, memory impairment, since NMDA receptors play an important role in the type of long-term synaptic plasticity that is believed to underlie memory (Ch. 25). Other effects produced by ethanol include an enhancement of the excitatory effects produced by activation of nicotinic acetylcholine receptors and 5-HT_3 receptors. The relative importance of these various effects in the overall effects of ethanol on CNS function is not clear at present.

The effects of acute ethanol intoxication in man are well known, and include slurred speech, motor incoordination, increased self-confidence and euphoria. The effect on mood varies among individuals, most becoming louder and more outgoing, but some becoming morose and withdrawn. At higher levels of intoxication, the mood tends to become highly labile, with euphoria and melancholy, aggression and submission, often occurring successively.

Intellectual and motor performance and sensory discrimination (which can be measured in many different ways) show uniform impairment by ethanol, but subjects are generally unable to judge this for themselves. In tests on bus drivers, for example, in which subjects were asked to drive through a gap which they considered to be the minimum for their bus to pass through, ethanol caused them not only to hit the barriers more often at any given gap setting, but also to set the gap to a narrower dimension, often narrower than the bus.

Much effort has gone into measuring the effect of ethanol on driving performance in real life, as opposed to artificial tests under experimental conditions. In one American study, large numbers of city drivers were tested for plasma ethanol concentration, including drivers who had been involved in an accident and those that had not. This allowed the relative probability of being involved in an accident to be calculated as a function of ethanol concentration. It was found that no significant change occurred up to 50 mg/100 ml (10.9 mmol/l); by 80 mg/100 ml (17.4 mmol/l) the probability was increased about fourfold and by 150 mg/100 ml (32.6 mmol/l) about 25-fold. In the UK, driving with a blood ethanol concentration greater than 80 mg/100 ml constitutes a legal offence.

The relationship between plasma ethanol concentration and effect is highly variable. A given concentration produces a larger effect when the concentration is rising than when it is steady or falling. A substantial degree of tissue tolerance develops in habitual drinkers with the result that a higher plasma ethanol concentration is needed to produce a given effect (see below). In a large American study, 'gross intoxication' (assessed by a battery of tests that measured speech, gait and so on) occurred in 30% of subjects between 50 and 100 mg/100 ml and in 90% of subjects with more than 150 mg/100 ml. Coma generally occurs at about 300 mg/100 ml and death from respiratory failure is likely at 400–500 mg/100 ml.

In addition to the acute effects of ethanol on the nervous system, chronic administration also causes several irreversible neurological syndromes (see Charness et al. 1989). These may be due to ethanol itself, or to metabolites such as acetaldehyde or fatty acid esters. The majority of chronic alcoholics show a degree of dementia associated with ventricular enlargement detectable by brain-imaging techniques. Degeneration in the cerebellum and other specific brain regions can also occur, as well as peripheral neuropathy and myopathy. Some of these changes are not due to ethanol itself, but to accompanying thiamine deficiency which is common in alcoholics.

Effects on other systems

The main cardiovascular effect of ethanol is to produce cutaneous vasodilatation, central in origin, which causes a warm feeling but actually increases heat loss.

Ethanol increases salivary and gastric secretion. This is partly a reflex effect produced by the taste and irritant action of ethanol. However, heavy consumption of spirits causes damage directly to the gastric mucosa, causing chronic gastritis. Both this and the increased acid secretion are factors in the high incidence of gastric bleeding in alcoholics.

Ethanol produces a variety of endocrine effects. In particular, it increases the output of adrenal steroid hormones, by stimulating the anterior pituitary gland to secrete ACTH. However, the increase in plasma hydrocortisone usually seen in alcoholics is due partly to inhibition by ethanol of hydrocortisone metabolism in the liver.

Diuresis is a familiar effect of ethanol. It is caused by inhibition of ADH secretion, and tolerance develops rapidly, so that the diuresis is not sustained. There is a similar inhibition of oxytocin secretion, which can cause postponement of parturition at term. Attempts have been made to use this effect to delay premature labour, but the dose needed is large enough to cause obvious drunkenness in the mother. If the baby is born prematurely in spite of the ethanol, it too may be intoxicated at birth, sufficiently for respiration to be depressed. The procedure evidently has serious disadvantages.

Chronic male alcoholics often show signs of feminisation, which is associated with impaired testicular steroid synthesis, but induction of hepatic microsomal enzymes by ethanol, and hence an increased rate of testosterone inactivation, also contributes.

Effects of ethanol on the liver

Together with brain damage, liver damage is the most serious long-term consequence of excessive ethanol consumption (see Lieber 1988 for a detailed review). In the sequence of effects, increased fat accumulation (fatty liver) progresses to hepatitis (i.e. inflammation of the liver) and eventually to irreversible hepatic necrosis and fibrosis. Diversion of portal blood flow around the fibrotic liver often causes oesophageal varices to develop, which can bleed suddenly and catastrophically. Increased fat accumulation in the liver occurs, in rats or in man, after a single large dose of ethanol. The mechanism is complex, the main factors being:

- increased release of fatty acids from adipose tissue, which is the result of increased stress, causing sympathetic discharge
- impaired fatty acid oxidation, because of the metabolic load imposed by the ethanol itself.

With chronic ethanol consumption, many other factors contribute to the liver damage. One is malnutrition, for an alcoholic may satisfy much of his calorie requirement from ethanol itself. 200 grams of ethanol, which is approximately the content of one bottle of whisky, provides about 1400 kcal, but, unlike a normal diet, it provides no vitamins, amino acids or fatty acids. Thiamine deficiency is an important factor in causing chronic neurological damage (see above). The hepatic changes occurring in alcoholics are partly due to chronic malnutrition, but mainly to the cellular toxicity of ethanol, which promotes inflammatory changes in the liver.

The overall incidence of chronic liver disease seems to be a function of cumulative ethanol consumption over many years. Thus, overall consumption, expressed as g/kg body weight per day multiplied by years of drinking, provides an accurate predictor of the incidence of cirrhosis.

Effects on lipid metabolism, platelet function and atherosclerosis

There is evidence that ethanol drinking has the effect of reducing the incidence of coronary heart disease. Two mechanisms have been proposed. The first involves the effect of ethanol on the plasma lipoproteins which are the carrier molecules for cholesterol and other lipids in the bloodstream (see Ch. 15). Various epidemiological studies, and also some experimental studies on volunteers, have shown that ethanol, in daily doses too small to produce obvious CNS effects, can over the course of a few weeks increase plasma HDL concentration, thus exerting a protective effect against atheroma formation.

Ethanol may also protect against ischaemic heart disease by inhibiting platelet aggregation. This effect occurs at ethanol concentrations in the range achieved by normal drinking in man (10–20 mmol/l) and probably results from inhibition of arachidonic acid formation from phospholipid. In man, the magnitude of the effect depends critically on dietary fat intake, and it is not yet clear how important it is clinically.

The effect of ethanol on foetal development

It was demonstrated convincingly in the early 1970s that ethanol consumption during pregnancy has an adverse effect on foetal development. Foetal alcohol syndrome (FAS) is the term used to describe the effects commonly seen in the children of mothers who drink heavily in pregnancy (see reviews by Clarren & Smith 1978, Streissguth et al. 1980, Ciba Foundation Symposium 1984). The full-blown picture is relatively uncommon, but it is estimated that smaller degrees of ethanol-related abnormality may occur very frequently. Indeed, one survey suggests that ethanol is responsible for about 8% of cases of mild mental retardation.

The characteristic features of the foetal alcohol syndrome are:

- abnormal facial development, with wide-set eyes, short palpebral fissures and small cheek bones
- reduced cranial circumference
- retarded growth
- mental retardation and behavioural abnormalities, often taking the form of hyperactivity and difficulty with social integration
- other anatomical abnormalities, which may be major or minor (e.g. congenital cardiac abnormalities, malformation of the eyes and ears).

The overall incidence of FAS is estimated at 1–2 per thousand live births. The incidence correlates strongly with maternal ethanol consumption during pregnancy, being about 19% in mothers who drink (on average) at least 4 units per day during pregnancy. Though there is no clearly defined threshold amount for producing FAS, it is generally agreed that the syndrome results only from regular heavy drinking by alcohol-addicted mothers, or from heavy 'binge' drinking. It is uncertain whether there is a critical period during pregnancy when ethanol consumption is likely to lead to FAS. One study (Hanson et al. 1978) suggests that FAS incidence correlates most strongly with ethanol consumption very early in pregnancy, even before pregnancy is recognised, implying that not only pregnant women, but also women who are likely to become pregnant, must be advised not to drink heavily.

Effects of ethanol

- Ethanol consumption is generally expressed in units of 8 ml pure ethanol. Consumption in Britain has increased steadily since mid-1950s.
- Ethanol acts as a general CNS depressant, similar to volatile anaesthetic agents, producing the familiar effects of acute intoxication.
- Several cellular mechanisms are postulated: inhibition of calcium-channel opening, enhancement of GABA action and inhibitory action at NMDA-type glutamate receptors.
- Effective plasma concentrations:
  —threshold effects: about 40 mg/100 ml (5 mmol/l)
  —severe intoxication: about 150 mg/100 ml
  —death from respiratory failure: about 500 mg/100 ml.
- Main peripheral effects are: self-limiting diuresis (reduced ADH secretion), cutaneous vasodilatation and delayed labour (reduced oxytocin secretion).
- Neurological degeneration occurs in heavy drinkers, causing dementia and peripheral neuropathies.
- Long-term ethanol consumption causes liver disease, progressing to cirrhosis and liver failure.
- Moderate ethanol consumption has a protective effect against ischaemic heart disease.
- Ethanol in pregnancy causes impaired foetal development, associated with small size, abnormal facial development and other physical abnormalities, and mental retardation.
- Tolerance, physical dependence and psychological dependence all occur with ethanol.

The mechanism by which ethanol produces these effects is unknown (see p. 808). Both ethanol and its metabolite, acetaldehyde, inhibit cell division and migration in culture, so it is possible that the same mechanism operates in vivo. From experiments on rats and mice, it is suggested that the effect on facial development may be produced very early in pregnancy (up to 4 weeks in man), while the effect on brain development is produced rather later (up to 10 weeks).

PHARMACOKINETIC ASPECTS

Ethanol, being uncharged and highly lipid soluble, is rapidly absorbed, an appreciable amount being absorbed from the stomach. A substantial fraction is removed from the portal vein blood by first-pass hepatic metabolism. Because the rate of hepatic metabolism of ethanol shows the property of saturation at quite low ethanol concentrations, the fraction of ethanol removed is greatest when the concentration is low, and decreases as the concentration increases. Thus, if ethanol absorption is rapid and portal vein concentration is high, most of the ethanol escapes into the systemic circulation, whereas with slow absorption, more is removed by first-pass metabolism. This is one reason why drinking ethanol on an empty stomach produces a much greater pharmacological effect. Ethanol is quickly distributed throughout the body water, the rate of its redistribution depending mainly on the blood flow to individual tissues, as with volatile anaesthetics (see Ch. 26).

Ethanol is about 90% metabolised in the body, 5–10% being excreted unchanged in expired air and in urine. This fraction is not pharmacokinetically significant, but provides the basis for estimating blood ethanol concentration from measurements on breath or urine. The ratio of ethanol concentrations in blood and alveolar air is taken to be 21% (i.e. 1 ml of blood contains as much ethanol as 2.1 litres of alveolar air). The concentration in urine is more variable, and provides a less accurate measure of blood concentration.

Ethanol metabolism occurs almost entirely in the liver, and mainly by a pathway involving successive oxidations, first to acetaldehyde and then to acetic acid. Since ethanol is often consumed in large quantities (compared with most drugs), 1–2 moles daily being by no means unusual, it constitutes a substantial load on the hepatic oxidative systems. The oxidation of 2 moles of ethanol consumes about 1.5 kg of the cofactor NAD^+. This means that ethanol oxidation can only proceed at a limited rate irrespective of the concentration that is presented to the liver (i.e. it shows *zero-order*, or *saturating, kinetics*; see Ch. 4). It also means that competition occurs between the ethanol and other metabolic substrates for the available NAD^+ supplies, which may be a factor in ethanol-induced liver damage (see Ch. 43). The intermediate metabolite, acetaldehyde, is a reactive and toxic compound and this may also contribute to the hepatotoxicity. A small degree of esterification of ethanol with various fatty acids also occurs in the tissues, and these esters may also contribute to long-term toxicity.

Alcohol dehydrogenase is a soluble cytoplasmic enzyme, confined mainly to liver cells, which oxidises ethanol at the same time as reducing NAD^+ to NADH (Fig. 33.4). Even after a small intake of ethanol, the plasma concentration is enough to saturate the enzyme, so that ethanol elimination takes place at a rate that is virtually independent of the plasma concentration (Fig. 33.5), corresponding in man to about 0.1 g/kg body weight/hour, or about 10 ml/hour in a normal subject. This rate is actually

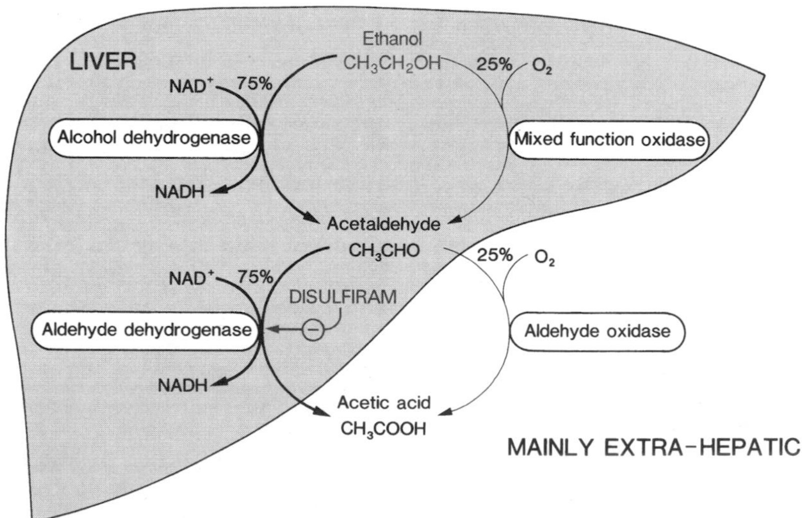

Fig. 33.4 Metabolism of ethanol.

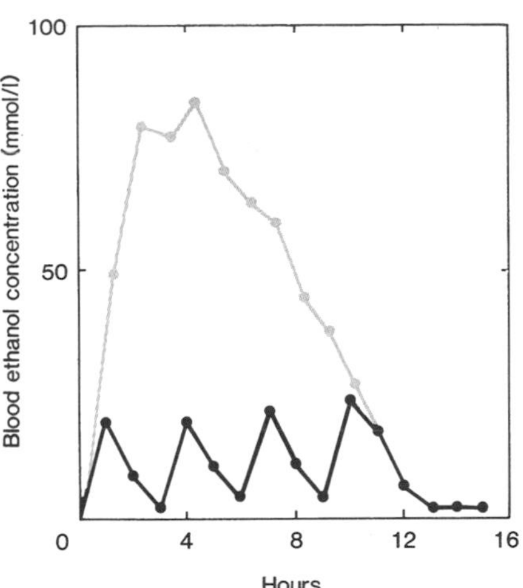

Fig. 33.5 Zero-order kinetics of ethanol elimination in rats. Rats were given ethanol orally (104 mmol/kg) either as a single dose, or as four divided doses. The single dose results in a much higher and more sustained blood ethanol concentration than the same quantity given as divided doses. Note that, after the single dose, ethanol concentration declines linearly, the rate of decline being similar after a small or large dose, because of the saturation phenomenon. (From: Kalant H et al. 1975 Biochem Pharmacol 24: 431)

limited by NAD^+ availability rather than by enzyme saturation. Ethanol metabolism causes the ratio of NAD^+ to NADH to fall, and this has other metabolic consequences (e.g. increased lactate, and slowing down of the Krebs cycle). The limitation on ethanol metabolism imposed by the limited rate of NAD^+ regeneration has led to attempts to find a 'sobering-up' agent that works by regenerating NAD^+ from NADH. One such agent is fructose, which is reduced by an NADH-requiring enzyme. In large doses it causes a small but measurable increase in the rate of ethanol metabolism, but the effect is not large enough to cause a significant increase in the rate of return to sobriety.

Some ethanol (about 25%) is metabolised by the microsomal mixed function oxidase system (see Ch. 4). This may be responsible for some reported drug interactions involving ethanol. Ethanol often seems to produce a dual effect on the metabolism of the many other drugs that are metabolised by the mixed function oxidase system (e.g. **phenobarbitone**, **warfarin** and **steroids**), with an initial inhibitory effect produced by competition, followed by enhancement due to enzyme induction.

Nearly all of the acetaldehyde produced is converted to acetate in the liver, by aldehyde dehydrogenase (Fig. 33.4). Normally, only a little acetaldehyde escapes from the liver, giving a blood acetaldehyde concentration of 20–50 μmol/l after an intoxicating dose of ethanol in man, the remainder being converted to acetic acid by *aldehyde oxidase*. The circulating acetaldehyde usually has little or no effect, but the concentration may become much larger under certain circumstances, and produce toxic effects. This occurs if aldehyde dehydrogenase is inhibited by drugs such as **disulfiram**. In the presence of disulfiram, which produces no marked effect when given alone, ethanol consumption is followed by a severe reaction, comprising flushing, tachycardia, hyperventilation and considerable panic and distress, which is due to excessive acetaldehyde accumulation in the bloodstream. This reaction is extremely unpleasant, but not harmful, and disulfiram can be used as aversion therapy to discourage people from taking ethanol. Some other drugs, notably oral hypoglycaemic agents of the sulphonylurea class (e.g. **chlorpropamide**; see Ch. 20) and certain antibacterial drugs (e.g. **metronidazole**; see Ch. 37) also occasionally produce similar reactions to ethanol. In 50% of Asians, an inactive genetic variant of one of the aldehyde dehydrogenase isoforms (ALDH-1) is expressed; these individuals experience a disulfiram-like reaction after alcohol, and the incidence of alcoholism in this group is extremely low. Interestingly, a Chinese herbal medicine, used traditionally to cure alcoholics, contains **daidzin**, recently shown to be a specific inhibitor of ALDH-1. In hamsters (which spontaneously consume alcohol in amounts that would defeat even the hardest two-legged drinker while remaining, as far as one can tell, completely sober), daidzin markedly inhibits alcohol consumption (see Keung & Vallee 1993).

Methanol is metabolised in the same way as ethanol, but produces formaldehyde instead of acetaldehyde from the first oxidation step. Formaldehyde is more reactive than acetaldehyde, and reacts rapidly with proteins, causing the inactivation of enzymes involved in the tricarboxylic acid cycle. It is converted to another toxic metabolite, formic acid. This, unlike acetic acid, cannot be utilised in the tricarboxylic acid cycle, and is liable to cause tissue damage. Conversion of alcohols to aldehydes occurs not only in the liver, but also in the retina, where the dehydrogenase responsible for the retinol–retinal conversion also oxidises exogenous alcohols. Formation of formaldehyde in the retina accounts for one of the main toxic effects of methanol, namely blindness, which can occur after ingestion of as little as 10 g. Formic acid production, and derangement of the tricarboxylic acid cycle, also produce severe acidosis. Methanol is used as an industrial solvent, and also to adulterate industrial ethanol in order to make it unfit to drink. Methanol poisoning is none the less quite common, and it is treated by administration of large doses of ethanol, which acts to retard methanol metabolism by competition for alcohol dehydrogenase.

TOLERANCE AND DEPENDENCE

Tolerance to the effects of ethanol can be demonstrated in both man and experimental animals, to the extent of a two- to threefold reduction in potency occurring over 1–3 weeks of continuing ethanol administration. A small component of this (up to about 30% decrease in potency) is due to pharmacokinetic tolerance resulting from more rapid elimination of ethanol. The major component is tissue tolerance, which accounts for a roughly twofold decrease in potency and which can be observed in vitro (e.g. by measuring the inhibitory effect of ethanol on transmitter release from synaptosomes) as well as in vivo. The mechanism of this tolerance is not known for certain (see Little 1991), but it is known that ethanol tolerance is associated with tolerance to many anaesthetic agents, and alcoholics are often difficult to anaesthetise with drugs such as halothane.

Chronic ethanol administration produces various changes in CNS neurons, which tend to oppose the acute cellular effects that it produces (see above). There is a small reduction in the density of $GABA_A$ receptors, and a proliferation of voltage-gated Ca^{2+} channels and NMDA receptors. The effect on Ca^{2+} channels has received particular attention (see Littleton 1984, Charness et al. 1989). Studies on brain synaptosomes and isolated neurons from ethanol-tolerant rats have revealed various changes. The acute effect of ethanol (see above) is to reduce Ca^{2+} entry through voltage-gated Ca^{2+} channels, and thus to reduce transmitter release. During chronic exposure to ethanol, Ca^{2+} entry recovers due to a proliferation of Ca^{2+} channels, and when ethanol is withdrawn, depolarisation-evoked Ca^{2+} entry and transmitter release are increased above normal, which is possibly associated with the physical withdrawal symptoms. Consistent with this explanation, Ca^{2+}-channel-blocking drugs of the dihydropyridine type (see Ch. 14) reduce the effects of ethanol withdrawal in experimental animals (see Little 1991).

A well-defined physical abstinence syndrome develops in response to ethanol withdrawal. As with most other dependence-producing drugs, this is probably important as a short-term factor in sustaining the drug habit, but other (mainly psychological) factors are more important in the longer term. The physical abstinence syndrome usually subsides in a few days, but the craving for ethanol and the tendency to relapse last for very much longer.

The physical abstinence syndrome in man, in severe form, develops after about 8 hours. In the first stage, the main symptoms are tremor, nausea, sweating, fever and, sometimes, hallucinations. These last for about 24 hours. This phase may be followed by tonic–clonic convulsions ('rum fits'), indistinguishable from grand mal epilepsy. Over the next few days, the condition of '*delirium tremens*' develops, in which the patient becomes confused, agitated and often aggressive, and may suffer much more severe hallucinations. A similar syndrome of central and autonomic hyperactivity can be produced in experimental animals by ethanol withdrawal. The most effective treatment of delirium tremens in man is the use of **chlormethiazole** or **benzodiazepines** (see Ch. 27), though **clonidine** and β-adrenoceptor antagonists, such as **propranolol**, are also useful. Clonidine, an α_2-adrenoceptor

Metabolism of ethanol

- Ethanol is metabolised mainly by the liver, first by alcohol dehydrogenase to acetaldehyde, then by aldehyde dehydrogenase to acetate. About 25% of the acetaldehyde is metabolised extra-hepatically.
- Small amounts of ethanol are excreted in urine and expired air. Hepatic metabolism shows saturation kinetics, mainly due to limited availability of NAD^+. Maximal rate of ethanol metabolism is about 10 ml/hour. Thus, plasma concentration falls linearly rather than exponentially.
- Acetaldehyde may produce toxic effects. Inhibition of aldehyde dehydrogenase by disulfiram accentuates nausea, etc., caused by acetaldehyde, and can be used in aversion therapy.
- Methanol is similarly metabolised to formic acid, which is toxic, especially to retina.

agonist, is believed to act by inhibiting the exaggerated transmitter release thought to occur during the withdrawal phase, while propranolol blocks the effects of excessive sympathetic activity.

CANNABIS

Extracts of the hemp plant, *Cannabis sativa*, which grows freely in temperate and tropical regions, contain the active substance **Δ¹-tetrahydrocannabinol (THC**; Fig. 33.6). **Marijuana** is the name given to the dried leaves and flower heads, prepared as a smoking mixture; **hashish** is the extracted resin. For centuries, these substances have been used for various medicinal purposes and as intoxicant preparations. Marijuana was brought to North America by immigrants, mainly in the nineteenth century, and began to be regarded as a social problem in the early years of this century; it was legally banned during the 1930s. Its use increased dramatically in the 1960s, and recent figures suggest that about 15% of the adult population in America and Western Europe have taken cannabis at some time, with a much higher proportion (close to 50%) among teenagers and young adults.

CHEMICAL ASPECTS

Cannabis extracts contain numerous related compounds, called cannabinoids, most of which are insoluble in water. The most abundant cannabinoids are Δ¹-THC (which is often called **Δ⁹-THC**, according to a different ring-numbering system), **Δ⁶-THC**, which is more weakly active than Δ¹-THC, and **cannabinol**, which is formed spontaneously from Δ¹-THC. Δ¹-THC is the most important from a biological point of view, and constitutes roughly 1–10% by weight of marijuana and hashish preparations. Various radioimmunoassays have been developed for cannabinoids, but they lack sufficient chemical specificity to be able to distinguish Δ¹-THC from the numerous other cannabinoids found in crude extracts, and from the various metabolites that are formed in vivo. Thus, the assay of pharmacologically active Δ¹-THC in biological fluids still presents a problem.

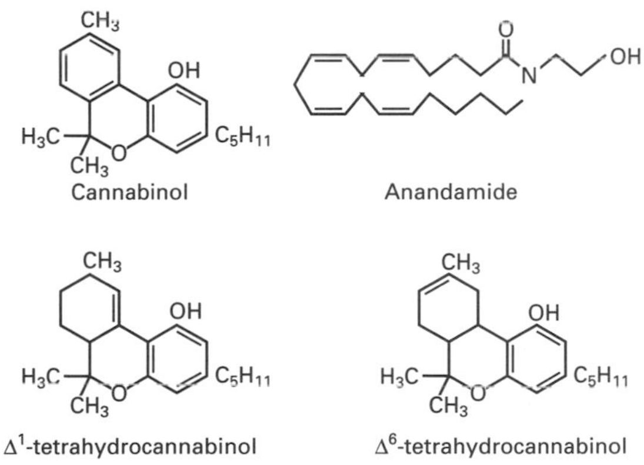

Cannabinol

Anandamide

Δ¹-tetrahydrocannabinol

Δ⁶-tetrahydrocannabinol

Fig. 33.6 Structure of cannabinoids. Anandamide is a recently discovered arachidonic acid derivative which is present in the brain and believed to be an endogenous agonist for cannabinoid receptors.

PHARMACOLOGICAL EFFECTS

Δ¹-THC acts mainly on the central nervous system, producing a mixture of psychotomimetic and depressant effects, together with various centrally mediated, peripheral autonomic effects (see review by Dewey 1986).

The main subjective effects in man consist of:

- a feeling of relaxation and well-being, not unlike that produced by ethanol
- a feeling of sharpened sensory awareness, with sounds and sights seeming more intense and fantastic.

These effects are similar to, but usually less pronounced than, those produced by psychotomimetic drugs such as LSD (see Ch. 32). Subjects report that time passes extremely slowly. The alarming sensations and paranoid delusions that often occur with LSD are seldom experienced after cannabis. Cannabis also increases appetite, an effect seen in experimental animals as well as human subjects. Objective tests of psychomotor performance show general impairment after cannabis. For example, subjects perform less well in simple learning and memory tasks, as well as in more complex tests of motor coordination, such as driving. The subjective feelings of confidence and heightened creativity are not reflected in actual performance. Aggressive behaviour is not enhanced after cannabis, nor is sexual activity, contrary to popular belief. Other effects that have been demonstrated include analgesia (which shows up in hot-plate tests on experimental animals), catalepsy (the adoption of a fixed immobile posture) which occurs in rats and mice, and an anti-emetic effect.

The main peripheral effects of cannabis are:

- tachycardia, which can be prevented by drugs that block sympathetic transmissions
- vasodilatation, which is particularly marked on the scleral and conjunctival vessels, producing a characteristic bloodshot appearance
- reduction of intraocular pressure
- bronchodilatation.

RECEPTORS AND ENDOGENOUS LIGANDS

Cannabinoids were originally thought to act as non-specific lipophilic agents, similar to general anaesthetic agents, but the identification of specific cannabinoid receptors in the brain and in the periphery suggest that they act on a specific signalling mechanism. Cannabinoid receptors have now been isolated and cloned (see Howlett et al. 1990, Munro et al. 1993), and shown to belong to the class of G-protein-coupled receptors (see Ch. 2). They exert an inhibitory effect on adenylate cyclase, as well as directly inhibiting calcium channel function (see Devane 1994), cellular effects which closely resemble those of opioids. The distribution of cannabinoid receptors in the brain conforms roughly to the pharmacological effects. They occur particularly in the hippocampus (memory impairment), cerebellum and *substantia nigra* (motor disturbance) and mesolimbic dopamine pathways (reward), as well as in the cortex. The peripheral cannabinoid receptor shows only limited amino acid homology with the CNS receptor, and is located mainly in the lymphoid system. This was an unexpected finding, but may account for the inhibitory effects on immune function that have been reported with cannabis. The discovery of specific cannabinoid receptors in the brain naturally led to a search for an endogenous chemical mediator, and the discovery of **anandamide**, an amide derivative of arachidonic acid (see Fig. 33.6), which produces short-lasting cannabinoid-like effects when injected into the brain. The physiological role of this system, and the mechanism of synthesis and release of anandamide are currently attracting much interest. The peripheral cannabinoid receptor may show a different pharmacological specificity from the CNS receptor, but so far very little is known about its function.

The effects of cannabis on intraocular pressure, bronchial smooth muscle, pain perception and the vomiting reflex are of potential therapeutic value, and certain cannabinoid derivatives (e.g. **nabilone**) have been developed as therapeutic agents (see Hollister 1986).

TOLERANCE AND DEPENDENCE

Tolerance to cannabis occurs only to a minor degree. Physical dependence, manifest as rather weak withdrawal symptoms, has been demonstrated. The symptoms are similar to those of ethanol or opiate withdrawal, namely nausea, agitation, irritability, confusion, tachycardia, sweating and so on, but are relatively mild and do not result in a compulsive urge to take the drug. Psychological dependence does not seem to occur with cannabis, and overall it cannot be classified as addictive (see review by Abood & Martin 1992).

PHARMACOKINETIC ASPECTS

The effect of cannabis, taken by smoking or by intravenous injection, takes about 1 hour to develop fully, and lasts for 2–3 hours, Δ^1-THC being converted to inactive metabolites. It is partly conjugated, and undergoes enterohepatic recirculation.

ADVERSE EFFECTS

Δ^1-THC is relatively safe in overdose, producing drowsiness and confusion, but not respiratory or cardiovascular effects that threaten life. In this respect it is safer than most abused substances, particularly opiates and ethanol. Even in low doses, Δ^1-THC and synthetic derivatives such as nabilone produce euphoria and drowsiness, sometimes accompanied by sensory distortion and hallucinations. These effects, together with the legal restrictions on the use of Δ^1-THC, preclude the widespread therapeutic use of cannabinoids.

Δ^1-THC has been shown to produce a teratogenic and mutagenic effect in rodents, and an increased incidence of chromosome breaks in circulating white cells has been reported in humans. Such breaks are, however, by no means unique to cannabis, and epidemiological studies have not shown any increased risk of foetal malformation or cancer among cannabis users.

Certain endocrine effects occur in man, notably a decrease in plasma testosterone and a reduction of sperm count. One study showed a reduction of more than 50% in both plasma testosterone and sperm count in subjects smoking 10 or more marijuana cigarettes per week.

It is very difficult to assess the evidence that cannabis causes long-term psychological changes. It has been suggested that it can cause schizophrenia, and that it leads to a gradually developing state of apathy and underachievement, but it is very difficult to prove causation even where a positive association has been found.

The long-running argument over the legalisation of cannabis centres mainly on the seriousness of these adverse effects. Opponents of legalisation argue that it would be folly to change the law in favour of the use by the public at large of a substance which could turn out to have serious toxic effects. Proponents of a change argue that the present law is clearly ineffective and encourages crime, and that cannabis is undoubtedly safer than either ethanol or tobacco.

Cannabis

- Main active constituent is Δ^1-tetrahydrocannabinol (THC), though pharmacologically active metabolites may be important.
- Actions on CNS include both depressant and psychotomimetic effects.
- Subjectively, subjects experience euphoria and a feeling of relaxation, with sharpened sensory awareness.
- Objective tests show impairment of learning, memory and motor performance.
- THC also shows analgesic and anti-emetic activity, as well as causing catalepsy and hypothermia in animal tests.
- Peripheral actions include vasodilatation, reduction of intraocular pressure and bronchodilatation.
- A cannabinoid receptor, coupled to adenylate cyclase, has been identified in the CNS by labelling and cloning studies. A peripheral cannabinoid receptor, mainly in lymphatic tissue, has also been identified.
- Anandamide, an arachidonic acid derivative, may be an endogenous ligand for the CNS cannabinoid receptor; its function has not yet been ascertained.
- Cannabinoids appear less liable than opiates, nicotine or alcohol to cause dependence, but may have long-term psychological effects.
- Nabilone, a THC analogue, has been developed for its anti-emetic property; otherwise, cannabinoids are not generally available for clinical use.

REFERENCES AND FURTHER READING

Abood M E, Martin B R 1992 Neurobiology of marijuana abuse. Trends Pharmacol Sci 13: 201–206

Benowitz N L 1988 Pharmacological consequences of cigarette smoking and nicotine addiction. N Engl J Med 319: 1318–1330

Benowitz N L 1993 Nicotine replacement therapy. Drugs 45: 157–170

Charness M E, Simon R P, Greenberg D A 1989 Ethanol and the nervous system. N Engl J Med 321: 442–454

Ciba Foundation Symposium 1984 Mechanisms of alcohol damage in utero. Pitman, London

Clarren S K, Smith D W 1978 The fetal alcohol syndrome. N Engl J Med 298: 1063–1067

Devane W A 1994 New dawn of cannabinoid pharmacology. Trends Pharmacol Sci 15: 40–41

Dewey W L 1986 Cannabinoid pharmacology. Pharmacol Rev 38: 151–178

Goldstein D B 1983 Pharmacology of alcohol. Oxford University Press, New York

Grenhoff J, Svensson T H 1989 Pharmacology of nicotine. Br J Addict 84: 477–492

Hanson J W, Streissguth A P, Smith D W 1978 The effects of moderate alcohol consumption during pregnancy on fetal growth and morphogenesis. J Pediatr 92: 457–460

Hewlett A C, Bidaut-Russell M, Devane W A, Melvin L S, Ross Johnson M, Herkenham M 1990 The cannabinoid receptor: biochemical, anatomical and behavioural characterization. Trends Neurosci 13: 420–423

Hofmann F 1983 A handbook on drug and alcohol abuse. Oxford University Press, New York

Hollister L E 1986 Health aspects of cannabis. Pharmacol Rev 38: 2–20

Keung W-M, Vallee B L 1993 Daidzin and daidzein suppress free-choice ethanol intake by Syrian golden hamsters. Proc Natl Acad Sci USA 90: 10 008–10 012

Koob G F 1992 Drugs of abuse: anatomy, pharmacology and function of reward pathways. Trends Pharmacol Sci 13: 177–184

Lee W L, D'Alonzo G E 1993 Cigarette smoking, nicotine addiction, and its pharmacologic treatment. Arch Int Med 153: 34–38

Lieber C S 1988 Biochemical and molecular basis of alcohol-

induced injury to liver and other tissues. N Engl J Med 319: 1639–1650
Lister R G, Nutt D J 1987 Is Ro 15–4513 a specific alcohol antagonist? Trends Neurosci 6: 223–225
Little H J 1991 Mechanisms that may underlie the behavioural effects of ethanol. Prog Neurobiol 36: 171–194
Littleton J M 1984 Biochemical pharmacology of ethanol tolerance and dependence. In: Edwards G, Littleton J M (eds) Pharmacological treatments for alcoholism. Croom-Helm, London
Mottram D 1988 Drugs in sport. E & F N Spon, London
Royal College of Physicians Reports 1971, 1977 Smoking or health. Pitman Medical Publishing, Tunbridge Wells
Munro S, Thomas K L, Abu-Shaar M 1993 Molecular characterization of a peripheral receptor for cannabinoids. Nature 365: 61–65
Nestler E J 1993 Cellular responses to chronic treatment with drugs of abuse. Crit Rev Neurobiol 7: 23–39
Pratt J 1991 The biological basis of drug tolerance and dependence. Academic Press, London
Samson H H, Harris R A 1992 Neurobiology of alcohol abuse. Trends Pharmacol Sci 13: 206–211
Sellers E M, Higgins G A, Sobell M B 1992 5-HT and alcohol abuse. Trends Pharmacol Sci 31: 69–75
Stolerman I P, Shoaib M 1991 The neurobiology of tobacco addiction. Trends Pharmacol Sci 12: 467–473
Streissguth A P, Landesman-Dwyer S, Martin J C, Smith D W 1980 Teratogenic effects of alcohol in humans and laboratory animals. Science 209: 353–361
Uhl G, Blum K, Noble E, Smith S 1993 Substance abuse vulnerability and D_2 receptor genes. Trends Neurosci 16: 83–88
US Department of Health & Human Services Reports 1981, 1982, 1983. The health consequences of smoking. US Government Publication, Washington, DC
Winger G, Hofmann F G, Woods J H 1992 A handbook on drugs and alcohol abuse. Oxford University Press, New York
Wonnacott S, Russell M A H, Stolerman I P (eds) 1990 Nicotine psychopharmacology: molecular, cellular and behavioural aspects. Oxford University Press, Oxford

34

LOCAL ANAESTHETICS AND OTHER DRUGS THAT AFFECT EXCITABLE MEMBRANES

INTRODUCTION

The property of electrical excitability is what enables the membranes of nerve and muscle cells to generate propagated action potentials, which are essential for communication in the nervous system and for the initiation of mechanical activity in cardiac and striated muscle. Electrical excitability depends on the existence of voltage-gated ion channels in the cell membrane, most importantly on Na^+ channels that are gated in such a way that they open, and the membrane becomes selectively permeable to Na^+, when the membrane is depolarised. Also important are the voltage-dependent K^+ channels and Ca^{2+} channels, which function in basically the same way. These channels are membrane proteins, and they all possess a basically similar molecular structure (see below). Their distinct ion selectivity, however, means that they have quite different physiological functions; Na^+, K^+ and Ca^{2+} channels are also selectively affected by quite different classes of drugs. The pharmacology of Ca^{2+} channels, which are particularly important in relation to the heart and vascular smooth muscle, is discussed in Chapters 13 and 14. This chapter focuses on the function and pharmacology of Na^+ and K^+ channels. The most important group of drugs discussed are the **local anaesthetics**, which act mainly by blocking Na^+ channels. Also in the category of Na^+-channel blockers are the class I antidysrhythmic drugs (see Ch. 13), certain anticonvulsants, such as **phenytoin** (see Ch. 30), and two neurotoxins, **tetrodotoxin** and **saxitoxin** (see below). Drugs that act selectively on K^+ channels include blocking agents, such as **4-aminopyridine**, and those that open K^+ channels, such as **cromokalim** and **pinacidil**, which act mainly on smooth muscle cells and are discussed in Chapter 14.

There are, broadly speaking, two ways in which channel function may be modified, namely *block of the channels* and *modification of gating behaviour*. Either mechanism can cause an increase or a decrease of electrical excitability. Thus, blocking Na^+ channels reduces excitability, whereas block of K^+ channels tends to increase it. Similarly, an agent that affects Na^+-channel gating so as to increase channel opening will tend to increase excitability and vice versa.

Na^+ AND K^+ CHANNELS OF EXCITABLE MEMBRANES

Our present understanding of electrical excitability—the ability of a cell to generate a short-lasting, all-or-nothing depolarisation or reversal of the membrane potential (known as an *action potential*) in response to electrical stimulation—rests firmly on the work of Hodgkin, Huxley & Katz, published in 1949–1952. Before then it was known that the resting cell membrane was selectively permeable to K^+, that the potential of the interior of the cell was negative to the outside by 60–90 mV, and that the action potential was associated with a large increase in membrane conductance. Hodgkin and his colleagues, in a remarkable tour de force (at a time when valve-operated amplifiers, and even oscilloscopes, had to be painstakingly designed and built by the scientists themselves) devised the *voltage-clamp technique* and applied it successfully to study the mechanism of action potential generation in the squid giant axon. For accounts of these experiments, see Katz (1966), Hille (1984), Nicholls et al. (1992). Their analysis showed that the action potential is generated by the interplay of two separate ionic permeability changes:

- a rapid, transient increase in Na^+ permeability which occurs when the membrane is depolarised beyond about –50 mV
- a slower, sustained increase in K^+ permeability.

Because of the inequality of Na^+ and K^+ concentrations on the two sides of the membrane, an increase in Na^+ permeability causes an inward current of Na^+ ions, whereas an increase in K^+ permeability causes an outward current. The separate nature of these two currents can be most clearly demonstrated by the use of Na^+ and K^+ channel-blocking drugs, as shown in Figure 34.1, depicting the currents that flow through the membrane of a single node of Ranvier of a frog axon when the membrane potential is suddenly stepped from –120 mV to a more depolarised level. Stepping to –45 mV produces a transient inward current which decays in about 10 ms. With larger depolarisations, this inward current gets smaller, and a later, sustained outward current is seen. If the membrane is depolarised even further, the transient current reverses in direction. This happens when the internal potential is made positive to the sodium equilibrium potential (E_{Na}) which is a function of the intracellular and extracellular Na^+ concentrations, and is about +40 mV under normal conditions. The explanation for this complex behaviour is that the sodium current at any moment depends on two factors:

- the *state of activation* of the channels (i.e. the fraction of channels that is open), which is a function of both membrane potential and time
- the *driving force* for Na^+ ions ($E_m - E_{Na}$).

At potentials negative to about –60 mV, no channels are activated, so no current flows. Between about 50 mV and –30 mV (the activation range for Na^+ channels) the channels progressively open. With further depolarisation, the peak current decreases because, though activation is complete, $E_m - E_{Na}$ decreases. When the membrane is made more positive than E_{Na} (normally about +40 mV), the driving force changes in direction and the current flows outward.

The Na^+ current can be seen uncomplicated by

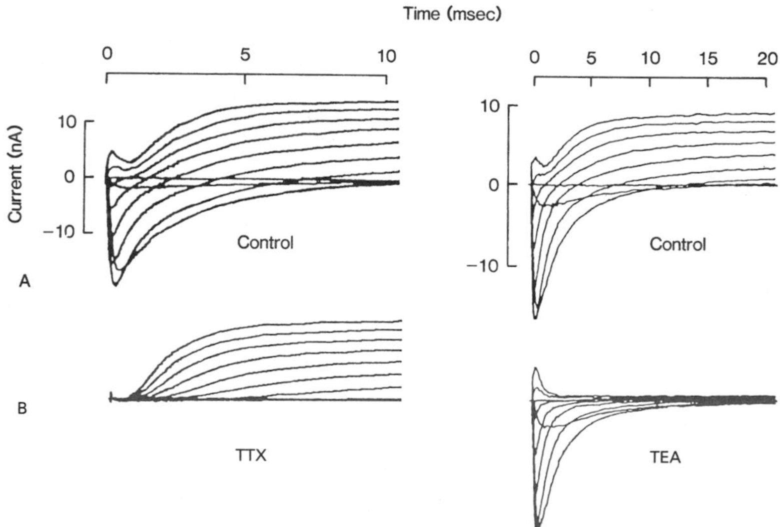

Fig. 34.1 Separation of Na^+ and K^+ currents in nerve membrane. Voltage-clamp records from the node of Ranvier of a single frog nerve fibre. At time 0 the membrane potential was stepped to a depolarised level, ranging from –60 mV (lower trace in each series) to +60 mV (upper trace in each series) in 15 mV steps. **A.** Control records from two fibres. **B.** Effect of TTX (left) abolition of Na^+ currents. Effect of TEA (right) abolition of K^+ currents. (TTX = tetrodotoxin; TEA = tetraethylammonium) (From: Hille B 1970 Prog Biophys 21: 1)

K^+ current (Fig. 34.1) if the K^+ channels are blocked with **tetraethylammonium** (**TEA**; see below). The Na^+ current is transient, even if the membrane depolarisation is sustained, and decays to zero in 5–10 ms. This spontaneous closure of the channels, known as *inactivation*, is an important property of the Na^+ channel. During the physiological initiation or propagation of a nerve impulse, the first event is a small depolarisation of the membrane, produced either by transmitter action or by the approach of an action potential passing along the axon. This opens Na^+ channels, allowing an inward current of Na^+ ions to flow, which depolarises the membrane still further. The process is thus a regenerative one, and the increase in Na^+ permeability is enough to bring the membrane potential close to E_{Na}.

In many types of cell, including most nerve cells, the process of repolarisation is assisted by the opening of voltage-dependent K^+ channels. These function in much the same way as Na^+ channels (i.e. they open when the cell is depolarised), but differ in two important ways. Firstly, their activation kinetics are about 10 times slower; secondly, their inactivation is less pronounced. This means that the K^+ channels open later than the Na^+ channels (Fig. 34.2). Because of the high intracellular and low extracellular K^+ concentrations, E_K is about −100 mV, so opening K^+ channels causes an outward (repolarising) current, which occurs later than the Na^+ current, and contributes to the rapid termination of the action potential. The behaviour of the Na^+ and K^+ channels during an action potential is shown in Figure 34.2, and an overall scheme showing the various regulatory processes and sites of drug action is shown in Figure 34.3.

The function of these voltage-gated ion channels has been intensively studied with the help of molecular biology techniques (see reviews by Pongs 1992; Catterall 1993). The three main types of channel show considerable sequence homology, and all have the same basic structure (Fig. 34.4). Each channel consists of an aggregate of four identical or very similar protein domains, which exist either as regions of a single very long peptide chain (as in the Na^+ channel) or as independent subunits (as in the K^+ channel). Each of the four domains contains six membrane-spanning α-helices (S1–S6) stacked like sticks of gelignite, and the four domains are arranged symmetrically around a central aqueous pore—the ion channel. The functional organisation of these complex proteins has been elucidated largely by making selective mutations, and observing their effects on the function and pharmacology of the channels. Part of the lining of the channel is formed

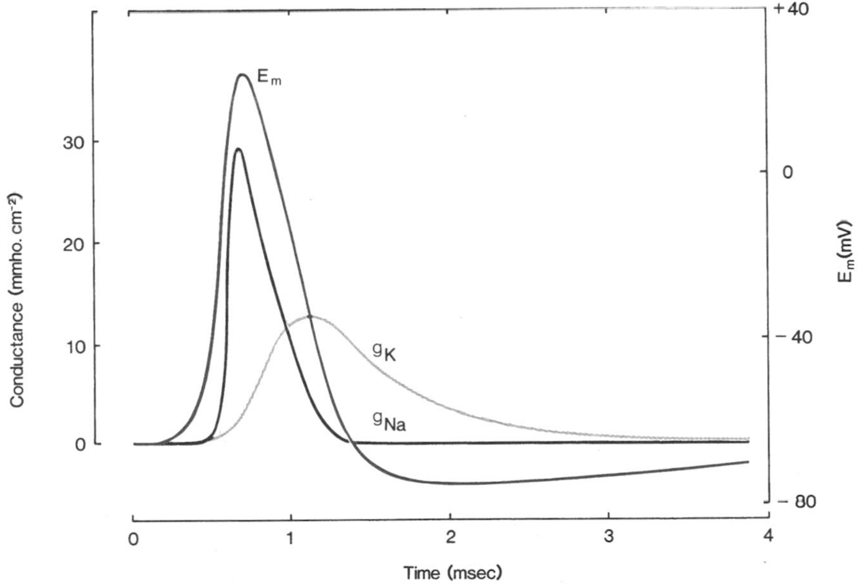

Fig. 34.2 Behaviour of Na^+ and K^+ channels during a conducted action potential. Rapid opening of Na^+ channels occurs during the action potential upstroke. Delayed opening of K^+ channels, and inactivation of Na^+ channels, causes repolarisation.

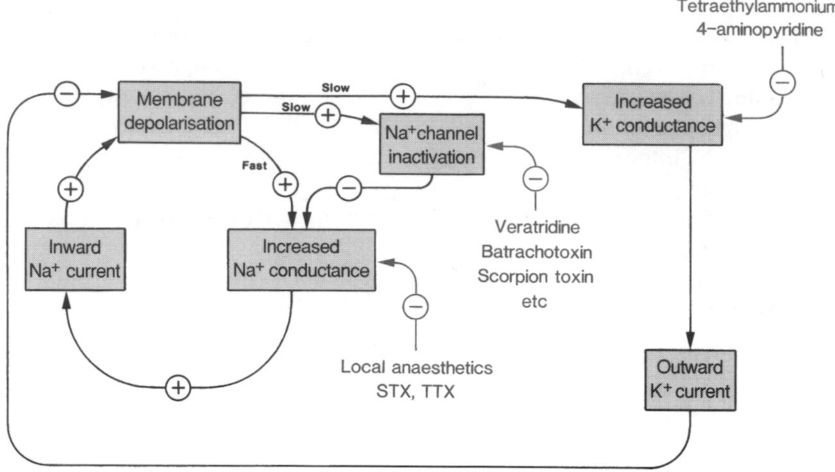

Fig. 34.3 Sites of action of drugs and other agents which affect membrane excitability.

by the loops linking S5 and S6 in each of the four domains, and this forms the binding site for some channel-blocking drugs, as well as conferring the ion-selectivity of the channel. The S4 helix contains positively charged residues, and is believed to be the voltage sensor. Depolarisation of the membrane causes this helix to move outwards, and probably to twist like a screw-thread. The net charge displacement associated with this gating process can be detected, independently of the ion movement though the channel, as a *gating current* (see Armstrong 1981); measurements of these gating currents have added greatly to the understanding of channel function. Exactly how the shift of the S4 helix results in channel opening remains uncertain. Inactivation of the channel results from the movement of an intracellular stretch of the protein, which physically blocks the channel, like a tethered stopper. In the case of the K^+ channel (Fig. 34.4), the stopper is made from the intracellular C-terminal region of each of the four subunits; in the Na^+ channel, it is formed by one of the intracellular loops linking two adjacent domains.

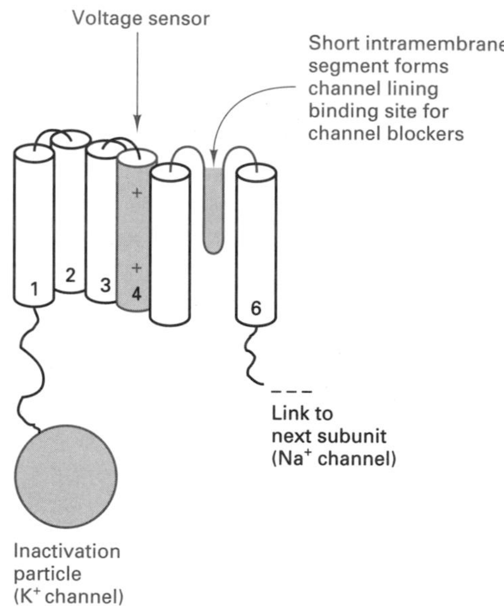

Fig. 34.4 Structure of voltage-gated ion channels. The diagram shows one of the four domains of the channel. In Na^+ channels, the four domains are linked as a single chain; in K^+ channels, they are separate subunits. Movement of helix 4 (voltage sensor) is responsible for channel activation. Inactivation occurs when the intracellular inactivation particle blocks the channel (in the Na^+ channel, the inactivating particle is formed from one of the intracellular loops; see text). The channel pore is formed from the short intramembrane segment, plus adjacent helices; channel-blocking drugs bind in this region.

DRUGS THAT AFFECT Na^+ CHANNELS

Though many drugs are able to block voltage-sensitive Na^+ channels, and inhibit the generation of the action potential, the only drugs in this category

Ionic basis of electrical excitability

- An electrically excitable cell is one that generates an all-or-nothing action potential in response to depolarisation of the membrane.
- In nerve and striated muscle cells, electrical excitability is due to the existence of voltage-activated Na^+ channels, which open transiently when the membrane is depolarised. Opening of Na^+ channels causes an inward current of Na^+ ions across the membrane, which further depolarises it.
- Recovery of the membrane potential is due to:
  —inactivation of Na^+ channels
  —delayed opening of voltage-activated K^+ channels, through which outward K^+ current flows, causing repolarisation.
- The refractory period represents the time taken for Na^+ channels to recover from inactivation.
- Drugs may reduce membrane excitability by:
  —blocking Na^+ channels (mainly neurons)
  —activating K^+ channels (more important in smooth muscle and myocardium than in neurons).
- Drugs may enhance membrane excitability by:
  —blocking inactivation of Na^+ channels
  —blocking K^+ channels.

that are clinically useful are the local anaesthetics, various anticonvulsant drugs (see Ch. 30) and class I antidysrhythmic drugs (see Ch. 13). The group of neurotoxins, exemplified by **tetrodotoxin** (TTX) and **saxitoxin** (STX), are the most potent agents that are known for blocking these channels. Agents that affect the gating properties of Na^+ channels include **veratridine**, neurotoxins such as **batrachotoxin**, and various insecticides such as **pyrethroids**.

LOCAL ANAESTHETICS

History

Coca leaves have been consumed for their psychotropic effects (see Ch. 32) by South American Indians for thousands of years, and the numbing effect of chewing these leaves on the mouth and tongue was known long before **cocaine** was isolated in 1860 and proposed as a local anaesthetic for surgical procedures. Sigmund Freud sought to make use of its 'psychic energising' power for psychiatric purposes. This was not a success, but his ophthalmologist friend in Vienna, Carl Köller, obtained some cocaine from Freud and showed in 1884 that reversible corneal anaesthesia could be produced by dropping cocaine into the eye. The idea was rapidly taken up, and within a few years cocaine anaesthesia was introduced into dentistry and general surgery. A synthetic substitute, **procaine**, was discovered in 1905, and many other useful compounds were later developed.

Chemical aspects

Local anaesthetic molecules consist of an aromatic part linked by an ester or amide bond to a basic side-chain (Fig. 34.5). They are weak bases, with pK_a values mainly in the range 8–9, so that they are mainly, but not completely, ionised at physiological pH. This is important in relation to their ability to penetrate the nerve sheath and axon membrane; quaternary derivatives, which are fully ionised irrespective of pH, are ineffective as local anaesthetics. **Benzocaine**, an atypical local anaesthetic, has no basic group.

The presence of the ester or amide bond in local anaesthetic molecules is important because of its susceptibility to metabolic hydrolysis. The ester-containing compounds are usually inactivated in the plasma and tissues (mainly liver) by non-specific esterases. Amides are more stable, and these anaesthetics generally have longer plasma half-lives.

Mechanism of action

Local anaesthetics block the initiation and propagation of action potentials by preventing the voltage-dependent increase in Na^+ conductance (Fig. 34.3). They appear to act in two main ways:

- by acting non-specifically on membranes, by virtue of their surface activity, somewhat in the manner of volatile anaesthetics
- by specifically plugging Na^+ channels.

Non-specific ('anaesthetic-like') actions are suggested because local anaesthetics (in sufficient concentration) affect various membrane functions, not only Na^+ conductance, and because local anaesthesia can be partly reversed by raising the hydrostatic pressure (as with volatile anaesthetics; see Ch. 26)—which can be interpreted to mean that volume expansion of the membrane plays a part in affecting function. This type of non-specific effect is probably significant for some local anaesthetics

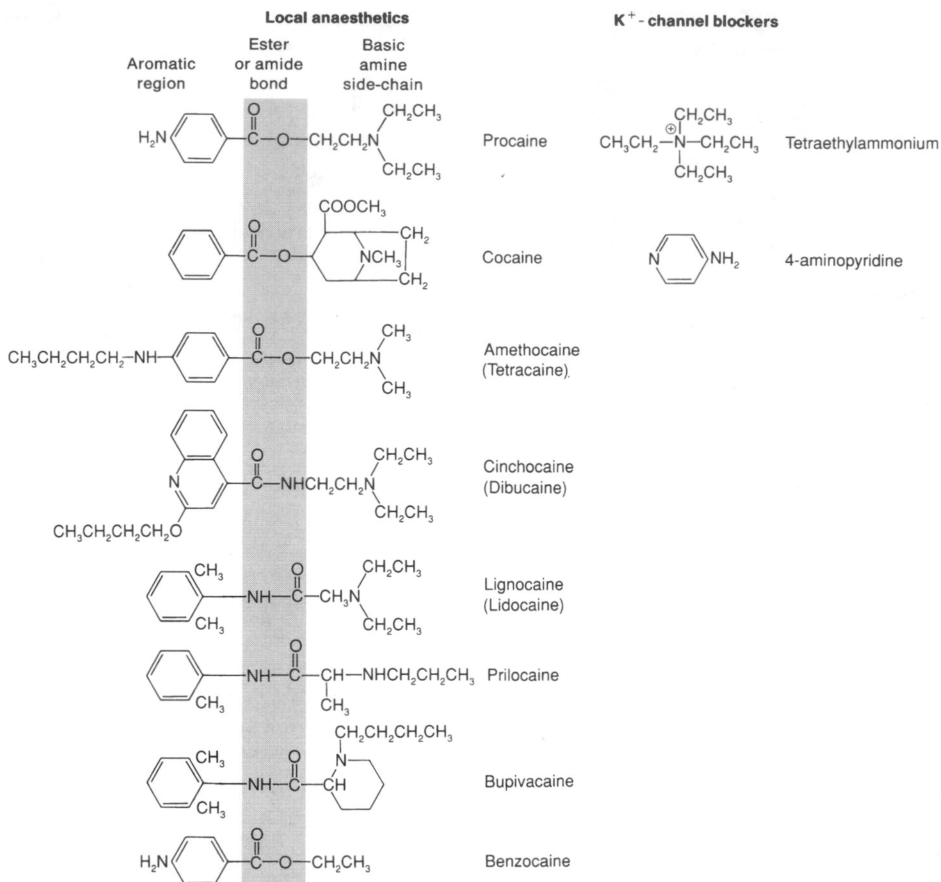

Fig. 34.5 Structures of local anaesthetics and drugs that block K^+ channels. The general structure of local anaesthetic molecules consists of aromatic group (left), ester or amide group (shaded) and amine group (right).

(especially benzocaine), but Na^+-channel block is predominant for most. For a detailed discussion of the Na^+-channel hypothesis, see Hille (1984), Strichartz & Ritchie (1987).

Local anaesthetic activity is strongly pH-dependent, being increased at alkaline pH (i.e. when the proportion of ionised molecules is low) and vice versa. This was first taken to mean that the *uncharged* molecule was the biologically active species, but it was later shown (see Ritchie & Greengard 1966, Narahashi & Frazier 1971) that the cationic species is the active form. In order to penetrate the nerve sheath and the axon membrane, however, to reach the inner end of the sodium channel (where the local anaesthetic binding site resides), the molecule must exist in its uncharged, membrane-permeant form, which accounts for the unexpected pH-dependence. This pH-dependence can be clinically important, since inflamed tissues are often acidic, and thus somewhat resistant to local anaesthetic agents.

Further analysis of local anaesthesic action (Strichartz 1973, Hille 1977, Strichartz & Ritchie 1987) has shown that many drugs exhibit the property of 'use-dependent' block of Na^+ channels, as well as affecting, to some extent, the gating of the channels. Use-dependence means that the more the channels are opened, the greater the block becomes. It is a prominent feature of the action of many class I antidysrhythmic drugs (Ch. 13), and occurs because the blocking molecule enters the channel much more readily when the channel is open than when it is closed. With quaternary local anaesthetics working from the inside of the membrane, the channels must be cycled through their

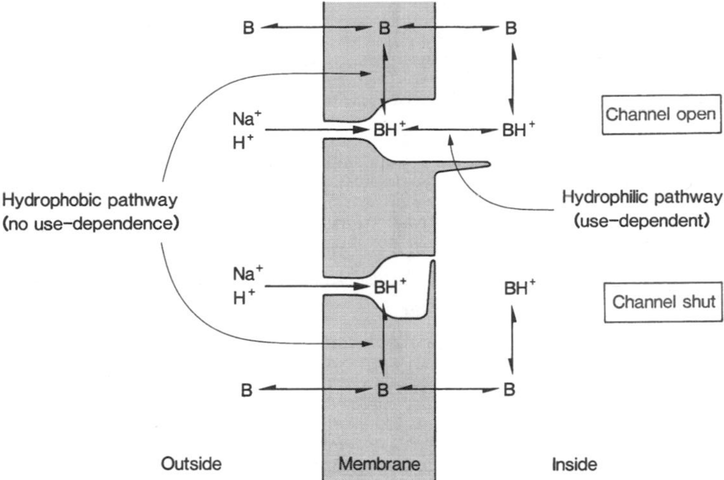

Fig. 34.6 Interaction of local anaesthetics with Na^+ channels. The blocking site within the channel can be reached via the open channel gate on the inner surface of the membrane by the charged species, BH^+ (hydrophilic pathway), or directly from the membrane by the uncharged species, B (hydrophobic pathway).

open state a few times before the blocking effect appears. With tertiary local anaesthetics, on the other hand, block can develop even if the channels are not open, and it is likely that the blocking molecule (uncharged) can enter the channel either directly from the membrane phase or via the open gate (Fig. 34.6). The relative importance of these two blocking pathways—the hydrophobic pathway via the membrane, and the hydrophilic pathway via the inner mouth of the channel—varies according to the lipid solubility of the drug, and the degree of use-dependence varies correspondingly.

As discussed earlier, the channel can exist in three functional states—resting, open and inactivated. Many local anaesthetics have been shown to bind most strongly to the inactivated state of the channel. Thus, at any given membrane potential the equilibrium between resting and inactivated channels will, in the presence of a local anaesthetic, be shifted in favour of the inactivated state, and this factor contributes to the overall blocking effect. The passage of a train of action potentials causes the channels to cycle through the open and inactivated states, both of which are more likely to bind local anaesthetic molecules than the resting state; thus, both mechanisms contribute to 'use-dependence'.

In general, local anaesthetics block conduction in small-diameter nerve fibres more readily than in large fibres. However, the smallest fibres in peripheral nerve are unmyelinated C-fibres, and these are rather less susceptible than the smallest myelinated (Aδ) fibres. Since nociceptive impulses are carried by Aδ- and C-fibres, pain sensation is blocked

Action of local anaesthetics (LAs)

- LAs block action potential generation by blocking Na^+ channels.
- LAs are amphiphilic molecules, with a hydrophobic aromatic group, and a basic amine group.
- LAs probably act in their cationic form, but must reach their site of action by penetrating the nerve sheath and axonal membrane as unionised species; they therefore have to be weak bases.
- Many LAs show use-dependence (depth of block increases with action potential frequency). This arises:
  - —because anaesthetic molecules gain access to the channel more readily when the channel is open
  - —because anaesthetic molecules have higher affinity for inactivated than for resting channels.
- Use-dependence is mainly of importance in relation to antidysrhythmic and anticonvulsant effects of LAs.
- LAs block conduction in the following order: small myelinated axons, non-myelinated axons, large myelinated axons. Nociceptive and sympathetic transmission is thus blocked first.

more readily than other sensory modalities (touch, proprioception, etc.). Motor axons, being large in diameter, are also relatively resistant. The differences in sensitivity among different nerve fibres, though easily measured experimentally, are not of much practical importance, and it is rarely possible to produce a block of pain sensation without affecting other modalities and causing local paralysis.

Local anaesthetics, as their name implies, are mainly used to produce local nerve block. In concentrations too low to cause nerve block, however, they are able to suppress the spontaneous discharge in sensory neurons that is believed to be responsible for *neuropathic pain* (see Ch. 31). Drugs undergoing trial for oral use as analgesics in such pain states include two antidysrhythmic drugs, **tocainide** and **mexiletine** (see Ch. 13).

Unwanted effects

The main unwanted effects of local anaesthetics involve the central nervous and cardiovascular systems, and they constitute the main source of hazard when local anaesthetics are used clinically. The main effect of local anaesthetics on the central nervous system is, paradoxically, to cause stimulation. This produces restlessness and tremor, with subjective effects ranging from confusion to extreme agitation. The tremor can progress to actual convulsions, and further increasing the dose produces CNS depression. The main threat to life comes from respiratory depression in this phase. The only local anaesthetic with markedly different CNS effects is **cocaine** (see Ch. 32), which produces marked euphoria at doses well below those that cause convulsions. This relates to its specific effect on monoamine uptake, an effect not shared by other local anaesthetics. **Procaine** is particularly liable to produce unwanted central effects, which is one reason for its replacement in clinical use by agents such as **lignocaine** and **prilocaine**, whose central effects are much less pronounced.

The cardiovascular effects of local anaesthetics are due mainly to myocardial depression and vasodilatation. Reduction of myocardial contractility probably results indirectly from an inhibition of the Na^+ current in cardiac muscle (see Ch. 13). The reduction of Na^+ entry leads to a decrease of $[Na^+]_i$, which in turn reduces intracellular Ca^{2+} stores (the opposite of the effect of cardiac glycosides; see Ch. 13), and this reduces the force of contraction. The antidysrhythmic effect of some local anaesthetics (especially **lignocaine**) is clinically useful.

Vasodilatation, mainly affecting arterioles, is due partly to a direct effect on vascular smooth muscle, and partly to inhibition of the sympathetic nervous system. The combined myocardial depression and vasodilatation leads to a fall in blood pressure, which may be sudden and life-threatening. **Cocaine** is an exception in respect of its cardiovascular effects, because of its ability to inhibit noradrenaline reuptake (see Ch. 7). This produces an enhancement of sympathetic activity, leading to tachycardia, increased cardiac output, vasoconstriction and increased arterial pressure.

Though local anaesthetics are usually administered in such a way as to minimise their spread to other parts of the body, they are ultimately absorbed into the systemic circulation. They may also be injected into veins or arteries by accident. The most dangerous unwanted effects result from actions on the central nervous and cardiovascular systems discussed above, namely restlessness and convulsions followed by respiratory depression, and hypotension, or even cardiac arrest. Hypersensitivity reactions sometimes occur with local anaesthetics, usually in the form of allergic dermatitis, but rarely as an acute anaphylactic reaction. Other unwanted effects that are specific to particular drugs include mucosal irritation (**cocaine** and **dibucaine**) and methaemoglobinaemia (which occurs after large doses of **prilocaine**, because of the production of a toxic metabolite).

Pharmacokinetic aspects

Local anaesthetics vary a good deal in the rapidity with which they penetrate tissues, and this affects the rate at which they cause nerve block when injected into tissues and the rate of onset of, and recovery from, anaesthesia (Table 34.1). It also affects their usefulness as surface anaesthetics for application to mucous membranes. **Procaine**, for example, penetrates tissues poorly and is unsuitable for surface anaesthesia.

Most of the ester-linked local anaesthetics (e.g. **procaine** and **amethocaine**) are rapidly hydrolysed by plasma cholinesterase, so their plasma half-life is short. Procaine is hydrolysed to p-aminobenzoic acid, a folate precursor which interferes with the antibacterial effect of sulphonamides (see Ch. 35), a fact which may occasionally be of clinical significance. The amide-linked drugs (e.g. **lignocaine** and **prilocaine**) are metabolised mainly in the liver,

Table 34.1 Pharmacokinetic properties of local anaesthetics

Drug	Rate of onset	Duration	Tissue penetration	Plasma $t_{½}$ (approx)
Procaine	Moderate	Short	Slow	30 min
Lignocaine	Rapid	Moderate	Rapid	2 h
Amethocaine	Slow	Long	Moderate	1 h
Dibucaine	Moderate	Long	Moderate	3 h
Bupivacaine	Slow	Long	Moderate	3 h
Prilocaine	Moderate	Moderate	Moderate	2 h

Unwanted effects and pharmacokinetics of LAs

- LAs are either esters or amides. Esters are rapidly hydrolysed by plasma cholinesterase, and amides are metabolised in the liver. Plasma half-lives are generally short, about l–2 hours.
- Unwanted effects are due mainly to escape of LAs into systemic circulation.
- Main unwanted effects are:
  - —CNS effects, agitation, confusion, tremors progressing to convulsions and respiratory depression
  - —cardiovascular effects, namely myocardial depression and vasodilatation, leading to fall in blood pressure
  - —occasional hypersensitivity reactions.
- LAs vary in the rapidity with which they penetrate tissues, and in their duration of action. Lignocaine penetrates tissues readily, and is suitable for surface application; bupivacaine has a particularly long duration of action.

usually by N-dealkylation rather than cleavage of the amide bond, and the metabolites are often pharmacologically active.

Benzocaine is an unusual local anaesthetic of very low solubility, which was used as a dry powder to dress painful skin ulcers. The drug is slowly released and produces long-lasting surface anaesthesia. It is also used in throat lozenges.

The *routes of administration*, *uses* and *main adverse effects* of local anaesthetics are summarised in Table 34.2.

TETRODOTOXIN AND SAXITOXIN

We should not be surprised that nature, rather than medicinal chemistry, has provided the most potent and selective agents that block Na^+ channels of excitable tissues. **Tetrodotoxin** (TTX) is produced in the tissues of a poisonous Pacific fish, the puffer fish, so called because when alarmed it inflates itself to an almost spherical spiny ball. It is evidently a species highly preoccupied with defense, but the Japanese are not easily put off and the puffer fish is regarded by them as a special delicacy. To serve it in public restaurants, however, the chef must be registered as sufficiently skilled in removing the toxic organs (especially liver and ovaries) so as to make the flesh safe to eat. Accidental tetrodotoxin poisoning is quite common, nonetheless. Historical records of long sea-voyages often contained reference to attacks of severe weakness, progressing to complete paralysis and death, caused by eating puffer fish. The same toxin is produced by a poisonous newt, a remarkable example of convergent evolution.

Saxitoxin (STX) is produced by a marine microorganism, which sometimes proliferates in very large numbers and even colours the sea, giving the 'red tide' phenomenon. At such times, marine shellfish can accumulate the toxin and become poisonous to humans.

These toxins, unlike conventional local anaesthetics, act exclusively from the outside of the membrane. Both are complex molecules, containing a *guanidinium* moiety (Fig. 34.7).The guanidinium ion is able to permeate voltage-sensitive Na^+ channels, and this part of the TTX or STX molecule lodges in the channel, leaving the rest of the molecule blocking its outer mouth. In contrast to the local anaesthetics, there is no interaction between the gating and blocking reactions with TTX or STX—their association and dissociation are independent of whether the channel is open or closed.

Table 34.2 Methods of administration, uses and adverse effects of local anaesthetics (LAs)

Method	Uses	Drugs	Notes and adverse effects
Surface anaesthesia	Nose, mouth, bronchial tree (usually in spray form), cornea, urinary tract Not effective for skin*	Lignocaine, tetracaine, dibucaine, cocaine	Risk of systemic toxicity when high concentrations and large areas are involved
Infiltration anaesthesia	Direct injection into tissues to reach nerve branches and terminals Used in minor surgery	Most	**Adrenaline** or **felypressin** often added as vasoconstrictors (not with fingers or toes, for fear of causing ischaemic tissue damage) Only suitable for small areas; otherwise, serious risk of systemic toxicity
Intravenous regional anaesthesia	LA injected intravenously distal to a pressure cuff to arrest blood flow; remains effective until the circulation is restored Used for limb surgery	Mainly lidocaine, prilocaine	Risk of systemic toxicity when cuff is released prematurely. Risk is small if cuff remains inflated for at least 20 minutes
Nerve-block anaesthesia	LA is injected close to nerve trunks (e.g. brachial plexus, intercostal or dental nerves) to produce a loss of sensation peripherally Used for surgery, dentistry, analgesia	Most	Less LA needed than for infiltration anaesthesia. Accurate placement of the needle is important Onset of anaesthesia may be slow Duration of anaesthesia may be increased by addition of vasoconstrictor Highly specialised use
Spinal anaesthesia	LA injected into the subarachnoid space (containing CSF) to act on spinal roots and spinal cord Used for surgery to abdomen, pelvis or leg, mainly when general anaesthesia cannot be used	Mainly lignocaine, tetracaine	Main risks are bradycardia and hypotension (due to sympathetic block), respiratory depression (due to effects on phrenic nerve or respiratory centre). Avoided by minimising cranial spread Postoperative urinary retention (block of pelvic autonomic outflow) is common
Epidural anaesthesia†	LA injected into epidural space, blocking spinal roots Uses as for spinal anaesthesia; also for painless childbirth	Mainly lignocaine, bupivacaine	Unwanted effects similar to those of spinal anaesthesia, but less probable, because longitudinal spread of LA is reduced Postoperative urinary retention common

* Surface anaesthesia does not work well on the skin, though recently a non-crystalline mixture of lignocaine and prilocaine (**eutectic mixture of local anaesthetics** or **EMLA**) has been developed for application to the skin, producing complete anaesthesia in about 1 hour.

† Intrathecal or epidural administration of LA in combination with an opiate (see Ch. 31) produces more effective analgesia than can be achieved with the opiate alone. Only a small concentration of LA is needed, insufficient to produce appreciable loss of sensation or other side effects. The mechanism of this synergism is unknown, but the procedure is proving useful in pain treatment.

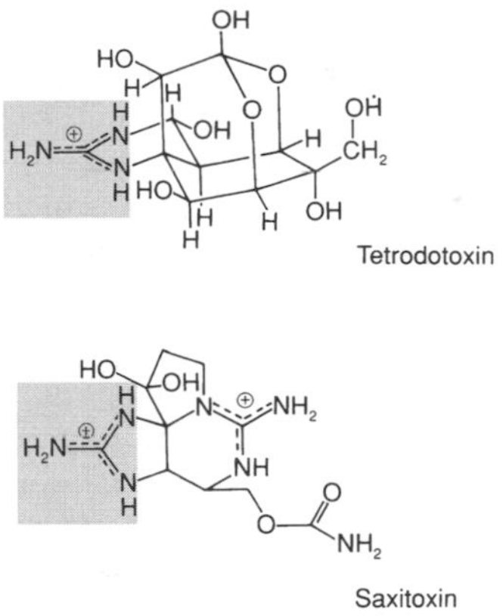

Tetrodotoxin

Saxitoxin

Fig. 34.7 Structure of tetrodotoxin and saxitoxin. The guanidinium residues are shown in light pink.

TTX and STX are quite unsuitable for clinical use as local anaesthetics, being expensive to obtain from their exotic sources and very poor at penetrating tissues because of their very low lipid solubility. They have, however, been important as experimental tools for the isolation and cloning of Na^+ channels (see Catterall 1993).

AGENTS THAT AFFECT Na^+-CHANNEL GATING

Various substances, mostly molecules of a highly Baroque nature, are known which modify Na^+-channel gating in such a way as to increase the probability of opening of the channels (see Hille 1984). They include various toxins, mainly from frog skin (e.g. **batrachotoxin**), scorpion or sea anemone venoms; plant alkaloids such as **veratridine**; and insecticides such as **DDT** and the **pyrethrins**. They facilitate Na^+-channel activation, so that Na^+ channels open at the normal resting potential; they also inhibit inactivation, so that the channels fail to close if the membrane remains depolarised. The membrane thus becomes hyperexcitable, and the action potential is prolonged (Fig. 34.8). Spontaneous discharges occur at first, but the cells eventually become permanently depolarised and inexcitable. All of these substances affect the heart, producing extrasystoles and other dysrhythmias, culminating in fibrillation; they also cause spontaneous discharges in nerve and muscle, leading to twitching and convulsions. The very high lipid solubility of substances like DDT makes them effective as insecticides, for they are readily absorbed through the integument. Drugs in this class are useful as experimental tools for studying Na^+ channels, but have no clinical uses.

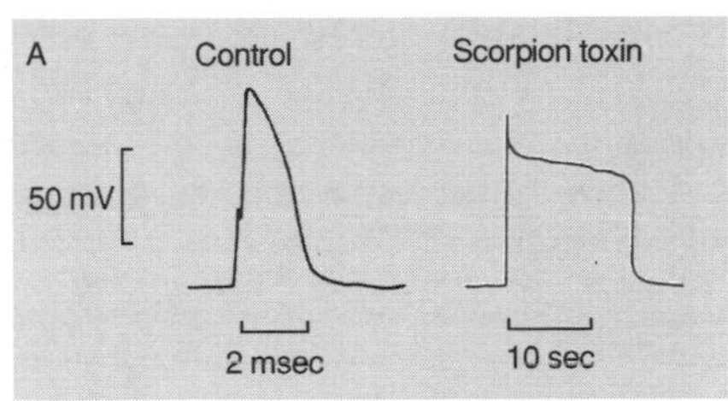

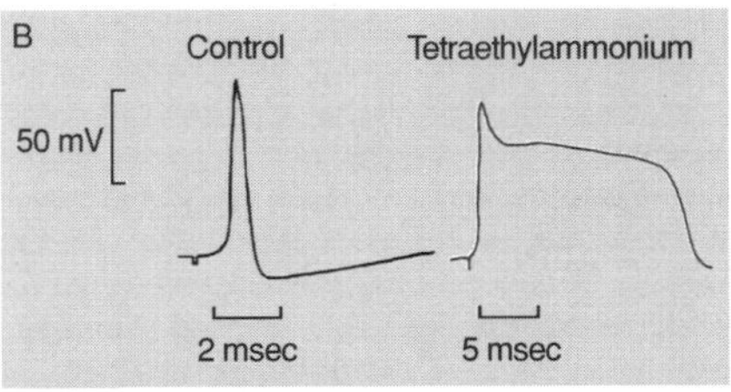

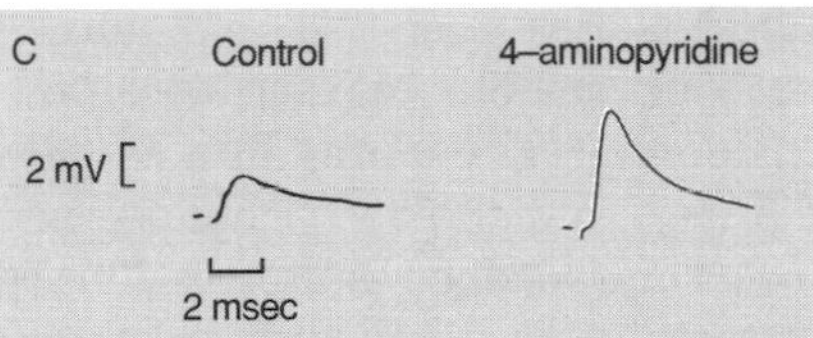

Fig. 34.8 Effects of scorpion toxin and K^+-channel-blocking drugs on action potential configuration. **A.** Scorpion toxin on the frog node of Ranvier. Scorpion toxin impedes Na^+-channel inactivation (see Fig. 34.3) and prolongs the action potential from 2 milliseconds to nearly 15 seconds. **B.** Tetraethylammonium on squid axon. TEA blocks K^+ channels, and thus delays membrane repolarisation. **C.** Effect of 4-aminopyridine on the endplate potential in frog muscle. Enhancement of the endplate potential is due to an increase in the amount of acetylcholine released from the nerve terminals, which results mainly from the increased action potential duration in the terminals. (From: (A) Schmitt O, Schmitt H 1972 Pflugers Arch 333: 51; (B) Tasaki I, Hagiwara S 1957 J Gen Physiol 40: 859; (C) Molgo J et al. 1977 J Pharmacol Exp Ther 203: 653)

AGENTS THAT AFFECT K^+ CHANNELS

The pharmacology of K^+ channels has recently

attracted considerable interest (see reviews by Cook & Quast 1990, Pongs 1992), mainly because of the discovery of many different K^+ channel types in different tissues. Other aspects of K^+ channel pharmacology are discussed elsewhere in this book (e.g. Chs 2, 14 and 20). The main types of K^+ channel are:

- Those activated by changes in membrane potential (voltage-activated channels). Four or five different subtypes are known, some of which have been cloned and characterised at the molecular level, and shown to belong to the structural type shown in Figure 34.4.
- Those activated by an increase in intracellular calcium concentration (calcium-activated channels).
- Various other K^+ channels. Examples of particular pharmacological significance include the ATP-sensitive K^+ channels in the pancreatic islets, on which hypoglycaemic drugs of the **sulphonylurea** type act (see Ch. 20), the K^+ channels of smooth muscle cells on which vasodilators such as **cromokalim** and **diazoxide** act (Ch. 14), and the acetylcholine-sensitive K^+ channels controlled by muscarinic receptors in the heart (Ch. 13). Similar types of K^+ channel also occur in neurons (see Halliwell 1990); one in particular, the M-channel (see Adams et al. 1982), which is susceptible to block by various neurotransmitters and modulators, may be important as a mechanism through which many such mediators can affect neuronal function.

In general, though K^+ channels clearly play an important role in controlling membrane excitability and the firing pattern of neurons, the details of which channels do what are still very unclear, and the casual observer may wonder weakly why so many are necessary. At present, the pharmacological manipulation of neuronal K^+ channels is of little clinical importance, and interest centres mainly on the use of channel-blocking agents, which include various snake toxins, as experimental tools.

Many substances are able to block voltage-sensitive K^+ channels of excitable membranes (see Cook & Quast 1990). They prolong the action potential (Fig. 34.8), since the delayed increase in K^+ conductance in response to depolarisation (Figs 34.1 and 34.3) is one of the mechanisms that causes the membrane to depolarise following the action potential.* Repetitive firing can also occur, the overall effect being similar to that of drugs that block Na^+-channel inactivation. Drugs that have this effect include **tetraethylammonium** (TEA) and **4-aminopyridine** (4AP), which act non-selectively on most types of K^+ channel. Their effects on nerve conduction, though much studied and revealing in relation to the mode of gating of K^+ channels, are not of much clinical use. Such drugs might be useful in multiple sclerosis, a demyelinating disease of the central nervous system in which conduction fails because of the loss of myelin. Blocking K^+ channels might enable action potentials to propagate successfully through the demyelinated segments of affected axons. However, 4AP produces severe side effects (nausea and convulsions), and more selective drugs will be needed.

The most striking effect seen with K^+-channel blockers is an enhancement of transmitter release at many central and peripheral synapses. This can be a very large effect (Fig. 34.8), and it probably results mainly from prolongation of the action potential in the nerve terminals. In theory, this could be useful for restoring neuromuscular transmission following the use of neuromuscular-blocking agents (Ch. 6), or in disorders of neuromuscular transmission such as myasthenia gravis, but existing compounds are unsatisfactory because of severe side effects.

The other main group of K^+-channel-blocking agents consists of various polypeptide toxins, which act much more selectively than TEA or 4AP. The first to be discovered was **apamin**, isolated from bee venom, which blocks specifically one of the several types of Ca^{2+}-activated K^+ channels in smooth muscle and liver cells. The toxin causes convulsions when injected into the brain. Another type of Ca^{2+}-activated K^+ channel is blocked by a toxin from scorpion venom, **charybdotoxin**. One type of voltage-activated K^+ channel is blocked by a component of the venom of the green mamba snake, known as **dendrotoxin**. Toxins of this kind

*Work by Ritchie and his colleagues has shown, rather surprisingly, that K^+ channels are not present in the nodal membrane of mammalian myelinated nerve fibres, and that K^+-channel-blocking agents have little effect on the action potential. They do affect mammalian nerve terminals, however.

are very useful in determining the function and biochemical characteristics of the various K^+ channels, but they have no clinical uses.

The therapeutic possibilities of blocking or activating specific types of K^+ channel are only just beginning to be explored.

REFERENCES AND FURTHER READING

Adams P R, Brown D A, Constanti A 1982 Pharmacological inhibition of the M-current. J Physiol 332: 223–262

Armstrong C M 1981 Sodium channels and gating currents. Physiol Rev 61: 644–683

Catterall W A 1993 Structure and function of voltage-gated ion channels. Trends Neurosci 16: 500–506

Cook N S 1988 The pharmacology of potassium channels and their therapeutic potential. Trends Pharmacol Sci 9: 21–28

Cook N S, Quast U 1990 Potassium channel pharmacology. In: Cook N S (ed) Potassium channels: structure, classification, functions and therapeutic potential. Ellis-Horwood, Chichester

Halliwell J V 1990 K^+ channels in the central nervous system. In: Cook N S (ed) Potassium channels: structure, classification, function and therapeutic potential. Ellis-Horwood, Chichester, p 348–381

Hille B 1977 Local anesthetics: hydrophilic and hydrophobic pathways for the drug–receptor interaction. J Gen Physiol 69: 497–515

Hille B 1984 Ionic channels of excitable membranes. Sinauer, Sunderland, MA

Hodgkin A L 1967 The conduction of the nervous impulse. Liverpool University Press, Liverpool

Katz B 1966 Nerve, muscle and synapse. McGraw Hill, New York

Narahashi T, Frazier D T 1971 Site of action and active form of local anaesthetics. Neurosci Res 4: 65

Nicholls J G, Martin A R, Wallace B G 1992 From neuron to brain. Sinauer, Sunderland, MA

Pongs O 1992 Structural basis of voltage-gated K^+-channel pharmacology. Trends Pharmacol Sci 13: 359–365

Ritchie J M, Greengard P 1966 On the mode of action of local anaesthetics. Annu Rev Pharmacol 6: 405–430

Strichartz G R 1973 The inhibition of sodium currents in myelinated nerve by quaternary derivatives of lidocaine. J Gen Physiol 62: 35–57

Strichartz G R, Ritchie J M 1987 The action of local anaesthetics on ion channels of excitable tissues. In: Strichartz G R (ed) Local anaesthetics. Handbook of experimental pharmacology. Springer-Verlag, Berlin, vol 81: 21–52

Weston A H, Edwards G 1992 Recent progress in potassium channel opener pharmacology. Biochem Pharmacol 43: 47–54

CHEMOTHERAPY

35

BASIC PRINCIPLES OF CHEMOTHERAPY

The development of chemotherapy during the past half-century constitutes one of the most important therapeutic advances in the history of medicine.

The term '**chemotherapy**' was coined by Ehrlich at the beginning of the century to describe the use of synthetic chemicals to destroy infective agents. In recent years the definition of the term has been broadened to include '**antibiotics**'—substances produced by some microorganisms that kill or inhibit the growth of other microorganisms. The term chemotherapy is now also applied to the use of chemicals (either natural or synthetic) used to inhibit the growth of malignant or cancerous cells within the body. Ehrlich had assumed that the development of completely selective agents was an unattainable goal and that the most that could be hoped for was the production of substances that were maximally 'parasitotropic' and minimally 'organotropic'. This view has turned out to be rather more pessimistic than was warranted because some totally selective antibacterial agents have been produced.

THE MOLECULAR BASIS OF CHEMOTHERAPY

Chemotherapeutic agents are chemicals which are intended to be toxic for the parasitic cell but innocuous for the host. The feasibility of such selective toxicity depends on the existence of exploitable biochemical differences between the parasite and the host cell. The extent of this difference depends mainly on how far apart host and parasite are in terms of evolutionary development. Parasitic cells may be prokaryotes (cells *without* nuclei—the *bacteria*) or eukaryotes (cells *with* nuclei). This second category of parasites includes both some single-celled organisms (e.g. *protozoa*) and some multicellular organisms (e.g. *helminths*). In general, the cells of these latter organisms are likely to be more similar biochemically to the cells of the host, which are also, of course, eukaryotic.

In a separate category are the *viruses*, which are not, properly speaking, cells at all because they do not have their own biochemical machinery for generating energy or for any sort of synthesis. Viruses need to utilise the metabolic machinery of the host cell and they thus present a particular kind of problem for chemotherapeutic attack.

In yet another category are *cancer* cells—host cells that have become malignant, i.e. they have escaped from the regulating devices which control normal cells. Cancer cells can be considered to be, in a special sense, 'foreign' or 'parasitic', but are clearly more similar to normal host cells than are any of the categories considered above, and constitute an especially difficult problem for selective toxicity.

In approaching the question of chemotherapy and the biochemical differences between parasite and host cell, it is easier, for simplicity, to start with a bacterial cell and to ask what such a cell has to do in order to grow and divide. Figure 35.1 shows in simplified diagrammatic form the main structures and functions of a 'generalised' bacterial cell. Surrounding the cell is the *cell wall*, which characteristically contains *peptidoglycan* in all forms of bacteria except mycoplasma. (Peptidoglycan is *unique* to prokaryotic cells and has no counterpart in eukaryotes.) Within the cell wall is the *plasma membrane*, which is similar to that of the eukaryotic cell, consisting of a phospholipid bilayer and pro-

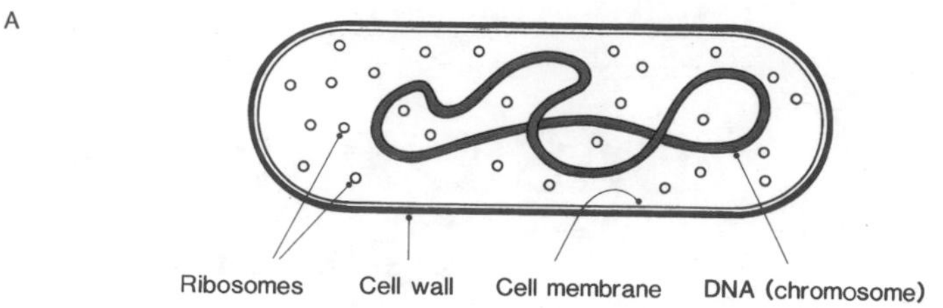

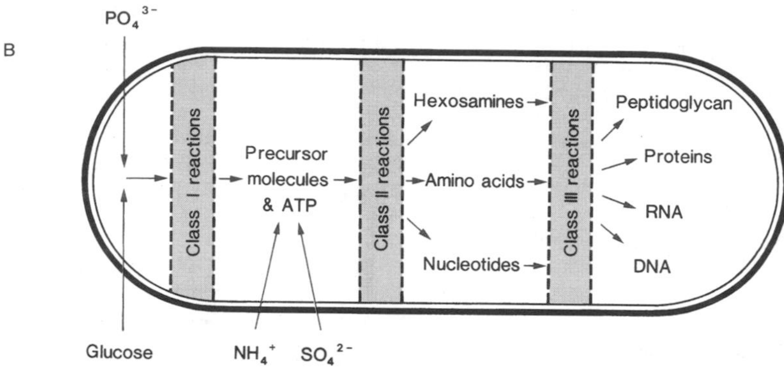

Fig. 35.1 Diagrams of structure and metabolism of a bacterial cell. A. Schematic representation of a bacterial cell. **B.** Flow diagram showing the synthesis of the main types of macromolecules of a bacterial cell. Class I reactions result in the synthesis of the precursor molecules necessary for class II reactions, which result in the synthesis of the constituent molecules, which are then assembled into macromolecules by class III reactions. (Modified from: Mandelstam, McQuillen & Dawes 1982)

teins. However, in bacteria the plasma membrane does not contain any sterols and this may result in differential penetration of chemicals. It functions as a selectively permeable membrane with specific transport mechanisms for various types of nutrients. The function of the cell wall is to support this underlying plasma membrane, which is subject to an internal osmotic pressure of about 5 atmospheres in Gram-negative organisms, and about 20 atmospheres in Gram-positive organisms.* The plasma membrane and cell wall together comprise the envelope.

Within the plasma membrane is the *cytoplasm*. As in eukaryotic cells, this contains all the soluble proteins (most having enzymic functions), the ribosomes involved in protein synthesis, all the small molecule intermediates involved in metabolism and all the inorganic ions. However, the bacterial cell, unlike the eukaryotic cell, has no nucleus; instead, the genetic material, in the form of a single chromosome that holds all the genetic information of the cell, lies loose in the cytoplasm. In further contrast to eukaryotic cells, the chromosome of the bacterial cell contains no histones, and there are no mitochondria—all the energy generation goes on in the plasma membrane.

These, then, are the essential structures of the generalised bacterial cell. Some bacteria have additional components such as a capsule and/or one or more flagella, but the only additional structure with relevance for chemotherapy is the *outer membrane*, outside the cell wall, which is found in Gram-negative bacteria and which may prevent penetration of antibacterial agents (see Ch. 37, p. 718). It also prevents easy access of lysozyme (an enzyme that can break down cell wall structures and is found in white blood cells and tissue fluids) to the peptidoglycan of the cell wall.

Having outlined the essential structures of the

*The terms Gram-positive and Gram-negative refer to whether or not the cell stains with a particular combination of dyes. More detail of the differences between Gram-positive and Gram-negative organisms is given in Chapter 37 (p. 718).

bacterial cell, the next step is to consider the biochemical reactions involved in their formation (Fig. 35.1). One can classify these reactions into three general categories:

- *Class I.* The utilisation of glucose or some alternative carbon source for the generation of energy (ATP) and of simple carbon compounds (such as the intermediates of the citric acid cycle) which are used as precursors in the next class of reactions.
- *Class II.* The utilisation of the energy and precursors to make all the necessary small molecules: amino acids, nucleotides, phospholipids, amino sugars, carbohydrates and growth factors.
- *Class III.* Assembly of the small molecules into macromolecules: proteins, RNA, DNA, polysaccharides and peptidoglycan.

These reactions are potential targets for attack by chemotherapeutic agents. Other potential targets are the formed structures of the cell, for example the cell membrane, or, in higher organisms, the microtubules (targets in fungi and cancer cells). Specific types of cells may be targets in some higher organisms (e.g. muscle tissue in helminths).

In considering these targets, emphasis will be placed on bacteria, but reference will also be made to protozoa, helminths, fungi, cancer cells and, where possible, viruses. The classification that follows is clearly not a rigid one; a drug may affect reactions in more than one class or more than one subgroup of reactions within a class.

> **The molecular basis of chemotherapy**
>
> - To be effective, chemotherapeutic drugs should be toxic for invading organisms and innocuous for the host; such selective toxicity depends on there being exploitable biochemical differences between the parasite (e.g. a bacterium) and the host.
> - The three general classes of biochemical reactions are potential targets for chemotherapy. The characteristics of each class are as follows:
>   - —*Class I*, glucose and other carbon sources are used to produce simple carbon compounds.
>   - —*Class II*, energy and class I compounds are used to make small molecules, e.g. amino acids, nucleotides, etc.
>   - —*Class III*, small molecules are built into larger molecules, e.g. peptidoglycan, proteins, nucleic acids, etc.

BIOCHEMICAL REACTIONS AS POTENTIAL TARGETS

Class I reactions

Class I reactions are not promising targets, for two reasons. First, there is no very marked difference between bacteria and human cells in the mechanism for obtaining energy from glucose, since both use the Embden–Meyerhof pathway and the citric acid cycle. Second, even if the glucose pathways were to be blocked, a large variety of other compounds (amino acids, lactate, etc.) could be used by bacteria as alternatives.

Class II reactions

Class II reactions are better targets since some pathways involved in class II reactions exist in parasitic but not in human cells. For instance, human cells have in the course of evolution lost the ability, possessed by bacteria, to synthesise some amino acids—the so-called 'essential' amino acids—and also the growth factors or vitamins. Any such difference represents a potential target. Another type of target occurs when a pathway is identical in both bacteria and man but has differential sensitivity to drugs.

Folate

The *synthesis* of folate is an example of a metabolic pathway found in bacteria but not in man. Folate is required for DNA synthesis in both bacteria and in man (see Chs 23 and 36). Man obtains it from the diet and has evolved a transport mechanism for taking it up into the cells. Man does not need to synthesise it and indeed cannot do so. By contrast, most species of bacteria, as well as the asexual forms of malarial protozoa, have not evolved the necessary transport mechanisms and they cannot make use of preformed folate. They must, of necessity, synthesise their own folate. This difference has proved to be useful for chemotherapy. **Sulphonamides** contain the sulphanilamide moiety—a structural analogue of p-aminobenzoic acid (PABA), which is essential in the synthesis of folate (see Figs 23.4 and 37.1). Sulphonamides compete with PABA for the enzyme involved in folate synthesis and thus inhibit the metabolism of the bacteria. They are consequently

Table 35.1 Specificity of inhibitors of dihydrofolate reductase

	IC_{50} (µmol/l) for FH_2 reductase		
Inhibitor	Human	Protozoal	Bacterial
Trimethoprim	260	0.07	0.005
Pyrimethamine	0.7	0.0005	2.5
Methotrexate	0.001	approx. 0.1*	Inactive

* Tested on *P. berghei*, a rodent malaria.

bacteriostatic not *bactericidal* and are therefore only really effective in the presence of adequate host defences (which are discussed in Ch. 11).

The *utilisation* of folate, in the form of tetrahydrofolate, as a cofactor in thymidylate synthesis (see Figs 23.7 and 36.8) is an example of a pathway in which there is differential sensitivity of human and bacterial enzymes to chemicals (Table 35.1). This pathway is virtually identical in microorganisms and man, but one of the key enzymes, dihydrofolate reductase, which reduces dihydrofolate to tetrahydrofolate (Fig. 23.5), is many times more sensitive to the folate antagonist **trimethoprim** in bacteria than in man. In some malarial protozoa this enzyme is somewhat less sensitive to trimethoprim than is the bacterial enzyme. The relative IC_{50} values (the concentration causing 50% inhibition) for bacterial, malarial, protozoal and mammalian enzymes are given in Table 35.1, as are those for **pyrimethamine**, primarily an antimalarial agent (Ch. 40). Another antimalarial drug which inhibits the protozoal enzyme specifically is **proguanil**. The human enzyme on the other hand is very sensitive to the effect of the folate analogue **methotrexate** (Table 35.1), and this compound is used in the chemotherapy of certain cancers (see Ch. 36). Methotrexate is inactive in bacteria because, being very similar in structure to folate, it requires active uptake by cells. Trimethoprim and pyrimethamine enter the cells by diffusion.

The use of sequential blockade with a combination of two drugs which, in parasite cells, affect the same pathway at different points, for example **sulphonamides** and the **folate antagonists** (Fig. 37.1, p. 721), is more successful than the use of either alone. Furthermore, lower concentrations of each drug are effective when the two are used together. A formulation that contains both a sulphonamide and trimethoprim is **co-trimoxazole** (p. 722).

Pyrimidine and purine analogues

The pyrimidine analogue, **fluorouracil**, which is used in cancer chemotherapy (Ch. 36) is converted to a fraudulent nucleotide that interferes with thymidylate synthesis. Other cancer chemotherapy agents that give rise to fraudulent nucleotides are the purine analogues **mercaptopurine** and **thioguanine**. **Flucytosine**, an antifungal drug (Ch. 39), is deaminated to fluorouracil within the cell; selectivity for fungal cells is due to the fact that this deamination occurs to a much lesser extent in man.

Class III reactions

Class III reactions are particularly good targets for selective toxicity because every cell *has* to make its own macromolecules—these cannot be picked up from the environment and there are very distinct differences between mammalian cells and parasitic cells in the pathways involved in class III reactions.

The synthesis of peptidoglycan

Peptidoglycan constitutes the cell wall of bacteria and does not occur in eukaryotes. It is the equivalent of a non-stretchable string bag enclosing the whole bacterium. For some bacteria (the Gram-negative organisms), the bag consists of a single thickness, but for others (Gram-positive organisms), it is up to 40 layers thick. Each layer consists of multiple backbones of amino sugars—alternating N-acetylglucosamine and N-acetylmuramic acid residues (Fig. 35.2)—the latter having short peptide side-chains which are cross-linked to form a latticework. The cross-links differ in different species. In staphylococci they consist of five glycine residues (Fig. 35.2). This cross-linking is responsible for the strength that allows the cell wall to resist the high internal osmotic pressure. The peptidoglycan is in fact one gigantic molecule with a molecular weight of many millions, constituting up to 10–15% of the dry weight of the cell.

In synthesising the peptidoglycan layer, the cell has the problem of using cytoplasmic components to build up this very large insoluble structure on the outside of the cell membrane. To do this it is necessary to transport the components, which are synthesised within the cell, and which are individually hydrophilic, through the hydrophobic cell membrane. This is accomplished by linking the

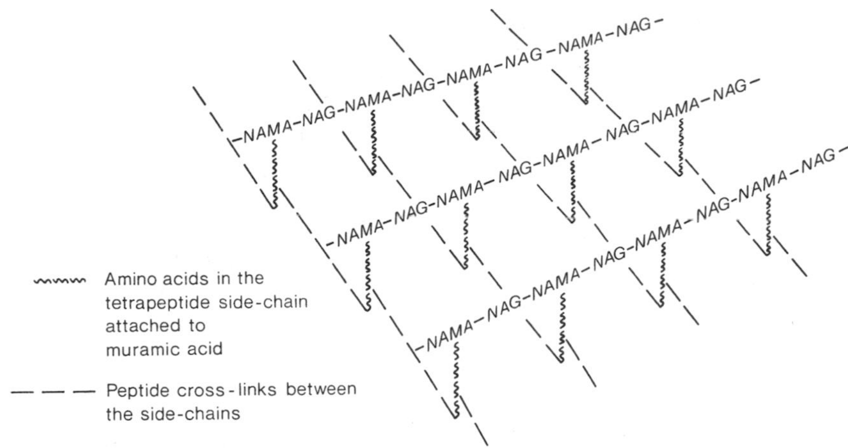

Fig. 35.2 Schematic diagram of a single layer of peptidoglycan from a bacterial cell (e.g. *Staph. aureus*). (NAMA = N-acetylmuramic acid; NAG = N-acetylglucosamine). In *Staph. aureus* the peptide cross-links consist of five glycine residues. Gram-positive bacteria have several layers of peptidoglycan.

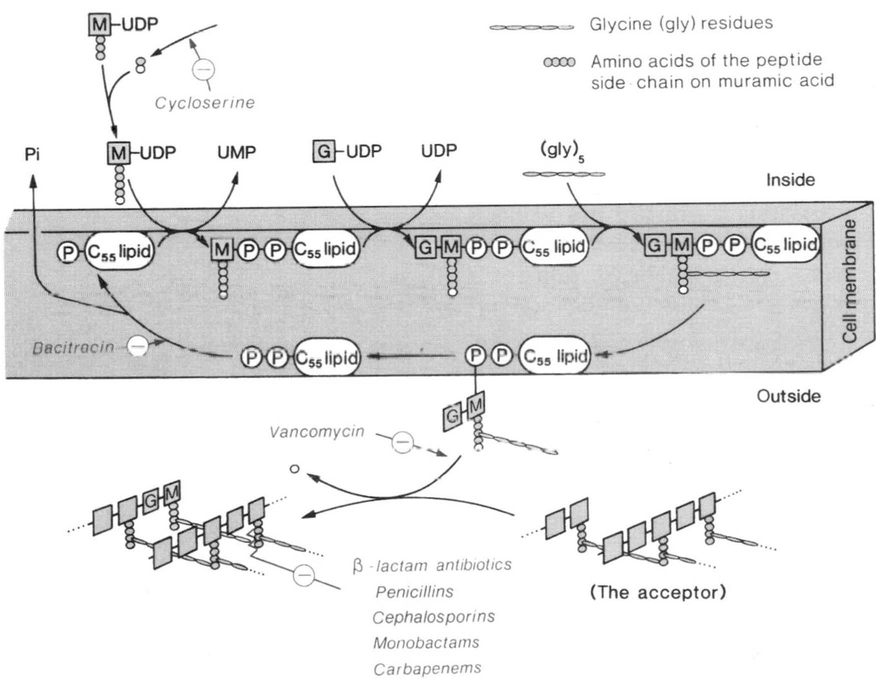

Fig. 35.3 Schematic diagram of the biosynthesis of peptidoglycan in a bacterial cell (e.g. *Staph. aureus*) with the sites of action of various antibiotics. The hydrophilic disaccharide–pentapeptide is transferred across the lipid cell membrane attached to a large lipid (C_{55} lipid) by a pyrophosphate bridge (–P–P–). On the outside, it is enzymically attached to the 'acceptor' (the growing peptidoglycan layer). The final reaction is a transpeptidation, in which the loose end of the (gly)5 chain is attached to a peptide side-chain of an M in the acceptor and during which the terminal amino acid (alanine) is lost. The lipid is regenerated by loss of a phosphate group (Pi) before functioning again as a carrier.
(M = N-acetylmuramic acid; G = N-acetylglucosamine)

components to a very large lipid carrier, consisting of 55 carbon atoms, which 'tows' them across the membrane. The process of synthesis of peptidoglycan is outlined in Figure 35.3. First, N-acetylmuramic acid, which has attached to it both UDP and a pentapeptide, is transferred to the C_{55} lipid carrier in the membrane, with the release of UMP. This is followed by a reaction with UDP-N-acetylglucosamine, resulting in the formation of a disaccharide carrying the pentapeptide and attached to the carrier. This disaccharide with peptide attached is the basic building block of the peptidoglycan. In *Staph. aureus*, the five glycine residues are attached to the peptide chain at this stage, as is shown in Figure 35.3. The 'building block' is now transported to the outside of the cell and added to the growing end of the peptidoglycan, the 'acceptor', with the release of the C_{55} lipid, which still has two phosphates attached. The lipid then loses one phosphate group and thus becomes available for another cycle. Cross-linking between the peptide side-chains of the sugar residues in the peptidoglycan layer then occurs, the hydrolytic removal of the terminal alanine supplying the requisite energy.

This synthesis of peptidoglycan can be blocked at several points by antibiotics (Fig. 35.3 and Ch. 37). **Cycloserine**, which is a structural analogue of D-alanine, prevents the addition of the two terminal alanines to the initial tripeptide side-chain on N-acetylmuramic acid, by competitive inhibition. **Vancomycin** inhibits the release of the building block unit from the carrier, thus preventing its addition to the growing end of the peptidoglycan. **Bacitracin** interferes with the regeneration of the lipid carrier by blocking its dephosphorylation. **Penicillins, cephalosporins** and other β-lactams inhibit the final transpeptidation that establishes the cross-links.

Protein synthesis

The ribosomes are cytoplasmic nucleoprotein structures that are the basic units of machinery for the synthesis of proteins on messenger RNA templates. They are different in eukaryotes and prokaryotes and this provides the basis for the selective antimicrobial action of some antibiotics. The bacterial ribosome consists of a 50S subunit and a 30S subunit (Fig. 35.4). In this respect it differs from the mammalian ribosome, which has a 60S and a 40S subunit.

A simplified version of protein synthesis in bacteria is as follows:

- Messenger RNA (mRNA), which is transcribed from DNA (see below), becomes attached to the 30S subunit of the ribosome, which moves along the mRNA so that successive codons of the messenger pass along the ribosome from the right, the A position, to the left, the P position, as shown in Figure 35.4. (A codon is a triplet consisting of three nucleotides that codes for a specific amino acid.)
- The 'P site' contains the growing peptide chain attached to a molecule of transfer RNA (tRNA). The next amino acid residue to be added—linked to its specific tRNA, with its distinctive anticodon—moves into the A site, being bound to the site by a codon : anticodon recognition, which occurs by complementary base-pairing (Fig. 35.4A and B).
- A transpeptidation reaction occurs which links the peptide chain on the tRNA at the P site to the amino acid on the incoming tRNA at the A site (Fig. 35.4C).
- The tRNA from which the peptide chain has been removed is now ejected from the P site (Fig. 35.4D).
- The tRNA at the A site is translocated to the P site, and the ribosome moves on one codon, relative to the messenger (Fig. 35.4D).
- A new tRNA, with amino acid attached and with the relevant anticodon, now moves into the A site, and the whole process is repeated.

Antibiotics may affect protein synthesis at any one of the above stages (Fig. 35.4 and Ch. 37).

Nucleic acid synthesis

The nucleic acids of the cell are DNA and RNA. There are three types of RNA: messenger RNA (mRNA), transfer RNA (tRNA) and ribosomal RNA (rRNA). (The ribosomal RNA is an integral part of the ribosome, being necessary for its assembly and having a role in the binding of mRNA.) All are involved in protein synthesis (see above).

DNA is the template for the synthesis of both DNA and RNA. It exists in the cell as a double helix. Each chain or strand is a linear polymer of nucleotides. Each nucleotide consists of a base linked to a sugar (deoxyribose) and a phosphate. The bases are adenine (A), cytosine (C), guanine (G) or thymine

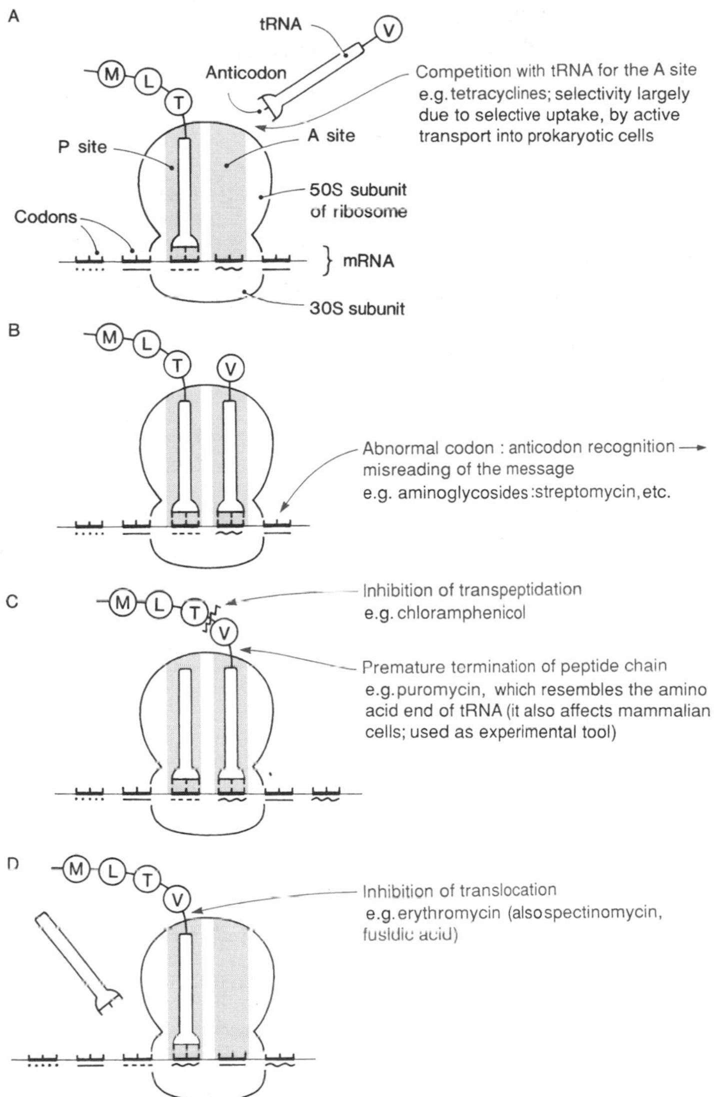
A
tRNA
V
M
L
T
Anticodon
Competition with tRNA for the A site
e.g. tetracyclines; selectivity largely
due to selective uptake, by active
transport into prokaryotic cells
P site
A site
50S subunit
of ribosome
Codons
mRNA
30S subunit
B
Abnormal codon : anticodon recognition →
misreading of the message
e.g. aminoglycosides: streptomycin, etc.
C
Inhibition of transpeptidation
e.g. chloramphenicol
Premature termination of peptide chain
e.g. puromycin, which resembles the amino
acid end of tRNA (it also affects mammalian
cells; used as experimental tool)
D
Inhibition of translocation
e.g. erythromycin (also spectinomycin,
fusidic acid)

Fig. 35.4 Antibiotics which inhibit bacterial protein synthesis.
A. Ribosome with messenger RNA (mRNA). The different mRNA codons (triplets of three nucleotides which code for specific amino acids) are represented by dots, dashes and straight or wavy lines. A transfer RNA with peptide chain Met–Leu–Trp (MLT) attached is in the P site, bound by codon : anticodon recognition (i.e. by complementary base-pairing). The incoming transfer RNA (tRNA) carries valine (V), covalently linked.
B. The incoming tRNA binds to the A site by complementary base-pairing.
C. Transpeptidation occurs. The peptide chain attached to the tRNA in the new A site now consists of Met–Leu–Trp–Val (MLTV). The tRNA in the P site has been 'discharged', i.e. has lost its peptide. **D.** The discharged tRNA is ejected from the P site. The tRNA with the peptide chain attached is translocated from the A to the P site leaving the A site free for the next tRNA. The ribosome moves to the next codon on the mRNA, shown as moving to the right along the codons.

(T). The chain is made up of alternating sugar and phosphate groups with the bases attached rather like beads on a necklace. Specific hydrogen bonding between G and C and between A and T on each strand (i.e. complementary base-pairing) is the basis of the double-strand structure of DNA (Fig. 35.5). The DNA helix is itself twisted, resulting in 'supercoiling' (Figs 35.6 and 37.7).

Initiation of DNA synthesis necessitates the prior activity of an enzyme that produces local unwinding of the positive 'supercoil' and introduction of a negative supercoil. This enzyme is DNA gyrase (also called topoisomerase II).

During the synthesis of DNA, the units, which are added by base-pairing with the complementary residues in the template, consist of a base linked to a sugar and three phosphate groups. Condensation occurs with the elimination of two of the phosphate groups, the enzyme responsible being DNA polymerase (Fig. 35.7).

RNA, like DNA, is a polymer of purine and pyrimidine nucleotides, but it exists as a single, not a double strand. The sugar moiety is ribose, and the ribonucleotides contain the bases adenine, guanine, cytosine and uracil (U).

It is possible to interfere with nucleic acid synthesis in five different ways:

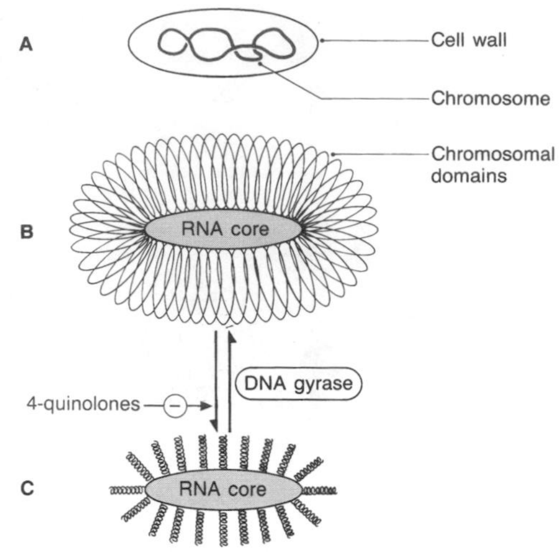

Fig. 35.6 Site of action for quinolone antibacterials. **A.** Conventional diagram used to depict a bacterial cell and chromosome (e.g. *Escherichia coli*). Note that the *Esch. coli* chromosome is 1300 μm long and is contained in a cell envelope of 2 μ × 1 μ; this is approximately equivalent to a 50-metre length of cotton folded into a matchbox. **B.** Chromosome folded around RNA core, and then **C.** supercoiled by DNA gyrase (topoisomerase II). Quinolone antibacterials interfere with the action of this enzyme. (Modified from: Smith J T 1985 In: Greenwood D, O'Grady F (eds), Scientific basis of antimicrobial therapy. Cambridge University Press, p. 69)

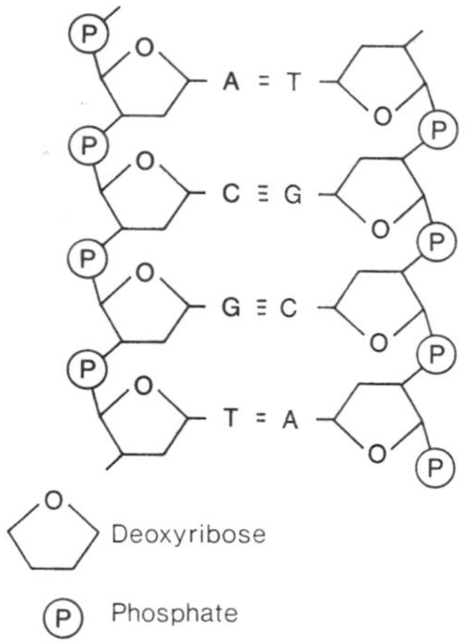

Fig. 35.5 Structure of DNA. Each strand of DNA consists of a sugar–phosphate backbone with purine or pyrimidine bases attached. The purines are adenine (A) or guanine (G) and the pyrimidines are cytosine (C) or thymine (T). The sugar is deoxyribose. Complementarity between the two strands of DNA is maintained by hydrogen bonds (either 2 or 3) between bases.

- *By inhibiting the synthesis of the nucleotides.* This can be accomplished by an effect on reactions earlier in the metabolic pathway. Examples of agents that have such an effect have been described under class II reactions.
- *By altering the base-pairing properties of the template.* Agents that intercalate in the DNA have this effect. Examples are the acridines (**proflavine, acriflavine**), which are used topically as antiseptics, and **chloroquine**, which is an antimalarial drug (Ch. 40). The acridines double the distance between adjacent base-pairs and cause a *frame-shift* mutation (Fig. 35.8). Some purine and pyrimidine analogues cause mispairing. One example is the antiviral drug **adenine arabinoside** (Ch. 38).
- *By inhibiting either DNA or RNA polymerase.* **Actinomycin D** binds to the guanine residues in DNA and blocks the movement of RNA polymerase, thus preventing transcription and consequently inhibiting protein synthesis. It is

used in cancer chemotherapy in man (Ch. 36) and as an experimental tool, but not as an antibacterial agent. Specific inhibitors of bacterial RNA polymerase that act by binding to this enzyme in prokaryotic but not in eukaryotic cells include **rifamycin** and **rifampicin**, which are active, in particular, against *Mycobacterium tuberculosis*, the tubercle bacillus (Ch. 37). **Acyclovir** (an analogue of guanine; see Fig. 38.5) is phosphorylated, in cells infected with herpes virus, to acyclovir triphosphate, which has a relatively selective inhibitory action on the DNA polymerase of the herpes virus (Ch. 38). **Cytarabine** (cytosine arabinoside) is used in cancer chemotherapy (Ch. 36). Its triphosphate derivative is a potent inhibitor of DNA polymerase in mammalian cells. **Hycanthone** intercalates in DNA in schistosomes, preventing transcription and the synthesis of essential enzymes.

- *By inhibiting DNA gyrase* (also called topoisomerase II; see Fig. 35.6). This is the mechanism of action of the 4-quinolones: **cinoxacin, ciprofloxacin, nalidixic acid** and **norfloxacin**—chemotherapeutic agents used in urinary tract infections with Gram-negative organisms (Ch. 37). These drugs are selective for the bacterial enzyme because it is structurally different from the mammalian enzyme. Some anticancer agents, for example doxorubicin (p. 709), act on the mammalian topoisomerase II.
- *By direct effects on DNA itself. Alkylating agents* form covalent bonds with bases in the DNA and prevent replication. Compounds with this action are used only in cancer chemotherapy and include **nitrogen mustard derivatives** and **nitrosoureas** (Ch. 36). **Mitomycin** also binds covalently to DNA. No antibacterial agents work by these mechanisms.

A pyrimidine analogue, **idoxuridine**, which is phosphorylated and incorporated into DNA, inhibits the replication of some DNA viruses (Ch. 38).

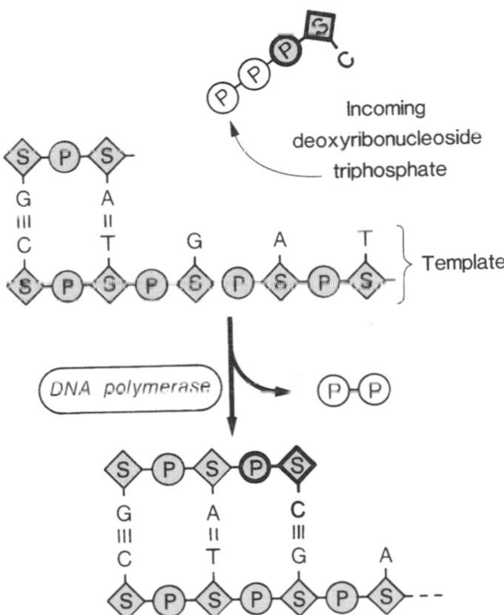

Fig. 35.7 DNA replication. Nucleotides are added, one at a time, by base-pairing to an exposed template strand and are then covalently joined together in a reaction catalysed by DNA polymerase. The units which pair with the complementary residues in the template consist of a base linked to a sugar and three phosphate groups. Condensation occurs with the elimination of two phosphates.
(P = phosphate; S = sugar; A = adenine; T = thymine; G = guanine; C = cytosine)

mRNA (normal)	UCU Ser	UUU Phe	CUU Leu	AUU Ile	GUU Val	UCU... Ser
mRNA (mutant)	UCU Ser	UUG Leu	UCU Ser	UAU Tyr	UGU Cys	UUC... Phe

Fig. 35.8 An example of the effect on RNA and protein synthesis of a frame-shift mutation in the DNA. A frame-shift mutation is one that involves an *insertion* of an extra base (cytosine in this example). The result is that when messenger RNA is formed, it has an additional guanine (G), as indicated in the light pink box. The effect is to alter that codon and all the succeeding ones (shown in red), so that a completely different protein is synthesised, as indicated by the different amino acids (Leu instead of Phe, Ser instead of Leu, etc.). (G = guanine; C = cytosine; A = adenine; U = uracil)

THE FORMED STRUCTURES OF THE CELL AS POTENTIAL TARGETS

The membrane

The plasma membrane of bacterial cells is fairly similar to that in mammalian cells in that it consists of a *phospholipid* bilayer in which proteins are embedded. Nevertheless, this structure can be more easily disrupted in certain bacteria and some fungi than in mammalian cells.

Polymixins are cationic detergent antibiotics that have a selective effect on bacterial cell membranes. They are peptides that contain both hydrophilic and lipophilic groups separated within the molecule. They interact with the phospholipids of the cell membrane and disrupt its structure and they are therefore bactericidal (Ch. 37).

Polyene antibiotics (e.g. **nystatin** and **amphotericin**; Ch. 39) are active against some fungi but have little action on mammalian cells and no action on bacteria. This is because of the different overall organisation of the plasma membrane of the protozoal and fungal cells and because the membrane of these cells contains large amounts of ergosterol, which facilitates the attachment and the subsequent effect of the polyenes. These antibiotics act as ionophores and cause leakage of cations.

Imidazoles, such as **miconazole**, have antifungal action and also affect Gram-positive bacteria, their selectivity being associated with the presence of high levels of free fatty acids in the membrane of susceptible organisms (Ch. 39).

DNA

Bleomycin, an anticancer antibiotic, causes fragmentation of the DNA strands following free radical formation (Ch. 36).

Microtubules and/or microfilaments

In high doses, **griseofulvin** interferes with microtubule function in mammalian cells and thus with mitosis and cell division. This may be the basis for its antifungal action (Ch. 39).

Colchicine and the vinca alkaloids, **vinblastine** and **vincristine**, are anticancer agents which disrupt the functioning of microtubules during cell division (Ch. 36). Colchicine is also used to treat gout (Ch. 12).

Muscle fibres

Some anthelminthic drugs have a selective action on muscle cells in helminths. **Piperazine** hyperpolarises muscle fibre membranes and paralyses the worm; **levamisole** has a nicotinic-like action on the muscle, causing contraction followed by paralysis (Ch. 41).

Potential targets for chemotherapy

Biochemical reactions

- *Class I reactions* are poor targets.
- *Class II reactions* are better targets:
  - —Folate synthesis in bacteria is inhibited by sulphonamides. Folate utilisation is inhibited by folate antagonists, e.g. trimethoprim in bacteria, pyrimethamine in the malarial parasite, methotrexate (an anticancer drug) in man.
  - —Pyrimidine analogues, e.g. fluorouracil, and purine analogues, e.g. mercaptopurine, give rise to fraudulent nucleotides; they are used to treat cancer.
- *Class III reactions* are important targets:
  - —Peptidoglycan synthesis in bacteria can be selectively inhibited by β-lactam antibiotics, e.g. penicillin.
  - —Protein synthesis can be selectively inhibited in bacteria by antibiotics that prevent binding of tRNA (e.g. tetracyclines), cause misreading of mRNA (e.g. aminoglycosides), inhibit transpeptidation (e.g. chloramphenicol), inhibit translocation of tRNA from A site to P site (e.g. erythromycin).
  - —Nucleic acid synthesis can be inhibited by: (a) altering base-pairing of DNA template (e.g. vidarabine), (b) inhibiting DNA polymerase (e.g. acyclovir), (c) inhibiting DNA gyrase (e.g. ciprofloxacin).

Formed structures of the cell

- These can be targets, e.g. amphotericin affects fungal but not human cell membranes.

RESISTANCE TO ANTIBIOTICS

During the last 40 years the development of effective and safe drugs to deal with bacterial infections has revolutionised medical treatment, and the morbidity and mortality from microbial disease has been dramatically reduced. Unfortunately, along with the development of man's chemotherapeutic defences against bacteria has gone the development of bacterial defences against chemotherapeutic agents, resulting in the emergence of *resistance*. This is not unexpected, it being an evolutionary principle that organisms adapt genetically to changes in their environment. Since the doubling time of bacteria can be as short as 20 minutes, there will be many generations in even a few hours and thus plenty of opportunity for evolutionary adaptation. The phenomenon of resistance can impose serious constraints on the options available for the medical treatment of many bacterial infections. Resistance to chemotherapeutic agents can also develop in protozoa, in multicellular parasites and in populations of malignant cells. However, in this chapter, discussion will be confined mainly to the mechanisms of resistance in bacteria.

Antibiotic resistance in bacteria spreads at three levels:

- by transfer of bacteria between people
- by transfer of resistance genes between bacteria (usually on plasmids)
- by transfer of resistance genes between genetic elements within bacteria, on transposons. (Transposons are defined and explained below.)

Understanding the mechanisms involved in antibiotic resistance is of importance both for the sensible use of these drugs in clinical practice and for the development of new antibacterial drugs to circumvent resistance. One result of the studies of resistance, R plasmids and resistance genes has been the development of new techniques for the cloning of foreign DNA. This cloning has been used rewardingly in many branches of biology and also in the production, by bacteria, of biologically active peptides such as mammalian hormones.

GENETIC DETERMINANTS OF ANTIBIOTIC RESISTANCE

Chromosomal determinants—mutations

The spontaneous mutation rate in bacterial populations for any particular gene is very low—about 1 per 10^6–10^8 cells per cell division, i.e. the probability is that 1 cell in, say, 10 million will, on division, give rise to a daughter cell containing a mutation in a particular gene. However, since in an infection there are likely to be very many more cells than this, the probability of a mutation causing a change from drug sensitivity to drug resistance may be quite high with some species of bacteria and with some drugs. Fortunately, with most infective species and with most antibiotics, a few mutants are not sufficient to produce resistance; if they were, the problem of resistance would be even more widespread than it is already. If an infecting bacterial population containing some mutants resistant to a particular antibiotic is exposed to that antibiotic, the mutants will have an enormous selective advantage. Luckily, in most cases the drastic reduction of the population by the antibiotic enables the host's natural defences (see Ch. 11) to deal effectively with the invading pathogens. However, this will not occur if the infection is caused by a population of microorganisms that are all resistant to the drug.

For most organisms, resistance due to chromosomal mutation is not of great clinical relevance, possibly because the mutants often have reduced pathogenicity. Nevertheless, it is important in mycobacterial infections, particularly tuberculosis, and it is also a significant factor in leprosy.

Extrachromosomal determinants—plasmids

Many species of bacteria contain, in addition to the chromosome, extrachromosomal genetic elements called *plasmids* that exist free in the cytoplasm. These are genetic elements *other* than the chromosome, which can replicate on their own. They consist of closed loops of DNA about 1–3% of the size of the chromosome. There may be 1–40 copies of a particular plasmid present, depending on the type, and there may be more than one type of plasmid in each bacterial cell. Plasmids that carry genes for resistance to antibiotics ('r genes') are referred to as R plasmids. Much of the drug resistance encountered in clinical medicine is plasmid determined. It is not known how the genes arose.

THE TRANSFER OF RESISTANCE GENES BETWEEN GENETIC ELEMENTS WITHIN THE BACTERIUM

Some stretches of DNA can be fairly readily transferred (transposed) from one plasmid to another and also from plasmid to chromosome or vice versa. This is because integration of these segments of DNA, which are called *transposons*, into the acceptor DNA can occur independently of the normal mechanism of genetic recombination (i.e. cross-over), which normally requires extensive homology. During the process of integration, the transposon can replicate (Fig. 35.9) and this results in a copy in both the donor and the acceptor DNA molecules. (Note that transposons, unlike plasmids, are not able to replicate on their own and that some transposons do not replicate during transfer.) Transposons may carry one or more resistance genes. They can 'hitch-hike' on a plasmid to a new species of bacterium and even if the plasmid is unable to replicate in the new host, the transposon may transfer to the new host's chromosome or to its indigenous plasmids. This probably accounts for the widespread distri-

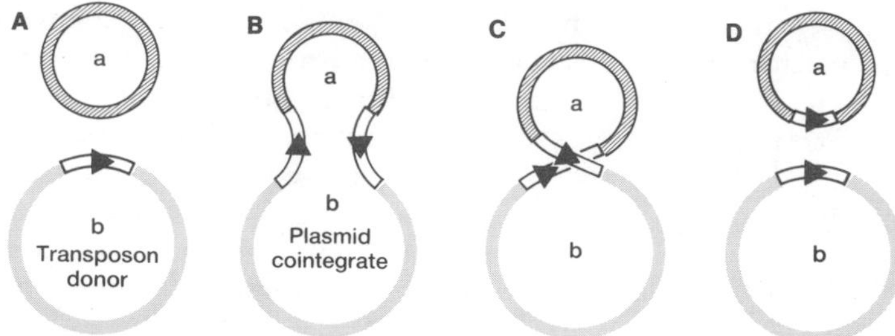

Fig. 35.9 An example of the transfer and replication of a transposon (which may carry genes coding for resistance to antibiotics).
A. Two plasmids, a and b, with plasmid b containing a transposon (shown in red). **B.** An enzyme encoded by the transposon cuts DNA of both donor plasmid and target plasmid a, to form a 'cointegrate'. During this process the transposon replicates. **C.** An enzyme encoded by the transposon 'resolves' the cointegrate. **D.** Both plasmids now contain the transposon DNA.

bution of certain of the resistance genes on different R plasmids and among unrelated bacteria.

THE TRANSFER OF RESISTANCE GENES BETWEEN BACTERIA

The transfer of resistance genes between bacteria of the same species and of different species is of fundamental importance in the spread of resistance to antibiotics. There are three mechanisms for gene transfer: conjugation, transduction and transformation.

Conjugation

Conjugation involves cell-to-cell contact during which chromosomal or extrachromosomal DNA is transferred from one bacterium to another. It is the main mechanism for the spread of resistance. The ability to conjugate is encoded in *conjugative plasmids*; these are plasmids that contain *transfer genes* which, in coliform bacteria, code for the production, by the host bacterium, of surface tubules of protein that connect the two cells—'sex pili'. The conjugative plasmid then passes across from one bacterium to the other, which is usually of the same species. Many Gram-negative and some Gram-positive bacteria can conjugate. Some plasmids cross the species barrier and, accepting one host as readily as another, are eloquently described as *promiscuous plasmids*. Many R plasmids are conjugative.* Non-conjugative plasmids can make use of the sex pili if they coexist in the 'donor' cell with conjugative plasmids. The transfer of resistance by conjugation is significant in populations of bacteria that are normally found at high densities, as in the gut.

Transduction

Transduction is a process by which plasmid DNA is enclosed in a bacterial virus (or phage) and transferred to another bacterium of the same species. It is a relatively ineffective means of transfer of genetic material, but there is evidence that it is clinically important in the transmission of resistance genes between strains of staphylococci and between strains of streptococci.

Transformation

In a few species, a bacterium can, under natural conditions, undergo transformation by taking up naked DNA from its environment and incorporating it into its genome through the normal cross-over mechanism. This is possible only when the incoming DNA comes from a cell belonging to the same strain as the host bacterium or one that is very closely related. Transformation is probably not of importance in the clinical problem of drug resistance.

*The combination of resistance genes with the stretch of DNA which encodes for the sex pilus, which is often referred to as the 'resistance transfer factor' or 'RTF', is sometimes called the 'R factor'.

Resistance to antibiotics

- Resistance in bacterial populations can be spread from person to person by bacteria, from bacterium to bacterium by plasmids, from plasmid to plasmid (or chromosome) by transposons.
- *Plasmids* are extrachromosomal genetic elements that can replicate independently and can carry genes coding for resistance to antibiotics (r genes).
- The main method of transfer of r genes from one bacterium to another is by *conjugative* plasmids, which can cause the bacterium to make a connecting tube between bacteria, through which the plasmid itself (and other plasmids) can pass.
  A less common method of transfer is by transduction, i.e. the transmission of an r-gene-carrying plasmid into a bacterium by a bacterial virus (phage).
- *Transposons* are stretches of DNA that can be transposed from one plasmid to another, and also from plasmid to chromosome and vice versa. For example an r-gene-carrying transposon in one plasmid codes for enzymes that cause integration of that plasmid into another plasmid, followed by their separation; during this the transposon replicates so that both plasmids will then contain the r-gene-carrying transposon.

BIOCHEMICAL MECHANISMS OF RESISTANCE TO ANTIBIOTICS

The production of an enzyme that inactivates the drug

Inactivation of β-lactam antibiotics

The most important example of resistance due to inactivation is that of β-lactams. The enzymes concerned are *β-lactamases*, which cleave the β-lactam ring of **penicillins** and **cephalosporins** (see Ch. 37). Cross-resistance between the two classes of antibiotic is not complete because some lactamases have a preference for penicillins and some for cephalosporins.

Staphylococci are the principal bacteria producing β-lactamase, and the genes which code for the enzymes are on plasmids that are transferred by transduction. In staphylococci the enzyme is inducible, i.e. its synthesis is at a very low level in the absence of the drug, but minute, subinhibitory, concentrations derepress the gene and result in a 50- to 80-fold increase in production. The enzyme may diffuse through the envelope and inactivate antibiotic molecules in the surrounding medium. The serious clinical problem posed by the staphylococci with resistance due to β-lactamase production was tackled by developing semisynthetic penicillins (such as **methicillin**) and new β-lactam antibiotics (**monobactams** and **carbapenems**), which were not susceptible, and cephalosporins (such as **cephamandole**), which were less susceptible to inactivation by these enzymes. (But see p. 694 for 'methicillin-resistant' staphylococci.)

Gram-negative organisms can also produce β-lactamases, which are a significant factor in their resistance to the semisynthetic **broad-spectrum β-lactam antibiotics**. In these organisms, the enzymes may be determined by either chromosomal genes or by plasmid genes. In the former case, the enzymes may be inducible. In the latter they are produced constitutively (i.e. they are synthesised even when the substrate is absent) and remain attached to sites in the cell wall, preventing access of the drug to the membrane-associated target site; they do not inactivate the drug in the surrounding medium. Many of these β-lactamases are encoded by transposons, some of which may also carry resistance determinants to several other antibiotics.

Inactivation of chloramphenicol

Chloramphenicol inactivation is brought about by *chloramphenicol acetyltransferase* produced by resistant strains of both Gram-positive and Gram-negative organisms, the resistance gene being plasmid borne. In Gram-negative bacteria the enzyme is produced constitutively, which results in levels of resistance fivefold higher than in Gram-positive bacteria, in which the enzyme is inducible.

Inactivation of aminoglycosides

Inactivation of aminoglycosides may be brought about by phosphorylation, adenylation or acetylation and the requisite enzymes have been found in both Gram-negative and Gram-positive organisms. The resistance genes are carried on plasmids and several are found on transposons.

Alteration of drug-sensitive site or drug-binding site

The protein on the 30S subunit of the ribosome, which is the binding site for **aminoglycosides**, may be altered as the result of a chromosomal mutation. A plasmid-mediated alteration of the binding-site protein on the 50S subunit underlies resistance to **erythromycin**, and decreased binding of **fluoro-**

quinolones because of a point mutation in the DNA gyrase A protein has recently been described. An altered DNA-dependent RNA polymerase determined by a chromosomal mutation is the basis for resistance to **rifampicin**.

Some staphylococci carry an altered penicillin-binding protein which is coded for by a mutated chromosomal gene; this confers 'intrinsic resistance'.

Decreased drug accumulation in the bacterium

An important example of decreased drug accumulation is the plasmid-mediated resistance to **tetracyclines** in both Gram-positive and Gram-negative bacteria. The resistance genes in the plasmid code for inducible 'resistance' proteins in the membrane, which promote energy-dependent efflux of the tetracyclines and hence resistance. This type of resistance is common and has reduced the value of the tetracyclines in human and veterinary medicine. A recently described *Staph. aureus* gene has also been shown to code for a membrane-associated protein that causes active efflux of **fluoroquinolones** from the cell. There is also recent evidence of plasmid-determined inhibition of 'porin' synthesis, which could affect those hydrophilic antibiotics that enter the bacterium by these water-filled channels in the outer membrane.

Altered permeability due to chromosomal mutations involving the polysaccharide components of the outer membrane of Gram-negative organisms may confer enhanced resistance to **ampicillin**.

Mutations affecting envelope components have been reported to affect the accumulation of **aminoglycosides, β-lactams, chloramphenicol, peptide antibiotics** and **tetracycline**.

The development of an alternative pathway that bypasses the reaction inhibited by the antibiotic

Recently, resistance to **trimethoprim** has developed, the mechanism being plasmid-directed synthesis of a dihydrofolate reductase with low or zero affinity for trimethoprim. It is transferred by transduction and may be spread by transposons.

Sulphonamide resistance in many bacteria is plasmid-mediated and is due to the production of a form of dihydropteroate synthetase with a low affinity for sulphonamides but no change in affinity for PABA. Disturbingly, bacteria causing serious infections have recently been found to carry plasmids with resistance genes to both sulphonamides and trimethoprim.

Note that some strains of staphylococci, in addition to producing β-lactamase, have become resistant even to some β-lactams that are not significantly inactivated by β-lactamase (e.g. **methicillin**). This is due to altered β-lactam-binding sites.

Staphylococci may also manifest resistance to many other antibiotics as follows:

- to **streptomycin** (due to chromosomally determined alteration of target site)
- to **aminoglycosides** in general (due to altered target site and plasmid-determined inactivating enzymes)
- to **chloramphenicol** and the **macrolides** (due to plasmid-determined enzymes)
- to **trimethoprim** (due to transposon-encoded drug-resistant dihydrofolate reductase)
- to **sulphonamides** (due to chromosomally determined increased production of PABA)
- to **rifampicin** (thought to be due to chromosomally determined and plasmid-determined increases in efflux of the drug)
- to **fusidic acid** (due to chromosomally determined decreased affinity of the target site or a plasmid-encoded decreased permeability to the drug)
- to **quinolones**, for example ciprofloxacin, norfloxacin (due to chromosomally determined reduced uptake).

Infections with these organisms which are referred to as ***'methicillin-resistant staphylococci'*** have become a serious problem, particularly in hospitals, where they can spread rapidly among elderly and/or seriously ill patients, and patients with burns or wounds. In a number of hospitals, surgical wards have had to be closed because of the high rates of infection among patients. Methicillin resistance is discussed by Lyons & Skurray (1987) and Brumfitt & Hamilton-Miller (1989).

But it is not just the staphylococci that are rapidly developing resistance to chemotherapeutic agents; enterococci have emerged as the second most common nosocomial* pathogen. Non-pathogenic enterococci are ubiquitously present in the intestine, have intrinsic resistance to many antibacterial drugs and can readily become resistant to other agents by taking up plasmids and transposons carrying the relevant resistance genes; this resistance is easily

*Nosocomial infections are those acquired in hospital.

transferred to invading pathogenic enterococci. Furthermore, many other pathogens are developing, or have developed; resistance to commonly used drugs. The list includes, among others, *P. aeruginosa*, *Strep. pyogenes*, *Strep. pneumoniae*, *N. meningitidis*, *N. gonorrhoeae*, *H. influenzae*, *H. ducreyi* as well as *Mycobacterium*, *Campylobacter*, and *Bacteroides* species (see Jacobi & Archer 1991). Nature has endowed microorganisms with fiendishly effective methods for dealing with our pharmaceutical defences against them and they are effortlessly keeping pace with our attempts to eradicate them. It may be that the eventual answer will lie not in the hands of pharmacologists but of molecular geneticists (discussed by Jacobi & Archer 1991). But it should be appreciated that one reason for our current inability to win the war is that antibiotics are often used indiscriminately and to excess.

Biochemical mechanisms of resistance to antibiotics

- Production of enzymes that inactivate the drug: e.g. β-lactamases, which inactivate penicillin; acetyltransferases, which inactivate chloramphenicol; kinases and other enzymes, which inactivate aminoglycosides.
- Alteration of the drug-binding sites: this occurs with aminoglycosides, erythromycin, penicillin.
- Reduction of drug uptake by the bacterium: e.g. tetracyclines.
- Alteration of enzymes: e.g. dihydrofolate reductase becomes insensitive to trimethoprim.
- Some strains of staphylococci have multiple resistance to virtually all current antibiotics involving the above mechanisms, resistance being transferred by transposons and/or plasmids.

REFERENCES AND FURTHER READING

Brumfitt W, Hamilton-Miller J 1989 Methicillin-resistant *Staphylococcus aureus*. N Engl J Med 320: 1188–1196

Datta N (ed) 1984 Antibiotic resistance to bacteria. Br Med Bull 40(1): 1–106

Franklin T J, Snow G A, Barrett-Bee K J, Nolan R D 1989 Resistance to antimicrobial drugs. In: Franklin T J, Snow G A (eds) Biochemistry of antimicrobial action, 4th edn. Chapman & Hall, London, ch 8

Frieden T R, Munsiff S S, Low D E et al. 1993 Emergence of vancomycin-resistant enterococci in New York City. Lancet 342: 76–79

Gale E F, Cundliffe E, Reynolds P E, Richmond M H, Waring M J 1981 The molecular basis of antibiotic action, 2nd edn. John Wiley & Sons, London, p 1–62

Greenwood D, O'Grady F (eds) 1985 The scientific basis of antimicrobial chemotherapy. Symposium 38 of The Society of General Microbiology, Cambridge University Press, Cambridge

Harai K, Mitsuhashi S 1992 Mechanisms of resistance to quinolones. Prog Drug Res 38: 107–120

Jacobi G A, Archer G L 1991 Mechanisms of disease: new mechanisms of bacterial resistance to antimicrobial agents. N Engl J Med 324: 601–612

Levy S B 1992 Active efflux mechanisms for antimicrobial resistance. Antimicrob Agents Chemother 36: 695–703

Lyons B R, Skurray R 1987 Antimicrobial resistance of *Staphylococcus aureus:* genetic basis. Microbiol Rev 57: 88–134

Mandelstam J, McQuillen K, Dawes I (eds) 1982 Biochemistry of bacterial growth, 3rd edn. Blackwell Scientific Publications, Oxford (especially Part 1, by eds)

Murray B E 1992 β-lactamase-producing enterococci. Antimicrob Agents Chemother 36: 2355–2359

O'Brien T F 1992 Global surveillance of antibiotic resistance. N Engl J Med 326: 339–340

Sato K, Hoshino K, Mitsuhashi S 1992 Mode of action of the new quinolones: the inhibitory action on DNA gyrase. Prog Drug Res 38: 121–132

Shaw K J, Rather P N, Hare R S, Miller G H 1993 Molecular genetics of the aminoglycoside resistance genes and familial relationships of the aminoglycoside-modifying enzymes Microbiol Rev 57: 138–163

Silver L S, Bostian K A 1993 Discovery and development of new antibiotics: The problem of antibiotic resistance. Antimicrob Agents Chemother 37: 377–383

Smith J T 1985 The 4-quinolone antibacterials. In: Greenwood D, O'Grady F (eds) The scientific basis of antimicrobial therapy. Cambridge University Press, Cambridge, p 69–94

36

CANCER CHEMOTHERAPY

Cancer can be defined very broadly as a disease in which there is uncontrolled multiplication and spread within the body of abnormal forms of the body's own cells. It is one of the major causes of death in the developed nations—one in five of the population of Europe and North America can expect to die of cancer. Figures for the last 100 years or so give the impression that the disease is increasing in these countries, but allowance has to be made for the fact that cancer is largely a disease of the later age groups, and with the advances in public health and medical science during this time many more people live to the age where they are likely to get cancer.

Strictly speaking one should use the term 'neoplasm' (meaning a 'new growth') rather than the term 'cancer'. Neoplasms that have only the characteristic of localised growth are classified as *benign*. Neoplasms with the additional characteristics of invasiveness and/or the capacity to metastasise are classified as *malignant*. The term 'cancer' is usually applied only to this latter type of growth. The word 'tumour', though in reality meaning 'a local swelling', is also often used interchangeably with 'cancer' and will be so used here. In this chapter we shall be concerned only with the therapy of malignant neoplasia or cancer.

There are three main approaches to dealing with established cancer—*surgical excision*, *irradiation*, and *chemotherapy*—and the role of each of these depends on the type of tumour and the stage of its development. Chemotherapy with cytotoxic drugs is the main method of treatment for only a few cancers but it is increasingly used as an adjunct to surgery or irradiation in a range of common types of tumour. The efficacy of other approaches to cancer treatment—immunotherapy and use of biological response modifiers (e.g. interferons, haemopoietic growth factors, etc.)—is being investigated.

Compared with chemotherapy of bacterial diseases, chemotherapy of cancer presents a difficult problem. It has been possible to find agents with selective toxicity for many microorganisms because in addition to being quantitatively different in biochemical terms from human cells, microorganisms are also qualitatively different (see Ch. 35); but it has proved difficult to find *general, exploitable, biochemical* differences between cancer cells and normal body cells.

THE BIOLOGY OF CANCER

In the past few years there has been a prodigious advance in the understanding of cell proliferation, which has led to better understanding of the biology of the cancer cell (discussed by Murray, 1992, Lane 1992); this in turn is beginning to lead to new approaches to the development of anticancer agents (Powis 1991). To understand how present anticancer drugs act (and how future agents will act), it is important to consider the special charateristics of the cancer cell.

THE SPECIAL CHARACTERISTICS OF CANCER CELLS

Cancer cells manifest four characteristics that distinguish them from normal cells:

- uncontrolled proliferation
- loss of function
- invasiveness
- metastases.

Uncontrolled proliferation

The proliferation of cancer cells is not controlled by the processes that normally regulate cell division and tissue growth. It is this, rather than their *rate* of proliferation, that distinguishes them from normal cells. Some normal cells (such as neurons) have little or no capacity to divide and proliferate, but others, for example in the bone marrow and the epithelium of the gastrointestinal tract, have the property of continuous rapid division. Some cancer cells multiply slowly (e.g. those in plasma cell tumours) and some fast (e.g. the cells of Burkitt's lymphoma). It is therefore not generally true that cancer cells proliferate faster than normal cells. Consider, for example, the cells of the liver. Under normal conditions only a very small proportion of these are undergoing division at any one time. However, if two-thirds of the liver is removed, the remaining cells will divide fast and continuously until (in 2 weeks in the rat) the liver regains its original size. Growth then stops, because it is controlled by regulatory processes which are as yet ill understood. The significant point about cancer cells is that their proliferation is not subject to these regulatory processes.

In discussing the difference between the proliferation of normal cells and that of cancer cells, one needs to consider the cell cycle of dividing cells. This starts with the cell gearing up for division by synthesising the components necessary for DNA replication. Figure 36.1 shows the various phases

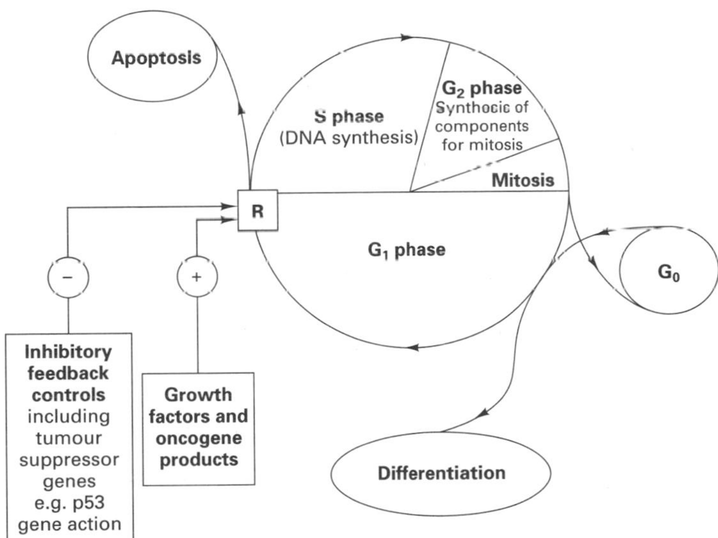

Fig. 36.1 The cell cycle. A dividing cell starts in G_1 phase, tooling up for DNA synthesis. R = a restriction point or check point. Progression signals, provided by growth factors, are necessary for the cycle to progress beyond the check point. Inhibitory feedback controls hold up DNA synthesis if there is DNA damage, allowing time for repair. If repair fails, apoptosis (cell suicide) may occur. In cancer cells there is (1) abnormally increased growth factor function and/or abnormal DNA synthesis as a result of oncogene activity and/or (2) abnormal decrease in feedback control due to functional disturbance of tumour suppressor genes. G_0 represents a phase in which cells are not dividing but can re-enter the cell cycle. As a cell differentiates, it leaves the cycle.

of the cycle. There is a check point (also termed 'restriction point') before DNA replication. Progression signals are necessary for the cell to cross this check point and it is here that growth factors (see Table 11.2 and Fig. 23.10) exert their effects. At this point also, various feedback controls operate to stop progression if there is damage to the DNA; this allows for DNA repair. If repair is unsuccessful, cell suicide by apoptosis may occur (Fig. 36.1). Apoptosis is a programmed series of events leading to cell death. It is a physiological process by which the body removes old or damaged cells, as for example in the shedding of the intestinal lining, the regression of mammary gland cells after lactation or the death of time-expired neutrophils. It is also the process that removes abnormal cells which could become malignant.

In cancer cells, uncontrolled proliferation can be due to abnormal production of, or response to, growth factors or to altered feedback controls or both.

Loss of function

This is due to lack of differentiation. The multiplication of normal cells involves division of the stem cells in a particular tissue to give rise to daughter cells. These daughter cells eventually differentiate to become the mature cells of the relevant tissue and carry out their programmed functions. Thus fibroblasts become capable of secreting and organising collagenous extracellular matrix, muscle cells become capable of contraction and relaxation, and so on. One of the main characteristics of cancer cells is the loss—to a varying degree—of the capacity to differentiate. In general, poorly differentiated cancers multiply fast, and have a poorer prognosis than well-differentiated cancer cells.

Invasiveness

Normal cells during differentiation and during the growth of tissues and organs develop certain spatial relationships with respect to each other, and these are continuously maintained even when the cells are involved in repair processes. Thus, although the cells of the normal mucosal epithelium of the rectum proliferate continuously as the lining is shed, they remain as a lining epithelium. A cancer of the rectal mucosa, on the other hand, invades the tissues in the other layers of the rectum and may invade the tissues of other pelvic organs. Recent work is elucidating the factors involved in the regulation of cell adhesion and motility and the changes in these characteristics which allow cancerous cells to invade and migrate through the extracellular matrix (discussed by Liotta et al. 1991, Weiner et al. 1993).

Metastases

These are secondary tumours formed by cells that have been released from the initial or primary tumour and have reached other sites through blood vessels or lymphatics, or as a result of being shed into body cavities. Cancer cells which have the ability to metastasise have undergone a series of genetic changes to the regulatory factors that control the position of normal cells—both positive factors (involving adhesion receptors, motility cytokines, proteases) and negative factors (involving metastasis suppressor genes, protease inhibitors). See Aznavoorian et al. (1993).

THE GENESIS OF A CANCER CELL

A normal cell turns into a cancer cell because of an alteration in its DNA. This is a multistage process; it takes place in a series of steps.

There are two main categories of genetic change which lead to cancer:

- the inactivation of tumour-suppressor genes
- the activation of proto-oncogenes to oncogenes.*

INACTIVATION OF TUMOUR SUPPRESSOR GENES

The fact that normal cells contain genes which have the ability to suppress malignant change was first described by Harris et al. (1969), and there is now good evidence that mutations of these genes (also termed anti-oncogenes, recessive oncogenes) are involved in many different cancers.

The precise role of these genes in normal functioning is gradually being elucidated. Gene p53 can be taken as an example. There is evidence that p53 acts as a molecular policeman in the nucleus, triggering a feedback control mechanism. If the DNA is damaged, p53 gene products accumulate and arrest DNA replication at the check point, allowing time for repair (see Fig. 36.1). If the repair fails, p53 activity triggers cell suicide by apoptosis.

*Oncogenes are genes which confer malignancy on a cell.

Cells in which p53 is altered by mutation, or by binding to viral or altered host proteins, cannot stop the abnormal DNA replicating. Such cells will accumulate mutations and chromosomal translocations undisturbed, leading eventually, if other genetic changes occur, to cancer. Mutations in p53 are the most commonly found mutations in human cancer cells.

It is possible that the critical event in carcinogenesis is the loss of function of tumour suppressor genes.

ACTIVATION OF PROTO-ONCOGENES

As explained above, one reason why cancer cells manifest uncontrolled proliferation is to do with the abnormal production of and response to growth factors—proteins that stimulate DNA synthesis and cell proliferation. The basis for this ability appears to be the presence of oncogenes in the DNA of the cancer cell.

These genes were originally thought to originate only through the insinuation of viral genetic material into the host cell. It is now known that the host's own genes can promote malignancy when suitably activated. These genes, termed 'proto-oncogenes', are almost certainly those that are involved in normal cell growth and differentiation. They can be converted into active oncogenes not only by certain viruses but also as a result of point mutations, gene amplification or chromosomal translocation. It is probable that the change from normal cell to malignant cell can, in many tumours, be traced back to distorted function of central growth regulator genes. Cells in multicellular organisms divide in response to the following:

- *extracellular signals* (growth factors), which act on
- *cell surface receptors* (see Ch. 2), which in turn trigger
- *intracellular transduction events* (stimulus–activation coupling events), which lead to
- *DNA synthesis and the processes involved in mitosis.*

Oncogenes can confer autonomy of growth on cells by affecting one or more of the above elements of growth control, i.e. by producing abnormalities in:

- the production of autocrine growth factors
- the receptors for growth factors
- the stimulus–activation coupling mechanisms for proliferation (important examples are the receptor protein tyrosine kinase pathway and the protein kinase C activating pathway; see Ch. 2)
- nuclear products involved in the response to the signals from the proliferation pathways.

For a simple summary of this topic see Hackford (1993). Oncogenes interfere not only with proliferation but also with differentiation, inducing defects in the execution of differentiation programmes. And it may well be that one of the fundamental effects of oncogene products is to interfere with the action of tumour suppressor genes.

GENERAL PRINCIPLES OF ACTION OF CYTOTOXIC ANTICANCER DRUGS

In experiments with rapidly growing transplantable leukaemias in mice it has been found that a given therapeutic dose of a cytotoxic drug destroys a constant fraction of the malignant cells. Thus a dose which kills 99.99% of cells, if used to treat a tumour with 10^{11} cells, will still leave 10 million (10^7) viable malignant cells. As the same principle holds for similar fast-growing tumours in man, schedules for chemotherapy of these tumours are necessarily aimed at producing as near a total cell kill as possible, because in contrast to the situation with microorganisms, very little reliance can be placed on the host's immunological defence mechanisms against the remaining cancer cells.

One of the major difficulties in the use of cancer chemotherapy is that a tumour is usually far advanced before it is diagnosed. Let us suppose that a tumour arises from a single cell and that the growth is exponential—as it may well be in the initial stages. Doubling times vary with different tumours, for example being, very roughly, 24 hours with Burkitt's lymphoma, 2 weeks with some leukaemias, and 3 months with mammary cancers. Approximately 30 doublings would be required to produce a cell mass with a diameter of 2 cm, containing 10^9 cells. A tumour that size is within the limits of diagnostic procedures, though it might be unnoticed in many organs, such as the liver. Another 10 doublings would produce 10^{12} cells—a tumour mass which is likely to be lethal, and which would measure about 20 cm in diameter if it were all in one clump. The

Cancer cell biology and cancer chemotherapy: general principles

- The term 'cancer' refers to a malignant neoplasm (new growth).
- Cancer cells can manifest:
  - —uncontrolled proliferation
  - —loss of function due to lack of the capacity to differentiate
  - —invasiveness
  - —the ability to metastasise.
- Cancer arises as a result of a series of genetic changes in the cell, the main genetic lesions being:
  - —inactivation of tumour suppressor genes
  - —the activation of oncogenes.
- Most anticancer drugs are antiproliferative and will also affect rapidly dividing normal cells; they are thus likely to depress bone marrow, impair healing, depress growth, cause sterility and hair loss, and be teratogenic. Most cause nausea and vomiting.

neoplasm would therefore be silent for the first three-quarters or more of its existence, and the problem of stopping its development after diagnosis, when there are very large numbers of malignant cells, would be considerable.

However, continuous exponential growth of this sort does not usually occur. With most solid tumours (for example of lung, stomach, uterus and so on, as opposed to leukaemias—the tumours of white blood cells) the growth rate falls as the neoplasm gets larger. This is partly because the tumour tends to outgrow its blood supply with resultant necrosis or death of part of its bulk, and partly because not all the cells proliferate continuously. The cells of a solid tumour can be considered as belonging to three compartments: compartment A consists of dividing cells, possibly being continuously in cell cycle (Fig. 36.1); compartment B consists of resting cells (in G_0 phase)—cells which, though not dividing, are potentially able to do so; and compartment C consists of cells that are no longer able to divide but which contribute to the tumour volume. Essentially only cells in compartment A, which may form as little as 5% of some solid tumours, are susceptible to the main currently available drugs, as is explained below. The cells in compartment C do not constitute a problem—it is the existence of cells in compartment B that makes cancer chemotherapy difficult, because these cells are not very sensitive to cytotoxic drugs, but are liable to re-enter compartment A following a course of chemotherapy.

Most currently used anticancer drugs, in particular those which are 'cytotoxic', affect only the first of the characteristics of cancer cells outlined previously—the process of cell division, i.e. they are antiproliferative; they have no specific effect on invasiveness, the loss of differentiation or the tendency to metastasise. (Their antiproliferative action is now thought to result not only from a direct effect on the G_1 and S phases of the cell cycle, but also on the events leading to apoptosis.) Furthermore, because their main effect is on cell division, they will affect all rapidly dividing normal tissues and thus they are likely to produce, to a greater or lesser extent, the following general toxic effects:

- *bone marrow toxicity* with decreased leucocyte production and thus decreased resistance to infection
- *impaired wound healing*
- *depression of growth* in children
- *sterility*
- *teratogenicity*
- *loss of hair* (alopecia)
- *damage to gastrointestinal epithelium.*

They can also, in certain circumstances, be *carcinogenic* (i.e. they may themselves cause cancer). In addition, if there is rapid cell destruction with extensive purine catabolism, urates may precipitate in the renal tubules and cause *kidney damage*. Finally, virtually all cytotoxic drugs produce *severe nausea and vomiting*, which has been called 'the inbuilt deterrent' to patient compliance in completing a course of treatment with these agents (see p. 395). Some compounds have particular toxic effects which are specific for them. These will be dealt with under the individual drugs.

DRUGS USED IN CANCER CHEMOTHERAPY

The term 'cytotoxic drug' applies to any drug that can damage or kill cells. In practice, it is used more restrictively to mean drugs that inhibit cell division and are potentially useful in cancer chemotherapy.

The main anticancer drugs can be divided into the following general categories:

- Cytotoxic drugs:

— **alkylating agents and related compounds** which act by forming covalent bonds with DNA and thus impeding DNA replication
— **antimetabolites**, which block or subvert one or more of the metabolic pathways involved in DNA synthesis
— **cytotoxic antibiotics**, i.e. substances of microbial origin which prevent mammalian cell division
— **vinca alkaloids and related compounds**—substances of plant origin that specifically affect microtubule function and hence the formation of the mitotic spindle.

The mechanism of action of these drugs is discussed more fully below and summarised in Figure 36.2.

- Hormones—of which the most important are steroids, namely **glucocorticoids**, **oestrogens** and **androgens**—and drugs that suppress hormone secretion or antagonise hormone action.

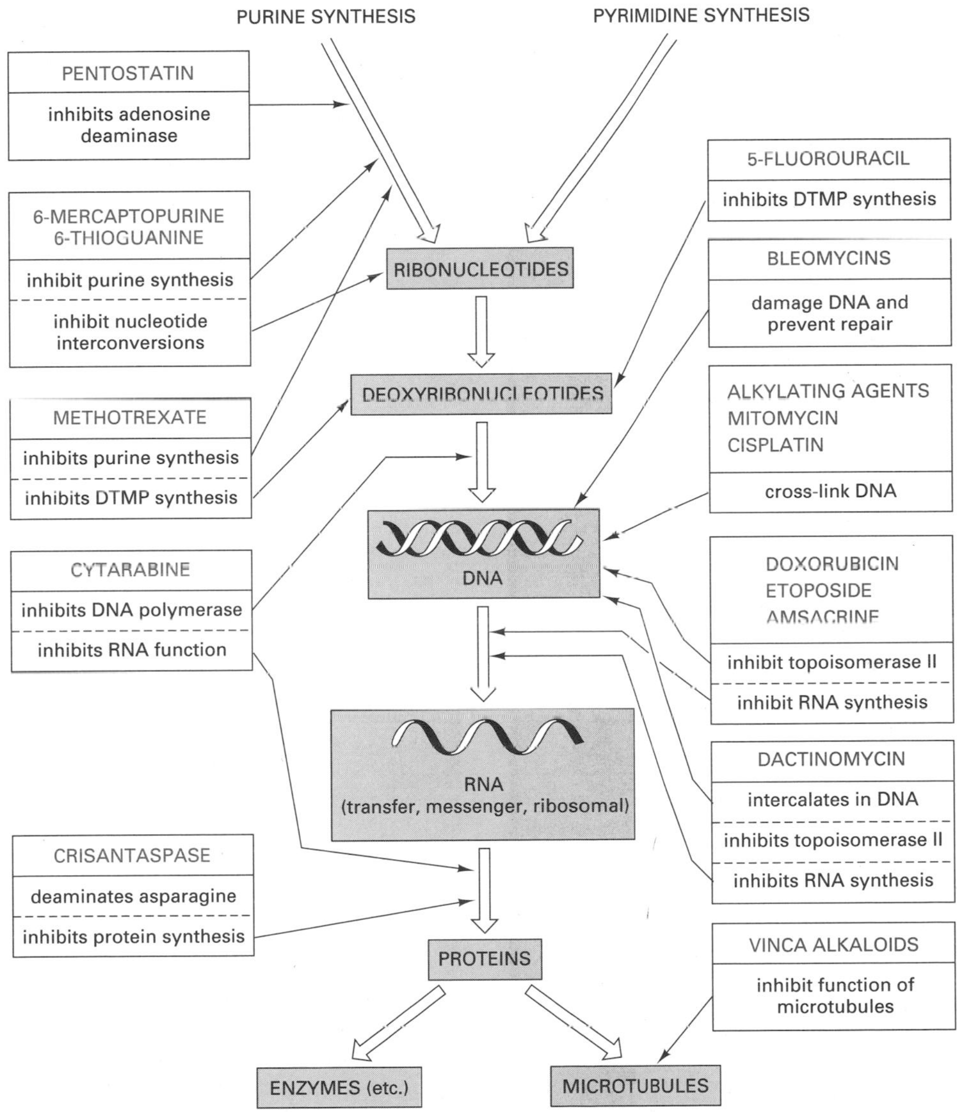

Fig. 36.2 Summary of the sites of action of cytotoxic agents that act on dividing cells. (DTMP = 2′deoxythymidylate) (Adapted from: Calabresi P, Parks R E 1980. In: Gilman A G, Goodman L S, Gilman A (eds) The pharmacological basis of therapeutics, 6th edn. Macmillan, New York)

Table 36.1 Examples of malignant diseases in which drug therapy has an important place*

Disease	Drugs (often used in combinations)	Comment
Hodgkin's disease	Mustine, Vincristine, Prednisolone, Procarbazine [†] Doxorubicin, Bleomycin, Vinblastine, Dacarbazine [†]	Radiotherapy curative in limited disease; combination chemotherapy sometimes curative in advanced disease
Non-Hodgkin's lymphomas	Prednisolone, Vinca alkaloids, Cyclophosphamide [†]	
Low grade lymphoproliferative disorders including chronic lymphocytic leukaemia	Chlorambucil Fludarabine 2-chlorodeoxyadenosine	
Chronic granulocytic leukaemia	Hydroxyurea Busulphan α-interferon	
Acute myeloid leukaemia	Cytarabine Doxorubicin	
Acute lymphocytic leukaemia	Vinca alkaloids Prednisolone Cristantaspase	Methotrexate for maintenance and (intrathecally) to prevent CNS relapse
Hairy cell leukaemia	Pentostatin	
Myeloma	Melphalan Prednisolone α-interferon Cyclophosphamide	
Breast cancer	Tamoxifen Cyclophosphamide, Fluorouracil, Methotrexate [†] Doxorubicin Mitoxanthrone Mitomycin C	Often used as an adjunct to surgery or radiotherapy. Tamoxifen and other endocrine treatments are used separately from cytotoxic drugs and there is no good case for combining them. Bisphosphonates are important in palliation of bone metastases (see Ch. 21)
Germ cell (testis, ovary)	Cisplatinum-based combinations	Can be curative even in metastatic disease
Choriocarcinoma	Methotrexate	Can be curative even in metastatic disease
Prostate cancer	GnRH analogues (e.g. leuprorelin, Ch. 22) and anti-androgen (e.g. cyproterone acetate)	Improve symptoms and prolong life
Thyroid cancer	Radio-iodine	Not all tumours retain capacity for iodine uptake

* This list is not exhaustive. Other cancers where drug therapy may be of value in selected cases include epithelial ovarian cancer, uterine body carcinoma, uterine cervix carcinoma, small cell lung cancer, colorectal cancer and gastric cancer.
[†] Drugs used concurrently in combination chemotherapy regimes

Further examples are given briefly under the heading 'Miscellaneous agents'.

The clinical use of the drugs is the province of the specialist oncologist and is not covered in detail here; however, Table 36.1 gives examples of malignant disease in which drug therapy has an important place. In the following sections we concentrate on basic pharmacology and outline the main unwanted effects of commonly used anticancer agents.

ALKYLATING AGENTS AND RELATED COMPOUNDS

Alkylating agents and related compounds contain chemical groups which have the property of forming covalent bonds with suitable nucleophilic substances in the cell. With alkylating agents themselves, the main step is the formation of a carbonium ion—a carbon atom with only six electrons in its outer shell (see Fig. 36.4). Such ions are highly reactive and react instantaneously with an electron donor such as an amine, –OH or –SH group. Most of the cytotoxic anticancer alkylating agents are bifunctional, i.e. they have two alkylating groups. (Monofunctional alkylating agents are, on the whole, more mutagenic and carcinogenic than cytotoxic.)

The 7 nitrogen (N7) of guanine, being strongly nucleophilic, is probably the main molecular target for alkylation in DNA, although N1 and N3 of adenine and N3 of cytosine may also be affected. A bifunctional agent, being able to react with two groups, can cause intra- or interchain cross-linking (Figs 36.3 and 36.4). This can interfere not only

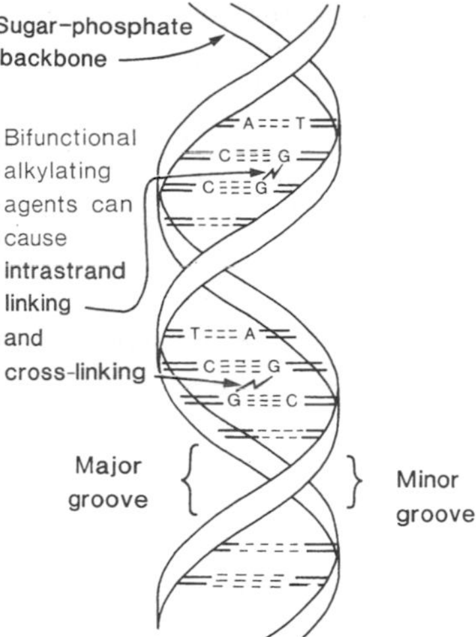

Fig. 36.3 The possible effects of bifunctional alkylating agents on DNA. (G = guanine; C = cytosine; A = adenine; T = thymine)

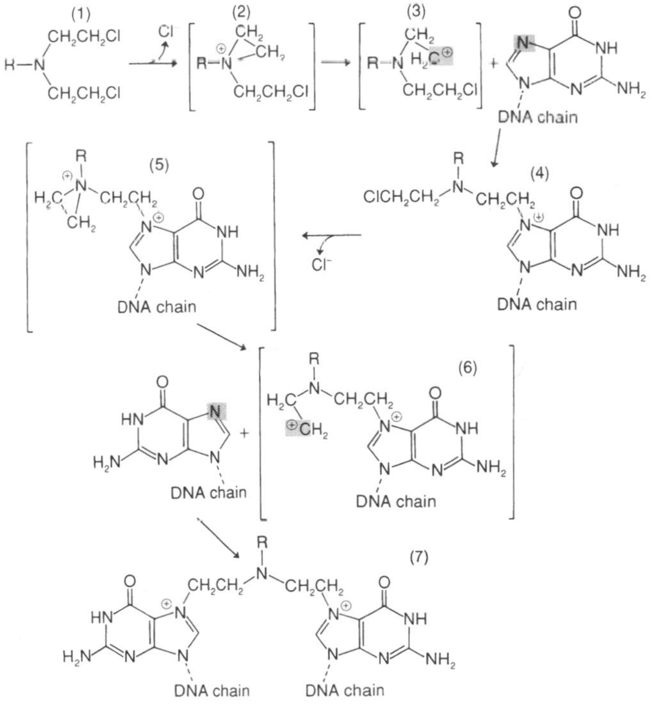

Fig. 36.4 An example of alkylation and cross-linking of DNA by a nitrogen mustard. A bis (chloroethyl) amine (1) undergoes intramolecular cyclisation forming an unstable ethylene immonium cation and releasing a chloride ion (2), the tertiary amine being transformed to a quaternary ammonium compound. The strained ring of the ethylene immonium intermediate opens to form a reactive carbonium ion (in light pink box) (3), which reacts immediately with N7 of guanine (in grey box) to give 7-alkylguanine (bond shown in red), the N7 being converted to a quaternary ammonium nitrogen (4). A bifunctional alkylating agent may undergo a second cyclisation (5), with carbonium ion formation—in light pink box (6), and interact with another guanine residue—in grey box—thus linking two bases as shown in Figure 36.3 (7).

with transcription but with replication, which is probably the critical effect of anticancer alkylating agents. Other effects of alkylation at guanine N7 are excision of the guanine base with main chain scission, or pairing of the alkylated guanine with thymine instead of cytosine and eventual substitution of the GC pair by an AT pair.

The main action occurs during replication, when some parts of the DNA are unpaired and more susceptible to alkylation; but the effects are made manifest during S phase, resulting in a block at G_2 (see Fig. 36.1) and subsequent cell death.

All alkylating agents depress bone marrow function and cause gastrointestinal disturbances. With prolonged use, two further unwanted effects are likely to occur: depression of gametogenesis (particularly in men) leading to permanent sterility, and an increased risk of acute non-lymphocytic leukaemia.

A large number of alkylating agents are available for use in cancer chemotherapy. Only a few commonly used ones will be dealt with here.

Nitrogen mustards

Nitrogen mustards are related to sulphur mustard, the 'mustard gas' used during the First World War, and their basic formula is R-N-bis-(2-chloroethyl). Examples are given in Figure 36.5. In the body, each 2-chloroethyl side-chain undergoes an intramolecular cyclisation with the release of a chloride ion. The highly reactive ethylene immonium derivative so formed can interact with DNA (see Fig. 36.4) and other molecules.

Cyclophosphamide is probably the most commonly used alkylating agent. It is inactive until metabolised in the liver by the P-450 mixed function oxidases. Details are given in Figure 36.6. Cyclophosphamide has a pronounced effect on lymphocytes and is used as an immunosuppressant (see Ch. 12). It is usually given orally or by intravenous injection but may also be given intramuscularly or into the pleural or peritoneal cavities. Important toxic effects are nausea and vomiting, bone marrow depression and haemorrhagic cystitis. This latter effect (which also occurs with the related drug, **ifosfamide**) is due to acrolein and can be ameliorated by increasing fluid intake and administering compounds that are sulphydryl donors, such as N-acetylcysteine or **mesna** (sodium-2-mercaptoethane sulphonate). These agents interact specifically with acrolein, forming a non-toxic compound.

Estramustine is a combination of mustine (the prototype nitrogen mustard; see Fig. 36.5) with an oestrogen. The intention underlying the use of this agent is that the mustine group will be effective after uptake of the oestrogen into the relevant cells.

Other nitrogen mustards used are **melphalan** and **chlorambucil**.

Nitrosoureas

The nitrosoureas are effective against a wide range of tumours, acting both by alkylation and by other as yet ill-understood mechanisms. The active alkylating moieties are formed by spontaneous, non-enzymatic degradation. Also liberated are organic isocyanates, which can carbamoylate lysine residues in proteins and may inactivate DNA repair enzymes. Examples are the chloroethylnitrosoureas, **lomustine** and **carmustine** (see Fig. 36.5), which, because they are lipid soluble and can thus cross the blood–brain barrier, may be used against tumours of the brain and meninges. However, most nitrosoureas have a severe cumulative depressive effect on the bone marrow that starts 3–6 weeks after initiation of treatment.

Busulphan

Busulphan has a selective effect on the bone marrow, depressing the formation of granulocytes and platelets in low dosage and red cells in higher dosage. It has little or no effect on lymphoid tissue or the gastrointestinal tract. It is accordingly used in chronic granulocytic leukaemia, in which it may increase the very short life expectancy by about a year, the thrombocytopenia constituting a hazardous toxic effect.

Other alkylating agents are **ethoglucid, thiotepa** and **treosulphan**.

Cisplatin

Cisplatin is a water-soluble planar coordination complex containing a central platinum atom surrounded by two chlorine atoms and two ammonia groups (Fig. 36.5). Its action is analogous to that of the alkylating agents. When it enters the cell, chloride ions dissociate leaving a reactive diamine–platinum complex which reacts with water and then interacts with DNA. It causes intrastrand cross-linking—probably between N7 and O6 of adjacent guanine molecules—which results in the breaking of the hydrogen bonds between the guanine and cytosine bases and thus local denaturation of the DNA chain.

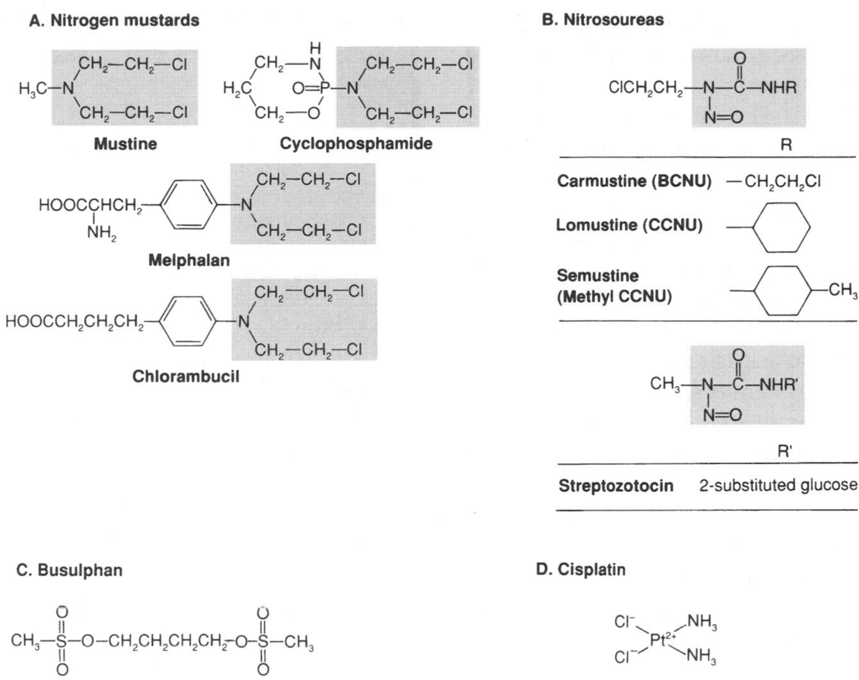

Fig. 36.5 Alkylating agents and related drugs used in anticancer therapy. **A.** Nitrogen mustards; the portion of the molecule within the light pink box is the nitrogen mustard group. **B.** Nitrosoureas; the portion within the grey box is the nitrosourea group. **C.** Busulphan (an alkylsulphonate). **D.** Cisplatin.

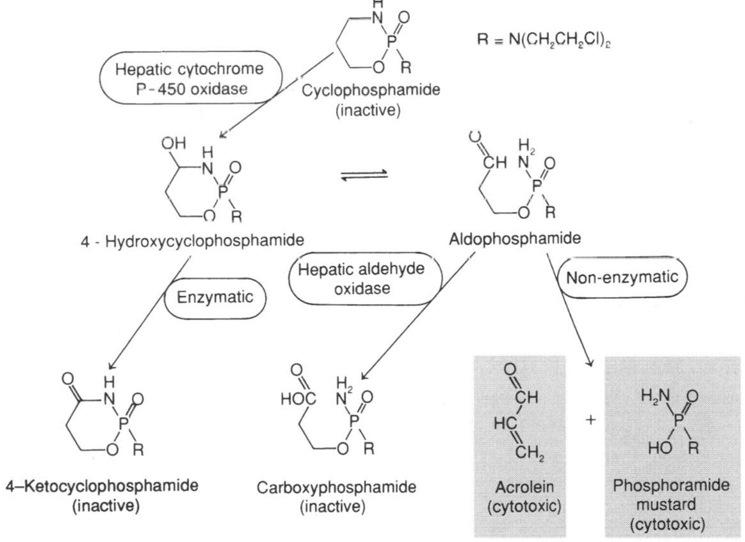

Fig. 36.6 The metabolism of cyclophosphamide. It is inactive until metabolised in the liver by the P-450 mixed function oxidases to 4-hydroxycyclophosphamide, which forms aldophosphamide reversibly. Aldophosphamide is conveyed to other tissues, where it is converted to phosphoramide mustard (the actual cytotoxic molecule) and acrolein, which is responsible for unwanted effects. The active metabolites are shown in the light pink boxes.

Cisplatin is given by slow intravenous injection or infusion. After 3 hours it is concentrated in the kidney, and after 40 hours in the liver and intestine as well. In the plasma most of it is bound to protein. Its clearance from the plasma is biphasic, with a $t_{1/2}$ of minutes for the first phase and days for the second phase. It is seriously nephrotoxic unless regimes of hydration and diuresis are instituted. It has low myelotoxicity but causes very severe nausea and vomiting. (5–HT_3-receptor antagonists, e.g. **ondansetron**, are extremely effective in preventing this and have transformed cancer chemotherapy with this compound.) Tinnitus and hearing loss in the high frequency range may occur, as may peripheral neuropathies, hyperuricaemia and anaphylactic reactions.

It has revolutionised the treatment of solid tumours of the testes and ovary.

Carboplatin is a derivative of cisplatin. It causes less nephrotoxicity, neurotoxicity and ototoxicity, and less severe nausea and vomiting than cisplatin, but is more myelotoxic.

Dacarbazine is activated by N-demethylation in the liver, and the resulting compound is subsequently cleaved in the target cell to release an alkylating derivative. It is given parenterally. *Unwanted effects* include myelotoxicity and severe nausea and vomiting.

Anticancer drugs: alkylating agents and related compounds

- **Alkylating agents** have alkyl groups which can form covalent bonds with cell substituents; a carbonium ion is the reactive intermediate.
- Most have two alkylating groups and can cross-link two nucleophilic sites such as the N7 of guanine in DNA. Cross-linking can cause:
  - —defective replication
  - —pairing of alkylguanine with thymine, and then substitution of AT for GC
  - —excision of guanine and chain breakage.
- Their principal effect occurs during DNA synthesis.
- *Unwanted effects* include myelosuppression, sterility and risk of non-lymphocytic leukaemia.
- The main alkylating agents are:
  - —*Nitrogen mustards:* e.g. **cyclophosphamide**, which is activated to give aldophosphamide, which is then converted to phosphoramide mustard (the cytotoxic molecule) and acrolein (which causes bladder damage that can be ameliorated by mesna). Cyclophosphamide myelosuppression affects particularly the lymphocytes. Given orally.
  - —*Nitrosoureas:* e.g. **lomustine** may act on non-dividing cells; can cross the blood–brain barrier; causes delayed, cumulative myelotoxicity. Given orally.
- **Cisplatin** causes intrastrand linking in DNA; it has low myelotoxicity but causes severe nausea and vomiting and can be nephrotoxic. Given intravenously, it has revolutionised the treatment of germ cell tumours.

ANTIMETABOLITES

Folate antagonists

The main folate antagonist is **methotrexate**: it is one of the most widely used antimetabolites in cancer chemotherapy.

Folates are essential for the synthesis of purine nucleotides and thymidylate, which in turn are essential for DNA synthesis and cell division. (This topic is also dealt with in Chs 23, 35 and 40.) In structure, folates consist of three elements: a hetero-bicyclic pteridine, p–aminobenzoic acid (PABA) and glutamic acid (Fig. 36.7). Folates in the blood have a single glutamate residue, but most intracellular folates are converted to polyglutamates. These polyglutamates are preferentially retained within the cells. In order to act as coenzymes, folates must be reduced to tetrahydrofolate (FH_4). This reaction

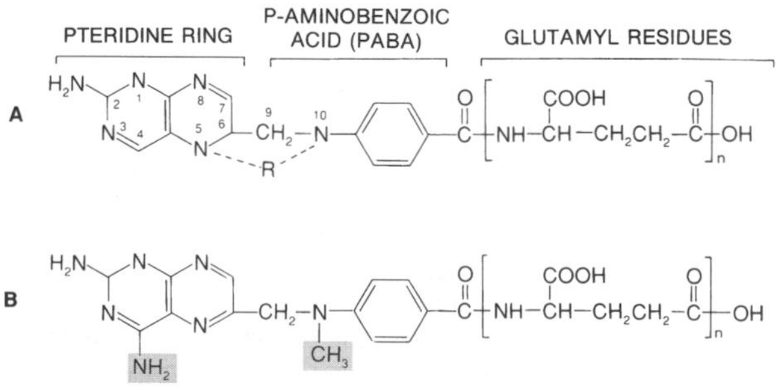

Fig. 36.7 Structure of (A) folic acid and (B) methotrexate. Both compounds are shown as polyglutamates. In tetrahydrofolate, one-carbon groups (R) are transported on N5 or N10 or both (shown dotted). See Figure 23.7.

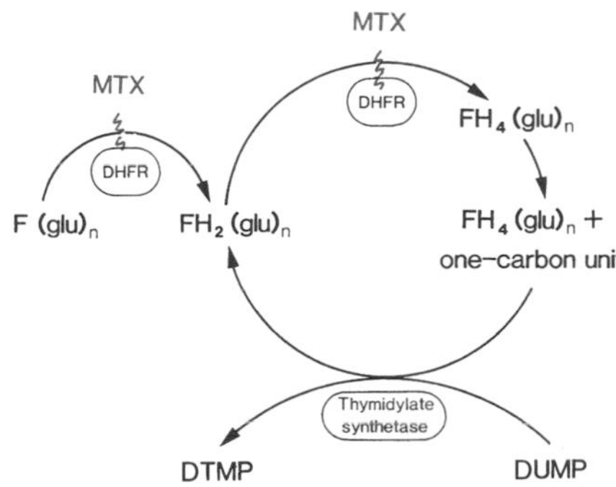

Fig. 36.8 Simplified diagram of action of methotrexate on thymidylate synthesis. Tetrahydrofolate polyglutamate [$FH_4(glu)_n$] functions as a carrier of a one-carbon unit, providing the methyl group necessary for the conversion of 2′deoxyuridylate (DUMP) to 2′deoxythymidylate (DTMP) by thymidylate synthetase. This one-carbon transfer results in the oxidation of $FH_4(glu)_n$ to $FH_2(glu)_n$.
(DHFR = dihydrofolate reductase; MTX = methotrexate)

is catalysed by *dihydrofolate reductase* and occurs in two steps, first to dihydrofolate (FH_2), then to FH_4 (Fig. 36.8). Folate polyglutamates have a much higher affinity for dihydrofolate reductase than does folate monoglutamate. FH_4 functions as a cofactor in the transfer of one-carbon units, a process which is essential both for the methylation of uracil in 2-deoxyuridylate (DUMP) to form thymidylate (DTMP) and thus for the synthesis of DNA, and also for the de novo synthesis of purines (see also Fig. 23.7).

During the formation of DTMP from DUMP, FH_4 is converted back to FH_2 (Fig. 36.8). Dihydrofolate reductase has a crucial role in maintaining the level of intracellular FH_4 by reduction of the FH_2 produced from folate reduction and that generated during thymidylate synthesis. **Methotrexate** inhibits dihydrofolate reductase and depletes intracellular FH_4 (Fig. 36.8). Methotrexate is an analogue of folate (see Fig. 36.7) and has a higher affinity for the enzyme than has FH_2. The binding of methotrexate to dihydrofolate reductase involves an additional hydrogen bond or ionic bond not present when FH_2 binds. The reaction most sensitive to FH_4 depletion is thymidylate synthesis, which is inhibited at a methotrexate concentration of 1 nmol/l, whereas inhibition of purine synthesis requires 10 times this concentration.

Pharmacokinetic aspects

Methotrexate is usually given orally. The peak blood concentration occurs 1–5 hours after administration and remains high for about 6 hours. It may also be given intramuscularly, intravenously or intrathecally.

About 50% of the drug is bound to plasma protein. It is distributed throughout the body fluids, including exudates and effusions. The drug has low lipid solubility and thus does not readily cross the blood–brain barrier. It is actively taken up into cells by the transport system used by folate, the rate of uptake of methotrexate being higher than that of the endogenous substance. A second uptake system, which probably involves diffusion, comes into play at high blood levels of the drug (in excess of 20 μmol/l); this may be important in overcoming that mechanism of resistance to methotrexate which involves decreased active transport (see later section). As with folic acid, intracellular methotrexate is metabolised to polyglutamate derivatives. These polyglutamates are retained in the cell for some time (weeks or months in some tissues) in the absence of extracellular drug.

Nearly half of a small dose and about 90% of a large dose is excreted unchanged in the urine, mostly within 12 hours, the $t_{½}$ being 2–3 hours. Renal excretion involves both glomerular filtration and tubular secretion.

Resistance to methotrexate may develop in tumour cells, a variety of mechanisms being involved: decreased membrane transport, altered dihydrofolate reductase with reduced affinity for the drug, increased amounts of the enzyme, and, possibly, decreased polyglutamation of the drug.

Unwanted effects are depression of the bone marrow and damage to the epithelium of the gastrointestinal tract; pneumonitis can occur. In addition, when high dose regimes are used, there may be nephrotoxicity, due to precipitation of the drug or a metabolite in the renal tubules. High dose regimes (doses 10 times greater than the standard doses), sometimes used in cases of methotrexate resistance, must be followed by 'rescue' with **folinic acid** (a form of tetrahydrofolate).

Pyrimidine analogues

Fluorouracil interferes with thymidylate synthesis and therefore with synthesis of DNA. Its structure is given in Figure 36.9. It is converted into a 'fraudulent' nucleotide fluorodeoxyuridine monophosphate (FDUMP). This interacts with thymidylate synthetase and the folate cofactors, but cannot be

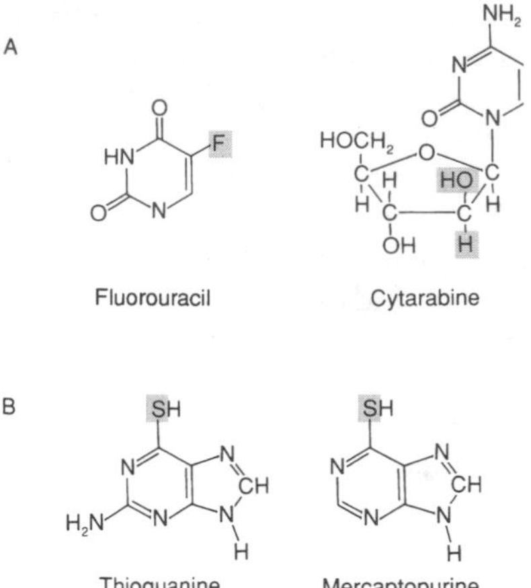

Fig. 36.9 Structural formulae of some cytotoxic antimetabolites. A. Pyrimidine analogues. **B.** Purine analogues. The points at which the drugs differ from endogenous compounds are shown in the light pink boxes.

converted into thymidylate because, in FDUMP, fluorine has replaced hydrogen at C5 where methylation would take place, and this carbon–fluorine bond is less susceptible to enzymic cleavage than the carbon–hydrogen bond. The result is inhibition of DNA synthesis but not RNA or protein synthesis.

Fluorouracil may be given orally or intravenously. After absorption it is rapidly distributed throughout the body water, and it readily crosses the blood–brain barrier. It undergoes rapid conversion to the nucleotide in the liver, only 20% of a dose being excreted unchanged in the urine. The $t_{½}$ is 11 minutes.

The main *unwanted effects* are gastrointestinal epithelial damage and myelotoxicity. Cerebellar disturbances can occur.

Cytarabine (cytosine arabinoside; Fig. 36.9) is an analogue of the naturally occurring nucleoside, 2′deoxycytidine. It differs from cytidine only in that, on the 2′ carbon of the pentose, the hydroxyl group is in the opposite configuration, that of arabinose instead of ribose. Cytarabine enters the target cell and undergoes the same phosphorylation reactions as the physiological nucleoside, to give the triphosphate. The drug is incorporated into both RNA and DNA to a limited extent, but its main cytotoxic action is the inhibition of DNA polymerase by its triphosphate. (The DNA polymerases require the triphosphates of the four deoxyribonucleosides for DNA synthesis—illustrated in Fig. 35.7.) Both replication and repair synthesis are inhibited by cytosine arabinoside triphosphate, the former more than the latter.

Cytarabine is given by intravenous or subcutaneous injection. It is metabolised in the liver and has a half-life of 30 minutes. It is able to cross the blood–brain barrier with moderate efficiency, giving CSF levels that are 40% of the plasma concentration. The main *unwanted effects* are on the bone marrow and the gastrointestinal tract. It causes nausea and vomiting.

Purine analogues

The main purine analogues used are **mercaptopurine** and **thioguanine** (Fig. 36.9). They are the 6-thiol analogues of the endogenous 6-OH purine bases, hypoxanthine and guanine, respectively. They are converted, in the cell, to the ribonucleotides: 6-thioguanosine-5′-phosphate and 6-thioinosine-5′-phosphate. These 'fraudulent' nucleotides produce their cytotoxic actions by many different mechanisms. They have several inhibitory actions on de novo purine synthesis and they may themselves be incorporated into DNA.

Mercaptopurine is well absorbed when given orally. It undergoes first-pass metabolism, being inactivated by xanthine oxidase in the liver; the products are excreted in the urine. The *unwanted*

Anticancer drugs: antimetabolites

- These drugs block or subvert pathways in DNA synthesis.
- *Folate antagonists:* **Methotrexate** inhibits dihydrofolate reductase, preventing generation of tetrahydrofolate; the main result is interference with thymidylate synthesis. Methotrexate is taken up into cells by the folate carrier, and, like folate, converted to the polyglutamate form. Given orally. Normal cells affected by high doses can be 'rescued' by folinic acid.
  Unwanted effects: myelosuppression, possible nephrotoxicity.
- *Pyrimidine analogues:* **Fluorouracil**, given orally or intravenously, is converted to a fraudulent nucleotide and inhibits thymidylate synthesis. **Cytarabine**, given intravenously or subcutaneously; its triphosphate form inhibits DNA polymerase; potent myelosuppressive.
- *Purine analogues:* **Mercaptopurine**, given orally, is converted into a fraudulent nucleotide.

effects are bone marrow depression, damage to the epithelium of the gut, pancreatitis and, rarely, liver damage. Thioguanine is given orally. The main unwanted effect is bone marrow depression.

A purine analogue with a different mechanism of action is **pentostatin**. It inhibits adenosine deaminase, the enzyme that catalyses deamination of adenosine to inosine. This action can interfere with critical pathways in purine metabolism and have significant effects on cell proliferation. It is very effective in hairy cell leukaemia.

Other purine analogues—the immunosuppressant **azathioprine**, which gives rise to mercaptopurine in vivo (see Fig. 12.3) and the xanthine oxidase inhibitor, **allopurinol** (see Fig. 12.2)—are used for non-malignant conditions. Allopurinol inhibits the breakdown of mercaptopurine and increases both its effect and its toxicity.

CYTOTOXIC ANTIBIOTICS

Antitumour antibiotics produce their effects mainly by direct action on DNA.

The anthracyclines

The main anticancer anthracycline antibiotic is **doxorubicin**. Others are **epirubicin, aclarubicin, mitozantrone** and **idarubicin**. Doxorubicin has several cytotoxic actions. It binds to DNA and inhibits both DNA and RNA synthesis, but its main cytotoxic action appears to be mediated through an effect on *topoisomerase II* (a DNA gyrase; see Ch. 35, p. 688), the activity of which is markedly increased in proliferating cells. The significance of the enzyme lies in the fact that during replication of the DNA helix in mammalian cells, reversible swivelling needs to take place around the replication fork in order to prevent the daughter DNA molecule becoming inextricably entangled during mitotic segregation. The swivel is produced by topoisomerase II, which nicks both DNA strands and subsequently reseals the breaks. Doxorubicin intercalates in the DNA and its effect is, in essence, to stabilise the DNA–topoisomerase II complex after the strands have been nicked, thus causing the process to seize up at this point (see Epstein 1988).

It is given by intravenous infusion and is rapidly taken up by most tissues, but does not cross the blood–brain barrier. Extravasation at the injection site can cause local necrosis. It is excreted mainly in the bile.

In addition to the general *unwanted effects* (p. 700), doxorubicin can cause cumulative, dose-related cardiac damage, leading to dysrhythmias and heart failure. This action may be due to generation of free radicals. Marked hair loss frequently occurs.

This drug is an effective cancer chemotherapy agent and is widely used, not only for leukaemias and lymphomas, but also for many solid tumours.

Epirubicin and **mitozantrone** are structurally related to doxorubicin. Mitozantrone has dose-related cardiotoxicity and causes bone marrow suppression. Epirubicin is less cardiotoxic than doxorubicin.

Dactinomycin is one of a series of antibiotics obtained from *Streptomyces* microorganisms. It intercalates, in the minor groove of DNA, between adjacent guanosine–cytosine pairs, interfering with the movement of RNA polymerase along the gene and thus preventing transcription. There is also evidence that it has a similar action to the anthracyclines on topoisomerase II. It has effects on cells in all phases of the cell cycle, but is particularly potent on rapidly proliferating cells. It can have all the toxic effects outlined previously at the beginning of this chapter. It is usually given by injection and rapidly disappears from the plasma, but it does not cross the blood–brain barrier.

The **bleomycins** are a group of metal-chelating glycopeptide antibiotics that degrade preformed DNA, causing chain fragmentation and release of free bases. Their action on DNA is thought to involve chelation of ferrous iron and interaction with oxygen, resulting in the oxidation of the iron and generation of superoxide and/or hydroxyl radicals. Bleomycin is most effective in the G_2 phase of the cell cycle and mitosis, but is also active against non-dividing cells, i.e. cells in the G_0 phase (Fig. 36.1). It is given by injection, is rapidly distributed and is cleared by renal excretion with a half-life of 120 minutes. In contrast to most anti-cancer drugs, bleomycin causes little myelosuppression. Its most serious toxic effect is pulmonary fibrosis, which occurs in 10% of patients treated and is reported to be fatal in 1%. Allergic reactions can occur. About half the patients manifest mucocutaneous reactions (the palms are frequently affected) and many develop hyperpyrexia.

Mitomycin, after enzymic activation in the cells, functions as a bifunctional alkylating agent, alkylating preferentially at O6 of guanine. It cross-links DNA and may also degrade DNA through the generation of free radicals. It is given intravenously,

Anticancer drugs: cytotoxic antibiotics

- **Doxorubicin** inhibits DNA and RNA synthesis; the DNA effect is due to interference with topoisomerase II action. Given by intravenous infusion, it is excreted mainly in bile. *Unwanted effects:* nausea and vomiting, myelosuppression, hair loss; it is cardiotoxic in high doses.
- **Bleomycin** causes fragmentation of DNA chains. It can act on non-dividing cells. Given by injection. *Unwanted effects:* fever, allergies, mucocutaneous reactions, pulmonary fibrosis. Virtually no myelosuppression.
- **Dactinomycin** intercalates in DNA, interfering with RNA polymerase and inhibiting transcription. It also interferes with the action of topoisomerase II. Given by injection. *Unwanted effects:* nausea and vomiting, myelosuppression.
- **Mitomycin** is activated to give an alkylating metabolite. Given intravenously.

is widely distributed in the body and is metabolised in the liver. It causes marked myelosuppression and can also cause kidney damage and fibrosis of lung tissue.

PLANT DERIVATIVES

Vinca alkaloids

Vinca alkaloids are derived from the periwinkle plant, the main alkaloids being **vincristine**, **vinblastine** and **vindesine**. They act by binding to tubulin and inhibit its polymerisation into microtubules preventing spindle formation in mitosing cells, and causing arrest at metaphase. Their effects only become manifest during mitosis. They also inhibit other cellular activities that involve the microtubules, such as leucocyte phagocytosis and chemotaxis as well as axonal transport in neurons.

They are all given by injection and extravasation may cause local damage. The drugs are rapidly sequestered in cells, particularly the white blood cells and platelets, which together may contain nearly half of the drug content of the blood. Vincristine has a longer half-life than the other two alkaloids—at 48 hours the tissues still contain more than 50% of the administered drug. Excretion of breakdown products is primarily into the bile.

The vinca alkaloids are relatively non-toxic. Vincristine has very mild myelosuppressive activity, but causes paraesthesias (sensory changes) and neuromuscular abnormalities fairly frequently. Vinblastine is less neurotoxic but causes leucopenia, while vindesine has both moderate myelotoxicity and neurotoxicity.

Etoposide is derived from mandrake root. Its mode of action is not clearly known but may be due to inhibition of mitochondrial function and of nucleoside transport, as well as to an effect on topoisomerase II similar to that seen with doxorubicin (p. 709). It may be given orally or intravenously and is widely distributed but does not cross the blood–brain barrier. It is excreted mainly in the urine.

Unwanted effects include nausea and vomiting, myelosuppression and hair loss.

Taxol is a derivative of yew tree bark which acts on microtubules, stabilising them (in effect 'freezing' them) in the polymerised state. This has repercussions similar to those described above for the vinca alkaloids. Unwanted effects include bone marrow suppression and paraesthesias. In early trials it has proved effective in ovarian cancer and drug-resistant breast cancer.

Anticancer drugs: plant derivatives

- **Vincristine** inhibits mitosis at metaphase by binding to tubulin. Given by injection. Relatively non-toxic, but can cause unwanted neuromuscular effects.
- **Etoposide** inhibits DNA synthesis by an action on topoisomerase II, and also inhibits mitochondrial function. Given orally or intravenously. Common unwanted effects include vomiting, myelosuppression and alopecia.

HORMONES

Tumours derived from hormone-sensitive tissues may be hormone-dependent. Their growth can be inhibited by hormones with opposing actions, by hormone antagonists or by agents that inhibit the synthesis of the relevant hormones. Hormones or hormone analogues which themselves have inhibitory actions on particular tissues can be used in treatment of tumours of those tissues.

Glucocorticoids have inhibitory effects on

lymphocyte proliferation (see Ch. 11) and are used in leukaemias and lymphomas. They are also used in a supportive role in other cancers on the basis of their effect on calcium metabolism and on raised intracranial pressure.

Oestrogens, such as **fosfestrol** (a prodrug, activated by acid phosphatase in prostatic tissue to yield stilboestrol), block the effect of androgens in androgen-dependent prostatic tumours. Oestrogens are also occasionally used in postmenopausal women with breast cancer.

One use of oestrogens in anticancer therapy is to employ these steroids to *recruit* resting mammary cancer cells (i.e. cells in compartment B; see p. 700) into the proliferating pool of cells (i.e. into compartment A), thus allowing a greater killing efficacy of the cytotoxic drugs which are then given.

Progestogens have been useful in endometrial neoplasms and hypernephromas. The main agents used are **megestrol** and **medroxyprogesterone**.

The hormone-dependency of tumours treated with steroids is, in general, related to the presence of steroid receptors in the malignant cells. The number of receptors can be estimated in biopsy specimens and this provides a guide to the potential efficacy of hormone therapy.

Gonadotrophin-releasing hormone analogues

As explained in Chapter 22 (p. 465) analogues of the gonadotrophin-releasing hormones, such as **goserelin**, can, under certain circumstances, inhibit gonadotrophin release. This can be made use of in prostate cancer and in some cases of advanced breast cancer in premenopausal women. When used for prostate tumours there is often, during the first week of treatment, a surge of gonadotrophin and testosterone secretion; the effect of the testosterone can be prevented by an antiandrogen such as **cyproterone** (p. 465).

An analogue of somastatin, **octreotide** (see pp. 420, 468), is used to treat the hormone-mediated effects of VIPomas, glucagonomas, carcinoid syndrome and gastrinomas.

Hormone antagonists

Hormone antagonists can be effective in several hormone-sensitive tumours.

Anti-oestrogens

An antioestrogen, **tamoxifen** (p. 460), is remarkably effective in some cases of hormone-dependent breast cancer, and may have a role in preventing these cancers. It has also proved effective against endometrial cancer.

In breast tissue, tamoxifen competes with endogenous oestrogens for the oestrogen receptors and inhibits the transcription of oestrogen-responsive genes. It may also have other anticancer actions in that it induces production of transforming growth factor-β (see Table 11.2), which can inhibit the growth of some malignant cells.

Tamoxifen is given orally and metabolised in the liver to produce an active metabolite. It takes several weeks for this metabolite to reach steady-state levels. Some of the drug is excreted in the faeces after enterohepatic cycling and some is excreted in the urine. Tamoxifen is also reported to have cardioprotective effects, partly by virtue of its ability to protect low density lipoproteins against oxidative damage.

It is estimated that five million women will develop breast cancer in the 1990s decade and large, double-blind, placebo-controlled trials of the preventive effect of tamoxifen are underway in the UK, the USA, Australia and parts of Europe.

Antiandrogens

Androgen antagonists, **flutamide** and **cyproterone** are used in prostate tumours.

Adrenal hormone synthesis inhibitors

Several agents which inhibit synthesis of adrenal hormones have effects in postmenopausal breast cancer. The drugs used are **formestane**, which acts

Anticancer agents: hormones and radioactive isotopes

- Hormones or their antagonists are used in hormone-sensitive tumours:
  - —**Glucocorticoids** for leukaemias and lymphomas
  - —**Oestrogens** for prostate tumours
  - —**Tamoxifen** for breast tumours
  - —**GnRH analogues** for prostate and breast tumours
  - —**Antiandrogens** for prostate cancers
  - —**Inhibitors of sex hormone synthesis** for postmenopausal breast cancer.
- Radioactive isotopes can be targeted at specific tissues, e.g. ^{131}I for thyroid tumours.

at a late stage of sex hormone synthesis, inhibiting the enzyme, aromatase, which metabolises androgens to oestrogens (see Fig. 22.3), and **trilostane** and **aminoglutethimide** (see Fig. 21.4) which inhibit sex hormone synthesis at an early stage. Replacement of corticosteroids is necessary with these latter two agents.

RADIOACTIVE ISOTOPES

Radioactive isotopes have a place in the therapy of certain tumours; e.g. **radioactive iodine** (^{131}I) is used in treating thyroid tumours (discussed in Ch. 21).

MISCELLANEOUS AGENTS

Procarbazine inhibits DNA and RNA synthesis and interferes with mitosis at interphase. Its effects may be due to the production of active metabolites. It is given orally.

It can be leukaemogenic, carcinogenic and teratogenic. It interacts with some agents: it causes disulfiram-like actions with alcohol (see Ch. 42), exacerbates the effects of CNS depressants and, because it is a weak monoamine oxidase inhibitor, can produce hypertension if given with certain sympathomimetic agents (Ch. 42). It causes the usual unwanted effects—nausea, myelosuppression, etc; allergic skin reactions may require cessation of treatment.

Hydroxyurea is a urea analogue that inhibits ribonucleotide reductase, thus interfering with the conversion of ribonucleotides to deoxyribonucleotides. It is given orally. It has the usual unwanted effects (p. 700), bone marrow depression being significant.

Crisantaspase is a preparation of the enzyme asparaginase, given intramuscularly or intravenously. It breaks down asparagine to aspartic acid and ammonia. It is active against tumour cells which, having lost the capacity to synthesise asparagine, now require an exogenous source of it, e.g. acute lymphoblastic leukaemia cells. Most normal body cells are able to synthesise asparagine, and the drug thus has a fairly selective action on certain tumours. It has very little suppressive effect on the bone marrow, or the mucosa of the gastrointestinal tract or hair follicles. It causes nausea and vomiting and it can cause CNS depression, anaphylactic reactions and liver damage.

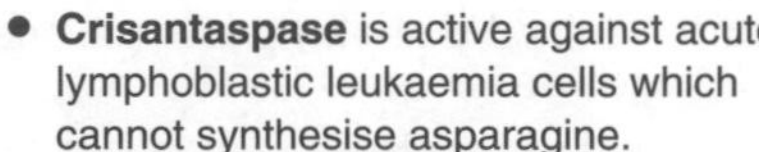

Anticancer drugs: miscellaneous agents

- **Crisantaspase** is active against acute lymphoblastic leukaemia cells which cannot synthesise asparagine.
- **Hydroxyurea** inhibits ribonucleotide reductase.
- **Amsacrine** acts on topoisomerase II.
- **Mitozantrone** causes DNA chain breakage.
- **Mitotane** stops synthesis of adrenocortical steroids.

Mitotane interferes with the synthesis of adrenocortical steroids (p. 436) having eventually a cytotoxic action on cells in the adrenal cortex. It is used solely for tumours of these cells. It is given orally and tends to accumulate in fatty tissue, from which it is released slowly.

Amsacrine has a mechanism of action similar to that of doxorubicin (p. 709). It is given intravenously, metabolised in the liver and excreted in the urine and the bile. Bone marrow depression and cardiac toxicity have been reported.

Mitozantrone binds to DNA causing chain breakage and inhibiting DNA and RNA synthesis. It has the usual toxic effects, bone marrow depression being particularly important.

DRUG RESISTANCE

The resistance which neoplastic cells may manifest to cytotoxic drugs may be primary (present when the drug is first given) or acquired (developing during treatment with the drug). Acquired resistance may be due either to adaptation of the tumour cells or to mutation, with the emergence of cells which are less affected or unaffected by the drug and which consequently have a selective advantage over the sensitive cells. Examples of various mechanisms of resistance are:

- Decreased accumulation of drugs in cells due to the increased expression of a cell surface, energy-dependent drug transport protein, termed P-glycoprotein. The transporter is coded for by the *mdr* gene and is responsible for *multidrug resistance* to many structurally dissimilar anticancer drugs (doxorubicin, vinblastine, dactinomycin, etc.). The physiological role of P-glycoprotein is thought to be the protection of cells against environmental toxins. The transporter consists of 12 transmembrane domains round a central core or barrel. It functions as a hydrophobic 'vacuum cleaner', picking up drugs as they enter the cell membrane and expelling them through the barrel to the outside. Several non-cytotoxic agents can reverse multidrug resistance (see p. 715).

- A decrease in amount of drug taken up by the cell (methotrexate).
- Insufficient activation of the drug (mercaptopurine, fluorouracil, cytarabine). By this is meant that there may be decreased metabolism of these agents so that they do not enter the pathways where they would normally exert their effects. Thus, fluorouracil may not be converted to FDUMP, cytarabine may not undergo phosphorylation, mercaptopurine may not be converted into a 'fraudulent' nucleotide.
- Increase in inactivation (cytarabine, mercaptopurine).
- Increased concentration of target enzyme (methotrexate).
- Decreased requirement for substrate (crisantaspase).
- Increased utilisation of alternative metabolic pathways (antimetabolites).
- Rapid repair of drug-induced lesions (alkylating agents).
- Altered activity of target, for example modified topoisomerase II (doxorubicin).

CELL CYCLE: DRUG EFFECTS AND THEIR POSSIBLE CLINICAL APPLICATIONS

The mitotic cycle of dividing cells can be considered to consist of four phases (see Fig. 36.1). Cells that are constantly in cell cycle constitute the 'growth fraction' of the tumour.

Anticancer drugs can be classified in terms of their actions on the cycle as:

- *Phase-specific agents*, i.e. acting at a specific phase of the cell cycle. The vinca alkaloids act in mitosis. Cytarabine, hydroxyurea, thiouracil, methotrexate and mercaptopurine act in S phase. Some of these compounds have some action during G_1 phase and thus may slow the entry of a cell into S phase, where it would be more susceptible to the drug.
- *Cycle-specific agents*, i.e. acting at all stages of the cell cycle and not having much effect on cells out of cycle: alkylating agents, actinomycin D, doxorubicin and cisplatin.
- *Cycle non-specific agents*, i.e. acting on cells whether in cycle or not: bleomycins and nitrosoureas.

It has been proposed that this information could be of value in selecting agents for clinical use. Tumours with a high growth fraction should respond to phase-specific and cycle-specific agents. For tumours with a small growth fraction the use of cycle non-specific agents (together with surgery or X-ray) could be considered. It has been suggested that combinations of cytotoxic drugs should be based on the above classification, but it has not been clearly established that treatment schedules based on these principles are better than purely empirical schedules.

TREATMENT SCHEDULES

Treatment with combinations of several anticancer agents increases the cytotoxicity against cancer cells without necessarily increasing the general toxicity. Thus, for example, **methotrexate**, with mainly myelosuppressive toxicity, may be used in a regime with **vincristine**, which has mainly neurotoxicity. The few drugs with low myelotoxicity, such as **cisplatin** and **bleomycin**, are good candidates for combination regimes. Treatment with combinations of drugs also decreases the possibility of the development of resistance to individual agents. Detailed consideration of the combination schedules used in the clinic can be found in Clinical Pharmacology manuals; the subject is beyond the scope of this book but some combination regimes are given in Table 36.1.

Drugs are often given in large doses intermittently, in several courses with intervals of 2–3 weeks between courses, rather than in small doses continuously. This is because such a regime permits the bone marrow to regenerate during the intervals. Furthermore, it has been shown that the same total dose of an agent is more effective when given in one or two large doses than in multiple small doses.

POSSIBLE FUTURE STRATEGIES FOR CANCER CHEMOTHERAPY

Some of the main drawbacks of the current chemotherapy of cancer are as follows:

- the severe toxic effects of many agents, particularly bone marrow suppression and nausea and vomiting
- the lack of selectivity of the drugs against tumour cells as compared with normal cells
- the fact that, with many tumours, total elimination of malignant cells is not possible with therapeutic doses, and the host's immune response is often not adequate to deal with the remaining cells
- the development of resistance (particularly multidrug resistance) to anticancer drugs
- the fact that current anticancer drugs are aimed at the destruction of the cancer cell rather than at the basic changes which make a cell malignant.

Attempts are being made to overcome these problems—the first by the use of more effective anti-emetics and the development of regimes for dealing with myelosuppression, the second by using selective targeting of anticancer compounds, the third by boosting or augmenting the host's immune responses to the tumour, the fourth by developing agents which reverse multidrug resistance and the fifth by developing new approaches based on the advances in knowledge of the biology of the cancer cell.

TECHNIQUES FOR DEALING WITH EMESIS AND MYELOSUPPRESSION

Emesis

The nausea and vomiting induced by many cancer chemotherapy agents constitutes an 'inbuilt deterrent' to patient compliance (see also Ch. 19, p. 395). It is a particular problem with cisplatin, but also complicates therapy with many other compounds, such as the alkylating agents. 5-HT_3-receptor antagonists such as **ondansetron** or **granesitron** (see Ch. 19) have proved, in double-blind clinical trials, to be extremely effective against cytotoxic-drug-induced vomiting. Of the other anti-emetic agents available (see p. 395), **metoclopramide**, given intravenously, has proved useful for chemotherapy-induced nausea and vomiting, and it is often combined with therapy with **dexamethasone** (Ch. 21) or **lorazepam** (Ch. 27). The extrapyramidal side effects of metoclopramide (common in children and young adults) seem to be reduced by giving concomitant **diphenhydramine** (Ch. 12).

Myelosuppression

Myelosuppression limits the use of many anti-cancer agents. Regimes to overcome the problem have included removing some of the patient's bone marrow prior to giving the chemotherapy agent, and replacing it afterwards. This has been combined with purging of the bone marrow in vitro (see below). The use of colony-stimulating agents, for example **G-CSF** (see p. 485), after replacement of the marrow has been successful in some cases. A new possibility is the introduction, into the extracted bone marrow, of the mutated gene which confers multidrug resistance, so that when replaced the *marrow cells* (but not the cancer cells) will be resistant to the cytotoxic action of the anticancer drugs.

THE TARGETING OF TOXINS AGAINST CANCER CELLS

In those instances when tumour-specific or tumour-associated antigens can be identified, attempts have been made to raise *monoclonal antibodies* against the antigens. The intention is that either these antibodies, or else *growth factors* which preferentially bind to cancer cells, could be used to direct *radioactive isotopes* or *toxic molecules*, specifically to the malignant cells. Toxic molecules so used include ricin, diphtheria toxin, and *Pseudomonas aeruginosa* exotoxin A.

Another use of monoclonal antibodies with bound toxins is to *purge* tumour cells from bone marrow taken from a patient, prior to the use of radiation and/or megadose chemotherapy regimes. Purging can also be accomplished by the use of complement (see pp. 216 and 223) after adding monoclonal antibodies against tumour cell antigens to the marrow in vitro. The purged marrow is then re-injected to reconstitute the bone marrow of the patient.

Progress with monoclonal antibodies against tumour antigens has been slow, in part at least because of the heterogeneity of antigen expression in tumour cells. A more fruitful approach has been to prepare recombinant chimeric toxins by fusing the genes which code for growth factors that act on cancer cells with the genes which code for the toxins (reviewed by Pastan et al. 1992).

Another approach which has been successful in experimental animals is the use of a monoclonal antibody against an angiogenesis factor spontaneously produced by tumour cells. This prevents the proliferation of new blood vessels without which a tumour is unable to grow.

ENHANCEMENT OF THE HOST'S RESPONSE TO CANCER

Agents which enhance the host's response are referred to as **biological response modifiers**. Various cytokines which enhance or otherwise modify host response against tumour cells (see Ch. 11, Table 11.2) are being tested as anticancer agents.

α-interferon has shown promise in hairy cell leukaemia, melanoma, some lymphomas, and Kaposi's sarcoma. It has anti-proliferative as well as immunoregulatory effects and this, in addition to stimulating a response ab initio, can augment an existing response. The main unwanted effect is a flu-like syndrome.

Aldesleukin, a preparation of interleukin 2 (see Table 11.2), given with lymphokine-activated killer lymphocytes, has had some action on solid tumours (notably renal cell carcinomas) unresponsive to other therapy at the expense of profound toxic effects due to vascular leakage. It is less toxic on its own.

Tretinoin, and its isomer, **isotretinoin**, derivatives of Vitamin A used topically for acne, can induce differentiation of a variety of tumour cells in vitro. These agents, given orally, have been shown to have action against acute promyclocytic leukaemia (see Warrell et al. 1993). An international clinical trial comparing their effects with that of standard chemotherapy is at present under way.

The anthelminthic, **levamisole** (p. 780), is reported to have an immunostimulant effect, and there is evidence that, combined with **fluorouracil**, it is effective in some cases of colon cancer.

Tumour necrosis factor (Table 11.2) has powerful anti-cancer action in experimental systems but has been less successful in human tumours. Possible synergy with other cytokines is being investigated.

REVERSAL OF MULTIDRUG RESISTANCE

Several non-cytotoxic drugs can reverse multidrug resistance. Examples are: calcium-channel blockers, some anti-arrhythmics (e.g. quinidine), some antihypertensives (e.g. reserpine), some antihistamines (e.g. terfenadine), some immunosuppressants (e.g. cyclosporine), some steroid hormones (e.g. progesterone), some antipsychotic drugs (e.g. phenothiazines). Development of related compounds could make it feasible to overcome this type of resistance. In addition, the use of antibodies, immunotoxins, antisense oligonucleotides (see below) or liposome-encapsulated agents could be useful in the elimination of cells with multidrug resistance (reviewed by Gottesman & Pastan 1993).

APPROACHES BASED ON THE BIOLOGY OF THE CANCER CELL

As outlined above on page 698, there have been significant advances in our understanding of the basis of malignancy, particularly as regards the role of oncogenes and tumour suppressor genes. A variety of agents which modify the various ways by which oncogenes confer autonomy of growth on cells are under investigation (reviewed by Powis 1991).

One example is the development of compounds which block the capacity of mutant *ras* genes to make cells malignant. Mutations of the *ras* gene contribute to 20–30% of all human cancers, to more than 50% of some common tumours such as colon cancer and to 80% of pancreatic tumours. The normal *ras* gene codes for the production of G-proteins. These proteins have a central role in the signal transduction pathways used by cells to proliferate in response to growth factors. In cells in which the *ras* gene has mutated, the G-proteins can be perpetually 'turned on', continuously giving the signal for cell division even in the absence of growth factors. In normal cells, the G-proteins, after synthesis, move to the cell membrane to which they become attached by a sort of molecular 'hook'—a farnesyl group. This group is added to the protein by the enzyme, farnesyl transferase. Compounds that inhibit this enzyme have recently been produced. They have been shown, in in vitro tests, to reverse the malignant transformation in cancer cells containing the *ras* oncogene, restoring normal growth patterns. They did not interfere with cell division in normal cells (see Travis 1993).

Perhaps the most exciting new developments are those involving gene therapy. As a result of the advances in recombinant DNA technology there are now vectors that can deliver new genetic information into living cells in the body. One such vector is a modified retrovirus which can become integrated into dividing human cells. Vectors can be used to introduce into cancer cells antisense oligonucleotides. These are short pieces of DNA (usually 15–30 base pairs) that are complementary to a portion of mRNA and which can bind to their opposite number on the mRNA molecule; this now double-stranded section prevents the action of the mRNA and thus blocks expression of the particular oncogene. Furthermore, ribozymes—short sequences of RNA that behave like enzymes and have the ability to cleave RNA—can also be introduced into vectors carrying antisense oligomers and could be even more effective in preventing oncogene expression.

The use of a retroviral vector to deliver antisense oligomers to block expression of a *ras* oncogene is being tested as a treatment of adenocarcinoma of the lung in the USA.

Another approach under investigation is the introduction into the body of a vector that contains the promoter region of an oncogene coupled to a non-mammalian enzyme with the capacity to activate a pro-drug to a cytotoxic agent. A useful enzyme for this purpose would be the cytosine deaminase of fungi which converts the antifungal drug flucytosine to the anticancer drug fluorouracil.

It is likely that dramatic advances in the treatment of cancer will occur during the coming decade.

REFERENCES AND FURTHER READING

Aznavoorian S, Murphy A N, Stetler-Stevenson W G, Liotta L A 1993 Molecular aspects of tumour invasion and metastasis. Cancer 71: 1368–1382

Boon T 1993 Teaching the immune system to fight cancer. Scientific American March: 32–39

Bunce K, Tyers M, Beranek P 1991 Clinical evaluation of 5-HT_3 receptor antagonists as anti-emetics. Trends Pharmacol Sci 12: 46–48

Carbone D P, Minna J D 1993 Antioncogenes and cancer. Annu Rev Med 44: 451–464

Carmichael J 1994 Cancer chemotherapy: identifying novel anticancer drugs. Br Med J 308: 1288–1290

Carson D A, Ribiero J M 1993 Apoptosis and disease. Lancet 341: 1251–1254

Cheson B D 1992 The maturation of differentiation therapy. N Engl J Med 327: 422–424

de Wet M, Falkson G, Rapoport B L 1993 Repeated use of granisotron in patients receiving cytostatic agents. Cancer 71: 4043–4048

Druker B J, Mamon H J, Roberts T M 1989 Oncogenes, growth factors and signal transduction. N Engl J Med 321: 1383–1391

Editorial 1988 DNA topoisomerases—new twists to tumour therapy. Lancet 1: 511–513

Editorial 1989 Interleukin-2: sunrise for immunotherapy. Lancet 2: 308

Editorial 1989 Multidrug resistance in cancer. Lancet 2: 1075–1076

Editorial 1990 Molecular targets for cancer therapy. Lancet 1: 826

Editorial 1991 Ondansetron *vs* dexamethosone for chemotherapy-induced emesis. Lancet 338: 478–479

Epstein R J 1988 Topoisomerases in human disease. Lancet 1: 521–524

Ferry D R, Kerr D J 1994 Multidrug resistance in cancer. Br Med J 308: 148–149

Ford J M, Hait W N 1990 Pharmacology of drugs that alter multidrug resistance in cancer. Pharmacol Rev 42: 156–198

Gelber R D, Coates A S, Goldhirsch A 1992 Adjuvant treatment of breast cancer: the overview. Ovarian ablation, chemotherapy, and tamoxifen all work. Br Med J 304: 859–860

Gottesman M M, Pastan I 1993 Biochemistry of multidrug resistance mediated by the multidrug transporter. Ann Rev Biochem 62: 385–427

Gutterman J 1988 Overview of advances in the use of biological proteins in human cancer. Semin Oncol 15: 2–6

Hackford A W 1993 Biochemical markers for colorectal cancer. Surg Clin North Am 73: 85–102

Harris C C, Holstein M 1993 Clinical implications of the p53 tumor suppressor gene. N Engl J Med 329: 1318–1327

Harris H 1990 The role of differentiation in the suppression of malignancy. J Cell Science 97: 5–10

Harris H, Miller O, Klein G, Worst P, Tachibana T 1969 Suppression of malignancy by cell fusion. Nature 233: 363–368

Hickman J A, Tritton T 1992 Cancer chemotherapy. Blackwells Scientific Publications, Oxford, p 1–288

Holyoake T L, Franklin I M 1994 Bone marrow transplants from peripheral blood: set to transform medical oncology. Br Med J 309: 4–5

Horwitz K B 1992 The molecular biology of RU486. Is there a role for antiprogestins in the treatment of breast cancer? Endocr Rev 13: 146–165

Iggo R, Gatter K et al. 1990 Increased expression of mutant forms of p53 oncogene in primary lung cancer. Lancet 2: 675–679

Jolivet J, Cowan K H, Curt G A, Clendinnin N J, Chabner B A 1983 The pharmacology and clinical use of methotrexate. N Engl J Med 309: 1094–1104

Jordan V C, Murphy C S 1990 Endocrine pharmacology of antiestrogens as antitumour agents. Endocr Rev 11: 578–610

Karp J E, Broder S 1992 Oncology. J Amer Med Assoc 268: 391–393

Kedar R P, Bourne T H et al. 1994 Effects of tamoxifen on uterus and ovaries of postmenopausal women in a randomised breast cancer prevention trial. Lancet 343: 1318–1321

Kinzler K W, Vogelstein B 1994 Cancer therapy meets p53. Br Med J 331: 49–50

Klohs W, Kraker A J 1992 Pentostatin: future directions. Pharmacol Rev 44: 459–479

Lane D P 1992 p53, guardian of the genome. Nature 358: 15–16
Lemoine N R, Sikora K 1993 Interventional genetics and cancer treatment: gene therapy predicted to join the therapeutic menu within the decade. Br Med J 306: 306–307
Liotta L A, Steeg P S, Stetler-Stevenson W G 1991 Cancer metastasis and angiogenesis: an imbalance of positive and negative regulation. Cell 64: 327–336
Macara I G 1989 Oncogenes and cellular signal transduction. Physiol Rev 69: 797–820
McVie J G 1988 DNA topo-isomerases in cancer treatment. Br Med J 296: 1145–1146
Magrath I (ed) 1989 New directions in cancer treatment. Springer-Verlag, Berlin
Malik S, Waxman J 1992 Cytokines and cancer. Br Med J 305: 265–267
Malone T, Sharpe R J 1990 Development of angiogenesis inhibitors for clinical applications. Trends Pharmacol Sci 11: 457–461
Morstyn G, Lieschke G J et al. 1989 Pharmacology of the colony-stimulating factors. Trends Pharmacol Sci 10: 154–158
Murray A W 1992 Creative blocks: cell-cycle check points and feedback controls. Nature 359: 599–604
Powis G 1991 Signalling targets for anticancer drug development. Trends Pharmacol Sci 12: 188–194
Pastan I, Chaudhary V, FitzGerald D J 1992 Recombinant toxins as novel therapeutic agents. Ann Rev Biochem 61: 331–354
Perren T, Selby P 1992 Current issues in cancer: biological therapy. Br Med J 304: 1621–1623
Sikora K 1994 Genes, dreams, and cancer. Br Med J 308: 1217–1221
Sporn M B, Roberts A B 1985 Autocrine growth factors and cancer. Nature 313: 745–747
Sporn M B, Roberts A B 1991 Autocrine growth factors and the regulation of tumour growth. In Broder S (ed) Molecular foundations of oncology. Williams & Wilkins, Baltimore, ch 9
Steel C M 1989 Peptide regulatory factors and malignancy. Lancet 1: 30–34
Steel G G, Stephens T C 1979 The relationship of cell kinetics to cancer chemotherapy. Adv Pharmacol Ther 10: 137–145
Travis J 1993 Novel anticancer agents move closer to reality. Science 260: 1877–1878
Twycross R 1992 Corticosteroids in advanced cancer. Br Med J 305: 969–970
Warrell R P, de The H, Wang Z-Y, Degros L 1993 Acute promyelocytic leukemia. N Engl J Med 329: 177–189
Waxman J 1987 Gonadotrophin hormone releasing analogues open new doors in cancer treatment. Br Med J 295: 1084–1085
Weiner T M, Liu E T, Craven R J, Cance W G 1993 Expression of focal adhesion kinase gene and invasive cancer. Lancet 342: 1024–1025
Wiseman H 1994 Tamoxifen: new membrane-mediated mechanisms of action and therapeutic advances. Trends Pharmacol Sci 15: 83–89

37
ANTIBACTERIAL AGENTS

A detailed classification of the bacteria of medical importance is beyond the scope of this book. However, a short list of the commoner and/or more important microorganisms which cause disease is given in Table 37.1. Individual chemotherapeutic agents are dealt with briefly in this chapter and a general indication of their main antibacterial actions is given in Table 37.1. Some of the diseases that may be caused by the organisms are included in the table but it should be understood that most of the organisms may, on occasion, produce other pathological conditions.

Certain principles should be borne in mind when choosing an antibiotic to treat a bacterial infection (see Moellering 1985, Geddes 1988). In general, two important requirements are to identify the infecting organism (if practicable) and to determine its susceptibility to antibacterial agents. In addition, certain host factors should be taken into account, such as previous exposure to antibiotics, age, renal and hepatic function, site of infection, concurrent administration of other drugs that might interact with the antibiotic, and whether the patient is pregnant or has a compromised immune system.

It will be seen from the table that many of the organisms cited are classified as either Gram-positive or Gram-negative. This classification is based on whether the organisms do or do not stain with Gram's stain, but has a significance far beyond that of an empirical staining reaction. Gram-positive and Gram-negative organisms are different in several respects, not least in the structure of the cell wall, which has implications for the action of antibiotics.

The cell wall of Gram-positive organisms is a relatively simple structure, 15–50 nm thick. It consists of about 50% peptidoglycan (see p. 684), about 40–45% acidic polymer (which results in the cell surface being highly polar and carrying a negative charge) and about 5–10% proteins and polysaccharides. The strongly polar polymer layer influences the penetration of ionised molecules, and favours the penetration of positively charged compounds, such as **streptomycin**, into the cell.

The cell wall of Gram-negative organisms is much more complex. From the plasma membrane outwards it consists of the following:

Table 37.1 General outline of the action of antibiotics against common or important microorganisms

Microorganism*	Antibiotics: First choice†	Second choice†
Gram-positive cocci		
Staphylococcus (infections of wounds, boils, etc.)		
Non-β-lactamase-producing	Penicillin G‡ or V‡	A cephalosporin, vancomycin (imipenem)
β-lactamase-producing	A β-lactamase-resistant penicillin, e.g. flucloxacillin	A cephalosporin, amoxycillin + clavulanic acid, vancomycin, erythromycin
Methicillin-resistant	Vancomycin, teicoplanin	Co-trimoxazole,§ ciprofloxacin, a macrolide + or – fusidic acid, rifampicin
Streptococcus, haemolytic types (septic infections)	Penicillin G or V,‡ + or – an aminoglycoside	A cephalosporin, a macrolide, vancomycin
Pneumococcus (pneumonia)	Penicillin G or V‡ ampicillin or a macrolide¶	A cephalosporin, vancomycin
Gram-negative cocci		
Neisseria gonorrhoeae (gonorrhoea)	Amoxycillin + clavulanic acid ceftriaxone, ciprofloxacin	Spectinomycin, cefoxitin, cefuroxime
Neisseria meningitidis (meningitis)	Penicillin G,‡ cefotaxime + ampicillin	Chloramphenicol, cotrimoxazole§
Gram-positive rods		
Corynebacterium (diphtheria)	A macrolide	Penicillin G
Clostridium (tetanus, gangrene)	Penicillin G‡	A tetracycline, a cephalosporin, clindamycin
Listeria (rare cause of meningitis and generalised infection in neonates)	Amoxycillin + or – an aminoglycoside	A tetracycline, erythromycin + or – an aminoglycoside, co-trimoxazole§
Gram-negative rods		
Enterobacteriaceae (coliform organisms)		
Escherichia coli, Enterobacter, Klebsiella		
— infections of urinary tract	Oral cephalosporin, trimethoprim, nitrofurantoin	Extended-spectrum penicillin, ciprofloxacin
— septicaemia	Aminoglycoside i.v.	Cephalosporin i.v.
Shigella (dysentery)	Ciprofloxacin	Ampicillin, a tetracycline, co-trimoxazole§
Salmonella (typhoid, paratyphoid)	Ciprofloxacin	Co-trimoxazole§
Haemophilus (infections of respiratory tract, ear, sinuses; meningitis)	Chloramphenicol, third-generation cephalosporin	Co-trimoxazole, ciprofloxacin
Bordetella (whooping cough)	A macrolide	Ampicillin
Brucella (brucellosis)	A tetracycline + or – streptomycin	Rifampicin and tetracycline, co-trimoxazole,§ chloramphenicol and/or streptomycin
Yersinia pestis (plague)	Streptomycin + or – a tetracycline	Chloramphenicol
Vibrio (cholera)	A tetracycline	Co-trimoxazole,§ ciprofloxacin
Legionella (pneumonia)	A macrolide + or – rifampicin	Co-trimoxazole,§ ciprofloxacin
Helicobacter pylori (peptic ulcer?)	Metronidazole,‖ amoxycillin‖	Ciprofloxacin, erythromycin
Pseudomonas aeruginosa (infection of burns, etc.)	Antipseudomonal penicillins + tobramycin,** quinolone	Ceftazidime, imipenem + or – aminoglycoside, aztreonam
Bacteroides fragilis (internal abscesses)	Clindamycin, metronidazole	Cefoxitin, imipenem, antipseudomonal penicillins + penicillinase inhibitor
Gram-negative anaerobic rods other than *B. fragilis*	Penicillin G,‡ metronidazole	Clindamycin, a tetracycline, a cephalosporin
Campylobacter (*diarrhoea*)	A macrolide, ciprofloxacin	A tetracycline, gentamicin

continued

Table 37.1 continued

Microorganism*	Antibiotics: First choice†	Second choice†
Spirochaetes		
Treponema (syphilis, yaws)	Penicillin G‡	A macrolide, a tetracycline
Borrelia (relapsing fever)	A tetracycline	Penicillin G‡
Borrelia (Lyme disease)	A tetracycline	Penicillin G,‡ doxycycline
Leptospira (Weil's disease)	Penicillin G‡	A tetracycline
Rickettsiae (typhus, Q fever, tick-bite fever, etc.)	A tetracycline	Chloramphenicol, co-trimoxazole§
Other organisms		
Mycoplasma pneumoniae	A macrolide, a tetracycline	Ciprofloxacin
Chlamydia (psittacosis, trachoma, urogenital infections)	A tetracycline, a macrolide	A sulphonamide
Actinomyces (abscesses)	Penicillin G‡	A tetracycline
Nocardia (lung disease)	Sulphonamide	Co-trimoxazole,§ minocycline
Mycobacteria (see text for details)		

* Only the main diseases caused by each organism are mentioned (in brackets).
† The agents given are alternatives; if they are to be used concomitantly, this is specified by a plus sign; if with *or* without another agent, this is signified by '+ or –'.
‡ Penicillin G = benzylpenicillin; Penicillin V = phenoxymethylpenicillin
§ Co-trimoxazole is trimethoprim and a sulphonamide; authorities now recommend using trimethoprim on its own for urinary and respiratory infections.
¶ In the absence of Gram stain
‖ Usually in combination with other drugs, e.g. bismuth chelate, omeprazole
** Not in same syringe
Note: This is not meant to be a definitive guide for clinical treatment, but a general indication of the main antimicrobial actions and thus of the overall usefulness of commonly used antibiotics. (For a more comprehensive list, see Laurence D R, Bennett P N 1992 Clinical pharmacology, Churchill Livingstone.) The selection of antibiotics to treat an infection will change as resistance occurs and as new agents are introduced. Susceptibility tests should be performed if possible.

- A periplasmic space containing enzymes and other components.
- A peptidoglycan layer 2 nm in thickness and comprising 5% of the cell wall mass; this is often linked to lipoprotein molecules which project outwards.
- An outer membrane consisting of a lipid bilayer similar in some respects to the plasma membrane. It contains protein molecules and on its inner aspect has lipoprotein that is linked to the peptidoglycan. Complex polysaccharides are important components on its outer surface. They are different in different strains of bacteria and are the main determinants of the antigenicity of the organism. They constitute the 'endotoxins' which, in vivo, trigger various aspects of the inflammatory reaction activating complement, causing fever, etc. (see Ch. 11). Recent studies have shown that there are proteins in the outer membrane that form transmembrane water-filled channels, termed 'porins', through which hydrophilic antibiotics may move freely.

Difficulty in penetrating this complex outer layer is probably the reason why some antibiotics are less active against Gram-negative than Gram-positive bacteria. This is of particular relevance in determining the extraordinary insusceptibility to most antibiotic drugs of *Pseudomonas aeruginosa*, a pathogen which can cause life-threatening infections of burns and wounds. Antibiotics for which penetration is a problem include **penicillin G, methicillin, the macrolides, rifampicin, fusidic acid, vancomycin, bacitracin** and **novobiocin.**

There is evidence that the lipopolysaccharide of the cell wall is the major barrier to penetration.

ANTIMICROBIAL AGENTS WHICH INTERFERE WITH THE SYNTHESIS OR ACTION OF FOLATE

SULPHONAMIDES

In the 1930s Domagk first demonstrated that a chemotherapeutic agent could influence the course of a bacterial infection. The drug was **prontosil**, a dye, and it was shown not only to protect mice against several thousand times the lethal dose of haemolytic streptococci but also to be effective in similar infections in man.* However, prontosil proved to be a pro-drug, inactive in vitro and needing to be metabolised in vivo to give the active product—**sulphanilamide** (Fig. 37.1). A large number of sulphonamides have been developed since, and although their therapeutic importance has declined somewhat they are still useful drugs. Furthermore, they are of considerable historical and theoretical interest, not least because chemical modification of the sulphonamide structure has given rise to several important groups of drugs, especially diuretics (acetazolamide and the thiazides; see Ch. 18), tuberculostatic and antileprotic agents (the sulphones; see below) and oral hypoglycaemic drugs (sulphonylureas; see Ch. 20).

The clinically useful antibacterial sulphonamides are derived from sulphanilamide (Fig. 37.1), by substitution on the amide moiety (SO_2NHR). Compounds in which the amino group (NH_2) has been substituted are pro-drugs that must be activated in the body, since a free amino group is necessary for antimicrobial activity.

The sulphonamides are usually used as their sodium salts, which are readily soluble in water.

Examples of sulphonamides in clinical use are:

- **sulphadiazine** (Fig. 37.1), **sulphadimidine**, **sulphamethoxazole**; short-acting, well absorbed in the gastrointestinal tract

*For an interesting history of the introduction of sulphonamides and its relevance to modern regulations for marketing new drugs see Lerner (1991).

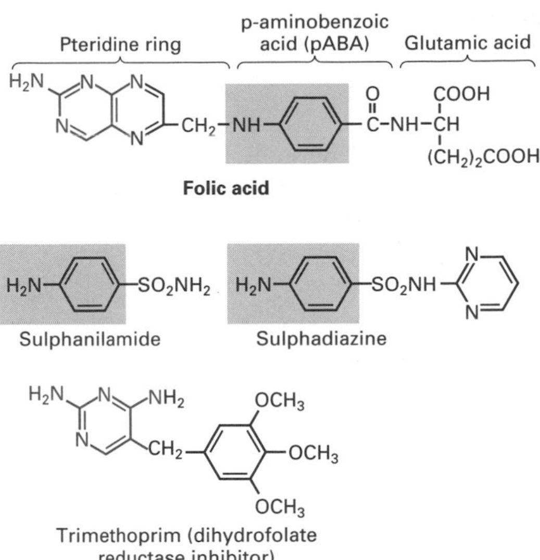

Fig. 37.1 Structures of two representative sulphonamides and trimethoprim. The structures illustrate the relationship between the sulphonamides and the pABA moiety in folic acid (light pink box), and the possible relationship between the antifolate drugs and the pteridine moiety (red). Co-trimoxazole is a mixture of sulphamethoxazole and trimethoprim. (See also Fig. 40.5.)

- **sulfametopyrazine**; long-acting, well absorbed in the gastrointestinal tract
- **sulphasalazine**; poorly absorbed in the gastrointestinal tract
- **sulphamethoxazole**; given with trimethoprim, the combination constitutes **co-trimoxazole** (see below).

Mechanism of action

Sulphanilamide is a structural analogue of p-aminobenzoic acid (see Fig. 37.1) which is essential for the synthesis of folic acid in bacteria. As explained in Chapter 35, folate is required for the synthesis of the precursors of DNA and RNA in both bacteria and mammals, but mammals obtain their folic acid in their diet and do not need to synthesise it, whereas bacteria do. The main mechanism of antibacterial action of the sulphonamides is by competing with p-aminobenzoic acid (pABA) for the enzyme *dihydropteroate synthetase*, and the effect of the sulphonamide may be overcome by adding excess pABA. This is why some local anaesthetics, for example **procaine** (see Ch. 33), which are pABA esters, can antagonise the antibacterial effect of these agents. The action of a sulphonamide is to inhibit growth of the bacteria, not to kill them, i.e. it is *bacteriostatic* rather than *bactericidal*. The bacteriostatic action is negated by the presence of pus and the products of tissue breakdown since these contain thymidine and purines, which bacteria use to bypass the need for folic acid. Resistance, which is common, is plasmid-mediated (see Ch. 35) and due to the synthesis of an enzyme insensitive to the drug.

Pharmacokinetic aspects

Because the action of sulphonamides is bacteriostatic, successful treatment necessitates maintaining an adequate concentration for long enough to allow cellular defence mechanisms (see Ch. 11) to destroy the pathogenic bacteria. Most sulphonamides are readily absorbed in the gastrointestinal tract and reach maximum concentrations in the plasma in 4–6 hours.

Sulphonamides are usually not given topically, mainly because of the risk of sensitisation and allergic reactions. An exception is **silver sulphadiazine** which is used topically in the treatment of infected burns.

Distribution depends partly on plasma protein binding, which varies with different compounds. The drugs pass into inflammatory exudates, and cross the placental barrier; most reach an effective concentration in the CSF.

They are metabolised mainly in the liver, the major product being an acetylated derivative which lacks antibacterial action. They are excreted in the urine.

The clinical use of sulphonamides is given on page 723.

Antimicrobial agents which interfere with the synthesis or action of folate

- **Sulphonamides** are bacteriostatic; they act by interfering with folate synthesis and thus with nucleotide synthesis. Unwanted effects include crystalluria and hypersensitivities.
- **Trimethoprim** is bacteriostatic. It acts by folate antagonism.
- **Co-trimoxazole** is a mixture of trimethoprim with sulphamethoxazole, which affects bacterial nucleotide synthesis at two points.

Unwanted effects

Mild to moderate side effects, which do not necessarily warrant withdrawal of the drug, are nausea and vomiting, headache and mental depression. Cyanosis due to methaemoglobinaemia may occur and is a lot less alarming than it looks. Serious toxic effects that necessitate cessation of therapy include hepatitis, hypersensitivity reactions (rashes, fever, anaphylactoid reactions), bone marrow depression and crystalluria. This last results from the precipitation of acetylated metabolites in the urine. It can be prevented by giving plenty of fluids and keeping the urine alkaline, and is less likely to occur with the more water-soluble preparations.

TRIMETHOPRIM

In structure, trimethoprim (Fig. 37.1) has some resemblance to the pteridine moiety of folate. The similarity is close enough to confuse the relevant bacterial enzyme. Trimethoprim is chemically related to the antimalarial drug, **pyrimethamine** (Fig. 40.4); both are *folate antagonists*. The metabolic importance of folate has been outlined in Chapters 23 and 35, and, as explained in Chapter 35, bacterial dihydrofolate reductase is many times more sensitive to trimethoprim than is the equivalent enzyme in man (Table 35.1).

Trimethoprim is active against most common bacterial pathogens, and it too is bacteriostatic. It is sometimes given as a mixture with sulphamethoxazole in a combination called **co-trimoxazole** (Fig. 37.1). Since sulphonamides affect an earlier stage in the same metabolic pathway in bacteria, i.e. folate synthesis, they can potentiate the action of trimethoprim. This is illustrated in Figure 37.2. When given in combination, trimethoprim and sulphonamides are effective at doses one-tenth or less of what would be needed if each drug were used on its own, so the use of co-trimoxazole should greatly reduce the incidence of unwanted effects. However, the hypersensitivity reactions that can be caused by sulphonamides are not dose-related, and can and do occur with the low dose of sulphamethoxazole in co-trimoxazole. Furthermore, there is evidence that, certainly in urinary infections, there may be no synergy between the two drugs and that trimethoprim alone is effective. On the other hand, the use of the combination appears to have slowed the development of resistance.

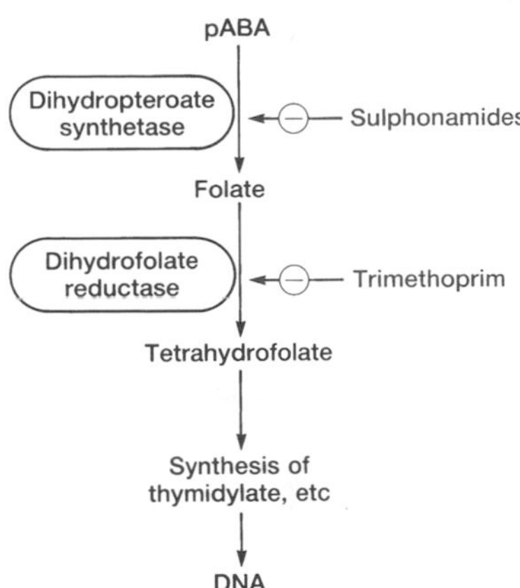

Fig. 37.2 The action of sulphonamides and trimethoprim on bacterial folate synthesis. See Figure 23.5 and Figure 36.8 for more detail of tetrahydrofolate synthesis, and Table 35.1 for comparisons of antifolate drugs.

Pharmacokinetic aspects

Trimethoprim is given orally, is fully absorbed in the gastrointestinal tract and widely distributed throughout the tissues and body fluids. It reaches high concentrations in the lungs and the kidneys and relatively high concentrations in the CSF. When given with sulphamethoxazole, about two-thirds of each is protein-bound and about half of each is excreted within 24 hours. Since trimethoprim is a weak base, its elimination by the kidney increases with decreasing urinary pH.

> **Clinical use of sulphonamides**
>
> - Absolute indications are very few
> - Acute urinary tract infection (now seldom used)
> - Respiratory infections; use now confined to a few special problems (e.g. infection with *Nocardia*)
> - Some sexually transmitted infections (e.g. trachoma, chlamydia, chancroid)
> - Combined with trimethoprim (co-trimoxazole), especially for *Pneumocystis carinii* (p. 771)
> - Combined with pyrimethamine for drug resistant malaria (Table 40.1, p. 764), and for toxoplasmosis
> - Sulphasalazine (sulphapyridine-salicylate combination) is used in inflammatory bowel disease and as an anti-inflammatory drug (p. 257)
> - Silver sulphadiazine is used topically for infected burns

> **Clinical use of trimethoprim/co-trimoxazole**
>
> The main uses are as follows:
> - for urinary tract and respiratory infections; trimethoprim, used on its own, is now usually preferred.
> - for infection with *Pneumocystis carinii*, which causes pneumonia in patients with AIDS, co-trimoxazole is used, in high dose.
>
> See also Table 37.1.

The clinical use of trimethoprim is given above.

Unwanted effects

Unwanted effects of trimethoprim include nausea, vomiting and skin rashes. Folate deficiency, with resultant megaloblastic anaemia (see Ch. 23)—a toxic effect related to the pharmacological action of trimethoprim—can be prevented by giving **folinic acid**. The sulphonamide moiety in co-trimoxazole can cause serious unwanted effects.

BETA-LACTAM ANTIBIOTICS

PENICILLIN

In 1928, Alexander Fleming, working at St Mary's Hospital in London, observed that a culture plate on which staphylococci were being grown had become contaminated with a mould of the genus *Penicillium*, and that bacterial growth in the vicinity of the mould had been inhibited. He isolated the mould in pure culture and demonstrated that it produced an antibacterial substance which he called **penicillin**. This substance was subsequently extracted and its antibacterial effects analysed by Florey & Chain and their colleagues at Oxford in 1940. They showed that it had powerful chemotherapeutic properties in infected mice and that it was non-toxic (see Hare 1970). Its remarkable antibacterial effects in man were clearly demonstrated in 1941. A small amount of penicillin extracted laboriously from crude cultures in the laboratories of the Dunn School of Pathology in Oxford was tested on a policeman who had staphylococcal and streptococcal septicaemia with multiple abscesses,

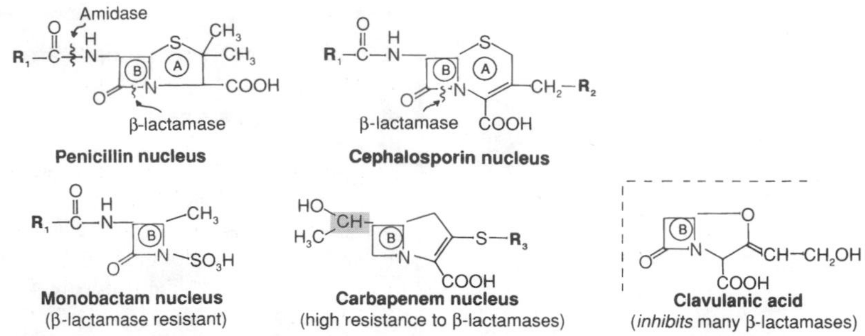

Penicillin nucleus

Cephalosporin nucleus

Monobactam nucleus (β-lactamase resistant)

Carbapenem nucleus (high resistance to β-lactamases)

Clavulanic acid (*inhibits* many β-lactamases)

Fig. 37.3 Basic structures of four groups of β-lactam antibiotics and clavulanic acid. The structures illustrate the β-lactam ring (marked B), and the sites of action of bacterial enzymes that inactivate these antibiotics (A = thiazolidine ring). Various substituents are added at R_1, R_2, R_3, to produce agents with different properties. In carbapenems the stereochemical configuration of the part of the β-lactam ring shown shaded in light pink here is different from the corresponding part of the penicillin and cephalosporin molecules; this is probably the basis of the β-lactamase resistance of the carbapenems. The β-lactam ring of clavulanic acid is thought to bind strongly to β-lactamase, meanwhile protecting other β-lactams from the enzyme. (More details of the structure/activity relationships of β-lactam antibiotics may be found in Donowitz & Mandell 1988.)

and osteomyelitis with discharging sinuses. He was in great pain and was desperately ill. (Sulphonamides were available but would have had no effect in the presence of pus; see p. 722.) Intravenous injections of penicillin were given every 3 hours. All the patient's urine was collected and each day the excreted penicillin was extracted and used again. After 5 days the patient's condition was vastly improved; his temperature was normal, he was eating well and there was obvious resolution of the abscesses. Furthermore, there seemed to be no toxic effects of the drug. Then the supply of penicillin ran out, his condition gradually deteriorated and he died a month later. This was the first evidence of the dramatic antibacterial effect of penicillin given *systemically* in man.* It is not generally known that *topical* penicillin had been used with success in five patients with eye infections 10 years previously by Paine—a graduate of St Mary's—who had obtained some penicillin mould from Fleming (see Howie 1986). The penicillins are extremely effective antibiotics and are very widely used.

Chemistry of penicillin

Penicillin is one of the group of β-lactam antibiotics which also includes cephalosporins, monobactams and carbapenems (Fig. 37.3). The basic nucleus of penicillin is 6-aminopenicillanic acid, which consists of a thiazolidine ring (A) linked to a β-lactam ring (B). This latter ring carries a secondary amino group. The side-chain substituents at R_1 determine the main antibacterial and pharmacological characteristics of each particular penicillin (see Table 37.2).

Penicillins may be destroyed by enzymes—amidases and β-lactamases (penicillinases) (see Fig. 37.3).

Mechanisms of action

All β-lactam antibiotics interfere with the synthesis of the bacterial cell wall peptidoglycan (see Ch. 35, p. 685). After attachment to binding sites on the bacterium (of which there may be up to six types, termed *penicillin-binding proteins*), they inhibit the transpeptidation enzyme that cross-links the peptide chains attached to the backbone of the peptidoglycan (see Fig. 35.3). The final bactericidal event is the inactivation of an inhibitor of the autolytic enzymes in the cell wall; this leads to lysis of the bacterium. Some organisms have defective autolytic enzymes and are inhibited but not lysed—they are referred to as 'tolerant'.

Resistance to penicillin may be due to different causes, the main ones being:

- *The production of β-lactamases* (see p. 693), of which there are about 50 different types. The process is genetically controlled, the gene some-

*See Fletcher 1984 for a brief description of this first clinical use of parenteral penicillin.

Table 37.2 Penicillins*

Name	Absorption in GI tract	Important properties and similar drugs
Benzylpenicillin and congeners		*Active against most Gram-positive cocci and some Gram-negative bacteria. See Table 37.1. Destroyed by β-lactamases; many staphs now resistant*
Benzylpenicillin (penicillin G)	Poor	The treatment of choice for many infections (see Table 37.1). Given i.m. or i.v.; $t_{½}$ after i.m. is 30 min. Life-saving in meningococcal meningitis caused by *Neisseria meningitidis*. Repository i.m. preparations which give more continuous, though lower, plasma concentrations are procaine penicillin (given once daily; drug of choice for syphilis) and benzathine penicillin (given 1- to 4-weekly)
Phenoxymethyl-penicillin (penicillin V)	Good	Less potent than benzylpenicillin, especially in gonorrhoea and meningococcal meningitis
β-lactamase-resistant penicillins		*Spectrum as for benzylpenicillin, but less potent. Many staphs now resistant*
Cloxacillin, Flucloxacillin, Oxacillin[†], Dicloxacillin[†]	Adequate	Used mainly in infections with β-lactamase-producing staphylococci. Given orally (except methicillin) or i.m. Cloxacillin adsorbed on food, $t_{½}$ 30–60 min. Excretion: mostly renal, some in bile
Methicillin	Poor	Nafcillin is the most active of the β-lactamase-resistant penicillins against organisms other than benzylpenicillin-resistant *Staph. aureus*; it reaches reasonable concentration in CSF. Excretion: 80% in bile, 20% in urine
Nafcillin[†]	Variable	
Temocillin		Temocillin is effective against penicillinase-producing Gram-negative bacteria but not pseudomonads
Broad-spectrum penicillins		*Destroyed by β-lactamases produced by* Staph. aureus *and many Gram-negative organisms. Spectrum as for benzylpenicillin (though less potent), plus some Gram-negative bacteria*
Ampicillin	Fairly good	All staphs, many *Esch. coli* strains and some *H. influenzae* strains now resistant, mainly due to production of β-lactamase. Given orally; food decreases absorption, $t_{½}$ 80 min. Excreted in bile and urine. May cause diarrhoea
Pivampicillin, Talampicillin, Bacampicillin	Good	All are pro-drugs releasing ampicillin in liver. Absorption not decreased by food. Less diarrhoea than with ampicillin
Amoxycillin	V. good	Higher blood levels than ampicillin and less GI tract disturbance. Can be given parenterally; $t_{½}$ 80 min. Is available in combination with β-lactamase inhibitor clavulanic acid
Extended-spectrum[‡] penicillins		*Susceptible to β-lactamases. Spectrum as for broad-spectrum drugs, plus pseudomonads. Most strains of* Staph. aureus *are resistant. Tend to inactivate aminoglycosides in vitro*
Carbenicillin	V. poor	Also active against *Proteus*. Given i.v. or i.m., $t_{½}$ 80 min. Renal excretion
Ticarcillin	V. poor	More potent against pseudomonads. Is available in combination with β-lactamase inhibitor, clavulanic acid
Azlocillin	V. poor	Very active against pseudomonads, also some strains of *Klebsiella*. Given i.v., $t_{½}$ 60 min. Excreted in bile and urine; clearance in bile decreased as dose increases
Piperacillin	V. poor	Has increased potency against common Gram-negative organisms

continued

Table 37.2 continued

Name	Absorption in GI tract	Important properties and similar drugs
Reversed-spectrum penicillins		
Pevmecillinam	Poor	More potent against Gram-negative enteric bacteria than against Gram-positive organisms. Hydrolysed by β-lactamase. Pevmecillinam is a pro-drug, given orally, hydrolysed to mecillinam

* The penicillins are bactericidal; they interfere with peptidoglycan synthesis. They are first choice for many infections.
† These may not be generally available in pharmacies in the UK.
‡ Extended to include pseudomonads

times residing in the chromosome but more commonly in a plasmid which can be transferred from one bacterium to another, even across the boundaries of species. β-lactamase production is particularly important in staphylococci, though other organisms (*Neisseria gonorrhoeae*, *Haemophilus* spp., etc.) also produce these enzymes: streptococci do not. Since the introduction of penicillin, staphylococcal resistance due to β-lactamase production has spread progressively, occurring first in staphylococcal strains in hospitals and then in strains in the community at large. In developed countries, at least 80% of staphylococci now produce β-lactamase. One solution to the problem of the susceptibility of penicillin to β-lactamases is the concomitant use of β-lactamase inhibitors. One such is **clavulanic acid** (Fig. 37.3), which was isolated from a strain of *Streptomyces*. Clavulanic acid, a 'suicide' inhibitor of the enzyme, contains a β-lactam ring and is thought to bind covalently to the enzyme at or near its active site. Some enzyme molecules are irreversibly inactivated; in others, the complex is cleaved only very slowly to release the enzyme and this meanwhile protects the penicillin from the enzyme. Other β-lactamase inhibitors are **sulbactam** and **tazobactam**.

- *A reduction in the permeability of the outer membrane* and thus a decreased ability of the drug to penetrate to the target site. This occurs with Gram-negative organisms, which have an outer membrane that limits the penetration of hydrophilic antibiotics (see p. 720).
- *The occurrence of modified penicillin-binding sites.*

See Chapter 35, pages 693–694, for discussion of methicillin-resistant staphylococci.

Types of penicillin and their antimicrobial activity

The first penicillins were the naturally occurring benzylpenicillin and its congeners. Benzylpenicillin is active against a wide range of organisms and is the drug of first choice for many infections (Table 37.1). Its main drawbacks are poor absorption in the gastrointestinal tract (which means it must be given by injection) and its susceptibility to bacterial β-lactamases.

Various semisynthetic penicillins have been prepared by adding different side-chains to the penicillin nucleus (at R_1 in Fig. 37.3). In this way **β-lactamase-resistant penicillins** and **broad spectrum penicillins** have been produced. More recently, **extended-spectrum penicillins** with antipseudomonal activity have been developed and have gone some way to overcoming the problem of serious infections caused by *Pseudomonas aeruginosa* (see p. 720). Details of the various types of penicillin are given in Table 37.2.

Pharmacokinetic aspects

When given orally, different penicillins are absorbed to differing degrees (see Table 37.2) depending on their stability in acid and their adsorption on to food. Parenteral administration can be intramuscular or intravenous. Intrathecal administration is inadvisable, particularly with **benzylpenicillin**, as it can cause convulsions. The drugs are widely distributed in the body fluids, passing into joints, into pleural and pericardial cavities, into the bile, the saliva and the milk and across the placenta. Being lipid insoluble they do not enter mammalian cells. They therefore do not readily cross the blood–brain barrier unless the meninges are inflamed, in which case they may reach therapeutically effective concentrations in the CSF (see Fig. 4.11).

Elimination of most penicillins is mainly renal and occurs rapidly, 90% being by tubular secretion. The relatively short plasma half-life is one of the main problems in the clinical use of **benzylpenicillin**, which can be overcome—either by frequent dosage or by substitution with a slow-release preparation, such as **procaine penicillin** or **benzathine penicillin**. For those penicillins the excretion of which is largely renal, tubular secretion can be partially blocked by **probenecid**, which raises the plasma concentration and prolongs the action (see Chs 42 and 18). The fact that penicillin is excreted in the urine was made use of when the drug was first tested in the first human patient (see above).

Clinical use

The main clinical uses of the penicillins are shown in Tables 37.1 and 37.2. (Note that since different β-lactam antibiotics may bind to different binding proteins it may be feasible to combine two or even more of these agents and achieve synergistic action between them.)

Unwanted effects

One of the remarkable features of the penicillins is their relative freedom from direct toxic effects. However, **carbenicillin** can produce hypokalaemia and, because it contains 4.7 mEq Na^+ per gram, it should perhaps be used with circumspection in cardiac disease. Haemostatic defects have been reported with this drug and with **benzylpenicillin**.

The main unwanted effects of the penicillins are hypersensitivity reactions, the basis of which is the fact that degradation products of penicillin combine with host protein and become antigenic. There are cross-reactions between various types of penicillin. *Skin rashes* of various sorts and fever are the most common manifestations of hypersensitivity; a delayed type of *serum sickness* with fever, urticarial skin eruptions and, in severe cases, generalised oedema, multiple joint effusions and enlargement of spleen and lymph glands occurs infrequently. Much more serious is *acute anaphylactic shock* which may, in some cases, be fatal but is fortunately very rare. Other hypersensitivity reactions seen occasionally are *vasculitis*, *interstitial nephritis* and various *haematologic disturbances*.

The occurrence of these allergic reactions is unpredictable, but in general if an individual does not react to penicillin when it is first given, the chance of a reaction to subsequent administration is low. About 10–15% of individuals who have had a reaction to penicillin will react if given penicillin again.

A side effect of the penicillins, particularly the broad-spectrum type given orally, is alteration of the bacterial flora in the gut. This can be associated with gastrointestinal disturbances and, in some cases, with suprainfection by microorganisms not sensitive to penicillin.

CEPHALOSPORINS AND CEPHAMYCINS

Cultures of a *Cephalosporium* fungus obtained from the sea near a sewer outlet in Sardinia were found to yield extracts which inhibited the growth of *Staphylococcus aureus*. Subsequent work by Abraham & Newton in Oxford resulted in the identification of three distinct antibiotics, cephalosporins N and C, which are chemically related to penicillin, and cephalosporin P, a steroid antibiotic that resembles fusidic acid (see below).

The nucleus of cephalosporin C (see Fig. 37.3) has been isolated and a very large number of semisynthetic **broad-spectrum cephalosporins** have been produced by the addition to this nucleus of different side-chains at R_1 and/or R_2. These agents are water soluble and relatively acid stable. They vary in susceptibility to β-lactamases.

The cephamycins are β-lactam antibiotics produced by *Streptomyces* organisms and they are closely related to the cephalosporins. **Latamoxef** is a synthetic cephamycin compound.

There are now a very large number of cephalosporins and cephamycins available for clinical use. They are usually classified arbitrarily in terms of the chronological order in which they were produced—the first generation compounds begat the second generation compounds which begat the third generation and so on. In Table 37.3 we eschew this biblical approach and classify them in terms of the method of administration, merely mentioning their genealogy in passing.

Table 37.3 Cephalosporins and cephamycins

Categories (with examples)	Important properties and similar drugs
Oral drugs	
Cephalexin ($t_{1/2}$ 1 h)	An example of the *first-generation compounds* which have reasonable activity against Gram-positive organisms and modest activity against Gram-negative organisms *Similar drugs:* Cephradine ($t_{1/2}$ 0.8 h). Cefachlor ($t_{1/2}$ 0.8 h) is a *second-generation compound* and has greater potency against Gram-negative organisms, but can cause unwanted cutaneous lesions. Cephdinir is under investigation
Parenteral drugs	
Cefuroxime ($t_{1/2}$ 1.5 h)	An example of the *second-generation compounds* which show only moderate activity against most Gram-positive organisms but reasonable potency against Gram-negative organisms. Effective against Enterobacteriaceae, also *Haemophilus influenzae* and *Neisseria gonorrhoeae*, but not pseudomonads. Resistance of the compounds to plasmid-mediated and chromosomal β-lactamases has decreased. An oral preparation, cefuroxime axetil, is available *Similar drugs:* Cephamandole ($t_{1/2}$ 0.8 h); cefoxitin ($t_{1/2}$ 0.7 h), good activity against Gram-negative organisms, resistant to β-lactamase from Gram-negative rods, good potency against anaerobes especially *Bacteroides fragilis*
Cefotaxime ($t_{1/2}$ 1 h)	An example of the *third-generation compounds* which are less active against Gram-positive bacteria than those of the second generation, but more active against Gram-negative bacteria. Has some activity against pseudomonads; resistance of the compounds to β-lactamases is decreasing *Similar drugs:* Ceftizoxime ($t_{1/2}$ 1.5 h); latamoxef ($t_{1/2}$ 2.5 h) — but not flomoxef — may interfere with haemostasis; cefotetan ($t_{1/2}$ 3 h), less active against pneumococci, no action against pseudomonads; ceftriaxone ($t_{1/2}$ 8.5 h), excreted largely in bile. Cefoperazone ($t_{1/2}$ 2 h), excreted mainly in bile, can cause decrease in vitamin-K-dependent clotting factors
Parenteral drugs with antipseudomonal activity Cefsoludin ($t_{1/2}$ 1.5 h)	An example of a subgroup of the *third-generation compounds* with activity similar to cefotaxime though less potent, and with additional action against *P. aeruginosa*. Poor activity against *B. fragilis*

Some of the above (e.g. cefuroxime, cefotaxime, ceftazidime, latamoxef) cross the blood–brain barrier and reach therapeutic concentrations in the CNS.

Mechanism of action

The mechanism of action of these agents is the same as that of the penicillins—interference with peptidoglycan synthesis after binding to the β-lactam antibiotic binding proteins. This is described in detail in Chapter 35 and illustrated in Figure 35.3. Resistance to this group of drugs has increased due to plasmid-encoded or chromosomal β-lactamase. (Nearly all Gram-negative bacteria have a chromosomal gene which codes for a β-lactamase that is more active in hydrolysing cephalosporins than penicillins; in several organisms a single-step mutation can result in high level constitutive production of this enzyme.) Resistance also occurs if there is decreased penetration of the drug due to alterations to outer membrane proteins or mutations of the binding-site proteins.

The **antibacterial spectrum** of these agents is summarised briefly in Table 37.3.

Pharmacokinetic aspects

Some cephalosporins may be given orally (see Table 37.1) but most are given parenterally, intramuscularly (which may be painful with some agents) or intravenously. After absorption they are widely distributed in the body, passing into the pleural, pericardial and joint fluids and across the placenta. Some, such as **cefoperazone, cefotaxime, cefuroxime**, **ceftriaxone** and **latamoxef** also cross the blood–brain barrier and are drugs of choice for meningitis due to Gram-negative intestinal bacteria. Excretion is mostly via the kidney, largely by tubular secretion, but 40% of ceftriaxone and 75% of cefoperazone is eliminated in the bile.

Clinical use

The clinical use of the cephalosporins is given in Table 37.1. (Note that since different β-lactam antibiotics may bind to different binding proteins it may be feasible to combine two or even more of these agents and achieve synergistic action between them.)

Unwanted effects

Hypersensitivity reactions, very similar to those that occur with penicillin, may be seen. Some cross-reactions occur; about 10% of penicillin-sensitive individuals will have allergic reactions to cephalosporins. Nephrotoxicity has been reported (especially with cephradine), as has intolerance to alcohol. Diarrhoea can occur with oral cephalosporins and cefoperazone.

OTHER β-LACTAM ANTIBIOTICS

Carbapenems and monobactams

Carbapenems and monobactams (see Fig. 37.3) were developed to deal with β-lactamase-producing Gram-negative organisms which were resistant to broad-spectrum and extended-spectrum penicillins.

The carbapenems are derived from *Streptomyces* species and one example is the semisynthetic **imipenem**, which acts in the same way as the other β-lactams (see Fig. 37.3). It has a very broad spectrum of antimicrobial activity, being active against many aerobic and anaerobic Gram-positive and Gram-negative organisms, including *Listeria*, pseudomonads and most Enterobacteriaceae. However many of the 'methicillin-resistant' staphylococci (see p. 694) are less susceptible, and resistant strains of *P. aeruginosa* have emerged during therapy. Imipenem was originally resistant to all β-lactamases but a few organisms now have chromosomal genes which code for specialised imipenem-hydrolysing β-lactamases (see Jacoby & Archer 1991).

Imipenem is given intravenously. In the kidney it is partly broken down by a dehydropeptidase in the proximal tubule and is therefore given in combination with **cilastatin**, a specific inhibitor of this enzyme.

Unwanted effects are similar to those seen with other β-lactams, nausea and vomiting being the most frequently seen. With high plasma concentrations, neurotoxicity can occur.

Panipenem is under test.

The main monobactam is **aztreonam**, a simple monocyclic β-lactam with a complex substituent at R_3 (see Fig. 37.3), which is resistant to most β-lactamases. This has an unusual spectrum—being active only against Gram-negative aerobic rods, including pseudomonads, *Neisseria meningitidis* and *Haemophilus influenzae*; it has no action against Gram-positive organisms or anaerobes.

It is given parenterally and has a plasma half-life

Beta-lactam antibiotics

Bactericidal by interference with peptidoglycan synthesis.

- **Penicillins:** First choice for many infections. Types of penicillin:
  - —Benzylpenicillin: This is given by injection, has a short $t_{1/2}$ and is destroyed by β-lactamases. Spectrum: Gram-positive and Gram-negative cocci and some Gram-negative bacteria. Many staphylococci are now resistant.
  - —β-lactamase-resistant penicillin: e.g. flucloxacillin. These are given orally. Spectrum: as for benzylpenicillin but less potent. Many staphylococci are now resistant.
  - —Broad-spectrum penicillins: e.g. amoxycillin. These are given orally. They are destroyed by β-lactamases. Spectrum: as for benzylpenicillin (though less potent); they are also active against Gram-negative bacteria.
  - —Extended-spectrum penicillins: e.g. ticarcillin. These are given orally. They are susceptible to β-lactamases. Spectrum: as for broad-spectrum penicillins; they are also active against pseudomonads.

  Unwanted effects: mainly hypersensitivities. A combination of clavulanic acid plus amoxycillin or ticarcillin is effective against many β-lactamase-producing organisms.
- **Cephalosporins and cephamycins:** Second choice for many infections.
  Oral drugs: e.g. cefachlor. These are used in urinary infections.
  Parenteral drugs: cefuroxime is active against *Staph. aureus*, *H. influenzae*, Enterobacteriaceae. Cefsoludin has antipseudomonal activity.
  Unwanted effects: mainly hypersensitivities.
- **Carbapenems:** e.g. imipenem (used with cilastin which blocks its breakdown in the kidney). A broad-spectrum antibiotic, resistant to many, but not all, β-lactamase-producing organisms.
- **Monobactams:** e.g. aztreonam. This is active only against Gram-negative aerobic bacteria and is resistant to most β-lactamases.

of 2 hours. *Unwanted effects* are, in general, similar to those of other β-lactam antibiotics, but it is possible that this agent will not cross-react immunologically with penicillin and its products, and so may not cause allergic reactions in penicillin-sensitive individuals. New injectable monobactams under test are **carumonam** and **tigemonam**.

ANTIMICROBIAL AGENTS AFFECTING BACTERIAL PROTEIN SYNTHESIS

TETRACYCLINES

Tetracyclines are broad-spectrum antibiotics that have a polycyclic structure. The first tetracyclines used, **chlortetracycline** (now superseded), **oxytetracycline**, and **demeclocycline** were derived from cultures of *Streptomyces*. More recently developed compounds, **tetracycline**, **methacycline**, **doxycycline**, **minocycline**, **clomocycline** and **lymecycline** are synthetic or semisynthetic.

Mechanism of action

Tetracyclines act by inhibiting protein synthesis after uptake into susceptible organisms by active transport. This action is described in detail in Chapter 35, p. 686 and Fig. 35.4. The tetracyclines are bacteriostatic, not bactericidal.

Antibacterial spectrum

The spectrum of antimicrobial activity of the tetracyclines is very wide and includes Gram-positive and Gram-negative bacteria, *Mycoplasma*, *Rickettsia*, *Chlamydia*, some spirochaetes and some protozoa (e.g. amoebae). Minocycline is also effective against *Neisseria meningitidis* and has been used to eradicate this organism from the nasopharynx of carriers; it does not penetrate the blood–brain barrier and is not used to treat meningitis.

However, many strains of organisms have become resistant to these agents, decreasing their usefulness. Resistance is transmitted mainly by plasmids and since the genes controlling resistance to tetracyclines are closely associated with genes for resistance to other antibiotics, organisms may become resistant to many drugs simultaneously. The basis of resistance is the development of energy-dependent efflux mechanisms which transport the tetracyclines out of the bacterium (see p. 694), but alteration of the target (the bacterial ribosome) also occurs.

Pharmacokinetic aspects

The tetracyclines are usually given orally but can be given parenterally. The absorption of most preparations from the gut is irregular and incomplete, and is improved in the absence of food. **Minocycline** and **doxycycline** are virtually completely absorbed. Since tetracyclines chelate metal ions (calcium, magnesium, iron, aluminium), forming non-absorbable complexes, absorption is decreased in the presence of milk, certain antacids and iron preparations. The drugs have a wide distribution, entering most fluid compartments, crossing the placenta to the foetus and appearing in the milk. Minocycline is found in high concentrations in tears and saliva. Excretion of most tetracyclines is by two routes—via the bile and via the kidney by glomerular filtration. Most tetracyclines will accumulate if renal function is impaired and this may exacerbate renal failure. Doxycycline is an exception, being excreted largely into the gastrointestinal tract. Minocycline is partly metabolised.

The clinical use of the tetracyclines is given in the box below.

Unwanted effects

The commonest unwanted effects are gastrointestinal disturbances, due initially to direct irritation and later to modification of the gut flora. Vitamin B complex deficiency can occur as can

Clinical use of the tetracyclines

The main uses are as follows:

- They are drugs of first choice for rickettsial, mycoplasma and chlamydial infections, brucellosis, cholera, plague and Lyme disease.
- They are drugs of second choice for infections with several different organisms (see Table 37.1).
- They are useful in mixed infections of the respiratory tract and in acne.

An unusual use of **demeclocycline** is for chronic hyponatraemia due to inappropriate secretion of antidiuretic hormone—the antibiotic is probably effective because it renders the renal tubule cells unresponsive to the hormone.

suprainfection. If the latter is due to *Clostridium difficile* or staphylococci it should be treated with oral **vancomycin**.

Because they chelate calcium, tetracyclines are deposited in growing bones and teeth, causing staining and sometimes dental hypoplasia and bone deformities. They should therefore not be given to children, pregnant women or nursing mothers. Another hazard in pregnant women is hepatotoxicity.

Phototoxicity (sensitisation to sunlight) has been seen, more particularly with **demeclocycline**. **Minocycline** can produce vestibular disturbances (dizziness and nausea), the frequency of these reactions being dose-related. High doses of tetracyclines can decrease protein synthesis in host cells—an anti-anabolic effect—which could result in renal damage and increased blood urea. Long-term therapy may cause disturbances of the bone marrow.

CHLORAMPHENICOL

Chloramphenicol was originally isolated from cultures of *Streptomyces* but is now synthesised commercially for clinical use. Its structure is illustrated in Figure 37.4. (**Thiamphenicol** is a related compound in which the *p*-NO_2 group of chloramphenicol has been replaced with SO_2CH_3.)

The *mechanism of action* is by inhibition of protein synthesis as described in Chapter 35 (p. 686 and Fig. 35.4). Chloramphenicol binds to the 50S subunit of the bacterial ribosome at the same site as do **erythromycin** and **clindamycin**. The drugs may compete and thus interfere with each other's actions if given concurrently.

Antibacterial spectrum

Both chloramphenicol and thiamphenicol have a wide spectrum of antimicrobial activity, including Gram-negative and Gram-positive organisms and rickettsiae. They are bacteriostatic for most organisms but bactericidal to *H. influenzae*. As with other bacteriostatic antibiotics, they will interfere with the action of bactericidal antimicrobials if used concurrently.

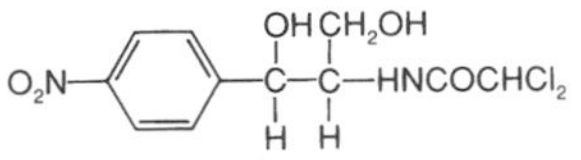

$$O_2N-C_6H_4-\underset{H}{\overset{OH}{C}}-\underset{H}{\overset{CH_2OH}{C}}-HNCOCHCl_2$$

Fig. 37.4 Chloramphenicol.

Resistance is due to the production of chloramphenicol acetyl-transferase (see p. 693) and is plasmid mediated. R plasmids containing determinants for multiple drug resistance for chloramphenicol, streptomycin, tetracyclines, etc. may be transferred from one bacterial species to another by 'promiscuous plasmids' (plasmids that can cross species barriers). The R genes coding for chloramphenicol acetyl-transferase may occur on transposons (see p. 691). Derivatives of chloramphenicol and thiamphenicol with the terminal OH on the side-chain replaced by fluorine are likely not to be susceptible to acetylation and thus to retain antibacterial activity.

Pharmacokinetic aspects

Given orally, chloramphenicol is rapidly and completely absorbed and reaches its maximum concentration in the plasma within 2 hours; it can also be given parenterally. It is widely distributed throughout the tissues and body fluids including the CSF, in which its concentration may be 60% of that in the blood. In the plasma it is 30–50% protein-bound and its half-life is approximately 2 hours. About 10% is excreted unchanged in the urine, and the remainder is inactivated in the liver.

The clinical use of chloramphenicol is given in the following box.

Clinical use of chloramphenicol

Clinical use of chloramphenicol should be reserved for serious infections in which the benefit of the drug is greater than the risk of toxicity (see below), such as:

- infections caused by *H. influenzae* resistant to other drugs
- meningitis in patients in whom penicillin cannot be used

It is also safe and effective in:

- bacterial conjunctivitis (given topically).

It is effective in typhoid fever but **ciprofloxacin** or **amoxycillin** and **co-trimoxazole** are similarly effective and less toxic. Other possible uses are given in Table 37.1.

Unwanted effects

The most important unwanted effect of chloramphenicol is depression of the bone marrow resulting in pancytopenia (a decrease in all blood cell elements)—an effect which, though rare, can occur even with very low doses in some individuals. In a small proportion of patients, fatal aplastic anaemia may occur, the incidence being approximately 1 in 50 000. This unwanted effect is believed to be related to the *p*-NO_2 group of chloramphenicol, which has been replaced with SO_2CH_3 in **thiamphenicol**. A dose-related disturbance in red cell maturation sometimes associated with some degree of leucopenia and/or thrombocytopenia occurs in many individuals taking chloramphenicol for 2 weeks or more; it disappears when treatment is stopped.

Chloramphenicol should be used with great care in newborns because inadequate inactivation and excretion of the drug (see Ch. 42) can result in the 'grey baby syndrome'—vomiting, diarrhoea, flaccidity, low temperature and an ashen-grey colour—which carries a 40% mortality; if its use is essential, plasma concentrations should be determined and the dose reduced. Hypersensitivity reactions can occur, as can gastrointestinal disturbances and other sequelae of alteration of the intestinal microbial flora.

AMINOGLYCOSIDES

The aminoglycosides are a group of antibiotics of complex chemical structure, resembling each other in antimicrobial activity, pharmacokinetic characteristics and toxicity. The main agents are **gentamicin**, **streptomycin**, **amikacin**, **kanamycin**, **tobramycin**, **netilmicin**, **neomycin** and **framycetin**. The structure of streptomycin is given in Figure 37.5 as an example of the group.

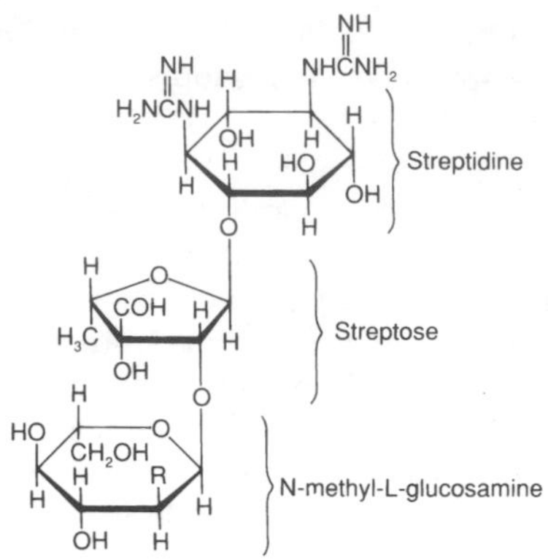

Fig. 37.5 Structure of streptomycin (R = CH_3NH–).

Mechanism of action

Aminoglycosides inhibit bacterial protein synthesis. All bind to sites on the 30S subunit of the bacterial ribosome, causing an alteration in codon : anticodon recognition (Fig. 35.4). This results in misreading of the messenger RNA and hence in the production of defective bacterial proteins. This action does not entirely explain their rapid lethality, so there may be a second target. Their penetration through the cell membrane of the bacterium depends partly on oxygen-dependent active transport by a polyamine carrier system and they have minimal action against anaerobic organisms. Chloramphenicol blocks this transport system. Their effect is bactericidal and is enhanced by agents that interfere with cell wall synthesis.

Resistance

Resistance to aminoglycosides is becoming a problem. It may occur by several different mechanisms (see pp. 693–694), the most important being inactivation by microbial enzymes, the genes for which are carried on plasmids. **Amikacin**, developed from its parent compound, **kanamycin**, was designed as a poor substrate for these enzymes; but there are recent reports of amikacin resistance due to modified, and now effective, inactivating enzymes. Other mechanisms of resistance include failure of penetration (this can be largely overcome by the concomitant use of **penicillin** and/or **vancomycin**, which synergise with the aminoglycosides) and lack of binding of the drugs to the ribosome due to a mutation that alters the binding-site on the 30S subunit. This last affects mainly streptomycin and is a rare reason for resistance.

Antibacterial spectrum

The aminoglycosides are effective against many aerobic Gram-negative and some Gram-positive organisms (see Table 37.1). Streptomycin is also active against *Mycobacterium tuberculosis* (see below).

Aminoglycosides are most widely used against Gram-negative enteric organisms and in sepsis. They may be given together with a **penicillin** in infections caused by *Streptococcus*, *Listeria* or *Pseudomonas aeruginosa* (see Table 37.1). **Gentamicin** is the aminoglycoside most commonly used, though **tobramycin** is the preferred member of this group for *P. aeruginosa* infections. **Amikacin** has the widest antimicrobial spectrum and along with **netilmicin** can be effective in infections with organisms resistant to gentamicin and tobramycin. **Neomycin** and **framycetin** are too toxic for parenteral use and are only used topically.

Pharmacokinetic aspects

The aminoglycosides are polycations and highly polar. They are not absorbed in the gastrointestinal tract. They are usually given intramuscularly or intravenously. Binding to plasma proteins is minimal. They do not enter cells, nor do they cross the blood–brain barrier into the CNS, penetrate the vitreous humor of the eye or reach high concentrations in secretions and body fluids, though high concentrations can be attained in joint and pleural fluids. They may, however, cross the placenta. The plasma half-life is 2–3 hours. Elimination is virtually entirely by glomerular filtration in the kidney, 50–60% of a dose being excreted unchanged within 24 hours. Tissue concentrations increase during treatment and can reach toxic levels after about a week of continuous unmodified dosage (Fig. 37.6). If renal function is impaired, accumulation occurs even more quickly with a resultant increase in those toxic effects (such as ototoxicity and nephrotoxicity) which are dose-related.

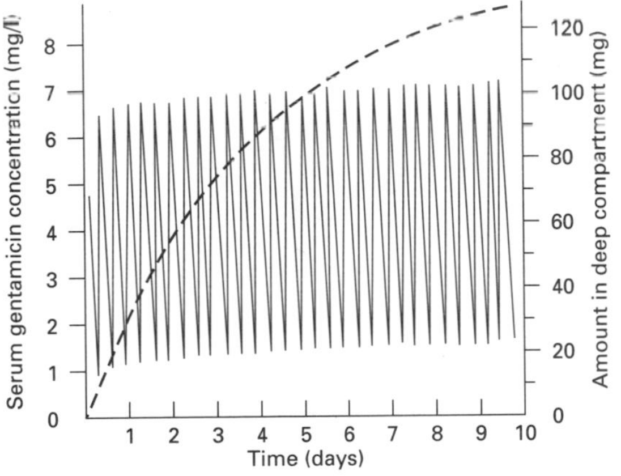

Fig. 37.6 Graph of serum and tissue concentrations of aminoglycoside antibiotics during repeated administration. The concentration in the tissues (dotted line) increases while the serum concentration (solid line) does not rise progressively. (Adapted from: Aronson & Reynolds 1992)

Clinical use

Clinical uses of the aminoglycosides are given in Table 37.1. **Streptomycin** is almost entirely reserved for the treatment of tuberculosis.

Unwanted effects

Serious, dose-related toxic effects, with the potential for increasing with length of treatment, can occur with the aminoglycosides, the main hazards being ototoxicity and nephrotoxicity.

Ototoxicity involves progressive damage to and destruction of the sensory cells in the cochlea and vestibular organ of the ear. The result, usually irreversible, may be vertigo, ataxia and loss of balance in the case of vestibular damage, and auditory disturbances, including deafness, in the case of cochlear damage. Any aminoglycoside may produce both types of effect, but **streptomycin** and **gentamicin** are more likely to interfere with vestibular function whereas with **kanamycin**, **neomycin** and **amikacin** the side effects are mostly on hearing. **Netilmycin** is less ototoxic than other aminoglycosides and is preferred when prolonged use is necessary. Ototoxicity is potentiated by the concomitant use of other ototoxic drugs (e.g. loop diuretics, p. 379).

The *nephrotoxicity* consists of damage to the kidney tubules and can be reversed if the use of the drugs is stopped. Nephrotoxicity is more likely to occur in patients with pre-existing renal disease or in conditions in which urine volume is reduced; concomitant use of other nephrotoxic agents (e.g. **cephalosporins**) increases the risk. Note that as the elimination of these drugs is almost entirely renal, their nephrotoxic action can impair their own excretion and a vicious cycle can be set up. Plasma concentrations must be monitored regularly.

A rare but serious toxic reaction is paralysis due to neuromuscular blockade, usually only seen if the agents are given concurrently with neuromuscular-blocking agents. It is due to inhibition of the calcium uptake necessary for the exocytotic release of acetylcholine (see Ch. 6).

Optic nerve dysfunction has been reported after **streptomycin**.

Spectinomycin

Spectinomycin is related to the aminoglycosides

in structure. Its use is confined to the treatment of gonorrhoea in patients allergic to penicillin or those whose infections are caused by penicillin-resistant gonococci.

MACROLIDES

For 40 years, **erythromycin** has been the only macrolide antibiotic in general clinical use. (The term 'macrolide' relates to the structure—a many-membered lactone ring to which one or more deoxy sugars are attached.) Recently a host of new macrolide antibiotics have become available, the two most important of which are **clarithromycin** and **azithromycin**. (The latter is an azalide—closely related to the macrolides and so included here.)

Mechanism of action

The mechanism of action of the macrolides is inhibition of bacterial protein synthesis by an effect on translocation (Fig. 35.4). Their action may be bactericidal or bacteriostatic, the effect depending on the concentration and on the type of micro-organism. The drugs are bound to the 50S subunit of the bacterial ribosome. The binding site is the same as that of **chloramphenicol** and **clindamycin** and the three types of agent could compete, if given concurrently.

Antimicrobial spectrum

The antimicrobial spectrum of **erythromycin** is very similar to that of penicillin and it has proved to be a safe and effective alternative for penicillin-sensitive patients. Erythromycin is effective against Gram-positive bacteria and spirochaetes but not against most Gram-negative organisms, exceptions being *N. gonorrhoeae* and, to a lesser extent, *H. influenzae*. *Mycoplasma pneumoniae*, *Legionella* and some chlamydial organisms are also susceptible. See Table 37.1. *Resistance* can occur and is due to a plasmid-controlled alteration of the binding site for erythromycin on the bacterial ribosome (p. 693).

Azithromycin is less active against Gram-positive bacteria than erythromycin, is considerably more effective against *H. influenzae* and may be more active against *Legionella*. It has shown excellent action against *Toxoplasma gondii* (p. 774), appearing to kill the cysts. It is reported that chlamydial urethritis can be treated with a single dose.

Clarithromycin is as active, and its metabolite is twice as active, against *H. influenzae* as erythromycin; it is also effective against *Mycobacterium avium cellulare* (which can infect immunologically compromised individuals and elderly patients with chronic lung disease) and may be useful in leprosy. Both these macrolides are effective in Lyme disease.

Pharmacokinetic aspects

The macrolides are administered orally, **azithromycin** and **clarithromycin** being more acid-stable than **erythromycin**. Erythromycin can also be given parenterally, though intravenous injections can be followed by local thrombophlebitis. They all diffuse readily into most tissues, including prostatic fluid and the placenta, but do not cross the blood–brain barrier and there is poor penetration into the synovial fluid. The plasma half-life of erythromycin is about 90 minutes; that of clarythromycin is 3 times longer and that of azithromycin 8 to 16 times longer. This latter agent persists at high concentrations in the tissues (which could be significant in some infections) but its peak plasma concentration can be quite low (which needs to be taken into account in infections such as pneumococcal pneumonia which can be complicated by septicaemia). Macrolides are able to enter and concentrate within phagocytes—azithromycin concentrations in phagocyte lysosomes can be 40 times higher than in the blood—and there is evidence that they can enhance phagocyte killing of bacteria.

Erythromycin is partly inactivated in the liver; azithromycin is more resistant to inactivation and clarithromycin is converted to an active metabolite. (Effects on the P-450 cytochrome system can affect the bioavailability of other drugs; see Ch. 42.) The major route of elimination is in the bile.

Clinical use

The clinical use of the macrolides is given in Table 37.1.

Unwanted effects

Gastrointestinal disturbances are common and unpleasant but not serious; on present evidence these occur less often with the two newer agents. With erythromycin, the following have also been reported: hypersensitivity reactions such as skin rashes and fever, transient hearing disturbances, and, rarely, with treatment longer than a fortnight, cholestatic jaundice.

Opportunistic infections of the gastrointestinal tract or vagina can occur.

LINCOSAMIDES

Clindamycin is a lincosamide antibiotic active against Gram-positive cocci, including penicillin-resistant staphylococci, and many anaerobic bacteria such as *Bacteroides* species.

Its *mechanism of action* involves inhibition of protein synthesis similar to that of the macrolides and chloramphenicol (Fig. 35.4).

Clindamycin can be given orally or parenterally and is widely distributed in tissues (including bone) and body fluids but does not cross the blood–brain barrier. There is active uptake into leucocytes. Its $t_{½}$ is 21 hours. Some is metabolised in the liver, and the metabolites, which are active, are excreted in the bile and the urine. *Unwanted effects* consist mainly of gastrointestinal disturbances. A potentially lethal condition, *pseudomembranous colitis*, can occur; this is an acute inflammation of the colon due to a necrotising toxin produced by a clindamycin-resistant organism, *Clostridium difficile*, which may be part of the normal faecal flora.* Vancomycin, given orally, and metronidazole (see below) are effective in the treatment of this condition.

Its *clinical use* is in infections caused by *Bacteroides* organisms and for staphylococcal infections of bones and joints. It is also used topically, as eye drops, for staphylococcal conjunctivitis.

Antimicrobial agents affecting bacterial protein synthesis

- **Tetracyclines:** e.g. **minocycline**. These are orally active, bacteriostatic, broad-spectrum antibiotics. Resistance is increasing. GIT disorders are common. They chelate calcium and are deposited in growing bone. They are contraindicated in children and pregnant women.
- **Chloramphenicol:** This is an orally active, bacteriostatic, broad-spectrum antibiotic. Serious toxic effects are possible, including bone marrow depression, grey baby syndrome. It should be reserved for life-threatening infections.
- **Aminoglycosides:** e.g. **gentamicin**. These are given by injection. They are bactericidal, broad-spectrum antibiotics (but with low activity against anaerobes, streptococci and pneumococci). Resistance is increasing. The main unwanted effects are dose-related nephrotoxicity and ototoxicity. Serum levels should be monitored. (**Streptomycin** is an antituberculosis aminoglycoside.)
- **Macrolides:** e.g. **erythromycin**. Can be given orally and parenterally. They are bactericidal/ bacteriostatic. The antibacterial spectrum is the same as for penicillin. Erythromycin can cause jaundice. Newer agents are **clarithromycin** and **azithromycin**.
- **Clindamycin:** Can be given orally and parenterally. It can cause pseudomembranous colitis.
- **Fusidic acid:** This is a narrow-spectrum antibiotic which acts by inhibiting protein synthesis. It penetrates bone. Unwanted effects include GIT disorders.

FUSIDIC ACID

Fusidic acid is a narrow-spectrum steroid antibiotic active mainly against Gram-positive bacteria. It acts by inhibiting protein synthesis (Fig. 35.4).

Sodium fusidate is well absorbed from the gut and is distributed widely in the tissues. Some is excreted in the bile and some metabolised.

Unwanted effects such as gastrointestinal disturbances are fairly common. Skin eruptions and jaundice can occur. It is used in combination with other drugs (e.g. **flucloxacillin**) mainly for serious staphylococcal infections caused by penicillin-resistant organisms, especially osteomyelitis, since sodium fusidate is concentrated in bone.

*This can also occur with some penicillins and cephalosporins.

ANTIMICROBIAL AGENTS AFFECTING TOPOISOMERASE II

FLUOROQUINOLONES

The fluoroquinolones are synthetic antibiotics recently introduced into clinical practice. They include the broad-spectrum agents **ciprofloxacin**, **ofloxacin**, **norfloxacin**, **acrosoxacin** and **pefloxacin**, and the narrower-spectrum drugs used in urinary tract infections—**cinoxacin**, and **nalidixic acid**. (The last named was the first quinolone and

A

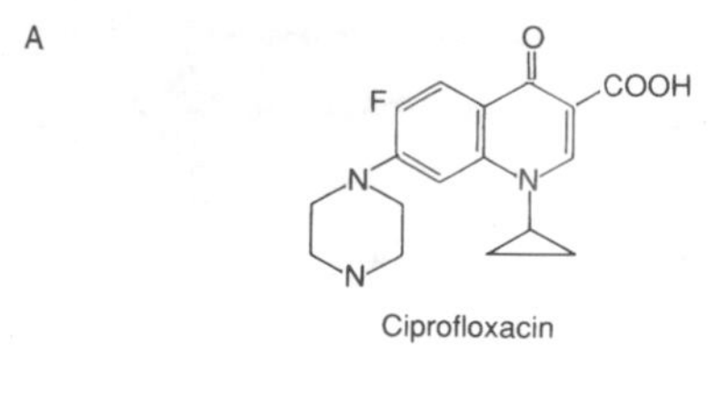

B

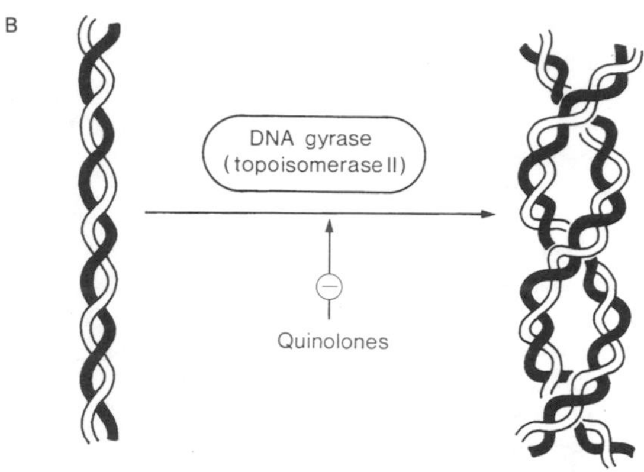

Fig. 37.7 A simplified diagram of the mechanism of action of the fluoroquinolones. A. An example of a quinolone (the quinolone moiety is shown in red).
B. Schematic diagram of (left) the double helix; and (right) the double helix in supercoiled form. (See also Fig. 35.6.) In essence, the DNA gyrase unwinds the RNA-induced positive supercoil (not shown) and introduces a negative supercoil.

is not fluorinated.) As explained on page 688 these agents inhibit topoisomerase II (a DNA gyrase), the enzyme that produces a negative supercoil in DNA, permitting transcription or replication (Fig. 37.7).

Antibacterial spectrum and clinical use

Ciprofloxacin is the most commonly used fluoroquinolone at present* and will be described as the type agent. It is a broad-spectrum antibiotic, effective against both Gram-positive and Gram-negative organisms, being especially active against the latter. It has excellent activity against the Enterobacteriaceae (the enteric Gram-negative bacilli), including many organisms resistant to penicillins, cephalosporins and aminoglycosides, and is also effective against *H. influenzae*, penicillinase-producing *N. gonorrhoeae*, *Campylobacter* and pseudomonads.

*It is estimated that in 1989 this drug was prescribed for 1 in 44 Americans.

Of the Gram-positive organisms, streptococci and pneumococci are only weakly inhibited and there is a high incidence of staphylococcal resistance. Ciprofloxacin should be avoided in methicillin-resistant staphylococcal infections. Intracellular pathogens, such as *Mycobacterium tuberculosis*, *Mycoplasma*, *Chlamydia*, *Legionella* and *Brucella* species are inhibited to a variable extent and there is only low activity against anaerobic bacteria.

Clinically the fluoroquinolones are best used for infections with facultative and aerobic Gram-negative rods and cocci. (Some clinical pharmacologists have suggested, sensibly, that to prevent emergence of resistance, ciprofloxacin should be reserved for organisms resistant to other drugs; but it looks as if the horse has not only left the stable but has bolted; see footnote. Resistant strains of *Staph. aureus* and *P. aeruginosa* have already emerged.)

Pharmacokinetic aspects

Given orally, the fluoroquinolones are well absorbed. The half-life of ciprofloxacin and norfloxacin is 3.3 hours, that of ofloxacin is 5 hours and that of perfloxacin is 10.5 hours. The drugs concentrate in many tissues, particularly in the kidney, prostate and lung. All quinolones are concentrated in phagocytes. Most do not cross the blood–brain barrier except for pefloxacin and ofloxacin which reach, in the CSF, respectively 40% and 90% of their serum concentrations. **Aluminium** and **magnesium antacids** interfere with the absorption of the quinolones. Elimination of ciprofloxacin, norfloxacin and enofloxacin is due partly to hepatic metabolism and partly to renal excretion. Perfloxacin is metabolised to norfloxacin. Ofloxacin is excreted in the urine.

The clinical use of the fluoroquinolones is given on page 737.

Unwanted effects

Unwanted effects are infrequent, usually mild and disappear if the agents are withdrawn. They consist mainly of gastrointestinal disorders and skin rashes. (Most antacids cannot be used to treat the gastric symptoms; see above.) Arthropathy has been reported, particularly in young individuals. CNS symptoms—headache, dizziness—have occurred and, less frequently, convulsions, which have been

Antimicrobial agents affecting DNA topoisomerase II

- These drugs—the fluoroquinolones, e.g. ciprofloxacin—interfere with the supercoiling of DNA.
- Ciprofloxacin has a wide antibacterial spectrum, being especially active against Gram-negative enteric coliform organisms including many organisms resistant to penicillins, cephalosporins and aminoglycosides; it is also effective against *H. influenzae*, penicillinase-producing *N. gonorrhoeae*, *Campylobacter* and pseudomonads. There is a high incidence of staphylococcal resistance. It is active orally with a $t_{1/2}$ of 4.5 hours.
- Unwanted effects include GI tract upsets and hypersensitivity reactions and, rarely, CNS disturbances.
- Newer agents include ofloxacin, norfloxacin.

associated with CNS pathology or concurrent use of theophylline or a non-steroidal anti-inflammatory drug. (Note that fluoroquinolones have been shown to inhibit the binding of GABA to its receptor.) Photosensitivity and hypersensitivity reactions (sometimes involving the blood cells) have been seen, as have renal disorders.

There is a clinically important interaction between **ciprofloxacin** and **theophylline** which can lead to theophylline toxicity in asthmatics treated with the fluoroquinolones (theophylline toxicity is discussed in Ch. 17).

Clinical use of the fluoroquinolones

The main uses are as follows:
- for complicated urinary tract infections (norfloxacin, ofloxacin)
- for *P. aeruginosa* respiratory infections in patients with cystic fibrosis
- for invasive external otitis caused by *P. aeruginosa*
- for chronic Gram-negative bacillary osteomyelitis
- for eradication of *S. typhi* in carriers
- for gonorrhoea (norfloxacin, ofloxacin)
- for bacterial prostatitis (norfloxacin)
- for cervicitis (ofloxacin).

In patients in whom penicillin cannot be used, a single dose of **acrosoxacin** can cure gonorrhoea.

MISCELLANEOUS ANTIBACTERIAL AGENTS

GLYCOPEPTIDE ANTIBIOTICS

The main glycopeptide antibiotic is **vancomycin**; others are **teicoplanin**, ramoplanin, decaplanin.

Vancomycin is bactericidal (except against streptococci) and acts by inhibiting cell wall synthesis (see Fig. 35.3). It is effective mainly against Gram-positive bacteria, including methicillin-resistant staphylococci, and has been used for resistant enterococci. Resistance in these latter microorganisms, rare during the 35 years that this agent has been used, is now emerging rapidly world-wide. It synergises with some **aminoglycoside** antibiotics against some organisms which vancomycin, on its own, does not kill.

It is not absorbed from the gut and is only given by the oral route for treatment of gastrointestinal infections. For parenteral use it is given intravenously (and if infused too fast causes a histamine-induced reddening of the skin). It is widely distributed. Elimination is virtually entirely by glomerular filtration into the urine and thus it could cumulate if renal function is impaired. Its plasma half-life is about 8 hours.

The *clinical use* of vancomycin is limited mainly to pseudomembranous colitis (see under 'Clindamycin', p. 735) and the treatment of some multi-resistant staphylococcal infections. It is also valuable in severe staphylococcal infections in patients allergic both to **penicillins** and **cephalosporins**, and in some forms of endocarditis.

Unwanted effects include fever, rashes and local phlebitis at the site of injection. Ototoxicity and nephrotoxicity can occur and hypersensitivity reactions are seen occasionally.

Teicoplanin, given intramuscularly or intravenously, is similar but is longer-acting.

POLYMIXIN ANTIBIOTICS

The polymixin antibiotics in use are **polymixin B** and **colistin** (polymixin E). They have cationic detergent properties and their *mechanism of action* involves interaction with the phospholipids of the cell membrane and disruption of its structure

(Ch. 35, p. 690). They have a selective, rapidly bactericidal action on Gram-negative bacilli, especially pseudomonads and coliform organisms. They are not absorbed from the gastrointestinal tract.

Unwanted effects may be serious and include neurotoxicity and nephrotoxicity. Their use is limited by their toxicity and is confined largely to gut sterilisation and topical treatment of ear, eye or skin infections caused by susceptible organisms.

BACITRACIN

Bacitracin is a polypeptide antibiotic with a range of activity similar to that of penicillin, being most active against Gram-positive organisms including staphylococci producing β-lactamase. Its mechanism of action involves inhibition of cell-wall formation (see Fig. 35.3).

Bacitracin has serious toxic effects on the kidney and is therefore only used topically for infections of mouth, nose, eye and skin.

METRONIDAZOLE

Metronidazole was introduced as an antiprotozoal agent (and is dealt with in more detail on p. 772) but it is also active against anaerobic bacteria such as *Bacteroides*, clostridia and some streptococci. It is effective in the therapy of *pseudomembranous colitis*, a clostridial infection sometimes associated with antibiotic therapy (see p. 735).

NITROFURANTOIN

Nitrofurantoin is a synthetic compound active against a range of Gram-positive and Gram-negative organisms. The development of resistance in susceptible organisms is rare and there is no cross-resistance. Its mechanism of action is not known.

It is given orally and is rapidly and totally absorbed from the gastrointestinal tract and very rapidly excreted by the kidney by both glomerular filtration and tubular secretion; thus it reaches antibacterial concentrations in the urine but not in the plasma. In renal failure, toxic blood levels ensue.

The *clinical use* of nitrofurantoin is confined to the treatment of urinary tract infections, and the drug is more active in acid urine.

Miscellaneous antibacterial agents

- **Glycopeptide antibiotics:** e.g. vancomycin. Vancomycin is bactericidal, acting by inhibiting cell wall synthesis. It is used intravenously for multiresistant staphylococcal infections and orally for pseudomembranous colitis. Unwanted effects include ototoxicity and nephrotoxicity.
- **Polymixins:** e.g. colistin. They are bactericidal, acting by disrupting bacterial cell membranes. They are seriously neurotoxic and nephrotoxic and are only used topically.
- **Bacitracin** inhibits bacterial cell wall formation. It is used topically for superficial infections.
- **Nitrofurantoin** is orally active and is used for urinary tract infections.

Unwanted effects such as gastrointestinal disturbances are relatively common and hypersensitivity reactions involving the skin and the bone marrow (e.g. leucopenia) can occur. Hepatotoxicity and peripheral neuropathy have been reported. (Note that nitrofurantoin interferes with the therapeutic action of some quinolones.)

ANTIMYCOBACTERIAL AGENTS

The main mycobacterial infections in man are *tuberculosis* and *leprosy*—both typically chronic infections, caused, respectively, by *Mycobacterium tuberculosis* and *Mycobacterium leprae*. A particular problem with both these conditions is that after phagocytosis, the microorganism can survive inside macrophages, unless these are 'activated' by T cell lymphokines (see Ch. 11, p. 223).

DRUGS USED TO TREAT TUBERCULOSIS

Tuberculosis was once a major killer disease. Then new drugs were developed and put to use and for the last 25 years or so it has been regarded as an easily curable condition. This is so no longer—the mycobacterium which causes it has come back to haunt us. A recent article in *Nature* gives the picture—it was entitled 'Tuberculosis. Back to a frightening future' (Bloom 1993). In May 1993, the World Health Organization took what it called the extraordinary step of declaring tuberculosis to be a 'global emergency'. To quote from the *British Medical Journal*—'The disease is out of control in many parts of the world, infecting more than a third of the world's population. More than 30 million people are expected to die of tuberculosis in the next decade, and the WHO predicts that there will be 90 million more cases worldwide by the year 2000. . . . It is now the world's leading cause of death from a single agent' (Godlee 1993). In the developed world, several interacting factors would have contributed to this situation, particularly the emergence of multidrug-resistant strains which have spread rapidly in prisons, shelters for the homeless, and among persons infected with HIV. Inadequate drug treatment in these cases and, in the Third World, no treatment at all, have compounded the problem.

Against this background we will now consider the antituberculosis drugs. The first-line drugs are, **isoniazid**, **rifampicin**, **ethambutol** and **pyrazinamide**. Some second-line drugs available are **capreomycin**, **cycloserine** and **streptomycin** (see p. 732); these are used for infections with tubercle bacilli likely to be resistant to first-line drugs or when the first-line agents have to be abandoned due to unwanted reactions.

To decrease the possibility of the emergence of resistant organisms, *compound drug therapy* is employed, involving the following:

- a first phase of about 2 months consisting of three drugs used concomitantly: isoniazid, rifampicin, pyrazinamide (plus ethambutol if the organism is suspected to be resistant)
- a second, continuation phase, of 4 months, consisting of two drugs: isoniazid and rifampicin; longer treatment is needed in some situations, for example meningitis, bone/joint involvement, drug-resistant cases.

ISONIAZID

The antibacterial activity of isoniazid is limited to mycobacteria. It is bacteriostatic on resting organisms but can kill dividing bacteria. It passes freely into mammalian cells and is thus effective against intracellular organisms and it is actively taken up by tubercle bacilli. The mechanism of its action is not clearly known. There is evidence that it inhibits the synthesis of mycolic acids, important constituents of the cell wall and peculiar to mycobacteria. It is also reported to combine with an enzyme that is uniquely found in isoniazid-sensitive strains of mycobacteria; this results in disorganisation of the metabolism of the cell. Resistance can occur and is due to reduced penetration of the drug. Cross-resistance with other tuberculostatic drugs does not occur.

Pharmacokinetic aspects

Isoniazid is readily absorbed from the gastrointestinal tract or after parenteral injection and is widely distributed throughout the tissues and body fluids, including the cerebrospinal fluid, where it reaches about 20% of the plasma concentration. An important point is that it penetrates well into 'caseous' tuberculous lesions (i.e. necrotic lesions, with a cheese-like consistency). Metabolism, which involves largely acetylation, depends on genetic factors that determine whether a person is a 'slow' or 'rapid' acetylator of the drug (see Ch. 42, p. 788), slow inactivators having a better therapeutic response.

The half-life in slow inactivators is 3 hours and in rapid inactivators, 1½ hours. Isoniazid is excreted in the urine partly as unchanged drug and partly in the acetylated or otherwise inactivated form.

Unwanted effects

Unwanted effects depend on the dosage and occur in about 5% of individuals, the commonest being allergic skin eruptions. A variety of other adverse reactions have been reported, including fever, hepatotoxicity, haematological changes, arthritic symptoms and vasculitis. Toxic effects involving the central or peripheral nervous systems are largely due to a deficiency of pyridoxine (see Fig. 37.8

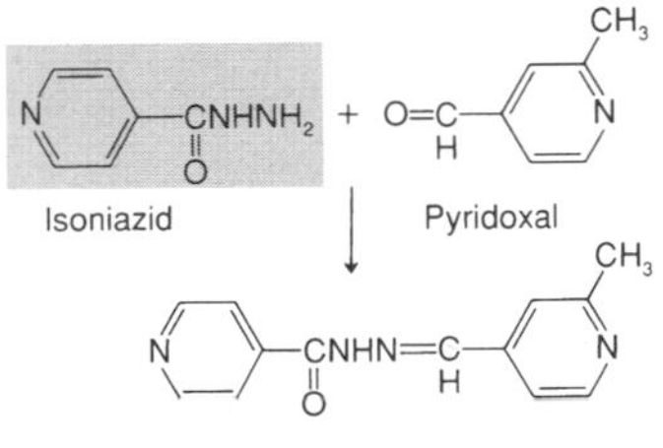

Isoniazid + Pyridoxal → Pyridoxal-hydrazone

Fig. 37.8 Isoniazid, a tuberculostatic drug. In some circumstances it can cause pyridoxine deficiency by spontaneously forming a hydrazone with pyridoxal (as shown), the complex being rapidly excreted in the urine.

for explanation) and are common in malnourished patients unless prevented by administration of this substance. Pyridoxal-hydrazone formation occurs mainly in slow acetylators. Isoniazid may cause haemolytic anaemia in individuals with glucose-6-phosphate deficiency and it decreases the metabolism of the antiepileptic agents, **phenytoin**, **ethosuximide** and **carbamazepine**, resulting in an increase in the plasma concentration and toxicity of these drugs.

RIFAMPICIN (RIFAMPIN)

Rifampicin acts by binding to, and inhibiting, DNA-dependent RNA polymerase in prokaryotic but not in eukaryotic cells (p. 689). It is one of the most active antituberculosis agents known. It is also active against most other Gram-positive bacteria as well as many Gram-negative species. It enters phagocytic cells and can kill intracellular micro-organisms including the tubercle bacillus. Resistance can develop rapidly in a one-step process and is thought to be due to chemical modification of microbial DNA-dependent RNA polymerase, resulting from a chromosomal mutation (see p. 691).

Pharmacokinetic aspects

Rifampicin is given orally and is widely distributed in the tissues and body fluids, giving an orange tinge to saliva, sputum, tears and sweat. In the CSF it reaches 10–40% of its serum concentration. It is excreted partly in the urine and partly in the bile, some of it undergoing enterohepatic cycling. There is progressive metabolism of the drug by deacetylation during its repeated passages through the liver. The metabolite retains antibacterial activity but is less well absorbed from the gastrointestinal tract. The half-life is 1½–5 hours, becoming shortened during treatment due to induction of the hepatic microsomal enzymes.

Unwanted effects are relatively infrequent, occurring in fewer than 4% of individuals. The commonest are skin eruptions, fever and gastrointestinal disturbances. Liver damage with jaundice has been reported and has proved fatal in a very small proportion of cases, the incidence being approximately 1 in 3000 treated patients and being mainly associated with prior liver disease. An influenza-like syndrome and a variety of symptoms of CNS disturbances have been recorded (dizziness, tiredness and confusion), as have various allergic manifestations such as urticaria and haemolysis. Rifampicin causes induction of hepatic metabolising enzymes resulting in an increase in the degradation of warfarin, glucocorticoids, narcotic analgesics, oral antidiabetic drugs, dapsone and oestrogens, the last leading to a decreased efficacy of oral contraceptives.

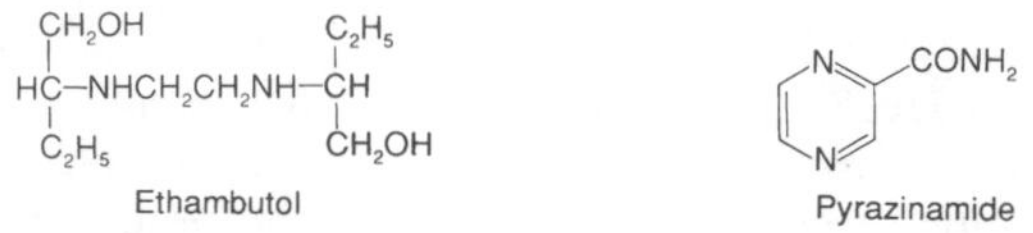

Fig. 37.9 Structures of ethambutol and pyrazinamide.

ETHAMBUTOL

Only the dextrorotatory isomer of ethambutol (Fig. 37.9) has antituberculosis activity, and the drug has no effect on organisms other than mycobacteria. It is taken up by the bacteria and after a period of 24 hours it inhibits their growth. The mechanism of action is unknown. Resistance emerges rapidly if the drug is used on its own.

Ethambutol is given orally and is well absorbed, reaching therapeutic plasma concentrations within 4 hours. In the blood it is taken up by erythrocytes and slowly released. It is partly metabolised and is excreted in the urine (50% of a dose as unchanged drug and 15% as metabolites). 20% appears in the faeces. The half-life is 3–4 hours. It can reach therapeutic concentrations in the CSF in tuberculous meningitis.

Unwanted effects are uncommon, the most important being optic neuritis, which is likely to occur if renal function is decreased. It results in visual disturbances such as red/green colour blindness and a decrease in visual acuity. This effect is dose-related, and if it occurs the drug should be stopped to prevent blindness.

Other unwanted effects are gastrointestinal disturbances, arthralgia, headache, giddiness and mental disturbances. About half the patients treated have an increased blood urate concentration due to reduced uric acid excretion.

PYRAZINAMIDE

Pyrazinamide is related to nicotinamide and its chemical structure is given in Figure 37.9. It is inactive at neutral pH but tuberculostatic at acid pH. It is effective against the intracellular organisms in macrophages, since, after phagocytosis, the

Antituberculosis drugs

First-line drugs

- **Isoniazid** kills actively growing mycobacteria within host cells; mechanism of action unknown. Given orally it penetrates necrotic lesions, also the CSF. 'Slow acetylators' (genetically determined) respond well. It has low toxicity. Pyridoxine deficiency increases risk of neurotoxicity. No cross-resistance with other agents.
- **Rifampicin** is a potent, orally active drug, which inhibits mycobacterial RNA-polymerase. It penetrates CSF. Unwanted effects are infrequent (but serious liver damage has occurred). It induces hepatic drug-metabolising enzymes. Resistance can develop rapidly.
- **Ethambutol** inhibits growth of mycobacteria by unknown mechanism. It is given orally and can penetrate CSF. Unwanted effects are uncommon; optic neuritis can occur and there may be reduced urate excretion. Resistance can emerge rapidly.
- **Pyrazinamide** is tuberculostatic against intracellular mycobacteria by an unknown mechanism. Given orally, it penetrates CSF. Resistance can develop rapidly. Unwanted effects: increased plasma urates, liver toxicity with high doses.

Second-line drugs

- **Capreomycin** is given intramuscularly. Unwanted effects include damage to kidney and to VIIIth nerve.
- **Cycloserine** is broad spectrum. It inhibits an early stage of peptidoglycan synthesis. Given orally it penetrates the CSF. Unwanted effects affect mostly CNS.
- **Streptomycin**, an aminoglycoside antibiotic, acts by inhibiting bacterial protein synthesis. Given i.m. Unwanted effects: ototoxicity (mainly vestibular) and nephrotoxicity. Infrequently used now.

To avoid emergence of resistant organisms, compound therapy is used, e.g. three drugs initially, then two drugs later.

organisms will be contained in phagolysosomes in which the pH is low. Resistance is rather readily developed but cross-resistance with isoniazid does not occur.

The drug is well absorbed after oral administration, and is widely distributed, penetrating well into the meninges. It is excreted through the kidney, mainly by glomerular filtration.

Unwanted effects include arthralgia, which is associated with high concentrations of plasma urates. Gastrointestinal upsets, malaise and fever are reported. With the high doses previously used, serious hepatic damage was a possibility; this is now less likely with lower doses and shorter courses.

CAPREOMYCIN

Capreomycin is a peptide antibiotic given by intramuscular injection. There is some cross-reaction with the aminoglycoside, **kanamycin**.

Unwanted effects are kidney damage and injury to the eighth nerve with deafness and ataxia. (The drug should not be given at the same time as **streptomycin** or other drugs that may damage the eighth nerve.)

CYCLOSERINE

Cycloserine is a broad-spectrum antibiotic inhibiting many bacteria including coliforms and myco-

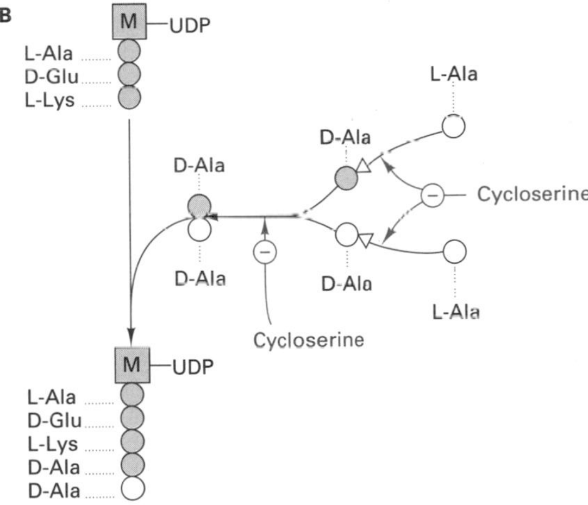

Fig. 37.10 Cycloserine. A. The relationship of cycloserine to D-alanine (D-Ala). **B.** Cycloserine inhibits an early stage of peptidoglycan synthesis; it inhibits the conversion of L-alanine (L-Ala) to D-Ala and also the conversion of two molecules of D-Ala to D-alanile-D-alanine. This is an enlarged section of Figure 35.3 and shows the peptide chain of *Staph. aureus*; N-acetylmuramic acid (M) and the four amino acids which make up the basic building block of the peptidoglycan are shown in light pink. (D-Glu = D-glutamic acid; L-Lys = L-lysine; UDP = uridine diphosphate)

bacteria. It is water soluble and destroyed at acid pH. It is a structural analogue of D-alanine (Fig. 37.10A) and competitively inhibits cell wall synthesis by preventing the formation both of D-alanine and of the D-Ala–D-Ala dipeptide which is added to the initial tripeptide side-chain on N-acetylmuramic acid, i.e. it prevents completion of the major building block of peptidoglycan (see Figs 37.10B and 35.3). After being given orally it is rapidly absorbed and reaches peak concentrations within 4 hours. It is distributed throughout the tissues and body fluids, concentrations in the CSF being equivalent to the concentration in the blood. Most of the drug is eliminated in active form in the urine, but some (approximately 35%) is metabolised.

Unwanted effects affect mainly the central nervous system. A wide variety of disturbances may occur, ranging from headache and irritability to depression, convulsions and psychotic states.

Its use is limited to tuberculosis that is resistant to other drugs.

DRUGS USED TO TREAT LEPROSY

There are estimated to be 10–12 million cases of leprosy in the world, most being in Africa and Asia. Multidrug treatment regimes initiated by WHO in 1982 are improving the outlook for this disease. Paucibacillary leprosy—leprosy with few bacilli, which is mainly *tuberculoid** in type—is treated for 6 months with **dapsone**, and **rifampicin**. Multi-bacillary leprosy—leprosy with numerous bacilli, which is mainly *lepromatous** in type—is treated for at least 2 years with rifampicin, dapsone and **clofazamine**. The effect of therapy with **minocycline** or the **fluoroquinolones** is being investigated.

DAPSONE

Dapsone (Fig. 37.11) is chemically related to the **sulphonamides** (Fig. 37.1) and, since its action is antagonised by PABA, probably acts by inhibition of folate synthesis.

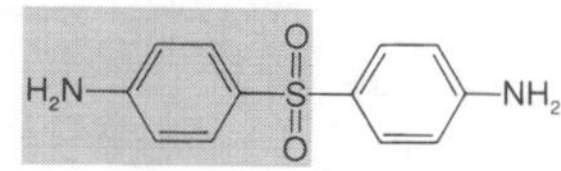

Fig. 37.11 Dapsone. The relationship with sulphanilamide (Fig. 37.1) is indicated by the light pink box.

Resistance to dapsone is increasing and treatment with combinations of drugs is now recommended.

Dapsone is given orally and is well absorbed and widely distributed through the body water and all tissues. The plasma half-life is 24–48 hours but some dapsone remains in certain tissues (liver, kidney, and, to some extent, skin and muscle) for much longer periods. There is enterohepatic recycling of the drug but some is acetylated and excreted in the urine. Dapsone is also used to treat dermatitis herpetiformis, a chronic blistering skin condition associated with coeliac disease.

Unwanted reactions occur fairly frequently and include haemolysis of red cells (usually not severe enough to lead to frank anaemia), methaemoglobinaemia, anorexia, nausea and vomiting, fever, allergic dermatitis and neuropathy. Lepra reactions (an exacerbation of lepromatous lesions) can occur and a syndrome resembling infectious mononucleosis, but which can be fatal, has occasionally been seen.

RIFAMPICIN

See page 740, under 'Drugs used to treat tuberculosis'.

Anti-leprosy drugs

- For tuberculoid leprosy: dapsone and rifampicin.
- For lepromatous leprosy: dapsone, rifampicin and clofazimine.
- **Dapsone** is sulphonamide-like and may inhibit folate synthesis. It is given orally. Unwanted effects are fairly frequent, a few are serious. Resistance is increasing.
- **Clofazimine** is a dye which is given orally and can cumulate by sequestering in macrophages. Action is delayed for 6–7 weeks. $t_{1/2}$ 8 weeks. Unwanted effects: red skin and urine, sometimes GIT upsets.
- **Rifampicin** (see box on p. 741).

*The basis of the difference appears to be that the T cells of patients with tuberculoid leprosy vigorously produce γ-interferon which enables macrophages to kill intracellular microbes, whereas in lepromatous leprosy, the immune response is dominated by interleukin-4 which blocks the action of γ-interferon. See Chapter 11.

CLOFAZIMINE

Clofazimine is a dye of complex structure. It has anti-inflammatory activity and is also therefore useful in patients in whom dapsone causes inflammatory side effects. Its mechanism of action against leprosy bacilli may involve an action on DNA.

It is given orally and tends to cumulate in the body, being sequestered in the mononuclear phagocyte system. The antileprotic effect is delayed and is usually not seen for 6–7 weeks. The plasma half-life may be as long as 8 weeks.

Unwanted effects may be related to the fact that clofazimine is a dye. Thus the skin and urine can develop a reddish colour and the lesions a blue-black discoloration. Dose-related nausea, giddiness, headache and gastrointestinal disturbances can also occur.

REFERENCES AND FURTHER READING

Aronson J K, Reynolds D J M 1992 Aminoglycoside antibiotics. Br Med J 305: 1421–1424

Ballow C H, Amsden G W 1992 Azithromycin; the first azide antibiotic. Ann Pharmacother 26: 1253–1261

Bloom B R 1992 Tuberculosis. Back to a frightening future. Nature 358: 538–539

Brumfitt W, Hamilton-Miller J 1989 Methicillin-resistant *Staphylococcus aureus*. N Engl J Med 320: 1188–1195

Donowitz G R, Mandell G L 1988 β-lactam antibiotics. N Engl J Med 318: 419–425, 490–500

Dooley S W, Jarvis W R, Martone W J, Snider D E 1992 Multidrug-resistant tuberculosis. Ann Intern Med 117: 257–258

Editorial 1988 Chemotherapy of leprosy. Lancet 2: 487–488

Eykyn S J 1988 Staphylococcal sepsis. Lancet 1: 286–289

Finch R 1990 The penicillins today. Br Med J 300: 1289–1290

Fletcher C 1984 First clinical use of penicillin. Br Med J 289: 1721–1723

Franklin T J, Snow G A 1989 Biochemistry of antimicrobial action, 4th edn. Chapman & Hall, London

Geddes A M 1988 Antibiotic therapy: a resumé. Lancet 1: 286–289

Godlee F 1993 Tuberculosis—a global emergency. Br Med J 306: 1147

Hare R 1970 The birth of penicillin and the disarming of microbes. Allen & Unwin, London

Hastings R C, Franzblau S G 1988 Chemotherapy of leprosy. Ann Rev Pharmacol Toxicol 28: 231–245

Heym B, Honoré N et al. 1994 Implications of multidrug resistance for the future of short-course chemotherapy of tuberculosis: a molecular study. Lancet 344: 293–298

Hooper D C, Wolfson J S 1991 Fluoroquinolone antimicrobial agents. N Engl J Med 324: 384–394

Howie J 1986 Penicillin: 1929–1940. Br Med J 293: 158–159

Iseman M D 1993 Treatment of multidrug-resistant tuberculosis. N Engl J Med 329: 784–791

Jacoby G A, Archer G L 1991 Mechanisms of disease: new mechanisms of bacterial resistance to antimicrobial agents. N Engl J Med 324: 601–612

Jacoby G A, Medeiros A 1991 More extended-spectrum β-lactamases. Antimicrob Agents Chemother 35: 1697–1704

Just P M 1993 Overview of the fluoroquinolone antibiotics. Pharmacotherapy 13: 4S–17S

Lerner B H 1991 Scientific evidence versus therapeutic demand: the introduction of the sulphonamides revisited. Ann Intern Med 115: 315–320

Mandell G L, Douglas R G, Bennett J E (eds) 1985 Principles and practice of infectious disease, 2nd edn. Section E: Anti-infective therapy. John Wiley & Sons, New York

Moellering R C 1985 Principles of anti-infective therapy. In: Mandell G L, Douglas R G, Bennett J E (eds) Principles and practice of infectious disease. John Wiley & Sons, New York

Moellering R C Jr 1993 Meeting the challenges of β-lactamases. J Antimicrob Chemother 31 (Suppl A): 1–8

Neu H C 1992 New macrolide antibiotics: azithromycin and clarithromycin. Ann Intern Med 116: 517–518

Peters D H, Friedel H A, McTavish D 1992 Azithromycin: a review of its antimicrobial activity, pharmacokinetic properties and clinical efficacy. Drugs 44: 750–799

Raoult D, Drancourt M 1994 Antimicrobial therapy of rickettsial diseases. Antimicrob Agents Chemother 35: 2457–2462

Sato K, Hoshino K, Mitsuhashi S 1992 Mode of action of the new quinolones: the inhibitory action on DNA gyrase. Prog Drug Res 38: 121–132

Shimada J, Hori S 1992 Adverse effects of fluoroquinolones. Prog Drug Res 38: 133–143

Siporin C, Heifetz C L, Domagala J M (eds) 1990 The new generation of quinolones. Marcel Dekker, New York

Smith J T 1985 The 4-quinolone antibacterials. In: Greenwood D, O'Grady F (eds) The scientific basis of antimicrobial therapy. Cambridge University Press, Cambridge, p 69–94

Sturgill M G 1992 Clarithromycin. Ann Pharmacother 26: 1099–1108

Tai P C, Davis B D 1985 The actions of antibiotics on the ribosome. In: Greenwood D, O'Grady F (eds) The scientific basis of antimicrobial therapy. Cambridge University Press, Cambridge, p 41–68

Toshihiko U, Nakashima M 1992 Pharmacokinetic aspects of the newer quinolones. Prog Drug Res 38: 39–58

Wise R 1987 Antimicrobial agents: a widening choice. Lancet 2: 1251–1254

Wood M J 1991 More macrolides. Br Med J 303: 594–595

Yunis A A 1988 Chloramphenicol: relation of structure to activity and toxicity. Ann Rev Pharmacol Toxicol 28: 83–100

38
ANTIVIRAL DRUGS

VIRAL INFECTION

Viruses are the smallest infective agents, consisting essentially of nucleic acid (either RNA or DNA) enclosed in a protein coat or capsid (Fig. 38.1). The proteins can be antigenic. The coat plus the nucleic acid core is termed the nucleocapsid. Some viruses have, in addition, a lipoprotein envelope which may contain antigenic viral glycoproteins, as well as host phospholipids acquired when the virus nucleocapsid buds through the nuclear membrane or plasma membrane of the host cell. Certain viruses also contain enzymes which initiate their replication in the host cell. The whole infective particle is termed a virion. In different types of virus the nucleic acids may be double-stranded or single-stranded.

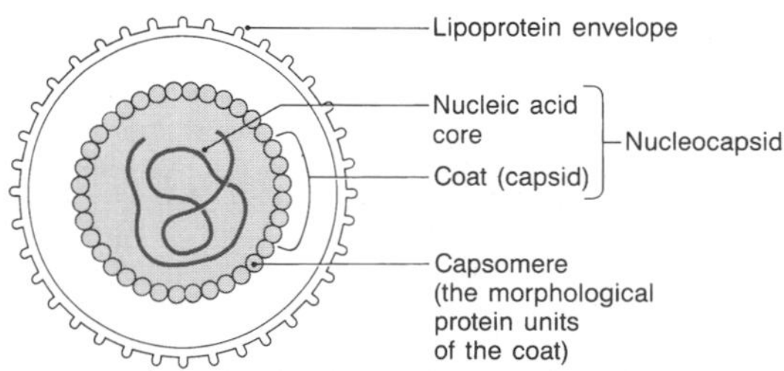

Fig. 38.1 Schematic diagram of the components of a virus particle or virion.

EXAMPLES OF PATHOGENIC VIRUSES

Some important examples of viruses and the diseases they cause are as follows:

- *DNA viruses:* poxviruses (smallpox), herpesviruses (chickenpox, shingles, herpes, glandular fever), adenoviruses (sore throat, conjunctivitis) and papillomaviruses (warts).
- *RNA viruses:* orthomyxoviruses (influenza), paramyxoviruses (measles, mumps), rubella virus (German measles), rhabdoviruses (rabies), picornaviruses (colds, meningitis, poliomyelitis), retroviruses (AIDS, T-cell leukaemia), arenaviruses (meningitis, Lassa fever), hepadnaviruses (serum hepatitis) and arboviruses (arthropod-borne encephalitis and various fevers, e.g. yellow fever).

Viruses are intracellular parasites with no metabolic machinery of their own. In order to replicate they have to attach to and enter a living host cell—animal, plant or bacterial—and use its metabolic processes. The binding sites on the virus are polypeptides on the envelope or capsid. The virus-specific receptors on the host cell, to which the virus attaches, are normal membrane constituents—ion channels, receptors for neurotransmitters or hormones, integral membrane glycoproteins, etc. (Some possible host cell receptors for particular viruses are listed in Table 38.1.) The receptor/virus complex enters the cell by receptor-mediated endocytosis during which the virus coat may be removed. The nucleic acid of the virus then uses the cell's machinery for synthesising nucleic acid and protein and the manufacture of new virus particles.

Viral replication requires DNA or RNA synthesis, synthesis of viral proteins and glycosylation. A simplified account of viral replication is given here.

In *DNA viruses*, there is generally entry of the viral DNA into the host cell nucleus,* transcription of

*The pox virus is an exception. It has its own RNA polymerase; it replicates in the host cytoplasm.

Table 38.1 Some host cell structures that may function as receptors for viruses

Host cell structure	Virus
Acetylcholine receptor on skeletal muscle	Rabies virus
Complement C3d receptor on B lymphocytes	Glandular fever virus
CD4 (T_4) molecule on T lymphocytes	AIDS virus
Interleukin-2 receptor on T lymphocytes	T-cell leukaemia viruses
β-adrenoceptors	Infantile diarrhoea virus
HLA histocompatibility molecules	Adenoviruses causing sore throat, conjunctivitis; T-cell leukaemia viruses

this viral DNA into mRNA by host cell RNA polymerase and translation of the mRNA into virus-specific proteins. Some of these proteins are enzymes which then synthesise more viral DNA as well as proteins of the coat and envelope. After assembly of coat proteins around the viral DNA, complete virions are released by budding or after cell lysis. An example of the replication of a DNA virus is given in Figure 38.2.

In *RNA viruses*, either enzymes in the virion synthesise its mRNA or the viral RNA serves as its own mRNA. This is translated into various enzymes, including RNA polymerase (which directs the synthesis of more viral RNA) and also into structural proteins of the virion. Assembly and release of virions occurs as explained above. With these viruses the host cell nucleus is normally not involved in viral replication (however, some RNA viruses, e.g. those causing influenza, have a requirement for active cellular transcription in the nucleus).

In *RNA retroviruses*, the virion contains a *reverse transcriptase* which makes a DNA copy of the viral RNA. This DNA copy is integrated into the host genome and it is termed a 'provirus'. This provirus DNA is transcribed into both new genomic RNA

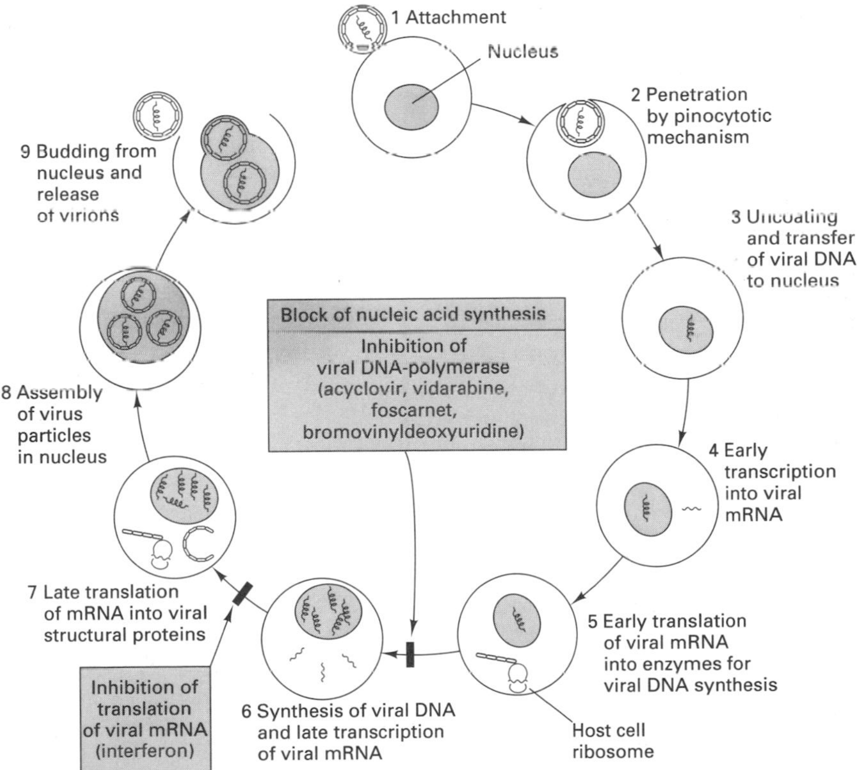

Fig. 38.2 Schematic diagram of replication of a DNA virus (e.g. herpes simplex) in a host cell with the probable sites of action of antiviral agents. Viral components are shown in red. In some viruses, assembly (stage 8) takes place in the host cell cytoplasm.

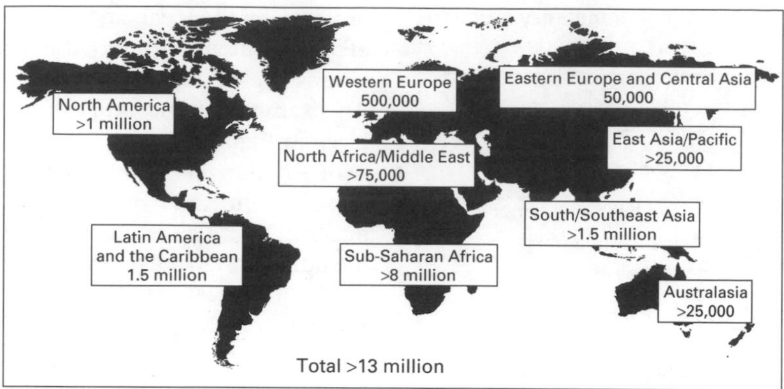

Fig. 38.3 Distribution of cumulative HIV infections since the start of the pandemic, estimated in mid-1993. (Adapted from Merson M H 1993 Science 260: 1266–1268)

and mRNA for translation into viral proteins. These viruses are released by budding and many can replicate without killing the host cell. Some RNA retroviruses can transform normal cells into malignant cells. The AIDS virus is an RNA retrovirus; it is discussed in more detail below.

THE HUMAN IMMUNODEFICIENCY VIRUS (HIV) AND AIDS

Infection with HIV* results in the acquired immune deficiency syndrome (AIDS), a syndrome first recognised in 1981. The World Health Organization estimated that, by mid-1993, over 13 million individuals had become infected with the virus since the start of the pandemic, and the disease continues to spread (Fig. 38.3). For a recent comprehensive review of the pathogenesis of AIDS, see Levy (1993).

The usual course of events after infection with HIV is shown in Figure 38.4. There is an initial acute illness (fever, headache, myalgia, swollen lymph glands, rash) associated with an increase in the number of virus particles in the blood, their widespread dissemination through the tissues and the seeding of lymphoid tissue with the virion particles. Within a few weeks the viraemia is reduced; this is thought to be the result of an antiviral immune response.

A variety of host cells are susceptible to the virus but interaction with cells having CD4 surface proteins (mainly helper T cells, but also macrophages, dendritic cells and neuroglial cells) determines the outcome of the infection. The coat of the virus has numerous spikes which contain a glycoprotein termed gp120, which has a 13-amino-acid sequence that mimics human major histocompatibility complex (MHC) molecules. This protein binds tightly to the CD4 receptor on host cells; the complex then enters the cell by endocytosis, and the sequence of events outlined above is initiated.

Viruses

- Viruses, the smallest infective agents, consist essentially of nucleic acid (RNA or DNA) enclosed in a protein coat.
- They are not cells and, having no metabolic machinery of their own, they are obligate intracellular parasites, i.e. they have to use the metabolic processes of the host cell which they enter and infect.
- DNA viruses normally enter the host cell nucleus and direct the generation of new viruses (the pox virus is an exception in that it does not enter the nucleus).
- RNA viruses direct the generation of new viruses, normally without involving the host cell nucleus (the 'flu' virus is an exception in that it does involve the host cell nucleus).
- RNA retroviruses (e.g. AIDS virus) contain an enzyme, reverse transcriptase, which makes a DNA copy of the viral RNA. This DNA copy is integrated into the host cell genome and directs the generation of new virus particles.

*Strictly speaking there are two viruses associated with AIDS—HIV-1 and HIV-2.

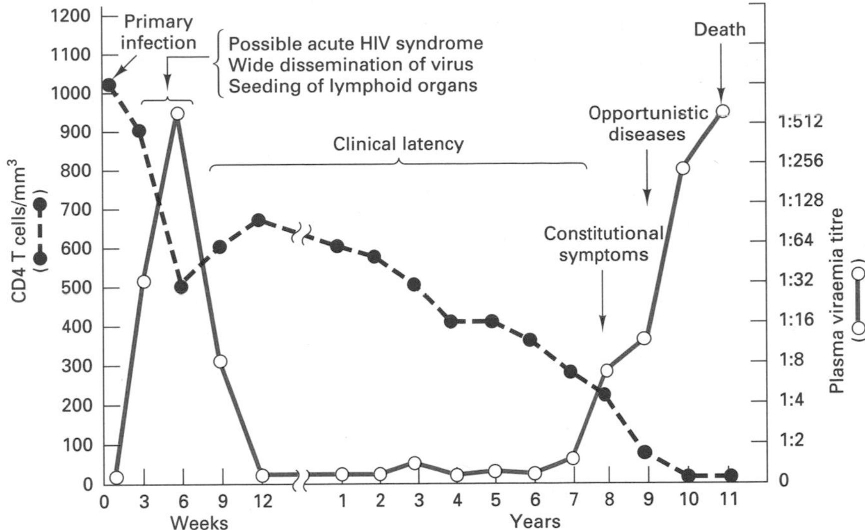

Fig. 38.4 Schematic outline of the course of HIV infection. (Adapted from Pantaleo et al. 1993 N Engl J Med 328: 327–335)

The acute illness is followed by a symptom-free period during which there is reduction in the viraemia accompanied by silent virus replication in the lymph nodes. This replication is associated with loss of CD4-positive lymphocytes and dendritic cells (probably due to apoptosis*) and damage to lymph node architecture. It is thought that there is an autoimmune component in these changes in host cells. After this period of clinical latency (median, 10 years) the signs and symptoms of AIDS appear—opportunistic infections (e.g. with *Pneumocystis carinii* or the tubercle bacillus), neurological disease (e.g. confusion, paralysis, dementia), bone marrow depression and cancers. Chronic gastrointestinal infections are probably the cause of the severe weight loss. Cardiovascular damage and kidney damage can also occur. Death usually follows within 2 years.

GENERAL ACTIONS OF ANTIVIRAL DRUGS

Because viruses share many of the metabolic processes of the host cell it is difficult to find drugs that are selective for the pathogen. However, there are some virus-specific enzymes that are potential targets for drugs. Most currently available antiviral agents are only effective while the virus is replicating. An additional problem is that by the time a viral infection becomes clinically detectable, the process of viral replication is usually far advanced and chemotherapeutic intervention is very difficult.

The main mechanisms of action of antiviral agents and the relevant drugs are given below.

INHIBITION OF NUCLEIC ACID SYNTHESIS

Acyclovir

The era of effective selective antiviral therapy began with acyclovir. This agent is a guanosine derivative (Fig. 38.5) with a high specificity for herpes simplex and varicella-zoster viruses (reviewed by Whiteley & Gnann 1992). Herpes simplex is more susceptible than varicella-zoster. (Varicella or chickenpox is caused by the same virus that causes varicella-zoster or shingles). Epstein–Barr virus (a herpes virus which causes glandular fever) is also slightly sensitive. Acyclovir has a small but reproducible effect against cytomegalovirus (CMV)—a herpes virus which can affect the foetus, and can cause a glandular-fever-like syndrome in adults and severe disease (e.g. retinitis, which can result in blindness) in individuals with decreased immune responses due to AIDS.

*See Chapter 36, Fig. 36.1.

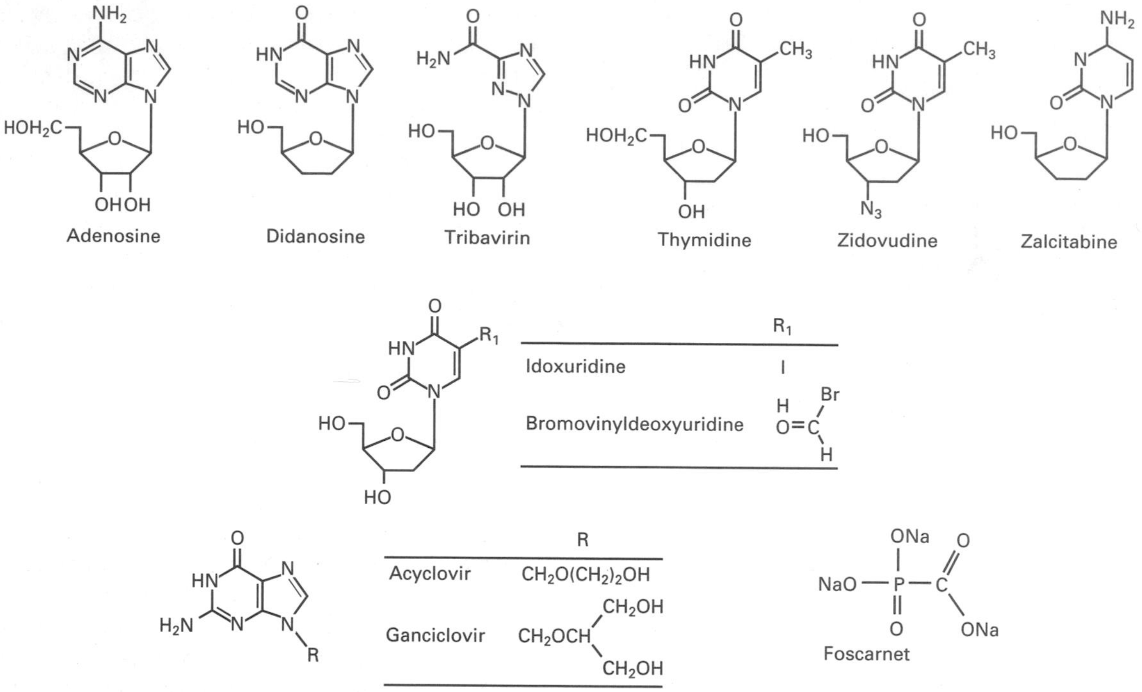

Fig. 38.5 **Structures of some antiviral agents.** The structures in black are found normally in vivo, those in red are drugs.

Mechanism of action

Acyclovir is converted to the monophosphate by thymidine kinase—the virus-specific form of this enzyme being very much more effective in carrying out the phosphorylation than the host cells' thymidine kinase—and is subsequently converted to the triphosphate by the host cell kinases. It is therefore only adequately activated in infected cells. Acyclovir triphosphate inhibits viral DNA-polymerase (Fig. 38.2), terminating the chain. It is 30 times more potent against the herpes virus enzyme than the host enzyme. Acyclovir triphosphate is fairly rapidly broken down within the host cells, presumably by cellular phosphatases. Resistance due to changes in the viral genes coding for thymidine kinase or DNA polymerase has been reported and acyclovir-resistant herpes simplex virus has been the cause of pneumonia, encephalitis and mucocutaneous infections in immunocompromised patients.

Pharmacokinetic aspects

Acyclovir can be given orally, intravenously and topically. When it is given orally, only 20% of the dose is absorbed and peak plasma concentrations are reached in 1–2 hours; intravenous infusion results in a plasma concentration 10- to 20-fold higher. The drug is widely distributed, reaching concentrations in the CSF which are 50% of those in the plasma. It is excreted by the kidneys partly by glomerular filtration and partly by tubular secretion.

The clinical use of acyclovir is given on page 749.

Unwanted effects

Unwanted effects are minimal. Local inflammation can occur during intravenous injection if there is extravasation of the solution, which is very alkaline (pH 10–11). Renal dysfunction has been reported when acyclovir is given intravenously; slow infusion reduces the risk. Nausea and headache can occur and, rarely, encephalopathy.

Ganciclovir

Ganciclovir (Fig. 38.5), a synthetic nucleoside analogue, is 100 times more active than acyclovir against cytomegalovirus (CMV) in vitro. Like acyclovir it has to be activated to the triphosphate and in this form is competes with guanosine triphosphate for incorporation into viral DNA. It suppresses viral DNA replication, but unlike acyclovir it does not

Clinical use of acyclovir

Acyclovir is used:

- to treat varicella-zoster infections (shingles), orally in immunocompetent patients, intravenously in immunocompromised patients
- to treat herpes simplex infections (genital herpes, mucocutaneous herpes and herpes encephalitis)
- to treat varicella (chicken pox) in immunocompromised patients
- *prophylactically* in patients who are to be treated with immunosuppressant drugs or radiotherapy and who are at risk of herpes virus infection due to reactivation of a latent virus
- *prophylactically* in individuals who suffer from frequent recurrences of genital infection with herpes simplex virus.

act as a chain terminator, nor is it rapidly broken down, being shown to persist in cells infected with cytomegalovirus for 18–20 hours. The initial phosphorylation of ganciclovir is carried out by a recently identified protein kinase encoded in human cytomegalovirus. Human cytomegalovirus differs from other human herpesviruses in that it does not encode a virus-specific thymidine kinase.

Ganciclovir is given intravenously, excreted in the urine and has a half-life of 4 hours. It has serious unwanted actions, including bone marrow depression and potential carcinogenicity. It is used for life- or sight-threatening cytomegalovirus infections in patients who are immunocompromised (see p. 747). (It is difficult to give ganciclovir with zidovudine since both cause granulocytopaenia.)

Vidarabine

Vidarabine (adenine arabinoside) is a purine nucleoside analogue with activity against herpes simplex and varicella-zoster virus. It is a second-line drug for these infections; in general acyclovir is preferred.

Vidarabine is phosphorylated by cellular kinases to the triphosphate, which acts as a relatively selective inhibitor of viral DNA polymerase (see Figs 35.7 and 38.2).

It is given in a large volume by slow intravenous infusion; it can also be applied topically. It is widely distributed in the body, and the CSF concentration is about 30–50% that in the plasma. It is excreted mainly in the urine, mostly as the deaminated metabolite.

Unwanted effects include nausea, vomiting and diarrhoea. Neurotoxicity can occur late in therapy with high doses, and is usually reversible. Bone marrow disturbances have been reported after high doses. Vidarabine can be mutagenic and carcinogenic.

Idoxuridine and bromovinyldeoxyuridine

Idoxuridine is an analogue of thymidine (see Fig. 38.5). It inhibits replication of DNA viruses. It is phosphorylated by cellular kinases and the triphosphate is incorporated into both viral and host DNA. Being mutagenic, it is too toxic for systemic use, and is therefore only used topically. It needs to be dissolved in dimethylsulphoxide—a solvent that can cause irritation.

Its main use is in the treatment of herpes simplex and varicella-zoster infections in the eye. It can cause contact dermatitis.

Bromovinyldeoxyuridine (BVDU; Fig. 38.5), is a potent inhibitor of herpes simplex and varicella-zoster viruses in vitro, its inhibitory action (Fig. 38.2) being correlated with its selective incorporation into viral DNA. It is not mutagenic. A congener of BVDU, namely **bromovinyldeoxyuridine arabinoside**, is undergoing clinical trials for varicella-zoster.

Tribavirin (ribavirin)

Tribavirin (Fig. 38.5) is a synthetic nucleoside, similar in structure to guanosine. Its mechanism of action is not clearly defined but there is some evidence that, in addition to altering virus nucleotide pools, it interferes with the synthesis of viral mRNA (Fig. 38.2). It inhibits a wide range of DNA and RNA viruses including many that affect the lower airways. In aerosol form it has been used to treat influenza and infections due to respiratory syncytial virus (an RNA paramyxovirus).

It has been shown to be effective in Lassa fever, an extremely serious arenavirus infection; given intravenously within the first 6 days of onset it has been shown to reduce to 9% a case-fatality rate previously 76%.

Foscarnet (phosphonoformate)

Foscarnet (Fig. 38.5) is a synthetic non-nucleoside analogue of pyrophosphate which inhibits viral DNA polymerase by binding directly to the pyrophosphate-binding site. It can have serious nephrotoxicity. Given by intravenous infusion, it is a second-line drug in cytomegalovirus eye infection in immunocompromised patients; (its toxic effects do not overlap with those of zidovudine).

Zidovudine (azidothymidine, AZT)

Zidovudine (Fig. 38.5) is an analogue of thymidine. In retroviruses—such as the HIV virus—it is an active inhibitor of reverse transcriptase (see Table 38.1). It is phosphorylated by cellular enzymes to the triphosphate form, in which it competes with equivalent cellular triphosphates which are essential substrates for the formation of proviral DNA by viral reverse transcriptase (viral RNA-dependent DNA polymerase); its incorporation into the growing viral DNA strand results in chain termination. Mammalian alpha DNA polymerase is relatively resistant to the effect. However, gamma DNA polymerase in the host cell mitochondria is fairly sensitive to the compound and this may be the basis of unwanted effects. The use of zidovudine in the prevention and treatment of AIDS is discussed in the box below. This topic is reviewed by Hirsch & D'Aquila (1993), Bartlett (1993).

Pharmacokinetic aspects

Given orally, the bioavailability of zidovudine is 60–80% due to first-pass metabolism, and the peak plasma concentration occurs at 30 minutes. It can also be given intravenously. Its half-life is 1 hour, and the intracellular half-life of the active triphosphate is 3 hours. There is little plasma protein binding so there are no drug interactions due to displacement by other drugs. Zidovudine enters mammalian cells by passive diffusion and in this is unlike most other nucleosides which require active uptake. The drug passes into the CSF and brain. Most of the drug is metabolised to inactive glucuronide in the liver, only 20% of the active form being excreted in the urine. **Probenecid** inhibits both the hepatic inactivation and the renal excretion and prolongs the plasma half-life. Other agents which also undergo glucuronidation may modify the metabolism of zidovudine.

Clinical use of zidovudine

- *In patients with AIDS*, it reduces the incidence of opportunistic infections (such as *Pneumocystis carinii* pneumonia), stabilises weight, reverses HIV-associated thrombocytopenia, stabilises HIV-associated dementia and reduces viral burden.
- *If given in HIV-positive individuals before the onset of AIDS*, it delays the progression of the disease, providing a time-limited benefit of 12–18 months. However, it may make no difference to the median survival time, which is usually 3 years from the diagnosis of AIDS, and there is debate as to when, in HIV infection, the drug should be given and whether and when it should be combined with other nucleoside analogues. It is clear that zidovudine and other nucleoside analogues are poorly tolerated and not very effective in late-stage disease.
- *In HIV-positive mothers* it reduces by 66% the risk of transmission of the virus to the foetuses.
- *After specific exposure to the HIV virus*—e.g. after needle-stick injury—it is recommended that zidovudine be given, but it is not yet clear whether this is effective in preventing disease.

The final place of zidovudine in the therapy and prevention of AIDS has still to be decided.

Unwanted effects

Unwanted effects are likely to occur when zidovudine is used to treat AIDS, mainly anaemia and neutropenia, the incidence of which has decreased as the doses of zidovudine used in therapy have been reduced. These complications are, however, still common with long-term administration.* Other unwanted effects sometimes seen are gastrointestinal disturbances, paraesthesia, skin rash, insomnia, fever, headaches, abnormalities of liver function and, more particularly, myopathy. Confusion, anxiety, depression and a flu-like syndrome are also reported. The prophylactic use of the drug, short-term, in fit individuals, after specific exposure to the virus, is associated with only minor, reversible unwanted effects.

Resistance to the antiviral action of zidovudine

In most patients, the therapeutic response to zidovudine wanes with long-term use, particularly in late-stage disease. It is known that the virus develops resistance to the drug due to mutations resulting in amino acid substitutions in the viral reverse transcriptase and that these genetic changes accumulate progressively. Thus, the virus is a constantly moving target. Resistant strains can be transferred between individuals. Other factors which could underlie the loss of efficacy of the drug are decreased activation of zidovudine to the triphosphate, increased virus load due to reduction in

*Administration of erythropoietin and GM-CSF (see Ch. 23, p. 485, and Table 11.2) may alleviate these problems.

immune mechanisms and increased virulence of the pathogen.

Didanosine (dideoxyinosine, ddI)

Didanosine is a synthetic purine dideoxynucleoside analogue. It is phosphorylated in the host cell to the triphosphate, dideoxyadenosine, in which form it acts as a chain terminator and inhibitor of the viral reverse transcriptase. It has been used to treat AIDS. Switching to didanosine after a period of zidovudine therapy has been shown to be beneficial. Drug resistance has occurred after prolonged therapy but is less than with zidovudine.

Pharmacokinetic aspects

Didanosine is given orally, rapidly absorbed (particularly if given with an antacid), and is actively secreted by the kidney tubules. The plasma half-life is 30 minutes but the intracellular half-life is more than 12 hours. The cerebrospinal fluid/plasma ratio is 0.2.

Unwanted effects

The main unwanted effect—occurring in >30% of patients—is dose-related peripheral neuropathy (pain and sensory loss in the feet). Dose-related pancreatitis occurs in 5–10% of patients and has been fatal in a few cases. Headache and gastrointestinal disturbance are also common and insomnia, skin rashes, bone marrow depression (less marked than with AZT) and alterations of liver function have been reported.

Zalcitabine (dideoxycytidine, ddC)

Dideoxycytidine, a synthetic nucleoside analogue, is used in combination with zidovudine for the therapy of AIDS. It is a reverse transcriptase inhibitor activated in the T cell by a different phosphorylation pathway from zidovudine. It is given orally, its plasma half-life is 20 minutes, its intracellular half-life is nearly 3 hours and its cerebrospinal fluid/plasma ratio is ~ 0.2.

Unwanted effects

The most important unwanted effect is a dose-related neuropathy (which can increase for several weeks after the drug has been stopped). Other unwanted effects include gastrointestinal disturbances, headache, mouth ulcers, nail changes, oedema of the lower limbs and general malaise. Skin rashes occur but may resolve spontaneously. Pancreatitis has been reported.

INHIBITION OF ATTACHMENT TO OR PENETRATION OF HOST CELLS

Amantadine

Amantadine is active against influenza A virus (an RNA virus) but has no action against influenza B virus. (It has an unrelated action in improving symptoms in Parkinson's disease; Ch. 25.) **Rimantadine** is similar in its effects. Used prophylactically, amantadine gives 50–80% protection against influenza A virus infection.

Mechanism of action

At two stages of viral replication within the host cell, a viral membrane protein, M_2, functions as an ion channel. The stages are: (i) the fusion of viral membrane and endosome membrane and (ii) the later stage of assembly and release of new virions at the host cell surface. Amantadine blocks this ion channel (Skehel 1992).

Pharmacokinetic aspects and unwanted effects

Given orally, amantadine is well absorbed, reaches high levels in secretions (e.g. saliva) and most is excreted unchanged via the kidney. Aerosol administration is also feasible.

Unwanted effects are relatively infrequent, occurring in 5–10% of patients, and are not serious. Dizziness, insomnia and slurred speech are the most commonly seen side effects.

Gamma globulin

Pooled gamma globulin contains antibodies against various viruses present in the population. The antibodies are directed against the virus envelope and can 'neutralise' some viruses and prevent their attachment to host cells. If used before the onset of signs and symptoms it may attenuate or prevent measles, infectious hepatitis, German measles, rabies or poliomyelitis. Hyperimmune globulin, specific against particular viruses, is used against hepatitis B, varicella-zoster and rabies.

Other putative inhibitors of viral attachment to the host cell are listed in Table 38.2.

Table 38.2 The sites of action of currently used and some potential anti-AIDS agents

Stages in the replication of the AIDS virus (HIV)	Currently used and potential anti-AIDS agents*
1 Attachment to host cell	Soluble recombinant CD4 (sCD4);† competitive CD4-receptor-specific synthetic peptides;† CD4 linked to pseudomonas toxin (kills the infected cells);‡ agents which damage the viral envelope (? amphotericin analogues); sulphated polysaccharides
2 Penetration by pinocytosis, and uncoating of virus	—
3 DNA copy of viral RNA made by virus reverse transcriptase	Reverse transcriptase inhibitors (RTIs): (i) nucleoside RTIs: **zidovudine**, **didanosine**, **zalcitabine**, 3-thiacytidine (3TC),§ 9-(2-phosphonomethoxyethyl)adenine (PMEA);§ (ii) various non-nucleoside reverse transcriptase inhibitors (NNRTIs)‡¶ including: foscarnet, carbovir, TIBO, nivirapine, etc.
4 Integration of viral DNA into the host genome	Antisense oligonucleotides;‖§ inhibitors of the viral enzyme, integrase
5 Transcription of viral DNA into viral RNA and copies of parent retrovirus	Antisense oligonucleotides;‖§ inhibitors of TAT—the protein that regulates transcription and controls the rate of replication§
6 Translation of viral mRNA into viral proteins by host ribosomes	Myristic acid analogues (inhibit necessary transfer of myristate to HIV proteins, Nef and Gag)
7 Assembly of viral coat proteins and viral RNA into new virus particles	Proteinase inhibitors, e.g. Ro31-8959;‡§ inhibitors of glycosylation (e.g. catanospermine); interferons; avarol, avarone
8 Release of new virus particles from host cell by budding	Interferons; ampligen (an interferon inducer)

* Drugs currently used are shown in bold.
† Recombinant, truncated CD4 or synthetic CD4-receptor-specific peptides would bind to HIV-I envelope and prevent the virus interacting with cell-bound CD4.
‡ Additive with nucleoside reverse transcriptase inhibitors (RTIs)
§ Substances at present in clinical trial
¶ These do not require intracellular conversion to active drug; there is rapid decrease in sensitivity of HIV, and cross-resistance between NNRTs.
‖ Antisense oligonucleotides are synthetic nucleotides of short chain length (13–20) which bind to specific portions of the viral genome by complementary base-pairing; they inhibit viral replication in vitro.

IMMUNOMODULATORS

Interferon (IFN)

Interferons are a family of inducible proteins synthesised by mammalian cells and now produced by recombinant DNA technology. There are at least three types of interferon, α-, β-, and γ-interferon, constituting a family of hormones involved in cell growth and regulation and modulation of immune reactions. γ-interferon, termed 'immune interferon', is a cytokine (see Ch. 11, p. 242), produced mainly by T lymphocytes as part of an immunological response to both viral and non-viral antigens, the latter including bacteria and their products, rickettsiae, protozoa, fungal polysaccharides and a range of polymeric chemicals and other cytokines. α- and β-interferons are produced by B and T lymphocytes, macrophages and fibroblasts in response to the presence of viruses and cytokines. The general actions of the interferons are described briefly in Chapter 11 (p. 243).

Mechanism of antiviral action of interferons

Interferons work by inducing, in the ribosomes of the host's cells, the production of enzymes that inhibit the translation of viral mRNA into viral proteins and thus stop the reproduction of the viruses (Fig. 38.2). Interferons bind to specific receptors

Antiviral drugs

These act by the following mechanisms:

- Inhibition of penetration of host cell:
  - —Amantadine inhibits uncoating and is effective against influenza A virus.
  - —Gamma globulin 'neutralises' viruses.
- Inhibition of nucleic acid synthesis:
  - —Acyclovir, a guanosine derivative, selectively inhibits viral DNA polymerase; effective against herpes viruses; minimal unwanted effects.
  - —Ganciclovir, also a guanosine derivative, is phosphorylated and then incorporated into viral DNA, suppressing its replication; used in cytomegalovirus (CMV) infection, especially CMV retinitis in AIDS patients.
  - —Vidarabine, an adenosine derivative, is a relatively selective inhibitor of viral DNA polymerase; effective against herpes simplex and varicella-zoster; can have serious unwanted effects.
  - —Tribavirin is similar to guanosine and is thought to interfere with synthesis of viral mRNA; can inhibit many DNA and RNA viruses.
  - —Foscarnet inhibits viral DNA polymerase by attaching to the pyrophosphate binding site; possibly effective in cytomegalovirus infection.
  - —Zidovudine, an analogue of thymidine, inhibits reverse transcriptase and is relatively effective in HIV infection.
  - —Zalcitabine and didanosine are reverse transcriptase inhibitors used in HIV infection.
- Immunomodulators:
  - —Interferons induce, in the host cells' ribosomes, enzymes which inhibit viral mRNA; they are used in hepatitis B infection and may be useful in AIDS.

on cell membranes, which may be gangliosides. They can be shown to inhibit the replication of most viruses in vitro.

Pharmacokinetic aspects

Given intravenously, interferons have a half-life of 2–4 hours. With intramuscular injections, peak blood concentrations are reached in 5–8 hours. They do not cross the blood–brain barrier.

Clinical use

Alpha-interferon is used for treatment of hepatitis B infections and AIDS-related Kaposi sarcomas. There are reports that interferons can prevent reactivation of herpes simplex after trigeminal root section, and prevent spread of herpes zoster in cancer patients.

Alpha-interferon is also used in some types of cancer (Table 36.1). When used for both antiviral and anticancer chemotherapy, interferons act partly by augmenting the host's immune response (see Ch. 11). Gamma-interferon is showing promise in some forms of disseminated sclerosis.

Unwanted effects are common and include fever, lassitude, headache and myalgia. Repeated injections cause chronic malaise. Bone marrow depression, rashes, alopecia and disturbances in cardiovascular, thyroid and hepatic function can also occur.

Inosine

Inosine is reported to stimulate both B and T lymphocyte differentiation, to increase macrophage activity and to enhance the effect of interferon. It has been used for herpes simplex infections but its place in antiviral therapy has yet to be established.

POSSIBLE FUTURE DEVELOPMENTS IN ANTIVIRAL THERAPY

Approaches which may be of use in the future are given below.

Agents affecting viral attachment to host cells

This group includes drugs which interact with the sites on viruses which bind to host cells (Table 38.1). An important example is the envelope protein, gp120, of HIV (see Table 38.2).

Agents affecting uncoating

The three-dimensional structure of the capsid of the RNA virus causing the common cold, rhinovirus 14, is known. Some drugs presently in development can bind tightly one of the proteins in the shell, preventing uncoating of the virion.

Agents affecting early stages of viral replication

The activity of ribonucleotide reductase, which converts ribonucleotides to deoxyribonucleotides, is an essential first step in DNA synthesis. The enzyme consists of two subunits which must form a dimer before the enzyme can act. A **synthetic nonapeptide** that mimics the sequence involved in the interaction between the two subunits can be shown to bind competitively to one subunit and prevent dimer formation. A shortened version of this peptide might have effective antiviral activity. **Semithiocarbazones** have also been shown to inhibit ribonucleotide reductase and to inhibit varicella-zoster virus when used topically with **acyclovir** in experimental animals.

In HIV-1 viruses, the reverse transcriptase has to be released from a precursor polypeptide before it can act. The protease which performs this cleavage is a specific target for antiviral therapy; synthetic **peptide inhibitors** of HIV protease are being tested (see Table 38.2).

Antisense oligonucleotides are synthetic nucleotides of short chain length (13–20) which bind to specific portions of the viral genome by complementary base-pairing; they inhibit viral replication in vitro (see Table 38.2).

Agents affecting late stages in viral replication

A late step in viral replication is formation of the viral envelope, which involves glycosylation; glycosylation inhibitors are being developed and tested. Cytoskeletal processes are involved in assembly and release of virus particles; agents which interfere with these processes are being sought. **Avarol** and **avarone** are thought to have this action in HIV (Table 38.2).

Further potential approaches to the therapy of HIV infections are outlined in Table 38.2.

Immune-directed therapies

There is some evidence that there is an autoimmune component* in the damage caused by HIV infection; consequently, strategies directed at the activated T cell, the process of apoptosis or cytokine secretion are being considered. Some authorities think that an imbalance between different types of immune responses* and the associated cytokines* could underlie the progress to AIDS. There is a hypothesis that a strong cell-mediated immune response, associated with 'Type I' helper cell action and the production of cytokines IL-2, IL-12 and IFN-γ, could delay progression to AIDS; whereas 'Type II' helper cell action, which is associated with IL-4, IL-5, IL-6 and IL-10, and which results in a predominantly antibody response, might have no effect or even a deleterious effect on the progression of AIDS (see Horton 1993b). Recent evidence indicates that cell-mediated immune responses could be beneficial in HIV infection, and that the CD8-positive cells—the cytotoxic T cells which normally kill off virus-infected cells—produce a factor that blocks HIV RNA expression. The Type II cytokines (see above) inhibit the production of this factor, whereas the Type I cytokines (IL-2 and IFN-γ) increase CD8 cell antiviral activity.

*For more detail, see Chapter 11.

PRION INFECTION

Prion infection constitutes a new and unique therapeutic challenge. Prion diseases are characterised by degenerative changes in the CNS developing over a period of years. Examples are Creutzfeldt-Jakob disease and kuru in man, scrapie in sheep and goats, bovine spongiform encephalopathy in cattle, etc. These conditions were originally thought to be caused by 'slow viruses' (lentiviruses), but it is now clear that the infective agents are *prions* and infection occurs when these are ingested or inadvertently injected. Each prion, when purified, consists of protease-resistant protein *without detectable DNA or RNA*, and the mode of replication was until recently a longstanding puzzle in molecular biology. However, the solution—at least in the case of scrapie—has now been found. The infective particle, PrP^{SC}, is a *conformational* variant of a protein, PrP^{C}, that occurs naturally in sheep. The infective particle replicates by triggering the conversion $PrP^{C} \rightarrow PrP^{SC}$; i.e. by, as it were, distorting the normal protein into its own abnormal shape through a direct protein–protein interaction. What is so remarkable is that the reaction is *purely physical*—occurring in cell-free preparations and without synthesis or, indeed, any sort of metabolism (see Beyreuther and Masters 1994; Kocisko et al. 1994).

At present, it is still not known whether prions from animals can infect man. Furthermore, the replication of prions other than those causing scrapie has not yet been examined, though it seems likely that they too will be found to result from autocatalytic conformational conversions. The reader will realise that this new type of infective agent poses an unusual and qualitatively different problem in therapeutics.

REFERENCES AND FURTHER READING

Abrams D I, Goldman A I et al. 1994 A comparative trial of didanosine or zalcitabine after treatment with zidovudine in patients with human immunodeficiency virus infection. N Engl J Med 330: 657–662

Bartlett J G 1993 Zidovudine now or later. N Engl J Med 329: 351–352

Beyreuther K, Masters C L 1994 Neurobiology: catching the culprit prion. Nature 370: 419–420

Bisceglie A M 1994 Interferon therapy for chronic viral hepatitis. N Engl J Med 330: 137–138

Butler K M, Husson R N, Balis F M et al. 1991 Dideoxyinosine in children with symptomatic human immunodeficiency virus infection. N Engl J Med 324: 137–144

Chatis P A, Crumpacker C S 1992 Resistance of herpes viruses to antiviral drugs. Antimicrob Agents Chemother 36: 1589–1595

Cohen J S 1989 Designing antisense oligonucleotides as pharmaceutical agents. Trend Pharmacol Sci 10: 435–437

Connolly K J, Hammer S M 1992a Antiretroviral therapy: reverse transcriptase inhibition. Antimicrob Agents Chemother 36: 245–254

Connolly K J, Hammer S M 1992b Antiretroviral therapy: strategies beyond single-agent reverse transcriptase inhibition. Antimicrob Agents Chemother 36: 509–520

Corey L, Fleming T R 1992 Treatment of HIV infection—progress in perspective. N Engl J Med 326: 484–487

Crumpacker C S 1989 Molecular targets of antiviral therapy. N Engl J Med 321: 163–171

Davey P G 1990 New antiviral and antifungal drugs. Br Med J 300: 793–798

DeClercq E 1990 Targets and strategies for the antiviral chemotherapy of AIDS. Trends Pharmacol Sci 11: 198–205

Editorial 1994 Vaccine against AIDS? Lancet 343: 493–494

Galasso G J, Whitely R J, Merigan T C (eds) 1990 Antiviral agents and viral diseases in man. Raven Press, New York

Greene W C 1993 AIDS and the immune system. Scientific American 269: 66–73

Hirsch M S, D'Aquila T D 1993 Therapy for human immunodeficiency virus infection. N Engl J Med 328: 1686–1692

Hirsch M S 1994 The treatment of cytomegalovirus in AIDS—more than meets the eye. N Engl Med J 326: 264–265

Hirsch M S, Schooley R T 1989 Resistance to antiviral drugs: the end of innocence. N Engl J Med 320: 313–314

Horton R 1993a Uncertain future for AIDS therapy. Lancet 341: 1588–1589

Horton R 1993b 'Renegade' HIV immunity hypothesis gains momentum. Lancet 342: 1545

Jaffe H S 1992 The interferons: a clinical overview. In: Jaffe H S, Bucalco L R, Sherwin S A (eds) Anti-infective applications of interferon-gamma. Marcel Dekker, New York, ch 1: 1–7

Johnston M I, Hoth D F 1993 Present status and future prospects for HIV therapies. Science 260: 1286–1293

Kocisko D A, Come J H et al. 1994 Cell-free formation of protease-resistant prion protein. Nature 370: 471–474

Lambert H P, O'Grady F W 1992 Antiviral agents In: Lambert H P, O'Grady F W (eds) Antibiotic and chemotherapy. Churchill Livingstone, Edinburgh, ch 4: 49–71

Levy J A 1993 Pathogenesis of human immunodeficiency virus infection. Microbiol Rev 57: 183–289

Lipsky J L 1993 Zalcitabine and didanosine. Lancet 341: 30–32

Lipton S A 1994 HIV displays its coat of arms. Nature 367: 113

McLeod G X, Hammer S M 1992 Zidovudine: five years later. Ann Int Med 117: 487–501

Nicholson K G, Wiselka M J 1991 Amantadine for influenza A. Br Med J 302: 425–426

Pantaleo G, Graziosi C, Fauci A S 1993 The immunopathogenesis of human immunodeficiency virus infection. N Engl J Med 328: 327–335

Petteway S R, Lambert D M, Metcalf B W 1991 The chronically infected cell as a target for the treatment of HIV infection and AIDS. Trends Pharmacol Sci 12: 28–34

Richman D D 1993 HIV drug resistance. Annu Rev Pharmacol Toxicol 32: 149–164

Skehel J J 1992 Influenza virus: amantadine blocks the channel. Nature 358: 110–111

Saag M S 1994 What to do when zidovudine fails. N Engl J Med 330: 706–707

Taylor G 1993 Drug design: a rational attack on influenza. Nature 363: 401

Timbury M C 1986 Notes on medical virology. Churchill Livingstone, Edinburgh

Weiss R A 1993 How does HIV cause AIDS? Science 260: 1273–1278

Whitley R J, Arvin A, Prober C et al. 1991 A controlled trial comparing vidarabin with acyclovir in neonatal herpes simplex virus infection. N Engl J Med 324: 444–449

Whitley R J, Gnann J W 1992 Acyclovir: a decade later. N Engl J Med 327: 782–789

Wiselka M 1994 Influenza: diagnosis, management, and prophylaxis. Br Med J 308: 1341–1345

Wlodawer A, Erickson J W 1993 Structure-based inhibitors of HIV-protease. Annu Rev Biochem 62: 543–585

Yarchoan R, Mitsuya H, Broder S 1993 Challenges in the therapy of HIV infection. Trends Pharmacol Sci 14: 196–202

39 ANTIFUNGAL DRUGS

FUNGAL INFECTIONS

Fungal infections are termed *mycoses* and in general can be divided into superficial infections (affecting skin, nails, scalp or mucous membranes) and systemic infections (affecting deeper tissues and organs). Many of the fungi that can cause mycoses live in association with man as commensals or are present in his environment; but until recently, serious superficial infections were relatively uncommon and systemic infections very uncommon indeed—at least in cool and temperate climatic zones.

In the last 20–30 years there has been a steady increase in systemic fungal infections. One factor in this increase has been the widespread use of broad-spectrum antibiotics, which eliminate or decrease the non-pathogenic bacterial populations that normally compete with fungi. Another, and particularly important factor, has been the increase in the number of individuals with reduced immune responses due to AIDS or, in some cases, the action of immunosuppressant drugs and cancer chemotherapy agents; this has led to an increased prevalence of opportunistic infections, i.e. infections with fungi which are normally either innocuous or readily overcome in immunocompetent individuals.

Primary *systemic* fungal infections are rare and usually occur in defined endemic areas in the world. In the UK the commonest systemic fungal disease is systemic candidiasis—an infection with a yeast-like organism. Others are cryptococcal meningitis or endocarditis, pulmonary or cerebral aspergillosis, and rhinocerebral mucormycosis. In other parts of the world the commonest systemic fungal infections are blastomycosis, histoplasmosis, coccidiomycosis and paracoccidiomycosis.

Superficial fungal infections can be classified into the *dermatomycoses* and *candidiasis*. Dermatomycoses are infections of the skin, hair and nails, caused by dermatophytes. The commonest are due to *Tinea* organisms, which cause various types of 'ringworm'. *Tinea capitis* affects the scalp, *Tinea cruris*, the groin, *Tinea pedis*, the feet (causing 'athlete's foot'), and *Tinea corporis*, the body. In superficial candidiasis, the yeast-like organism infects the mucous membranes of the mouth ('thrush') or vagina, or skin.

The drugs used in fungal infections are described briefly below and their clinical use is outlined in Table 39.1.

DRUGS USED FOR FUNGAL INFECTIONS

ANTIFUNGAL ANTIBIOTICS

Amphotericin

Amphotericin is an amphoteric polyene antibiotic of complex structure, characterised by a many-membered ring of carbon atoms which is closed by the formation of an internal ester or lactone (Fig. 39.1). It is insoluble in water and unstable at 37°C.

Mechanism of action

Amphotericin binds to cell membranes (like other polyene antibiotics; see Ch. 35) and interferes with permeability and with transport functions. It forms a pore in the membrane, the hydrophilic core of the molecule creating a transmembrane ion channel. One of the repercussions of this is a loss of intracellular K^+ ions. Amphotericin has a selective action, binding avidly to the membranes of fungi and some protozoa, less avidly to mammalian cells and not at

Table 39.1 Outline of the uses of antifungal drugs

Disease	Drugs used
Systemic infections	
Systemic candidiasis	Amphotericin + or – flucytosine,* fluconazole
Cryptococcosis (meningitis)	Amphotericin + flucytosine,* fluconazole, itraconazole
Systemic aspergillosis	Itraconazole*
Blastomycosis	Itraconazole*
Histoplasmosis	Amphotericin, itraconazole, fluconazole, ketoconazole†
Coccidiomycosis	Fluconazole, itraconazole
Paracoccidiomycosis	Amphotericin, itraconazole, ketoconazole†
Mucormycosis	Amphotericin and/or flucytosine
Disseminated sporotrichosis	Amphotericin, itraconazole
Superficial infections	
Dermatomycosis	
Tinea pedis (athlete's foot)	A topical azole
Tinea corporis (skin ringworm), *Tinea cruris*	A topical azole, or griseofulvin if widespread
Tinea capitis	Oral griseofulvin
Tinea unguium (nail infection)	Oral griseofulvin, oral terbinafine
Candidiasis	
Skin	A topical azole, topical nystatin
Mouth (thrush)	Topical amphotericin or nystatin, oral fluconazole
Vagina	Topical miconazole, oral fluconazole
Chronic mucocutaneous candidiasis	Fluconazole, ketoconazole†

* Drugs of choice
† The potential benefits of treatment should be carefully weighed against the risk of liver damage.

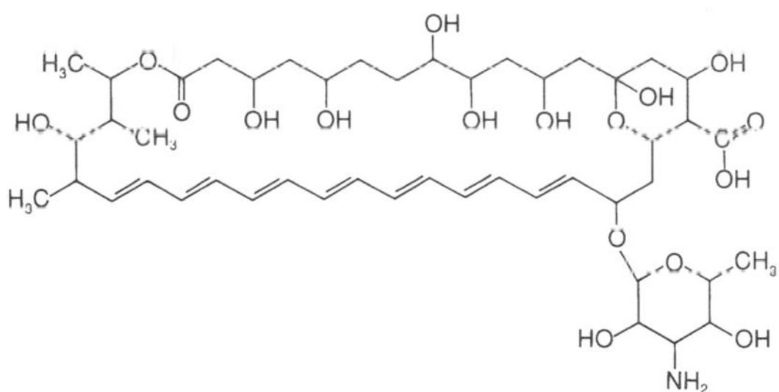

Fig. 39.1 The structure of amphotericin.

all to bacteria. The relative specificity for fungi may be due to the drug's greater avidity for ergosterol (the fungal membrane sterol) than for cholesterol, the main sterol in the plasma membrane of animal cells. It is active against most fungi and yeasts.

Amphotericin enhances the antifungal effect of **flucytosine** (see below) and may confer antifungal activity on **rifampicin**, an antibacterial antibiotic that does not otherwise have antifungal properties.

Pharmacokinetic aspects

Given orally, amphotericin is poorly absorbed, and it is therefore only given by this route for fungal infections of the gastrointestinal tract. For systemic infections it is given by slow intravenous injection. It can also be given topically. A preparation of amphotericin encapsulated in liposomes for intravenous infusion is available.

The drug is very highly protein-bound and is found in fairly high concentrations in inflammatory exudates. It normally crosses the blood–brain barrier poorly but penetration may be improved when the meninges are inflamed since intravenous amphotericin, used with flucytosine, is effective in cryptococcal meningitis. It is excreted very slowly via the kidney, traces being found in the urine for 2 months or more after administration has ceased.

Unwanted effects

The commonest and most serious unwanted effect of amphotericin is renal toxicity. Some degree of reduction of renal function occurs in more than 80%

of patients receiving the drug, and, though this is generally reversed after treatment is stopped, some impairment of glomerular filtration may remain. Hypokalaemia occurs in 25% of patients, requiring potassium chloride supplementation. Anaemia can also occur. Other unwanted effects include impaired hepatic function, thrombocytopenia, and anaphylactic reactions. Injection frequently results initially in chills, fever, tinnitus and headache, and about one in five patients vomit. The drug is irritant to the endothelium of the veins and local thrombophlebitis is sometimes seen after intravenous injection. Intrathecal injections can cause neurotoxicity, and topical applications a skin rash. The liposome-encapsulated preparation is said to be less toxic.

Nystatin

Nystatin is a polyene macrolide antibiotic similar in structure to amphotericin and with the same mechanism of action. There is virtually no absorption from the mucous membranes of the body or from skin and its use is limited to fungal infections of the skin and the gastrointestinal tract.

Griseofulvin

Griseofulvin (Fig. 39.2) is a narrow-spectrum antifungal agent isolated from cultures of *Penicillium griseofulvum*. It is fungistatic and its mechanism of action involves an interaction with microtubules which causes interference with spindle formation in dividing cells and therefore with mitosis. Impairment of microtubule function also interferes with the transport of material through the cytoplasm to the periphery, and this action is the basis of the inhibition of hyphal cell wall synthesis. In addition there is evidence that the drug binds to RNA and also that it inhibits nucleic acid synthesis. Resistance can be shown experimentally but has not been a problem in the clinic.

Pharmacokinetic aspects

Griseofulvin is given orally. It is poorly soluble in water and absorption varies with the type of preparation, in particular with particle size. Peak plasma concentrations are reached in about 5 hours. It is taken up selectively by newly formed skin and concentrated in the keratin. It is the drug of choice for extensive and intractable fungal infections of the skin.

The plasma half-life is 24 hours, but it is retained in the skin for much longer.

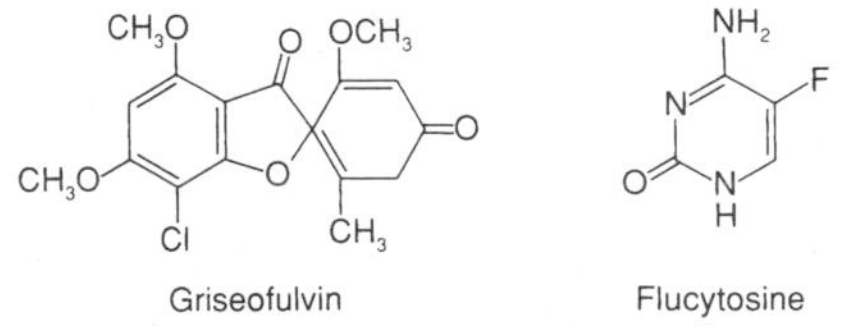

Unwanted effects

Unwanted effects with griseofulvin use are infrequent but the drug can cause gastrointestinal upsets, headache and photosensitivity. Allergic reactions (rashes, fever) may also occur.

CH₃O O OCH₃ O CH₃O O Cl CH₃ Griseofulvin

NH₂ N F O N H Flucytosine

Fig. 39.2 Griseofulvin and flucytosine.

SYNTHETIC ANTIFUNGAL AGENTS

Flucytosine

Flucytosine (Fig. 39.2) is a synthetic antifungal agent which, given orally, is active against a limited range of systemic fungal infections, being effective mainly in those caused by yeast.

Mechanism of action

The mechanism of action of flucytosine as an antimycotic is due to its conversion to 5-fluorouracil, an antimetabolite that inhibits thymidylate synthetase and thus DNA synthesis (see Chs 35 and 36). It is specific for fungal cells as compared with mammalian cells because in the latter very little of the enzyme activity is required for the conversion of the drug to its active metabolite. Some yeasts are naturally resistant to the drug, and, among sensitive strains, resistant mutants may emerge rapidly. Because of this, it is recommended that this drug should not be used alone.

Pharmacokinetic aspects

Given orally, flucytosine is rapidly and almost completely absorbed, and is widely distributed throughout the body fluids including the CSF. About 85% is excreted unchanged via the kidneys, and the plasma half-life is 3–5 hours. The dosage should be reduced if renal function is impaired. The drug is 20% protein-bound and it can be removed by haemodialysis.

Unwanted effects

Unwanted effects are infrequent and flucytosine has been well tolerated even when given in high dosage for a prolonged period. Such toxic effects as there are, are due to the active metabolite 5-fluorouracil. Gastrointestinal disturbances, anaemia, neutropenia, thrombocytopenia and alopecia have occurred, but these are usually mild and are reversed when therapy ceases. Uracil is reported to decrease the toxic effects on the bone marrow without impairing the antimycotic action. Hepatitis has been reported but is rare.

Azoles

The azoles are a group of synthetic antimycotic agents with a broad spectrum of activity. The main drugs available are **ketoconazole, miconazole, fluconazole, itraconazole, econazole**. For review, see Como & Dismukes (1994).

Mechanism of action of the azoles

The azoles block the synthesis of ergosterol, the main sterol in the fungal cell membrane, by interacting with the enzyme necessary for the conversion of lanosterol to ergosterol. The resulting depletion of ergosterol alters the fluidity of the membrane and this interferes with the action of membrane-associated enzymes. The overall effect is an inhibition of replication. A further repercussion is the inhibition of the transformation of candidal yeast cells into hyphae—the invasive and pathogenic form of the parasite.

Ketoconazole

Ketoconazole was the first azole that could be given orally to treat systemic fungal infections. It is effective against several different types of fungi (see Table 39.1). It is, however, toxic (see below) and relapse is common after apparently successful treatment. It is well absorbed from the gastrointestinal tract, being best absorbed in conditions of low pH. It is distributed widely throughout the tissues and tissue fluids but does not reach therapeutic concentrations in the CNS unless high doses are given. It is inactivated in the liver and excreted in bile and in urine. Its half-life in the plasma is 8 hours.

Liver toxicity has been reported with ketoconazole treatment, and has proved fatal in a few cases. Hepatic damage can occur without overt clinical evidence and may progress after stopping the drug. It is therefore recommended that any potential benefit of this drug be weighed against the risk of liver damage. Other side effects that occur are gastrointestinal disturbances and pruritus. Inhibition of adrenocortical steroid and testosterone synthesis has been recorded with high doses, the latter resulting in gynaecomastia in some male patients. There may be adverse interactions with other drugs. Cyclosporin, terfenadine and astemizole all interfere with the metabolising enzymes, causing increased plasma concentrations of the azole or the interacting drug or both. Rifampicin, H_2-receptor antagonists and antacids decrease the absorption of the azole and hence decrease its plasma concentration.

Miconazole

Miconazole is given by intravenous infusion for systemic infections and orally for infections of the gastrointestinal tract. It can also be given topically. It has a short plasma half-life and needs to be given every 8 hours. It reaches therapeutic concentrations in bone, joints and lung tissue but not in the CNS. For fungal infections in the CNS it has been given intrathecally in specialist centres. It is inactivated in the liver. Unwanted effects are relatively infrequent, those most commonly seen being gastrointestinal disturbances, but pruritus, blood dyscrasias and hyponatraemia are also reported. There can be problems during the process of injection—the occurrence of anaphylactic reactions, dysrhythmias and fevers. The drug can have an irritant action on the venous endothelium. Because of the possibility of adverse interactions, concomitant administration with terfenadine and astemizole should be avoided (see above, under 'Ketoconazole').

Fluconazole

Fluconazole can be given orally or intravenously. It reaches high concentrations in the cerebrospinal fluid and ocular fluids and may become the drug of first choice for most types of fungal meningitis. Fungicidal concentrations are also achieved in vaginal tissue, saliva and nails. It has a half-life of ~ 25 hours and is excreted unchanged in the urine.

Unwanted effects, which are generally mild, include nausea, headache and abdominal pain. However, exfoliative skin lesions (including, on occasion, Stevens–Johnson syndrome*) have been seen in some individuals—primarily in AIDS patients who are being treated with multiple drugs.

*This is a severe and usually fatal condition involving blistering of the skin, mouth, eyes and genitalia, often accompanied by fever, polyarthritis and kidney failure.

Hepatitis has been reported, though this is rare, and fluconazole, in the doses usually used, does not produce the inhibition of hepatic drug metabolism and of steroidogenesis which occurs with ketoconazole.

Itraconazole

Itraconazole is given orally and, after absorption (which is variable), undergoes extensive hepatic metabolism. Its half-life is ~36 hours and it is excreted in the urine. It does not penetrate the cerebrospinal fluid, but experimental data suggest that it could be effective in fungal meningitis if combined with flucytosine. Unwanted effects include gastrointestinal disturbances, headache and dizziness. Rare unwanted effects are hepatitis, hypokalaemia, hypertension and impotence. Allergic skin reactions have been reported (including Stevens–Johnson syndrome; see p. 759). Inhibition of steroidogenesis has not been reported.

Clotrimazole, econazole, tioconazole and sulconazole

Clotrimazole, econazole, tioconazole and sulconazole are azole antifungal agents used only for topical application. Clotrimazole interferes with amino acid transport into the organism by an action on the cell membrane. It is active against a wide range of fungi, including candida organisms.

Terbinafine

Terbinafine is an allylamine that is fungicidal for a wide range of skin pathogens. It acts by selectively inhibiting the enzyme, squalene epoxidase, which is involved in the synthesis of ergosterol from squalene in the fungal cell wall. The accumulation of squalene within the cell is toxic to the organism.

It is used to treat fungal infections of the nails. The drug is given orally, rapidly absorbed and is taken up by skin and adipose tissue. It is metabolised in the liver by a cytochrome P-450 and the metabolites excreted in the urine.

Unwanted effects occur in about 10% of individuals and are usually mild and self-limiting. They include gastrointestinal disturbances, rashes, pruritus, headache and dizziness. Joint and muscle pains have been reported and, more rarely, hepatitis.

Amorolfine is a morpholine derivative which interferes with fungal sterol synthesis. It is given locally as a lacquer and is reported to be effective against fungal infections of the nails.

REFERENCES AND FURTHER READING

Como J A, Dismukes W E 1994 Oral azoles as systemic antifungal chemotherapy. N Engl J Med 330: 263–272

Davy P G 1990 New antiviral and antifungal drugs. Br Med J 300: 793–798

Denning D W, Stevens D A 1989 New drugs for fungal infections. Br Med J 299: 407–408

Jawetz E, Melnick J L, Adelberg E A 1987 Medical mycology. In: Jawetz E, Melnick J L, Adelberg E A (eds) Review of medical mycology. Appleton & Lange, California, p 318–337

Lambert H P, O'Grady F W 1992 Antifungal agents. In: Lambert H P, O'Grady F W (eds) Antibiotic and chemotherapy. Churchill Livingstone, Edinburgh, ch 2

Polak A, Hartman P G 1991 Antifungal chemotherapy—are we winning? Prog Drug Res 37: 181–265

Ryley J F (ed) 1990 Chemotherapy of fungal diseases. Springer-Verlag, Berlin

Sobel J D 1988 Recurrent vulvovaginal candidiasis: a prospective study of the efficacy of maintenance ketoconazole therapy. N Engl J Med 315: 1455–1458

St Georgiev V 1992 Fungal cell envelope and mode of action of antimycotic drugs. In: Yamaguchi H, Kobayashi G S, Takahashi H (eds) Recent advances in antifungal chemotherapy. Marcel Dekker, New York, ch 2: 11–24

Walsh T J 1992 Invasive fungal infections: problems and challenges for developing new antifungal compounds. In: Sutcliffe J A, Georgopapadakou N H (eds) Emerging targets in antibacterial and antifungal therapy. Chapman & Hall, New York, ch 13

Yamaguchi H, Kobayashi G S, Takahashi H 1992 (eds) Recent progress in antifungal chemotherapy. Marcel Dekker, New York

40

ANTIPROTOZOAL DRUGS

The main protozoa that produce disease in man are those causing malaria, amoebiasis, leishmaniasis, trypanosomiasis and trichomoniasis.

MALARIA

Malaria is mosquito borne and is one of the major killer diseases of the world, causing an estimated one to two million deaths annually. It is also responsible for a staggering amount of chronic ill health. In some parts of Africa, 10% of the deaths of children under 5 years are due to the direct effects of malaria, and its contribution to the mortality from other diseases cannot be computed. During the 1950s and 1960s the World Health Organization attempted to eradicate malaria from most of the areas where it had been prevalent using the powerful 'residual' insecticides and the highly effective antimalarial drugs which had become available. By the end of the 1950s the incidence of malaria had dropped dramatically. However, during the 1970s it became clear that the attempt at eradication had failed—partly due to the increasing resistance of the mosquito to the insecticides and of the malarial parasite to the drugs—and by 1988 it was estimated that the number of new infections annually had reached the original level, i.e. about 250 million, many of these being 'malignant' malaria caused by the most dangerous of the malaria parasites, *Plasmodium falciparum*. At present about 46% of mankind lives in malarious areas (Fig. 40.2). Sporadic cases—the result of air travel—are seen even in areas such as Western Europe and the USA, where the risk of transmission is negligible. The incidence of this travellers' malaria is rising year by year; nearly 2500 cases were reported in the UK in 1990.

THE LIFE CYCLE OF THE MALARIA PARASITE

The life cycle consists of a *sexual cycle*, which takes place in the female anopheline mosquito, and an *asexual cycle*, which occurs in man (Fig. 40.1). With the bite of an infected female mosquito, *sporozoites*—usually few in number—are injected and reach the bloodstream. Within 30 minutes they disappear from the blood and enter the parenchymal cells of the liver, where, during the next 10–14 days they undergo a *pre-erythrocytic* stage of development and multiplication. At the end of this stage the liver cells rupture and a host of *merozoites* are released. These bind to and enter the red cells of the blood and form motile intracellular parasites termed *trophozoites*. The development and multiplication of the plasmodia

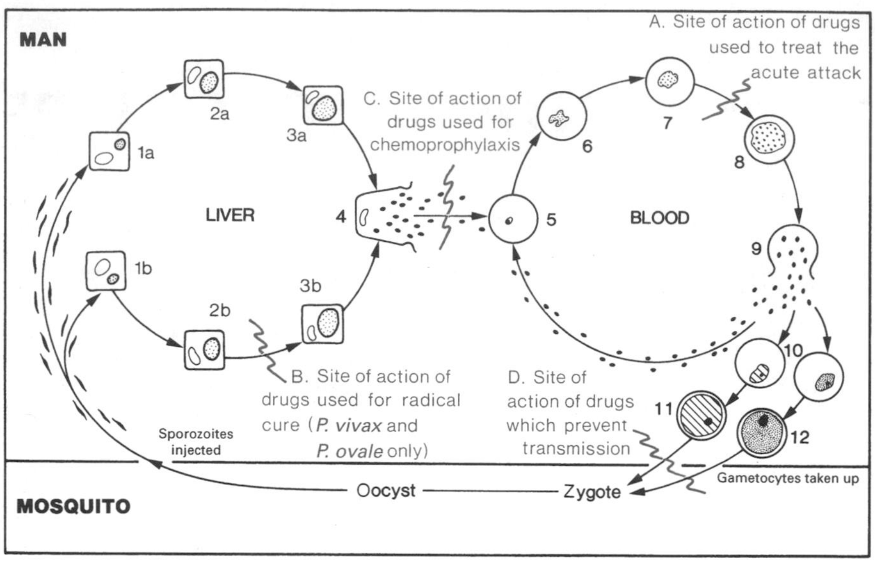

Fig. 40.1 The life cycle of the malarial parasite and the site of action of antimalarial drugs. The pre- or exo-erythrocytic cycle in the liver and the erythrocytic cycle in the blood are shown: **1a** Entry of sporozoite into liver cell (the parasite is shown as a small circle containing dots and the liver cell nucleus as a white oval); **2a** and **3a** Development of the schizont in liver cell; **4** Rupture of liver cell with release of merozoites (some may enter liver cells to give resting forms of the parasite, hypnozoites); **5** Entry of a merozoite into a red cell; **6** Trophozoite in red cell; **7** and **8** Development of schizont in red cell; **9** Rupture of red cell with release of merozoites, most of which parasitise other red cells; **10, 11** and **12** Entry of some merozoites into red cells and development of male and female gametocytes; **1b** Resting form of parasite in liver (hypnozoite); **2b** and **3b** Growth and multiplication of hypnozoites. *Sites of drug action:* **A.** Drugs used to treat the acute attack (also called 'blood schizonticidal agents' or 'drugs for suppressive or clinical cure'). **B.** Drugs that affect the exo-erythrocytic hypnozoites and result in *radical cure* of *P. vivax* and *P. ovale.* **C.** Drugs that block the link between the exo-erythrocytic stage and the erythrocytic stage; they are used for chemoprophylaxis (also termed 'causal prophylactics') and prevent the development of malarial attacks. **D.** Drugs that prevent transmission and thus prevent increase of the human reservoir of the disease.

within these cells constitutes the *erythrocytic* stage. During maturation within the red cell, the parasite remodels the host cell, a process that involves insertion of parasite proteins and phospholipids into the red cell membrane. The host's haemoglobin is digested and transported to the parasite's food vacuole where it provides a source of amino acids. This leads to the accumulation in the red cell of malarial pigment (haemozoin), which is thought to represent the residue from the haemoglobin digestion. Following mitotic replication of its nucleus, the parasite in the red cell is called a *schizont* and its rapid growth and division, *schizogony*, which is another phase of multiplication, results in the production of further merozoites which are released when the red cell ruptures. These merozoites then bind to and enter fresh red cells and the erythrocytic cycle starts all over again.

In certain forms of malaria, some sporozoites on entering the liver cells form *hypnozoites*, or resting forms of the parasite, which can be reactivated to continue an *exo-erythrocytic cycle* of multiplication.

Malaria parasites can multiply in the body at a phenomenal rate—a single parasite of *Plasmodium vivax* being capable of giving rise to 250 million merozoites in 14 days. In terms of the action required of an antimalarial drug, it should be appreciated that destruction of 94% of the parasites every 48 hours will only *maintain* equilibrium and will not reduce their number or their propensity for proliferation.

Some merozoites, on entering red cells, differentiate into male and female forms of the parasite, called *gametocytes*. These can only complete their cycle when taken up by the mosquito, when it sucks the blood of an infected host.

The cycle in the mosquito involves fertilisation of the female gametocyte by the male gametocyte with the formation of a zygote, which develops into an *oocyst* (sporocyst). A further stage of division and multiplication takes place leading to rupture of the sporocyst with release of sporozoites, which then migrate to the mosquito's salivary glands and enter another human host with the mosquito's bite.

The periodic episodes of fever that characterise malaria are due to the periodic synchronised rupture of red cells with release of merozoites and cell debris.

Relapses of malaria are likely to occur with those forms of malaria that have an exo-erythrocytic cycle, because the dormant hypnozoite form in the liver can emerge after an interval of weeks or months to start the infection again.

The chief species of human malaria parasites are as follows:

- *Plasmodium falciparum*, which has an erythrocytic cycle of 48 hours in man, produces *malignant tertian malaria*. The word 'tertian' refers to the fact that the fever recurs every third day, and it is called 'malignant' because clinically it is the most severe form of malaria and may be fatal. The plasmodium induces, on the infected red cell's membrane, receptors for the adhesion molecules on vascular endothelial cells (see Ch. 11, p. 218). These parasitised red cells then adhere to and pack the vessels of the microcirculation, interfering with tissue blood flow and causing organ dysfunction, for example renal failure and encephalopathy (cerebral malaria). *P. falciparum* does not have a significant exo-erythrocytic stage, so that if the erythrocytic stage is eradicated, relapses do not occur (Fig. 40.1).
- *Plasmodium vivax*, which has an erythrocytic cycle of 48 hours, produces *benign tertian malaria*, so-called because it is less severe and rarely fatal. Exo-erythrocytic forms may persist for years and cause relapses (Fig. 40.1).
- *Plasmodium ovale*, which has a 48-hour cycle, is the cause of a rare form of malaria. An exo-erythrocytic stage occurs (Fig. 40.1).
- *Plasmodium malariae*, which has a 72-hour cycle, causes *quartan malaria*. There is no exo-erythrocytic cycle (Fig. 40.1).

Malaria

- Malaria is caused by various species of plasmodia. The female anopheline mosquito injects sporozoites which can develop in the liver into:
  - —Schizonts (the pre-erythrocytic stage), which liberate merozoites. These infect red blood cells, forming motile trophozoites that, after development, release another batch of erythrocyte-infecting merozoites, causing fever; this constitutes the erythrocytic cycle.
  - —Dormant hypnozoites which may liberate merozoites later (the exo-erythrocytic stage).
- The main malarial parasites causing fever every third day (tertian malaria) are:
  - —*P. vivax*, which causes benign tertian malaria
  - —*P. falciparum* which causes malignant tertian malaria; unlike *P. vivax*, this plasmodium has no exo-erythrocytic stage.
- Some merozoites develop into gametocytes which, when ingested by the mosquito, give rise to further stages of the parasite's life cycle within the insect.

Immunity to malaria is known to occur and protects many individuals living in malarious areas, but little is known, for certain, of the immune mechanisms involved. The immunity is lost if the individual is absent from the area for more than 6 months. There is hope that it may be possible to make vaccines for immunisation against malaria.

The development of plasmodial resistance to antimalarial drugs

When WHO launched the Malaria Global Eradication Campaign in 1957 there were several safe, effective antimalarial drugs available. Chloroquine, a 4-aminoquinoline compound (see Fig. 40.3), was the most widely used agent both to prevent malaria and to treat the clinical attack. During the past 30 years, malarial parasites, especially *P. falciparum*, have rapidly developed resistance to chloroquine (Fig. 40.2), and resistance of this parasite to other agents has also been reported in many areas.

ANTIMALARIAL DRUGS

Antimalarial drugs are usually classified in terms of the action against the different stages of the life cycle of the parasite (Fig. 40.1).

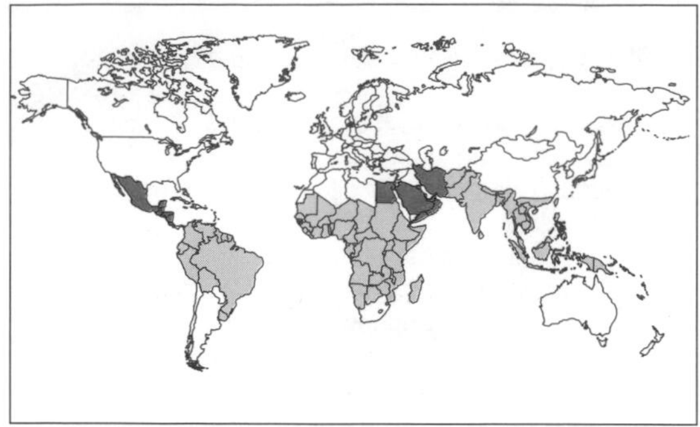

Fig. 40.2 Geographic distribution of malaria. Red areas show regions where *P. falciparum* strains are sensitive to chloroquine; shaded areas show where they are chloroquine-resistant. (Map from Centre for Disease Control and Prevention, USA; adapted from N Engl J Med 1993 329: 36.

Drugs used to treat the acute attack

Blood schizonticidal agents (Fig. 40.1, site A) are used to treat the acute attack—they are also known as drugs for suppressive or clinical cure. They are effective against the erythrocytic forms of the plasmodial organism. In infections with *P. falciparum* or *P. malariae*, which have no exo-erythrocytic stage, these drugs effect a cure; with *P. vivax* or *P. ovale* the drugs suppress the actual attack but exo-erythrocytic forms can cause later relapses.

This group of drugs includes quinoline–methanols (e.g. **quinine** and **mefloquine**), various 4-aminoquinolines (e.g. **chloroquine**), the phenanthrene, **halofantrine,** and agents which interfere either with the synthesis of folate (e.g. **sulphones**) or with its action (e.g. **pyrimethamine**). Combinations of these agents are frequently used. Some antibiotics, such as **tetracycline** and **doxycycline** (see Ch. 37), have proved useful when combined with the above agents. Compounds derived from quinhaosu, for example **artemether**, have also proved effective.

Some of these drugs are used for *'stand-by'* treatment, i.e. when chemoprophylaxis fails and the subject is out of reach of medical assistance.

For a brief summary of currently recommended treatment regimes see Table 40.1. A more detailed coverage of the treatment of malaria is given by Molyneux & Fox (1993).

Drugs which effect radical cure

Tissue schizonticidal agents effect a radical cure: they are effective against the parasites in the liver (Fig. 40.1, site B). Only the 8-aminoquinolines (**primaquine**) have this action. These drugs also

Table 40.1 Summary of drugs used for treatment and chemoprophylaxis of malaria*

Infections	Drugs for the treatment of the clinical attack†	Drugs for chemoprophylaxis‡
All plasmodial infections except chloroquine-resistant *P. falciparum*§	Oral chloroquine¶	Oral chloroquine or proguanil
Infection with chloroquine-resistant *P. falciparum**	Oral mefloquine or Oral quinine††† plus: (i) pyrimethamine–sulphadoxine‖ or (ii) doxycycline** or Oral halofantrine††	Oral mefloquine‡‡ (for short-term use) or Oral chloroquine plus (i) proguanil or (ii) pyrimethamine–dapsone§§ or (iii) doxycycline**

* The specific combinations of drug used vary in different malarious areas
† See Molyneux & Fox (1993) for more detail.
‡ See Bradley (1993), Wyler (1993) for more detail.
§ Note that chloroquine-resistant *P. falciparum* is now very widespread and there are reports of chloroquine resistance in *P. vivax*.
¶ If oral administration is not feasible, chloroquine can be given by infusion.
‖ Fansidar
** Contraindicated in children under 12, pregnant women and nursing mothers
†† Can cause cardiac problems
‡‡ Contraindicated in pregnancy, in females who might become pregnant within the next 3 months and in individuals undertaking precision tasks
§§ Maloprim
††† If patient is severely ill or unable to take tablets by mouth, quinine is given by slow intravenous infusion.

destroy gametocytes and thus reduce the spread of infection.

Drugs used for chemoprophylaxis

Drugs used for chemoprophylaxis (also known as *causal prophylactic* drugs) block the link between the exo-erythrocytic stage and the erythrocytic stage and thus prevent the development of malarial attacks. Note that true causal prophylaxis—the prevention of infection by the killing of the sporozoites on entry into the host—is not feasible with the drugs at present in use, though it may be achieved in the future with vaccines. Prevention of the development of clinical attacks can, however, be effected by chemoprophylactic drugs that kill the parasites when they emerge from the liver after the pre-erythrocytic stage (Fig. 40.1, site C). The drugs used for this purpose are mainly those listed above: **chloroquine**, **mefloquine**, **proguanil**, **pyrimethamine**, **dapsone** and **doxycycline**. They are often used in combinations.

Chemoprophylactic agents are given to individuals who intend travelling to an area where malaria is endemic. It is important that administration should start 1 week before entering the area and should be continued throughout the stay and for at least a month afterwards. No chemoprophylactic regime is 100% effective and the choice of drug is difficult. In addition to the normal criteria used in selecting a drug, the unwanted effects of some antimalarial agents need to be borne in mind and weighed against the risk of a serious, possibly fatal, parasitaemia. A further problem is the complexity of the regimes which require different drugs to be taken at different times* and the fact that different agents may be required for different travel destinations.**

For a brief summary of currently recommended regimes of chemoprophylaxis see Table 40.1. More detailed coverage is given by Bradley (1993) and Wyler (1993).

Drugs used to prevent transmission

Some drugs (e.g. **primaquine**, **proguanil** and **pyrimethamine**) have the additional action of destroying the gametocytes (Fig. 40.1, site D), preventing transmission by the mosquito and thus preventing the increase of the human reservoir of the disease—but they are rarely used for this action alone.

*Wyler (1993) heads his discussion on chemoprophylaxis 'High levels of confusion and low levels of compliance'.

**See details of malaria chemoprophylaxis, regimens for travellers in relevant copies of WHO: Weekly Epidemic Record.

Approaches to antimalarial therapy

- Drugs used to treat the *acute attack* of malaria (i.e. for suppressive or clinical cure) act on the parasites in the blood; they can cure infections with parasites (e.g. *P. falciparum*) which have no exo-erythrocytic stage.
- Drugs used for *chemoprophylaxis* (causal prophylactics), i.e. to prevent malarial attacks when in a malarious area, act on merozoites emerging from liver cells.
- Drugs used for *radical cure* are active against parasites in the liver.
- Some drugs act on gametocytes and *prevent transmission* by the mosquito.

4-AMINOQUINOLINE

The main 4-aminoquinoline used clinically is **chloroquine** (Fig. 40.3). Amodiaquine has been withdrawn because it causes agranulocytosis.

Chloroquine

Chloroquine is a very potent blood schizonticidal drug (Fig. 40.1, site A), effective against the erythrocytic forms of all four plasmodial species (if sensitive to the drug), but it does not have any effect on sporozoites, hypnozoites or gametocytes. It has a complex mechanism of action which is not fully understood. It is a weak base but its accumulation in the parasite lysosome is 1000-fold greater than is predicted on the basis of a weak base effect. This suggests that there are additional parasite-specific drug-concentrating mechanisms. Chloroquine inhibits digestion of haemoglobin by the parasite and thus reduces the supply of amino acids necessary for parasite viability; it is also said to cause fragmentation of the parasite RNA, and to be able to intercalate in the DNA. There is further evidence that chloroquine binds with high affinity to a component of the malarial pigment, haemozoin, which is left after the proteolysis of haemoglobin. The resulting complex is thought to be toxic to the parasite (see Ward 1988, Krogstad et al. 1992).

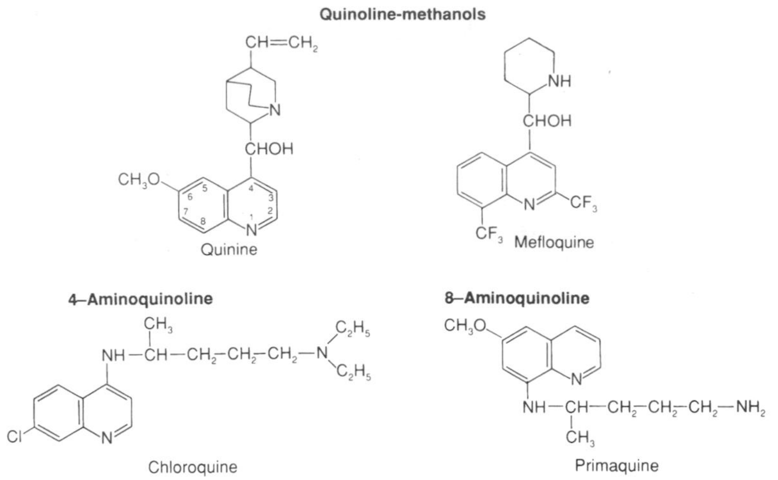

Quinoline-methanols

Quinine

Mefloquine

4–Aminoquinoline

Chloroquine

8–Aminoquinoline

Primaquine

Fig. 40.3 Structures of some quinoline antimalarial drugs. The quinoline moiety is shown in red.

Resistance

P. falciparum is now resistant to chloroquine in many parts of the world. Resistance appears to be due to increased efflux of the drug from parasitic vesicles and/or decreased uptake and/or increased metabolism of chloroquine by the parasite. There are reports of *P. vivax* resistance to chloroquine in some areas.

Pharmacological actions

Chloroquine has a fairly marked anti-inflammatory action (p. 257). It also has some quinidine-like actions on the heart.

The clinical use of chloroquine is given on page 770.

Administration and pharmacokinetic aspects

Chloroquine is given orally, is completely absorbed, is extensively distributed throughout the tissues and is concentrated in parasitised red cells. In severe falciparum malaria it may be given by frequent intramuscular or subcutaneous injection of small doses or by *slow* continuous intravenous infusion.

As explained above, chloroquine concentrates particularly in parasitised red cells. It is released slowly from the tissues and metabolised in the liver. It is excreted in the urine, 70% as unchanged drug and 30% as metabolites. Elimination is slow, the major phase having a half-life of 50 hours, and a residue persists for weeks or months.

Unwanted effects

Chloroquine has few side effects when given for chemoprophylaxis. With the larger doses used to treat the clinical attack of malaria, unwanted effects can occasionally occur, including nausea and vomiting, dizziness and blurring of vision, headache, and urticarial symptoms. Large doses have sometimes resulted in retinopathies (p. 72). Bolus intravenous injections of chloroquine can cause hypotension and, if high doses are used, fatal dysrhythmias.

Chloroquine is considered to be safe for use by pregnant women.

QUINOLINE–METHANOLS

The two most widely used quinoline–methanols are **quinine** and **mefloquine** (Fig. 40.3).

Quinine

Quinine is an alkaloid derived from cinchona bark. It is a blood schizonticidal drug, effective against the erythrocytic forms of all four species of plasmodia (Fig. 40.1, site A); it has no effect on exo-erythrocytic forms or on the gametocytes of *P. falciparum*. Its mechanism of action as an antimalarial agent is not understood, but, like chloroquine, it is known to bind to a component of the malarial pigment, haemozoin; it is also believed to intercalate in the DNA.

Quinine was relegated to a drug of second choice when chloroquine was introduced, but with the emergence and spread of **chloroquine** resistance, quinine has again assumed therapeutic importance; it is now the main chemotherapeutic agent for *P. falciparum*.

Pharmacological actions

Pharmacological actions on host tissue include a depressant action on the heart, a mild oxytocic effect on the uterus in pregnancy, a slight blocking action on the neuromuscular junction and a weak antipyretic effect.

The clinical use of quinine is given in the box on page 770.

Pharmacokinetic aspects

Quinine is usually given orally in a 7-day course, but may be given by slow intravenous infusion for severe *P. falciparum* infections. It may also be necessary to give it parenterally in patients who are vomiting. A loading dose may be required. Bolus intravenous administration is contraindicated because of the risk of cardiac dysrhythmias. It is well absorbed from the gastrointestinal tract, and 80% is bound to plasma protein. It is metabolised in the liver, the metabolites being excreted in the urine within about 24 hours. The $t_{1/2}$ is 10 hours.

Unwanted effects

Quinine is irritant to the gastric mucosa and oral doses can cause nausea and vomiting. If the concentration in the plasma exceeds 30–60 μmol/l, the syndrome of 'cinchonism' is likely to occur. This consists of nausea, dizziness, tinnitus, headache and blurring of vision. Excessive plasma levels of quinine can result in hypotension, cardiac dysrhythmias and severe CNS disturbances such as delirium and coma.

Other unwanted reactions that have been reported are hypoglycaemia, blood dyscrasias and hypersensitivity reactions.

Quinine can stimulate insulin release. Patients with marked falciparum parasitaemia might have low blood sugar for this reason and also because of glucose consumption by the parasite. This has clinical relevance in that 20–30% of patients thought to be in coma because of cerebral malaria may respond to intravenous glucose.

'Blackwater fever', a severe and often fatal condition in which acute haemolytic anaemia is associated with renal failure, is a rare result of treating malaria with quinine or of erratic and inappropriate use of quinine for a 'fever'.

Mefloquine

Mefloquine (Fig. 40.3) is a blood schizonticidal quinoline–methanol compound, active against *P. falciparum* and *P. vivax* (Fig. 40.1, site A); however, it has no effect on hepatic forms of the parasites, so treatment of *P. vivax* infections should be followed by a course of primaquine (see below) to eradicate the hypnozoites.

The *mechanism of action* is thought to be by interference with the transport of haemoglobin products and other substances from the host to the parasite's food vacuole. It may also bind to the malarial pigment, haemozoin.

Resistance has occurred in *P. falciparum* in some areas but cross-resistance with quinine or with chloroquine does not necessarily occur.

The clinical use of mefloquine is given in the box on page 770.

Pharmacokinetic aspects

Mefloquine is given orally and is rapidly absorbed. It has a slow onset of action and a very long plasma half-life (up to 30 days), which may be due to enterohepatic cycling or to tissue storage.

Unwanted effects

When mefloquine is used for treatment of the acute attack, about 50% of subjects complain of gastrointestinal disturbances. Transient CNS toxicity—giddiness, confusion, dysphoria, insomnia (and more rarely, psychosis and/or convulsions)—can occur and consequently the drug is contraindicated in individuals undertaking precision tasks. It is also contraindicated in pregnant women and in women liable to become pregnant within 3 months of stopping the drug, because of its long half-life and uncertainty about its possible teratogenicity.

When used for chemoprophylaxis the unwanted actions are usually mild and the risk of neurotoxicity is similar to that with chloroquine.

PHENANTHRENE–METHANOL

Halofantrine

Halofantrine is a blood schizonticidal drug. It is one of a group of compounds that was studied during the Second World War and found to have antimalarial activity but which were not developed when chloroquine was found to be successful. However, since plasmodia have become resistant to chloroquine, halofantrine has come in from the cold. It is active against strains of *P. falciparum* that are resistant to **chloroquine, pyrimethamine** and **quinine** and is also effective against the erythrocytic form of *P. vivax* (Fig. 40.1, site A) but not the hypnozoites. Cross-resistance with mefloquine in falciparum infections has been reported. Its mechanism of action is not known.

The clinical use of halofantrine is given in the box on page 770.

Pharmacokinetic aspects

Halofantrine is given orally. It is slowly and rather irregularly absorbed, with a peak plasma concentration approximately 4–6 hours after ingestion and a half-life of 1–2 days, though its main metabolite, which has equal potency, has a half-life of 3–5 days. Absorption is substantially increased by a fatty meal and elimination is in the faeces.

Unwanted effects

Halofantrine causes fewer unwanted effects than mefloquine. Abdominal pain, gastrointestinal disturbances, headache, a transient rise in hepatic enzymes and cough occur. Pruritus is reported but is less marked than with chloroquine. Halofantrine can produce changes in cardiac rhythm and should be used with caution in patients with a history of dysrhythmia; there have been reports of sudden cardiac death. More serious but rarer reactions are haemolytic anaemia and convulsions.

DRUGS AFFECTING THE SYNTHESIS OR UTILISATION OF FOLATE

The folate antagonists, **pyrimethamine** and **proguanil**, inhibit the utilisation of folate by inhibiting dihydrofolate reductase; the **sulphonamides** and the **sulphones** inhibit the synthesis of folate by competing with para-aminobenzoic acid (see Chs 35 and 37). Combinations of folate antagonists with drugs inhibiting folate synthesis cause sequential blockade, affecting the same pathway at different points and thus have synergistic action (see Fig. 37.2).

Pyrimethamine is a 2,4,diaminopyrimidine (see Fig. 40.4) and is similar in structure to trimethoprim (see Fig. 37.1). The structure of **proguanil** is different but it can assume a configuration similar to that of pyrimethamine (see Fig. 40.4). These compounds inhibit the formation of tetra-hydrofolate with the

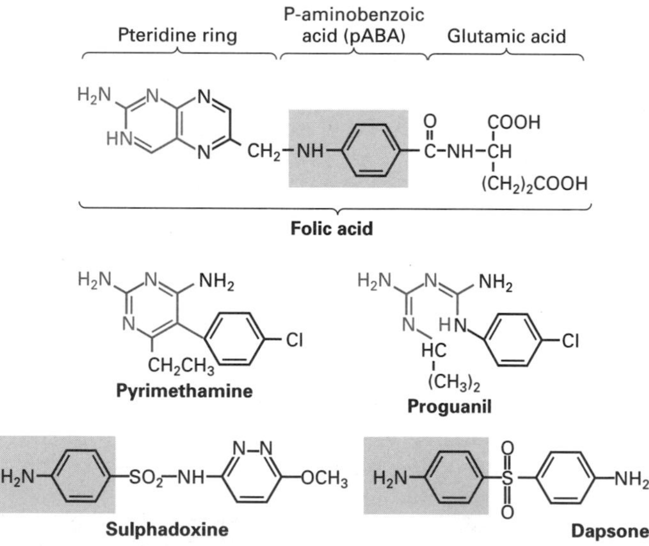

Fig. 40.4 Structures of some antimalarial drugs which act on the folic acid pathway of the plasmodia. Folate antagonists (pyrimethamine, proguanil) inhibit dihydrofolate reductase; the relationship between these drugs and the pteridine moiety is shown in red. Sulphones (e.g. dapsone) and sulphonamides (e.g. sulphadoxine) compete with p-aminobenzoic acid for dihydropteroate synthetase (relationship shown in light pink). (See also Fig. 37.1.)

consequences for DNA syn-thesis outlined in Chapter 36 (p. 706). As explained in Chapters 35 and 37, some agents (pyrimethamine, proguanil) have a greater affinity for the plasmodial enzyme than for the human enzyme. They have a slow action against the erythrocytic forms of the parasite (Fig. 40.1, site A) and proguanil is believed to have an additional effect on the initial hepatic stage (1a to 3a in Fig. 40.1) but not the hypnozoites of *P. vivax* (Fig. 40.1, Site B). Pyrimethamine is only used in combination with either dapsone or sulphadoxine.

The main sulphonamide used in malaria treatment is **sulphadoxine** and the only sulphone used is **dapsone** (see Figs 37.11 and 40.4). Details of these drugs are given in Chapter 37. The sulphonamides and sulphones are active against the erythrocytic forms of *P. falciparum* but are less active against those of *P. vivax*; they have no activity against the sporozoite or hypnozoite forms of the plasmodia.

The clinical use of these drugs is given on page 770.

Pharmacokinetic aspects

Both pyrimethamine and proguanil are given orally and are well absorbed, though the process is slow. Pyrimethamine has a plasma half-life of 4 days and effective 'suppressive' plasma concentrations may last for 14 days; it is taken once a week. The $t_{1/2}$ of proquanil is 16 hours. It is a pro-drug, metabolised in the liver to its active form—a triazine metabolite which is excreted mainly in the urine. It must be taken daily. Details of the pharmacokinetics of dapsone are given in Chapter 37 (p. 742).

Unwanted effects

These drugs have few untoward effects if used in therapeutic doses. Larger doses of the pyrimethamine–dapsone combination can cause serious reactions such as haemolytic anaemia and agranulocytosis. The pyrimethamine–sulphadoxine combination can cause serious skin reactions and blood dyscrasias and is no longer recommended for chemoprophylaxis. Pyrimethamine occasionally causes skin rashes, and in toxic doses, may affect mammalian dihydrofolate reductase and cause a megaloblastic anaemia (see Ch. 23); folic acid supplements should be given during pregnancy.

Antimalarial drugs

- Chloroquine is a blood schizonticide; it is usually given orally ($t_{1/2}$ 50 h); it is concentrated in the parasite. Unwanted effects include GI tract disturbances, dizziness, urticaria; bolus i.v. injections can cause dysrhythmias.
- Quinine is a blood schizonticide; it is given orally ($t_{1/2}$ 10 h); it can be given by i.v. infusion if necessary. Unwanted effects include GI tract upsets, tinnitus, blurred vision and, with large doses, dysrhythmias and CNS disturbances. Blackwater fever is very occasionally associated with its administration. It is usually given in combination therapy *with*:
- Pyrimethamine, a folate antagonist, a slow blood schizonticide, given orally ($t_{1/2}$ 4 days), *and*
- Dapsone, a sulphone, given orally ($t_{1/2}$ 24–48 h).
- Proguanil, a folate antagonist, is a slow blood schizonticide with some action on the primary liver forms of *P. vivax;* given orally ($t_{1/2}$ 16 h).
- Mefloquine is a blood schizonticidal agent active against *P. falciparum* and *P. vivax*; given orally, it acts by interfering with the transport of host material into the parasite's food vacuole; onset of action is slow, and $t_{1/2}$ is 30 days; main unwanted effects: neurotoxicity (e.g. convulsions), psychiatric problems.
- Halofantrine is a blood schizonticidal agent active against all species of malarial parasite, including multiresistant *P. falciparum*; it is given orally, is irregularly absorbed; $t_{1/2}$ of parent drug is 1–2 days, of active metabolite, 3–5 days; common unwanted effects (abdominal pain, GIT disturbances, headache) are fewer than with mefloquine, but serious cardiac problems sometimes occur.
- Primaquine is effective against the liver hypnozoites, and is also active against gametocytes. Given orally its $t_{1/2}$ is 36 hours. Unwanted effects are mainly GI tract disturbances and, with large doses, methaemoglobinaemia. Haemolysis is produced in individuals with genetic deficiency of erythrocyte glucose-6-phosphate dehydrogenase.

8-AMINOQUINOLINE

The only 8-aminoquinoline used is **primaquine** (see Fig. 40.3). This drug has been shown in tissue culture studies to affect the mitochondria of the exo-erythrocytic forms of an avian form of *P. falciparum*, but the details of its mechanism of action are not really known. It does not affect DNA transcription or replication.

Its antimalarial action is exerted against the liver hypnozoites. It is the only drug that can effect a *radical cure* of those forms of malaria in which the

Clinical use of antimalarial drugs

Chloroquine is used:

- To treat the clinical attack of chloroquine-sensitive malaria (i.e. for suppressive or clinical cure, see Table 40.1). It reduces the fever and clears the blood of parasites within about 24 hours; with sensitive *P. falciparum* strains, this results in radical cure since this parasite has no exo-erythrocytic cycle; with vivax or ovale malaria, a clinical attack can occur later because of the hypnozoites that may be present in the liver, unless primaquine is given subsequently. Chloroquine resistance now common.
- For chemoprophylaxis against *P. vivax* and *P. ovale* and sensitive strains of *P. falciparum* (see Table 40.1). It is given with proguanil for vivax or ovale infections to prevent a later clinical attack due to hypnozoites in the liver.
- For chemoprophylaxis against resistant strains of *P. falciparum*; it is given with pyrimethamine–dapsone.
- For rheumatoid arthritis (see Ch. 12).

Quinine is used:

- As the drug of choice for treating *the acute clinical attack* with *P. falciparum* resistant to chloroquine; it is given as a 7-day course followed by a course of tetracycline or pyrimethamine–sulphadoxine. (It is not used for chemoprophylaxis; see Table 40.1.)
- For stand-by treatment when chemoprophylaxis fails and an attack of malaria develops out of reach of medical assistance.

Mefloquine is used:

- For uncomplicated chloroquine-resistant falciparum malaria.
- For short-term chemoprophylaxis (less than 3 months) in chloroquine-resistant areas, given once a week. It is one of the drugs of choice for most subjects (except pregnant women and subjects carrying out precision tasks).

Halofantrine is used:

- For treatment of the acute attack of uncomplicated, multiresistant falciparum malaria.
- As a 'stand-by drug', i.e. a drug used if chemoprophylaxis fails and a traveller develops malaria when out of reach of medical assistance. (It is not used for chemoprophylaxis.)

Drugs that affect the folic acid pathway:

Pyrimethamine, proguanil, dapsone are used:

- For *chemoprophylaxis* against chloroquine-resistant *P. falciparum* infections. Either proguanil or pyrimethamine–dapsone is used, with a course of chloroquine.
- For *chemoprophylaxis* against *P. vivax* infections; pyrimethamine–dapsone is used, with a course of chloroquine.
- For treatment of the *acute attack* of chloroquine-resistant falciparum malaria after a course of quinine.
- For *preventing transmission* of malaria because, although not gametocytocidal, these drugs prevent the development of the parasite in the mosquito. (When used for chemoprophylaxis, the folic acid pathway agents should continue to be taken for at least 4 weeks after the individual leaves the malarious area since dormant hypnozoites are likely to be present in the liver.)

parasites have a dormant stage in the liver—*P. vivax* and *P. ovale*. It does not affect sporozoites and has little if any action against the erythrocytic stage of the parasite. However, it has a gametocidal action and is the most effective antimalarial drug for *preventing transmission* of the disease in all four species of plasmodia, thus reducing the human reservoir of malaria. It is almost invariably used in combination with another drug, usually **chloroquine**. Resistance to primaquine is rare, though evidence of a decreased sensitivity of some vivax strains has been reported.

Pharmacokinetic aspects

Primaquine is given orally and is well absorbed. Its metabolism is rapid and very little drug is present in the body after 10–12 hours. The $t_{1/2}$ is 3–6 hours.

Unwanted effects

Primaquine has few unwanted effects when used in normal therapeutic dosage for most patients. Dose-related gastrointestinal symptoms may occur and large doses may cause methaemoglobinaemia with cyanosis.

A particular side effect that is seen with primaquine is haemolysis, related to an X-chromosome-linked genetic metabolic condition—a deficiency of glucose-6-phosphate dehydrogenase in the red cells (see p. 789). This means that the cells are not able to regenerate NADPH, the concentration of which is reduced by the oxidant metabolic derivatives of primaquine and other drugs. As a consequence, the general metabolic functions of the red cells are impaired and haemolysis occurs. Primaquine metabolites have greater haemolytic activity than the parent compound. The deficiency of the enzyme is found in some black males and some white racial groups, and in these individuals, glucose-6-phosphate dehydrogenase levels should be estimated before giving primaquine and the drug must be used with great care.

Antibiotics used in malaria

Some antibiotics, for example **doxycycline**, have a place in the treatment of the acute attack of malaria; see page 764 above and Table 40.1. Details are given in Chapter 37 (p. 730).

POTENTIAL NEW ANTIMALARIAL DRUGS

Qinghaosu (artemisinin) and related compounds

These compounds are derived from the herb, *qing hao*, a traditional Chinese remedy for malaria. The scientific name, conferred on the herb by Linnaeus, is *Artemisia*.* **Artemesinin**, a chemical extract from *Artemisia*, poorly soluble in water, is a fast-acting blood schizonticide that has been effective in treating the acute attack of both vivax and falciparum malaria (including chloroquine-resistant and cerebral malaria). **Artesunate**, a water-soluble derivative and the synthetic analogues, **artemether** and **artether** have higher activity and are better absorbed. The compounds are concentrated in parasitised red cells. The mechanism of action is not known; it may involve damage to the parasite membrane by free radicals or covalent alkylation of proteins. These compounds do not have any effect on liver hypnozoites and are not useful for chemoprophylaxis. Artemisinin can be given orally, intramuscularly and by suppository; artemether orally and intramuscularly; artesunate intramuscularly and intravenously. They are rapidly absorbed and widely distributed, and are converted in the liver to the active metabolite, dihydroartemisinin. The half-lives are: artemesinin, about 4 hours; artesunate, 45 minutes; artemether, 4–11 hours.

There have been few *unwanted effects* in humans. Transient heart block, transient decrease in blood neutrophils and brief episodes of fever have been reported.

In rodent studies, artemisinin potentiated the effects of mefloquine, primaquine, and tetracycline, was additive with chloroquine and antagonised the sulphonamides and the folate antagonists.

In the randomised trials so far conducted the qinghaosu compounds have cured attacks of malaria, including cerebral malaria, more rapidly and with fewer unwanted effects than all other antimalarial agents. However, the pre-clinical and clinical data are at present insufficient to satisfy the drug regulatory requirements in many countries. Artemether may become available fairly soon.

For a review of this topic, see Hien & White (1993).

Pyronaridine is a new synthetic schizonticidal agent derived from mepacrine, developed in China. Atovaquone, a novel hydroxynapohoquinone is under test.

*The herbs are noted for their extreme bitterness and their name derives from Artemisia, wife and sister of the fourth century king of Halicarnassus; her sorrow on his death led her to mix his ashes with whatever she drank to make it bitter.

PNEUMOCYSTIS PNEUMONIA AND ITS TREATMENT

Pneumocystis carinii, previously considered to be an innocuous microorganism widely distributed in the animal kingdom without causing disease, has come into prominence in recent years as causing opportunistic infection in AIDS patients. Pneumocystis pneumonia is often the presenting symptom in an AIDS patient and it is a leading cause of death. First recognised in 1909, *Pneumocystis carinii* was presumed to belong to the protozoa, but recent studies have shown that it shares structural features with both protozoa and fungi, leaving its precise classification uncertain.

Many drugs have been used to treat *P. carinii* pneumonia. High-dose **co-trimoxazole** (Ch. 37, p. 722) is the drug of choice, with parenteral **pentamidine** (see above) as an alternative. Other treatment regimes include **trimethoprim–dapsone**, or **atovaquone** or **clindamycin–primaquine**. A combination of the folate antagonist, **trimethexate**, plus **folinic acid**, has been approved by the FDA for treatment of the pneumonia in the USA.

AMOEBIASIS AND AMOEBICIDAL DRUGS

Amoebiasis is an infection with *Entamoeba histolytica* produced by the ingestion of cysts of this organism. In the intestine the cysts develop into trophozoites. These adhere to colonic epithelial cells by means of a lectin on the parasite membrane that has similarity to host adherence proteins (Ch. 11, p. 218). The trophozoite then lyses the host cell (hence *histolytica*) and invades the submucosa, where it may secrete a factor that inhibits γ-interferon-activated macrophages (p. 243) which would otherwise kill it. These processes result in dysentery, though in most subjects there may be a chronic intestinal infection without dysentery. The parasite may invade the liver leading to the development of liver abscesses and in some subjects an amoebic granuloma (an amoeboma) develops in the intestinal wall. Some individuals are 'carriers'—they harbour the parasite without developing overt disease; however, the cysts are present in their faeces and they may infect other individuals. The cysts can survive outside the body for at least a week in a moist and cool environment.

The use of drugs in treating this condition depends largely on the site and type of infection, and different drugs may be effective in acute amoebic dysentery, in chronic intestinal amoebiasis, in extra-intestinal infection and in the carrier state.

The main drugs currently used are: **metronidazole, tinidazole** and **diloxanide**. The agents may be used in combination.

The drugs of choice for the various forms of amoebiasis are as follows:

- for acute invasive intestinal amoebiasis resulting in acute severe amoebic dysentery: metronidazole (or tinidazole) followed by diloxanide
- for chronic intestinal amoebiasis: diloxanide
- for hepatic amoebiasis: metronidazole followed by diloxanide
- for the carrier state: diloxanide.

Metronidazole

Metronidazole kills the trophozoites of *E. histolytica* but has no effect on the cysts. It is the most effective drug available for invasive amoebiasis involving the intestine or the liver, but it is less effective against organisms in the lumen of the gut.

The action of metronidazole is thought to be through damage to the DNA of the trophozoite by toxic oxygen products generated from the drug by the parasite.

Pharmacokinetic aspects

Metronidazole is usually given orally and is rapidly and completely absorbed, giving peak plasma concentration in 1–3 hours, with a $t_{1/2}$ of about 7 hours. Preparations for intravenous use are also available. It is distributed rapidly throughout the tissues, reaching high concentrations in the body fluids, including the cerebrospinal fluid. Some is metabolised but most is excreted in urine.

Unwanted effects

There are few unwanted effects with therapeutic doses. It has a metallic, bitter taste in the mouth. Minor gastrointestinal disturbances have been reported as have CNS symptoms (dizziness, headache, sensory neuropathies). The drug interferes with alcohol metabolism (cf disulfiram, p. 659) and alcohol should be strictly avoided. Metronidazole should not be used in pregnancy.

Other similar drugs are **tinidazole** and **nimorazole**. Tinidazole is eliminated more slowly than metronidazole, having a half-life of 12–14 hours. *Unwanted effects* are similar to those seen with metronidazole.

Diloxanide

Both diloxanide itself and, more particularly, an

Drugs used in amoebiasis

- Amoebiasis is due to infection with *Entamoeba histolytica*, which causes dysentery associated with invasion of the intestinal wall and, rarely, of the liver. The organism may be present in motile, invasive form, or as a cyst.
- Metronidazole ($t_{1/2}$ 7 h), given orally, is active against the invasive form in gut and liver but not the cysts. Unwanted effects, which are rare, include GIT disturbances and CNS symptoms.
- Diloxanide, given orally with no serious unwanted effects, is active, while unabsorbed, against the non-invasive form.

insoluble ester, **diloxanide furoate**, are effective against the non-invasive intestinal parasite. The drugs have a direct amoebicidal action, affecting the amoebae before encystment. Diloxanide furoate is given orally, the unabsorbed moiety being the amoebicidal agent. It has no serious adverse effects.

LEISHMANIASIS AND LEISHMANICIDAL DRUGS

There are a variety of *Leishmania* organisms that cause disease, mainly in tropical and subtropical regions. The World Health Organization estimates that there are about 1 million cases worldwide, with 400 000 new cases each year. With increasing international travel, leishmaniasis is being imported into areas where it was not previously seen and opportunistic infections are now being reported (particularly in AIDS patients).

The parasite exists in two forms—a flagellated form, which occurs in a sandfly (the insect vector) which feeds on warm-blooded animals, and a non-flagellated form, which occurs in the bitten mammalian host. In the latter, the parasite is taken up by the mononuclear phagocyte system and remains alive and viable within the host cells.

There are several clinical types of leishmaniasis—a simple skin infection which may heal spontaneously, a mucocutaneous form (in which there may be large ulcers of the mucous membranes) and a visceral form ('kala azar'). In this last, the parasite spreads through the bloodstream and causes hepatomegaly and splenomegaly, anaemia and intermittent fever.

The main drugs used in visceral leishmaniasis are pentavalent antimony compounds, **sodium stibogluconate**, and **meglumine antimoniate**, but resistance to these agents is increasing. Sodium stibogluconate is given intramuscularly or by slow intravenous injection in a 10-day course. It is rapidly eliminated in the urine—70% being excreted within 6 hours. More than one course may be required. Unwanted effects are anorexia, vomiting, bradycardia and hypotension. Coughing and substernal pain may occur during intravenous infusion. Combination of sodium stibogluconate with γ-interferon (Ch. 11, p. 243) is being investigated.

Pentamidine isethionate (see below) can be used in antimony-resistant leishmaniasis.

Other drugs used in leishmaniasis are liposomally-incorporated **amphotericin** (also used as an antifungal agent; p. 756) and **metronidazole** (see above), which is effective against cutaneous lesions. The leishmanicidal action of **paramomycin** (Ch. 37) and various **antifungal azoles** (p. 759) is being investigated.

Allopurinol (see Ch. 12) is reported to be converted to toxic metabolites in the unflagellated parasite, and since this does not happen in the host cells some selective toxicity may be achieved. It may be combined with sodium stibogluconate.

New approaches to the treatment of leishmaniasis are discussed by Olliaro & Bryceson (1993).

TRYPANOSOMIASIS AND TRYPANOSOMICIDAL DRUGS

There are three main species of trypanosome that cause disease in man—*T. gambiense* and *T. rhodesiense*, which cause sleeping sickness in Africa, and *T. cruzi*, which causes Chagas' disease in South America. In both types of disease there is an initial local lesion at the site of entry, followed by bouts of parasitaemia and fever. Damage to organs is caused by the toxins released, involving the CNS (in sleeping sickness), and the heart and sometimes liver, spleen, bone and the intestine (in Chagas' disease).

The main drugs used for African sleeping sickness are **suramin**, with **pentamidine** as an alternative, in the haemolymphatic stage of the disease and the arsenical, **melarsoprol**,* for the late stage with CNS involvement.

Drugs used in Chagas' disease include **primaquine** (see above), and **puromycin** (see Ch. 37), **nifurtimox*** and **benznidazole*** (the latter two used in the acute disease only), but there is, in essence, no really effective treatment for this condition.

Suramin

Suramin was introduced into the therapy of trypanosomiasis in 1920. It does not kill the parasites immediately but induces biochemical changes which result in the organisms being cleared from the circulation after an interval of 24 hours.

The drug binds firmly to host plasma proteins and the complex enters the trypanosome by endo-

*Not available in the UK.

cytosis; it is then liberated by lysosomal proteases. It has a selective action on trypanosomal enzymes.

It is given by slow intravenous injection. The blood concentration drops rapidly during the first few hours and then more slowly over the succeeding days. A low concentration remains for 3–4 months. It tends to accumulate, in the mononuclear phagocyte system of the host and is also found in the cells of the proximal tubule in the kidney.

Unwanted effects

Suramin is relatively toxic, particularly in a malnourished patient, the main toxic effect being on the kidney. Other slowly developing adverse effects reported include optic atrophy, adrenal insufficiency, skin rashes, haemolytic anaemia and agranulocytosis. A small proportion of individuals have an immediate idiosyncratic reaction to suramin injection—nausea, vomiting, shock, seizures, and loss of consciousness.

Pentamidine isethionate

Pentamidine has a direct trypanocidal action in vitro. It is rapidly taken up in the parasites by a high-affinity energy-dependent carrier and is thought to interact with the DNA. Pentamidine is given intramuscularly, usually daily for 10–15 days and, after absorption from the injection site, it soon leaves the circulation. It is eliminated slowly—only 50% of a dose being excreted over 5 days. Fairly high concentrations of the drug persist in the kidney, the liver and the spleen for several months. Its usefulness is limited by its unwanted effects—an immediate decrease in blood pressure, with tachycardia, breathlessness and vomiting, and later serious toxicity, such as kidney damage, hepatic impairment, blood dyscrasias and hypoglycaemia.

TRICHOMONIASIS AND TRICHOMONICIDAL DRUGS

The principal *Trichomonas* organism that produces disease in humans is *T. vaginalis*. Virulent strains cause inflammation of the vagina in females and sometimes of the urethra in males.

The main drug used in therapy is **metronidazole** (p. 772). **Tinidazole** is also effective.

TOXOPLASMOSIS AND ITS TREATMENT

Toxoplasma gondii is a protozoan that infects cats and other animals. Oocysts in the infected animal's faeces can infect humans, giving rise to sporozoites, then trophozoites and finally to cysts in the tissues. In many individuals, toxoplasmosis is self-limiting or even asymptomatic, but infection with the protozoan during pregnancy can cause serious disease in the foetus. Immunocompromised individuals (e.g. AIDS patients) are also very susceptible.

The treatment of choice is **pyrimethamine-sulphdiazine** (to be avoided in pregnant patients); **trimethoprim-sulfamethoxazole** or parenteral **pentamidine** is also used and, more recently, **azithromycin** has shown promise.

REFERENCES AND FURTHER READING

Adams S A, Robson S C et al. 1993 Immunological similarity between the 170 kD amoebic adherence glycoprotein and human β2 integrins. Lancet 341: 17–19

Bradley D et al. 1993 Prophylaxis against malaria for travellers from the United Kingdom. Br Med J 306: 1247–1252

Bryson H M, Goa K L 1992 Halofantrine. A review of its antimalarial activity, pharmacokinetic properties and therapeutic potential. Drugs 43: 236–258

Cook G C 1990 Parasitic disease in clinical practice. Springer-Verlag, Berlin

Cook G C 1992 Use of antiprotozoan and anthelmintic drugs during pregnancy: side-effects and contra-indications. J Infect 25: 1–9

Cox F E G 1992 Malaria: getting into the liver. Nature 359: 361–362

Editorial 1992 Desferrioxamine and cerebral malaria. Lancet 340: 1386–1387

Fu S, Xiao S-H 1991 Pyronaridine: a new antimalarial drug. Parasitol Today 7: 310–313

Greenwood D 1989 Antimicrobial chemotherapy. In: Antiprotozoal and anthelminthic agents. Oxford University Press, Oxford, ch 5: 65–74

Goldsmith R, Heyneman D (eds) 1989 Tropical medicine and parasitology. Appleton & Lange, Norwalk, Conn.

Herwaldt B, Krogstad D J, Schlesinger P H 1988 Antimalarial agents: specific chemoprophylaxis regimes. Antimicrob Agents Chemother 32: 953–956

Hien T T, White N J 1993 Qinghaosu. Lancet 341: 603–608

Howard R J 1992 Malaria: asexual deviants take over. Nature 357: 647–648

Hudson A T 1993 Atavoquone—a novel broad-spectrum anti-infective drug. Parasitol Today 9: 66–68
Hughes W, Leoung G et al. 1993 Comparison of atovaquone (556C80) with trimethoprim–sulfamethoxazole to treat *Pneumocystis carinii* pneumonia in patients with AIDS. N Engl J Med 328: 1521–1527
Kenter M, van Eijk A, Hoogstrate M et al. 1990 Comparison of chloroquine, pyrimethamine and sulfadoxine, and chloroquine and dapsone as treatment of falciparum malaria in pregnant and nonpregnant women, Katamega district, Kenya. Br Med J 301: 466–470
Knell A J (ed) 1991 Malaria. Oxford University Press, Oxford
Knight R 1980 The chemotherapy of amoebiasis. J Antimicrob Chemother 6: 577–593
Krogstad D J, Schlesinger P H, Gluzman I Y 1992 The specificity of chloroquine. Parasitol Today 8: 183–184
Lobel H O, Miani M et al. 1993 Long-term malaria prophylaxis with weekly mefloquine Lancet 341: 848–851
Martinez S, Marr J J 1992 Allopurinol in the treatment of American cutaneous leishmaniasis. N Engl J Med 326: 741–744
Masur H 1992 Prevention and treatment of Pneumocystis pneumonia. N Engl J Med 327: 1853–1860
Meshnick S R 1993 International congress for tropical medicine and malaria. Parasitol Today 9: 195–196
Mishra M, Biswas U K et al. 1992 Amphotericin versus pentamidine in antimony-unresponsive kala-azar. Lancet 340: 1256–1257
Molyneux M, Fox R 1993 Diagnosis and treatment of malaria. Br Med J 306: 1175–1180
Murphy G S, Basri H et al. 1993 Vivax malaria resistant to treatment and prophylaxis with chloroquine. Lancet 341: 96–100
Nosten F, ter Kuile F O et al. 1993 Cardiac effects of antimalarial treatment with halofantrine. Lancet 341: 1054–1056
Olliaro P L, Bryceson A D M 1993 Practical progress and new drugs for changing patterns of leishmaniasis. Parasitol Today 9: 323–328
Petri W A, Clark C G 1993 International seminar on amebiasis. Parasitol Today 9: 73–76
Salomone S, Godfreund T 1990 Drugs that reverse resistance in malaria. Trends Pharmacol Sci 11: 475–476
Simões A P, Roelofsen B, Op den Kamp J A F 1992 Lipid compartmentalization in erythrocytes parasitized by plasmodium spp. Parasitol Today 8: 18–21
Steffen R, Behrens R H 1992 Travellers' malaria. Parasitol Today 8: 61–66
Steffen R, Fuchs E et al. 1993 Mefloquine compared with other malaria chemoprophylactic regimens in tourists visiting East Africa. Lancet 341: 1299–1303
Ter Kuile F O, Dolan G et al. 1993 Halofantrine versus mefloquine in treatment of multidrug-resistant falciparum malaria. Lancet 341: 1044–1049
Thakar C P, Kumar M, Kumar P, Mishra B N, Pandey A K 1988 Rationalisation of regimes of treatment of kala-azar with sodium stibogluconate in India: a randomised study. Br Med J 296: 1557–1560
Vakil B J, Dala N J 1974 Comparative evaluation of amoebicidal drugs. Prog Drug Res 18: 353–364
Ward S A 1988 Mechanisms of chloroquine resistance in malarial chemotherapy. Trends Pharmacol Sci 9: 241–246
White N J 1994 Mefloquine in the prophylaxis and treatment of falciparum malaria. Br Med J 308: 286–287
WHO Expert Committee on Malaria 18th Report 1986 WHO Technical Report Series 735
Wyler D J 1993 Malaria chemotherapy for the traveller. N Engl J Med 329: 31–37

41 ANTHELMINTHIC DRUGS

A large proportion of mankind harbours helminths (worms) of one species or another. In some cases these infections result mainly in discomfort and do not cause substantial ill health (an example being threadworms in children). Other worm infections, such as schistosomiasis (bilharzia) and hookworm disease, can produce very serious morbidity. In many countries, particularly those in tropical and subtropical regions, almost all the indigenous population is infected with hookworms and/or other helminths and the problem of the treatment of helminthiasis is, therefore, one of very great practical importance.

HELMINTH INFECTIONS

There are two clinically important types of worm infections—those in which the worm lives in the host's alimentary canal, and those in which the worm lives in other tissues of the host's body.

The main examples of worms that live in the host's *alimentary canal* are:

- **Tapeworms (cestodes)**: *Taenia saginata, Taenia solium, Hymenolepis nana, Diphyllobothrium latum* (only the first two are likely to be seen in the UK, the latter of the two very rarely). In Asia, Africa and parts of America about 82 million people harbour one or other of these tapeworm species.

  The usual intermediate hosts—the hosts which harbour the larval stages—of the two most common tapeworms *(T. saginata and T. solium)* are cattle and pigs, respectively. Man becomes infected by eating raw or undercooked meat containing the larvae, which have encysted in the animals' muscle tissue. (In some circumstances, the larval stage of *T. solium* can develop in man, resulting in *cysticercosis*, a condition characterised by encysted larvae in the muscles and the viscera or, more seriously, in the eye or the brain.)

  Hymenolepis nana can have both the adult stage (the intestinal worm) and the larval stage in the same host, which may be man or rodent, though some insects (fleas, grain beetles) can also serve as intermediate hosts. The infection is usually asymptomatic.

  Diphyllobothrium latum has two sequential intermediate hosts—a freshwater crustacean and a freshwater fish. Man becomes infected by eating raw or incompletely cooked fish containing the larvae. Vitamin B_{12} deficiency sometimes occurs (see Ch. 23).
- **Intestinal roundworms (nematodes)**: *Ascaris lumbricoides* (common roundworm), *Enterobius vermicularis* (threadworm), *Trichuris trichiura* (whipworm), *Strongyloides stercoralis* (threadworm in USA), *Necator americanus, Ankylostoma duodenale* (hookworms). It is estimated that 1000 million people harbour *A. lumbricoides*, 500 million *T. trichiura*, and 500 million *E. vermicularis*, while at least 800 million have hookworm infection (Sharma 1987).

The main examples of worms that live in the *tissues* of the host are:

- **Trematodes or flukes:** *Schistosoma haematobium, Schistosoma mansoni, Schistosoma japonicum*. These cause schistosomiasis (bilharzia). The adult worms of both sexes live in the veins or venules of the gut wall or the bladder. The female lays eggs which pass into the bladder or gut and produce inflammation of these organs, resulting in haematuria in the former case and, occasionally, loss of blood in the faeces in the latter. The eggs hatch in water after discharge from the body and give rise to *miracidia*, which enter the secondary host—a particular species of snail. After a period of development in this host, free-swimming *cercariae* emerge. These are capable of infecting man by penetration of the skin. About 200 million people are infected with one of the schistosomes.

- **Tissue roundworms:** *Trichinella spiralis*, *Dracunculus medinensis* (guinea-worm) and the filariae which include *Wuchereria bancrofti*, *Loa loa*, *Onchocerca volvulus* and *Brugia malayi*.

  The adult filariae live in the lymphatics, connective tissues or mesentery of the host and produce live embryos or microfilariae, which find their way into the bloodstream. They may be ingested by mosquitoes or similar biting insects when they feed. After a period of development within this secondary host, the larvae pass to the mouthparts of the insect and are re-injected into man. Major filarial diseases are caused by *Wuchereria* or *Brugia*, which cause obstruction of lymphatic vessels producing elephantiasis; other related diseases are onchocerciasis (in which the presence of microfilariae in the eye causes 'river-blindness') and loaiasis (in which the microfilariae cause inflammation in the skin and other tissues).

  In guinea-worm infection, larvae released from crustaceans in wells and water-holes are ingested and migrate from the intestinal tract to mature and mate in the tissues; the gravid female then migrates to the subcutaneous tissues of the leg or the foot where she may protrude through an ulcer in the skin. The worm may be up to a metre in length and has to be removed surgically or by slow mechanical winding of the worm on to a stick over a period of days.

  T. spiralis causes trichinosis; the larvae from the viviparous female worms in the intestine migrate to skeletal muscle, where they become encysted.

- **Hydatid tapeworm:** *Echinococcus* species. These are cestodes for which canines are the primary (definitive) hosts, and sheep the intermediate hosts. The primary, intestinal stage does not occur in man, but under certain circumstances man can function as the intermediate host, in which case the larvae develop into *hydatid cysts* within the tissues.

Some nematodes that usually live in the gastrointestinal tract of animals may infect humans and penetrate tissues. A skin infestation, termed 'creeping eruption' or 'cutaneous larva migrans' is caused by the larvae of dog and cat hookworms. Toxocariasis or 'visceral larva migrans' is caused by larvae of cat and dog roundworms of the *Toxocara* genus.

ANTHELMINTHIC DRUGS

To be an effective anthelminthic,* a drug must be able to penetrate the cuticle of the worm or gain access to its alimentary tract.

An anthelminthic drug can act by causing narcosis or paralysis of the worm, or by damaging its cuticle, leading to partial digestion or to rejection by immune mechanisms. Anthelminthic drugs can also interfere with the metabolism of the worm, and since the metabolic requirements of these parasites vary greatly from one species to another, drugs that are highly effective against one type of worm are ineffective against others.

In most cases, anthelminthic drugs have to be tested by measuring their ability to eliminate worms from infected animals rather than by in vitro tests, since the efficacy of an anthelminthic agent may depend on its conversion by the host into a more active compound. Conversely, a drug which is active by in vitro tests may be inactivated by secretions in the alimentary tract of the host. Individual drugs are described briefly below; indications for their use are given in Table 41.1. For a review of clinical applications, see Cook (1991).

Benzimidazoles

The benzimidazole anthelminthics include **mebendazole, thiabendazole** and **albendazole**. These compounds are broad-spectrum agents and constitute one of the main groups of anthelminthics used clinically. They have a selective inhibitory action on helminth microtubular function, being 250–400 times more potent in helminth than in mammalian tissue in inhibiting colchicine binding. The effect takes time to develop and the worms may not be expelled for several days.

Only 10% of mebendazole is absorbed after oral administration; a fatty meal increases absorption. It is rapidly metabolised, the products being excreted in the urine and the bile within 24–48 hours. It is given as a single dose for threadworm and twice

*Helmins, helminthos = worm, hence 'anthelminthic' or 'anthelmintic': medicine acting against parasitic worms. (Concise Oxford Dictionary)

Table 41.1 Drugs used in helminth infections

Helminth	Drugs used
Threadworm (pinworm)* *Enterobius vermicularis*	Mebendazole,† albendazole† (piperazine, pyrantel)
Strongyloides stercoralis (called 'threadworm' in the USA)	Thiabendazole,† albendazole,† ivermectin‡
Common roundworm (*Ascaris lumbricoides*)	Mebendazole,† pyrantel, (piperazine) levamisole§
Other roundworms (filariae)	
Wuchereria bancrofti, Loa loa	Diethylcarbamazine, albendazole
Onchocerca volvulus	Ivermectin‡
Guinea-worm¶ (*Dracunculus medinensis*)	Praziquantel† (mebendazole, metronidazole‖)
Trichiniasis (*Trichinella spiralis*)	Thiabendazole,† mebendazole, (pyrantel)
Tapeworm (*Taenia saginata, Taenia solium*)	Praziquantel,† (niclosamide)
Cysticercosis (infection with larval *T. solium*)	Praziquatel,† albendazole
Hydatid disease** (*Echinococcus granulosus*)	Albendazole,† praziquantel
Hookworm (*Ankylostoma duodenale, Necator americanus*)	Mebendazole,† albendazole,† pyrantel
Whipworm (*Tricuris trichiura*)	Mebendazole,† albendazole,† diethylcarbamazine
Blood flukes	
S. haematobium	Praziquantel,† metriphonate‡†
S. mansoni	Praziquantel,† oxamnoquine
S. japonicum	Praziquantel†
Cutaneous larva migrans (*Ankylostoma caninum*); Visceral larva migrans (*Toxocara canis*)	Albendazole,† thiabendazole

* Combination of hygienic measures with anthelminthics is essential.
† Indicates drugs of first choice. Drugs less commonly used now are given in brackets.
‡ Available in the UK on a 'named patient' basis.
§ Not available in the UK.
¶ The worm should be extracted, whole, from the ulcer.
‖ See Chapter 40.
** Surgery may be needed for cysts.

daily for three days for hookworm and roundworm infestations. Thiabendazole is rapidly absorbed from the gastrointestinal tract, very rapidly metabolised and excreted in the urine in conjugated form. It is given twice-daily for 3 days for guinea-worm and strongyloides infestations, and for up to 5 days for trichinosis and for cutaneous larva migrans.

Unwanted effects are few with mebendazole though gastrointestinal disturbances can occasionally occur. Unwanted effects with thiabendazole are more frequent but usually transient, the commonest being gastrointestinal disturbances, though headache, dizziness and drowsiness are reported and allergic reactions (fever, rashes) can occur. More serious toxic effects (such as parenchymal liver damage) have been seen in a few cases.

Albendazole, the most recently introduced benzimidazole, is a broad-spectrum anthelminthic. Given orally it is rapidly absorbed and metabolised to the sulphoxide and sulphone which may be responsible for its anthelminthic actions. The plasma concentration of its active metabolite is 100 times greater than that of mebendazole.

Praziquantel

Praziquantel is a broad-spectrum anthelminthic drug (available but not marketed in the UK). It is the drug of choice for all species of schistosomes and is effective in cysticercosis, for which there was previously no effective therapy.

It acts by altering calcium homeostasis in the helminth cells (see Day et al. 1992). This interferes with the function of the musculature and eventually results in paralysis and death of the worm. The drug affects not only the adult schistosomes but also the immature forms and the cercariae—the form of the parasite that infects man by penetrating the skin (see above, pp. 776–777).

Praziquantel has no pharmacological effects in man in therapeutic dosage. Given orally it is rapidly absorbed; much of the drug is rapidly metabolised to inactive metabolites on first passage through the liver and the metabolites are excreted in the urine. The plasma half-life of the parent compound is 60–90 minutes.

Mild *unwanted effects* occur but are usually transitory and rarely of clinical importance. They include gastrointestinal disturbance, dizziness, aching in muscles and joints, skin eruptions and low-grade fever. Some effects are more marked in patients with a heavy worm load and may be due to products released from the dead worms. The therapeutic index is high; in experimental animals, serious toxicity only occurs with doses two orders of magnitude higher than those used for clinical treatment.

Piperazine

Piperazine can be used to treat infections with the common roundworm (*Ascaris lumbricoides*) and the threadworm (*Enterobius vermicularis*)—which is called 'pinworm' in the USA. It reversibly inhibits neuromuscular transmission in the worm, probably by acting like GABA, the inhibitory neurotransmitter. The paralysed worms are expelled alive.

Piperazine is given orally and some but not all is absorbed. It is partly metabolised and the remainder is eliminated, unchanged, via the kidney. The drug has singularly little pharmacological action in the host.

Unwanted effects are uncommon but gastrointestinal disturbances, urticaria and bronchospasm occur occasionally and some patients experience dizziness, paraesthesias, vertigo, incoordination.

Used to treat roundworm, piperazine is effective in a single dose. For threadworm, a longer course (7 days) at lower dosage is necessary. This drug has been largely superseded by the benzimidazoles.

Pyrantel

Pyrantel is a derivative of tetrahydropyrimidine that is thought to act by depolarising the helminth neuromuscular junction, causing spasm and paralysis. It also has some anticholinesterase activity. There is poor absorption from the gastrointestinal tract after oral dosing—more than 50% of the drug being eliminated in the faeces.

It is generally regarded as a safe drug. Unwanted effects are mild and transitory and involve mostly gastrointestinal upsets. Dizziness and fever have been reported, but no serious effects on blood, kidney or liver. It has been largely superseded by the benzimidazoles.

Niclosamide

Niclosamide was the drug of choice for tapeworm infections, but has now largely been superseded by praziquantel. The scolex (the head of the worm with the parts that attach to the host intestinal cells) and a proximal segment are irreversibly damaged by the drug, the worm separates from the intestinal wall and is expelled. Neither the larvae nor the ova are affected. For *T. solium* the drug is given in a single dose after a light meal, followed by a purgative 2 hours later. A purgative is necessary because the damaged tapeworm segments may release ova, which are not affected by the drug, so there is a theoretical possibility that cysticercosis may develop. For other tapeworm infections, it is not necessary to give a purgative after administration of niclosamide. There is negligible absorption of the drug from the gastrointestinal tract.

Unwanted effects are few, infrequent and transient. Nausea and vomiting can occur.

Oxamniquine

Oxamniquine is used for schistosomiasis; it is related chemically to hycanthone and lucanthone, previously used against these blood flukes. Oxamniquine is effective only against *Schistosoma mansoni*, affecting both mature and immature forms. Its mechanism of action may involve intercalation in the DNA and its selective action may be related to the ability of the parasite to concentrate the drug. Resistance has occurred in some geographical areas. It is given orally, is well absorbed, and is metabolised in the gut wall and in the liver to inactive metabolites that are excreted in the urine. It has a short half-life of 1–2 hours and is eliminated from the plasma by 10–12 hours.

Unwanted effects of transient dizziness and headache are reported in 30–95% of patients in various studies, and gastrointestinal disturbances in 10–20% of patients. Symptoms caused by CNS stimulation may occur and include hallucinations and convulsive episodes. Allergic manifestations and other symptoms, which appear several days after treatment has stopped, may be related to the release of products from the dead fluke.

Metriphonate

Metriphonate (only available in the UK on a 'named patient' basis) is an organophosphate anticholinesterase that was originally used as an insecticide. It was subsequently found to be effective against *Schistosoma haematobium* and is now one of the drugs of choice for infections with this blood fluke. It is a pro-drug, giving rise spontaneously to the active drug, **dichlorvos**, in vivo. Its action is thought to be due to an inhibitory effect on cholinesterases in the helminth, causing paralysis. The ova of the fluke are not affected. Given orally it is absorbed rapidly and the parent compound is cleared from the plasma within 8 hours. The serum concentration of active metabolite constitutes about 1% of that of the parent compound and both are cleared from the tissues within 1–2 days.

Effects on the host enzymes occur but do not usually result in serious physiological changes. Plasma cholinesterase activity is inhibited and there is a marked decrease in red cell acetylcholinesterase activity. Recovery from these effects takes 4–15 weeks, the plasma enzyme recovering more rapidly.

Unwanted effects occur in some patients (gastrointestinal disturbances, bronchospasm, dizziness) but usually last less than a day. Foetal damage has been reported in pregnancy.

Diethylcarbamazine

Diethylcarbamazine is a piperazine derivative that is active in filarial infections caused by *W. bancrofti* and *L. loa*. Diethylcarbamazine rapidly removes the microfilariae from the blood circulation and has a limited effect on the adult worms in the lymphatics, but it has little action on microfilariae in vitro. It has been suggested that it modifies the parasite so that it becomes susceptible to the host's normal immune responses.

The drug is given orally, is absorbed and is distributed throughout the cells and tissues of the body, excepting adipose tissue. It is partly metabolised and both the parent drug and its metabolites are excreted in the urine, being cleared from the body within about 48 hours.

Unwanted effects are common but transient, subsiding within a day or so even if the drug is continued. Side effects due to the drug itself are gastrointestinal disturbances, arthralgias, headache and a general feeling of weakness. Allergic side effects referable to the products of the filariae are common and vary with the species of worm. In general these start during the first day's treatment and last 3–7 days; they include skin reactions, enlargement of lymph glands, dizziness, tachycardia and gastrointestinal and respiratory disturbances. When these symptoms disappear, larger doses of the drug can be given without further problem. The drug is not used in patients with onchocerciasis in whom it can have serious unwanted effects.

Levamisole

Levamisole (not marketed in the UK) is effective in infections with the common roundworm (*Ascaris lumbricoides*). It has a nicotine-like action, stimulating and subsequently blocking the neuromuscular junctions. The paralysed worms are then passed in the faeces. Ova are not killed. The drug is given orally, is rapidly absorbed, and is widely distributed; it crosses the blood–brain barrier. It is metabolised in the liver to inactive metabolites, which are excreted via the kidney. Its plasma half-life is 4 hours. When single-dose therapy is used, *unwanted effects* are few and soon subside. They include gastrointestinal disturbances, dizziness and skin eruptions.

High concentrations can have nicotinic actions on autonomic ganglia in the mammalian host.

Niridazole, previously used to treat guinea-worm infection, has been superseded by praziquantel.

Ivermectin

Ivermectin (available in the UK on a 'named patient' basis) is a semisynthetic agent derived from a group of natural substances, the avermectins, obtained from an actinomycete. It has potent anthelminthic activity against filaria in man, being the drug of choice for onchocerciasis, which causes 'river blindness'; it has also given good results in early trials against *Wuchereria bancrofti*, which causes elephantiasis. A single dose kills the immature microfilariae of *Onchocerca volvulus* but not the adult worms. A well-controlled study has shown that annual treatment with ivermectin can reduce the incidence of onchocercal blindness by up to 80% (see Abiose et al. 1993). The drug also has activity against infections with some roundworms—the common roundworm, the whipworm, the threadworm, both the UK variety (*E. vermicularis*) and the US variety (*S. stercoralis*)—but not the hookworm (see Fisher et al. 1992).

It is given orally and has a half-life of 11 hours.

It is thought to paralyse the worm by opening chloride channels and increasing chloride conductance. Its binding site is different from that in mammalian species and distinct from that of all other effector molecules of the chloride channel.

Unwanted effects include skin rashes, fever, giddiness, headaches and pains in muscles, joints and lymph glands. In general, the drug is well tolerated (Whitworth 1992).

REFERENCES AND FURTHER READING

Abiose A, Jones B R et al. 1993 Reduction in incidence of optic nerve disease with annual ivermectin to control onchocerciasis. Lancet 341: 130–134

Bennett J L, Depenbusch J W 1984 The chemotherapy of schistosomiasis. In: Mansfield J M (ed) Parasitic diseases: the chemotherapy. Marcel Dekker, Basle, vol 2: 73–131

Cook G C 1991 Anthelminthic agents: some recent developments and their clinical applications. Postgrad Med J 67: 16–22

Cook G C 1992 Use of protozoan and anthelmintic drugs during pregnancy: side-effects and contra-indications. J Infect 25: 1–9

Day T A, Bennett J L, Pax R A 1992 Praziquantel: the enigmatic antiparasitic. Parasitol Today 8: 342–344

Fisher M H, Mrozik H 1992 The chemistry and pharmacology of the avermectins. Annu Rev Pharmacol Toxicol 32: 537–553

Ginger C D 1991 Filarial worms: targets for drugs. Parasitol Today 7: 262–264

Greene B M, Taylor H R, Cupp E W et al. 1985 Comparison of ivermectin and diethylcarbamazine in the treatment of onchocerciasis. N Engl J Med 313: 133–136

James, Dinah H, Gilles H M 1985 Human antiparasitic drugs: pharmacology and usage. Section C: Anthelmintic drugs. John Wiley, Chichester, p 189–268

Moodley M, Moosa A 1989 Treatment of neurocysticercosis: is praziquantel the new hope? Lancet 1: 262–263

Nutman T B, Miller K D, Mulligan M et al. 1988 Diethylcarbamazine prophylaxis for human loiasis. N Engl J Med 319: 750–751

Sharma S 1986 Advances in the treatment and control of tissue-dwelling helminth parasites. Prog Drug Res 30: 473–547

Sharma S 1987 Treatment of helminth diseases—challenges and achievements. Prog Drug Res 31: 9–55

Van den Bossche, Thienpont D, Janssens P G 1985 Chemotherapy of gastrointestinal helminths. In: Handbook of experimental pharmacology. Springer-Verlag, Berlin, vol 77

Weller P F, Liu L X 1990 Bancroftian filariasis and ivermectin. N Engl J Med 322: 1153–1154

Whitworth J 1992 Treatment of onchocerciasis with ivermectin in Sierra Leone. Parasitol Today 8: 138–140

GENERAL TOPICS

42

INDIVIDUAL VARIATION AND DRUG INTERACTION

Variability in the effect of a drug, given either to different individuals or to the same individual on different occasions, results from either differing concentrations of the drug at the site of action or from differing physiological responses to the same drug concentration. Variation of the first kind is often called *pharmacokinetic*, and may occur because of differences in absorption, distribution, metabolism or excretion of the drug. Variation of the second kind is called *pharmacodynamic*, and its possible causes are legion. In most cases, the variation is *quantitative* in the sense that the drug may produce a larger or smaller effect, or may act for a longer or shorter time, while still exerting qualitatively the same effect. In other cases, the action is qualitatively different (e.g. the haemolytic reaction that drugs such as **primaquine** cause in certain susceptible individuals with an inherited deficiency of glucose-6-phosphate dehydrogenase, p. 770). Such instances are known as *idiosyncratic* reactions (the OED defines an idiosyncrasy as 'the physical constitution peculiar to an individual or class'). A more common type of qualitatively different drug reaction occurs when individuals develop immunological *hypersensitivity* (allergic) reactions to particular drugs (see Chs 11 and 43).

Effects of various factors such as bioavailability, food intake, gastric and urinary pH, on the absorption and elimination of drugs were discussed in Chapter 4. All of these contribute substantially to quantitative variations in drug responses. In this chapter some other important factors responsible for variation in drug response are presented under five headings:

- age
- genetic factors
- idiosyncratic reactions
- disease
- drug interactions.

> **Individual variation**
>
> - Variability is a serious problem when drugs are used clinically; if not taken into account it can result in:
>   - —lack of efficacy
>   - —unexpected side effects.
> - Types of variability may be classified as:
>   - —pharmacokinetic
>   - —pharmacodynamic
>   - —idiosyncratic.
> - The main causes of variability are:
>   - —age
>   - —genetic factors
>   - —physiological states (e.g. pregnancy)
>   - —pathological states
>   - —drug interactions.

EFFECTS OF AGE

The main reason that age affects drug action is that drug metabolism and renal function are less efficient in babies and old people, so that, with some exceptions, drugs tend to produce greater and more prolonged effects at the extremes of life. Other age-related factors, such as variations in pharmacodynamic sensitivity or variation in plasma-protein binding, are also important with some drugs. Physiological factors (e.g. altered cardiovascular reflexes) and pathological factors (e.g. hypothermia) which are common in elderly people may influence drug effects. Body composition changes with age, fat contributing a greater proportion to body mass in the elderly with consequent changes in distribution volume of drugs (increased for lipid-soluble drugs, reduced for polar drugs in old people). Elderly people consume more drugs so the potential for drug interactions is also increased.

Renal excretion

Renal function in the newborn, measured either as glomerular filtration rate or as maximal tubular secretory rate, is only about 20% of the adult value (normalised to body surface area). Normally it develops to the adult level in less than a week, but in premature infants this process is rather slower. From the age of about 20 years, renal function begins to decline slowly, falling by about 25% at age 50 and by 50% at age 75. There is a corresponding change in the rate of renal elimination of drugs. The plasma half-life of various antibiotics that are mainly eliminated by the kidney is two to four times as long in the neonate as in the adult (Table 42.1); with other drugs, for example the diuretic **frusemide** (Ch. 18), the difference may be as great as 10- to 20-fold. Figure 42.1 shows the renal clearance of **digoxin** in young and old subjects, which is closely correlated with creatinine clearance. The tendency for the plasma digoxin concentration to increase steadily with age, even though the dose is not changed, is a well-recognised cause of glycoside toxicity (see Ch. 13). Renal immaturity in premature infants can have a very large effect on drug elimination. Thus, in newborn premature babies the antibiotic **gentamicin** has a plasma half-life of 18 hours, compared with about 2 hours for adults. In full-term newborn babies, the value is about 6 hours. It is therefore necessary to reduce and space out doses to avoid toxicity in the newborn. Glomerular filtration, normalised for body weight, although depressed in the neonate, rapidly increases to reach a maximum value at about 6 months of age when it is approximately twice that in the adult. Consequently if an infant of this age requires treatment with gentamicin the dose (per kilogram body weight) is greater than that needed by an adult.

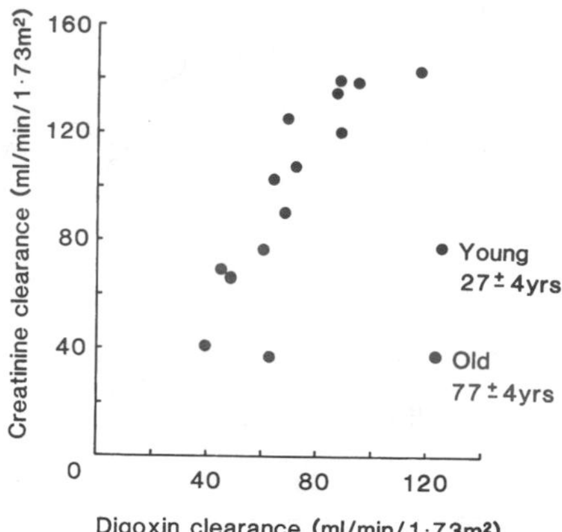

Fig. 42.1 Relationship between renal function (measured as creatinine clearance) and digoxin clearance in young and old subjects. (From: Ewy G A et al. 1969 Circulation 34: 452)

Table 42.1 Effect of age on plasma half-lives for various drugs

Drug	Neonate	Adult	Elderly
Drugs that are mainly excreted unchanged in the urine			
Ampicillin	4.0	1–2	
Methicillin	2.4	0.5	
Neomycin	5.4	2.0	
Kanamycin	9.0	2.0	
Streptomycin	7.0	2–3	
Gentamicin	18.0	2.0	
Drugs that are mainly metabolised			
Diazepam	25–100	15–25	50–150
Phenytoin	10–30	10–30	10–30
Sulphamethoxypyridazine	140	60	100

Data from: Reidenberg 1971 Renal function and drug action. Saunders, Philadelphia

Drug metabolism

In the neonate, and particularly in premature babies, the hepatic microsomal oxidase, glucuronyl transferase, and acetyl transferase, as well as the plasma esterases, have low activity compared with those in the adult. These enzymes take 8 weeks or longer to reach the adult level of activity. The relative lack of conjugating activity in the newborn can have serious consequences, as in *kernicterus* caused by drug displacement of bilirubin from its binding sites on albumin (see below) and in the 'grey baby' syndrome caused by the antibiotic **chloramphenicol** (see Ch. 37). At first thought to be a specific biochemical sensitivity to the drug in young babies, this sometimes fatal condition was shown to result simply from accumulation of very high tissue concentrations of chloramphenicol because of slow hepatic conjugation. If allowance is made for this, chloramphenicol is no more toxic to babies than to adults. Slow conjugation is also one reason

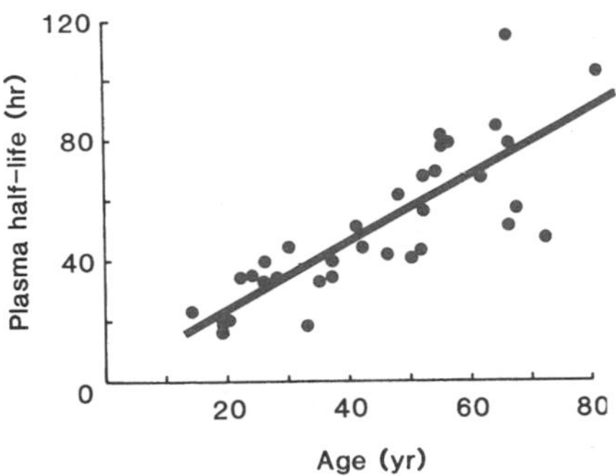

Fig. 42.2 Increasing plasma half-life for diazepam with age in 33 normal subjects. (From: Klotz U et al. 1975 J Clin Invest 55: 347)

why **morphine** (which is excreted mainly as the glucuronide) is not used as an analgesic in labour. Any drug transferred to the newborn baby will have a long plasma half-life ($t_{1/2}$), and can cause prolonged respiratory depression.

The activity of hepatic microsomal enzymes declines slowly (and very variably) with age, and the distribution volume of lipid soluble drugs increases. The steadily increasing plasma $t_{1/2}$ of the anxiolytic drug, **diazepam** (Fig. 42.2; see also Ch. 27), is one example of this. As can be seen the effect is large, amounting to a roughly fourfold change between the ages of 20 and 70 years, and requires a considerable adjustment of dosage to compensate for it. In other instances the effect of age is less marked. Even though the mean $t_{1/2}$ may not change much, there is a striking increase in the variability of $t_{1/2}$ between individuals with age, a fact of some clinical importance. Thus, a population of old people will contain some individuals with grossly reduced rates of drug metabolism, whereas a young population will not show such extremes. Apart from a decline in the intrinsic capacity of drug-metabolising systems in old age, hypothermia can markedly prolong the plasma $t_{1/2}$ for many drugs.

Variations in sensitivity

There are many examples where the same plasma concentration of a drug will cause different effects in young and old subjects. Thus, anxiolytic and hypnotic drugs such as **benzodiazepines** and **barbiturates** (Ch. 27) produce more confusion and less sedation in elderly than in young subjects. Hypotensive drugs tend to cause a larger fall in arterial pressure, together with giddiness, in old patients. **Amphetamine**, which causes excitement and sleeplessness in adults, tends to have the opposite effect in hyperactive children.

Effects of age

- At birth and in old age, renal and hepatic function are generally impaired relative to other ages, so drug effects are prolonged and accumulation tends to occur.
- Premature infants have particularly poor renal and hepatic function in relation to drug clearance. These functions mature in the first few weeks of life.
- Renal and hepatic function decline slowly and variably after middle age, so inter-individual variation is greater in the elderly.
- Body composition changes with age, fat contributing a greater proportion to body mass in the elderly with consequent changes in distribution volume of drugs (increased for lipid-soluble drugs like diazepam, reduced for polar drugs like digoxin in old people).
- Physiological factors in the elderly (e.g. impaired cardiovascular reflexes) may qualitatively alter drug effects.
- Pathological factors that influence drug metabolism (e.g. hypothermia) are commoner in the elderly.
- Elderly people consume more drugs, so the potential for drug interactions is increased.

GENETIC FACTORS

Drug metabolism

Studies on identical and non-identical twins have shown that much of the individual variability in plasma $t_{1/2}$ for various drugs is genetically determined. Thus $t_{1/2}$ values for **antipyrene**, a probe of hepatic drug oxidation, and for **coumarin** in pairs of identical twins are 6–22 times less variable than in fraternal twins. The effect of this kind of variation is to produce a continuous, roughly Gaussian, distribution of pharmacokinetic characteristics within a population. Figure 42.3 shows the distribution of plasma concentrations achieved 3 hours after an oral dose of **salicylate** in 100 subjects; genetic factors will contribute only a part of the variation seen, the rest being due to physiological factors affecting absorption or elimination of the drug (e.g. gastrointestinal motility, urine flow and urinary pH).

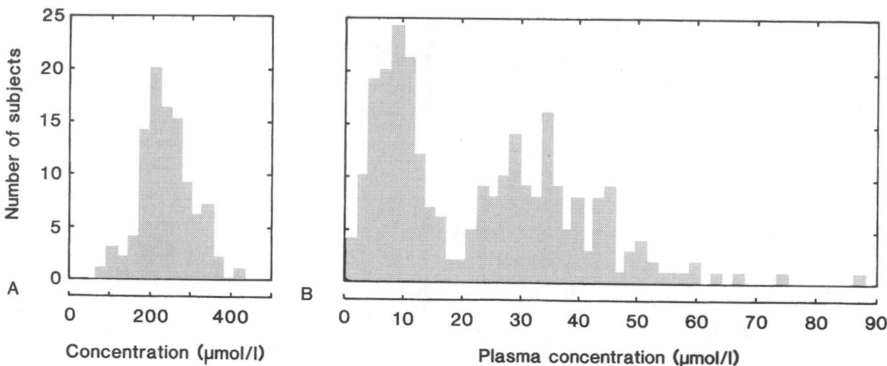

Fig. 42.3 Distribution of individual plasma concentrations for two drugs in man. **A.** Plasma salicylate concentration 3 hours after oral dosage with sodium salicylate at 0.19 mmol/kg. **B.** Plasma isoniazid concentration 6 hours after oral dosage at 71 mol/kg. Note the normally distributed values for salicylate, compared with the bimodal distribution with isoniazid. (From: (A) Curry S H 1980 Drug disposition and pharmacokinetics; (B) Price-Evans D A 1963 Am J Med 3: 639)

In some special cases, such population studies reveal two distinct subclasses, a well-studied example being the rate of acetylation of the antituberculosis drug, **isoniazid** (Fig. 42.3; see also Ch. 37). Given the same oral dose, about half the population shows a plasma concentration of <20 µmol/l, whereas in the other half it is >20 µmol/l. The elimination of isoniazid depends mainly on acetylation, involving acetyl-CoA and an acetyltransferase enzyme. The population contains roughly equal numbers of 'fast acetylators' and 'slow acetylators', and family studies have shown that this characteristic is controlled by a single recessive gene associated with low hepatic acetyltransferase activity. Isoniazid causes two distinct forms of toxicity. One is a peripheral neuropathy, produced by isoniazid itself, whose incidence is greater in slow than in fast acetylators. The other is hepatotoxicity which has been related to conversion of the acetylated metabolite to acetylhydrazine; its incidence is greater in fast acetylators, at least in some populations. This type of genetic variation thus produces a qualitative change in the pattern of toxicity seen with the drug. The same enzyme is important in the degradation of other drugs, such as **hydralazine** (see Ch. 14), **procainamide** (Ch. 13) and various **sulphonamides** (Ch. 37).

Another well-studied example of genetic variation in the rate of drug metabolism is that of **suxamethonium** hydrolysis. Suxamethonium (see Ch. 6) is a short-acting neuromuscular-blocking drug, widely used in anaesthesia, which is inactivated in a few minutes by hydrolysis catalysed by plasma cholinesterase. About 1 in 3000 individuals fail to inactivate suxamethonium rapidly. Suxamethonium causes neuromuscular block that lasts several hours in such individuals. This is due to a recessive gene that gives rise, in homozygotes, to an abnormal type of plasma cholinesterase. The abnormal enzyme has a modified pattern of substrate and inhibitor specificity; it handles many substrates quite normally, but not suxamethonium. It is most easily detected by measuring the effect of the inhibitor **dibucaine**, which inhibits the abnormal enzyme less than the normal enzyme. The enzyme in the heterozygote hydrolyses suxamethonium at a more or less normal rate, but has reduced sensitivity to dibucaine, intermediate between the normal and homozygous enzymes (Fig. 42.4). There are other, non-genetic, reasons why suxamethonium hydrolysis may be impaired in an individual patient (see p. 137), so in a patient who shows prolonged paralysis with this drug it is important to discover whether this genetic abnormality is present, and to test members of the family who may be similarly abnormal.

New examples of polymorphic variations of drug metabolism are being discovered all the time, and the list is now quite long. Drugs for which such variation is important include **phenytoin**, an antiepileptic drug (Ch. 30); **debrisoquine**, a hypotensive drug that is obsolete therapeutically but useful because it is a convenient indicator for several other drugs metabolised by the same form of cytochrome

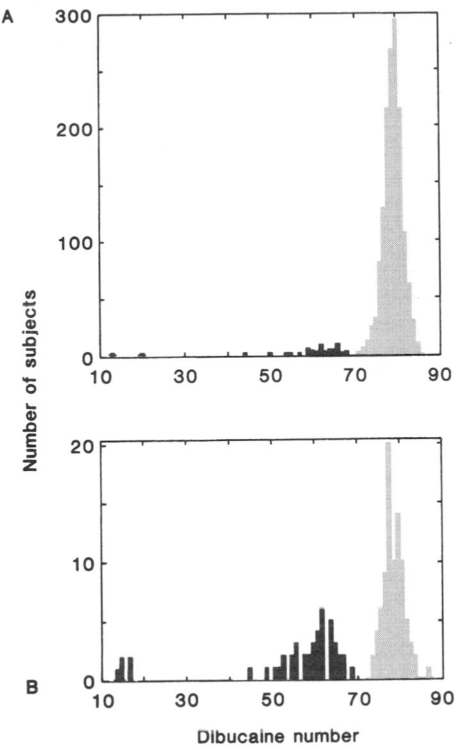

Fig. 42.4 Distribution of plasma cholinesterase phenotypes in man. Dibucaine number is a measure of the percentage inhibition of plasma cholinesterase by 10^{-5} mol/l dibucaine. The abnormal enzyme has, in addition to low enzymic activity, a low dibucaine number. **A.** Normal population. **B.** Families of subjects with low or intermediate dibucaine numbers. (From: Kalow 1962)

P-450 (Ch. 4); and **mercaptopurine**, an antitumour drug (Ch. 36).

Sex differences in the rate and pattern of drug metabolism are important in various animal species, but are seldom important in man.

Racial differences can be important. For example, ethnic Chinese differ from whites in the way in which they metabolise **ethanol** (Ch. 33), producing a higher plasma concentration of acetaldehyde which results in higher incidence of symptoms of flushing and palpitations. Chinese subjects are considerably more sensitive to the cardiovascular effects of **propranolol** (Ch. 7) than whites, whereas black subjects are less sensitive. Despite their increased sensitivity to β-adrenoceptor antagonists, Chinese subjects metabolise propranolol consistently *faster* than whites, so the cause of the difference relates to pharmacodynamic differences in sensitivity at or beyond the β-adrenoceptors.

Genetic factors

- Genetic variation is an important source of pharmacokinetic variability.
- There are several examples of clear-cut genetic polymorphism, including:
  —fast/slow acetylators (hydralazine, procainamide, isoniazid)
  —plasma cholinesterase variants (suxamethonium)
  —hydroxylase polymorphism (debrisoquin).
- Several racial differences in drug metabolism are known (ethanol, propranolol).

IDIOSYNCRATIC REACTIONS

An idiosyncratic reaction is a qualitatively abnormal, and usually harmful, drug effect that occurs in a small proportion of individuals. For example, chloramphenicol causes aplastic anaemia in approximately 1: 50,000 patients (p. 732). In many cases, genetic anomalies are responsible, though the mechanisms are often poorly understood. An interesting example concerns the antimalarial drug **primaquine** (Ch. 40) which is well tolerated in most individuals. However, in 5–10% of black males, the drug causes haemolysis leading to severe anaemia. This reaction, in sensitive individuals, also occurs with other aniline derivatives, including some **sulphonamide** drugs. The underlying abnormality consists of a deficiency of the enzyme *glucose-6-phosphate dehydrogenase* (G6PD) in the red cells, a trait that is inherited as a sex-linked recessive. This enzyme is necessary to maintain the content of reduced glutathione (GSH) in red cells, GSH being necessary to prevent haemolysis. Aniline derivatives cause GSH to drop, harmlessly in normal cells, but enough to cause haemolysis in G6PD-deficient cells. Interestingly, heterozygotic females, who show no tendency to haemolysis, have an increased resistance to malaria infection, providing a selective advantage that accounts for the persistence of the gene in malaria-endemic regions (balanced polymorphism).

Another clinically important example of an idiosyncratic reaction is the effect of many drugs (e.g. **barbiturates**, **griseofulvin**, **carbamazepine**, **oestrogens**) in precipitating attacks of acute *porphyria* in susceptible individuals. Hepatic porphyria

> **Idiosyncratic reactions**
>
> - Harmful, sometimes fatal, reactions that occur in a small minority of individuals.
> - Reactions may occur with low doses.
> - Genetic factors may be responsible (e.g. primaquine sensitivity, malignant hyperthermia), though often the cause is poorly understood (e.g. bone marrow depression).

is an inherited disorder in which one of the enzymes required for haem synthesis is lacking, with the result that various porphyrin-containing haem precursors accumulate, giving rise to acute attacks of gastrointestinal, neurological and behavioural disturbances. These porphyrins are synthesised from a precursor δ-amino laevulinic acid (ALA), formed in the liver by the action of an enzyme, ALA synthetase. This enzyme is induced, like various other hepatic enzymes, by drugs such as barbiturates, resulting in increased ALA production and, hence, increased porphyrin accumulation.

There are various other examples of genetically-determined idiosyncratic reactions. They include the condition of *malignant hyperpyrexia*, a dangerous metabolic reaction to drugs such as **halothane**, **suxamethonium** and various **neuroleptic** drugs, which is known to be an inherited trait though its biochemical basis is not well understood, and **alcohol**-induced flushing and nausea that occurs in a proportion of subjects treated for diabetes with **chlorpropamide** (Ch. 20).

EFFECTS OF DISEASE

Detailed consideration of the many diseases that are important as a cause of individual variation is beyond the scope of this book. Disease can cause altered handling of drugs by the body (pharmacokinetic variation) and/or altered sensitivity to drugs (pharmacodynamic variation) (see box opposite). Several such diseases are important because they are common, notably *impaired renal* or *hepatic function* which predispose to toxicity by causing unexpectedly intense or prolonged drug effects. Drug absorption is slowed in conditions causing *gastric stasis* (e.g. *migraine*), and may be incomplete in patients with *malabsorption* due to *ileal* or *pancreatic disease* or to *oedema* of the ileal mucosa caused by *heart failure* or *nephrotic syndrome*. Nephrotic syndrome (characterised by heavy proteinuria, oedema and reduced concentrations of plasma albumin) not only alters drug absorption due to oedema of intestinal mucosa, and drug disposition by altered binding to plasma albumin, but also causes insensitivity to diuretics such as **frusemide** that act on ion transport mechanisms on the luminal surface of tubular epithelium (Ch. 18) because of binding to albumin in tubular fluid. *Hypothyroidism* is associated with increased sensitivity to several widely used drugs (e.g. **pethidine**), for reasons that are poorly understood.

Other disorders, although unusual, are important because they illustrate mechanisms of variability of responsiveness to drugs that may prove to be of more general applicability. Examples include:

- *Diseases that influence receptors*, for example:
  - *myasthenia gravis*, an autoallergic disease characterised by antibodies to acetylcholine receptors at the neuromuscular junction (Ch. 6)

> **Variation due to disease**
>
> **Pharmacokinetic alterations**
> - In absorption:
>   - gastric stasis (e.g. migraine)
>   - malabsorption (e.g. steatorrhoea from pancreatic insufficiency)
>   - oedema of ileal mucosa (e.g. heart failure, nephrotic syndrome).
> - In distribution:
>   - altered plasma protein binding (e.g. of phenytoin in chronic renal failure)
>   - impaired blood–brain barrier (e.g. to penicillin in meningitis).
> - In metabolism:
>   - hepatic cirrhosis and portal hypertension
>   - hypothermia.
> - In excretion:
>   - acute and/or chronic renal failure.
>
> **Pharmacodynamic alterations**
> - In receptors (e.g. myasthenia gravis, nephrogenic diabetes insipidus, familial hypercholesterolaemia).
> - In signal transduction (e.g. pseudohypoparathyroidism, familial precocious puberty, functioning thyroid adenoma).
> - Mechanism unknown (e.g. increased sensitivity to pethidine in hypothyroidism).

- X-linked *nephrogenic diabetes insipidus*, characterised by an abnormality in vasopressin receptors
- *familial hypercholesterolaemia*, an inherited disease of LDL-receptors (Ch. 15).

- *Diseases that influence signal transduction mechanisms*, for example:
  - *pseudohypoparathyroidism*, a disease that stems from impaired coupling of receptors with adenylate cyclase
  - *familial precocious puberty*, and hyperthyroidism caused by *functioning thyroid adenomas*, which are each caused by mutations in G-protein-coupled receptors that result in the receptors remaining 'turned on' even in the absence of the hormones that are their natural agonists (Parma et al. 1993, Shenker et al. 1993).

DRUG INTERACTIONS

The administration of one drug (A) can alter the action of another (B) by one of two general mechanisms, namely modification of the pharmacological action of B without altering its concentration in the tissue fluid (i.e. *pharmacodynamic interactions*) or alteration of the concentration of B that reaches its site of action (i.e. *pharmacokinetic interactions*).* For such interactions to be important clinically it is necessary that the therapeutic range of drug B is narrow (i.e. that a small reduction in effect will lead to loss of efficacy and/or a small increase in effect will lead to toxicity). For pharmacokinetic interactions to be clinically important it is also necessary that the concentration–response curve of drug B is steep (so that a small change in plasma concentration leads to a substantial change in effect). For many drugs these conditions are not met: even quite large changes in plasma concentrations of relatively non-toxic drugs like **penicillin** are unlikely to give rise to clinical problems because there is usually a comfortable safety margin between plasma concentrations produced by usual doses and those resulting in either loss of efficacy or toxicity. Several cardiovascular drugs, in particular, do have steep concentration–response relationships and a narrow therapeutic margin, and drug interactions can cause major problems with **antithrombotic** and **antidysrhythmic** drugs, as well as **anticonvulsants**, **lithium** and several **antineoplastic** and **immunosuppressant** drugs.

*A third category of *pharmaceutical interactions* should be mentioned, in which drugs interact in vitro so that one or both are inactivated. No pharmacological principles are involved, just chemistry. An example is the formation of a complex between **thiopentone** and **suxamethonium**, which must not be mixed in the same syringe. **Heparin** is highly acidic and interacts in this way with many basic drugs; it is sometimes used to keep intravenous lines or cannulae open, and can interact with such drugs if they are injected without first clearing the line with saline.

Pharmacodynamic interaction

Pharmacodynamic interaction can occur in many different ways (including those discussed under 'Drug antagonism' in Ch. 1). There are many mechanisms, and some examples of practical importance are probably more useful than attempts at classification. Consider the following:

- **β-receptor antagonists** diminish the effectiveness of bronchodilators, such as **salbutamol** or **terbutaline**, that are β-receptor agonists (Ch. 7).
- Many **diuretics** lower plasma potassium concentration (see Ch. 18), and thereby enhance some actions of **cardiac glycosides** and predispose to glycoside toxicity (Ch. 13).
- **Monoamine oxidase inhibitors** increase the amount of noradrenaline stored in noradrenergic nerve terminals and thereby enhance the actions of drugs such as **ephedrine** and **tyramine**, which work by releasing stored noradrenaline.
- **Warfarin** works by competition with vitamin K, preventing hepatic synthesis of various coagulation factors (see Ch. 16). If vitamin K production in the intestine is inhibited (e.g. by **antibiotics**), the anticoagulant action of warfarin is increased. Drugs that cause bleeding by distinct mechanisms (e.g. **aspirin**, which inhibits platelet thromboxane A_2 biosynthesis and can cause gastric ulceration) increase the bleeding tendency caused by warfarin.
- **Sulphonamides** prevent the synthesis of folic acid by bacteria and other microorganisms; **trimethoprim** inhibits its reduction to tetrahydrofolate. Given together the drugs have a synergistic action of value in treating *Pneumocystis carinii* (Ch. 40).
- **Non-steroidal anti-inflammatory drugs** (NSAIDs; Ch. 12), such as **ibuprofen** or **indo-**

methacin, inhibit biosynthesis of prostaglandins, including renal vasodilator/natriuretic prostaglandins (PGE_2, PGI_2). If administered to patients receiving treatment for hypertension with any of a variety of drugs with quite different mechanisms of antihypertensive action (e.g. **β-adrenoceptor antagonists, diuretics, angiotensin-converting enzyme inhibitors**) they cause variable but sometimes marked loss of antihypertensive control.

- **H_1-receptor antagonists**, such as **mepyramine**, commonly cause drowsiness as an unwanted effect. This is more troublesome if such drugs are taken with **alcohol**, and may lead to accidents at work or on the road.

Pharmacokinetic interaction

All of the four major processes that determine the pharmacokinetic behaviour of a drug—absorption, distribution, metabolism and excretion—can be affected by co-administration of other drugs. Such interactions have received a great deal of attention, and examples have sprouted in the literature like mushrooms. Some of the more important mechanisms are given here, with examples.

Absorption phase

Gastrointestinal absorption may be slowed by drugs that inhibit gastrointestinal motility, such as **atropine** or **opiates**, or accelerated by drugs (e.g. **metoclopramide**; see Ch. 19) which hasten gastric emptying. Alternatively, drug A may interact with drug B in the gut in such a way as to inhibit absorption of B (cf. pharmaceutical interactions; see footnote, p. 791). Thus calcium (and also iron) forms an insoluble complex with **tetracycline** antibiotics and retards their absorption; **cholestyramine**, a bile acid binding resin used to treat hypercholesterolaemia (Ch. 15), binds several drugs (e.g. **warfarin, digoxin**) preventing their absorption if administered simultaneously. Another example is the addition of **adrenaline** to local anaesthetic injections for infiltration anaesthesia (Ch. 34). The vasoconstriction slows the absorption of the anaesthetic, thus prolonging its local effect.

Effects on drug distribution

One drug may alter the distribution of another, but such interactions are seldom clinically important. Displacement of a drug from binding sites in plasma or tissues transiently increases the concentration of *free* (unbound) drug, but this is followed by increased elimination so a new steady state results in which *total* drug concentration in plasma is reduced, and the free drug concentration is similar to that before introduction of the second 'displacing' drug. There are several direct consequences of potential clinical importance:

- toxicity from the transient increase in concentration of free drug, before the new steady state is reached
- if dose is being adjusted according to measurements of total plasma concentration, it must be appreciated that the target therapeutic range of concentrations will be altered by a second drug that displaces it from binding sites.
- when the displacing drug additionally reduces elimination of the first, so that not only is the free concentration increased acutely, but the free concentration is also increased chronically at the new steady state, severe toxicity may ensue.

Though many drugs have appreciable affinity for plasma albumin and therefore might potentially be expected to interact, there are rather few instances of clinically important interactions of this type. Protein-bound drugs that are given in large enough dosage to act as 'displacing agents' include **aspirin** and various **sulphonamides**, as well as **chloral hydrate** whose metabolite, trichloracetic acid, binds very strongly to plasma albumin. Displacement of *bilirubin* from albumin by such drugs in jaundiced premature neonates could have clinically disastrous consequences: bilirubin metabolism is undeveloped in the premature liver, and unbound bilirubin can cross the blood–brain barrier and cause *kernicterus* (staining of the basal ganglia by bilirubin, which causes a distressing disturbance of movement known as choreoathetosis, characterised by writhing and twisting involuntary movements in the child).

Phenytoin dose is adjusted according to measurement of its concentration in plasma, and such measurements do not routinely distinguish bound from free phenytoin (that is, they reflect the total concentration of drug). Introduction of a displacing drug in an epileptic patient stabilised on phenytoin (Ch. 30) will result in a reduction in total plasma phenytoin concentration due to increased elimination of free drug, but no loss of efficacy because the free concentration at the new steady state is unaltered. If it is not appreciated that the therapeutic range of plasma concentrations has been reduced in this way, an increased dose may be prescribed resulting in toxicity.

There are several instances where drugs that alter protein binding additionally reduce elimination of the displaced drug, causing clinically important interactions. **Phenylbutazone** displaces **warfarin** from binding sites on albumin and more importantly selectively inhibits metabolism of the pharmacologically active *S* isomer (see below), prolonging prothrombin time and resulting in increased bleeding (Ch. 16). **Salicylates** displace **methotrexate** from binding sites on albumin and reduce its secretion into the nephron by competition with the anion secretory carrier (Ch. 4). **Quinidine** and several other antidysrhythmic drugs including **verapamil** and **amiodarone** (Ch. 13) displace **digoxin** from tissue-binding sites while simultaneously reducing its renal excretion, and can consequently cause severe dysrhythmias due to digoxin toxicity.

Effects on drug metabolism

Some examples of drugs that inhibit or induce drug metabolism are shown in Table 42.2. Enzyme induction (e.g. by **barbiturates**, **ethanol** or **rifampicin**; see Ch. 4) is an important cause of drug interaction. At least 200 drugs are known that cause enzyme induction and can thereby decrease the pharmacological activity of a range of other drugs. Since the inducing agent is normally itself a substrate for the induced enzymes, the process can result in slowly developing tolerance, although this pharmacokinetic kind of tolerance is generally less important clinically than tolerance that results from pharmacodynamic adaptations (e.g. to **opioid analgesics**; Ch. 31), and the lethal dose of inducing drugs such as the barbiturates is only moderately increased in chronic users. Conversely, enzyme induction can increase toxicity of a second drug whose toxic effects are mediated via a metabolite. **Paracetamol** toxicity is a case in point (see Fig. 43.1): it is due to N-acetyl-benzoquinone imine, which is formed by cytochrome P-450. Consequently the risk of serious hepatic injury following paracetamol overdose is increased in patients whose cytochrome P-450 system has been induced by chronic use of **barbiturates** or **alcohol**.

There are many examples of clinically important drug interactions resulting from enzyme induction, a few of which are listed in Table 42.2. Figure 42.5 shows how the antibiotic **rifampicin**, given for 3

Table 42.2 Examples of drugs that induce or inhibit drug-metabolising enzymes

Drugs modifying enzyme action	Drugs whose metabolism is affected
Enzyme induction	
Phenobarbitone and other barbiturates Rifampicin Griseofulvin Phenytoin Ethanol Carbamazepine	Warfarin Oral contraceptives Corticosteroids Cyclosporin (as well as drugs listed in left-hand column)
Enzyme inhibition	
Disulfiram	Warfarin
Allopurinol	Mercaptopurine, azathioprine
Ecothiopate and other anticholinesterases	Suxamethonium, procaine, propanidid
Chloramphenicol	Phenytoin
Corticosteroids	Various drugs, e.g. tricyclic antidepressants, cyclophosphamide
Cimetidine	Many drugs, e.g. amiodarone, phenytoin, pethidine
MAO inhibitors	Pethidine
Erythromycin	Cyclosporin, theophylline
Ciprofloxacin	Theophylline

days, reduces the effectiveness of **warfarin** as an anticoagulant. It is likely that part of the variability in rates of drug metabolism between individuals results from varying exposure to environmental contaminants, some of which are strong enzyme inducers.

Enzyme induction can serve a useful purpose. Excessive neonatal jaundice can cause brain damage because unconjugated bilirubin penetrates the blood–brain barrier. Administration of **phenobarbitone** to induce glucuronyl transferase increases bilirubin conjugation and reduces this risk.

Enzyme inhibition, particularly of the P-450 system, occurs with a number of drugs. This can slow the metabolism, and hence increase the action, of various other drugs. The effects can be clinically important, but it is difficult to predict which drugs will interact in this way, because there is marked selectivity in the inhibition of different cytochromes P-450 by different agents. To make life even more difficult, several inhibitors of drug metabolism influence metabolism of different stereoisomers selectively. Examples of drugs that inhibit the metabolism of the active *S* and less active *R* isomers of warfarin in this way are shown in Table 42.3.

Table 42.3 Stereoselective and non-stereoselective inhibition of warfarin metabolism

Stereoselective inhibition of clearance of *S* isomer
Phenylbutazone
Metronidazole
Sulphinpyrazone
Trimethoprim–sulphamethoxazole
Disulfiram
Stereoselective inhibition of clearance of *R* isomer
Cimetidine*
Omeprazole*
Non-stereoselective inhibition of clearance of *R* and *S* isomers
Amiodarone

* Minor effect only on prothrombin time
From: Hirsh J 1991 N Engl J Med 324: 1865–1875

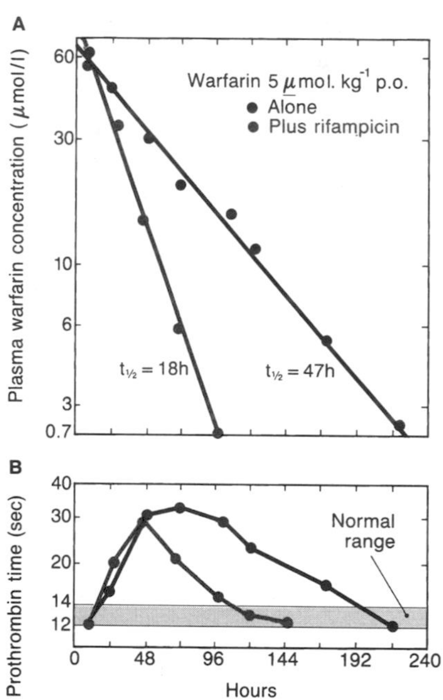

Fig. 42.5 Effect of rifampicin on the metabolism and anticoagulant action of warfarin. **A.** Plasma concentration of warfarin (log scale) as a function of time following a single oral dose. After the subject was given rifampicin (600 mg daily for a few days), the plasma half-life of warfarin decreased from the normal value of 47 hours (black curve) to 18 hours (red curve). **B.** The effect of a single dose of warfarin on prothrombin time under normal conditions (black curve) and after rifampicin administration (red curve). (Redrawn from: O'Reilly 1974 Ann Intern Med 81: 337)

The therapeutic effects of some drugs are a direct consequence of enzyme inhibition (e.g. the xanthine oxidase inhibitor, **allopurinol**, used in prevention of gout; Ch. 12), and it is coincidental that their target enzymes also play a role in the metabolism of other drugs. Xanthine oxidase also metabolises certain cytotoxic and immunosuppressant drugs, such as **mercaptopurine** (the active metabolite of **azathioprine**), whose action is thus potentiated and prolonged by allopurinol. Similarly, **disulfiram**, an inhibitor of aldehyde dehydrogenase used to produce an aversive reaction to **ethanol** (see Ch. 33), also inhibits metabolism of other drugs, such as **warfarin** and some **benzodiazepines**, and consequently prolongs their action. **Metronidazole**, an antimicrobial used to treat anaerobic bacterial infections and several protozoal diseases (Chs 37 and 40) also inhibits this enzyme, and patients prescribed it need to be advised to avoid alcohol for this reason.

In other cases the inhibition of drug metabolism is rather unexpected, since enzyme inhibition is not the main mechanism of action of the offending agents. Thus **steroids** and **cimetidine** enhance the actions of a range of drugs including some **antidepressants** and some **cytotoxic** drugs. The only rule for prescribers is: if in doubt about the existence of a possible interaction, look it up (e.g. in the British National Formulary).

Haemodynamic effects

If a drug (e.g. **lignocaine** or **propranolol**) is subject to extensive first-pass hepatic metabolism, then variations in hepatic blood flow significantly affect the rate at which it is inactivated. A reduction in cardiac output reduces hepatic blood flow, and negatively inotropic drugs (e.g. propranolol) reduce the rate of metabolism of lignocaine by this mechanism.

Effects on drug excretion

The main mechanisms by which one drug can affect the rate of renal excretion of another are:

- by altering protein binding, and hence rate of filtration
- by inhibiting tubular secretion
- by altering urine flow and/or urine pH.

Effects on protein binding have been discussed already (see Ch. 4). In general, reduction of protein binding has only a small effect on renal excretion, and it can be in either direction.

Table 42.4 Examples of drugs that inhibit renal tubular secretion

Drugs causing inhibition	Drugs whose $t_{½}$ may be affected
Probenecid Sulphinpyrazone Phenylbutazone Sulphonamides Aspirin Thiazide diuretics Indomethacin	Penicillin Azidothymidine Indomethacin
Verapamil Amiodarone Quinidine	Digoxin
Diuretics	Lithium
Indomethacin	Frusemide
Aspirin NSAID	Methotrexate

> **Drug interactions**
>
> - They are many and varied; the rule is: if in doubt, look it up.
> - Interactions may be pharmacodynamic or pharmacokinetic in origin.
> - Pharmacodynamic interactions are often predictable from the actions of the interacting drugs.
> - Pharmacokinetic interactions can involve:
>   —effects on drug absorption
>   —effects on distribution (e.g. competition for protein binding)
>   —effects on hepatic metabolism (induction or inhibition)
>   —effects on renal excretion.

Inhibition of tubular secretion. The clearest example is **probenecid** (Ch. 18), which was developed expressly to inhibit penicillin secretion and thus prolong its action. Other drugs have an incidental probenecid-like effect which can enhance the actions of substances that rely on tubular secretion for their elimination. Table 42.4 gives some examples.

Alteration of urine flow and pH. Not surprisingly, diuretic drugs tend to increase the urinary excretion of other drugs. Thus **frusemide** (see Ch. 18) increases the rate of excretion of **indomethacin** and lowers its plasma concentration. There are not many reported examples of accidental interactions based on this mechanism. Similarly, the effect of urinary pH on the excretion of weak acids and bases (see Ch. 4) is put to use in the treatment of poisoning, though it is not a cause of accidental interactions.

REFERENCES AND FURTHER READING

Caldwell J, Jakoby W B 1983 Biological basis of detoxication. Academic Press, London

Curry S H 1980 Drug disposition and metabolism. Blackwell, Oxford

du Sonich P, Lambert C 1983 What is the clinical meaning of the acetylator phenotype? In: Lamble J W (ed) Drug metabolism and distribution. Elsevier, Amsterdam

Gibaldi M 1984 Biopharmaceutics and clinical pharmacokinetics. Lea & Febiger, Philadelphia

Gibaldi M, Prescott L 1983 Handbook of clinical pharmacokinetics. ADIS Health Science Press, Sydney

Gorrod J W, Beckett A H 1978 Drug metabolism in man. Butterworth, London

Griffin J P, D'Arcy P F 1984 A manual of adverse drug interactions. Wright, Bristol

Hansten P D 1985 Drug interactions. Lea & Febiger, Philadelphia

Kalow W 1989 Race and therapeutic drug response. N Engl J Med 320: 588–590

Kalow W, Goedde H W, Agarwal D P (eds) 1986 Ethnic differences in reactions to drugs and xenobiotics. Liss, New York

Lamble J W (ed) 1983 Drug metabolism and distribution. Elsevier, Amsterdam

Montamat S C, Cusack B J, Vestal R E 1989 Management of drug therapy in the elderly. N Engl J Med 321: 303–309

Murray M, Reidy G F 1990 Selectivity in the inhibition of mammalian cytochromes P-450 by chemical agents. Pharmacol Rev 42: 85–101

Parma J, Duprez L, van Sande J, Cochaux P, Gervy C, Mockel J, Dumont J, Vassart G 1993 Somatic mutations in the thyrotropin receptor gene cause hyperfunctioning thyroid adenomas. Nature 365: 649–651

Patrono C, Dunn M J 1987 The clinical significance of inhibition of renal prostaglandin synthesis. Kidney Int 32: 1–12

Price-Evans D A 1993 Genetic factors in drug therapy, clinical and molecular pharmacogenetics. Cambridge University Press, Cambridge

Rane A 1985 Drug metabolism and disposition in neonates and infancy. In: Wilkinson G R, Rawlins D M (eds) Drug metabolism and disposition. MTP Press, Lancaster

Shenker A, Laue L, Kosugi S, Merendino J J Jr, Minegishi T, Cutler GB 1993 A constitutively activating mutation of the luteinising hormone receptor in familial male precocious puberty. Nature 365: 652–654

Smith S E, Rawlins M D 1973 Variability in human drug response. Butterworth, London

Stockley I H 1981 Drug interactions. Blackwell, Oxford

Vessell E S 1977 Genetic and environmental factors affecting drug disposition in man. Clin Pharmacol Ther 22: 659–679

Winstanley P A, Orme M L'E 1988 Which adverse drug interactions are really important? Adv Drug React Bull 130: 488–491

43

HARMFUL EFFECTS OF DRUGS

TYPES OF ADVERSE DRUG REACTION

All drugs are capable of producing harmful as well as beneficial effects. Such harmful effects are either: (a) related or (b) unrelated to the principal pharmacological action of the drug. Many of the adverse effects in the first category are predictable, at least if the pharmacodynamics are understood in sufficient detail, and are sometimes referred to as 'Type A' adverse reactions (Rawlins & Thompson 1981). Adverse effects in the second category may also occur predictably when the drug is taken in excessive dose (e.g. **paracetamol** hepatotoxicity, **aspirin**-induced tinnitus, **aminoglycoside** ototoxicity), during pregnancy (e.g. **thalidomide** teratogenicity), or in disease (e.g. **primaquine** haemolysis in patients with G6PD deficiency). In addition, unpredictable adverse effects unrelated to the principal pharmacological action of a drug can occur, albeit rarely (e.g. **chloramphenicol**: aplastic anaemia, **penicillin**: anaphylaxis, **practolol**: oculomucocutaneous syndrome). These are sometimes called idiosyncratic reactions (or 'Type B' reactions in the Rawlins & Thompson classification). These rare conditions are usually severe—otherwise they would go unrecognised, and their existence is important in establishing the safety of medicines. If the incidence of an adverse reaction is 1 in 6000 patients exposed approximately 30 000 patients would have to be exposed to the drug for three events to be detected even if there were no background incidence of the event in question. This sort of arithmetic shows that the possibility of such reactions cannot be excluded by early-phase clinical trials which usually expose only 1–2000 individuals to the drug, and it indicates the need for continued monitoring by regulatory authorities after drugs have been licensed and marketed. Different countries have responded to this need in different ways, and coordination of the different agencies involved is a major international challenge.

Many of the unwanted effects related to the principal pharmacological actions of drugs have been discussed in previous chapters. For example, postural hypotension occurs with **α_1-adrenoceptor antagonists**, bleeding with **anticoagulants** and cardiac dysrhythmias with **glycosides**. There are also examples in which the unwanted effect appears at first sight to be unrelated to the basic pharmacological action of the drug, but where it is, in fact, a direct consequence of its main action. One such example is gastric bleeding with **aspirin** (see p. 252). In most instances, this type of unwanted effect is reversible, and the problem can often be dealt with by reducing the dose or changing to a different drug. Sometimes, however, such effects can be fatal (e.g. intracerebral bleeding due to **anticoagulants**, hypoglycaemic coma from **insulin** or **sulphonylurea** drugs) and occasionally they are not easily reversible, for example in the case of tardive dyskinesia produced by **antipsychotic** drugs (see Ch. 28) or the syndromes of drug dependence produced by **opiate analgesics**, **alcohol**, **nicotine** and many other drugs (see Ch. 34).

The second category of adverse reactions (i.e. those that arise by a biochemical mechanism unrelated to the main pharmacological effect of the

Table 43.1 Examples of the diversity of organ systems involved in adverse drug reactions classified as to whether or not these are known to be related to the principal pharmacological action of the drug

Organ	Drug/clinical situation	Adverse effect	Mechanism			See Chapter
			Related*	Unrelated†	Unknown	
Heart	β-adrenoceptor antagonists	Heart failure	+			7, 13
	Doxorubicin	Heart failure		+		36
	Digoxin	Dysrhythmia	+			13
	Astemizole	Dysrhythmia		+		13
Brain	L-dopa, bromocriptine	Hallucinations	+, +			30
	Ethanol (alcohol withdrawal)	Hallucinations		+		33
	Muscarinic receptor antagonists	Memory impairment	+			25, 30
	Chlorpromazine	Malignant neuroleptic			+	28
	syndrome					
Sensory						
Eye	Ethambutol, chloroquine	Blindness (maculopathy)		+, +		37, 40
Ear	Aminoglycoside antibiotics	Deafness (sensorineural)		+		37
Taste	Captopril	Distortion		+		14
Touch/pain	Vincristine	Pain and numbness	+			36
Locomotor	β-adrenoceptor antagonists	Fatigue	+			7
	Fibrates (myositis)	Myalgia		+		15
	Diuretics	Gout		+		18
	Prednisolone	Osteoporosis		+		21
	Phenytoin	Osteomalacia		+		30
Gastrointestinal						
Stomach	NSAID	Peptic ulcer	+			12
Pancreas	Asparaginase	Pancreatitis		+		36
Colon	Clindamycin, amoxycillin (pseudomembranous colitis)	Diarrhoea	+			37
Liver	Phenytoin	Hepatitis		+		30
Gall bladder	Octreotide	Gallstones			+	21
Lung	β-adrenoceptor antagonists, NSAID	Worsening of asthma	+, +			7, 12
	Amiodarone	Interstitial fibrosis		+		13
Kidney	Angiotensin-converting enzyme inhibitors	Acute renal failure	+			14
	NSAID		+			12
	Aminoglycoside antibiotics			+		37
	Analgesic abuse	Chronic renal failure			+	31
	Methysergide (retroperitoneal fibrosis)			+		8
	Penicillamine, captopril	Nephrotic syndrome		+, +		12, 14
Genitourinary tract	Cyclophosphamide (haemorrhagic cystitis)	Haematuria		+		36
	Thiazide diuretics	Erectile impotence			+	14, 18

Table 43.1 continued

Organ	Drug/clinical situation	Adverse effect	Mechanism			See Chapter
			Related*	Unrelated†	Unknown	
Endocrine/ metabolism	Thiazide diuretics	Hyperglycaemia		+		14, 18
	Sulphonylureas	Hypoglycaemia	+			20
	Amiodarone	Thyroid dysfunction		+		13
	Dopamine antagonists, e.g. chlorpromazine, haloperidol, metoclopramide	Gynaecomastia/ galactorrhoea	+			28, 19
Blood—haemopoietic						
Red cells	Methyldopa	Haemolytic anaemia		+		14
White cells	Carbimazole	Neutropenia		+		21
Platelets	Quinine	Thrombocytopenia		+		40
All lineages	Chloramphenicol	Aplastic anaemia		+		37
Coagulation	Stilboestrol	Thrombosis		+		22
	Heparin, warfarin	Haemorrhage	+, +			16
Skin	Penicillins, many others	Minor measles-like ('morbilliform') rash		+		37
	Allopurinol, sulphonamides	Generalised potentially fatal erythema multiforme (Stevens–Johnson syndrome)		+, +		12, 37
Multisystem Joints/ muscles/ kidneys/ brain	Hydralazine	Drug-induced lupus syndrome		+		14
Foetal development	Etretinate	Teratogenesis		+		—
	Phenytoin			+		30
Carcinogenesis	Immunosuppressant and cytotoxic drugs	Cancer	+			36

* Probably related to principal pharmacological action of drug
† Probably unrelated to principal pharmacological action of drug

drug) often involve a chemically reactive metabolite rather than the parent drug, and are sometimes immunological in nature. Examples include liver or kidney damage, bone marrow suppression, carcinogenesis and disordered foetal development. Such effects (which are by no means confined to drugs, being liable to occur with any kind of chemical) fall conventionally into the area of toxicology rather than pharmacology.

The diversity of clinically important adverse drug reactions is very great. Any organ system can be the principal target, or several systems can be involved simultaneously. Examples that illustrate this diversity are shown in Table 43.1. Anticipating, avoiding, recognising and responding to adverse drug reactions are among the most important parts of clinical practice. A full account of this area of therapeutics is beyond the scope of the present work.

DRUG TOXICITY

TOXICITY TESTING

Toxicity testing in animals is carried out on new drugs to identify potential hazards. The basic premise is that toxic effects caused by a drug are similar in man and other animals. This is inherently reasonable in view of the similarities between higher organisms at the cellular and molecular levels. There are nevertheless wide interspecies variations, so that toxicity testing in animals is not always a reliable guide. Toxic effects can range from negligible to so severe as to preclude further development of the compound. Intermediate levels of toxicity are more acceptable in drugs intended for the more severe illnesses (for example AIDS or cancers) and decisions on whether or not to continue development are often difficult. If development does proceed, safety monitoring can be concentrated on the system 'flagged' as a potential target of toxicity by the animal studies. *Safety* (as opposed to toxicity) can only be established during use of a drug in man.

Important types of harmful drug effects of the toxicological kind are emphasised in this chapter rather than predictable pharmacodynamic effects, which are described in the chapters on systemic pharmacology.

Discussed here are:

- general mechanisms of toxin-induced cell damage and death
- mutagenesis and carcinogenesis
- teratogenesis
- allergic reactions to drugs.

The first three categories have a good deal in common, for they all involve biochemical damage to cellular constituents (proteins, membrane lipids or DNA) resulting principally from covalent reactions with reactive metabolites of the parent compound. If the affected biological molecules are lipid or protein, the effect is often to change the metabolism of the cell, or to kill it; if the target is DNA, the result may be mutation. This sometimes leads to malignancy (carcinogenesis) or foetal malformation (teratogenesis).

Types of drug toxicity

- Toxic effects of drugs can be:
  - —related to the principal pharmacological action, e.g. bleeding with anticoagulants
  - —unrelated to the principal pharmacological action, e.g. liver damage with paracetamol.
- Some adverse reactions that occur with ordinary therapeutic dosage are unpredictable, serious and uncommon (e.g. agranulocytosis with **carbimazole**). Such reactions are almost inevitably only detected after widespread use of a new drug.
- Adverse effects unrelated to the main action of a drug are often caused by reactive metabolites and/or immunological reactions.

GENERAL MECHANISMS OF TOXIN-INDUCED CELL DAMAGE AND DEATH

Although cell injury can be produced directly by some drugs, in most cases it is caused by reactive moieties formed during metabolism. Toxic metabolites can form covalent bonds with target molecules, or alter the target molecule by non-covalent interactions (Table 43.2). Some metabolites do both. An outline of non-covalent and covalent mechanisms implicated in cell damage is given below, followed by brief descriptions of specific types of damage affecting liver and kidney. The liver is of paramount importance in drug metabolism (Ch. 4), and hepatocytes are exposed to high concentrations of nascent metabolites as these are formed by cytochrome P-450-dependent drug oxidation. Drugs and their polar metabolites are concentrated in renal tubular fluid as water is reabsorbed from the nephron, so renal tubules are exposed to higher concentrations than are other tissues. Furthermore, renal vascular mechanisms are critical to the maintenance of glomerular filtration, and are vulnerable to drugs that interfere with the control of afferent and efferent arteriolar contractility. It is therefore not surprising that the occurrence of hepatic and/or renal damage is a common reason for abandoning a potential new drug during toxicity testing.

Non-covalent interactions

Reactive metabolites of drugs can be involved in several related, potentially cytotoxic, non-covalent interactions in the cell including:

- lipid peroxidation
- generation of toxic oxygen species

Table 43.2 Drugs whose reactive metabolites interact with target molecules causing potential cell damage and/or death*

Covalent interactions		Non-covalent interactions	
Drug	Dealt with in Chapter	Drug	Dealt with in Chapter
Paracetamol	12	Paracetamol	12
Hydrocortisone	21	Adriamycin	36
Stilboestrol	22	Bleomycin	36
Isoniazid	37	Nitrofurantoin	37
Iproniazid	29	Menadione	16
Paraoxon	6	Halothane†	26
Procainamide†	13		

* In many cases, though covalent binding can be demonstrated, the exact mechanism of cell damage/death is not clear.
† See also below, under 'Allergic reactions to drugs'.
From: Nelson S D, Pearson P G 1990 Annu Rev Pharmacol Toxicol 30: 169

- reactions causing depletion of glutathione (GSH)
- modification of sulphydryl groups.

Some of these effects are also produced by covalent reactions.

Lipid peroxidation of polyunsaturated lipids can be initiated either by reactive metabolites or by reactive oxygen species generated by such metabolites (see below). Lipid peroxyradicals (ROO$^\bullet$) can produce lipid hydroperoxides (ROOH), which produce further lipid peroxyradicals. This chain reaction—a peroxidative cascade—may eventually affect much of the membrane lipid. Cell damage and eventually cell death can result from alteration of membrane permeability or from reactions of the products of lipid peroxidation with proteins. However, lipid peroxides and peroxyradicals are usually dealt with effectively, for example by glutathione peroxidase and vitamin E, and lipid peroxidation may not, in itself, be sufficient as a cause of cell death.

Generation of toxic oxygen radicals by reactive metabolites involves reduction of molecular oxygen to superoxide anion (O_2^-) followed by dismutation to H_2O_2 and protonation to the hydroperoxyradical (HOO$^\bullet$). Hydroxyl radicals (OH$^\bullet$) and singlet oxygen ($^1O_2$) can also be formed. These oxygen species are cytotoxic, both directly and through lipid peroxidation (see above).

Reactions causing depletion of glutathione result in 'oxidative stress', which is a disturbance in the pro-oxidant/anti-oxidant balance in cells in favour of the pro-oxidant state. It can be caused by accumulation of the normal oxidative products of cell metabolism, or by the action of toxic chemicals. The glutathione (GSH) redox cycle is a protective system that minimises cell damage from oxidative stress. GSH acts as both a nucleophilic scavenger of reactive metabolites, and as a substrate in GSH-peroxidase-mediated detoxification of hydroperoxides produced during peroxidative reactions (see above).

GSH is normally maintained in a redox couple with its disulphide, GSSG. Oxidising species convert GSH to GSSG. GSH is usually regenerated by NADPH-dependent GSSG-reductase; but when the rate of GSH oxidation to GSSG exceeds the capacity of this enzyme, GSSG is removed from the cell by active transport (see Boobis et al. 1989). This, plus the fact that reactive metabolites form adducts with glutathione, depletes cellular GSH. Reduction of GSH to about 20–30% of normal impairs cellular defence against toxic compounds and results in cell death. A shift in the ratio of NADP/NADPH, and in the status of anti-oxidants such as vitamin E, are also implicated in oxidative stress.

Modification of sulphydryl (SH) groups can be produced either by oxidising species that alter SH groups reversibly or by covalent interaction. Free SH groups have a critical role in the catalytic activity of many enzymes, and modification of such SH groups results in inactivation. Important targets for SH-group modification by reactive metabolites include the cytoskeletal protein actin, glutathione reductase (see above) and Ca^{2+}-transporting ATPases in the plasma membrane and endoplasmic reticulum. These maintain cytoplasmic Ca^{2+} concentration at approximately 0.1 µmol/l, in the face of an external Ca^{2+} concentration of more than 1 mmol/l. A sustained rise in cell calcium occurs with inactivation of these enzymes (or with increased membrane permeability; see above), and compromises cell viability (reviewed by Nicotera et al. 1992). Lethal processes leading to cell death after acute calcium overload include activation of degradative enzymes (neutral proteases, phospholipases, endonucleases) and protein kinases, mitochondrial damage and cytoskeletal alterations (e.g. modification of association between actin and actin-binding proteins and activation of proteases). In *chronic* toxic injury altered cell signalling and programmed cell death ('apoptosis') appear to be involved.

Covalent interactions

Targets for covalent interactions include DNA, proteins/peptides, lipids and carbohydrates. Covalent bonding to DNA is a basic mechanism of action of mutagenic chemicals; this is dealt with below. Several non-mutagenic chemicals also form covalent bonds with macromolecules, but the relationship between this and cell damage is not clear. Some drugs with metabolites that form covalent bonds are listed in Table 43.2. For example, the cholinesterase inhibitor, **paraoxon**, binds acetylcholinesterase at the neuromuscular junction and causes necrosis of skeletal muscle. One toxin from the toadstool, *Amanita phalloides*, binds actin and another binds to RNA-polymerase, resulting in interference with actin depolymerisation and protein synthesis respectively. However, not all such reactions result in cytotoxicity. For example, **chloramphenicol** metabolites bind to lysine residues in proteins in liver cells, without causing hepatotoxicity.

General mechanisms of cell damage and cell death

- Drug-induced cell damage/death is usually due to reactive metabolites of the drug, involving non-covalent and/or covalent interactions with target molecules (Table 43.2).
- Non-covalent interactions include:
  - —lipid peroxidation; peroxyradicals produce hydroperoxides that produce further peroxyradicals and so on
  - —generation of cytotoxic oxygen radicals
  - —reactions causing depletion of GSH, resulting in 'oxidative stress'
  - —modification of SH groups on key enzymes (e.g. Ca^{2+}-ATPases, GSSG reductase) and structural proteins.
- Covalent interactions, e.g. adduct formation between NAPBQI and cellular macromolecules (Fig. 43.1). Covalent binding to protein can produce an immunogen; binding to DNA can cause carcinogenesis and teratogenesis.

HEPATOTOXICITY

Many therapeutic drugs cause liver damage, manifested clinically as hepatitis, or (in less severe cases) only as laboratory abnormalities (e.g. increased plasma aspartate transaminase activity). **Paracetamol**, **isoniazid**, **iproniazid** and **halothane** cause cell necrosis by the mechanisms of cell damage outlined above. Genetic differences in drug metabolism have been implicated in some instances (e.g. **isoniazid**, **phenytoin**). Mild drug-induced abnormalities of liver function are not uncommon but the mechanism of liver injury is often uncertain (e.g. **HMG-CoA reductase inhibitors**; Ch. 15). It is not always necessary to discontinue a drug when mild laboratory abnormalities occur, but the occurrence of end-stage liver disease (cirrhosis) as a result of long-term low-dose **methotrexate** treatment (Ch. 12) for psoriasis argues for caution on the part of prescribers. Hepatotoxicity of a different kind occurs with **chlorpromazine** (Ch. 28) and **androgens** (Ch. 21); in this type of toxicity, reversible obstructive jaundice occurs.

Hepatotoxicity caused by toxic doses of **paracetamol** is clinically important (paracetamol was the fourth most common cause of death following self-poisoning in the UK in 1989). An outline of the initial reactions in which this drug is involved is given in Chapter 12, page 254 and Figure 12.1. Because the body's handling of this drug exemplifies many of the general mechanisms of cell damage outlined above, the story is taken up again here. With toxic doses of paracetamol, the enzymes catalysing the normal conjugation reactions are saturated (see Ch. 12), and mixed-function oxidases convert the drug to the reactive metabolite *N-acetyl-p-benzoquinone imine* (NAPBQI). This compound can initiate several of the covalent and non-covalent interactions described above and illustrated in Figure 43.1, although the precise mechanisms critical for

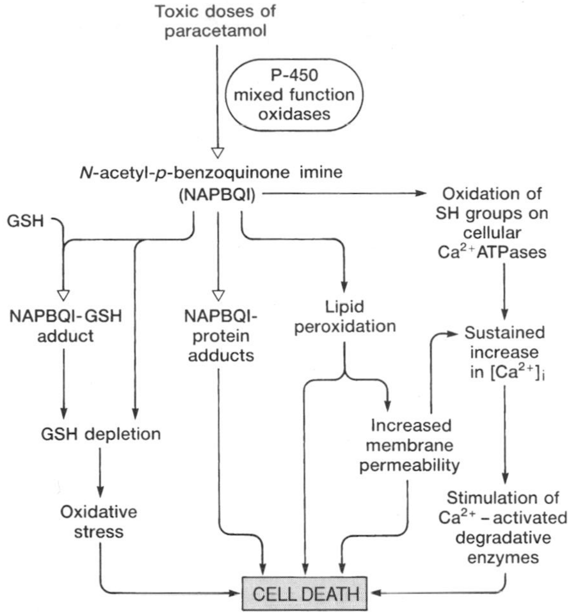

Fig. 43.1 Potential mechanisms of liver cell death resulting from the metabolism of paracetamol to N-acetyl-p-benzoquinone imine (NAPBQI).
(GSH = glutathione) (Based on data from: Boobis A R et al. 1989, and Nelson S D, Pearson P G 1990 Annu Rev Pharmacol Toxicol 30: 169) See also Figure 12.1.

cell death are not yet clear. Oxidative stress due to GSH depletion is clearly important. Synthesis of new GSH depends on the availability of cysteine, but the supply of this can be limiting. Agents such as **acetylcysteine** and **methionine** can, within limits, increase GSH synthesis and reduce mortality when used clinically in patients with severe paracetamol poisoning.

Liver damage can also be produced by immunological mechanisms (see below), which have been particularly implicated in **halothane** hepatitis (see Ch. 26).

Hepatotoxicity

- Liver damage can be produced by general mechanisms of cell injury; paracetamol exemplifies many of these (see Fig. 43.1).
- Some drugs (e.g. chlorpromazine can cause reversible cholestatic jaundice.
- Immunological mechanisms are sometimes implicated (e.g. halothane).

NEPHROTOXICITY

Drug-induced nephrotoxicity is a common clinical problem. Indeed, **non-steroidal anti-inflammatory drugs (NSAIDs**; Table 43.3) and **angiotensin-converting enzyme inhibitors (ACEIs**) are currently among the commonest causes of acute renal failure. This is usually a result of their principal pharmacological actions in patients whose underlying disease results in renal haemodynamics (blood flow and glomerular filtration) that are dependent on vasodilator prostaglandin biosynthesis (**NSAIDs**) or on angiotensin-II-mediated efferent arteriolar vasoconstriction (**ACEIs**). *Acute renal impairment* occurs on starting the drug and is reversible if it is discontinued promptly. NSAIDs and ACEIs are discussed further in Chapters 12 and 14 respectively. By reducing prostacyclin production **NSAIDs** can indirectly depress renin and aldosterone secretion thus predisposing to hyperkalaemia, especially if the glomerular filtration rate is also reduced. **ACEIs** also reduce aldosterone secretion and have a similar effect.

In addition to these effects related to their main pharmacological action, **NSAIDs** can also cause an *allergic-type interstitial nephritis*. This is rare but severe and usually occurs several months to one year after starting NSAID treatment. It manifests itself clinically as acute renal failure often accompanied by proteinuria, or sometimes by frank nephrotic

Table 43.3 Adverse effects of non-steroidal anti-inflammatory drugs on the kidney

Due to principal pharmacological action (i.e. inhibition of prostaglandin biosynthesis)
Acute ischaemic renal failure
Sodium retention (leading to or exacerbating hypertension and/or heart failure)
Water retention
Hyporeninaemic hypoaldosteronism (leading to hyperkalaemia)
Allergic-type interstitial nephritis (unrelated to principal pharmacological action)
Renal failure
Proteinuria
Analgesic nephropathy (unknown whether or not related to principal pharmacological action)
Papillary necrosis
Chronic renal failure

Adapted from: Murray & Brater 1993

syndrome (heavy proteinuria, hypoalbuminuria and oedema). **Fenoprofen** is particularly liable to cause this type of renal damage, possibly because its metabolites bind irreversibly to albumin.

Analgesic nephropathy is a third kind of renal damage in which **NSAIDs** are implicated. This consists of *renal papillary necrosis* leading to chronic interstitial nephritis and severe and irreversible *chronic renal failure*. It is associated with prolonged and massive abuse of analgesics (usually for their effects on mood rather than on pain), usually taken in combination preparations. **Phenacetin** has particularly been incriminated, but **paracetamol** and **NSAIDs** have not been exonerated. The role of **caffeine** (often included with analgesics and NSAIDs in abused preparations) is uncertain but could be important. It is possible that such analgesic-associated nephropathy is causally related to inhibition of renal prostaglandin synthesis, but its pathogenesis is not understood.

Captopril in higher doses than are currently recommended clinically can cause heavy proteinuria (Ch. 14). This is due to glomerular injury and is also caused by other drugs that contain a sulphydryl group (e.g. **penicillamine**), and it is believed that it is this chemical feature rather than ACE inhibition *per se* that is responsible for this adverse effect.

Cyclosporin, used to prevent transplant rejection (see Ch. 12), causes renal damage via a change in renal vascular dynamics—a persistent increase in renal vascular resistance with a marked decline in glomerular filtration rate, and systemic hypertension. It alters renal prostaglandin biosynthesis.

Many drugs that cause hepatotoxicity are also liable to cause toxic damage to the kidney, most commonly by producing necrosis of renal tubular cells. The mechanisms involved seem to be generally similar to those described above under 'General mechanisms of cell death'.

Nephrotoxicity

- Kidney damage can be produced by general mechanisms of cell injury, which can cause papillary and/or tubular necrosis.
- Reduction in compensatory vasodilator prostaglandins can result in increased renal vascular resistance and decreased renal function.

MUTAGENESIS AND CARCINOGENICITY

Mutation occurs through a change in the genotype of a cell, which is passed on when the cell divides. Chemical agents cause mutation by covalent modification of DNA. Certain kinds of mutation result in carcinogenesis, because the affected DNA sequence codes for a protein that is involved in growth regulation. It usually requires more than one mutation in a cell to initiate the changes that result in malignancy. The current view is that cancer arises when the function of 'proto-oncogenes' (which are probably normal growth-regulator genes) is altered by mutation. This can result in the expression of a protein that is not normally formed by the cell, or of a modified version of a normally expressed protein (see Ch. 36). Alteration of so-called tumour suppressor genes could also be involved; these genes code for products that inhibit the transcription of oncogenes. Some oncogenes code for modified growth factors or growth-factor receptors, or for elements of the intracellular transduction mechanism by which growth factors regulate cell proliferation (see Ch. 36, p. 699). Growth factors are polypeptide mediators that stimulate cell division; examples are *epidermal growth factor* (EGF) and *platelet-derived growth factor* (PDGF). The receptors for these growth factors regulate a number of cellular processes (see Ch. 2). Though there are many details to be filled in, the complex connection between exposure to a mutagenic chemical and the development of a cancer is beginning to be understood.

Biochemical mechanisms of mutagenesis

Most chemical carcinogens act by modification of the bases in DNA, particularly guanine. The O_6 and N_7 positions on the guanine molecule readily become covalently attached to reactive metabolites of chemical carcinogens (Fig. 36.4). Substitution at the O_6 position is the more likely to produce a permanent mutagenic effect, since N_7 substitutions are usually quickly repaired.

The accessibility of bases in DNA to chemical attack is greatest when DNA is in the process of replication (i.e. during cell division). The likelihood of genetic damage by many mutagens is therefore related to the frequency of cell division. The developing foetus is particularly susceptible, and mutagens are also potentially teratogenic (see later section). This is also important in relation to mutagenesis of *germ cells*, particularly in the female, because in humans the production of primary oocytes occurs by a rapid succession of mitotic divisions when the female baby is in utero—in fact very early in embryogenesis. Each of these primary oocytes then undergoes only two further divisions much later in life at the time of ovulation. It is thus during early pregnancy that germ cells of the developing female embryo are most likely to undergo mutagenesis. Mutations that occur in female germ cells as a result of exposure to chemical or other mutagens can be transmitted to progeny conceived many years after exposure to the mutagen. In the male, germ cell divisions occur throughout life, and sensitivity to mutagens is continuously present.

The importance of drugs, in comparison to other chemicals such as pollutants and food additives, as a causative factor in mutagenesis has not been established, and such epidemiological evidence as exists suggests that they are uncommon (but not unimportant) causes of foetal malformations and cancers.

Mutagenesis and carcinogenicity

- Mutagenesis involves alteration of the genotype of a cell by covalent modification of DNA.
- Carcinogenesis involves alteration of proto-oncogenes or tumour suppressor genes by mutation; more than one mutation is usually required.
- Carcinogens commonly act by binding to N, or O, of guanine during cell division; the former modification is likely to be repaired by DNA repair enzymes, the latter not.
- In the female embryo, the germ cells undergo several rapid divisions and are therefore very vulnerable to mutagens, but the effects will not be manifest till the next generation. Later in development (from infancy till reproductive adult life) female gametes are relatively resistant to mutagenesis, but if mutations do occur they can be transferred to progeny years afterwards.
- In the male, germ cell division occurs throughout life and sensitivity to mutagens is continuously present.
- Drugs are relatively uncommon (but not unimportant) causes of birth defects and cancers.

CARCINOGENESIS

The development of a cancer is a complex, multistage process. Alteration of DNA is the first step, but many later steps, at present only poorly understood, are also necessary. Carcinogens are chemical substances that cause cancer. The term is sometimes restricted to substances that interact directly with DNA. However, various substances act at a later stage to increase the likelihood that mutation will result in the production of a tumour (Fig. 43.2), and are also carcinogenic. Here we classify carcinogens by the scheme put forward by Weisburger & Williams (1984), by which carcinogens can be divided into:

- *Genotoxic carcinogens* (i.e. mutagens, as discussed above). These are also termed 'initiators' and can be further divided into:
  - — Primary carcinogens, which act on DNA directly.
  - — Secondary carcinogens, which must be converted to a reactive metabolite before they affect the DNA. Most important chemical carcinogens fall into this category.
- *Epigenetic carcinogens* (i.e. agents that do not themselves cause genetic damage, but increase the likelihood that such damage will cause cancer).

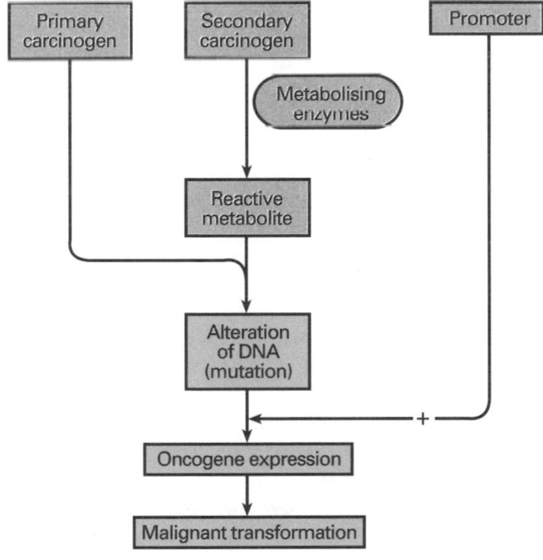

Fig. 43.2 Sequence of events in mutagenesis and carcinogenesis.

There are several different types of epigenetic carcinogen, the most important being:

- *Promoters*. These substances are not carcinogenic by themselves, but increase the likelihood of tumour development from genetically damaged cells; they can thus produce cancers when given *after* a genotoxic agent. Examples include **phorbol esters**, bile acids and saccharin. *Cigarette smoke* not only contains carcinogenic aromatic hydrocarbons, but also has promoter activity.
- *Co-carcinogens*. These substances are not carcinogens by themselves but enhance the effect of genotoxic agents when given simultaneously; examples include **phorbol esters** and various aromatic and aliphatic hydrocarbons. Note that some chemicals have both genotoxic and promoter/co-carcinogenic activity. *Urban polluted air* contains substances that have carcinogenic, co-carcinogenic and promoter actions.
- *Hormones*. Some tumours are hormone-dependent (see Ch. 36), the most important examples being **oestrogen**-dependent breast cancers and **androgen**-dependent prostatic cancers. Endometrial hyperplasia induced by prolonged **oestrogen** treatment increases the risk of uterine carcinoma unless countered by cyclical **progestogen** administration. This is probably due to a change in the DNA which is given expression when the cells proliferate. Hormone replacement therapy with oestrogen for postmenopausal women with an intact uterus is therefore accompanied by cyclical treatment with a progestogen (Ch. 22).

Measurement of mutagenicity and carcinogenicity

Much effort has gone into developing tests for detecting mutagenicity and carcinogenicity which can be broadly divided into:

- *In vitro tests for mutagenicity*. These rapid tests are suitable for screening large numbers of compounds, but they can give positive results on compounds that are not subsequently shown to be carcinogenic in tests on whole animals, and can miss known carcinogens.
- *Whole animals tests for carcinogenicity*. Such tests are expensive and time-consuming, but are usually required by drug regulatory authorities before a new drug is licenced for use in man. The main limitation of this kind of study is that there are important species differences, mainly to do with the metabolism of the foreign compound and the formation of reactive products.
- *Whole animal tests for teratogenesis*. These are required for drugs that are to be used by women of reproductive potential especially (obviously) if they are to be used during pregnancy. Similar limitations of such tests apply as with carcinogenicity testing.

In vitro tests for genotoxic carcinogens

Bacteria have great advantages as a test system for measuring mutagenicity because of their high replication rate. The most widely used assays are variations on the *Ames test*, which measures the rate of back-mutation (i.e. reversion from mutant to wild-type form) in a culture of *Salmonella typhimurium*. The normal, wild-type strain can grow in a medium containing no added amino acids, because it can synthesise all the amino acids it needs from simple carbon and nitrogen sources. The test makes use of the fact that a mutant form of the organism cannot make histidine and therefore only grows on a medium containing this amino acid. The test involves growing the mutant form on a medium containing a small amount of histidine, the drug to be tested being added to the culture. After several divisions, the histidine becomes depleted, and the only cells that continue dividing are those that have back-mutated to the wild-type. A count of colonies following subculture on plates deficient in histidine gives a measure of the mutation rate.

Primary carcinogens cause mutation by a direct action on bacterial DNA but most carcinogens have to be converted to an active metabolite (see above). Therefore it is necessary to include, in the culture, enzymes that catalyse the necessary conversion. An extract of liver from a rat treated with **phenobarbital** to induce liver enzymes is usually employed. Some of the many variants of the Ames test are described by Venitt (1981).

Other short-term in vitro tests for genotoxic chemicals include measurements of mutagenesis in mouse lymphoma cells, and assays for chromosome aberrations and sister chromatid exchanges in hamster ovary cells. However, all the in vitro tests give some false positives and some false negatives.

In vivo tests for carcinogenicity

In vivo tests for carcinogenicity entail detection of tumours in groups of test animals. Carcinogenicity tests are very slow, since there is usually a latency of months or years before tumours develop. Such tests may yield clear evidence of carcinogenic activity with a dose-related increase in malignant neoplasms (or of benign neoplasms with a known propensity to progress to malignancy), or no evidence of carcinogenic activity. Unfortunately, however, findings often provide only equivocal evidence of carcinogenicity, making it difficult for industry and regulatory authorities to decide on further development and possible licencing of a product. None of the tests so far described can reliably detect *epigenetic carcinogens*. To do this it is necessary to use an assay system that measures the effect of the test substance on tumour production with a non-carcinogenic dose of a genotoxic agent. Such tests are being evaluated.

The number of drugs associated with increased cancer risk in man is small, the most important group being those that are known to act on DNA, i.e. **cytotoxic** and **immunosuppressant** drugs. Few drugs with positive carcinogenicity tests are used therapeutically. **Pyrimethamine** (Ch. 40) is mutagenic in high concentrations, and carcinogenicity testing in strain A mice (but not other strains or species) was positive for a threefold increase in lung tumours. **Methoxsalen** (a psoralen used together with ultraviolet light (PUVA) in special centres for treatment of the skin disease, psoriasis) is a positive mutagen and carcinogen, and may increase the incidence of skin cancer.

Carcinogens

- Carcinogens can be:
  - —*Genotoxic*, i.e. causing mutations directly (primary carcinogens) or after conversion to reactive metabolites (secondary carcinogens)
  - —*Epigenetic*, i.e. increasing the possibility that a mutagen will cause cancer, though not themselves mutagenic. Epigenetic carcinogens include 'promoters' which increase cancer rate if given after the mutagen, and 'co-carcinogens' which increase the rate if given with it. Phorbol esters have both actions.
- New drugs are tested for mutagenicity and carcinogenicity.
- The main test for mutagenicity measures back-mutation, in histidine-free medium, of a mutant *Salmonella typhimurium* (which, unlike the wild type, cannot grow without histidine) in the presence of:
  - —the chemical to be tested
  - —a liver microsomal enzyme preparation for generating reactive metabolites. Colony growth indicates that mutagenesis has occurred. Some false positives and false negatives occur.
- Carcinogenicity testing involves chronic dosing of groups of animals. It is expensive and time-consuming.
- There is no really suitable test for epigenetic carcinogens.

TERATOGENESIS AND DRUG-INDUCED FOETAL DAMAGE

The term 'teratogenesis' is usually used to mean the production of gross structural malformations during foetal development, to distinguish it from other kinds of drug-induced foetal damage such as growth retardation, dysplasia (e.g. *iodide-associated goitre*) or *asymmetric limb reduction* due to vasoconstriction caused by **cocaine** (see Ch. 33) in an otherwise normally developing limb. A list of drugs that can affect foetal development adversely is given in Table 43.4.

It has been known that external agents can affect foetal development since about 1920, when it was discovered that X-irradiation during pregnancy could cause foetal malformation or death. Nearly 20 years later the importance of *rubella* infection was recognised, but it was not until 1960 that drugs were implicated as causative agents in teratogenesis: the shocking experience with **thalidomide** led to a widespread reappraisal of many other drugs in clinical use, and led to the setting up of drug regulatory bodies in many countries. The majority of birth defects (about 70%) occur with no recognisable causative factor. Drug or chemical exposure during pregnancy are believed to account for only about 1% of all foetal malformations. While this percentage may appear small, the total numbers are substantial and result in appalling suffering as well as major social and economic effects on families and the community.

Table 43.4 Drugs reported to have adverse effects on human foetal development

Agent	Effect	Teratogenicity*	See Chapter
Thalidomide	Phocomelia, heart defects, gut atresia, etc.	K	43
Penicillamine	Loose skin, etc.	K	12
Warfarin	Saddle nose, retarded growth, defects of limbs, eyes, CNS	K	16
Corticosteroids	Cleft palate and congenital cataract — rare		21
Androgens	Masculinisation in female		22
Oestrogens	Testicular atrophy in male		22
Stilboestrol	Vaginal adenosis in female foetus, also vaginal or cervical cancer 20+ years later		22
Anticonvulsants			
Phenytoin	Cleft lip/palate, microcephaly, mental retardation	K	30
Valproate	Neural tube defects, e.g. spina bifida	K	30
Carbamazepine	Retardation of foetal head growth	S	30
Cytotoxic drugs (esp. folate antagonists)	Hydrocephalus, cleft palate, neural tube defects, etc.	K	36
Aminoglycosides	8th cranial nerve damage		37
Tetracycline	Staining of bones and teeth, thin tooth enamel, impaired bone growth	S	37
Ethanol	Foetal alcohol syndrome	K	33
Retinoids	Hydrocephalus, etc.	K	43
Angiotensin-converting enzyme inhibitors	Oligohydramnios, renal failure		14

* K = known teratogen (in experimental animals and/or humans); S = suspected teratogen (in experimental animals and/or humans)
Adapted from: Juchau 1989 Annu Rev Pharmacol Toxicol 29: 165

Mechanism of teratogenesis

The timing of the teratogenic insult in relation to the stage of foetal development is critical in determining the type and extent of damage produced. Mammalian foetal development passes through three phases (Table 43.5):

- blastocyst formation
- organogenesis
- histogenesis and maturation of function.

Cell division is the main process occurring during *blastocyst formation*. During this phase, drugs can cause death of the embryo by inhibiting cell division, but provided the embryo survives, its subsequent development does not generally seem to be com-

Table 43.5 The nature of drug effects on foetal development

Stage	Gestation period in man	Main cellular processes	Affected by
Blastocyst formation	0–16 days	Cell division	Cytotoxic drugs
Organogenesis	17–60 days approx.	Division Migration Differentiation Death	Teratogens
Histogenesis and functional maturation	60 days to term	As above	Miscellaneous drugs, e.g. alcohol, nicotine, antithyroid drugs, steroids

promised, although there is evidence that **ethanol** may affect development at this very early stage (see Ch. 33).

It is during *organogenesis*, which occurs during the first trimester of pregnancy, that drugs can cause gross malformations. The structural organisation of the embryo occurs in a well-defined sequence: eye and brain, skeleton and limbs, heart and major vessels, palate, genitourinary system. The type of malformation produced thus depends on the time of exposure to the teratogen.

The cellular mechanisms by which teratogenic substances produce their effects are not at all well understood. There is a considerable overlap between mutagenicity and teratogenicity. In one large survey, among 78 compounds, 34 were both teratogenic and mutagenic, 19 were negative in both tests and 25 (among them **thalidomide**) were positive in one but not the other. It therefore seems that damage to DNA is important, but, as with carcinogenesis, it is certainly not the only factor. The control of morphogenesis is poorly understood; vitamin A derivatives (**retinoids**) are believed to be involved and are potent teratogens. Known teratogens also include a number of drugs (e.g. **methotrexate** and **phenytoin**) that do not react directly with DNA, but inhibit its synthesis by their effects on folate metabolism. Administration of **folate** during pregnancy *reduces* the frequency of both spontaneous and drug-induced malformations.

In the final stage of *histogenesis and functional maturation*, the foetus is dependent on an adequate supply of nutrients, and development is regulated by a variety of hormones. Gross structural malformations do not arise from exposure to mutagens at this stage, but drugs that interfere with the supply of nutrients or with the hormonal milieu may have deleterious effects on growth and development. Exposure of a female foetus to androgens at this stage can cause masculinisation. **Stilboestrol** was commonly given to pregnant women with a history of recurrent miscarriage during the 1950s (for unsound reasons) and causes dysplasia of the vagina of the infant and an increased incidence of carcinoma of the vagina in the teens and twenties.

Testing for teratogenicity

The **thalidomide** disaster dramatically brought home the need for routine teratogenicity studies on potential new therapeutic drugs. Assessment of teratogenicity in man is a particularly difficult problem, for various reasons. One is that the 'spontaneous' malformation rate is high (3–10% depending on the definition of a significant malformation) and highly variable between different regions, age groups and social classes. Large-scale studies are required, which take many years and much money to perform, and usually give suggestive, rather than conclusive, results.

In vitro methods, based on the culture of cells, organs or whole embryos, have not so far been developed to a level where they satisfactorily predict teratogenesis in vivo, and most regulatory authorities require teratogenicity testing in one rodent (usually rat or mouse) and one non-rodent (usually rabbit) species. Pregnant females are dosed at various levels during the critical period of organogenesis, and the foetuses are examined for structural abnormalities. However, poor cross-species correlation means that tests of this kind are not reliably predictive in man, and it is usually recommended that new drugs are not used in pregnancy unless it is essential.

Some definite and probable human teratogens

Though many drugs have been found to be teratogenic in varying degrees in experimental animals, relatively few are known to be teratogenic in humans (see Table 43.4). Some of the more important are discussed below.

Thalidomide

Thalidomide is virtually unique in producing, at modest clinical dosage, virtually 100% malformed infants when taken in the first 3–6 weeks of gestation. It was introduced in 1957 as a hypnotic and sedative with the special feature that it was extremely safe in overdosage, and it was even recommended specifically for use in pregnancy. As was then normal, it had been subjected only to acute toxicity testing, and not to chronic toxicity* or

*A severe peripheral neuropathy, leading to irreversible paralysis and sensory loss, was reported within a year of the drug's introduction and subsequently confirmed in many reports. The drug company responsible was less than punctilious in acting on these reports (see Sjostrom & Nilsson 1972), which were soon eclipsed by the discovery of teratogenic effects, but the neurotoxic effect was severe enough in its own right to necessitate withdrawal of the drug from general use, although it still has a few highly specialised applications under tightly controlled and restricted conditions.

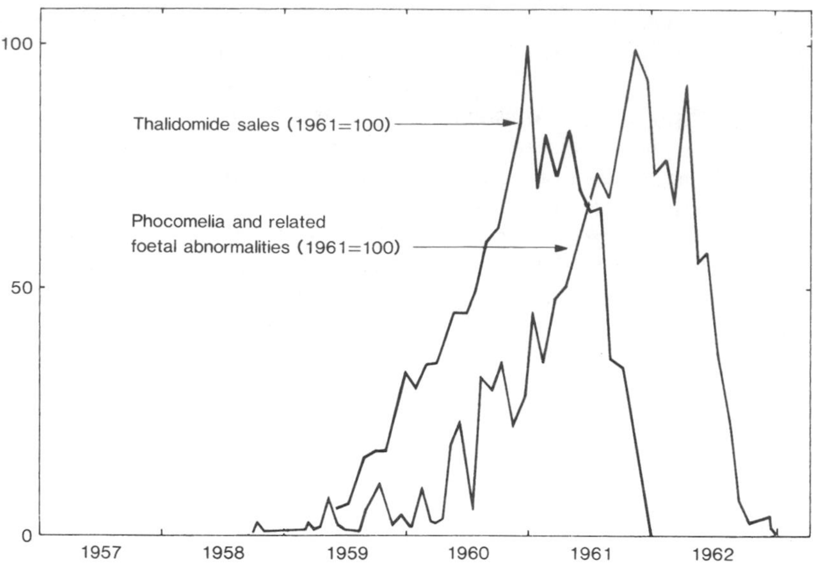

Fig. 43.3 Incidence of major foetal abnormalities in Western Europe following the introduction and withdrawal of thalidomide.

teratogenicity testing. Thalidomide was marketed energetically and successfully, and the first suspicion of its teratogenicity arose early in 1961 with reports of a sudden increase in the incidence of *phocomelia* ('seal limbs'; an absence of development of the long bones of the arms and legs) which had hitherto been virtually unknown. At this time approximately 1 000 000 tablets were being sold daily in West Germany. Reports of phocomelia came simultaneously from Hamburg and Sydney, and the connection with thalidomide was made. The drug was withdrawn late in 1961, by which time an estimated 10 000 malformed babies had been born (Fig. 43.3). In spite of intensive study, its mechanism of action remains very poorly understood. Study of the many cases of thalidomide teratogenesis in man showed very clearly the correlation between the time of exposure and the type of malfunction produced (Table 43.6).

Table 43.6 Thalidomide teratogenesis

Day of gestation	Type of deformity
21–22	Malformation of ears Cranial nerve defects
24–27	Phocomelia of arms
28–29	Phocomelia of arms and legs
30–36	Malformation of hands Anorectal stenosis

Cytotoxic drugs

Many alkylating agents (e.g. **chlorambucil** and **cyclophosphamide**) and antimetabolites (e.g. **azathioprine** and **mercaptopurine**) can cause malformations when used in early pregnancy, but more often lead to abortion (see Ch. 36). Folate antagonists (e.g. **methotrexate**) produce a much higher incidence of major malformations, evident in both live-born and still-born foetuses.

Retinoids

Etretinate, a retinoid (i.e. vitamin A derivative), with marked effects on epidermal differentiation is a known teratogen and causes a high proportion of serious abnormalities (notably skeletal deformities) in exposed foetuses. It is used by dermatologists to treat severe psoriasis and other skin diseases. It accumulates in subcutaneous fat and in consequence is eliminated extremely slowly, detectable amounts persisting for many months after chronic dosing is discontinued. Because of this, women should avoid pregnancy for at least 2 years after treatment. **Acitretin** is an active metabolite of

Teratogenesis and drug-induced foetal damage

- Teratogenesis means production of gross structural malformations of the foetus, e.g. the absence of limbs after thalidomide. Less comprehensive damage can be produced by many other drugs (see Table 43.4). < 1% of congenital foetal defects are attributed to drugs given to the mother.
- Gross malformations can be produced only if teratogens act during organogenesis. This occurs during the first 3 months of pregnancy but after blastocyst formation. Drug-induced foetal damage is rare during blastocyst formation (exception: foetal alcohol syndrome) and after the first 3 months.
- The mechanisms of action of teratogens are not clearly understood, though DNA damage is a factor in many cases.
- New drugs are tested in pregnant females of one rodent and one non-rodent (e.g. rabbit) species.

etretinate. It is equally teratogenic, but tissue accumulation is less pronounced and elimination may therefore be more rapid.

Heavy metals

Lead, *cadmium* and *mercury* all cause foetal malformations in man. The main evidence comes from Minamata disease, named after the locality in Japan where an epidemic occurred when the local population ate fish contaminated with methylmercury that had been used as an agricultural fungicide. The effect was impaired brain development, resulting in cerebral palsy and mental retardation, often with microcephaly. Mercury, like other heavy metals, inactivates many enzymes by forming covalent bonds with sulphydryl and other groups, and this is presumed to be responsible for the developmental abnormality.

Anticonvulsant drugs

Congenital malformations are two to three times more frequent in babies born to epileptic as compared with normal mothers, and there is evidence that this is associated with the use of anticonvulsant drugs (see Ch. 30) rather than with the epilepsy itself. The drugs that are implicated include **phenytoin** (particularly cleft lip/palate), **valproate** (neural tube defects) and **carbamazepine** (spina bifida and hypospadias — a malformation of the male urethra).

Warfarin

Administration of warfarin (see Ch. 16) in the first trimester is associated with nasal hypoplasia and various central nervous system abnormalities, affecting roughly 25% of babies. In the last trimester it must not be used because of the risk of intracranial haemorrhage in the baby during delivery.

Anti-emetics

Anti-emetics have been widely used in treating morning sickness in early pregnancy, and some are teratogenic in animals. Results of surveys in humans are inconclusive, providing no clear evidence of teratogenicity. Nevertheless, it is prudent to avoid the use of these drugs in pregnant patients if possible.

ALLERGIC REACTIONS TO DRUGS

Allergic reactions of various kinds are a very common form of adverse response to drugs. Most drugs, being low-molecular weight substances, are not immunogenic in themselves. A drug or its metabolites can, however, interact with protein to form a stable conjugate that can function as an *immunogen* which sensitises the individual. Sensitisation means essentially the induction of an immune response, as described on page 221 and illustrated in Figures 11.3 and 11.4. Subsequent administration of the drug can then evoke a variety of the unwanted effects described in Chapter 11 (p. 224). In some instances, the immunological basis for such responses has been well worked out, but very often it is inferred from the clinical characteristics of the reaction, and direct evidence of an immunological mechanism is lacking. The main criteria that are suggestive of an immune-type response are:

- The reaction has a time-course different from that of the pharmacodynamic effect, i.e. it is either delayed in onset, occurring a few days after administration of the drug, or occurs only with repeated exposure to the drug.
- Sensitisation and/or the subsequent allergic reaction may occur with doses that are too small to elicit pharmacodynamic effects.
- The reaction conforms to one of the clinical

syndromes associated with allergy—the hypersensitivity reactions (Ch. 11, p. 224, and below) and is unrelated to the pharmacodynamic effect of the drug.

The overall incidence of allergic drug reactions is variously reported as being between 2 and 25%. The great majority are relatively harmless skin eruptions. Serious reactions (e.g. *anaphylaxis*, *haemolysis* and *bone marrow depression*) which may be life-threatening, are rare. The incidence of death from allergic reactions among hospital patients is estimated at 1 : 10 000. **Penicillins**, which are the commonest cause of drug-induced anaphylaxis, produce this response in an estimated 1 in 50 000 patients exposed.

Immunological mechanisms

The formation of an immunogenic conjugate between a small molecule and an endogenous protein requires covalent bonding. In most cases, reactive metabolites, rather than the drug itself, are able to bind covalently. Such reactive metabolites can be produced during drug oxidation or by photoactivation in the skin. They may also be produced by the action of toxic oxygen metabolites generated by activated leucocytes. Rarely (e.g. in *drug-induced lupus erythematosus*) the reactive moiety interacts with nuclear components (DNA, histone) rather than proteins to form an immunogen (see below). The mechanism for covalent coupling of **benzylpenicillin** to protein is shown in Figure 43.4. Metabolites of penicillin such as *benzylpenicillenic acid* also couple to proteins, forming immunogens.

The types of allergic response that drugs can

Benzylpenicillin

Protein

Protein conjugate

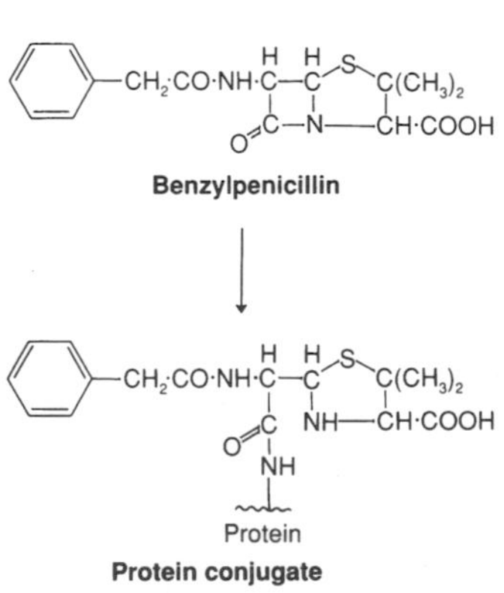

Fig. 43.4 Mechanism of formation of protein conjugate by penicillin.

produce conform broadly to types I, II, III and IV of the Gell & Coombs classification (see Ch. 11, p. 224).

In nearly all of these reactions, conjugation with a carrier appears to be essential, not only for the primary sensitisation process, but also, frequently, for the secondary response. One possible exception is penicillin, which can form dimers and polymers in solution, forming sufficiently large conglomerates of antigenic determinants to elicit an anaphylactic reaction in a sensitised individual, without conjugation to protein (De Weck 1983).

Clinical types of allergic response to drugs

In the Gell & Coombs classification of hypersensitivity reactions (Ch. 11), types I, II and III are antibody-mediated and type IV is cell-mediated. Unwanted reactions with drugs, in which specific antibody-mediated or cell-mediated immune reactions have been implicated as wholly or partly responsible, are given in Table 43.7. The more important clinical manifestations of hypersensitivity are considered below.

Anaphylactic shock

Anaphylactic shock—a type I hypersensitivity response—is a sudden and life-threatening reaction that results from the release of *histamine* and *other mediators* (Ch. 11). The main features include urticarial rash, swelling of soft tissues, bronchoconstriction and hypotension.

The drugs most likely to cause anaphylactic reactions are the **penicillins**, which account for about 75% of anaphylactic deaths, reflecting the frequency with which they are used in clinical practice. Other drugs that can cause anaphylaxis include: various enzymes, for example **streptokinase** (Ch. 16), **asparaginase** (Ch. 36); hormones, for example **ACTH** (Ch. 21), **insulin** preparations (Ch. 20); **heparin** (Ch. 16); **dextrans**; **radiological contrast agents**; **vaccines**; and **serological products**. Anaphylaxis with **local anaesthetics** (Ch. 34) and the surface antiseptic, **chlorhexidine**, and with many other drugs has been reported but is uncommon. Acute anaphylactic attacks are treated by injection of **adrenaline** (which is life-saving in this circumstance), **corticosteroids** and **antihistamines**.

It is feasible to carry out a skin test for the presence of anaphylactic hypersensitivity, by injecting

Table 43.7 Drug toxicity in which specific humoral and cellular immunity have been implicated

Drug	Toxicity	Immunological mechanisms		
		Humoral	Cellular	See Chapter
Probenecid	Haemolytic anaemia	+		4, 12, 18
Gallamine Suxamethonium Tubocurarine	Anaphylaxis	+		6
Paracetamol	Thrombocytopenia	+		12
Allopurinol	Dermatitis, urticaria		+	12
Penicillamine	Neutropenia	+		12
Salicylates	Anaphylaxis	+		12
Procainamide	Drug-induced lupus erythematosus	+		13
Captopril	Urticaria, dermatitis, nephritis	+	+	14
Hydralazine	Drug-induced lupus erythematosus	+		14
Methyldopa	Haemolytic anaemia, neutropenia, hepatitis	+		14
Tolbutamide	Haemolytic anaemia	+		20
Halothane	Hepatitis	+	+	26
Thiopentone	Anaphylaxis	+		26
Mianserin	Thrombocytopenia, neutropenia	+		29
Phenytoin	Hepatitis	+		30
Cyclophosphamide	Anaphylaxis, urticaria	+		36
Amoxicillin	Haemolytic anaemia	+		37
Cephamandole	Thrombocytopenia	+		37
Cloxacillin	Hepatitis	+		37
Erythromycin	Hepatitis		+	37
Isoniazid	Drug-induced lupus erythematosus	+		37
Penicillins	Asthma, serum sickness, dermatitis, urticaria, anaphylaxis	+	+	37
Sulphonamides	Drug-induced lupus erythematosus	+		37
Quinine	Thrombocytopenia	+		40

Adapted from: Pohl et al. (1988)

a minute dose of the drug intradermally. This is sometimes done if a patient reports that he or she is allergic to a particular drug. However, the test is not completely reliable, and false negative results are not uncommon. Furthermore, the test dose itself may elicit a severe reaction. The use of *penicilloylpolylysine* as a skin test reagent for penicillin allergy appears to be an improvement over the use of penicillin itself, because it bypasses the need for conjugation of the test substance, thereby reducing the likelihood of a false negative. Other specialised tests are available to detect the presence of specific IgE in the plasma, or to measure histamine release from the patient's basophils, but these are not used routinely.

Other drug-induced type I hypersensitivity reactions include *bronchospasm* (see Ch. 17) and *urticaria*.

Haematological reactions

Drug-induced haematological reactions can be produced by type II, III or IV hypersensitivity (see p. 224). Type II hypersensitivity involves the antibody binding to an antigen (constituted by the drug–macromolecule complex) which is part of a cell surface. The antigen–antibody reaction can activate complement leading to lysis (Fig. 11.1) or attack by killer lymphocytes or phagocytic leucocytes with receptors for the projecting Fc portion of antibody.

Type II reactions to drugs can affect any or all of the formed elements of the blood, which may be destroyed by effects either on the circulating blood cells themselves or on their progenitors in the bone marrow.

Haemolytic anaemia can occur with many drugs, but has been most commonly reported with **sulphonamides** and related drugs (Ch. 37) and with the antihypertensive drug, **methyldopa** (see Ch. 7). With methyldopa, significant haemolysis occurs in less than 1% of patients, but the appearance of antibodies directed against the surface of red cells is detectable in 15% by the Coombs' test. The antibodies are directed against Rh antigens, but it is not known how methyldopa produces this effect.

Drug-induced agranulocytosis (complete absence of circulating neutrophils) is usually delayed in onset (2–12 weeks after beginning drug treatment) and may then be sudden in onset. The condition often presents as mouth ulcers or a severe sore throat or other infection. Serum from the patient causes leucocyte death in blood samples from other individuals, and circulating antileucocyte antibodies can usually be detected immunologically. The main groups of drugs associated with agranulocytosis are **NSAIDs** (especially **phenylbutazone**; Ch. 12), **carbimazole** (Ch. 21) and **clozapine** (Ch. 28). **Sulphonamides** and related drugs (e.g. **thiazide diuretics** and **oral hypoglycaemic drugs**) are uncommon but well-documented causes of agranulocytosis. This is a rare, but highly dangerous condition, because recovery when the drug is stopped is often absent or incomplete and the marked reduction of blood granulocytes makes the patient extremely vulnerable to bacterial infections. This type of antibody-mediated leucocyte destruction must be distinguished from the direct effect of **cytotoxic drugs** (see Ch. 36), most of which cause granulocytopenia. With these latter drugs, however, the effect is rapid in onset, predictably related to dose and usually reversible.

Thrombocytopenia (reduction in platelet numbers) is caused (albeit rarely) by **quinine** (Ch. 40), **heparin** (Ch. 16) and **thiazide diuretics** (Ch. 18).

Some drugs (notably **chloramphenicol**) can suppress all three haemopoietic cell lineages giving rise to *aplastic anaemia* (anaemia with associated agranulocytosis and thrombocytopenia).

The distinction between type III and type IV hypersensitivity reactions in the causation of haematological reactions is not clear-cut, and it is likely that either or both mechanisms are often involved.

Allergic liver damage

Most drug-induced liver damage is due to the direct toxic effects of drugs or their metabolites as described above. However, hypersensitivity reactions are sometimes involved, a particular example being **halothane**-induced hepatic necrosis (see Ch. 26). *Trifluoracetyl chloride*, a reactive metabolite of halothane, couples to a macromolecule to form an

Allergic reactions to drugs

- Drugs or their reactive metabolites can bind covalently to tissue proteins to form immunogens (see Table 43.7). Penicillin (which can also be immunogenic by forming polymers) is an important example.
- Drug-induced allergic (hypersensitivity) reactions may be antibody-mediated (types I, II, III) or cell-mediated (type IV). Important clinical manifestations include:
  - —*Anaphylactic shock* (type I). This is life-threatening, by obstructing respiration. Many drugs can cause the condition; most deaths are due to penicillin.
  - —*Haematological reactions* (type II, III or IV). These, along with examples of causative drugs, are: haemolytic anaemia (sulphonamides and methyldopa), agranulocytosis, which can be irreversible (sulphonamides, chloramphenicol and carbimazole) and thrombocytopenia (quinine, heparin and thiazide diuretics).
  - —*Allergic liver damage* (type II, III). The reactive metabolite of halothane couples to liver proteins to form an immunogen.
  - —*Skin rashes* (type I, IV). These occur with many drugs, are usually type IV and usually mild, though some can be life-threatening.
  - —*Drug-induced systemic lupus erythematosus* (mainly type II). This involves antibodies to nuclear material.

immunogen. There are several polypeptide carriers; one is a liver *carboxylesterase*, another a protein *disulphide isomerase*. Most patients with halothane-induced liver damage have antibodies that react with halothane–carrier conjugates. There is evidence from rabbit experiments that the halothane–protein antigens can be expressed on the surface of the liver cells. Destruction of the cells occurs by type II hypersensitivity reactions involving killer T cells. If antigen–antibody complexes are released by damaged cells, type III reactions can contribute.

Enflurane may also cause antibody-mediated liver damage, and apparent cross-sensitisation with halothane is reported.

Other hypersensitivity reactions

The clinical manifestations of type IV hypersensitivity reactions are many and varied, ranging from minor skin rashes to generalised autoimmune disease. Fever may accompany these reactions.

Skin rashes can be antibody-mediated, but are usually cell-mediated. They range from mild eruptions to fatal exfoliation. In some cases the lesions are photosensitive, probably because of degradation of the drug to reactive substances in the presence of UV light.

Some drugs (notably **hydralazine** and **procainamide**; see Table 43.7) can produce an autoimmune syndrome resembling *systemic lupus erythematosus* (SLE). This is a multisystem disorder in which there is immunological damage to many organs and tissues (joints, skin, lung, CNS and kidney) caused particularly, but not exclusively, by type III hypersensitivity reactions. The prodigious array of antibodies directed against 'self' components has been termed 'an autoimmune thunderstorm'. The antibodies react with determinants shared by many molecules, for example the phosphodiester backbone of DNA, RNA and phospholipids. In drug-induced SLE, the immunogen may result from the reactive drug moiety interacting with nuclear material, and in the effector phase, joint and pulmonary damage is common. The condition usually resolves when the drug is stopped.

REFERENCES AND FURTHER READING

Beckman D A, Brent R L 1984 Mechanisms of teratogenesis. Annu Rev Pharmacol Toxicol 24: 483–500

Boobis A R, Fawthrop D J, Davies D S 1989 Mechanisms of cell death. Trends Pharmacol Sci 10: 275–280

Bridges J W 1985 Frontiers in biochemical toxicology. Trends Pharmacol Sci FEST Suppl: 11–15

Davies D M (ed) 1981 Textbook of adverse drug reactions. Oxford University Press, Oxford

Dayan A D, Paine A J 1988 Advances in applied toxicology. Taylor & Francis, London, vol 1

De Weck A L 1983 Immunopathological mechanisms and clinical aspects of allergic reactions to drugs. In: De Weck A L, Bundgaard H (eds) Allergic responses to drugs. Handbook of experimental pharmacology. Springer-Verlag, Berlin, vol 63: 75–135

Gorrod J W (ed) 1981 Testing for toxicity. Taylor & Francis, London

Hanson J W, Streissguth A P, Smith D W 1978 The effects of moderate alcohol consumption during pregnancy on fetal growth and morphogenesis. J Paediatr 92: 457–460

Hathway D E 1984 Molecular aspects of toxicology. Royal Society of Chemistry, London

Hawkins D F (ed) 1987 Drugs and pregnancy: human teratogenesis and related problems. Churchill Livingstone, Edinburgh

Hay A 1988 How to identify a carcinogen. Nature 332: 782–783

Hinson J A, Roberts D W 1992 Role of covalent and noncovalent interactions in cell toxicity: effects on proteins. Annu Rev Pharmacol Toxicol 32: 471–510

Huff J, Haseman J, Rall D 1991 Scientific concepts, value, and significance of chemical carcinogenesis studies. Annu Rev Pharmacol Toxicol 31: 621–652

Juchau M R 1989 Bioactivation in chemical teratogenesis. Annu Rev Pharmacol Toxicol 29: 165–187

Kenna J G, Knight T L, van Pelt F N A M 1993 Immunity of halothane metabolite-modified proteins in halothane hepatitis. Ann NY Acad Sci 685: 646–661

Lohman P H M, Bean R A et al. 1985 Molecular dosimetry of genotoxic damage: biochemical and immunochemical methods to detect DNA damage. Trends Pharmacol Sci FEST Suppl: 21–25

Loomis T A 1978 Essentials of toxicology, 3rd edn. Lea & Febiger, Philadelphia

Lutz W K, Maier P 1988 Genotoxic and epigenetic chemical carcinogens: one process, different mechanisms. Trends Pharmacol Sci 9: 322–326

Murray M D, Brater D C 1993 Renal toxicity of the nonsteroidal anti-inflammatory drugs. Annu Rev Pharmacol Toxicol 33: 435–465

Nicotera P, Bellomo G, Orrenius S 1992 Calcium-mediated mechanisms in chemically-induced cell death. Annu Rev Pharmacol Toxicol 32: 449–470

Pohl L R, Satoh H, Christ D D, Kenna J G 1988 The immunologic and metabolic basis of drug hypersensitivities. Annu Rev Pharmacol 28: 367–387

Rawlins M D, Thomson J W 1981 In: Davies D M (ed) Textbook of adverse drug reactions. Oxford University Press, Oxford

Reed D J 1990 Glutathione: toxicological implications. Annu Rev Pharmacol Toxicol 30: 603–631

Scales M D G 1993 Toxicity testing. In: Griffin J P, O'Grady J, Wells F O (eds) The textbook of pharmaceutical medicine. Queen's University Press, Belfast, p 53–79

Schreiner C A, Holden H E 1983 Mutagens as teratogens: a correlative approach. In: Johnson E M, Kochhar D M (eds) Teratogenesis and reproductive toxicology. Handbook of experimental pharmacology. Springer-Verlag, Berlin, vol 65: 135–170

Sjostrom H, Nilsson R 1972 Thalidomide and the power of the drug companies. Penguin Books, London

Styles J A 1981 Other short-term tests in carcinogenesis studies. In: Gorrod J W (ed) Testing for toxicity. Taylor & Francis, London

Timbrell J A 1982 Principles of biochemical toxicology. Taylor & Francis, London

Uetrecht J 1989 Mechanism of hypersensitivity reactions: proposed involvement of reactive metabolites generated by activated leucocytes. Trends Pharmacol Sci 10: 463–467

Venitt S 1981 Microbial tests in carcinogenesis studies. In: Gorrod J W 1981 Testing for toxicity. Taylor & Francis, London

Vroomen L H, Berghmans M C et al. 1988 Reversible interaction of a reactive intermediate derived from furazolidone with glutathione and protein. Toxicol Appl Pharmacol 95: 53–60

Weinberg R A 1984 Cellular oncogenes. Trends Biochem Sci 9: 131–133

Weisburger J H, Williams G M 1984 New, efficient approaches to tests for carcinogenicity of chemicals based on their mechanisms of action. In: Zbinden et al. (eds) Current problems in drug toxicology. Libbey, Paris

Wilson J G 1973 Present status of drugs as teratogens in man. Teratology 7: 3–15

INDEX

B

C

D

E

F

G

H

I

J

K

L

M

N

O

P

Q

R

S

T

U

V

W